PHILIP L. HILLSMAN, M. D.

Contributors

GENE G. ABEL, M.D.
Professor of Clinical Psychiatry, Department of Psychiatry, Emory University School of Medicine, Atlanta, Georgia; Clinical Professor of Psychiatry, Morehouse School of Medicine, Atlanta, Georgia; Director, Center for Behavioral Medicine, West Paces Medical Center, Atlanta, Georgia; Director, Behavioral Medicine Institute of Atlanta, Atlanta, Georgia.
Sexual Disorders

HAGOP S. AKISKAL, M.D.
Professor, Department of Psychiatry, University of California at San Diego, La Jolla, California.
The Mental Status Examination; Mood Disturbances

BRUCE ALEXANDER, PHARM. D.
Clinical Pharmacist Specialist, Psychiatry, Departments of Pharmacy and Psychiatry, Iowa City Department of Veterans Affairs Medical Center, Iowa City, Iowa; Clinical Associate Professor, College of Pharmacy, University of Iowa College of Medicine, Iowa City, Iowa.
Genetics of Psychiatric Disorders

NANCY C. ANDREASEN, M.D., PH.D.
Professor, Department of Psychiatry, Director of Mental Health Research Center, University of Iowa College of Medicine, Iowa City, Iowa; Attending Physician, University of Iowa Hospitals and Clinics, University of Iowa, Iowa City, Iowa.
Thought Disorder

GAIL A. BERNSTEIN, M.D.
Academic Associate Professor, Division of Child and Adolescent Psychiatry, Department of Psychiatry, University of Minnesota School of Medicine, Minneapolis, Minnesota; Director of Outpatient Services for Child and Adolescent Psychiatry, University of Minnesota Hospitals and Clinics, Minneapolis, Minnesota.
Anxiety, Phobia and Obsessive Disorders in Children

REMI CADORET, M.D.
Professor, Department of Psychiatry, University of Iowa College of Medicine, Iowa City, Iowa; Attending Physician, University of Iowa Hospitals and Clinics, University of Iowa, Iowa City, Iowa.
Antisocial Personality

DENNIS P. CANTWELL, M.D.

Joseph Campbell Professor of Child Psychiatry, Department of Psychiatry and Biobehavioral Sciences, University of California Los Angeles Neuropsychiatric Institute, Los Angeles, California
The Disruptive Behavior Disorders: Attention Deficit Disorders, Oppositional Disorder, and Conduct Disorder

PAULA J. CLAYTON, M.D.

Professor and Head, Department of Psychiatry, University of Minnesota School of Medicine, Minneapolis, Minnesota.
Bipolar Illness

C. ROBERT CLONINGER, M.D.

Wallace Renard Professor and Head, Department of Psychiatry, Washington University School of Medicine, St. Louis, Missouri; Washington University Medical Center, St. Louis, Missouri.
Somatoform and Dissociative Disorders

WILLIAM CORYELL, M.D.

Professor, Department of Psychiatry, University of Iowa College of Medicine, Iowa City, Iowa. Attending Physician, University of Iowa Hospitals and Clinics, University of Iowa, Iowa City, Iowa.
Schizoaffective and Schizophreniform Disorders

THOMAS J. CRAIG, M.D., M.P.H.

Professor of Psychiatry and Behavioral Science, State University of New York at Stony Brook College of Medicine; Health Science Center, Stony Brook, New York; Northport Veterans Administration Medical Clinic, Northport, New York.
Epidemiology of Psychiatric Illness

RAYMOND R. CROWE, M.D.

Professor, Department of Psychiatry, University of Iowa College of Medicine, Iowa City, Iowa; Attending Physician, University of Iowa Hospitals and Clinics, Iowa City, Iowa.
Delusional (Paranoid) Disorders

ELKE D. ECKERT, M.D.

Professor, University of Minnesota School of Medicine, Minneapolis, Minnesota; Medical Director of Inpatient and Day Treatment Programs for Eating Disorders, University of Minnesota Hospital, Minneapolis, Minnesota.
Anorexia Nervosa and Bulimia Nervosa

STEPHEN V. FARAONE, PH.D.

Assistant Professor of Psychology, Department of Psychiatry, Harvard Medical School at the Brockton/West Roxbury Veterans Administration Medical Center, Brockton, Massachusetts.
Schizophrenia

BARRY D. GARFINKEL, M.D.

Associate Professor, Division of Child and Adolescent Psychiatry, Department of Psychiatry, University of Minnesota School of Medicine, Minneapolis, Minnesota; Attending Psychiatrist, University of Minnesota Hospital and Clinics, Minneapolis, Minnesota.
Major Affective Disorders in Children and Adolescents.

MICHAEL J. GARVEY, M.D.

Professor, Department of Psychiatry, University of Iowa College of Medicine, Iowa City, Iowa; Staff Physician, University of Iowa Hospitals and Clinics; Staff Physician, Veterans Administration Medical Center, Iowa City, Iowa.
Clinical Psychopharmacology and Other Somatic Therapies

ELLIOT S. GERSHON, M.D.
Chief, Clinical Neurogenetics Branch, National Institute of Mental Health, Bethesda, Maryland. Attending Physician, Clinical Center, National Institute of Health, Bethesda, Maryland. Attending Physician, Suburban Hospital, Bethesda, Maryland.
Genetics of Psychiatric Disorders

LYNN R. GOLDIN, PH.D.
Research Geneticist, Clinical Neurogenetics Branch, National Institute of Mental Health, Bethesda, Maryland.
Genetics of Psychiatric Disorders

DONALD W. GOODWIN, M.D.
Professor, Department of Psychiatry, Kansas University School of Medicine, Kansas City, Kansas; Kansas City Medical Center, Kansas City, Kansas.
Alcoholism

FRITZ A. HENN, PH.D., M.D.
Professor and Chairman, Department of Psychiatry and Behavioral Sciences, State University of New York at Stony Brook College of Medicine; Psychiatrist in Chief, State University Hospital at Stony Brook, Stony Brook, New York.
The Neurobiologic Basis of Psychiatric Illnesses

CRAIG S. HOLT, Ph.D.
Assistant Professor, Department of Psychiatry, University of Iowa College of Medicine, Iowa City, Iowa

BARRY LISKOW, M.D.
Professor, Department of Psychiatry, University of Kansas School of Medicine, Kansas City, Kansas; Chief of Psychiatry, Kansas City Veterans Administration Medical Center, Kansas City, Missouri.
Alcoholism

THOMAS B. MACKENZIE, M.D.
Professor, Department of Psychiatry, University of Minnesota School of Medicine, Minneapolis, Minnesota; Attending Psychiatrist, University of Minnesota Hospitals, Minneapolis, Minnesota.
Obsessive Compulsive Neurosis

RONALD L. MARTIN, M.D.
Professor and Chairman, Department of Psychiatry, University of Kansas School of Medicine, Wichita, Kansas.
Use of the Laboratory in Psychiatry

JAMES E. MITCHELL, M.D.
Professor and Director of Adult Psychiatry, Department of Psychiatry, University of Minnesota School of Medicine, Minneapolis, Minnesota; Attending Psychiatrist, University of Minnesota Hospitals, Minneapolis, Minnesota.
Anorexia Nervosa and Bulemia Nervosa

GEORGE E. MURPHY, M.D.
Professor Emeritus, Department of Psychiatry, Washington University School of Medicine, St. Louis, Missouri; Barnes Hospital, Emeritus, St. Louis, Missouri.
Suicide and Attempted Suicide

RUSSELL NOYES, JR., M.D.
Professor, Department of Psychiatry, University of Iowa College of Medicine, Iowa City, Iowa.
Attending Physician, University of Iowa Hospitals and Clinics, Iowa City, Iowa.
Anxiety Disorders

JOHN I. NURNBERGER, JR., M.D., PH.D.
Professor of Psychiatry and Medical Neurobiology and Director, Institute for Psychiatric Research,
Indiana University School of Medicine, Indianapolis, Indiana.
Genetics of Psychiatric Disorders

CANDICE A. OSBORN, M.A.
Director of Sexual Offender Treatment, Behavioral Medicine Institute of Atlanta, Atlanta, Georgia.
Sexual Disorders

PAUL J. PERRY, PH.D.
Professor, Department of Psychiatry, University of Iowa College of Medicine, Iowa; Professor,
College of Pharmacy, University of Iowa, Iowa; Attending Physician, University of Iowa Hospitals
and Clinics, Iowa City, Iowa.
Clinical Psychopharmacology and Other Somatic Therapies

BRUCE PFOHL, M.D.
Professor, Department of Psychiatry, University of Iowa College of Medicine, Iowa City, Iowa;
Attending Physician, University of Iowa Hospitals and Clinics, University of Iowa, Iowa City, Iowa.
Personality Disorders

MICHAEL K. POPKIN, M.D.
Professor of Psychiatry and Medicine, Department of Psychiatry, University of Minnesota School
of Medicine, Minneapolis, Minnesota; Chief of Psychiatry, Hennepin County Medical Center,
Minneapolis, Minnesota.
*Syndromes of Brain Dysfunction Presenting With Cognitive Impairment or Behavioral Disturbance: Delerium,
Dementia and Secondary Disorders*

SHELDON H. PRESKORN, M.D.
Professor and Vice Chairman, Department of Psychiatry, University of Kansas School of Medicine,
Witchita, Kansas; President and Director, Psychiatric Research Institute, Saint Francis Regional
Medical Center, Wichita, Kansas.
Use of the Laboratory in Psychiatry

ROBERT G. ROBINSON, M.D.
Professor and Head, Department of Psychiatry, University of Iowa College of Medicine, Iowa City,
Iowa; Attending Physician, University of Iowa Hospitals and Clinics, Iowa City, Iowa.
Phenomenology of Coarse Brain Disease

KEITH L. ROGERS, M.D., PH.D.
Assistant Professor, Department of Psychiatry, University of Washington, Seattle, Washington;
Attending Psychiatrist, Seattle Veterans Administration Medical Center, Seattle, Washington.
Motor Symptoms in Psychiatric Illnesses

JOANNE L. ROULEAU, PH.D.
Associate Professor, Department of Psychology, University of Montreal, Montreal, Quebec, Can-
ada; Director, Centre d'etude et de recherche de l'Université de Montreal, Montreal, Quebec,
Canada.
Sexual Disorders

MARC-ANDRÉ ROY, M.D.
Centre de Recherche Université Lavel Robert-Giffard, Pavillon Landry-Poulin, Beauport, Quebec

LUKE Y. TSAI, M.D.
Professor of Child Psychiatry and Pediatrics, Department of Psychiatry, University of Michigan Medical Center, Ann Arbor, Michigan; Director, Developmental Disorders Clinic, University of Michigan Medical Center, Ann Arbor, Michigan.
Autistic Disorder and Schizophrenia in Childhood

MING T. TSUANG, M.D., PH.D., D.SC.
Stanley Cobb Professor of Psychiatry, Department of Psychiatry, Harvard Medical School, Boston, Massachusetts; Professor, Department of Epidemiology, Harvard School of Public Health, Boston, Massachusetts; Head, Department of Psychiatry, Harvard Medical School at Brockton/West Roxbury Veterans Administration Medical Center, Brockton, Massachusetts; Chief of Psychiatry, Brockton/West Roxbury Veterans Administration Medical Center, Brockton, Massachusetts.
Schizophrenia

CHARLES VAN VALKENBURG, M.D.
Clinical Associate Professor, Health Sciences Center, Texas Tech University School of Medicine, El Paso, Texas; Staff Psychiatrist, Veterans Administration Outpatient Clinic, El Paso, Texas. Consultant, William Beaumont Army Hospital, El Paso, Texas.
Anxiety Symptoms

RAFIQ WAZIRI, M.D.
Associate Professor, Department of Psychiatry, University of Iowa College of Medicine, Iowa City, Iowa; Attending Physician, University of Iowa Hospitals and Clinics, Iowa City, Iowa.
The Amnestic Syndrome

JOSEPH WESTERMEYER, M.D., M.P.H., PH.D.
Department of Psychiatry, University of Minnesota, Minneapolis, Minnesota; Chief of Psychiatry, Veterans Administration Medical Center, Minneapolis, Minnesota.
Drug Abuse

GEORGE WINOKUR, M.D.
Professor, Department of Psychiatry, University of Iowa College of Medicine, Iowa City, Iowa; Department of Psychiatry Administration, University of Iowa Hospitals and Clinics, Iowa City, Iowa.
Unipolar Depression

WILLIAM R. YATES, M.D.
Associate Professor, Department of Psychiatry, University of Iowa College of Medicine, Iowa City, Iowa; Attending Physician, University of Iowa Hospitals and Clinics, Iowa City, Iowa.
Other Psychiatric Syndromes: Adjustment Disorders, Factitious Disorder, Illicit Steroid Abuse

Preface

WHY A SECOND EDITION?

Seven years have elapsed since the first edition of this book. Considerable progress in the way of new data have emerged on the subjects that comprise the chapters. In the 1930s up to the end of the 1960s, new textbooks arrived on the scene and older textbooks were revised. With a few exceptions, the reason for this was that opinions and practices had changed, but these additions were not fueled by changes in the data or in enlarged knowledge. The field of psychiatry was heavily dependent on new words that were introduced and many bright, creative people were convinced that new words meant new insights, and that the reading professionals should be knowledgeable about these new words as they might herald important theories about psychiatric problems.

Since the 1970s, there has been a revolution in both thinking and behavior in psychiatry. Specific criteria for the diagnoses of our major mental disorders emerged. Less credence is given to people sitting around a table coming up with new words to explain the same time worn observations. Instead there has been an explosion of data, often biological in nature, but sometimes psychological and social. Psychiatry in the last third of the 20th century has become an expanding field with the promise of new discoveries in the cause of the mental illnesses and the yearly accretion of important advances in treatment. Perhaps the words which might best describe the charged current atmosphere in psychiatry are those of Wordsworth, written in the early days of the French Revolution, "Bliss was it in that dawn to be alive." It is our intention to assess new contributions to the data base and present them in the description of the clinical picture, the course, the etiology, and the treatment of the psychiatric illnesses.

We believe that there is a place for new chapters in the book. The chapter on special and unusual psychiatric syndromes has been replaced with a chapter on uncommon psychiatric problems which include new psychiatric syndromes that have become important in our western civilization through the use of new drugs and new evidence about the cause of the disease. The data on anxiety disorders in children have reached a critical mass and deserve a special place of their own in the book. In psychopharmacology and other somatic treatments, there has been a large advance in knowledge and we believe that a special chapter on these subjects will assist the reader, although each chapter contains that information perhaps presented in a different way. Other chapters have been revised in order to bring material up to date.

How often should a revision of such a text book occur? Probably five years is too soon and 15 years is too long. We have adopted the range of seven to 13 years in order to circumvent being considered either radical or reactionary. In fact, we have no idea how much time should elapse between a book and its revision.

We have included the first edition preface because we have not changed as regards viewpoint. We still think that there is a place for a book based on the idea that psychiatric illnesses should be regarded similarly to other illnesses in the field of medicine. We believe this adherence to the medical model was correct in 1986 and is still correct at the present time. Could we be wrong? It's possible, but we think not.

Who should use the book? It is presented with the idea that it will be useful to medical students in their psychiatry clerkships, to psychiatric residents during their period of training, to practicing physicians and psychiatrists who need an up-to-date evaluation of the status of the psychiatric illnesses that they see daily in their offices. Should it be used by psychologists and social workers? As a reference for diagnosis, classification, and the biological aspects of psychiatric illnesses, we believe it could be useful.

This book is somewhat different from other and earlier textbooks of psychiatry. Previous efforts were often clearly presented with an adherence of a specific way of thinking, a school of psychological or biological thought or an attempt to influence the teaching of psychiatry. Certainly, there is a diversity of orientations in psychiatric residencies and medical school programs and some of these views may be more useful than others. It is true that this book has been written from the vantage point of the medical model but it is not our intent to downgrade other positions or schools. What is in this second edition are data that every psychiatrist, physician, or mental health worker should know. To paraphrase the Latin "ignorantia juris Neminem excusat" we might say that ignorance of the data excuses no one. We realize that in any patient, there are many options for treatment. Also, there may be differences about diagnosis and classification but we think that these subjects may be presented as a concrete foundation for the major psychiatric conditions. That is what this book is about.

George Winokur, M.D.
Paula J. Clayton, M.D.

October 29, 1992

Preface
to the First Edition

One dictionary defines psychiatry as the branch of medicine that deals with mental, emotional, and behavioral disorders, but another defines it as the branch of medicine that relates to brain, gland, and nerve diseases. The one thing that the definitions have in common is that they both note that psychiatry is relevant to *disease* or *disorders*. Psychiatry is a branch of medicine and a psychiatrist is a specialist in that field. The practice of psychiatry is related to the diagnosis and treatment of people with disorders that fit a definition of a medical illness and are associated with emotional or behavioral changes of sufficient severity as to cause a disruption of the person's life and behavior.

For practical purposes our definition of what constitutes a psychiatric illness is simply a medical illness with major emotional and behavioral aspects. The definition of an illness is always arguable, of course, but beyond that it is generally true that the study of medicine in the literature divides its presentation of illness and disease into a definition, epidemiology, signs and symptoms, etiology, and treatment. Because an overlap of symptoms occurs, there is usually a section on differential diagnosis. The presentation of material in this text will therefore assume that psychiatric problems are analogous to other medical problems and will follow the familiar paradigm.

What then is the role of psychosocial factors in medicine and in psychiatry? They are of considerable importance if the evidence indicates that illnesses in themselves create social disturbances or social incapacities, or that social problems are relevant to the etiology or the cause of the illness. In other words, they can be quite significant depending on the circumstances.

Likewise, consider the role for psychotherapy in medicine and in psychiatry. If psychotherapy is nonspecific and applicable to a wide range of medical and psychiatric problems, it probably does not need to be discussed in a text concerned with the medical bases of diseases. However, when it proves to be an effective treatment for any of the reasonably well-defined illnesses it is included in the discussion.

One additional issue needs to be considered. How does one best present the illnesses that are seen in psychiatry? We have found it most useful for the mode of presentation to parallel the way in which a person learns clinical medicine. Similar to the idea that ontogeny recapitulates phylogeny, a medical student or resident learns clinical medicine by seeing patients as well as reading books. One starts to learn by seeing patients and then categorization occurs. This is the way in which clinical material becomes alive for the student who then returns to the text to read about an illness. Rather than present introductory chapters on etiology and classification and then launch into the pictures of the clinical states, we believe that the best way to present the material is to describe the clinical entities first. After that, chapters dealing with specific kinds of circumstances, such as symptom clusters or various biological or psychosocial etiologies, become far more meaningful. These realities have contributed to the organization of this book.

In the final analysis we are interested in specific psychiatric illnesses or entities. The frontispiece of this book, which comes from Hobbes' *Leviathan*, describes this very well. We are not interested in *Leviathan* per se. We are not interested in the "psyche." We are interested in specific psychiatric illnesses; that is, what is inside the *Leviathan*. As with medicine, psychiatry deals not on the basis of "soma" or symptoms but on the basis of specific diagnoses.

G.W.
P.C.

Contents

UNIT I

Syndromes—Adult

CHAPTER 1
THE MENTAL STATUS EXAMINATION 3
Hagop S. Akiskal

CHAPTER 2
**SYNDROMES OF BRAIN DYSFUNCTION PRESENTING WITH
COGNITIVE IMPAIRMENT OR BEHAVIORAL DISTURBANCE:
DELIRIUM, DEMENTIA, AND MENTAL DISORDERS DUE TO A
GENERAL MEDICAL CONDITION** 17
Michael K. Popkin

CHAPTER 3
THE AMNESTIC SYNDROME 39
Rafiq Waziri

CHAPTER 4
BIPOLAR ILLNESS 47
Paula J. Clayton

CHAPTER 5
UNIPOLAR DEPRESSION 69
George Winokur

CHAPTER 6

SCHIZOPHRENIA **87**

Ming T. Tsuang & Stephen V. Faraone

CHAPTER 7

SCHIZOAFFECTIVE AND SCHIZOPHRENIFORM DISORDERS **115**

William Coryell

CHAPTER 8

DELUSIONAL (PARANOID) DISORDERS **131**

Raymond R. Crowe & Marc-André Roy

CHAPTER 9

ANXIETY DISORDERS **139**

Russell Noyes, Jr. & Craig S. Holt

CHAPTER 10

OBSESSIVE-COMPULSIVE NEUROSIS **161**

Thomas B. Mackenzie

CHAPTER 11

SOMATOFORM AND DISSOCIATIVE DISORDERS **169**

C. Robert Cloninger

CHAPTER 12

ANOREXIA NERVOSA AND BULIMIA NERVOSA **193**

Elke D. Eckert & James E. Mitchell

CHAPTER 13

ANTISOCIAL PERSONALITY **205**

Remi Cadoret

CHAPTER 14

ALCOHOLISM **219**

Barry Liskow & Donald W. Goodwin

CHAPTER 15

DRUG ABUSE **237**

Joseph Westermeyer

CHAPTER 16
SEXUAL DISORDERS **253**
Gene G. Abel, Joanne L. Rouleau & Candice A. Osborn

CHAPTER 17
OTHER PSYCHIATRIC SYNDROMES: ADJUSTMENT DISORDER, FACTITIOUS DISORDER, ILLICIT STEROID ABUSE **273**
William R. Yates

UNIT II

Child Psychiatry

CHAPTER 18
THE DISRUPTIVE BEHAVIOR DISORDERS: ATTENTION DEFICIT DISORDERS, OPPOSITIONAL DISORDER, AND CONDUCT DISORDER **289**
Dennis P. Cantwell

CHAPTER 19
MAJOR AFFECTIVE DISORDERS IN CHILDREN AND ADOLESCENTS **301**
Barry D. Garfinkel

CHAPTER 20
AUTISTIC DISORDER AND SCHIZOPHRENIA IN CHILDHOOD **321**
Luke Y. Tsai

CHAPTER 21
ANXIETY, PHOBIA, AND OBSESSIVE DISORDERS IN CHILDREN ... **349**
Gail A. Bernstein

UNIT III

Symptoms Clusters

CHAPTER 22
MOOD DISTURBANCES **365**
Eagop S. Akiskal

CHAPTER 23
ANXIETY SYMPTOMS **381**
Charles Van Valkenburg

CHAPTER 24
THOUGHT DISORDER **393**
Nancy C. Andreasen

CHAPTER 25
PHENOMENOLOGY OF COARSE BRAIN DISEASE **403**
Robert G. Robinson

CHAPTER 26
MOTOR SYMPTOMS IN PSYCHIATRIC ILLNESSES **417**
Keith L. Rogers

CHAPTER 27
PERSONALITY DISORDERS **425**
Bruce Pfohl

UNIT IV

Special Areas

CHAPTER 28
THE NEUROBIOLOGIC BASIS OF PSYCHIATRIC ILLNESSES **439**
Fritz A. Henn

CHAPTER 29
GENETICS OF PSYCHIATRIC DISORDERS **459**
John I. Nurnberger

CHAPTER 30
USE OF THE LABORATORY IN PSYCHIATRY **493**
Ronald L. Martin & Sheldon H. Preskorn

CHAPTER 31
EPIDEMIOLOGY OF PSYCHIATRIC ILLNESS **511**
Thomas J. Craig

CHAPTER 32

SUICIDE AND ATTEMPTED SUICIDE **529**

George E. Murphy

CHAPTER 33

CLINICAL PSYCHOPHARMACOLOGY AND OTHER SOMATIC THERAPIES **545**

Paul J. Perry, Bruce Alexander, & Michael J. Garvey

UNIT 1

Syndromes—Adult

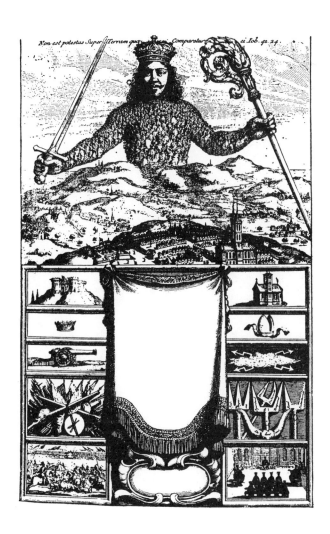

ability. The presence of a positive family history

CHAPTER 1

The Mental Status Examination

HAGOP S. AKISKAL

This chapter is devoted to the science and art of eliciting the specific signs and symptoms of mental disorders. The systematic perusal of these manifestations during the psychiatric interview constitutes the mental status examination, which can be viewed as analogous to physical examinations in other branches of medicine (Kraepelin, 1904).

Consider, as an example of this process, the mental examination of a 26-year-old single, male Caucasian engineering student who was brought to the hospital because of "acute sinus trouble." He had locked himself in his apartment for a week and refused to speak to anyone. When asked about his reasons for this behavior, he stated that he did not wish other people to hear the "noise emanating from my sinuses." The patient looked disheveled and had a frightened facial expression. Despite the psychotic content of his verbalizations, associations were grossly intact. Upon further questioning, he admitted that the "sinus noise" actually consisted of "voices, as if a transistor was installed up there in my head." The voices that were of the greatest concern to him argued in the third person about whether or not he was a "female." He was tremulous and restless during the interview, and on one occasion, he walked to a mirror and began to examine his facial features; he reluctantly admitted that he felt he was "transforming into a female," as the voices implied. At one point he became hostile and threatened to take legal action against a surgeon who, he believed, had "implanted a device" into his sinuses during an operation for deviated nasal septum 8 months previously; he added that subsequent to this operation he had intermittently experienced "foul smells" which, like his thoughts, had been "implanted from outside." All these manifestations occurred in clear consciousness, without evidence of disorientation or memory disturbances.

To arrive at a diagnostic formulation, the examiner considers the signs and symptoms observed during the mental status examination in combination with information obtained from the psychiatric

history. In this case, the diagnosis of paranoid schizophrenia was suggested by lifelong traits of seclusiveness, suspiciousness, and litigiousness; the absence of a history of substance abuse; and persistence of this clinical picture for longer than 6 months in the absence of major affective symptoms. Laboratory studies [e.g., negative urinary drug screen for stimulants and a normal sleep-deprived electroencephalogram (EEG)] were used to rule out, respectively, the remote possibility of stimulant-induced psychosis or complex partial (temporal lobe) seizures as the basis for his presenting complaints. Such physical workup to rule out somatic contributions is often a necessary step in psychiatric presentations with complex symptomatology, especially in patients with first psychotic breakdowns (Slater and Roth, 1977; Schiffer et al., 1988). The presence of a positive family history for schizophrenia in a paternal cousin provided further support for a schizophrenic diagnosis.

Thus the diagnostic process in psychiatry is analogous to that used in other branches of medicine: personal history, family history, examination, and laboratory tests constitute the essential steps. Because the raw data of psychopathology are often subjective and may elude precise characterization, the examination is of particular importance in psychiatry. Accurate description is difficult to obtain without careful and skillful probing during face-to-face interview. The faithful description of subjective experiences in psychiatry, known as *phenomenology*, was perfected by the German psychiatrist Karl Jaspers (1963). His approach differs from that of Freudian psychodynamics, which concerns itself with the unconscious meaning and interpretation of symptoms. In contrast to the Freudians, who focused on the *content* of psychopathology—which derived meaningfully from life situations—Jaspers believed that phenomenology, by its emphasis on the *form* of psychopathologic experiences, would eventually disclose "primary" symptoms, which are closest to the neurophysiologic substrate of the illness and which would therefore carry the greatest diagnostic weight. For instance, in the case of the young student, the fact that he heard voices arguing about him in the third person is more important diagnostically than what those voices said about him (that he was a female).

A detailed mental status examination constitutes an area of psychiatric expertise, but in briefer format, it is an essential tool for all physicians. A brief mental status examination should be performed as part of the routine physical examination on all patients. When indicated, this should be followed by a more detailed mental examination.

THE IMPORTANCE OF SIGNS AND SYMPTOMS IN PSYCHIATRY

Precision in the use of clinical terms to describe signs and symptoms is essential in all branches of medicine, promoting professional communication and preparing the ground for differential diagnostic workup. Imagine, for instance, what would happen if a patient with hemoptysis was erroneously described as having hematemesis. This would certainly confuse one's colleagues as to the medical status of the patient and could lead to an inappropriate series of diagnostic procedures. One can cite many other examples, such as jaundice versus pallor, ascites versus obesity, a functional versus an aortic stenosis murmur, which can all lead to difficulties in differentiation. In brief, genuine difficulties in eliciting, describing, and differentiating the myriad signs and symptoms that characterize diseases occur in all branches of medicine. Psychiatry is certainly not immune to such difficulties, but the belief—regrettably voiced by some medical educators—that differential diagnosis in psychiatry is haphazard and unproductive is both unfounded and dangerous. It is such attitudes that often lead patients with "functional" complaints to be labeled as "crocks," without the benefit of appropriate diagnostic evaluation. They may be viewed as having "imaginary" somatic complaints that waste the physician's time. The potential dangers of such attitudes can be seen in a study in the *Annals of Internal Medicine* (Murphy, 1975), which reported that the majority of a sample of completed suicides in St. Louis were seen by physicians within 6 months before their deaths; not only was the depressive nature of their ailment missed, but sedatives, in lethal quantities, were prescribed for their complaints of disordered sleep.

Although physicians typically spend many years mastering the art and science of physical diagnosis, little attention is given in medical education to the mental status examination. Many physicians are unaware that there exist systematic rules—analogous to those used in physical diagnosis—and which can serve to assess mental status. Moreover, it is seldom recognized that the failure to distinguish, for instance, whether a patient on reserpine is "sedated" or "depressed" can be as grave as the failure to distinguish between dyspepsia and angina: just as angina can be the prelude to myocardial infarction, reserpine-triggered depression can be the prelude to jumping out the hospital window.

The mental status examination is not just common sense or an expression of humane attitudes that assist the physician in empathizing with the patient while probing his inner experiences. Good judgment in complex human situations (an uncommon form of common sense) and an approach that considers the patient in his totality are not the sole prerogative of psychiatry: they are important in all branches of medicine. These attitudes merely set the stage for the practice of the clinical principles that constitute the body of scientific knowledge in any field. In psychiatry, there are established rules in the use of phenomenologic terms to arrive at diagnostic formulations that are the product of nearly 200 years of systematic clinical observation (Hamilton, 1974; Wing et al., 1974). International consensus and standardization have now been reached on the description and clinical probing of psychopathologic experiences as exemplified, most recently, in the World Health Organization (1992) development of the Schedule for Clinical Assessment in Neuropsychiatry (SCAN).

SPECIAL PROBLEMS IN PSYCHIATRIC PHENOMENOLOGY

Admittedly, there are many difficulties in the application of psychiatric terms and concepts. These fall into several categories.

1. Many psychiatric phenomena are subjective and do not easily lend themselves to objective description.

For instance, one of the author's patients described herself as being "transformed into a pig" while looking in the mirror. Here, the patient's verbal report is the only evidence for the occurrence of this experience. It is important to record such symptoms—in the patient's exact words—to decide whether the incident is indicative of incipient schizophrenia (psychotic depersonalization in which the self changes) or primary mood disorder (a depressive delusion that one is as ugly and dirty as a pig). This patient, who had no family or personal history of mental illness, suffered from a psychotic major depressive episode. She also saw herself in a coffin and heard voices commanding her to cut her throat with a butcher knife. She recovered fully with a course of electroconvulsive therapy (ECT).

2. The concepts used in psychiatry are not readily susceptible to the same kinds of external validation that are used in other branches of medicine (e.g., laboratory data). Psychiatrists heavily

rely on family history, pharmacologic response, and prospective course in validating diagnostic decisions made during cross-sectional examination. For instance, in the case just described, the response to ECT and the full recovery from the psychotic episode strongly favor the affective diagnosis. Recently there has been considerable momentum in attempting to link psychopathologic events with biologic correlates (Akiskal and Webb, 1978). Although no single biologic finding has yet been accepted universally as an unambiguous marker for a specific psychiatric syndrome, several sleep laboratory and neuroendocrine indices can now be used—along with more traditional approaches—in elucidating diagnostic dilemmas (Carroll, 1982; Kupfer and Thase, 1983; Akiskal and Lemmi, 1983). These biologic markers, then, are not meant to substitute for clinical judgment, but to supplement it in difficult differential diagnostic decisions.

3. Mental health professionals themselves have, at times, been imprecise in the use of psychopathologic terms and concepts. This situation, however, has improved with the advent of modern pharmacotherapy and biologic psychiatry, in which syndrome-specific treatments, such as lithium carbonate, dictate precise diagnostic evaluation.

Being awarded a doctorate in medicine does not automatically confer to the recipient the art of communication. Given the life-and-death nature of their endeavor, medical students—perhaps more than any other group of professional students—should endeavor to develop the proper habits of precise expression.

RECORDING SIGNS AND SYMPTOMS IN PSYCHIATRY

Signs refer to the clinician's observations of the patient. *Symptoms*, on the other hand, represent the subjective complaints of the patient based on his verbal report. For instance, agitation is a sign, based on the observation of motor restlessness, pacing, pulling one's hair, and so on. Auditory hallucination is a symptom typically based on patient report. Signs assume major significance when the patient is mute, stuporous, confused, or reluctant to talk.

Whenever feasible, one should try to corroborate symptoms with other observations. There are several ways to accomplish this.

- *Recording overt behavior that is consistent with the symptom.* For instance, does the patient who reports hearing voices appear preoccupied—perhaps mumbling to himself in an attempt to answer the voices? More serious, the patient may obey the commands given by voices. Likewise, the presence of a delusion can be inferred from behavior that results from it. For instance, a patient who believes himself to be persecuted

by the Mafia may decide to move to another town.

- *Recording historical data consistent with the symptoms.* Often patients' reports suggest corollary data that can be confirmed or refuted by other information obtained from patient or significant others. For instance, in the case of a patient who reports loss of ability to derive pleasure from life (anhedonia), one may question his wife as follows: Does he indulge in his hobbies? Does he engage in sexual activities that he previously enjoyed? For the patient who complains of loss of appetite, one might inquire whether he had lost weight or whether his clothes are large on him.

- *Recording other subjective experiences correlated with the symptom.* In some situations this is indeed the best validation. For instance, the avowal of homosexual orientation or preoccupation can be assessed in terms of masturbatory fantasies. In this instance, it is known that homosexual masturbatory fantasies may be more valid indicators of homosexuality than, say, incidental same-sex activity.

- *Physiologic monitoring.* In some situations, a precise physiologic measure can be recorded to substantiate a symptom. The subjective complaint of insomnia, for instance, can be measured with all-night sleep polygraphy (Hauri, 1991). This is important because many complaints of insomnia are vague. Neurophysiologic evaluations in sleep laboratories have indeed found that some "insomniacs" actually sleep as long and consistently as people without sleep complaints. Other insomniacs manifest delayed latency to sleep and frequent awakening in the first part of the night (as is characteristic of anxiety disorders). Others manifest early appearance of the first period of rapid eye movement and frequent awakening in the middle and terminal part of sleep (as is characteristic of clinical depression). Finally, other insomniacs may exhibit specific physiologic changes that characterize specific sleep disorders such as restless leg syndrome and nocturnal myoclonus.

A cardinal rule in recording psychopathologic phenomena is to distinguish clearly those phenomena which are based on history, direct observation, or patient report from inferences that one may derive from such phenomena. For instance, the student should avoid describing a patient who says "Everybody hates me" as engaging in "massive projection." The patient's actual report should appear in quotes in the mental status proper, while the inference of "projection" (if made plausible by other evidence) is best reserved for psychodynamic formulation (Perry et al., 1987). Thus the mental status examination should be free from speculation: it should be a record of the patient's mental condition as described by him and as observed by the clinician.

Aristotle said that some phenomena, such as colors, can only be defined by pointing at them. This is also true of many manifestations of psychopathology that can be learned only in reference to actual patients. Hence the definitions offered in the following sections are merely a guide for a more intensive patient-based study. Moreover, this is not an exhaustive list of approaches and terms used in mental status examinations. The differential diagnoses of signs and symptoms discussed throughout this introductory chapter will selectively focus on those concepts which have special diagnostic significance and which appear to be particularly problematic for beginning students.

CONDUCT OF THE MENTAL EXAMINATION

The areas covered in the mental status examination are summarized in Table 1-1. Although flexibility is necessary to allow for special circumstances presented by individual patients, a complete psychiatric examination generally should cover all these areas and is conventionally written up (if not conducted) in the order outlined.

Patients' presenting problems generally dictate the types of questions asked and the length and depth of interview. Research clinicians often conduct extensive structured interviews using specific probes for a standardized assessment of individual signs and symptoms. Practicing clinicians have traditionally conducted more or less unstructured interviews that provide for flexibility to tailor questions to the particular situation of the individual patient. Current experience indicates that when major mental illness is suspected, much can be gained by combining the virtues of these two approaches in a semistructured format. This way one would conduct a full examination to inquire about areas that an unstructured interview could easily miss while at the same time providing flexibility to follow the patient's leads and to frame the questions as best understood by that patient. When conducting an interview, beginning students should have available for quick reference an outline of the mental status examination, as well as the specific signs and symptoms most relevant to the differential diagnosis at hand. A pocket copy of the "mini-DSM-IV" [*Diagnostic and Statistical Manual of Mental Disorders*, fourth edition (1994)] is useful for this purpose; another useful guide is Goodwin and Guze's *Psychiatric Diagnosis* (1990).

It is not necessary to conduct all parts of the interview with the same depth on all patients. For instance, one need not directly check the orientation, vocabulary, and calculating ability of a moderately anxious young university professor who appears to be in good contact. Nor is it necessary to inquire extensively about bizarre psychotic experience when interviewing a diabetic patient who presents with the chief complaint of difficulty in attaining erections. Experience teaches one when such shortcuts can be made. The examiner must at times forego inquiry into a given area out of consideration for the patient, who may be unwilling or too uncomfortable to talk about certain topics; if the omitted area is of major significance for differential diagnosis, one should endeavor to obtain collateral information from significant others and return to questioning the patient at a later time, using a more indirect approach. There are situations in which one should conduct the mental status in multiple brief encounters, as in the case of extremely disturbed, violent, psychotic, or semistuporous patients, attempting to glean the optimal amount of information necessary for a tentative diagnosis.

TABLE 1-1. *Mental Status Examination Outline*

Appearance and behavior
  Attire, grooming, appears stated age?, posture, facial expression, eye contact
Attitude toward interviewer
  Friendly, cooperative, seductive, ambivalent, hostile
Psychomotor activity
  Normal, retarded, accelerated, agitated, catatonic symptoms
Affect and mood (emotional state)
  Euthymic, irritable, anxious, labile, inappropriate, blunted or flat, depressed, elated
Speech and thinking
  Process or form: Coherent, circumstantial, pressure of speech, flight of ideas, derailment (loose associations)
  Content: Phobias, obsessions, compulsions, delusions
  Specific speech disorders: Echolalia, perseveration, mutism, aphonia, aphasia
Perceptual disturbances
  Illusions, hallucinations, depersonalization, derealization
Orientation
  Time, place, person, situation
Attention (concentration) and memory
  Digits forward and backward, serial 7, street address, recall of three objects, amnesia
Intelligence
  Abstraction, vocabulary, global clinical impression of IQ
Reliability, judgment, and insight

AREAS OF THE MENTAL STATUS

The mental status typically begins with a statement about the setting in which the examination was conducted (e.g., inpatient or outpatient, private or public institution) and the purpose for which it was done (e.g., initial evaluation for outpatient treatment, disability determination, consultation for another physician). It typically follows a careful review of all existing records and proceeds with the areas described below.

Appearance and Behavior

Although this is the first section of the mental examination, relevant data are gathered throughout the interview process. Attire, posture, facial expression, and the level of grooming are described in such a way that the person reading the narration can visualize the patient's physical appearance at the time of the examination. It is important to note any obvious physical signs or deformities that point toward medical disease. The chronically ill and those experiencing great suffering may look older than stated age; by contrast, hypomanic, histrionic, and hebephrenic individuals may look younger. Poor eye contact may indicate shame, embarrassment, anxiety, social phobia, or paranoia. In some cases, little will be revealed in this section beyond the fact that the patient's physical appearance was unremarkable compared with other individuals of same age, educational level, and socioeconomic status. In other instances, the general observation may provide important clues about the patient's personality, mood, thought, awareness of social conventions, and ability to function adequately within society.

Attitude Toward the Interviewer

The patient's attitude toward the interviewer is often evident without specific inquiry, simply by ongoing observing of the patient throughout the interview. Some patients relate easily, are open and cooperative, and reveal plenty of information without much probing. Others may be reticent, guarded, or even suspicious—too embarrassed, unwilling, or frightened to share personal experiences. Some may be overtly hostile, perhaps attempting to embarrass or humiliate the examiner; in the extreme, the patient may be uncommunicative or even openly belligerent. Some patients are obsequious, trying to flatter the examiner, emphasizing how competent he is compared with all previous doctors, who "do not seem to care." Others may display *ambivalence*, a term that refers to the simultaneous presence of incompatible emotions (positive and negative). Still others may be overtly seductive. Clinical experience teaches the student how to interview these different kinds of patients. The two extremes of aggressive and seductive behavior represent the greatest challenge for clinical interviewers. Faced with such behaviors, the interviewer must set limits and maintain objectivity without losing empathy.

Psychomotor Activity

Psychomotor activity refers to physical activity as it relates to psychological functioning. A patient who displays *psychomotor agitation* moves around constantly, cannot sit still, and often shows pressure to talk. One may observe hand wringing, shuffling of feet, crossing and uncrossing of knees, picking on scabs, scratching, nail biting, hair twisting, and even hair pulling. One must contrast this purposeless physical restlessness with the more patterned *psychomotor acceleration*, in which the patient is ex-

tremely "busy," engages in many activities, talks incessantly by jumping from topic to topic, and experiences rapid thought progression. In the extreme, both agitation and acceleration may lead to frenzied activity that can be debilitating. In fact, before the availability of electroconvulsive and neuroleptic treatments, some of these patients died of sheer exhaustion. In other patients, one observes *psychomotor retardation*, in which there is a general slowing of movement, speech, and thought progression. Here, the patient may sit in a slumped, often frozen posture; speech is slow, monosyllabic, and of low pitch, accompanied by few gestures; and facial expression is either sad or blank. For such patients, talking may seem to be an effort, and latency of response to questions is typically prolonged. In some conditions, such as mixed states of affective psychosis, psychomotor agitation and retardation can be present simultaneously (i.e., physical slowing with racing thoughts). Abnormal psychomotor activity on repeated examination is usually indicative of a major psychiatric disorder. Quantitative rating of psychomotor function is now possible through the use of a reliable scale recently developed by Widlöcher (1983) and his team at the Salpêtrière in France. Despite proposals to develop physiologic measures of speech pause time and abnormalities of facial expression of emotions (Greden and Carroll, 1981), this area still very much relies on qualitative judgments made by experienced clinicians. In other words, there is no objective test to determine whether the facial expression of a patient is one of fear, depression, anger, or elation.

Other forms of psychomotor disturbances that occur in psychotic states include *posturing, stereotyped movements, mannerisms, negativism* (doing the opposite of what is requested), *echopraxia* (imitating the movements of another person), and *waxy flexibility* (maintaining certain awkward positions despite apparent discomfort). In the extreme, such manifestations may progress to *stupor*, which represents an extreme degree of psychomotor retardation and mutism combined. The condition is sometimes observed on the battlefront or in civilian catastrophes, where the victim may be "paralyzed by fear." In the absence of such history, organic contributions should be excluded by EEG, various brain imaging techniques, lumbar puncture, and other laboratory tests. Once this is done, intravenous amytal may help in differentiating depressive from schizophrenic stupor; the schizophrenic patient will momentarily come out of his state of inactive mutism and express delusional thoughts, for example, that he dare not move because his weight "would tilt the balance of the earth and bring the end of the world." The two conditions may be further distinguished clinically by the presence of incontinence, *catalepsy* (increased muscle tension), and expressionless facies, all of which are more suggestive of catatonic schizophrenia than of depression.

Affect and Mood

Affect is the prevailing emotional tone during the interview, as observed by the clinician. One must describe whether the patient exhibits an appropriate range of affect, which varies with the theme of the conversation and may include fear, sadness, and joy. In the case of marked disparity between affect and thought content, one speaks of *inappropriate* or *incongruent affect*. Other commonly observed disturbances of affect include *tension* (or inability to relax), *panic* (a crescendo increase in fear), *anger* (a predominantly argumentative or hostile stance), *lability* (rapid shifts from happiness to sadness, often accompanied by giggling, laughing, or, conversely, sobbing and weeping), and *blunting* or *flattening* (minimal display of emotion, with little variation in facial expression). In addition to the observed disturbances of affect, the clinician also must record the *mood*, or subjective feeling state, reported by the patient over the preceding several days or weeks. The most common moods reported by patients are *depression* (i.e., feeling in "low spirits" or "down in the dumps") and *anxiety*, a feeling of apprehension whose source remains undefined. When *irritability* is the prevailing mood, the patient may report having a "short fuse." In *euphoria*, the mood is one of extreme happiness and jubilation that is not justified by objective circumstances. These self-reports will not necessarily coincide with the observed affect. For instance, some patients may have a gloomy, downcast expression yet vigorously deny experiencing depressed mood; conversely, patients who do not show prominent signs of emotional distress may report a pervasive gloom. Such lack of concordance between subjective report of mood and observable affect and behavior is not uncommon in both normal and psychopathologic states (Lader and Marks, 1971). In the absence of specific disturbance in affect or mood, the patient is described as *euthymic*.

Speech and Thought

In this section the examiner describes the patient's verbal communication and its disturbances. *Thought form* (or *thought process*) refers to how ideas are put together in an observed sample of speech and in what sequence and speed. A patient exhibiting no abnormality in the formal aspect of thought is said to have coherent thought that is clear, logical, and easy to follow and understand. In *circumstantiality*, there is a tendency to answer questions in terms of long-winded details. In *pressure of speech*, the patient seems to be compelled to talk, while in *flight of ideas*, thoughts actually race ahead of the patient's ability to communicate them; he skips from one idea or theme to another, and ideas may be connected by rhymes or puns (*clang association*), as shown in this address made by a patient to the psychiatrist in chief during the morning round:

"Let me part soon—to the moon—moonshine is for lovers—the cure for lovers' heart—the lure of poets—the doors of perception—a magnificent conception—on! on! Let me conquer the moon."

This form of thought is most characteristic of mania and tends to be *overinclusive*, with difficulty in excluding irrelevant, extraneous details from the association. In the extreme, it may be hard to draw the line between manic flight of ideas and schizophrenic *derailment* (literally, "off the track"), in which it is impossible for the observer to glean any logical sequence from the patient's speech. Patients with this degree of *loosening of associations* sometimes invent new words that have private meanings (*neologisms*). Associative slippage also may manifest in general vagueness of thinking, which is not grossly incoherent but conveys little information, even though many words may have been used. This disturbance, known as *poverty of thought*, is a major diagnostic sign of schizophrenia when known organic mental disorders have been ruled out (Andreasen, 1979b). Here is a sample from a letter a high school student wrote to the psychiatrist to explain why he was in the hospital:

I often contemplate. It is a general stance of the world. It is a tendency which varies from time to time. It defines things more than others. It is in the nature of habit. This is what I would like to say to explain everything that happened.

Bleuler (1950) coined the term *autism* to refer to the self-absorption that he believed characterized schizophrenic thought, feeling, and behavior. Thinking that is governed by inner drives and a "private logic" is therefore known as autistic thinking; *dereistic* thinking is a synonym for it. Current evidence indicates that such thinking may actually reflect, in some cases, measurable neurologic deficits (Andreasen, 1984).

Echolalia, most commonly observed in catatonia, is the irrelevant, sometimes playful, repeating of words used by the interviewer (e.g., "What day is today?" "Today.") In *perseveration*, also seen in catatonia, as well as in chronic organic mental disorders, the patient adheres to the same concept or words and appears unable to proceed to others. *Thought block* refers to the sudden arrest of thought in the middle of a sentence, often followed, after a momentary pause, with a new and unrelated thought. When mild, this experience may be caused by exhaustion, anxiety, or depression; severer degrees are seen in schizophrenia, where they may be the observable counterpart of the subjective experience of thought withdrawal. *Mutism* consists of the loss of speech and can be intentional in origin (as part of a dramatic cluster personality disorder) and limited to interactions with certain people (elective mutism) or involuntary (as part of catatonia or midline lesions of the brain). In *aphasia*, owing to dominant temporal lobe lesions, the patient has a specific memory disorder for words and language; even when unable to talk, the patient usually attempts to communicate by other methods. In *dysphonia*, the patient loses his voice and cannot raise it beyond a whisper, which, in the extreme, can proceed to *aphonia;* here, in contrast with mutism, one can observe lip movements or nonverbal attempts to communicate. Unless based on laryngeal pathology or excessive abuse of vocal cords (as seen in voluble manics), these deficits in phonation are almost always due to a conversion disorder, representing, for example, a compromise in an adolescent who feels conflicted between lying and telling her parents the truth about sexual behavior of which they would strongly disapprove.

Common abnormalities of thought content include *obsessions* (repetitive ideas, images, or impulses that intrude into consciousness unwanted, yet patients are aware that these thoughts are their own), *compulsions* (irresistible urges to engage in apparently meaningless acts), and *phobias* (irrational fears unjustified by objective circumstances). Phobias are usually categorized by the circumstances eliciting them, such as social phobia (a common form of which consists of fear of facing a group in a lecture situation), agoraphobia (fear of going out alone in public places), acrophobia (fear of heights), etc.

Two obsessions that commonly torment neurotic patients are the unwanted idea that one might inadvertently harm or kill loved ones and that one could be contaminated by germs, dirt, excreta, or other undesirable elements. The latter obsession is typically associated with cleaning compulsions or rituals to rid oneself of such elements. The unwanted idea (obsession) that one might (inadvertently) hurt loved ones does not ordinarily lead to taking action; instead, it may be associated with the ritual of hiding away knives, scissors, other sharp objects, etc. Thus obsessions with aggressive content should be distinguished from *homicidal ideation or threats*, which do carry some likelihood of being carried out. The clinician must likewise distinguish between an obsession with self-injury content and *suicidal ideation.* The former refers to the tormenting thought that one might, contrary to one's value system, hurt or kill oneself. However, in other patients, the pain of depression can be of such a magnitude that the normal barriers that prevent one from taking one's life do break down, and thus suicidal thoughts can lead to suicidal action; suicidal ideation is a particularly ominous symptom if associated with loss of hope for the future (*hopelessness*). Therefore, the clinician should always inquire about suicidal ideation; the notion that one thereby inadvertently "puts thoughts into the patients' head" is unfounded; on the contrary, patients are typically relieved that the physician is aware of their mental suffering and could provide appropriate measures to terminate it. It is also important to

realize that not all depressed patients actively contemplate suicide; instead, this propensity may be expressed more passively as a general feeling that life holds little meaning for them (*tedium vitae*) and that they would prefer not to wake up in the morning, or that they would welcome a fatal disease or an accident. It is incumbent upon the psychiatric examiner to explore such possibilities with circumspection and sensitivity.

Delusions are common abnormalities of thought content among psychotic patients. They are defined as false beliefs that are unshakable and idiosyncratic to the individual. Thus the beliefs of a delusional patient cannot be undone by logical arguments to the contrary, as illustrated in the following vignette.

A black female inpatient, admitted to an emergency psychiatric service, believed that she was Jesus Christ. When questioned how this was possible, given that Christ was male, white, and Jewish, the patient responded with a smile: "The Bible is wrong." The examiner in this instance was lucky to elicit a mere smile; delusional beliefs are often associated with more vehement affect. Therefore, they should be probed with the requisite tact and sensitivity on the part of the examiner, especially when they involve race, gender, and religion.

It is also important to keep in mind that the idiosyncratic nature of delusional beliefs means that they are not shared by members of the same culture or subculture. For instance, the belief that one is sexually "voodooed" and will not regain one's potency until the spell is lifted is not necessarily delusional; neither are beliefs in unusual health practices and folk remedies. The decision of whether one is dealing with a culturally accepted phenomenon must be based on a thorough knowledge of a given culture or subculture. To complicate matters, in cultures where voodoo and witchcraft are part of daily life, delusions may sometimes represent pathologic elaborations of such beliefs. The definitive test is whether an unusual belief is shared by members of the patient's subculture. Delusions also must be differentiated from *overvalued ideas*, which are fanatically maintained notions, such as the superiority of one sex, nation, or race over others, and while not necessarily an indication of clinical pathology, such ideas may, in the extreme, suggest the diagnosis of a personality disorder known as "fanatical psychopath" (Schneider, 1958).

Delusions are categorized as primary or secondary. Primary delusions cannot be understood in terms of other psychological processes. The most common examples of these are represented by Schneider's first-rank symptoms (1959), which consist of externally imposed influences in the spheres of thought (*thought insertion*), emotion, and somatic function (*passivity feelings*), as well as experiences of *thought withdrawal* and *thought broadcasting;* hence they are also known as *delusions of control* or *delusions of influence.* Primary delusions may arise in the setting of what is termed *delusional mood*, in which the patient is gradually losing his grasp of reality: neutral percepts may suddenly acquire special personal or revelatory significance of delusional proportion (e.g., a red car being seen as an indicator of imminent invasion by communist forces). This two-stage phenomenon, known as *delusional perception*, is also considered a first-rank symptom. Although one or two schneiderian symptoms may be seen in severely psychotic affective—especially manic—patients (Clayton et al., 1965; Carlson and Goodwin, 1973), the presence of a large number of such symptoms usually points toward schizophrenia (Mellor, 1970; Akiskal and Puzantian, 1979), provided that stimulant-induced psychosis, complex partial (temporal lobe) seizures, and alcoholic hallucinosis are excluded.

Secondary delusions derive from other psychopathologic experiences and occur in a variety of psychiatric disorders. Delusions may be secondary to

- *Hallucinations*—the patient hears the voice of his deceased mother and concludes that he must be dead too.
- *Other delusions*—the patient, believing that he is being persecuted by others, may decide that he must be the messiah.
- *Impaired memory*—a patient with general paresis of the insane who, unable to remember where she had placed her purse, repeatedly called the police to report that her neighbors were robbing her.
- *Morbid affective states*—These are sometimes referred to as *affective delusions* and arise from the prevailing mood—usually depression—and the associated guilt, low self-esteem, and insecurity (Akiskal and Puzantian, 1979). They can take the form of *delusions of guilt* or *sinfulness* (the belief that one has committed an unpardonable act), *delusions of jealousy* (false belief in infidelity of spouse or lover), *hypochondriacal* or *somatic delusions* (i.e., delusions of ill-health), *nihilistic delusions* (the belief that parts of one's body are missing), and *delusions of poverty* (the belief that one has lost all means and family members will starve).

Other secondary delusions include *delusions of reference* (the idea that one is being observed, talked about, laughed at, etc.), *erotomania* (in which the patient believes that a famous person is in love with him or her), and *grandiose delusions* (belief that one has unusual talents or powers or that one has the identity of a famous person). Although erotomania and grandiose delusions often arise in the setting of expansive mood, one can usually find clinical evidence for underlying low self-esteem or depression. Delusions of reference can occur in affective, schizophrenic, as well as organic psychoses. In *delusions of assistance*, the patient believes himself to be the object of benevolence from others or supernatural

powers; for example, a manic woman, who had run away from her ex-husband's harassment, stated that chariots were being sent to transport her and her children to heaven. In the more common *persecutory delusions*, the patient believes himself to be the target of malevolent action; this may be due to the conviction that one is somehow guilty and deserves punishment, or it may result from a grandiose self-concept; in other cases, the patient may be misattributing his hostile impulses to his presumed persecutors.

Perceptual Disturbances

The simplest form of perceptual aberration is represented by an *illusion*, often in the visual sphere, in which real stimuli are mistaken for something else (e.g., a belt for a snake in a dimly lit room). Such misinterpretation can be secondary to exhaustion, anxiety, altered states of consciousness, delirium, or a functional psychosis. *Hallucination*, a more serious perceptual disturbance, consists of a perception without external stimulus (Esquirol, 1965) (e.g., hearing voices when nobody is around, seeing things that are not there, or perceiving unusual odors and tastes). In *synesthesia*, observed in psychedelic intoxication, the perceptual disturbances are in more than one sensory modality, and the subject "hears" colors, "smells" music, and so on. For example, Baudelaire, the French poet whose drug experimentation was well known, wrote about the color of vowels: *"A noir, E blanc, I rouge, U vert, O bleu."*

Auditory hallucinations are classified as either elementary (noises) or complete (voices or words). They are commonly reported by schizophrenic patients but also occur in organic mental disorders and drug intoxication or withdrawal. Some patients in the initial stages of a psychotic breakdown report hearing their own thoughts spoken aloud (*écho de pensée*); at a later stage, voices lose their connection with the person and appear to be coming from outside, making a running commentary on the patient's behavior or arguing about him in the third person. These are all special categories of hallucinatory phenomena included in Schneider's list of first-rank symptoms (1959). They occur in a variety of psychotic disorders, but when they are extremely pronounced or continuous, they suggest schizophrenia. Schneiderian hallucinations are considered to be mood-incongruent, in that they have no plausible link to the patient's state of mood. Hallucinations also can be mood-congruent; these are observed in the affective psychoses, in which voices typically make derogatory statements about the patient, usually in the second person ("You are a jerk") or give self-destructive commands ("Slit your throat"). Perceptual disturbances that occur in affective illness tend to be transient and typically occur at the depth or height of an affective episode or during the unstable neurophysiologic transition (mixed state) from depression to mania. They also can arise from the exhaustion, dehydration, or superimposed drug or alcohol abuse that often complicates affective disorders; these complications explain in part why mood-incongruent psychotic experiences are occasionally seen in otherwise classic affective psychoses (Akiskal and Puzantian, 1979).

Visual hallucinations are most characteristic of organic mental disorders, especially acute delirious states. Sometimes they are lilliputian (less than lifesize); they may coexist with auditory hallucinations and can be frightening. Visual phenomena associated with psychedelic drugs can be pleasant or frightening, depending on mental set. Visual hallucinations are not characteristic of schizophrenia but can occur in normal grief (visions of a dead relative), in depressive psychoses (e.g., seeing oneself in one's casket), and in brief reactive psychoses observed in abnormal personalities. *Hypnagogic* and *hypnopompic hallucinations* are visual experiences that occur in twilight state between sleep and wakefulness, occurring respectively when falling asleep and waking up. Although their occasional occurrence is normal, repeated experiences, especially when associated with sleep paralysis and sudden loss of muscle tone under emotional arousal (cataplexy), are cardinal manifestations of narcolepsy, representing rapid eye movement intrusions into consciousness. Other circumstances that can provoke visual hallucinosis include sensory deprivation (e.g., after cataract surgery), delirium, and other organic mental disorders (Lipowski, 1990). Histrionic personalities may give flamboyant accounts of "perceiving" objects or events that fit their fantasies. All these manifestations must be distinguished from *dysmegalopsia*, in which objects may seem to get larger or closer (*macropsia*) or smaller and recede into space (*micropsia*), which are special forms of illusory phenomena that occur in retinal detachment, disorders of accommodation, posterior temporal lesions, and psychedelic drug intoxication. Finally, psychedelic drugs can produce impression of extremely vivid colors with geometric patterns (*kaleidoscopic hallucinations*).

Olfactory hallucinations may be difficult to distinguish from illusions. For example, a woman with low self-esteem might be preoccupied with vaginal odor and might misinterpret neutral gestures made by other people as indicative of olfactory disgust. In complex partial seizures of temporal lobe origin, hallucinations of burning paint or rubber present as auras.

Haptic hallucinations (hallucinations of touch) are usually experienced as insects crawling on one's skin (known as *formication*) and characteristically occur in cocaine intoxication, amphetamine psychosis, and delirium tremens owing to alcohol or sedative-hypnotic withdrawal. In schizophrenic disorders, they may take such bizarre forms as or-

gasms produced by invisible objects or creatures. *Tactile hallucinations* must be distinguished from extreme tactile sensitivity (*hyperesthesia*) and diminished sensitivity (*hypesthesia*), both of which can occur in peripheral nerve disease as well as in hysterical conditions.

Vestibular hallucinations (e.g., those of flying) are seen most commonly in organic states, such as delirium tremens and LSD psychosis, and may result in serious injuries when, for example, the subject attempts to fly off a roof. In *hallucinations of presence*, most commonly reported by schizophrenic, histrionic, or delirious patients, the subject senses the presence of another person or creature who remains invisible. In *extracampine hallucinations*, the patient sees objects outside the sensory field (e.g., behind his head), whereas in *autoscopy*, the patient visualizes himself projected into space. The latter phenomenon, which can occur in organic, conversion, depressive, and schizophrenic disorders, is also known as *Döppelganger*, or seeing one's double, and is skillfully portrayed in Dostoevski's novel, *The Double*.

Other perceptual disturbances that cannot be classified easily into specific sensory modalities include *depersonalization* (the uncanny feeling that one has changed), *derealization* (the feeling that the environment has changed), *déjà vu* (a sense of familiarity with a new perception), and *déjà entendu* (the feeling that a new auditory perception has been experienced before). As isolated findings, these can occur in normal people who are anxious, tired, or sleepy, but repeated experiences along these lines indicate the following differential diagnoses (Roth, 1959): complex partial seizures, panic disorder, schizophreniform psychosis, hysterical dissociation, and psychedelic intoxication.

Orientation

In this section the clinician records whether the patient knows who he is (orientation to person), where he is (orientation to place), why he is there and with whom he is interacting (orientation to situation), and what date and time of day it is (orientation to time). One who is orientated in all spheres is considered to have a *clear sensorium*. Patients with affective and schizophrenic psychoses are not typically disoriented (although, because of apathy, they may fail to keep track of daily routines), whereas patients who suffer from organic mental disorders are characteristically disoriented. In acute brain disease, patients often show remarkable fluctuation in orientation depending on time of day, with worsening disorientation at night. With increasing severity of brain impairment, the patient is totally confused as to orientation, and his sensorium may be *clouded* at all times to such an extent that in the extreme he may lapse into an *organic stupor*.

Attention (Concentration) and Memory

The patient who shows deficits in attention or concentration is, in the extreme, unable to filter relevant from irrelevant stimuli as they pertain to the interview material and thus may be easily distracted by the TV, telephone, and other background stimuli. A patient with milder disorder may be able to achieve the attention required for a successful interview but may complain that his mind is "not working." Care must be taken to distinguish between deficits in attention, which are involuntary, and lack of cooperation; an example of the latter would be a patient who whistles instead of answering questions posed to him. Attention and concentration are usually tested by digits forward and digits backward ("Can you repeat 7248 forward? Can you repeat it backward?"). A related test is serial sevens (i.e., subtracting 7 from 100 and from each successive remainder); in using this test, the observer needs to make some allowance for educational background.

Deficits in memory are conveniently grouped into four kinds: (1) immediate, when the patient cannot even register things he has just been told, (2) short-term, when he cannot retain information for 5 minutes or so, (3) recent, when he is unable to recall the events of the past months or years, and (4) long-term, or remote, when he is unable to recollect what took place many years ago. Deficits in immediate recall suggest serious acute brain impairment or stupor. Less severe brain insults tend to spare registration but can lead to deficits in short-term memory, which can be assessed by asking the patient to remember a street address or three unrelated items (e.g., "17, yellow, chair") in 5 to 7 minutes, after making sure that the patient fully understands the items to be remembered. Recent memory is most likely to be compromised by chronic organic impairment; its intactness can be tested by asking the patient about verifiable recent events in his life or current events. Remote memory is usually spared in the early course of dementing diseases, but at later stages, it may be impaired to such an extent that the patient may not recognize his own children. This is best tested by asking about several past historical events that someone with the patient's social background and intelligence can reasonably be expected to be familiar with.

Disturbances in attention, concentration, and memory are most characteristic of organic mental disorders, yet schizophreniform and acute affective psychoses also may exhibit reversible abnormalities in these functions. Although it is customary to use the term *pseudodementia* to refer to this phenomenon, it appears that reversible neurophysiologic derangements underlying these psychotic illnesses may well be responsible for the observed cognitive deficits (McHugh and Slavney, 1983). Finally, memory disturbances also can result from a combination of organic insults (e.g., head trauma) and emotional causes (e.g., hysterical dissociation) that could lead to amnesia for events before (retrograde) or after (anterograde) the injury. In general, the more psychogenic in origin, the more circumscribed is the amnesia, and the more organic, the more global. Retrograde amnesia for autobiographic events for variable periods can also occur after a course of electroconvulsive therapy.

Intelligence

Intelligence can be indirectly inferred from the patient's overall intellectual performance during the mental status examination. If deficits are grossly apparent, historical information should be used to decide whether they have always been present (intellectual subnormality) or developed after a certain age (intellectual impairment). Intelligence is commonly assessed by testing for abstracting ability. To do this, one inquires about similarities, going from simpler comparisons ("How are an airplane and a car alike?") to more difficult ones ("A painting and a poem?"). The examiner also must pay special attention to the patient's vocabulary. Vocabulary and performance on similarities testing depend not only on the patient's intellectual capacity but also on his age, social background, and educational level. For instance, the presence of a good vocabulary and abstracting ability, despite a third-grade education, indicates above-average intelligence. If vocabulary and abstracting ability are poor, allowance should be made for social deprivation. In the absence of such factors, and especially if the patient has a college education, the examiner must consider the possibility of intellectual impairment owing to an organic mental disorder.

Classically, organic mental disorders have been described as involving changes in orientation, attention, memory, and intelligence. When profound, such changes provide unequivocal clinical evidence for an underlying somatic disease. However, as indicated, subtle yet measurable deficits in these mental faculties often accompanies the so-called functional psychiatric disorders, and such data point to underlying disturbances in cerebral structures involved with these faculties, the precise nature of which continues to elude psychiatric research. The clinician also must keep in mind the not uncommon occurrence of moderate to severe subcortical pathology or disease with relatively intact intellectual function, manifesting instead in profound alterations in perception, mood, and psychomotor behavior; delusions, obsessions, phobias, depersonalization, derealization, and related bizarre psychopathologic disturbances often accompany such disease (Taylor 1993; Lishman, 1987).

Reliability, Judgment, and Insight

Every mental status examination should have a statement regarding the extent to which the patient's report of his experiences and behavior is to be considered reliable. This assessment is largely based on an estimate of the patient's intellectual ability, honesty, attention to detail, and motivation. Sociopathic and histrionic individuals are notoriously unreliable. *Retrospective falsification*, commonly observed in such patients, consists of distortion of real past experiences to conform with present emotional needs; at other times, they may lie to avoid personal responsibilities. A related type of unreliability is *pseudologia fantastica*, expansive storytelling such that the individual is unable to discern which of his statements are true and which are false. Psychotic patients and those with organic mental disorders also tend to be unreliable informants; here one sometimes observes *confabulation*, a spontaneous fabrication of responses to fill in memory gaps.

Judgment refers to the patient's ability to evaluate the proper course of action in difficult situations and is traditionally tested by asking what one would do if one were the first to observe smoke in a movie theater. The patient's history will often give clues as to whether he generally has good or poor judgment. Disturbances in judgment can be circumscribed to one or more areas (e.g., money, attire, sexual conduct), leaving other areas, like maternal role, intact. *Insight* pertains to a more complex form of judgment regarding the patient's awareness of his emotional state, its causes, its severity, and its impact on significant others. Psychotic patients, especially manics, notoriously lack insight and are often unaware of the painful consequences of their spending sprees and sexual promiscuity, which explains in part their frequent lack of cooperation with treatment regimens.

COMMON ERRORS IN MENTAL STATUS EXAMINATION

Eugen Bleuler's work on schizophrenia (1950) continues to exert a major influence in the description and differential diagnosis of schizophrenic manifestations. Bleuler believed that disturbances in associations, affect, ambivalence, and autism characterized this group of disorders. His ideas were, unfortunately, accepted before being empirically tested, leading to much confusion in mental status evaluations. This is particularly true for disturbance in affect and associations. Recent work, as exemplified by Andreasen (1979a, 1979b), has provided a fresh empirical perspective in regard to these two areas. This section examines affective and thinking disturbances in light of recent experience.

Disturbances in Affect

The examiner must distinguish between flat and depressed affect, which occur in disorders that seldom intersect (i.e., chronic schizophrenia versus primary mood disorder). *Shallow, blunted,* and *flat affect* refer to increasing degrees of emotional impoverishment—often accompanied by a subjective feeling that one cannot experience emotions, a classical disturbance of schizophrenia. By contrast, depression is a painful affect, what William James (1902) termed a psychical neuralgia.

EDITORS' COMMENT

Depressed patients given antipsychotics, usually for agitation, also appear to have flat or blunted affect.

Many depressed patients also experience anhedonia, best described by Shakespeare: "How weary, stale, flat, and unprofitable/Seem to me all the uses of this world" (Hamlet, Act I, Scene II). Diagnostic difficulties arise in severe depression, where the anhedonia may progress to a pervasive sense of emptiness, often accompanied by the inability to feel normal emotions; such patients may feel "dead inside" and see the world around them as lifeless. Differentiation can be accomplished as follows: First, the facial expression of the chronic schizophrenic is typically vacuous, whereas that of the depressive is one of pain, gloom, and dejection. Second, the schizophrenic tends to produce, in the observer, a cold feeling and an inability to empathize (the so-called praecox feeling), whereas the depressive's dejection and pain are usually communicated in such a way that the interviewer can empathize with him. Admittedly, this is a subjective criterion, but it is quite useful in the hands of experienced clinicians.

Labile affect (which changes quickly, often from one extreme to the other) must be distinguished from incongruent affect (which is inappropriate to the thought content or the context). Labile and incongruent affects should both be differentiated from *affective incontinence*, in which the patient laughs or cries for long periods with little or no provocation. Lability is encountered in the dramatic cluster of personality disorders; in mixed states of manic-depressive illness, where there are rapid shifts from elation to irritability to depression; and in acute organic brain disease, where the affect can quickly change from anxiety to terror to panic. Inappropriate affect (e.g., laughing while relating the gory details of a natural disaster) should raise the suspicion of schizophrenia. Emotional incontinence suggests organic states, such as arteriosclerotic dementia and multiple sclerosis.

Euphoria and elation, although characteristic of manic states, also can occur in organic mental disorders, such as general paresis of the insane and multiple sclerosis. The euphoria seen in mania has a warmth that is communicated to the observer (although manics, especially when crossed, can be irritable, hostile, and obnoxious); the interviewer should thus avoid direct confrontation with manic patients. A type of euphoria characteristic of chronic schizophrenia and frontal lobe lesions, known as *Witzelsucht*, consists of the patient relating silly jokes; these lack the empathic contagiousness of the humor of bipolar patients.

La belle indifference should be differentiated from *apathy*. In the former condition—seen in conversion reactions—the patient exhibits lack of concern or even smiles in the face of reported disability. Apathy, on the other hand, seen in many chronic psychiatric patients because of their overall dismal situation, is a feeling akin to demoralization.

Disturbances in Thinking

Unfortunately, "thought disorder" is often used rather loosely to refer to both formal thought disorder and delusional content. For the sake of clarity, the unqualified use of *thought disorder* should be discarded. Even the term *formal thought disorder* covers too wide a territory. It should always be made clear whether one is referring to derailment or loose associations, flight of ideas, or circumstantiality. The presence of a delusion cannot be considered evidence of underlying formal thought disorder because, as noted previously, delusions can be secondary to affective, perceptual, and memory disturbances.

Derailment refers to a disorder in associations whereby different thoughts are dissociated, disconnected, or rambling. If mild, it leaves the impression of vagueness; if the patient makes no sense at all, it is referred to as *word salad*. The phrase *loose associations* is used for an intermediate degree of severity, wherein one finds fragmented thoughts that do not seem to follow Aristotelian logic but may nevertheless have an inner, private (autistic) logic of their own. The incoherence that one observes in the thinking of organic patients is qualitatively distinct from the loose associations of the schizophrenic in that it lacks symbolism and autistic quality; however, in severe cases of schizophrenia, this distinction may be difficult to make. *Vorbeireden*, or talking past the point, also should be differentiated from incoherence. In vorbeireden, which occurs in the Ganser syndrome, the patient gives obvious indication that he has understood the question yet deliberately provides "approximate" answers.

For instance, a patient examined in 1977, when asked who the president was, replied, "Jerry Carter," and when asked who was president before him, he replied, "Jimmy Ford."*

It is often erroneously assumed that inability to abstract on testing of similarities or proverbs (i.e.,

---

* The Ganser syndrome seen among prisoners is best understood in terms of conscious and unconscious reasons for appearing psychotic or demented; hence it is also referred to as *hysterical pseudodementia*. To complicate matters, adolescent schizophrenic patients may find approximate answers amusing and may respond to an entire interview with a series of approximate answers; such patients may therefore *appear* to exhibit hysterical pseudodementia, but in reality, they have a *hysterical pseudopseudodementia*.

---

concrete thinking) has major diagnostic importance in schizophrenia. There is little scientific rationale for this belief. Concreteness correlates best with poor intellectual endowment, cultural impoverishment, and organic brain disease. Because all three of these factors not infrequently coexist with schizophrenia, to that extent, schizophrenics will have impaired ability in abstraction. The major value of testing abstraction in schizophrenia lies in the patient's tendency to give highly idiosyncratic and bizarre answers to proverb and similarities testing.

Pressure of speech, usually seen in agitated depression, refers to patients who feel pressured to talk and usually cannot be stopped.

Flight of ideas, a major diagnostic sign of mania, refers to a type of overproductivity wherein the patient rapidly skips from one idea or theme to another, often by resorting to rhyming or punning, but without totally abandoning logic. Pressure of speech and flight of ideas both should be distinguished from loose associations that do not follow Aristotelian logic. Circumstantiality is the unnecessary elaboration of detail and is seen in dullards (borderline IQ), pedantic obsessionals, and patients with severe somatization disorder, but in severe degree, it may be difficult to differentiate from schizophrenic looseness.

EDITORS' COMMENT

Some manic patients present when they are partially treated with antimanic drugs, so the triad of hyperactivity, flight of ideas, and pressure of speech is not as obvious as their delusional thinking.

The term *paranoid* is often used incorrectly to refer to suspiciousness or persecutory beliefs. *Paranoid* actually means "delusional" and should be restricted as a generic term for disorders characterized by prominent delusional formation (e.g., paranoid schizophrenia and paranoid states). Paranoid schizophrenia is a schizophrenic subtype in which delusions—not always persecutory in nature—occur in abundance. In paranoid states, usually one delusional theme predominates, with no evidence of schizophrenic formal thought disorder. For example, in conjugal paranoia, a man believes that his wife is having an affair and interprets all her behavior along those lines.

Delusions can be graded on the basis of their plausibility. For instance, the false belief that one's spouse is unfaithful is nevertheless a believable idea. The false belief that one's spouse is having multiple affairs simultaneously, although delusional, is not impossible. However, the belief that one's spouse is having an affair with a creature with green tentacles is patently absurd; such bizarre delusions are the hallmark of schizophrenia, although they also can sometimes be associated with organic mental disorders.

SUMMARY

The mental status examination represents the portion of the psychiatric interview that is devoted to a systematic elicitation of psychopathologic signs and symptoms that are important in diagnostic formulation. Consequently, it is essential that descriptive terms be used precisely and consistently. This will not only facilitate professional communication, but will also enhance the chances of formulating differential diagnosis in a cogent way, setting the stage for rational therapy.

REFERENCES

Akiskal HS, Lemmi H: Clinical, neuroendocrine, and sleep EEG diagnosis of "unusual" affective presentations: A practical review. Psychiatr Clin North Am 6:69–83, 1983.

Akiskal HS, Puzantian VR: Psychotic forms of depression and mania. Psychiatr Clin North Am 2:419–439, 1979.

Akiskal HS, Webb WL: Psychiatric Diagnosis: Exploration of Biological Predictors. New York, Spectrum Publications, 1978.

Andreasen NC: Affective flattening and the criteria for schizophrenia. Am J Psychiatry 136:944–947, 1979a.

Andreasen NC: The clinical assessment of thought, language, and communication disorders. Arch Gen Psychiatry 36:1315–1330, 1979b.

Andreasen NC: The Broken Brain. New York, Harper & Row, 1984.

Bleuler E: Dementia Praecox, or the Group of Schizophrenias, trans by J Zinkin. New York, International Universities Press, 1950.

Carlson G, Goodwin F: The stages of mania. Arch Gen Psychiatry 28:221–288, 1973.

Carroll J: Use of the dexamethasone suppression test in depression. J Clin Psychiatry 43:44–48, 1982.

Clayton PJ, Pitts FN, Winokur G: Affective disorder: V. Mania. Compr Psychiatry 6:313–322, 1965.

Esquirol JE: Mental Maladies: A Treatise on Insanity (1845). New York, Hafner Publishing Co, 1965.

Greden J, Carroll B: Psychomotor functioning in affective disorders: An overview of new monitoring techniques. Am J Psychiatry 11:1441–1448, 1981.

Goodwin DW, Guze SB: Psychiatric Diagnosis. New York, Oxford University Press, 1984.

Hamilton M (ed): Fish's Clinical Psychopathology: Signs and Symptoms in Psychiatry. Bristol, John Wright & Sons, 1974.

Hauri PJ (ed): Case Studies in Insomnia. New York, Plenum Press, 1991.

James W: Varieties of Religious Experience (1902). Glasgow, William Collins & Sons, 1982.

Jaspers K: General Psychopathology, trans by J Hoenig, MW Hamilton. Manchester, University Press, 1963.

Kraepelin E: Lectures on Clinical Psychiatry. London, Balliere, Tindall & Cox, 1904.

Kupfer DJ, Thase ME: The use of the sleep laboratory in the diagnosis of affective disorders. Psychiatr Clin North Am 6:3–21, 1983.

Lader M, Marks IM: Clinical Anxiety. New York, Grune & Stratton, 1971.

Lipowski, ZJ: Delirium: Acute Confusional States. New York, Oxford Universities Press, 1990.

Lishman WA: Organic Psychiatry: Psychological Consequences of Cerebral Disorder, second edition. Oxford, Blackwell Scientific Publications, 1987.

McHugh PR, Slavney PR: The Perspectives of Psychiatry. Baltimore, Johns Hopkins University Press, 1983.

Mellor CS: First rank symptoms of schizophrenia. Br J Psychiatry 117:15–23, 1970.

Murphy GE: The physician's responsibility for suicide. Ann Intern Med 82:301–309, 1975.

Perry S, Cooper AM, Michels R: The psychodynamic formulation: Its purpose, structure, and clinical application. Am J Psychiatry 144:543–550, 1987.

Quick Reference to Diagnostic Criteria from DSM-IV. Washington, American Psychiatric Press, 1994.

Roth M: The phobic anxiety-depersonalization syndrome. Proc R Soc Med 52:587–595, 1959.

Schiffer RB, Klein RF, Sider RC: The Medical Evaluation of Psychiatric Patients. New York, Plenum Medical Book Co., 1988.

Schneider K: Psychopathic Personalities, trans by MW Hamilton. London, Cassell, 1958.

Schneider K: Clinical Psychopathology, trans by MW Hamilton. New York, Grune & Stratton, 1959.

Slater E, Roth M: Mayer-Gross' Clinical Psychiatry, 3d ed, revised. Baltimore, Williams & Wilkins, 1977.

Taylor MA: The Neuropsychiatric Guide to Modern Everyday Psychiatry. New York: The Free Press, 1993.

Widlöcher DJ: Psychomotor retardation: Clinical, theoretical, and psychometric aspects. Psychiatr Clin North Am 6:27–40, 1983.

Wing JK, Cooper JE, Sartorius N: The Measurement and Classification of Psychiatric Symptoms. Cambridge, Cambridge University Press, 1974.

World Health Organization: Schedules for Clinical Assessment in Neuropsychiatry (SCAN). Geneva, Division of Mental Health, World Health Organization, 1992.

CHAPTER 2

Syndromes of Brain Dysfunction Presenting with Cognitive Impairment or Behavioral Disturbance: Delirium, Dementia, and Mental Disorders Due to a General Medical Condition

MICHAEL K. POPKIN

Hoping to achieve a new clarity in an area long beset by uncertainty and controversy, the developers of the *Diagnostic and Statistic Manual of Mental Disorders,* third edition (DSM-III), coined the broad rubric *organic mental disorders* (OMDs). The term was designed to span a heterogeneous group of disorders linked by two common elements: brain dysfunction and associated cognitive or behavioral abnormality. ICD-10 notwithstanding, those charged with the preparation of DSM-IV have proposed to eliminate the term *organic mental disorders* (DSM-IV Draft Criteria, 1993). To many observers, the term conveys the erroneous implication that the remainder of the diagnostic manual consists of ''nonorganic conditions,'' thus perpetuating a false dichotomy. Altered levels of neurotransmitters, changes in receptor affinities, neuroanatomic and computed tomographic (CT) scan aberrations, and genetic factors have been identified as associated features of many of the ''functional,'' or nonorganic, disorders. Nevertheless, several authorities have opined that the proposed ''demise'' of OMDs is premature and not without untoward consequences. The outcome of this debate seems a foregone conclusion. In DSM-IV, the syndromes of brain dysfunction presenting with cognitive impairment will be grouped as *delirium*, *dementia*, *amnestic*, and *other* cognitive disorders. They are to be grouped together with amnestic disorder as the *cognitive impairment disorders*. The remaining former OMDs (e.g., organic mood, organic delusional, organic anxiety, and organic personality disorders) will be returned to their respective phenomenologic home categories within the diagnostic manual and retitled *mental disorders due to a general medical condition*.

Nosology aside, these conditions are critically positioned at the interface of psychiatry and medicine. Only in this section of the diagnostic manual must the clinician address etiology together with descriptive features of thought and behavior. Here alone the clinician is expected to demonstrate ''by means of the history, the physical exam or laboratory tests, the presence of a specific organic factor judged to be etiologically related to the abnormal mental state'' (DSM-IIIR, p. 98).

Are these syndromes medical conditions or psychiatric conditions, or both? Clinical problems of this kind have been regarded historically as psychiatric until a specific pathophysiology has been established. After such clarification, the individual disorders have been perceived as within the province of medicine or neurology. Recently, however, psychiatry is changing course, displaying heightened interest in the clinical correlates and management of brain dysfunction, well explained or not. This development has been spurred in part by the rapid growth of technology concerned with imaging, visualizing, and understanding the brain. There is no hint of earlier proclivities to relinquish this realm to other medical disciplines.

DSM-III ''liberalized'' the concept of organicity, no longer requiring cognitive or intellectual impairment as a sine qua non (Lipowski, 1984). As a result, the OMDs framework was broadened to include a range of clinical presentations (affective, delusional, and altered personality) that may be caused by (1) brain dysfunction (primary or secondary), (2) ingestion of an exogenous toxic substance, or (3) withdrawal from certain abused substances. In short, DSM-III proposed that an OMD could simulate almost any psychiatric disorder. Work by investigators such as Hall et al. (1980) and Koranyi (1979) has underscored that psychiatric symptomatology is *nonspecific*. These authors have shown the high frequency with which physical illnesses take a psychiatric guise or contribute to psychiatric symptomatology. Their work exemplifies that clinicians have responsibility to consider carefully physiologic explanations for much, if not all, psychopathology. To overlook such factors may condemn the patient to inappropriate treatment and the risk that physical illness and its central nervous system (CNS) impact may become irreversible. Accordingly, the behavioral concomitants of brain dysfunction become the concern of all psychiatric practitioners, not only those who research or study specific cerebral disturbances.

Despite the apparent nosologic complexity, the universe of choices regarding a given syndrome of brain dysfunction is surprisingly limited. The clinician contemplating such a diagnosis must choose from among a short list of specific clinical syndromes. These can be divided into three major groups: (1) global disturbances of cognition (delirium and dementia), (2) a selective cognitive deficit (amnestic disorder), and (3) disorders due to a general medical condition (formerly these were organic mood, organic delusional, organic anxiety, and organic personality disorders; DSM-IV adds categories for catatonic and dissociative disorders as well). In addition to these specific syndromes, it is proposed in DSM-IV to have three residual ("not otherwise specified") categories and move the general syndromes of intoxication and withdrawal to the substance-related disorders section of the manual. In this chapter, the major two groups of syndromes of brain disturbances are examined in detail (amnestic disorder is considered elsewhere in the text).

SYNDROMES OF BRAIN DYSFUNCTION PRESENTING WITH GLOBAL COGNITIVE IMPAIRMENT: DELIRIUM AND DEMENTIA

Historical Perspective

Delirium and dementia are the two common neuropsychiatric syndromes manifested by global cognitive impairment; they have been appreciated since antiquity. The two terms first appear within the writings of Celsus, a Roman aristocrat of the first century A.D. Heralding an ironic pattern that persisted for centuries, Celsus used the term *delirium* "inconsistently" (Lipowski, 1980a). He identified it as a marker of the imminence of death and as an

unfavorable sign in small bowel disease (Lipowski, 1980a). Araetaeus, in the second century, distinguished "dotage," or senile dementia, as a chronic brain dysfunction (Lipowski, 1980a). Although descriptions of the two conditions appeared with some consistency in the writings of physicians through the centuries, constructs now in use did not emerge until recently. A series of twentieth-century theorists and investigators, including Bonhoeffer (1910), Wolff and Curran (1935), and Engel and Romano (1944), have shaped and refined earlier constructs leading to the present-day clinical entities as set forth in the most recent diagnostic manual. Structured cognitive examinations, such as M. Folstein, S. Folstein, and P. McHugh's Mini-Mental State (1975), offer a rapid screening instrument to heighten recognition of cognitive impairment. A screening battery for the detection of abnormal mental decline in older persons was shown in one study to classify correctly 89 percent of cases (Eslinger et al, 1985). The 15-minute battery combined tests of visual retention, controlled oral word association, and temporal orientation. Nonetheless, such disturbances are still best appreciated by the clinical examination, by the careful assessment of the mental status, and the benchmark cognitive decline. The diagnoses are more than academic exercises; they carry prognostic significance. The cognitively impaired, specifically those with delirium, have sharply increased fatality rates compared with cognitively intact persons (Guze and Cantwell, 1964; Rabins and Folstein, 1982).

Interest in cognitive impairment has grown since the 1970s. Investigations of dementia continue to predominate; delirium remains something of a "stepchild," studied infrequently, as Lipowski (1967) noted.

DELIRIUM

Definition

Delirium is *"a psychiatric syndrome characterized by a transient disorganization of a wide range of cognitive functions due to widespread derangement of cerebral metabolism"* (Lipowski, 1980a, p. 34). Perception, information processing, goal-directed thought, and memory function are disrupted. The stable, constant grasp of internal and external reality gives way to a sequence of fragmented experiences that cannot be successfully integrated by the patient. Abrupt in its onset and relatively brief in duration, delirium is marked by impairment of consciousness, changes in cognition, and an abrupt, fluctuating course. Difficulties in sustaining attention and reduced clarity of awareness of the environment are the hallmarks of the disorder (not simply disorientation, as is sometimes mistakenly assumed). The disorder shows wide variability from patient to patient and from moment to moment in the same individual. It is presumed to be fully reversible but entails diffuse dysfunction of the cerebral hemispheres, the reticular activating system, and the autonomic nervous system (Wells and Duncan, 1980).

The term *delirium* is derived from the Latin *de lira*, meaning "out of the furrow" or off the track. In their classic work (1959), Engel and Romano called delirium "a syndrome of cerebral insufficiency." They likened it to other medical insufficiencies: renal, cardiac, hepatic, and pulmonary. Lipowski's definitive monograph (1980a) is comparably titled *Delirium: Acute Brain Failure in Man*.

Etiology and Pathogenesis

Delirium can be evoked by any process, disorder, or agent that disrupts the integrity of the CNS and diffusely impairs its functioning at a cellular level. Thus the list of potential etiologic factors is extensive, if not nearly limitless (see Lipowski for a full accounting; 1980a). It is frequently difficult for the clinician to confirm a suspected etiology. Not only are most deliria short-lived, but they are also often the product of multiple factors converging to precipitate a final behavioral outcome. Causal disorders or factors may be either intrinsic to the CNS (tumor, trauma, bleeding, seizure disorder, or infection) or extracranial in origin. The latter group includes medical illnesses involving organs other than the CNS, medications, and toxic substances.

In my experience as a psychiatric consultant in a tertiary-care hospital, the most common causes of delirium are fluid and electrolyte disturbances, drug toxicity, infections, and vascular events. The first two predominate. In the case of fluid and electrolyte disturbances, the clinical picture of delirium may antedate by as much as 24 to 48 hours the emergence of aberrant electrolyte values. Behavioral resolution may then be accompanied by clearly abnormal electrolyte values, reflecting disparities between peripheral and central events (i.e., lags involving the blood–brain barrier). With particular reference to metabolic disorders, it is important to appreciate that the *rate of change* may be more crucial than the extent of laboratory abnormality involved. For example, cognitive dysfunction secondary to uremic changes may be expected with blood urea nitrogen (BUN) values greater than 60 mg/ml. Yet many patients with end-stage renal disease have BUN levels that are greater than or equal to 100 mg/ml without evidence of brain dysfunction. Conversely, with rapid elevation of the BUN, as in acute renal failure, delirium is common. Similarly, many patients with chronic obstructive lung disease (COPD) routinely have PCO_2 values that are greater than or equal to 55 mmHg. Were this range of values to result rapidly, delirium would be invariable. This capacity in metabolic and insufficiency disorders to obviate syndromes of brain dysfunction presenting with cognitive impairment and/or behavioral disturbance through gradual adjustment should not obscure the general principle that the more pronounced or severe the pathogenic factor, the greater is the likelihood that delirium will occur.

Although many theories have been propounded over the years, surprisingly little is understood of the pathogenesis of delirium. The known electroencephalographic (EEG) changes in delirium (to be reviewed later) have prompted some to argue that substrate deficiencies, particularly of glucose and oxygen, are crucial to pathogenesis. Other "speculations" have cited disrupted synaptic transmission, false transmitters, compromised blood–brain barrier, altered cerebral blood flow, and biochemical changes, particularly in those pathways subserving sleep–wake cycles. Lipowski (1980a) notes that delirium is not a failure of cerebral energy metabolism; rather, he suggests that it is a final common pathway for a variety of pathophysiologic processes and mechanisms. What these share appears to be a disruption, particularly in the usual relationship of cortical and subcortical structures. Given that delirium is principally a disorder of attention and arousal, it is difficult to minimize the role of the reticular activating system (RAS) in its pathogenesis. The RAS is responsible for alertness, wakefulness, and responsivity to external stimuli. Although delirium affects the brain as a whole, any proposed account of its pathophysiology must literally begin with the state of the RAS, which in turn influences the extent of cortical excitability.

Epidemiology

With the exception of dementia, the epidemiology of the syndromes of brain dysfunction presenting with cognitive and/or behavioral disturbances has received little systematic investigation. The majority of available data has emerged from studies of the population of medical–surgical patients referred for psychiatric consultation. In most settings, 20 to 25 percent of such referrals are assigned a psychiatric diagnosis of brain dysfunction (e.g., cognitive impairment or disorders due to a general medical condition) by the consultants. Not surprisingly, delirium and dementia account for upward of three-quarters of such cases. The prevalence of delirium and other syndromes of brain dysfunction in the larger (unreferred) medical–surgical inpatient population has been estimated at *10 to 15 percent* (Engel, 1967). Often a transient episode in a protracted illness course, delirium can be overlooked. It undoubtedly occurs with greater frequency in the elderly; estimates of the prevalence of delirium in the hospitalized elderly have ranged from one-third to one-half (Lipowski, 1983). Impaired hearing and vision, brain damage, increased vulnerability to hypoxia, and decreased drug metabolism all play a role.

Other groups at increased risk for developing delirium are those with preexisting CNS dysfunction or injury and those with substance-abuse problems. There is no substantial evidence to support the idea that certain personality features heighten the vulnerability to delirium. It is agreed, however, that certain factors, including sensory deprivation, immobilization, extreme psychological stress, and immaturity of the brain, can predispose to delirium.

Pathology

The neuropathologic changes associated with delirium are nonspecific and largely reversible in patients who survive. There may be evidence of cerebral edema with widening of perivascular and perineuronal spaces. On microscopic examination, there may be noted "swelling of the neurons of the cerebral cortex and hippocampus, some dissolution of the Nissl granules and generalized pallor" (Wells and Duncan, 1980). Such changes fail to point to a specific etiology.

Clinical Picture

Disturbances of attention and awareness are central to the clinical presentation of delirium. The delirious patient has difficulty shifting, focusing, and sustaining attention to environmental stimuli. Thus the usual capacity to regulate one's attention at will is impaired. All critical components of attention are altered; these include alertness and the readiness to respond to stimuli, directiveness, and selectiveness (Lipowski, 1980a). These core changes, directly linked to a reduced awareness of surroundings and self, have long been described as a "clouding of consciousness." This term was included in the A criteria for delirium in DSM-III, although it has been chastized as "obsolete, vague and redundant" (Lipowski, 1983). Lipowski alternatively suggested that the attentional deficits are best regarded as manifestations of a *disorder of wakefulness or arousal* (1983). A somewhat more speculative explanation of the attentional difficulties in delirium would emphasize that the barriers or psychological mechanisms normally used to screen and prioritize incoming stimuli are lowered or rendered inoperative (much as disinhibition may become apparent in areas of impulse control). As a consequence, the delirious individual is flooded with incoming stimuli that he or she can no longer structure by selectively attending to some of the input. The result is chaos, with the delirious patient focusing on seemingly inconsequential or inappropriate stimuli or ineffectually endeavoring to scan the suddenly overwhelming environment.

No matter what the explanation for the attentional disturbances or impairment of consciousness, the clinical encounter is likely to be thwarted by a patient who is unable to maintain meaningful engagement with the examiner. The patient's level of awareness may vary from modest deficits in recognizing details to stupor and, eventually, coma. Change in arousal and level of vigilance may range from lethargy to agitation. The delirious patient seems given to "drifting off" or apparently grasping and responding to only fragments of the dialogue. The persistent examiner usually finds it necessary to attempt repeatedly to refocus the patient's attentional process. This sequence is instructive in itself. Interviews with the delirious are often characterized by their brevity; this should not preclude adequate appreciation of the syndrome.

Often accompanying the difficulties in attention and awareness is *disturbance of the sleep–wake cycle*. The delirious patient commonly naps or sleeps during daytime hours and is awake "all night long." Nocturnal insomnia, bewilderment, and restlessness are often striking parts of a prodromal pattern.

Cognitive dysfunction is always heightened by fatigue and minimized by ample sleep. Patients with global cognitive impairment (delirium or dementia) are at their best after a good sleep. They are likely to be at their worst when they have been awake for many hours and the latter part of their day arrives. In this phenomenon, called *sundowning*, reduced sensory input and fatigue combine to unmask organicity in nighttime hours. The disturbance in the sleep–wake cycle also contributes to the lucid intervals that can be observed in delirium. Clinical features, especially early on, tend to fluctuate over the course of a day; this may relate to the intrinsic pathophysiology of the disturbance, but the sleep-cycle factor undoubtedly explains much of the variation.

Perceptual abnormalities are common in delirium. These encompass misperceptions, illusions, and hallucinations; none has been studied extensively, despite their apparent ubiquity in delirium. As the delirious patient sustains the attentional and awareness problems mentioned earlier, he or she struggles to achieve or regain a satisfactory grasp of the situation and is always at least mildly disoriented in time. In this sequence, the patient is also prone to misperceive and, specifically, to mistake the unfamiliar for the familiar. Confronted with an overwhelming experience, patients are often likely to mis-identify strangers as family members and the hospital room as home. This intriguing process seems to be quite adaptive—converting the threatening to the known. Less comforting are the propensities to perceive objects as too big, too small, moving or flowing together. Patients are also inclined to misread or mistake common objects: spots for insects, folds in the bedcovers for snakes, or a bedpost for a rifle. Finally, in terms of hallucinations, Lipowski (1980a) proposes that visual hallucinations occur in 40 to 75 percent of deliria. Auditory and tactile hallucinations are somewhat less common. Most important, hallucinations are neither diagnostic nor pathognomonic for delirium. In addition, they do not distinguish between delirium and dementia (Rabins and Folstein, 1982).

Disturbances of thinking are routinely posited as part of delirium. Thought is disorganized and fragmented; reasoning is defective. Generally, thought processes are slowed; they may be impoverished as well. The capacity to assess and problem-solve is dramatically reduced. Frequently, the patient experiences "oneiroid" or dreamlike imagery, which is disturbing and reinforces the disruption in the sleep–wake cycle. Ideas of persecution are possibly the most common form of delusions in delirium, although patients are perhaps equally inclined to believe that their hallucinations are real. As a rule, delusions are transient and not highly developed in delirium.

All delirious patients experience *memory impairment*. They manifest difficulties in receiving, retaining, and recalling; these are usually readily demonstrable deficits. Engel and Romano (1959) proposed that serial subtraction of numbers was the most valuable bedside test for the diagnosis. Remote memory is often relatively intact (to the examiner's surprise). Patients are subsequently able to recall only bits and pieces of their delirium.

Motor activity may be increased or decreased in delirium. This is associated with two clinical variants—hyperactive and hypoactive—which seem to occur in equal percentages (Lipowski, 1980a). In addition, speech and nonverbal behavior are often altered.

The clinical picture in delirium also normally entails affective lability, fine to coarse irregular tremor at 8 to 10 seconds, asterixis, multifocal myoclonus, and various signs of autonomic dysfunction (e.g., nausea, vomiting, flushing, blood pressure changes). Other neurologic signs are comparatively uncommon.

Clinical Course

Delirium has a sudden onset, involving no more than hours or a day or two at most. Prodromal symptoms may occur but are usually appreciated only in retrospect. These may include restlessness, impaired concentration, hyperacusis, insomnia, vivid dreams, and nightmares. Fluctuation in symptoms is a characteristic feature of the course. The severity of the symptoms varies, most often being greatest at night, with lucid intervals likely to be observed in the morning. These unpredictable fluctuations facilitate clinical diagnosis; they are not features of other syndromes of brain dysfunction.

Any variety of behavior can be encountered in delirium. In a given patient, the particular clinical presentation is probably determined by an interplay of four factors: (1) the premorbid personality, (2) the nature and locus of the insult rendered to the CNS, (3) the environment in which the delirious individual is placed, and (4) the reactive response to the recognition of the impairment. Although the insult rendered is possibly most important, there is little question that the mode of responding to cognitive disorganization often carries the day in terms of the resulting clinical picture. Many consultation requests are occasioned by consultees' dilemmas with agitated, paranoid, or depressed patients who in fact are suffering from an unrecognized delirium. Perceiving that their cognitive integrity has been violated or lost, patients respond in personalized, if not idiosyncratic, fashion. Some become despondent, others phobic, anxious, paranoid, or hysterical. Those who are conversant with altered consciousness may be less alarmed than those who have never experienced loss of control. In any case, the clinician is obligated to explore the question of reactive response. Hackett and Weisman (1960) have shown that dialogue anticipating the likelihood of delirium can clinically modify the resulting course. Delirium is marked by wide clinical variability, even in the same patient.

Most deliria are short-lived, on the order of a week. A longer process suggests that the syndrome has shifted to another, more enduring syndrome of brain dysfunction or that death is imminent. Recovery is usually complete unless the underlying disorder cannot be redressed. The issue of psychological outcome of delirium has recently been raised. Mackenzie and Popkin (1980) suggested that the patient's lack of clear and correct information about his or her delirium may impede assimilation of the event. Blank and Perry (1984) found that postdelirium psychological outcome was associated with psychological processes manifest during the delirium.

Laboratory Findings

The brain dysfunction underlying the clinical picture of delirium can be demonstrated by EEG. The typical abnormality is relative slowing of the EEG background activity (with or without superimposed fast activity—found in hyperactive delirium). The EEG can be useful diagnostically if serial tracings are done and the changes in background activity are consonant with changes in attention, awareness, and cognition (Lipowski, 1980a). A diffusely slow tracing can help to make the diagnosis, but a normal or fast record does not rule it out (Pro and Wells, 1977).

Organic causative factors are identified in perhaps 80 percent of cases (Lipowski, 1982). Specific laboratory studies must be directed to the evidence for associated physical illness or drug intoxication. In the absence of specific indications of etiology, initial measures should include electrolyte determinations, drug screen, hepatic and renal function studies, blood gas analyses, urinalysis, and an electrocardiogram.

Differential Diagnosis

Although some psychotic disorders may involve hallucinations, delusions, and the like, it is seldom difficult to recognize that one is dealing with a syndrome of brain dysfunction. Accordingly, the differential diagnosis for delirium primarily involves dementia. This distinction should center on the features of disordered attention and arousal, which are not expected to be at issue in dementia. Yet distinguishing the conditions can be problematic despite examining factors such as rate of onset, fluctuating course, and sleep–wake cycle alterations. Rabins and Folstein (1982) argue that "altered cognition and consciousness alone can validly distinguish them [delirium and dementia]." In some instances, delirium may be superimposed on dementia. Watchful waiting and a provisional diagnosis are occasionally indicated when the diagnoses cannot be immediately clarified. Factitious disorder with psychological symptoms must be included in the differential diagnosis of delirium. Likewise, "pseudodelirium" has to be considered (Lipowski, 1983).

Treatment

The first step after diagnosis of delirium should be the determination and correction of the underlying causes. Special attention must be directed to fluid and electrolyte status, hypoxia, anoxia, and diabetic problems. This search for an etiology is not always a rewarding process. While the workup proceeds, or after it has been effected, clinical management of the delirious patient requires attention to several points. The delirious patient should have a constant attendant both to monitor behavior and to provide reorientation and assurance. The room environment should ensure that the patient is neither excessively stimulated nor deprived of external stimuli. My preference is to avoid adding medications, especially when the etiology of the delirium is unclear. Additional agents may only compound the syndrome of brain dysfunction. However, the patient's agitation and penchant for pulling intravenous lines and assaulting the staff may force the issue. In such instances, low-dose neuroleptics— usually haloperidol—are effective. (If physical restraints are used, chemical restraints must be invoked as well.) In daily amounts between 2 and 15 mg orally (or half as much intramuscularly), most delirious patients become tractable. The elderly require the more modest doses. Generally, one-third to one-half of what would be used to contain a psychotic disorder works satisfactorily in agitated delirium, although larger amounts are needed occasionally. If possible, the neuroleptic should be administered at night so as to facilitate sleep and help restore the disrupted sleep–wake cycle. Orientation cues, night lights, the presence of family members, and a primary nurse are all helpful in management.

DEMENTIA

Definition

The term *dementia* is derived from the Latin *dement*, meaning "to be out of one's mind." Like delirium,

this syndrome is characterized by global dysfunction. Its essential feature is *broad-based intellectual decline;* the cognitive deficits in dementia must be of *sufficient severity to cause significant impairment in social or occupational functioning and represent a significant decline from a previous higher level of functioning.* Thus the DSM-IV definition permits or tolerates a modest degree of cognitive fall-away with advancing age—so long as it does not compromise the individual's overall functioning. The specific DSM-IV diagnostic criteria for dementia include the development of multiple cognitive deficits as manifested by *memory impairment* (inability to learn new information and inability to recall previously learned knowledge) and *cognitive impairment* (aphasia, apraxia, agnosia, or a disturbance in executive functioning). These deficits must occur in "a state of clear awareness" (Lipowski, 1984); this removes the question of delirium or intoxication from diagnostic consideration.

Dementia has traditionally signaled an irreversible and usually progressive process presumed to be associated with neuron loss. "Cell death" thus precluded the prospect of reversibility. DSM-III and its successors have chosen, however, to restrict the concept of dementia to descriptive parameters. As one of the syndromes of brain dysfunction, dementia is but a clinical constellation of symptoms devoid of the prior prognostic connotations. It may be transient, static, or progressive. Which of these courses is encountered will prove a function of the underlying pathology.

DSM-IV proposes to divide the dementias into six groups: (1) dementia of the Alzheimer's type (DAT), (2) vascular dementia, (3) dementias due to other general medical conditions, (4) substance-induced persisting dementia, (5) dementia due to multiple etiologies, and (6) dementia not otherwise specified. At present, the diagnosis of many of the dementing illnesses can be established definitely only at autopsy, and inaccuracies in antemortem diagnosis persist (Rebok and Folstein, in press). DSM-IV revisions of the diagnostic criteria for dementia have been developed with particular reference to the criteria set forth by the National Institute of Neurological and Communicative Disorders and Stroke (NINCDS; McKhann et al., 1984) and the Alzheimer's Disease and Related Disorders Association (ADRDA; McKhann et al., 1984).

Dementia of the Alzheimer's type (DAT) is the most common dementing illness. Although DSM-III and DSM-IIIR offered presenile and senile categories, such a distinction is unnecessary. Alzheimer's disease and "senile dementia" are now regarded as one disease. *Vascular dementia* is the DSM-IV term to replace "multi-infarct dementia" (MID). The remaining dementing illnesses span a wide range from processes primarily affecting brain tissue with or without observable features such as abnormal movements (e.g., normal-pressure hydrocephalus, Huntington's chorea, Creutzfeldt-Jakob disease, progressive supranuclear palsy, and Wilson's disease) to the dementias associated with diseases that do not usually attack the brain directly. The latter, formerly called "secondary dementias" and now *dementias due to other general medical conditions*, encompass the behavioral sequelae of, for example, infection, endocrine disorder, and drug toxicity. In some constructs, depression and pseudodementia fall within this category as well.

Etiology and Pathogenesis

DEMENTIA OF THE ALZHEIMER'S TYPE

Although considerable advances have recently been made in understanding the neurobiologic features of DAT, "the pathogenesis and aetiology of Alzheimer's disease remain *unknown territory*" (Deakin, 1983, my emphasis). Genetic factors have been shown to be instrumental in at least a portion of Alzheimer's cases. Heston et al. (1981) found in a study of 125 autopsy-proven cases of DAT that 40 percent were familial. Pick's disease is regarded as hereditary, most likely an autosomal dominant (Spar, 1982). Genetics, however, do not account for the majority of DAT. Efforts to identify causal factors have focused on neurotransmitters, viruses (especially slow viruses), aluminum toxicity, immune system dysfunction, and amyloid formation.

Since the 1970s, many studies have demonstrated that the amount of acetylcholine found in the brains of patients with DAT is substantially reduced (Kokmen, 1984). These changes, as reflected by marker enzymes (choline acetyltransferase and acetylcholinesterase), entail loss or destruction of cholinergic neurons in specific areas (especially the basal forebrain and the nucleus basalis of Meynert). It also has been shown that temporary memory deficits can be produced in healthy, young volunteers by interfering with CNS cholinergic activity. Physostigmine, a cholinomimetic, reverses such deficits. Together with the biochemical findings, these data have led to a cholinergic hypothesis concerning DAT (Coyle et al., 1983). Identification of cholinergic abnormalities gave promise of a ready treatment, but to date, trials of acetylcholine precursors have been unrewarding in DAT patients. More recently, other subcortical nuclei and their transmitter systems have been implicated in DAT (Besson, 1983). These include the locus ceruleus (noradrenergic), the raphe nucleus (serotonergic), and the substantia nigra (dopaminergic). The etiologic significance of these changes and associated biochemical abnormalities remains to be clarified.

The transmissibility of DAT has been at issue for some time. In one study, inoculation of scrapie (a slow virus) into the CNS of certain mice induced neuritic plaques akin to those of DAT (Bruce and Fraser, 1975). This study, however, stands alone in the literature. Yet Creutzfeldt-Jakob disease is a transmissible encephalopathy of humans with a long incubation period. Subacute sclerosing panencephalitis and postencephalitic Parkinson's disease can culminate in dementia. These examples serve to keep the issue of a viral etiology for DAT alive (if tenuously).

Aluminum toxicity has been suggested as a cause of DAT. An extremely small excess of aluminum has been found consistently in the brains of patients succumbing to DAT. Aluminum may induce in animals brain lesions similar to those in DAT, but these "tangles" are morphologically distinct (Wisniewski et al., 1970). As with other theories, the aluminum hypothesis is unresolved.

Defects in the immune system also have been proposed to underlie DAT. This prospect is linked to well-known declines of immunologic competence with aging, the immunologic origin of amyloid in senile plaques, and increased levels of brain-reactive antibodies in DAT (Watson and Seiden, 1984).

Hereditary or familial Alzheimer's disease has been identified as an autosomal dominant form of localized amyloidosis. Patients with hereditary DAT typically develop (1) senile plaques in the cerebral cortex with a central amyloid core, (2) neurofibrillary tangles, and (3) congophilic angiopathy of the leptomeningeal vessels. At present, a host of researchers are investigating the processes by which amyloid is made. Recent data (Murrell et al., 1991) suggest that a mutation in amyloid precursor proteins may be the inherited factor causing both amyloid fibril formation and dementia.

VASCULAR DEMENTIA

As a result of the elegant neuropathologic work of Tomlinson et al. (1970), it has been generally appreciated that cerebral atherosclerosis does not account for the typical, insidiously progressive dementia of old age. When vascular disease is responsible for dementia, it is through the occurrence of multiple small or large cerebral infarcts. Vascular dementia has been estimated to account for 10 to 20 percent of all cases of dementia. Complicating the situation is the fact that at autopsy, DAT and vascular dementia are found to coexist in perhaps 20 percent of cases (Tomlinson et al., 1970).

Most cerebral infarcts are caused by thromboembolism from extracranial arteries and the heart (Hachinski et al., 1974). Direct or in situ occlusion of cerebral vessels is a much less frequent event. In either case, the compromised blood supply results in the death of cells and subsequent encephalomalacia. Hypertension commonly underlies vascular dementia; Corsellis (1969) observed that it was unusual for autopsy to reveal an arteriosclerotic etiology for dementia unless there was hypertension exceeding 210/110 mmHg.

Early identification of vascular dementia is crucial because vigorous intervention should serve to minimize or retard progression of the condition. A single infarct seldom, if ever, yields a dementia;

rather, it is the cumulative impact of multiple, often small lesions (*état lacunaire*) that evokes the dementiform process. A minimal volume of brain destruction of 60 ml, with particular involvement of the corpus callosum and the temporal and occipital lobes, has been adequately defined (Torack, 1978). Arteriosclerosis is often more prominently developed in one part of the body than in another. Thus the status of the peripheral and retinal vasculature does not invariably coincide with the condition of the cerebral vessels.

REMAINING DEMENTIAS

More than 50 diseases have been identified that can cause dementia. The list of causes continues to grow and has been reviewed in detail by Haase (1977). Causes of dementing illnesses span a gamut that includes genetic, viral, traumatic, and toxic factors. As with delirium, etiology often may be multifactorial. Among the list of causes, special attention should be directed briefly to certain disorders. They underscore the fact that widely disparate pathogenetic mechanisms may each result in the final common pathway of dementia (as a clinical syndrome).

Huntington's chorea is a *hereditary* disorder characterized by dementia and choreiform movements. It is inherited as an autosomal dominant with high penetrance. Approximately half the offspring of an affected person will develop the disease. In 1973, the term *subcortical dementia* was introduced by McHugh and Folstein to characterize the cognitive difficulties in Huntington's patients. Subsequently, the term has been extended to Parkinson's disease, Wilson's disease, supranuclear palsy (Steele-Richardson syndrome), and multiple sclerosis, among others. The clinical validity of the subcortical versus cortical construct for dementias remains to be established. "Most diseases are neither purely cortical or subcortical" (Rebok and Folstein, in press).

Creutzfeldt-Jakob disease is an *infectious* disease caused by slow virus; it has been transmitted by corneal transplantation and by performing craniotomy or autopsy. Its clinical course is generally fulminant once it becomes manifest. Normal-pressure hydrocephalus is often a sequelae of *injury* to the brain, with resultant impaired absorption of cerebrospinal fluid. It presents with a clinical triad including dementia, ataxia, and incontinence. Finally, the *toxicity* of drugs and alcohol can be critical to the pathogenesis of dementia.

Epidemiology

Community surveys have found that 4 to 5 percent of the population over age 65 are severely demented (i.e., the extent of intellectual decline precludes independent living). An additional 10 to 15 percent suffer mild to moderate dementia. Prevalence rates for severe forms increase to approximately 20 percent by age 80 (Brody, 1982). Recent data also suggest that after age 85, the incidence of dementia plateaus or declines (Jarvik et al., 1980). In all major postmortem series, DAT has been reported as accounting for between 50 and 60 percent of cases of severe dementia (Terry and Katzman, 1983). Vascular dementias account for approximately another 20 percent of these severe cases. Under age 75, the prevalences of DAT and vascular dementia are nearly equal; by age 85, DAT is six times more common (Rebok and Folstein, in press).

DEMENTIA OF THE ALZHEIMER'S TYPE

At present, genetic factors are the only known risk for DAT. In a small number of families, DAT presents as though it were a straightforward autosomal dominant disorder (Cook et al., 1979). Jarvik et al. (1980) reported incomplete concordance among identical twins. In general, the risk to siblings of an affected person has been gauged at about 7 percent up to age 75 (Heston and White, 1980). Estimates of risk for children of DAT probands are not yet available because of the lack of long-term followup studies. Heston and White (1983) emphasize that the risks of developing DAT are age-specific. Since DAT "will eventually affect 20 to 30 percent of those living long enough" (Heston and White, 1983), the main impact of having an affected first-degree relative is an increased risk of developing the disease earlier in life (versus someone without a DAT-affected relative). Of considerable interest is that DAT occurs predictably in patients with Down syndrome (trisomy 21) who survive to age 40. Heston and Mastri (1977) found that relatives of probands with histologically confirmed DAT had an increased incidence of dementing illness, Down syndrome, and hematologic malignancies. Given the known 20-fold increased risk of leukemia in Down syndrome, the Heston–Mastri study suggested that the common denominator in the group of diseases (DAT, Down syndrome, and hematologic malignancies) may have been an inherited microtubular abnormality.

A case control study (Heyman et al., 1984) exploring epidemiologic aspects of DAT found a significantly higher frequency of prior thyroid disease among female patients versus controls and an increased history of severe head injury among patients versus controls. It did not corroborate differences in the frequency of hematologic malignancies in the families of patients and controls.

More uncommon than DAT, Pick's disease also has a different distribution of age at onset. Risks in terms of inheritability are much less defined than for DAT.

VASCULAR DEMENTIA

Vascular dementia occurs more frequently in men than in women. Genetic factors may contribute; the most significant predisposing factor is arterial hypertension. Although it can affect individuals in their forties, vascular dementia usually begins in the seventh or eighth decade of life.

REMAINING DEMENTIAS

Table 2-1 (Popkin MK, MacKenzie TB, 1984) presents data from six major studies conducted between 1972 and 1982. Subjects assigned provisional diagnoses of dementia were further examined by psychiatrists and neurologists. Specific etiologies were sought to account for the clinical presentations. Methodologies were not uniform in the studies; no postmortem examinations were conducted. Overall, 39 percent of the confirmed dementias were assigned a specific etiology according to criteria of inclusion. Fourteen percent of the confirmed dementias were attributed to vascular dementia; the remaining 47 percent were presumed to be cases of DAT. Table 2-2 (Popkin and Mackenzie, 1984) details those 15 percent of dementias identified as having a "potentially reversible" etiology. Seven specific medical disorders accounted for 90 percent of the reversible conditions. These were normal-pressure hydrocephalus (31 percent), tumors and cysts of the CNS (21 percent), drug toxicity (12 percent), subdural hematoma (9 percent), thyroid dysfunction (8 percent), alcoholism (5 percent), and general paresis (4 percent). Of nonreversible etiologies other than vascular dementia (formerly MID) and DAT, Huntington's chorea accounted for 3 percent; trauma, 2 percent; and Creutzfeldt-Jakob disease, Parkinson's disease, and encephalitis, 1 percent each. These distributions emerged in secondary and tertiary referral centers; those encountered in a primary-care setting may differ markedly.

Pathology

Beginning with work by Roth et al. (1967), much evidence has been gathered that establishes a direct relationship between the severity of the clinical picture of dementia and the severity of neuropathologic change. The extent of intellectual loss has been quantitatively associated with the density of senile plaques and neurofibrillary tangles, the volume of brain softening, and the mass of tissue loss (Wells and Duncan, 1980).

DEMENTIA OF THE ALZHEIMER'S TYPE

In 1907, Alois Alzheimer described neurofibrillary tangles and senile plaques in brain tissue from a 51-year-old woman who died after a 4-year course of profound intellectual decline and behavioral change. These classic features of the disease are most prominent in the hippocampus. The tangles are masses of neurofibers arranged as paired helical filaments (Terry and Katzman, 1983); the plaques are derived from degenerative neurites and granulovascular degeneration. The biochemical nature of the amyloid in these plaques is the subject of vigorous current study. The amyloid in hereditary DAT contains "fibril subunit protein of 39 to 43 amino acid residues, which is a portion of the carboxyl terminus of the amyloid precursor protein (APP)" (Murrell et al., 1991). Plaques and tangles are not unique to DAT. They are found in small numbers in normal aging. In most cases of DAT, there is generalized cortical atrophy, most marked in the frontal and temporal lobes. The ventricles may be enlarged.

The microscopic findings in Pick's disease are dramatically different from those in DAT. Affected cells have *Pick's bodies*, collections of the components of the normal cell in disarray. In most cases, plaques and tangles are conspicuous by their absence (Lishman, 1978). The gross appearance of the brain is characteristic, with marked reduction of frontal and temporal lobes. Involvement of the parietal and occipital lobes is unusual.

VASCULAR DEMENTIA

The brain may demonstrate generalized or localized atrophy. On microscopic examination, effects of ischemia and infarction are apparent. Cystic soften-

TABLE 2-1. *Evaluations for Provisional Diagnosis of Dementia*

	No. in original sample	Confirmed dementia	Specific etiology established (diagnosis by inclusion)	Diagnosis by exclusion	
				Vascular dementia	DAT
Marsden, Harrison (1972)	106	86 (81%)	40/86 (47%)	8/86 (9%)	38/86 (44%)
Freeman (1976)	60	59 (98%)	21/59 (36%)	5/59 (8%)	33/59 (56%)
Victoratos et al. (1977)	52	49 (94%)	25/49 (51%)	5/49 (10%)	19/49 (39%)
Smith, Kiloh (1981)	200	164 (82%)	62/164 (38%)	22/164 (13%)	80/164 (49%)
Rabins (1981)	41	41 (100%)	21/41 (51%)	8/41 (20%)	12/41 (29%)
Delaney (1982)	100	100 (100%)	27/100 (27%)	22/100 (22%)	51/100 (51%)
TOTALS	559	499 (89%)	196/499 (39%)	70/499 (14%)	233/499 (47%)

From Popkin MK, MacKenzie TB: The provisional diagnosis of dementia: Three phases of evaluation. In Hall RCW, Beresford TP (eds): The Handbook of Psychiatric Diagnostic Procedures. Jamaica, NY, Spectrum, 1984.

TABLE 2-2. *Etiologies Assigned to Potentially Reversible Dementias (n = 77 or 15 percent) and Their Actual Clinical Outcomes*

Studies	Marsden, Harrison (n = 86)	Freeman (n = 59)	Victoratos et al.* (n = 49)	Smith, Kiloh (n = 164)	Rabins* (n = 41)	Delaney (n = 100)	Total (%)	Cumulative (%)	Outcomes no change (%)	(If reported) partially improved (%)
Normal pressure hydrocephalus	5	7	1	8	1	2	24 (31)	31	12 (55)	6 (27)
Tumors/cyst of CNS	8	0	0	3	0	5	16 (21)	52	8 (50)	5 (31)
Drug toxicity	2	5	0	0	0	2	9 (12)	64	0 (0)	0 (0)
Subdural hematoma	0	2	1	0	1	3	7 (9)	73	0 (0)	5 (100)
Hypothyroidism	0	1	0	2	1	0	4 (5)	78	0 (0)	1 (33)
Alcoholism	0	0	1	0	0	3	4 (5)	83	0 (0)	0 (0)
General paresis	0	1	1	0	0	1	3 (4)	87	1 (50)	1 (50)
Hyperthyroidism	0	0	0	0	1	1	2 (3)	90	0 (0)	0 (0)
Hepatic encephalopathy	0	1	0	0	0	1	2 (3)	93	0 (0)	0 (0)
Fungus	0	0	0	0	0	2	2 (3)	96	0 (0)	2 (100)
Lead	0	0	0	0	0	1	1 (0.2)	96	0 (0)	0 (0)
Other	0	0	1	0	0	2	3 (4)	100	0 (0)	2 (100)
TOTAL	15	17	5	13	4	23	77 —	—	21 (27)	22 (29)

*Outcomes not reported by authors.
*From Popkin MK, Mackensie TB: The provisional diagnosis of dementia: Three phases of evaluation. In Hall RCW, Beresford TP (eds): The Handbook of Psychiatric Diagnostic Procedures. Jamaica, NY, Spectrum, 1984.

ings, reactive gliosis, and necrotic degeneration are common. The cerebral vasculature itself may show a range of changes.

REMAINING DEMENTIAS

The cellular pathology of dementia is a function of the underlying disease; given 50 or more etiologies, this topic is too extensive for the current chapter. The interested reader is referred to Tomlinson's review of the pathology of dementia (1977).

Clinical Picture

Memory impairment is the most prominent feature of a dementia. Often insidious in its presentation, it may begin with difficulties in short-term recall and in the acquisition and retrieval of new information. There is no problem with maintenance of attention, arousal, and awareness. As the dementing illness progresses, memory impairment becomes more pronounced and interferes with more remote memories. Early coping mechanisms may involve excessive use of lists, schedules, and notes to contend with forgetfulness in daily life. Cognitive impairment also is present, manifested by disturbance in language, motor function, and executive functioning. Loss of interest and initiative are also relatively early signs, resulting in less than usual standards of performance. Distractibility is increased, and the patient is prone to fatigue readily. Thinking is comparably impaired in dementia, with a poverty of associations and inability to generate new constructs. Perseveration is frequent; intellectual capacity/flexibility is compromised. Paranoid ideation is common, as is delusional thinking. Persecutory delusions are the most frequent psychotic feature of dementia and may be present in 30 to 40 percent of demented patients (Rebok and Folstein, in press). Speech shows similar deficits, with great reliance on clichés or "old tapes." Paraphasic errors and difficulty in word finding are common. Constructional ability is almost always disturbed.

As the dementing illness proceeds, impaired judgment and impulse control are often manifest, together with sweeping personality shifts. Because of changes in the frontal lobes, the individual becomes disinhibited; inappropriate sexual and social actions may first prompt medical attention. There is increasing inattention to the rudiments of self-care; incontinence may develop. When taxed beyond his or her cognitive capacity, the demented patient is prone to show marked, intense affective response. Emotional lability can dominate the later clinical picture. Memory dysfunction becomes profound; the individual loses the capacity to effect meaningful interchanges. Eventually behavior becomes "futile and aimless" (Lishman, 1978). Though data reflect that disruptive behaviors and psychiatric symptoms are commonly part of dementia, these facets of the illness have received surprisingly little systematic study. The extent of affective symptoms in dementia is not well established nor a point of consensus. Aggression, wandering, insomnia, and assaultiveness may be encountered in two-thirds of patients with dementia. DSM-IV proposes to incorporate categories of behavioral disturbances into the diagnostic framework of dementia.

Clinical Course

The initial presenting features and the ensuing course of a dementia are functions of the specific etiology of the disorder. DAT is, for the most part, insidious in its onset and steadily progresses to death over an interval of several years. Fifty percent of patients with DAT present between ages 65 and 69. Earlier onset is associated with severer illness and, subsequently, shorter courses. For DAT manifesting between the ages of 55 and 74, the average survival time is about 8.5 years (Heston and White, 1983). Pick's disease presents somewhat earlier, with a peak incidence at age 55. Average survival is slightly longer than 7 years. (In DAT and Pick's disease, dating onset with precision is clearly difficult.) During the early phase, the neurologic examination may remain normal. As cognitive and behavioral changes become more manifest, signs of neurologic dysfunction also emerge. Aphasia, apraxia, and agnosia usually appear. "Primitive reflexes" are characteristic of most diffuse brain disease and depend on the speed of the course and the extent of brain injury. In DAT, disturbances of posture, gait, muscle tone, and extensor plantar responses are common as the dementia proceeds. In the final phase of DAT, as the patient becomes bedridden, gross neurologic disability is often seen, together with grand mal seizures (reported in up to 75 percent of cases).

In vascular dementia, the onset is typically abrupt, earlier than in DAT, and the course shows stepwise decrements over time with an uneven progression. The cognitive deficits, especially early in the course, may be selective rather than diffuse. Focal neurologic signs are common, and associated features include dysarthria, dysphagia, and pseudobulbar palsy. Time to death varies widely (Lishman, 1978); generally, the course is slower than in DAT. The personality may be preserved until late in the course owing to the patchy nature of the insults. Seizures have been found in approximately 20 percent of cases. Birkett (1972) found that neurologic abnormalities predicted vascular dementia more accurately than any mental feature.

The courses of the remaining dementias are variable. Table 2-2 details the observed outcomes of a series of potentially reversible dementias. Only 44 percent of these cases proved reversible in fact as well as in theory. Duration of the dementing process and the time of its detection are crucial to outcome in the reversible cases. The longer a process remains uncorrected, the less likely full restitution becomes.

Systems for staging dementia have been detailed by Sjogren et al. (1980) and Reisberg et al. (1986).

Subcortical dementias are thought to be characterized by "marked slowness of mental processing, forgetfulness (failure of retrieval), apathy and depressed mood, and the relative lack of disorders of acquired knowledge (e.g., aphasia, apraxia, and agnosia)." In contrast, cortical dementias have as characteristics emotional lability, apraxia, aphasia paranoia, amnesia, and the preservation of gait (Rebok and Folstein, in press).

Finally, as with delirium, the course of any dementing illness is strongly colored by the patient's premorbid personality, the precise neuroanatomic location and extent of brain lesions, and the crucial element of reactive response to cognitive and neurologic impairment.

Laboratory Findings

Based on data from studies presented in Tables 2-1 and 2-2, it has been suggested that a battery consisting of a CT scan, drug screen, thyroid functions, and serology will suffice to identify 90 percent of the potentially reversible etiologies of dementing processes (Popkin and Mackenzie, 1984). Additional studies should proceed only from a combination of clinical acumen and the patient's individual history. Exhaustive laboratory testing is reserved for those few cases with decidedly atypical courses.

Two sets of investigators (Fox et al., 1975; Freeman and Rudd, 1982) have found that demented patients with lesser degrees of atrophy on CT scans had a greater likelihood of having a treatable disorder. A normal CT scan does not rule out dementia; neither do abnormalities on a scan establish a diagnosis of dementia. Scanning has shown differences between DAT and vascular dementia. Ventricular dilatation is greater in DAT; changes in temporal zones are more frequent in vascular dementia. Of note, positron emission tomography and nuclear magnetic resonance imaging both are capable of distinguishing DAT from vascular dementia (Besson, 1983). Oxygen utilization is reduced in both conditions, but this is more generalized in DAT. The value of positron emission tomography (PET) in distinguishing DAT from other forms of dementia and from normal aging has been shown in a few studies (Rebok and Folstein, in press).

One of the clearest physiologic correlates of DAT is symmetrical, usually diffuse slowing of the EEG (Terry and Katzman, 1983). If the diagnosis of dementia is uncertain, the EEG may prove useful if focal or diffuse dysfunction is found. However, dementia can be advanced and the EEG remain unremarkable (Wilson et al., 1977).

Differential Diagnosis

In the studies detailed in Table 2-1, presumed diagnoses of dementia were confirmed in 89 percent of cases. Restricting the data to those four studies with truly provisional diagnoses, dementia was confirmed in 86 percent of cases. The majority of patients receiving a primary psychiatric diagnosis other than dementia were diagnosed as depressed. Remaining diagnoses included a cadre of brain dysfunction syndromes (particularly delirium) and schizophrenia. These categories reflect the differential diagnoses for an apparent loss of intellectual abilities. The distinctions between dementia and delirium have been discussed earlier. Emil Kraepelin first called schizophrenia by the term *dementia praecox*. Cross et al. (1981) have demonstrated cognitive decline in type II schizophrenics; careful history should help to identify such patients. However, distinguishing dementia from depression can be difficult. Data from follow-up studies underscore the point. Ron et al. (1979) found that as many as 30 percent of original diagnoses of dementia cannot be supported on reexamination several years later. They concluded that unappreciated affective disorders chiefly explained the outcomes they observed.

The term *pseudodementia* has been used to describe cognitive dysfunction appearing in depressed patients (especially the elderly). This mimicry of dementia by an affective disturbance usually begins more discretely and progresses more rapidly than dementia. There may be a preceding history of affective illness, and performance on cognitive testing is often variable and marked by poor motivation. Mood disturbance is more pervasive in depression and accompanied by complaints of memory dysfunction. (The latter are uncommon in dementia.) In contrast to earlier work (McAllister, 1981), Rabins et al. (1984) reported in a 2-year follow-up study that patients with "the dementia syndrome of depression" can be readily identified (versus irreversibly demented patients) by a standard clinical history and examination. In those instances in which the question of depression versus dementia cannot be resolved, a trial of antidepressants is warranted. It also must be recalled that affective illness arises in as many as 25 percent of patients with progressive dementias. These secondary depressions are often benefited by antidepressant medication.

Although psychometric tests may identify mild cases of DAT (Storandt et al., 1984), dementia is a clinical diagnosis. Currently, there are no psychological test batteries or rating scales specific for DAT, vascular dementia, or other forms of dementia (Rebok and Folstein, a press). Evidence to establish the diagnosis is derived from clinical interview, a reliable corroborative history, physical examination, and laboratory workup. Within the hospital setting, memory dysfunction often goes unrecognized (Jacobs et al., 1977). Most memory-impaired patients defend vigorously against revelation of their deficits. Those with longer courses may become facile at evading the examiner's efforts. Careful review of the medical record usually provides indication of cognitive difficulties. This prospect can be confirmed by an examination that presumes that cognitive dysfunction is at issue and offers the patient a forum for sharing his or her concerns about this. Because the diagnosis of dementia is often revealed by changes in function over time, and because the patient often cannot provide such history, a corroborative history is crucial.

Treatment

Once the diagnosis of dementia has been confirmed, the clinician's focus must be first directed to the question of etiology. The foremost considerations are the identification and resolution of potentially reversible processes. Data from Tables 2-1 and 2-2 indicate that as few as 7 percent of dementias are actually reversed (e.g., restitution achieved). Yet the obligation to be circumspect remains; to miss a potentially reversible etiology borders on negligence. Ironically, the preoccupation with correcting treatable or reversible dementias may have contributed to a pattern/practice of "writing off" those patients with irreversible dementing disorders (Well, 1984).

The need for general supportive care of the demented has been long recognized. Provisions must be made for security, stimulation, patience, and nutrition. Symptomatic treatment should reduce reliance on lost functions and maximize use of residual functions. The history of drug therapy for dementia is replete with reports of initial success, eventually followed by observations of failure (Torack, 1978).

Although Hydergine (dihydrogenated ergot alkaloid) has been used extensively in dementia, resultant improvements are "generally modest and clinically unimportant" (Kokmen, 1984). As noted previously, drugs enhancing cholinergic activity in the CNS have not proven helpful in reversing the signs and symptoms of dementia. However, double-blind crossover studies have demonstrated that physostigmine can facilitate memory in some DAT patients but not others (Terry and Katzman, 1983). Work is currently underway using gangliosides in DAT; such agents may produce increased sprouting and regeneration of injured nerve cells.

Psychotropic medications in the demented should be reserved for (1) the control of agitated, assaultive behavior, (2) paranoid ideation and other psychotic features, (3) the improvement of mood state, and (4) facilitating impaired sleep, thereby minimizing organicity. Generally, low-dose neuroleptics should be used for all save number 3 and given at night in order to aid sleep. In the face of known CNS dysfunction, my preference is for thiothixene (Navane) or thioridazine (Mellaril), beginning with modest amounts and slowly increasing as needed. In terms of treating depressive disorders superimposed on dementia, nortriptyline works satisfactorily, in my experience, in doses between 50 and 75 mg daily. There is a significant risk of heightening the underlying cognitive dysfunction with this agent. Supportive psychotherapy can be of benefit to some demented patients (Wells and Duncan, 1980).

Increasing attention is being directed in the literature to the needs of the family of the demented patient. The family requires vigorous education regarding the dementing process; they likewise need assistance and support in implementing treatment plans. Caring for the demented patient is a full-time task. The increasing responsibilities as the disease evolves are likely to prove stressful. Caretakers require their own support systems and regular respite. Day care may assist patients and families alike (Fisk, 1983). While the search for pharmacologic treatments that can facilitate memory function continues, it is important to recall that demented patients can be helped in a variety of ways. Poor prognosis should not be equated with resignation or abdication of responsibility for vigorous care and management.

MENTAL DISORDERS DUE TO A GENERAL MEDICAL CONDITION

In a striking departure from prior nosologic constructs, DSM-III (1980) added a group of three organic brain syndromes that did not require cognitive impairment as an essential feature. These categories were revised and expanded in DSM-IIIR (1986). They included organic mood syndrome, organic delusional syndrome, organic personality syndrome, organic anxiety syndrome. For each, the manual specified that cognitive impairment, if present, be no more than mild. In DSM-IV, these entities are to be returned to their phenomenologic home groupings and called mental disorders due to a general medical condition. It is further proposed that the Axis III condition judged responsible for the behavioral syndrome be included *directly* on Axis I (e.g., depressive disorder due to cerebrovascular accident). The group will include mood disorder, psychotic disorder, anxiety disorder, and personality change due to a general medical condition, plus a new category—catatonic disorder due to a general medical condition.

Definitions and General Observations

Changes in mood, thinking, and personality have long been associated with cerebral disorders. It is briefly inviting to think of the brain syndromes presenting with little or no cognitive impairment as "functional equivalents," signaling the extent to which they may resemble and overlap with standard functional disorders. However, the diagnostic criteria for these disorders are not merely transpositions of the usual DSM criteria for affective disorder, schizophrenia, or personality disorder combined with the requirement to demonstrate an organic factor etiologically related to the abnormal mental state. Careful examination shows major differences; these extend well beyond the presence of criteria excluding delirium and dementia.

A diagnosis of secondary psychotic disorders requires that delusions attributed to an organic factor *predominate* in a clinical presentation without evidence of delirium, dementia, or hallucinosis. A diagnosis of depressive disorder (depressed) due to a general medical condition rests on the identification of *dysphoria* (attributed to an organic factor) as the *predominant* clinical feature. Parallel observations apply to the criteria for manic presentations of manic disorder due to a general medical condition as well. Even a cursory glance at the elements of secondary personality change due to a general medical condition suffices to indicate that it shares surprisingly little with any of the personality disorders coded on Axis II of DSM-III. It principally requires evidence of changes in behavior and personality (attendant to a specific organic factor or process).

The rationales that underlie the specific elements of these diagnostic criteria remain to be clarified in DSM-IV. DSM-III and DSM-IIIR failed to address what might satisfy the required etiologic relationship in these conditions. As a consequence, considerable latitude has been extended to the clinician's subjective judgment.

The category *mood disorder* due to a general medical condition is an outgrowth of the concept of "secondary depression," which appeared in the late 1960s. The original Feighner et al. criteria (1972) included among secondary depressive disorders those arising in the context of life-threatening or incapacitating medical illness. The major focus, however, was directed to those depressive syndromes beginning after the onset of other nonaffective psychiatric illness. The depression that follows the resolution of an acute schizophrenic episode is a ready example of such a secondary disorder.

EDITORS' COMMENT

An appropriate term for the syndromes following a disease affecting the central nervous system is an *induced* syndrome. Thus there would be an induced depression and induced anxiety disorder or an induced delusional disorder. An induced affective disorder should be differentiated from a secondary affective disorder to a medical disease which does not affect the brain, e.g., a secondary depression to a myocardial infarction or a secondary depression to a life-terminating illness. Such secondary depressions, in fact, may be reactive depressions, though more work needs to be done on the classification of such depressions (see Winokur G, *Mania and Depression: A Classification of Syndrome and Disease*, Baltimore, Johns Hopkins Press, 1991). Considerable data are available concerning an induced mania. Cook and others (*Acta Psychiatrica Scandinavica* 76:674–677, 1987) compared patients with an "organic" bipolar illness with those with a spontaneous bipolar illness. Those with a spontaneous illness had a significantly higher family history of affective disorder, were

less likely irritable when manic, were less likely assaultive when manic, were less likely to have an organic personality disorder when examined, and were more likely to show first-rank symptoms such as are seen in schizophrenia. Cook and his collaborators (*Journal of Affective Disorders* 11:147–149, 1986) also evaluated EEG abnormalities in bipolar illness and found that those patients who had an EEG abnormality were less likely to have a family history for affective illness. This has been found in almost all the studies that have looked at this phenomenon.

Andreasen and Winokur (1979) argued for excluding preexisting medical illnesses from the category of secondary affective disorder in order to achieve a more homogeneous clinical entity; Klerman (1981) favored expanding the concept to include "not only the affective states secondary in time to other well-defined psychiatric syndromes but also secondary to, or associated with, *concomitant* systemic medical disease or drug reactions." DSM-IV's mood disorder due to a general medical condition is an indirect product of this dialogue. It provides a discrete category for medical affective disturbances and has been designed with the assumption that physiologic or biologic variables engender these affective disturbances. It seems to look past the perplexing question of reactive or psychological response to medical illness.

As has been noted by Kathol and Petty (1981) and Klerman (1981), diagnosing affective disorder in the face of medical–surgical illness is a difficult task; many of the usual guideposts, particularly vegetative functions, are confounded by the physical illness process itself. One cannot rely with certainty on such parameters as impaired sleep, impaired appetite, weight loss, and reduced energy to diagnose mood disorder in the patient with malignancy, a collagen-vascular disease, or respiratory insufficiency. This led Stewart et al. (1965) to conduct their study of depression among the medically ill "based entirely on psychological symptoms." Such diagnostic dilemmas have impeded vigorous investigation of "medical depression." Few data aside from prevalence estimates are presently available to characterize these conditions; little is known of their natural course, outcome, and treatment response.

The category *psychotic disorder* due to a general medical condition addresses schizophrenia-like presentations associated with organic disorders. These disturbances may involve the CNS directly or indirectly. Kraepelin and Bleuler both viewed schizophrenia as the clinical outcome of an *organic* cerebral pathologic process. Studies using CT scanning (Luchins, 1982), brain electrical activity mapping (BEAM) (Morihisa et al., 1983), evoked potential (Morstyn et al., 1983), and positron emission tomography (PET) (Buchsbaum et al., 1982), together with the earlier work of Johnstone et al. (1976, 1978) and Cross et al. (1981), lend increasing credence to the early postulates. Without the technology for sophisticated brain imaging, the early German theorists could only look to presumed relationships between known organic disorders (including alcoholism) and paranoid or schizophrenia-like states. These "models" apparently served quite well. Over the ensuing years, the literature has documented any number of medical disorders, brain trauma, and drugs capable of evoking schizophrenic symptomatology. Substance-induced disorders have recently come to the fore and may be the most common cause of the syndrome (Lipowski, 1984).

The category personality change due to a general medical condition traces its origins to the nineteenth-century recognition of behavioral change in end-stage neurosyphilis. Subsequently, the outbreak of encephalitis in 1918 and the extensive number of World War I brain injuries focused attention on the question of specific lesions of the CNS and concomitant changes in personality and behavior (Lipowski, 1980c). The DSM-III category of organic personality syndrome was specifically constructed to encompass the frontal lobe syndromes (Blumer and Benson, 1975). These consisted of two types: (1) a "pseudodepressed" convexity syndrome with "negative symptoms," in which patients are impoverished in thought and action alike, and (2) "pseudopsychopathic"—with dysfunction in the orbitomedial areas of the frontal lobes—in which patients are disinhibited, impulsive, puerile, and often intensely labile. Focal brain lesions involving other areas of the cortex merit no special status as yet in the diagnostic manual, although other "regional cortical syndromes" are well described.

The category of *anxiety disorder* due to a general medical condition was added to the diagnostic manual in 1986 (as organic anxiety disorder). This followed formulation of diagnostic criteria and a definition by Mackenzie and Popkin (1983).

Etiology

An explicit goal of liberalizing this section of the manual in 1980 was to encourage reporting of associations of disturbances in mood, thinking, and personality with cerebral disorders. This, in turn, was expected to stimulate further investigation of causative and pathogenetic relationships (Lipowski, 1980b). These intentions remain to be fulfilled, but it is appreciated that a wide range of diseases, substances, and trauma can evoke each of the brain syndromes presenting with little or no cognitive impairment. In the tertiary-care setting, however, a modest number of physiologic factors account for the majority of cases. These have recently been reviewed in detail (Popkin and Tucker, 1992).

Endocrinopathies, drugs, direct lesions of the CNS, and infections are the causes for most mood disorders due to a general medical condition. This list of etiologies applies to both depressive and manic forms of their disorders (although the second is far less prevalent). Thyroid dysfunction and cortisol aberrations are both well known for evoking mood change; affective disturbances have been described in a full complement of endocrine conditions (Popkin and Mackenzie, 1980). Substance-induced mood disorders are encountered frequently in the hospital setting. For example, steroid-induced mood disorders respond promptly to neuroleptics but may be exacerbated by tricyclics (Hall et al., 1978). Only a small number of drugs (especially antihypertensives, oral contraceptives, barbiturates, and ethanol) precipitate depressive symptoms with any frequency (Whitlock and Evans, 1978). Other "offenders" in the tertiary-care hospital include steroids and several chemotherapeutic agents.

Work by Robinson and Rabins (1989) clarifies the association of stroke and affective disorder of the depressive type. Krauthammer and Klerman (1978) did not identify vascular events (e.g., hemorrhages, cerebrovascular accidents) as a significant etiologic factor in "secondary mania." Lishman (1978) noted the elevation of mood after at least one type of vascular event, the rupture of anterior communicating artery aneurysms. Associations of mood disorder with multiple sclerosis, viral illness, and pancreatic carcinoma are well described. The first is a point of controversy—Is the affective condition reactive or a direct function of demyelination? The last is a puzzle—Are neuropeptides the underlying mechanism?

Etiologic factors in psychotic disorder due to a general medical condition include drugs, metabolic disorders, a range of CNS conditions (e.g., encephalitis, head trauma, epilepsy, and tumor), and a number of other conditions, including systemic lupus erythematosus, vitamin B_{12} deficiency, porphyria, and Huntington's chorea. Substance-induced delusions are probably the most common etiology; stimulants dominate the clinical picture, although L-dopa and steroids are common offenders on medical–surgical services. In psychiatric consultation work, psychotic disorder due to a general medical condition is most likely to be encountered in patients with epileptic disorders. The emergence of schizophreniform features in patients who have had epilepsy for 15 or more years is well recognized (Davison and Bagley, 1969); considerable controversy still surrounds the pathogenesis of such clinical phenomenology.

In contrast to the other mental disorders due to a general medical condition, *personality* change is predominantly the result of head trauma or structural damage to the brain. The latter may involve vascular insults (particularly subarachnoid bleeds), tumors, poisoning, and psychosurgery. The diagnosis of personality change due to a general medical condition is commonly extended to numbers of hospitalized epilepsy patients as well.

Epidemiology

Epidemiologic studies using DSM-IIIR criteria and systematically examining the mental disorders due to a general medical condition are not yet available, to my knowledge. In the consultation psychiatry setting, such disorders account for approximately 15 to 20 percent of all brain syndrome cases. Technical problems of diagnosis aside, it can be expected that mood disorder due to a general medical condition is the most common and psychotic disorder due to a general medical condition is the least common. A number of investigators have estimated the prevalence of depression in the medically ill to range between 20 and 30 percent. Moffic and Paykel (1975) used the Beck Depression Inventory and found that 24 percent of a group of medical inpatients scored at or above a cutoff point of 14 within 1 week of admission to a teaching hospital. [A cutoff point of 14 has been reported by Beck (1967) to differentiate reliably between depressives and nondepressives.] Few of these patients were, however, identified by their physicians as depressed. Schwab et al. (1967) concluded that "at least 20 percent" of a series of medical inpatients were depressed. Few published studies of medical depression used DSM-III or DSM-IIIR criteria; nor did most preceding studies take pains to separate reactive processes from "purely" physiologic depressions, i.e., those with an identified (organic) etiology. The association of depression and medical illness need not imply an etiologic relationship. In reviewing the available studies of "medical depression," certain intriguing observations about risk factors appear with consistency. First, there is no evidence of the usual female preponderance in affective illness; rather, the incidence of depression in the medically ill appears independent of gender. Neither is there usually a prior history of mood disorder in the patient or in his or her family. In a similar vein, data regarding mania due to a general medical condition suggest a negative family history and late onset. The overall severity of these constellations appears less pronounced than that found in "functional" major depressive or manic episodes. Suicide is generally regarded as uncommon in the medically ill; however, there is evidence that patients with specific illnesses, particularly respiratory disorders, constitute high-risk groups for suicide (Mackenzie and Popkin, 1987).

In the absence of formal epidemiologic inquiries, the work of Hall et al. (1980) and Koranyi (1979) does offer some perspective. Hall et al. reported data from the exhaustive medical evaluation of 100 psychiatrically disturbed subjects of lower socioeconomic strata admitted to a research ward in lieu of commitment to a state mental hospital. Forty-six percent were judged to have medical illnesses that directly accounted for or greatly exacerbated their behavioral symptoms. Of this group, one-third had a schizophreniform presentation, another third presented with affective features, and less than one-tenth had personality disorders. (In retrospect, these would now be assigned per DSM-IV to the respective categories under discussion in this chapter.) Of the medical conditions manifesting

as psychiatric disease (or evoking psychiatric constellations), endocrinopathies were predominant. Disturbances of the CNS, hematologic disorders, and cardiovascular disturbances accounted for most of the remaining cases. Koranyi (1979) studied some 2000 subjects referred to his psychiatric clinic; 43 percent had major medical illness. In 18 percent of those with medical illness, the presenting psychopathology was judged to be caused by the physical disease. In 51 percent, the medical condition contributed substantially to the behavioral picture; in the remaining 31 percent, the two disorders were judged independent though concurrent. Koranyi found that the frequencies of medical conditions in psychiatric patients by organ system were as follows: (1) cardiovascular, (2) CNS, (3) endocrine/metabolic, and (4) gastrointestinal. Although Hall's work dealt with a specific socioeconomic population, Koranyi's data are more broad-based. Together they signal that the psychiatrist and the primary-care physician alike must conscientiously consider organic etiologies for a sizable fraction of psychiatric presentations in either the inpatient or outpatient setting.

Pathology

Investigators have pursued the neuroanatomic basis of psychiatric illness throughout the course of modern psychiatry, but precise anatomic correlates for psychiatric disorders have proven elusive (Ross and Rush, 1981). Studies of the psychopathology arising with "organic" disorders show that the *site* of CNS lesions and the *nature of the pathologic process* are crucial to resultant behavioral presentations. Flor-Henry and Koles (1980) proposed that both mood and thought disorder relate to alterations of the frontotemporal regions of the brain. Numerous studies of temporal lobe epileptics have led to the suggestion that right-sided lesions are more frequently associated with affective changes and those on the left, with schizophreniform presentations (Flor-Henry, 1976; Bear and Fedio, 1977). Studies of patients with unilateral brain damage have consistently indicated that left hemisphere lesions are associated with dysphoria, hopelessness, and self-depreciation; in contrast, right hemisphere damage is correlated with indifference, euphoria, social disinhibition, and placidity (Sackeim et al., 1982). While some argue for hemispheric asymmetry in the expression of positive and negative emotions (Sackeim et al., 1982), others (Ross and Rush, 1981) emphasize that both hemispheres participate in affective disorders, each modulating certain features. Studying brain-damaged patients, the latter authors observed that in the right hemisphere a loss of ability to express emotion correlated with more anterior lesions and a loss of emotional recognition with more posterior lesions. In contrast, Kiloh (1980) focused exclusively on the limbic system and its interconnections, viewing laterality issues with reservation and implying that no one nucleus has a monopoly on a specific behavior.

In this confusing picture, the work of Robinson and Rabins (1989) is noteworthy. Studying mood disorders in stroke patients without preceding psychiatric disorder, they found that behavioral changes were a function of the location of the hemispheric lesion. Severity of depression was greatest in patients with left anterior lesions or left basal ganglia lesions (versus all others). In addition, "the severity of depression correlated with the proximity of the lesion on CT scan to the frontal pole" in this group. In the group with right hemisphere lesions, the reverse trend was found. The more posterior the lesion, the more pronounced was the depression. Right anterior lesions were accompanied by apathy or undue cheerfulness. Thus intrahemispheric lesion location seems to be critical to mood disorder in stroke patients.

In analogous work, Levine and Grek (1984) studied patients manifesting delusions after right cerebral infarction. No particular site or size of lesion was associated with particular delusions; however, there was a relationship between delusions and all measures of brain atrophy. The authors concluded that the emergence of delusions depended on premorbid brain atrophy; thus they argue that the state of the left hemisphere determines the response to right cerebral infarction.

The literature includes a number of neuropathologic accounts of the psychiatric manifestations of cerebral tumors (Haberland, 1965; Malamud, 1967). Factors including site of the cerebral pathology, rate of tumor growth, and amount of tissue compromised are critical to the behavioral sequelae, which span a full gamut of psychopathology. [The interested reader is referred to Lishman's review (1978) of the psychopathology accompanying cerebral tumors.] Davison and Bagley (1969) compiled a comprehensive account of schizophrenia-like psychoses associated with CNS disorders. This work reflects how varied may be the pathology evoking what DSM-3-R called organic delusional syndrome.

Discussing personality changes with frontal and temporal lobe lesions, Blumer and Benson (1975) note that in addition to *localization*, the *nature of the lesion* is important. "Frontal personality disorders result from destructive lesions, whereas temporal personality changes are the product of *irritative* (epileptic) disorders." In addition to studies of war-injured and neurosurgical patients, the consequences of frontal lobe injury on personality can be appreciated by reviewing the psychosurgery or lobotomy literature. The "pseudodepressed" type of frontal lobe personality alteration appears to result from pathology affecting the prefrontal convexity and its connections to the basal ganglia and thalamus. These latter sites also have been implicated in subcortical dementia (e.g., Parkinson's disease, Huntington's chorea). The "pseudopsy-chopathic" presentation involves lesions of the orbital frontal lobe (Blumer and Benson, 1975). The personality changes appearing late in the course of temporal lobe epilepsy are associated with varied types of pathology (tumors, vascular insults, infections, scars from trauma). Blumer and Benson (1975), however, caution that in most cases of frontal lobe disorder, pathology "fails to respect anatomical boundaries."

Clinical Picture and Course

For two of the disorders at hand, the clinical picture is straightforward. The patient presenting with a psychotic disorder due to a general medical condition has overt delusions, an identified organic etiologic factor, and no evidence of delirium or dementia. Associated features of a schizophreniform process may be encountered. Hallucinations may be present, although Davison and Bagley (1969) noted that auditory and tactile hallucinations are less common in "organic" versus true schizophrenics. Catatonic symptoms were found to be more common in the organic group. Of interest, Davison and Bagley also comment on the low incidence of primary delusions in the organic group. Persecutory delusions are suggested (DSM-III, p. 114) to be the most common type of delusions.

The patient assigned a diagnosis of personality change due to a general medical condition is "not himself." Although not seriously cognitively impaired and not manifesting major mood or thought disorder, the individual will be recognized by family and friends as changed, different, particularly in terms of lifelong emotional responsivity and general demeanor. Emotional lability and incontinence (such as seen in pseudobulbar palsy patients), poor capacity for impulse control, and altered (usually reduced) initiative are prominent. Inattention and indifference are often striking contrasts to what has gone before. The spectrum ranges from those appearing lethargic and apathetic to those who have ostensibly lost all social graces (if once present). Although the clinician is unlikely to miss such features, the premorbid picture as described by family and friends is crucial to a full appreciation of the psychopathology.

Abnormal mood judged to be the consequence of an organic factor is the essential feature of a mood disorder due to a general medical condition. The disturbances of mood may closely resemble those in a depressive or manic episode, and clinical phenomenology may be the same as in a manic or depressive episode. Lipowski (1980b) argues that the presence of an organic factor should *antedate* the mood disturbance. In practice, the diagnosis is often less than straightforward; as noted earlier, assessing the presence and extent of affective symptomatology in the physically ill is problematic. The diagnostic manual has previously skirted this problem by its emphasis on the organic etiologic factor. More explicit criteria concerning the actual affective features of the diagnoses are needed. Endicott (1984) has proposed substituting alternative associated symptoms in order to diagnose major depressive episode in the patient with malignancy. (She suggests fearfulness or depressed appearance to replace the parameter of weight change/appetite, social withdrawal instead of sleep dysfunction, brooding or self-pity instead of the loss of energy criterion, and "cannot be cheered up" in place of the impaired concentration parameter.) Presumptively, these changes could apply to a diagnosis of mood disorder due to a general medical condition as well. They leave unaddressed the critical issues of reactive response to a physiologically induced mood disorder or how the clinician meaningfully distinguishes mood disorder due to a general medical condition in the cancer patient from major depressive episode or adjustment disorder with depressed mood.

The clinical course of the disorders due to a general medical condition depends predominantly on the etiology of the specific disorder. Drug-induced disturbances are perhaps the most likely to remit promptly; metabolic- and endocrine-related disturbances may do likewise when corrected. The conditions linked to destruction, permanent compromise of CNS tissue, are most likely to have ongoing behavioral sequelae. In general, mood disorders due to a general medical condition should be short-lived; in contrast, the non-drug-induced and personality change due to a general medical condition are more chronic states. Systematic data from cohort studies on the clinical course of these syndromes are needed.

Laboratory Findings

Evidence of CNS or systemic disease is required for any of the diagnoses involving "due to a general medical condition." No specific approach has been formulated to date. However, history and physical with neurologic examination, CT scan, sleep-deprived electroencephalography, electrocardiography, urinalysis, blood counts, and a battery of blood chemistry studies sufficed in Hall et al.'s study (1980) to identify 90 percent of cases in which unrecognized medical illness presented as psychiatric disease. Foster et al. (1976) demonstrated that patients with medical-associated depression had significantly less rapid eye movement (REM) activity during REM sleep compared with patients with primary depression. Such quantification of REM density has not yet been used as a marker for mood disorder due to a general medical condition. Clinical acumen must guide routine investigations in the search for an organic etiology. When the patient is age 35 or older and without a personal or familial history of psychiatric illness, the search for an organic factor should be more extensive.

Differential Diagnosis

The diagnosis of personality change due to a general medical condition can be confused primarily with dementia and secondary mood disorder. Personality changes may be among the initial features of a dementing illness, but in time the intellectual decline serves to distinguish the two. Likewise, the patient with a mood disorder due to a general medical condition may display personality alteration; the predominance of mood disturbance is the diagnostic "cutting edge." Psychotic disorder due to a general medical condition must be distinguished from such processes as schizophrenia and paranoid disorder. This may prove problematic at times. Delusions may arise in mood disorder due to a general medical condition as well, but they are mood-congruent and not the predominant feature. The dilemmas of differentiating these mood disorders from primary affective disorders have been discussed previously. Lipowski (1980c) suggests not diagnosing organic (secondary) personality change unless behavioral changes have persisted for 1 month. No duration criteria presently apply in any of the secondary disorders under discussion.

Treatment

CORRECTING THE MEDICAL PROBLEM

The treatment of medical disorders due to a general medical condition has been largely neglected in the literature. Once an etiologic factor has been identified, efforts to resolve or minimize the pathophysiologic process must follow. In some instances, correcting the medical disorder alone may suffice. For example, behavioral changes caused by a parathyroid adenoma can be expected to abate with surgical removal of the tumor and restoration of eucalcemia. In other instances, medical treatment may not redress the psychiatric disturbance. Time may be a critical variable in this process. Vitamin B_{12} deficiency takes more than a year to develop, but if it is permitted to go uncorrected, at some point irreversible neuronal loss will result. In perhaps the only such study extant, Tonks (1964) found that three factors predicted whether restoration of euthyroid status would result in cessation of affective changes associated with hypothyroidism. He observed that full clearing of the psychiatric picture was likely if (1) the patient was over age 60, (2) the presentation involved cognitive impairment, and (3) the process was less than 2 years in duration.

MANAGEMENT OF THE PSYCHOPATHOLOGY PER SE

Treatment of the mental disorders due to a general medical condition has not been well researched. Little specific therapy is available for personality change due to a general medical condition; one can treat the underlying disease, structure the environment, support and educate family members, and reserve neuroleptics for agitation or psychotic outbursts. There is evidence that agents, including lithium (Dale, 1980; Williams and Goldstein, 1979) and propranolol (Yudofsky et al., 1981; Elliot, 1976), may be useful in the management of patients with CNS damage and problems in impulse control. Patients with psychotic disorder due to a general medical condition benefit from neuroleptic medication to attenuate delusional ideation and preclude flagrant decompensation. My clinical experience has found thiothixene (Navane) the best choice in patients with known CNS lesions or dysfunction. [In contrast, haloperidol (Haldol) has seldom been helpful in such patients.] No clear explanation for these observations is available; however, it is interesting to note that Navane has not to date been associated with increased seizure activity. I find that two-thirds of standard amounts (e.g., dose for schizophrenia) will contain delusional thinking and schizophreniform behavior in brain syndrome patients, especially epileptics.

Perhaps most distressing is the absence of guidelines regarding the treatment of mood disorders due to a general medical condition. Davies et al. (1971) found that 13 percent of psychiatric patients treated with antidepressants became confused. When tricyclics are used in the medically ill, one-third of drug trials must be discontinued owing to side effects, principally delirium (Popkin et al., 1985). Falk et al. (1979) reported that lithium prophylactically averted steroid-induced affective disorders in a group of multiple sclerosis patients. Veith et al. (1982) and Glassman et al. (1983) have demonstrated that tricyclics will not significantly alter left ventricular function in patients with known cardiac disease; Lipsey et al. (1987) reported that nortriptyline proved useful in some mood disorders associated with stroke. (The study has numerous limitations and requires replication with a larger sample.) Fava et al. (1988) have noted that to date the efficacy of antidepressants in treating mood disorders due to a general medical condition remains unclear. Prospective studies with more specific diagnostic criteria and newer antidepressants (e.g., selective serotonin reuptake inhibitors) are needed; the clinician is often confronted with dilemmas that demand choices be made despite diagnostic impasses.

REFERENCES

Andreasen NC, Winokur G: Secondary depression—Familial, clinical and research perspectives. Am J Psychiatry 136:62–66, 1979.

Bear D, Fedio P: Quantitative analysis of interictal behavior in temporal lobe epilepsy. Arch Neurol 34:454–467, 1977.

Beck AT: Depression: Clinical, Experimental and Therapeutic Aspects. New York, Hoeber Medical Division, Harper & Row, 1967.

Besson J: Dementia: Biological solution still a long way off. Br Med J 287:926–927, 1983.

Birkett DP: The psychiatric differentiation of senility and arteriosclerosis. Br J Psychiatry 120:321–325, 1972.

Blank K, Perry S: Relationship of psychological processes during delirium to outcome. Am J Psychiatry 141:843–847, 1984.

Blumer D, Benson DF: Personality changes with frontal and temporal lobe lesions. In Benson DF, Blumer D (eds): Psychiatric Aspects of Neurologic Disease. New York, Grune & Stratton, 1975, pp 51–170.

Bonhoeffer K: Exogenous psychoses (1910). Reprinted in Hirsch SR, Shepherd M (eds): Themes and Variations in European Psychiatry. Bristol, John Wright, 1974, pp. 47–52.

Brody JA: An epidemiologist views senile dementia: Facts and fragments. Am J Epidemiol 115:155–162, 1982.

Bruce ME, Fraser H: Amyloid plaques in the brains of mice infected with scrapie: Morphological variation and staining properties. Neuropathol Appl Neurobiol 1:189–202, 1975.

Buchsbaum MS, Ingvar DH, Kessler R, et al: Cerebral glucography with positron tomography: Use in normal subjects and in patients with schizophrenia. Arch Gen Psychiatry 39: 251–259, 1982.

Cook RH, Ward BE, Austin JH: Studies in aging of the brain: IV. Familial Alzheimer's disease: Relation to transmissible dementia aneuploidy and microtubular defects. Neurology (NY) 29:1402–1412, 1979.

Corsellis JAN: The pathology of dementia. Br J Hosp Med 2:695–702, 1969.

Coyle JT, Price DL, DeLong MR: Alzheimer's disease: A disorder of cortical cholinergic innervation. Science 219:1184–1190, 1983.

Cross AJ, Crow TJ, Owen F: ³H-Flupenthixol binding in post-mortem brains of schizophrenics: Evidence for a selective increase in dopamine D_2 receptors. Psychopharmacology (Berl) 74:122–124, 1981.

Dale PG: Lithium therapy in aggressive mentally subnormal patients. Br J Psychiatry 137:469–474, 1980.

Davies RK, Tucker GJ, Harrow M, et al: Confusional episodes and antidepressant medication. Am J Psychiatry 128:95–99, 1971.

Davison K, Bagley C: Schizophrenia-like psychoses associated with organic disorders of the CNS: A review of the literature. Br J Psychiatry, special publication 4: Current Problems of Neuropsychiatry, ed by RN Herrington, 1969, pp 113–184.

Deakin JFW: Alzheimer's disease: Recent advances and future prospects. Br Med J 287:1323–1324, 1983.

Delaney P: Dementia: The search for treatable causes. South Med J 75:707–709, 1982.

Diagnostic and Statistical Manual of Mental Disorders, 3d ed. Washington, American Psychiatric Association, 1980.

Diagnostic and Statistical Manual of Mental Disorders, 3d ed, revised. Washington, American Psychiatric Association, 1986.

DSM-IV Draft Criteria (3/1/93). Task Force on DSM-IV. Washington, American Psychiatric Association, 1993.

Elliot FA: The neurology of explosive rage. Practitioner 217:51–60, 1976.

Endicott J: Measurement of depression in patients with cancer. Cancer 53:2243–2248, 1984.

Engel GL: Delirium. In Freedman AM, Kaplan HI (eds): Comprehensive Textbook of Psychiatry. Baltimore, Williams & Wilkins, 1967, pp 711–716.

Engel G, Romano J: Studies of delirium: II. Reversibility of the encephalogram with experimental procedure. Arch Neurol Psychiatry 51:378–392, 1944.

Engel G, Romano J: Delirium: A syndrome of cerebral insufficiency. J Chronic Dis 9:260–277, 1959.

Eslinger P, Damasio A, Benton A, Van Allen M: Neurologic detection of abnormal mental decline in older persons. JAMA 253:670–674, 1985.

Falk WE, Mahnke MW, Poskanzer DC: Lithium prophylaxis of corticotropic induced psychosis. JAMA 241:1011–1012, 1979.

Fava GA, Sonino N, Wise TN: Management of depression in medical patients. Psychother Psychosom 49:81–102, 1988.

Feighner JP, Robins E, Guze SB, et al: Diagnostic criteria for use in psychiatric research. Arch Gen Psychiatry 26:57–63, 1972.

Fisk AA: Management of Alzheimer's disease. Postgrad Med 73: 237–241, 1983.

Flor-Henry P: Lateralized temporal-limbic dysfunction and psychopathology. Ann NY Acad Sci 280:777–795, 1976.

Flor-Henry P, Koles ZJ: EEG studies in depression, mania and normals: Evidence for partial shifts of laterality in the affective psychoses. Adv Biol Psychiatry 4:21–43, 1980.

Folstein M, Folstein S, McHugh P: "Mini-mental state": A practical method for grading the cognitive state of patients for the clinician. J Psychiatr Res 12:189–198, 1975.

Foster FG, Kupfer DJ, Coble P, et al: Rapid eye movement sleep density: An objective indicator in severe medical-depressive syndromes. Arch Gen Psychiatry 33:1119–1123, 1976.

Fox JH, Topel JL, Huckman MS: Use of computerized tomography in senile dementia. J Neurol Neurosurg Psychiatry 38:948–953, 1975.

Freeman FR: Evaluation of patients with progressive intellectual deterioration. Arch Neurol 33:658–659, 1976.

Freeman FR, Rudd SM: Clinical features that predict potentially reversible progressive intellectual deterioration. J Am Geriat Soc 7:449–451, 1982.

Glassman AH, Johnson LL, Giardina EGV, et al: The use of imipramine in depressed patients with congestive heart failure. JAMA 250:1997–2001, 1983.

Guze SB, Cantwell DP: The prognosis in organic brain syndromes. Am J Psychiatry 120:878–881, 1964.

Haase GR: Diseases presenting as dementia. In Wells CE (ed): Dementia, 2d ed. Philadelphia, FA Davis, 1977.

Haberland C: Psychiatric manifestations in brain tumors. Akt Frasen Psychiatr Neurol 2:65–86, 1965.

Hachinski VC, Lassen NA, Marshall J: Multi-infarct dementia: A cause of mental deterioration in the elderly. Lancet 2:207–209, 1974.

Hackett TP, Weisman AD: Psychiatric management of operative syndromes: I. The therapeutic consultation and the effect of noninterpretive interventions. Psychosom Med 23:267–282, 1960.

Hall RCW, Gardner ER, Stickney SK, et al: Physical illness manifesting as psychiatric disease: II. Analysis of a state hospital inpatient population. Arch Gen Psychiatry 37:989–995, 1980.

Hall RCW, Popkin MK, Kirkpatrick B: Tricyclic exacerbation of steroid psychosis. J Neur Ment Dis 166:738–743, 1975.

Heston LL, Mastri AR: The genetics of Alzheimer's disease. Arch Gen Psychiatry 34:976–981, 1977.

Heston LL, White J: A family study of Alzheimer's disease and senile dementia: An interim report. In Cole JO, Barrett JE (eds): Psychopathology in the Aged. New York, Raven Press, 1980.

Heston LL, White JA: Dementia: A Practical Guide to Alzheimer's Disease and Related Illnesses. New York, WH Freeman, 1983.

Heston LL, Mastri AR, Anderson E, White J: Dementia of the Alzheimer type: Clinical genetics, natural history and associated conditions. Arch Gen Psychiatry 38:1085–1090, 1981.

Heyman A, Wilkinson WE, Stafford JA, et al: Alzheimer's disease: A study of epidemiological aspects. Ann Neurol 15:335–341, 1984.

Jacobs JW, Bernhard MR, Delgado A, Strain JJ: Screening for organic mental syndromes in the medically ill. Ann Intern Med 86:40–46, 1977.

Jarvik LF, Ruth V, Matsuyama SS: Organic brain syndrome and aging: A six-year follow-up of surviving twins. Arch Gen Psychiatry 37:280–286, 1980.

Johnstone EC, Crow TJ, Frith CD, et al: Cerebral ventricular size and cognitive impairment in chronic schizophrenia. Lancet 2:924–926, 1976.

Johnstone EC, Crow TJ, Frith CD, et al: The dementia of dementia praecox. Acta Psychiatr Scand 57:305–324, 1978.

Kathol RG, Petty F: Relationship of depression to medical illness. J Affective Disord 3:111–121, 1981.

Kiloh LG: Psychiatric disorders and the limbic system. In Girgis M, Kiloh LG (eds): Limbic Epilepsy and the Dyscontrol Syndrome. New York, Elsevier, 1980.

Klerman GL: Depression in the medically ill. Psychiatr Clin North Am 4:301–317, 1981.

Kokmen E: Dementia—Alzheimer type. Mayo Clin Proc 59:35–42, 1984.

Koranyi EK: Morbidity and rate of undiagnosed physical illness in a psychiatric clinic population. Arch Gen Psychiatry 36:414–419, 1979.

Krauthammer C, Klerman GL: Secondary mania. Arch Gen Psychiatry 35:1333–1339, 1978.

Levine DN, Grek A: The anatomic basis of delusions after right cerebral infarction. Neurology (NY) 34:577–582, 1984.

Lipowski ZJ: Delirium: Clouding of consciousness and confusion. J Nerv Ment Dis 145:227–255, 1967.

Lipowski ZJ: Organic brain syndromes: A reformulation. Compr Psychiatry 19:309–322, 1978.

Lipowski ZJ: Delirium: Acute Brain Failure in Man. Springfield, IL, Charles C Thomas, 1980a.

Lipowski ZJ: A new look at organic brain syndromes. Am J Psychiatry 137:674–678, 1980b.

Lipowski ZJ: Organic mental disorders: Introduction and review of syndromes. In Kaplan HI, Freedman AM, Saddock BJ (eds): Comprehensive Textbook of Psychiatry, 3d ed. Baltimore, Williams & Wilkins, 1980c.

Lipowski ZJ: Differentiating delirium from dementia in the elderly. Clin Gerontol 1:3–10, 1982.

Lipowski ZJ: Transient cognitive disorders (delirium, acute confusional states) in the elderly. Am J Psychiatry 140:1426–1436, 1983.

Lipowski ZJ: Organic mental disorders—An American perspective. Br J Psychiatry 144:542–546, 1984.

Lipsey JR, Robinson RG, Pearlson GD, et al: Nortriptyline treatment of poststroke depression: A double-blind study. Lancet 1:297–299, 1984.

Lishman WA: Organic Psychiatry. Oxford, Blackwell, 1978.

Luchins DJ: Computed tomography in schizophrenia. Arch Gen Psychiatry 39:859–860, 1982.

Mackenzie TB, Popkin MK: Organic Anxiety Syndrome. Am J Psychiatry 140:342–344, 1983.

Mackenzie TB, Popkin MK: Stress-response syndrome occurring after delirium. Am J Psychiatry 137:1433–1435, 1980.

Mackenzie TB, Popkin MK: Suicide in the medical patient. Int J Psychiatr Med 17:3–22, 1987.

Malamud N: Psychiatric disorder with intracranial tumors of limbic system. Arch Neurol 17:113–123, 1967.

Marsden CD, Harrison MJC: Outcome of investigations of patients with presenile dementia. Br Med J 2:249–252, 1972.

McAllister TW: Cognitive functioning in the affective disorders. Compr Psychiatry 22:572–586, 1981.

McHugh PR, Folstein MF: Subcortical Dementia. Address to the American Academy of Neurology, Boston, MA, April 1973.

McKhann G, Drachman D, Folstein M, et al: Clinical diagnosis of Alzheimer's disease: Report of the NINCDS-ADRA Work Group under the auspices of the Department of Health and Human Services Task Force on Alzheimer's Disease. Neurology 34:939–944, 1984.

Moffic HS, Paykel ES: Depression in medical inpatients. Br J Psychiatry 126:346–353, 1975.

Morihisa JM, Duffy FH, Wyatt RJ: Brain electrical activity mapping (BEAM) in schizophrenic patients. Arch Gen Psychiatry 40:719–728, 1983.

Morstyn R, Duffy FH, McCarley RW: Altered P300 topography in schizophrenia. Arch Gen Psychiatry 40:729–734, 1983.

Murrell J, Farlow M, Ghett B, Benson MD: A mutation in the amyloid precursor protein associated with hereditary Alzheimer's disease. Science 254:97–99, 1991.

Popkin MK, Tucker GJ: Secondary and drug-induced mood, anxiety, psychotic, catatonic and personality syndromes: A review of the literature. J Neuropsychiatry and clinical neurosciences 4(4):369–385, 1992.

Popkin MK, Mackenzie TB: The provisional diagnosis of dementia: Three phases of evaluation. In Hall RCW, Bereford TP (eds): The Handbook of Psychiatric Diagnostic Procedures. Jamaica, NY, Spectrum, 1984.

Popkin MK, Mackenzie TB: Psychiatric presentations of endocrine dysfunctions. In Hall RCW (ed): Psychiatric Presentations of Medical Illness. Jamaica, NY, Spectrum, 1980, pp 139–156.

Popkin MK, Callies A, Mackenzie T: The outcome of antidepressant use in the medically ill. Arch Gen Psychiatry 42:1160–1163, 1985.

Pro JD, Wells CE: The use of the electroencephalogram in the diagnosis of delirium. Dis Nerv Syst 38:804, 1977.

Rabins PV: The prevalence of reversible dementia in a psychiatric hospital. Hosp Community Psychiatry 32:490–492, 1981.

Rabins PV, Folstein MF: Delirium and dementia: Diagnostic criteria and fatality rates. Br J Psychiatry 140:149–153, 1982.

Rabins PV, Merchant A, Nestadt G: Criteria for diagnosing reversible dementia caused by depression. Br J Psychiatry 144:488–492, 1984.

Rebok G, Folstein M: Dementia: A review. In DSM-IV Sourcebook (in press).

Reisberg B, Ferris SH, Shulman E, et al: Longitudinal course of normal aging and progressive dementia of the Alzheimer's type: A prospective study of 106 subjects over 3.6 year mean interval. Progr Neuropsychoparamacol Biol Psychiatry 10:571–578, 1986.

Robinson RG, Rabins PV: Aging and Clinical Practice: Depression and Co-Existing Disease. New York, Igaku-Shoin, 1989.

Ron MA, Toone BK, Garralda ME, Lishman WA: Diagnostic accuracy in presenile dementia. Br J Psychiatry 134:161–168, 1979.

Ross ED, Rush AJ: Diagnosis and neuroanatomical correlates of depression in brain-damaged patients. Arch Gen Psychiatry 38:1344–1353, 1981.

Roth M, Tomlinson BE, Blessed G: The relationship between quantitative measures of dementia and of degenerative changes in the cerebral grey matter of elderly subjects. Proc R Soc Med 60:254–259, 1967.

Sackeim HA, Greenberg MS, Weiman AL, et al: Hemispheric asymmetry in the expression of positive and negative emotions: Neurologic evidence. Arch Neurol 32:210–218, 1982.

Schwab JJ, Bialow M, Brown JM, et al: Diagnosing depression in medical inpatients. Ann Intern Med 67:695–707, 1967.

Sjögrent H, and Lindgren AGH: Morbus Alzheimer and Morbus Picks: A genetic, clinical, and pathoanotomical study. Acta Psychiatrica et Neurologica Suppl 82:1–152, 1952.

Smith JS, Kiloh LG: The investigation of dementia: Results in 200 consecutive admissions. Lancet 1:824–827, 1981.

Spar JE: Dementia in the aged. Psychiatr Clin North Am 5:67–86, 1982.

Storandt M, Botwinick J, Danziger WL, et al: Psychometric differentiation of mild senile dementia of the Alzheimer type. Arch Neurol 41:497–499, 1984.

Stewart MA, Drake F, Winokur G: Depression among medically ill patients. Dis Nerv Syst 26:479–485, 1965.

Taylor MA: DSM-III organic mental disorders. In Tischler G (ed): Diagnosis and Classification in Psychiatry. Cambridge, Cambridge University Press.

Terry RD, Katzman R: Senile dementia of the Alzheimer type. Ann Neurol 14:497–506, 1983.

Tomlinson BE: The pathology of dementia. In Wells CE (ed): Dementia, 2d ed. Philadelphia, FA Davis, 1977.

Tomlinson BE, Blessed G, Roth M: Observations on the brains of demented old people. J Neurol Sci 11:205–242, 1970.

Tonks CM: Mental illness in hypothyroid patients. Br J Psychiatry 110:706–710, 1964.

Torack RM: Pathologic Physiology of Dementia. Berlin, Springer-Verlag, 1978.

Veith RC, Raskind MA, Caldwell JH, et al: Cardiovascular effects of tricyclic antidepressants in depressed patients with chronic heart disease. N Engl J Med 306:954–959, 1982.

Victoratos GC, Lemmon JAR, Herzeberg L: Neurological investigation of dementia. Br J Psychiatry 130:131–133, 1977.

Watson WJ, Seiden HS: Alzheimer's disease: A current review. Can Fam Physician 30:595–599, 1984.

Wells CE: Diagnosis of dementia: A reassessment. Psychosomatics 25:183–188, 1984.

Wells CE, Duncan GW: Neurology for Psychiatrists. Philadelphia, FA Davis, 1980.

Whitlock FA, Evans LEJ: Drugs and depression. Drugs 15:53–71, 1978.

Williams KH, Goldstein G: Cognitive and affective responses to lithium in patients with organic brain syndrome. Am J Psychiatry 136:800–803, 1979.

Wilson WP, Musella L, Short MJ: The EEG in dementia. In Wells CE (ed): Dementia, 2d ed. Philadelphia, FA Davis, 1977.

Wisniewski H, Terry RD, Hirano P: Neurofibrillary pathology. J Neuropathol Exp Neurol 29:163–176, 1970.

Wolff HG, Curran D: Nature of delirium and allied states: The dysergastic reaction. Arch Neurol Psychiatry 51:378–392, 1935.

Yudofsky S, Williams D, Gorman J: Propranolol in the treatment of rage and violent behavior in patients with chronic brain syndromes. Am J Psychiatry 138:218–220, 1981.

CHAPTER 3

The Amnestic Syndrome

RAFIQ WAZIRI

DEFINITION

The amnestic syndrome is characterized by (1) moderate to severe degree of inability to remember recently observed or experienced events after the onset of brain disease (anterograde amnesia), (2) mild to moderate inability to remember minor or important and significant events or both that occurred before the onset of brain disease (retrograde amnesia), and (3) a relative absence of significant other cerebral dysfunctions, such as aphasias, apraxias, clouding of consciousness, and impairment of abstractive abilities. Originally, this term applied to the alcohol-induced Wernicke-Korsakoff syndrome.

ETIOLOGY AND PATHOGENESIS

The most common causes of the amnestic syndrome are (1) alcoholism in association with thiamine deficiency, (2) brain trauma (by concussion, crush, or penetration), (3) cerebral anoxemia, especially associated with carbon monoxide poisoning, (4) vascular occlusions leading to brain infarct, (5) viral encephalitis affecting specific brain areas, (6) tumors involving diencephalic structures, (7) seizures—especially those of the temporal lobe origin, and (8) degenerative diseases, such as Alzheimer's, when affecting predominantly the temporal lobes.

ANATOMIC PATHOLOGY

With such diverse etiologic correlates, it would be unlikely that a single, discrete locus for a brain lesion leading to the syndrome will be uncovered. In the first half of this century, brain autopsies done on alcoholics who had suffered a Wernicke's en-

cephalopathy with the resultant amnestic symptoms (Korsakoff syndrome) implicated pathology of the mammillary bodies (Brierly, 1977) either solely or in conjunction with other lesions in the diencephalic structures (fornix and the gray matter in the walls of the third ventricle). Since the 1950s, the limbic structures, especially the hippocampus and the amygdaloid nucleii, have been the subject of intense research as sites for the pathology of memory processes. The studies of Scoville and Milner (1957) on the memory defects produced in subject H.M., by bilateral removal of amygdaloid nucleii and the hippocampal formation, led to the hypothesis that the hippocampal formation was essential in the mediation of learning and short-term memory. Studies on similarly operated subjects, who developed moderate to severe defects in memory processes (Milner, 1970), appeared to confirm the original observations. Occlusion of posterior cerebral artery, which results in hippocampal damage and Korsakoff-type of memory defect (Van Buren and Borke, 1972), provided further support for this idea. The studies of Victor et al. (1971) raised serious questions about the role of the hippocampus as the main site for memory processing. The authors reported elaborately on 245 alcoholics who had suffered from the Wernicke-Korsakoff syndrome. Eighty-one of these patients died either about a week after the onset of their encephalopathy (44 patients) or an average of 3.2 years after the onset of the illness (37 patients). In 62 of these patients, brain autopsies revealed gross neuropathologic changes in various parts of the brain, the majority (74 percent) having abnormalities in the mammillary bodies. Fifty-three had microscopic brain examinations, and of these, 43 had sections through the dorsomedial thalamic nucleii and the mammillary bodies. Of these 43 subjects, 5 had no memory problems in their postencephalopathy period. The brains of these 5 subjects all showed lesions in the mammillary bodies but not in the dorsomedial thalamus. Few had extensive hippocampal lesions. Victor et al. (1971, 1989) have proposed the idea that lesions of the dorsomedial nucleii were essential in the pathogenesis of Korsakoff's syndrome. Support for a role for the dorsomedial thalamus as an important station for memory processing has come from surgical lesions placed specifically in this locus, resulting in severe memory disturbances of the Korsakoff type (Spiegel et al., 1955). Victor et al. (1971) found no consistent lesions in the limbic structures, other than in the mammillary bodies, that correlated with Korsakoff's syndrome. Recent studies on Korsakoff and non-Korsakoff amnestics by Squire et al. (1990) using magnetic resonance imaging (MRI) and computed tomographic (CT) scan techniques have shown definitive evidence that in the alcohol-induced (Korsakoff) amnestics there is a virtual absence of mammillary bodies and loss in thalamic tissue density, while the non-Korsakoff amnestics have mainly damage in the hippocampal formation.

If the diencephalic dorsomedial nucleus of the thalamus is the site for memory processing, then what is the explanation for the severe recent memory and learning deficits that ensue after surgical removal of the hippocampal formation in humans? Horel (1978), in a careful review of the pathologic neuroanatomy associated with memory disturbances, considered neither the limbic system nor the dorsomedial nucleus of the thalamus as structures that mediate short-term memory and learning. He postulated that the anterior portion of the inferior temporal gyri sending fibers by way of the temporal stem to the dorsomedial nucleii are involved in short-term memory and learning. In monkeys, where selective lesions of the hippocampal formation are easily accomplished without the destruction of the temporal stem, no memory deficits (for certain tasks) are noted when this site is removed. The only defects noted postoperatively are disturbances of spatial orientation. Similarly, lesions of the mammillary bodies or the fornices have led to no defects in learning or memory in animals. Fibers from the inferior temporal cortex traverse through the temporal stem to end up partially in the dorsomedial nucleus (pars magnocellularis); hippocampectomy in humans destroys the temporal stem, severing the input from the inferior temporal cortex to the diencephalic structures. In animals, lesions of the thalamus that involve the magnocellular part of the dorsomedial nucleus result in learning deficits. In monkeys with cooling probes placed in the temporal lobes, the hippocampal formation, and the amygdaloid nucleii, learning and memory show severe decrements only when the anterior part of the inferior temporal gyrus or the fibers emanating from this area are cooled to 6°C. These functions return to normal levels of performance when the temperature is raised back to normal (Horel and Pytko, 1982). Zola-Morgan and Squire (1984) studied monkeys with lesions either in the temporal stem or conjointly in the hippocampus–amygdaloid complex. They showed that in learning tasks modeled on human memory for reward–nonreward discrimination, only lesions of the conjoint hippocampus–amygdaloid complex produce memory deficits; lesions in the temporal stem were associated with defects of visual pattern discrimination. It appears that lesions at different sites in the brain lead to different types of memory disturbance. As yet, evidence that pathology of the inferior temporal gyrus by itself can cause memory disturbances in humans is scanty. Evidence that in humans damage to the inferior temporal cortices and the basal forebrain structures (Damasio et al., 1985) produces amnestic symptoms provides support for a role of these structures in the mediation of memory processes. Also, the observations of Penfield and Jasper (1954) that electrical stimulations of the cortex of the temporal lobe evokes memories and those of Bickford et al. (1958) that stimulation of white matter of the middle temporal gyrus produces amnesia are of interest and provide further support for the importance of the temporal lobe and its cortex in memory mechanisms. Thus the controversy as to what is the essential locus of memory pathology in the brain remains unresolved. Figure 3-1 is a coronal section of the brain in which pathologic anatomy of several structures (their names in capital letters) have been implicated with the amnestic syndrome.

Other neuropathologic conditions associated with memory disturbances of the Korsakoff type in the presence or absence of various degrees of cognitive dysfunction also have been associated mostly with lesions of the limbic or diencephalic structures. Tumors most commonly produce amnestic symptoms when they are located in the walls or floor of the third ventricle. Craniopharyngiomas and cysts in the third ventricle that exert pressure on dorsomedial nucleii and the hypothalamus produce anterograde amnesia, as well as retrograde amnesia and confabulation in the presence of relatively intact cognitive functions.

Head trauma, resulting in either negative or positive acceleration of the brain and consequent posttraumatic amnesia, probably affects the axial structures of the brain more than it affects the outer structures. The pathology may be due to localized hemorrhage, edema, or actual shearing of connecting fibers important in the mediation of memory. In the majority of cases, posttraumatic amnesias are not permanent, and various degrees of restitution of functions occur in the months or years after the trauma. Generally, with the passage of time the extent of retrograde amnesia shrinks more quickly than that of the anterograde amnesia (Russell, 1971; Whitty and Zangwill, 1977).

Occlusion of posterior cerebral arteries, which supply the hippocampi, part of globus pallidus, and

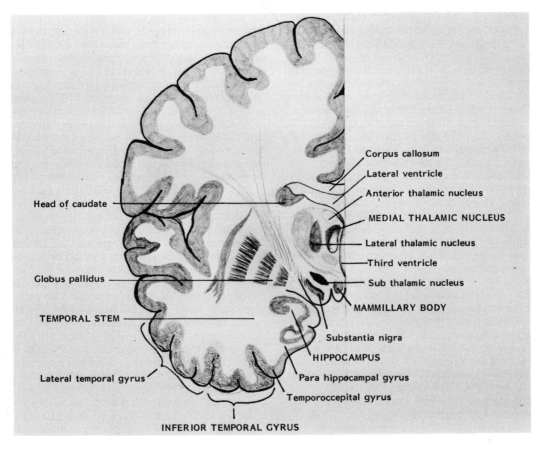

Head of caudate

Corpus callosum

Lateral ventricle

Anterior thalamic nucleus

MEDIAL THALAMIC NUCLEUS

Lateral thalamic nucleus

Third ventricle

Globus pallidus

Sub thalamic nucleus

MAMMILLARY BODY

TEMPORAL STEM

Substantia nigra

HIPPOCAMPUS

Lateral temporal gyrus

Para hippocampal gyrus

Temporoccepital gyrus

INFERIOR TEMPORAL GYRUS

FIGURE 3-1   *Coronal section passing through the mammillary bodies. Capital letters are used for structures putatively important in mediating memory processes.*

the area through which temporal lobe fibers traverse to midline structures, can produce an amnesia similar to that of Korsakoff's syndrome. Viral encephalitis resulting in variable degrees of Korsakoff's syndrome is sometimes associated with neuropathology in the limbic and diencephalic structures (Glaser and Pincus, 1969).

In the initial stages of Alzheimer's disease, when the temporal lobes are more affected, amnesia and learning problems are the salient features. This occurs before the pathology becomes extensive and other cognitive dysfunctions become predominant. In these cases, the entorhinal cortices of temporal lobes, in addition to the hippocampal formation, are the main sites of degeneration (Van Hoesen et al., 1987). Temporal lobe seizures and electroconvulsive treatment (ECT) produce transient amnesias of both the retrograde and the anterograde type. In the first instance, in addition to a pathophysiology of temporal lobes, resulting in localized seizure activity, there may be structural pathology. In the case of ECT, only a pathophysiologic state

exists, which affects not only the temporal lobes locally but also the whole nervous system in a global fashion.

CLINICAL PICTURE

Chronic alcohol intoxication associated with thiamine deficiency manifesting as an acute confusional state (Wernicke's encephalopathy) is accompanied by (1) ocular dysfunction and nystagmus, paralysis of lateral and conjugate gaze with strabismus and diplopia, (2) various degrees of cerebellar dysfunction with wide-based stance and short-stepped gait, and (3) polyneuropathy with disturbance of sensory and motor function. The confusional state is characterized by disturbances of awareness, attention, and motivation; disorientation to time, place, and person; and inability to recall recent or remote occurrences. Before the advent of thiamine therapy, a majority of these patients died within 10 days of the onset of symptoms. Brain autopsies in these cases showed lesions in the cerebellum, the dorsal motor nucleii, the paraventricular structures of the thalamus, and the hypothalamus. Lesions of the mammillary bodies were quite severe (Victor et al., 1971). Questions have arisen as to what brings about this pathology in the brain. Severe thiamine deficiency, as seen in Wernicke's encephalopathy, does lead to diencephalic lesions in monkeys without being associated with alcohol intoxication. Parkin et al. (1991) have described a case of Wernicke-Korsakoff amnesia in a patient who had been fed with parenteral fluids without thiamine for about a month. However, chronic alcoholics not having suffered overt Wernicke's encephalopathy end up having memory disturbances that are intermediate between those of normals and those of the Korsakoff's patients (Butters and Cermak, 1980). Thus it would appear that the concomitant deficiency of thiamine and the toxic levels of alcohol may be synergistic in the pathogenesis of the amnestic syndrome.

Those who survive the acute period of the Wernicke's encephalopathy end up with memory problems of various degrees and duration. The description of amnesia with polyneuritis in alcoholics (and some nonalcoholics) by Korsakoff (1889) still is unsurpassed. The memory difficulties are manifested by a decreased or lack of ability to learn and recall new information for more than a few minutes in the post-illness period. Also, there is difficulty in recalling experiences and events that have occurred before the onset of the illness.

In anterograde amnesia, immediate or instantaneous (as tested by recall within several seconds) memory may be relatively intact, indicating that registration of perceptions is fairly normal. Recent memory, dating back from a few minutes or hours to weeks, is moderately or severely deficient. This is sometimes referred to as "rapid forgetting." A patient may not remember that an hour earlier he had undergone a painful lumbar puncture or that he had eaten breakfast or shaken hands with a doctor, whom he greets again as if he has seen him for the first time. He may be repeatedly shown the way to his house or room and yet cannot find his way back where he came from or loses his way in the streets or the hospital corridors. This disorientation to place and person extends to time and date. The patient may be reading the newspaper with apparent interest and attention and a few minutes later not remember what he had read and start reading the same item again with interest. The patient may remember his name and recognize his close relatives if he lives with them but may not know what their occupation is, how many children they have, or when he last saw them. His memory may show less deficiency if he is given cues about what he has learned recently, i.e., he shows "responsiveness to recognition probes." Such patients may or may not have insight into their memory defects. Some, being aware of their problems, complain about their inability to remember and are upset about it. Others are partially aware and mostly deny any disability, while still others are totally unaware and express puzzlement when confronted with evidence for their memory deficits. Insight into illness generally diminishes as the postillness period of amnesia is prolonged. However, despite the severity of amnesia, patients are still able to learn with frequent practice, even under limited conditions, certain specified tasks (Piercy, 1977; Hirst, 1982). They are better at learning skills than learning facts. Memories of events or experiences antecedent to the illness are generally better preserved than those of recent events or experiences.

The nearer retrograde amnesia is temporally to the illness, the severer it is. Habitual functions, such as speech, reading, writing, getting dressed, or riding a bicycle, that were learned in childhood and adolescence remain intact. Memory for remote events may be fairly good but may show various degrees of disorganization in the temporal and spatial context. A patient may remember that the four presidents before Nixon were Johnson, Kennedy, Eisenhower, and Truman, but he might not remember the temporal order in which they occupied the office. He may remember that there were two wars after World War II but might say that the war in Korea came after the war in Vietnam, or he may think that General McArthur was in the war in Vietnam. He may remember that his children were married but may not remember their spouses' names or their wedding dates. He may know the names of the states bordering his own state but may make mistakes in their geographic relationships to one another. Significant and dramatic events in his life many years before the onset of the illness may be remembered but with embellishment from other events in the life of the patient. When the patient recounts these events, there is a fictional and, at times, fantastic tinge to the story.

Patients with severe or moderate anterograde amnesia and with partial or complete loss of insight, when asked questions about their recent activities or experiences, will not state that they cannot remember but will embark on long, circumlocutory stories that are not factual. The stories may contain elements of actual events experienced by the patient in the past. This confabulatory tendency is manifested generally without any element of doubt; when confronted with the facts, the patient may either express puzzlement, show anger, or accuse the interviewer of trying to confuse or persecute him. It is this lack of insight that gives such patients the designation of having a "psychosis." Confabulations also can be prompted in patients by asking them leading questions. The examiner may ask the patient who has been in the hospital for weeks, "Didn't I see you in the park yesterday?" The patient could respond, "Sure, wasn't it a beautiful day? Oh, the kids flying kites and playing with their Frisbees! My friend Johnny and I were playing with our dog, Snapper, and he was such a card . . . '' and so on. While telling this story, the patient may express facial emotions appropriate to the content of what he is recounting. It is quite likely that this fictitious presentation is made up from fragments of a repository of old memories or events that may have been experienced by the patient.

The following case is an example of the amnesic syndrome:

The patient is a 37-year-old married white male house painter who had abused alcohol since his teenage years. In the past 4 to 5 years he had shown signs of alcohol addiction and had suffered twice from withdrawal (delirium tremens). About 3 months before his hospitalization, while drinking heavily for weeks, he had undergone a period of confusion, hallucinations, inability to walk without holding onto objects and had complained of seeing double and having visions. He had been admitted to a local hospital for about 3 weeks, treated with vitamins, enriched diet, benzodiazepines, and thioridazine. When he went home, his wife noted that he did not know his way around the house, did not remember names, and could not recognize some of his friends and relatives. An hour after having been served breakfast, he would ask if he were going to have breakfast soon. He had no memory of the events that led to his hospitalization or of his hospital stay. He had no memory about his job. Two or 3 weeks after discharge from the local hospital, he was able to find his way around the house and was able to remember the names of his children but could not remember their ages or birthdays. Sometimes he would misidentify one of his children with another. At times his memory would be slightly better than at other times. Two weeks before admission he and his children had gone to the park, which was a few blocks from his house. While the children were playing, he walked away and then could not find his way to them or to his house. Two hours later he was found many blocks away from the park and had no memory of where he had been. He was readmitted to the hospital. In the hospital he was noted to appear older than his stated age. He was casually dressed, pleasant, and sociable. He was not oriented to time, place, or person. He had no insight as to why he was in the hospital. He knew the town from which he had come but could not remember the address of his house. His memory for recent events was practically nil. His memory of events before the onset of his illness was severely diminished for up to 3 to 4 years antecedent to the illness. He could not remember what he had done as a house painter, where he had lived, and what kinds of cars he had driven. His memory for remote events was patchy; e.g., he knew the year of his marriage but did not remember what church he was married in. When asked how was it that he could not remember the name of the church, he answered, ''Oh, I am not interested in churches. Why don't you go and find out from the records?''

In the hospital he continued to be disoriented and was not able to find his bed or the bathroom unassisted. He could not retain the names of nursing staff, medical students, or doctors for more than a few minutes. When the doctor who had introduced himself to the patient and had shaken hands with him an hour earlier saw him and asked him if he had known the doctor before, he would say, ''Sure, you are Dr. Johnson, who mended my broken knee after the car accident.'' (His wife reported that indeed about 12 years ago he had had a car accident and a Dr. Johnson had taken care of him.) Every time the doctor saw the patient, the patient would behave as if he had seen the doctor for the first time in his life. A few days after admission, this conversation took place between the doctor and the patient:

Doctor (D): Hi, Mr. McD. Do you remember me?
Patient (P): Sure, you are Dr. Barry. [Not the correct name.]
D: Where did we meet?
P: You are David's brother, aren't you? And David is a good friend of mine.
D: How are you feeling today?
P: Oh, fine . . .
D: Do you have any memory problems?
P: No.
D: Can you tell me what you did since you woke up this morning?
P: [Hesitates for several seconds] Sure. I woke up, took a good shower, and then had breakfast.
D: What did you have for breakfast?
P: Oh, I had two eggs sunny side up, two pancakes with bacon, a glass of orange juice, and a cup of coffee. [Actually, he had a boiled egg, cereal with milk, orange juice, and coffee.]
D: What did you do after breakfast?
P: Oh, I was here and there.
D: Did you go out of here?
P: Yep.
D: Did you drive a car?
P: Yep.
D: Can you tell me where you went?
P: [He hesitates, as if searching his memory.] Sure. My friend Bill and I got into the car and were driving around, when we came to a crossing. The light was still yellow when we tried to cross, but sure as heck, here comes a Cadillac driven by a dame with a flowered hat on top of her head, bearing down on us as if she owned the damn street. Before you know it, her car has taken off half the front of our car. A few minutes later there are policemen and they take us to the hospital, where they take care of my broken knee and my friend's broken nose and shoulder. Then we end up in front of the judge, who gives me a lecture on how to drive my car. The judge is actually the same one who sent one of my friends to jail for twenty years. Now, jails weren't for sissies and perverts. A lot of good, hardworking people ended up there because they wanted to be unionized . . . [The wife later corroborated part of the story of the car accident at the crossing and the court appearance about 12 years ago.]
D: Then how did you get here?
P: Why, on my own steam.
D: What would you say if I told you that in the past few days you have never left the hospital?
P: [Looking puzzled] Then I won't believe you.

After 3 weeks of hospitalization, the patient's condition remained essentially unchanged, although he was able to recognize some of the staff better than others and was able to find his way in the ward. He lived as if in a perpetual present time, where everything around him was novel and worthy of interest. If in the past hour he had suffered frustrations and had burst out in tears, he had no memory of them and behaved as if nothing was wrong and nothing was bothering him.

This case is illustrative of a severe amnestic syndrome. The amnesia in patients who have suffered from the Wernicke-Korsakoff illness is graded from severe to mild. The more severe the amnesia, the greater is the probability that other cognitive functions also will be disturbed to some degree.

The amnestic syndromes resulting from other pathogenetic causes also will manifest themselves with various degrees of intensity and associations with other cognitive dysfunctions.

After the acute state of Wernicke's alcoholic encephalopathy has subsided with vigorous vitamin therapy, progressive improvement in midbrain, cerebral, and cerebellar dysfunctions occurs in a period ranging from a few hours to several weeks in most cases. Neurologic signs, such as ophthalmoplegia, disequilibrium, and nystagmus, disappear within a few weeks. The delirious–confusional state lasts somewhat longer and may take a few months to clear. When the confusional state has cleared up, the signs of amnestic syndrome become evident in more than 80 percent of patients who have survived the acute state. Of these subjects, about 50 percent improve completely or significantly within the next year, while the other 50 percent have minor or no improvement in their amnestic syndrome (Victor et al., 1971). The extent of residual memory deficits depends on the extent of structural changes in the brain brought about by thiamine deficiency in association with other nutritional deficiencies that result when alcohol is chronically abused.

The clinical picture of amnesia secondary to trauma differs in accordance with the degree and site of damage. A concussive episode that results in a short- or long-term period of unconsciousness also may result in anterograde and retrograde amnesia of various intensities. Confabulation may not be as frequent, and the rate of recovery from the amnesia may be faster than what is observed in Korsakoff's psychosis (Russell, 1971). Carbon monoxide poisoning and other hypoxic states produce amnesias that are rarely pure, since other than diencephalic structures may be involved and other cognitive dysfunctions are also manifest. These observations are true also of amnesias secondary to encephalitis. Tumors in the region of the third ventricle tend to produce a purer form of the amnestic syndrome. In these cases, the onset of the illness is gradual and the removal of tumor leads to a quicker amelioration of the memory problems than observed with the Wernicke's-Korsakoff syndrome.

Amnesias caused by temporal lobe seizures and ECTs manifest themselves during the ictal and postictal periods, lasting for a few minutes to a few hours or several days. In these cases, too, other cognitive functions may be impaired to a certain extent, although for a shorter time than the memory functions. Occasionally, patients who have received ECT have relatively extensive retrograde amnesias and tend to have less problem with anterograde amnesia.

LABORATORY FINDINGS

In the last decade, significant advances have been made in our ability to use correlative neuromorphologic techniques such as CT scans and MRI with a variety of sophisticated neuropsychological tests. It has become evident that although amnestic symptoms may resemble each other in cases where there are disparate neuropathologic findings, there are certain brain structures that tend to be more associated with one type of amnesia than with another (e.g., Squire et al., 1990). These advances are helping us increasingly with the differential diagnosis of the amnestic syndrome. Clinical examination and neuropsychological testing are at present the mainstays of diagnosis.

DIFFERENTIAL DIAGNOSIS

Amnesias of the psychogenic type (Ganser's syndrome, fugue states, conversion reactions, malingering, multiple personality) are generally differentiated from organic amnesias by their relationship to traumatic and stressful situations, by their being either of the purely retrograde or purely anterograde type, and by their rather abrupt onset after a traumatic psychological experience occasionally associated with mild head trauma. In Ganser's syndrome, memory defects are manifested by the subject, who in response to questions will give approximate answers; for example, a man age 26 who is in prison, whose wife's name is Mary, and who has three children (two sons and one daughter) will say that he is 25 years old, that his wife's name is Miriam, and that he has four children (one son, three daughters). In fugue states, the individual has no memory of his past; he maintains that he does not remember his name, family, address, job, or age. When confronted with evidence about these aspects of his past life, he appears puzzled and confused. He is able to assume and remember a new name; his recent memory is generally intact. He learns new information and retains it normally. The fugue state is frequently due to an untenable situation facing the patient, and it seems to provide him with an escape mechanism by which he "wanders away" from unpleasant circumstances. Fugue states of shorter duration are known to occur as a postictal complication of temporal lobe epilepsy. Fugue states are most often observed in soldiers facing battles or in those who have been defeated or who have suffered shell shock. Dysfunctions of memory as a conversion reaction are akin to the disturbances of motor or sensory functions in hysterical subjects. In malingering, where memory losses are simulated, these losses are patchy and at times exaggerated. Such subjects would claim that they cannot read or write because they have forgotten how to. Malingering in such cases is generally associated with circumstances in which the subject gains financially or avoids punishment. Subjects with multiple personalities, while assuming a new personality, may say that they do not remember what the "other" person has said or done. Whereas in fugue state the subject loses his past identity, in the case of multiple personality the subject gains new identity and memories. The subject may have some inkling into the identity of the other person or persons; however, he seems to be somewhat forgetful of what the others have done. The memory for the others may become clearer with hypnosis or suggestion.

TREATMENT

The brain lesions that produce the amnestic syndrome are various; hence treatment would include, initially, the removal, if possible, of the causative process, be it vitamin deficiency and alcoholism or a growing tumor exerting pressure on the paraventricular structures. The long-term treatment of patients with amnestic syndrome is mostly ameliorative rather than curative. Once brain structures have been damaged and their functions impaired, it is unlikely that complete restitution of function will occur, especially in the older individual. Nevertheless, with passage of time, slow progress in many cases has been observed. If no improvement of memory function has occurred within the first year or two with memory-enhancing psychological maneuvers, it is unlikely that significant further progress in memory functions will ensue. Repetition of tasks in a fairly uniform and relaxed environment, avoidance of frustrating experiences, and provision of appropriate rewards and incentives as psychological aids may help the patient. Drugs to enhance memory, such as cholinergics, magnesium pemoline, and, more recently, neuropeptides, have not been tested rigorously enough to be used routinely in patients with the amnestic syndrome. The memory-enhancing status of these drugs at this time is still equivocal at best.

REFERENCES

Bickford RG, Mulder DW, Dodge HW, et al: Changes in memory function produced by electrical stimulations of the temporal lobe in man. Res Publ Assoc Res Nerv Ment Dis 36:227–243, 1958.

Brierly JB: Neuropathology of amnestic states. In Whitty CWM, Zangwill OL (eds): Amnesia. London, Butterworth, 1977, pp 199–223.

Butters N, Cermak LS: Alcoholic Korsakoff's Syndrome: An Information-Processing Approach to Amnesia. New York, Academic Press, 1980.

Damasio AR, Eslinger P, Damasio H, Van Hoesen GW, et al: Multimodal amnestic syndrome following bilateral temporal and basal forebrain damage. Arch Neurol 42:252–259, 1985.

Glaser GH, Pincus JH: Limbic encephalitis. J Nerv Ment Dis 149:59–66, 1969.

*Hirst W: The amnesic syndrome: Descriptions and explanations. Psychol Bull 91:435–460, 1982.

*Horel JA: The neuroanatomy of amnesia. A critique of the hippocampal memory hypothesis. Brain 101:403–445, 1978.

Horel JA, Pytko DE: Behavioral effects of local cooling in temporal lobe of monkey. J Neurophysiol 47:11–22, 1982.

*Korsakoff SS: Psychic disorders in conjunction with peripheral neuritis (1889). Trans by M. Victor, PI Yakovlev. Neurology 5:394–406, 1955.

*Milner B: Memory and the medial temporal regions of the brain. In Pribram KH, Broadbent DE (eds): Biology of Memory. New York, Academic Press, 1970, pp 29–50.

Parkin AJ, Blunden J, Reece JE, Hunkin MN: Wernicke-Korsakoff syndrome of nonalcoholic origin. Brain Cogn 15:69–82, 1991.

Penfield W, Jasper HH: Epilepsy and the Functional Anatomy of the Human Brain. Boston, Little, Brown, 1954.

Piercy MF: Experimental studies of the organic amnesic syndrome. In Whitty CWM, Zangwill OL (eds): Amnesia. London, Butterworth, 1977, pp 1–51.

Russell WR: The Traumatic Amnesias. Oxford, Oxford University Press, 1971.

Scoville WB, Milner B: Loss of recent memory after bilateral hippocampal lesions. J Neurol Neurosurg Psychiatry 20:11–21, 1957.

Spiegel EA, Wycis HT, Orchinik LW, Freed H: The thalamus and temporal orientation. Science 121:770–772, 1955.

Squire LR, Amaral DG, Press GS: Magnetic resonance imaging of the hippocampal formation and mammillary nuclei distinguish medial temporal lobe and diencephalic amnesia. J Neurosci 10:3106–3117, 1990.

Van Buren JM, Borke RC: The medial temporal substratum of memory: Anatomical study in three individuals. Brain 95:599–632, 1972.

Van Hoeson GW, Damasio AR: Neural correlates of the cognitive impairment of Alzheimer's disease. In Mountcastle VB, Plum F (eds): The Handbook of Physiology: Higher Functions of the Nervous System. Bethesda, MD, American Physiological Society, 1987, pp 871–989.

*Victor M, Adams RD, Collins GH: The Wernicke-Korsakoff Syndrome. Philadelphia, FA Davis, 1971.

Victor M, Adams RO, Collins GH: The Wernicke-Korsakoff Syndrome and Related Neurological Disorders due to Alcoholism and Malnutrition, 2d ed. Philadelphia, FA Davis, 1989.

Whitty CWM, Zangwill OL: Traumatic amnesia. In Whitty CWM, Zangwill OL (eds): Amnesia. London, Butterworth, 1977, pp 118–135.

Zola-Morgan S, Squire LR: Preserved learning in monkeys with medical temporal lesions: Sparing of motor and cognitive skills. J Neurosci 4:1072–1085, 1984.

*References with asterisks are important in terms of understanding the description, history, neuropathology, and neuropsychology of the amnestic syndrome.

CHAPTER 4

Bipolar Illness

PAULA J. CLAYTON

The affective disorders are disorders of mood. In the past, numerous terms, usually dichotomous, have been used to distinguish these disorders. One major separation made on the basis of genetic and clinical differences that seemed viable was the separation into unipolar disorder and bipolar mood disorders. *Unipolar affective disorder* refers to patients who have depression only. *Bipolar affective disorder* refers to patients who have episodes of both mania and depression or episodes of mania only.

Mania is derived from a Greek word meaning "to be mad." Hippocrates is credited with introducing psychiatric diagnoses into medical nomenclature. Two of the six diagnoses that he proposed were mania and melancholia. In his classification, *mania* referred to acute mental disorders without fever, and *melancholia* referred to a wide variety of chronic mental illnesses. In the first century, Aretaeus noted that depression and excitement often alternated in the same person and therefore might represent different aspects of the same illness. Although it is difficult to tell from the classification systems how pervasive this idea of cycling became in the centuries thereafter, the term *mania* remained prominent in all. For hundreds of years, the diagnosis of mania seemed to have been used primarily for an illness with an acute onset and with a mood of merriment or rage or fury (Menninger et al., 1977).

In 1686, Bonet used the term *maniacomelancholicus* to characterize a group of patients. In the 1850s, Falret adopted the term *circular insanity*, and Baillarger used *double-form insanity* for similar patients (Sedler, 1983). In 1874, Kahlbaum referred to patients with *cyclothymia*. Kraepelin (1921) drew on and synthesized the various approaches to nosology bequeathed to him from the preceding centuries. Beginning in 1883, he published nine editions of his textbook on psychiatry, and it was he who sepa-rated dementia praecox from manic-depressive illness using clinical descriptions and the natural history of the illnesses.

If we could assume that names are given to illnesses in an attempt to organize clinical observations, then it must be said, from the long history of the term *mania*, that the recognition of mania and the occurrence of mania were apparent to clinicians throughout history.

Schou (1927) maintained that Lange (1895) first suggested the separation of unipolar from bipolar illness. He and coworkers (Pederson et al., 1947) noted that "periodical depression has no manic phases and differs from manic-depressive psychoses with regard to heredity as well as distribution of somatic types and prognosis." They added that manic-depressive patients were more likely chronic and disabled in contradistinction to periodic depressives, who were more likely to be discharged and recovered. Leonhard (1957), Perris (1966), and Angst (1966) solidified this point of view. The first American researchers to place emphasis on this distinction were Winokur et al. (1969). Although bipolar illness was separated from unipolar illness on the basis of differences in age of onset, course, family history, and response to treatment, this separation may not, in the end, prove valid. This author believes that data are beginning to accumulate that suggest, as Kraepelin (1921) did, that the two illnesses may be different forms of the same disorder, with bipolar illness being a more severe, earlier-onset form than *recurrent* unipolar illness.

DEFINITION

Manic-depressive disease, or *manic-depressive illness*, is the old term in the *Diagnostic and Statistical Manual of Mental Disorders*, revised third edition (DSM-IIIR), for bipolar affective disorder, which includes patients with mania and depression or mania only. Each episode is classified as mixed, manic, or depressed. DSM-IIIR lists the following symptoms for a diagnosis of mania: a distinct elevated, expansive, or irritable mood and three of the following symptoms (four if the mood is only irritable): (1) inflated self-esteem or grandiosity, (2) decreased need for sleep, (3) more talkative than usual or pressure to keep talking, (4) flight of ideas or subjective experience that thoughts are racing, (5) distractibility, (6) increase in goal-directed activity or psychomotor retardation, and (7) excessive involvement in pleasurable activities which have a high potential for painful consequences, plus marked social impairment and no organic factor to initiate the disturbance, except somatic antidepressant treatment. DSM-IIIR lists the same symptoms for a diagnosis of hypomanic syndrome, absent marked social impairment. An episode requires no duration of symptoms and can be characterized with or without psychotic features. The psychotic features can be further characterized as either mood-congruent, with delusions or hallucinations that are consistent with inflated worth, power, and knowledge, or mood-incongruent, with delusions and hallucinations that are not consistent with this elevated mood, such as persecutory delusions, thought insertion or delusions of being controlled, and catatonic symptoms, such as stupor, mutism, negativism, and posturing. The depressive episode also has a mood change, distinct features, and a 2-week duration. These characteristics are outlined in Chapter 5. For either diagnosis, there is no requirement of disability or hospitalization.

DSM-IV is undecided as to where to place bipolar II disorder, either as a new category in the bipolar spectrum or as another specifier of course in recurrent major depressive disorder. Despite where it will be placed, the definition is solid. Bipolar II illness requires that the individual have a history of one or more episodes of major depressive disorder and hypomanic episodes that do not meet the criteria for mania in impairment or severity. The unreliability of the retrospective determination of the occurrence of hypomania makes this diagnosis confusing. Patients with personality disorders endorse brief previous hypomanic symptoms, and patients with chronic depression sometimes confuse hypomania with euthymia. Course and family history do not help to clarify the disorder. Coryell et al. (1984) suggested that bipolar II illness is seen in families of bipolar and unipolar depressive probands. There is also a set of bipolar II patients who breed true within families. Rice et al. (1986) reported that all bipolar II probands come from families with bipolar I or bipolar II members. The disorder is heterogeneous and needs to be further delineated before it can qualify as a valid diagnosis. Unipolar and bipolar II patients with family histories of bipolar I disorder probably should be considered part of the bipolar I spectrum.

ETIOLOGY

At present, it is evident that genetic factors play a significant role in the etiology of bipolar affective disorder. There are no other data as strong as those in the genetic area, although they are currently of limited predictive value. With new genetic techniques, it seems likely that the entire human genome will be mapped. With this map and DNA probes for linkage markers, transmission and linkage to specific chromosomal markers will be possible (see Chap. 29).

In addition to the genetic factors, biochemical, neuroendocrine, neurophysiologic, and sleep abnormalities have been reported, but whether these are specific to bipolar affective disorder or overlap with recurrent unipolar disorder findings is questionable. Besides the confusion of always including some not-yet-identified bipolar patients in unipolar studies (at least 10 percent), one must always consider if the abnormalities described in any particular report occurred during a unipolar or bipolar depression, during a mania, pure or mixed, or during a well state and under what conditions (e.g., on lithium maintenance). Because there are few unequivocal findings, a limited discussion of these issues, as well as of animal models or other disease models that mimic mania, follows.

Genetics

There is no doubt that bipolar affective disorder is familial; that is, it runs in families, with close relatives being more likely to be affected than unrelated subjects. Three types of studies contribute to the extent of the genetic knowledge of this illness: (1) family studies of patients with affective disorder, (2) adoption studies, and (3) twin studies.

FAMILY STUDIES

Family studies were originally anecdotal. Falret's 1854 article on circular insanity (Sedler, 1983) noted that by interviewing the parents of patients, he obtained compelling evidence as to the hereditary disposition in the illness. He concluded that circular insanity was very heritable. He could not decide, however, whether it was more heritable than any other type of mental illness, although he was inclined to think so.

Based on studies by Angst and Perris and his own work, Winokur (1978) summarized the literature and reported that in bioplar patients, 52 percent could be expected to have a parent with an affective disorder, 54 percent could be expected to have two generations of members affected, and 63 percent could be expected to have an affective illness in the parents or an extended family member. He reported the incidence of mania in the first-degree relatives as between 4 and 10 percent. Thus, even in bipolar patients, the majority of affected relatives have unipolar depression.

Gershon et al. (1982) looked at schizoaffective, bipolar I, bipolar II, and unipolar patients and normal controls. The authors concluded that the most common disorder in the relatives of all probands was unipolar affective disorder and that since there was bipolar illness in the relatives of all ill probands, there was probably genetic overlap between types. In the bipolar probands, the morbid risk in parents and offspring for schizoaffective disorder was 1.2 percent; for bipolar affective disorder, 9.2 percent; and for unipolar disorder, 12.3 percent. Similar figures in siblings were 0.8 percent for schizoaffective disorder, 6.9 percent for bipolar affective disorder, and 18.1 percent for unipolar disorder. The normal individuals had little illness except unipolar affective disorder (5.7 percent in siblings, parents, and children). The authors also looked at how the number of affected parents related to illness in the adult children. To do this, they combined the schizoaffective, bipolar I and II, and unipolar patients. If one parent was ill, the risk of having an ill child was 27 percent, compared with 57 percent if both parents were ill. Among the siblings of probands, the risk was 24 percent if no parents were ill and 32 percent if one parent was ill (not significantly different). They found no significant differences in illness in the relatives when the probands and controls were separated by sex and no increase in alcoholism, drug abuse, or sociopathy in the relatives of patients with these affective disorders as compared with controls. Winokur et al. (1969) noted the occurrence of compulsive gambling in the fathers and brothers of some bipolar patients, but without control rates, they could not comment further.

Goodwin and Jamison (1990) summarized all family studies to date. Although prevalence rates varied, it was still clear that unipolar depression was the most frequent illness in relatives of bipolar probands, usually comparable with its frequency in relatives of unipolar probands, and bipolar disorder appeared more frequently in relatives of unipolar probands than in the controls gathered simultaneously. The conclusion must be that embedded in unipolar disorder are "bipolar-like" or silent bipolar patients. Akiskal et al. (1989) suggested using cyclothymic and hyperthymic temperament in families as a marker for the bipolar diathesis. Using their criteria, they concluded one of every three primary depressives belongs to the bipolar spectrum (Cassano et al., 1989). Blacker and Tsuang (1992) also recommended ways to identify in family members potential bipolars nested in unipolar groups and how to use this information in linkage analysis.

If the confusion over how to clarify probands and relatives with bipolar II disorder is added, it is little wonder that segregation studies and linkage analysis have yielded no reproducible results. This author recommends that psychotic depressives, schizoaffective depressives with previous hypomania, and treated postpartum depressives could

be considered "silent bipolars." Other groups who probably are bipolar are uncomplicated treated depressives under 20 years of age and those who have a somatic therapy–induced mania (antidepressant drugs, sleep deprivation, light treatment, ECT). All these cross-sectionally diagnosed "unipolar" patients should be considered bipolar.

Studies of *children* (age varies from 6 to 17 years) of bipolar parents have yielded conflicting results. Even the best studies that included children of bipolars and controls assessed blindly and with strict criteria do not lend themselves to clear interpretation, although in the most negative study (Gershon et al., 1985), out of 76 children, there were 3 with mania or hypomania (by National Institute of Mental Health criteria), and all were from bipolar families. A recent nonblind controlled longitudinal study of high-risk children (Hammen et al., 1990) reported that offspring of bipolar mothers had higher rates of psychiatric disorders than children of mothers with chronic medical illnesses or normal mothers but somewhat less than children of unipolar mothers. Children of bipolar mothers had surprisingly high rates of anxiety disorders.

As with the studies of children, studies of assortative mating have produced variable results. Here, too, blind structured assessment of spouses of bipolar patients and controls is essential. Also, because bipolar studies probably will have equal numbers of male and female spouses and affective disorder rates are always higher in women, sex of spouses must be controlled for. Merikangas (1982) summarized the literature and concluded that there probably was assortative mating in affective disorder (not separated by polarity) but that the magnitude of the problem was unknown. Later, Merikangas et al. (1983) indicated that when assortative mating occurred, it predicted a poorer outcome at follow-up. Waters et al. (1983) confirmed an increased prevalence of affective disorders in spouses of bipolar patients, although their interpretation of results was unduly guarded.

ADOPTION STUDIES

There is only one study of adoptees with bipolar illness. Mendlewicz and Rainer (1977) reported that 31 percent of biologic parents and 12 percent of adopted parents of hospitalized bipolar adoptees had an affective disorder. This percentage in biologic parents was comparable with the risk they reported in parents of nonadopted bipolar patients. There are studies of unipolar adoptees and of completed suicide in adoptees that are not specific to bipolar illness.

TWIN STUDIES

Nurnberger and Gershon (1982) summarized the twin studies on affective disorders, although not by polarity. The best study that dealt with bipolar illness was that of Bertelsen et al. (1977), who reported that starting with a bipolar twin, the concordance for 55 pairs of monozygotic twins was 0.67 and for 52 pairs of dizygotic twins was 0.20. Concordance was higher in bipolar than in unipolar monozygotic twins. As an extension of that study, Fischer (1980) dealt in greater detail with bipolar illness in 28 pairs of monozygotic and 35 pairs of dizygotic twins. When the monozygotic twins were looked at for concordance for affective psychosis only, the concordance was 75 percent for monozygotic twins compared with 20 percent for dizygotic twins. However, when other psychosis, severe affective personality disorder, or completed suicide was added as "illness," the concordance for monozygotic twins rose to 96 percent and for dizygotic twins to 49 percent. There was thus only one pair of monozygotic twins who were discordant. Fischer also discussed the issue of discordance in monozygotic twins with one being bipolar and the other being schizophrenic. There were only two pairs from two studies that reported such twins, and Fischer reported these case histories in detail.

To summarize, bipolar affective disorder is a genetic illness. The extent of assortative mating and the extent of illness in children are unclear. Genetic analyses will probably not be productive until we decide how to identify "silent bipolars" in both unipolar patients and bipolar II probands and family members. Schizoaffective manics are already included. Since most genetic analyses already include these hidden bipolar patients as "affected," the first concern is to identify them as bipolar probands. Blacker and Tsuang (1992) extended the problem to relatives in order to also eliminate as "affected" reactive or nonbiologic depressives.

Biochemical and Neuroendocrine Parameters

The depressant effect of reserpine when given for hypertension and the euphoric effects of a monoamine oxidase inhibitor when given for tuberculosis led to the development of the "biogenic amine hypothesis" for the etiology of depression. The classic amine hypothesis stated that in depression, there was a functional deficit of either norepinephrine or serotonin at critical synapses in the central nervous system and implied that, conversely, an excess of such amines was associated with mania. Swann et al. (1983) reported that the only difference between the manics and the controls in cerebrospinal fluid monoamine metabolites was an elevated level of 3-methoxy-4-hydroxyphenylglycol (MHPG) in the manic patients, which also has been reported in depressed patients. An unreplicated study by Lewis and McChesney (1985) presented data showing significantly fewer tritiated [^{3}H]imipramine binding sites on platelet membranes in bipolar patients compared with controls. More recently, it has become evident that the third

biogenic amine, dopamine, is also important and that other neurotransmitters or neuromodulators, such as the cholinergic system, the GABAergic system, and the endorphin system, may be implicated in bipolar disorder. Janowsky et al. (1983) suggested that an affective state may represent a balance between central cholinergic and adrenergic neurotransmitters and that depression may be a disorder of cholinergic predominance and mania, the opposite. In keeping with this, there is reference to the use of pilocarpine to treat mania (Olfson, 1987). Petty and Sherman (1984), in a review, indicate a state of confusion concerning gamma-aminobutyric acid (GABA).

In summary, there is no consistent body of evidence to date to confirm that the two poles of illness (mania and depression) are biologic opposites of each other. Clinically, there are many mixed states that have not been dealt with from a putative biologic standpoint.

The fact that *all* antidepressant treatments [accepted antidepressants, novel drugs such as *S*-adenosylmethionine (Carney et al., 1987; Kagan et al., 1990), ECT, light therapy, and sleep deprivation] can precipitate mania has led investigators to expand postulations beyond neurotransmitters to membrane fluidity and functioning of ion channels and second messenger systems.

EDITORS' COMMENT

Not all studies support the idea that antidepressants precipitate manias in bipolar patients (Lewis and Winokur, *Arch Gen Psychiatry* 39:303–306, 1982; Angst, J Psychopharmacol 1:13–19, 1987; Kupfer, Carpenter, and Frank, Am J Psychiatry 145:804–808, 1988). Most of the studies supporting the concept of a precipitation are individual case reports or series of patients without controls. Bipolar illness is a highly episodic illness, and it would be reasonable to expect that mania following antidepressant therapy simply is a reflection of the natural history of bipolar illness.

One line of research is to study inositol incorporation (Banks et al., 1990) into phosphoinositides in cells from bipolar patients (treatment status not given). It was found to be less than in control cells. Another study (Kato et al., 1991) showed a brain increase in inositol-1-phosphate in lithium-treated bipolar patients. A different approach is to examine the involvement of G proteins in the pathogenesis of bipolar disorder. This approach is particularly convincing because it explains the difference between depression and mania by involving first one and then a second system. Untreated manic patients were found to have hyperactive functions of G proteins. Antibipolar treatments attenuated both receptor-coupled G_s and non-G_s protein function, whereas antidepressant treatment inhibited only G_s protein function (Avissar and Schreiber, 1992; Post et al., 1992).

In the same way, early observations of the affective state of patients with excesses or deficiencies of corticosteroids (Cushing's syndrome and Addison's disease) led to the measurement of corticosteroids in the plasma and urine of patients with depression. Some depressed patients had elevated levels of corticosteroids that returned to normal with recovery (Winokur et al., 1969). Capitalizing on the endocrine challenge test for the diagnosis of Cushing's disease, Carroll et al. (1981) began systematically to evaluate the dexamethasone suppression test in depressed patients. They reported that about 40 percent of depressed melancholic inpatients and outpatients given 1 mg of dexamethasone at 11:00 P.M. failed to suppress cortisol at either 4:00 or 11:00 P.M. the next day. In most of the studies, the bipolar and the unipolar depressed patients were similar, and manics were suppressors. Controversy over this test, owing to many difficulties, emerged. Stokes et al. (1984), for instance, using data from the collaborative study of the psychobiology of affective disorders, showed that patients in the manic state had the highest percentage of nonsuppression. This was not confirmed by Joyce et al. (1987), although they attributed the marked differences to individual variations and failure to assess or report dysphoria during mania. Use of this test by clinicians as a biologic marker for primary depression has been questioned, but everyone agrees that a significant minority of bipolar and unipolar depressed patients have elevated corticosteroid levels, that some (not necessarily the same) are nonsuppressors after dexamethasone, and that in these, with recovery, the test returns to normal. The manic state needs further clarification.

Amsterdam et al. (1983) looked at a full neuroendocrine test battery in bipolar patients and healthy subjects. They measured baseline levels of leutinizing hormone (LH), follicle-stimulating hormone (FSH), thyroid-stimulating hormone (TSH), prolactin (PRL), growth hormone (GH), cortisol, thyroxine (T_4), and triiodothyronine (T_3) in 22 bipolar outpatients (14 of whom were currently depressed and 8 of whom were hypomanic) and appropriate controls. They used four provocative tests (thyrotropin-releasing hormone, gonadotropin-releasing hormone, insulin tolerance, and dexamethasone suppression). All assays were measured by radioimmunoassay. For the most part, they found no difference between the depressed and the hypomanic patients at baseline and minimal differences at baseline between the subjects and the patients. Only when they looked at the distribution of abnormal responses did a highly significant difference emerge. Twelve patients (54.5 percent) but no normal subjects demonstrated abnormalities in two or more tests. The most useful tests in these patients were the dexamethasone suppression test and the measurement of TSH and PRL after protirelin administration. This last finding of a blunted response of TSH to protirelin has been observed in frankly manic patients and is the same as that which is reported in depressed patients (Extein et al., 1982).

Although further studies (Joyce et al., 1988) have been done, no clear picture emerges.

Because the neuroendocrine system is related to the amine and immune systems, attempts to integrate findings emerged. Noting a relationship between serotonin activity and production of anterior pituitary hormones, Meltzer et al. (1983) reported that serotonin activity in platelets in unipolar, bipolar, and schizoaffective depressed inpatients was significantly decreased but varied independently of those patients who were dexamethasone nonsuppressors. These findings have not been replicated. Goodwin and Jamison (1990) offer a complete discussion of all these controversial parameters. Suffice it to say that the central defect of bipolar illness is yet to be identified.

Another interesting avenue of research is emerging from the study of seasonal affective disorder. Thompson et al. (1990) reported that both bipolar and unipolar seasonal affective disorder (SAD) patients compared with controls displayed an abnormal seasonal variation in the suppression of melatonin by light. There was excessive sensitivity to bright light in the winter (less production of melatonin) and less than normal sensitivity in the summer. (It is interesting that bipolar patients may be less likely to use sun glasses than most people.) The authors postulated this change may be due to a serotonergic input to the suprachiasmatic nucleus. The psychoactive components of melantonin are unclear (Zetin et al., 1987). Lithium affects foveal dark adaptation perhaps through G proteins (Emrich et al., 1990), but how this all is related remains to be elucidated.

In conclusion, these studies indicate abnormalities and variability in biochemical, neuroendocrine, and second messenger system function, but they do not shed bright light on a specific neurobiology of bipolar illness, either mania or depression.

Sleep and Other Electrophysiologic Parameters

The sleep parameters of depressed patients are well known. Both unipolar and bipolar depressed patients have shortened rapid eye movement (REM) latency, higher REM density, and problems with sleep continuity (Kupfer, 1983). Giles et al. (1986) confirmed this and added that bipolar II depressed patients are similar. Hudson et al. (1988) reported exactly the same findings in nine unmediated manics. Sitaram (1983) reported that in remitted, mainly bipolar, depressed patients, arecoline (an acetylcholine agonist) induced REM sleep significantly more rapidly than in normal controls. Some of the remitted patients and normal controls also had an amphetamine challenge test. There was a negative correlation between arecolinergic REM induction and amphetamine-induced behavioral excitation. That is, those former patients who had REM induction sooner also were less likely to develop an elation or excitation with intravenous amphetamines, again suggesting a reciprocal relationship between the cholinergic and catecholamine systems even in the well state.

In depressed patients who received total sleep deprivation as treatment, 25 percent of nonbipolar and 30 percent of bipolar depressives became hypomanic or manic (Wu and Bunney, 1990). Although these authors advanced several hypotheses that may account for this, they proposed that during sleep, a substance is produced that is associated with depressed mood, and this is metabolized or stored during wakefulness. It explains the reported response of depressives to napping and the diurnal variation of depression. Although the authors do not address it, they must assume that the well-described sleep morphology of depression still allows for or enhances the production of this substance. How this substance relates to induction of mania is also not clarified. The precipitation of mania after a stressful life event (see Ambelas, 1987, p. 28) could be through sleep deprivation (Wehr and Sack, 1987).

Studies have shown that between 17 and 45 percent of bipolar patients have abnormal EEGs (Dewan et al., 1988b). Dewan et al. (1988a) also reported an increase in third ventricular size in remitted bipolar patients compared with controls. They found no correlation between this and any clinical, neurophysiologic, or neuropsychometric measures.

Using positron emission tomography, Baxter et al. (1989) reported that bipolar and unipolar depressives had similar lower left dorsal anterolateral prefrontal cortex blood flow compared with normal controls, obsessive compulsives without depression, and bipolar manics. Others (Silfverskiöld and Risberg, 1989) have reported normal cerebral blood flow in all affective disorder patients.

Animal Models

Robbins and Sahakian (1980) reviewed the animal models for mania, including a thoughtful discussion of how to relate clinical symptoms to animal behavior, criteria for the ideal animal model of a syndrome, and a discussion of models produced by drugs, lesions, and behavioral manipulations. Their own research emphasized the amphetamine-induced model and is particularly interesting in light of the clinical studies of amphetamine-induced symptoms and syndromes in humans (see next section).

Secondary Mania

Krauthammer and Klerman (1978) thoroughly reviewed the literature on secondary mania. They required specific criteria to include cases as mania. The major reported causes have been neurologic conditions such as neoplasm, epilepsy, head injury, cerebrovascular lesions, drugs, metabolic or endocrine disturbances, infections, or other systemic conditions.

EDITORS' COMMENT

Perhaps a better term than secondary mania might be *induced mania*. *Secondary mania* implies only that a mania occurs in relation to a temporal sequence. The Krauthammer and Klerman paper present a series of organic and neurologic factors that precede the mania, suggesting that some kind of abnormal metabolism, tumor, or other biologic disturbance caused the mania.

A number of recent articles (Shukla et al., 1987; Clark and Davison, 1987; Pope et al., 1988) have commented on the development of mania after a closed head injury. Some suggest that the intervening variable in head injury is seizures; others fail to confirm this. Mania developing after specific left and right intercerebral pathology (Jampala and Abrams, 1983) also has been reported with literature review.

Several recent reviews (Cook et al., 1987; Larson and Richelson, 1988; Starkstein et al., 1988) have tried to summarize the differences between organic and nonorganic mania. Patients with secondary mania are frequently older at their age of onset, their mood is more typically irritable rather than manic, they are less frequently psychotic, their family histories are more frequently negative, and they do not respond to the usual treatment but do well on anticonvulsants.

Black et al. (1988a, 1988b) reported on uncomplicated and complicated (either concurrent medical or psychiatric disorders) bipolar patients. These medical patients differed from those reported above, since despite being older, they had more prior psychiatric hospitalizations than the uncomplicated bipolars. Their death rate was surprisingly high. The psychiatrically comorbid bipolar patients also had poorer outcomes. The second psychiatric illness was alcoholism or drug abuse in 60 percent of the patients.

There also has been an emphasis on the co-occurrence of medical illness and typical manic depressive disease. These should be considered bipolar with second or additional diagnoses. There is a set of reports on the occurrence of bipolar illness in patients with mental retardation (McLaughlin, 1987; Glue, 1989; Arumainayagam and Kumar, 1990).

Besides the mania that is precipitated by somatic therapies for depression, mania also has been reported during treatment with corticosteroids, cocaine, and L-dopa, as well as during the spontaneous use of amphetamines and khat, a leaf used as part of the culture of people of North and South Yemen. Tatetsu (1963, 1972) reported on 131 Japanese patients who, because it was legal and available, used methamphetamine after World War II. The most common diagnoses in both the acute and stationary stages in these addicted patients (30 to 90 mg/day IV) were either manic-depressive illness or manic-depressive illness with schizophrenia-like features. The paranoid delusions that developed were compatible with a diagnosis of manic-depressive illness. Gough and Cookson (1984) reported that after the use of khat, a patient became manic with elation, hyperactivity, pressured speech, diminished appetite, poor sleep, and delusions. The patient was called *schizophreniform*. The drug screen was positive for amphetamines but negative for other drugs. Another report (Arnold et al., 1980) described a patient given baclofen, which is structurally related to GABA and presumably acts as a GABA agonist or as an inhibitor of substance P, for cervical myelopathy who developed a manic-like syndrome 1 day after he discontinued the drug. There are numerous other drugs and drug withdrawals reported to be associated with the onset of mania. These should be considered secondary manias and treated as such.

As with the neurobiology and electrophysiologic findings, these animal and human models provide evidence that this illness is a biologic brain disorder but emphasize the complexity, diffuseness, and variability of the syndrome rather than clarify the cause.

EPIDEMIOLOGY

Boyd and Weissman (1981), in reviewing studies of bipolar affective disorder, estimated that the lifetime risk for bipolar I disorder was between 0.2 and 0.9 percent. These estimates probably were not age-corrected. In the same way, the epidemiologic catchment area (ECA) study (Robins et al., 1984) estimated the lifetime risk to be 0.6 percent. Thus the frequency of illness is similar to schizophrenia. The incidence of bipolar disorder per 100,000 per year varies enormously between studies. Using modern diagnostic techniques, Myers et al. (1984) reported a 6-month prevalence for manic episode to be between 0.4 and 0.8 percent. In all these studies the distribution of males to females was about equal. The risk for mania seems to increase in more recent birth cohorts (Gershon et al., 1987; Rice et al., 1987; Lasch et al., 1990).

All calculations of bipolar affective disorder are underestimates, since to calculate the prevalence of lifetime risk requires that the patient have an identifiable mania, and a majority of patients, particularly women, begin with depressive episodes (Angst, 1978). Perris (1969), Angst (1974), and Angst et al., (1978) reported that 16, 13, and 16 percent, respectively, of their patients who had had three previous episodes of depression still became bipolar. A study of manic episodes in older people (Shulman and Post, 1980) indicated that a mean of 10 years elapsed between the first depressive episode and the first manic episode. Akiskal et al. (1983b), in a younger sample, reported that 20 percent of 206 depressed outpatients switched to bipolar I or II an average of 6.4 years after the initial identification. If the illness began at a younger age, the switch was earlier. Krauthammer and Klerman (1979) estimated a similar switch rate.

Factors besides young age found to be associated with a change of polarity from unipolar to bipolar (Akiskal et al., 1983b) were hypersomnic and retarded phenomenology, psychotic depression, and postpartum episodes. Also, a large percentage of young males who were depressed switched (Winokur and Wesner, 1987). A family history of bipolarity and a pharmacologic hypomania produced by antidepressants also were predictive of a bipolar outcome. The mean age at which the switch occurred was 32. The average number of previous episodes was two to four.

There are no data to suggest that unipolar mania differs from the bipolar disorder. Unipolar mania was said to be rare and to constitute only 2 to 5 percent of all the patients in this category. Nurnberger et al. (1979), however, reported that 16 percent of a group of bipolar patients had never been hospitalized or treated for depression, and Abrams et al. (1979) reported that 18 percent of patients hospitalized for affective disorder (not necessarily bipolar) were unipolar manics. Pfohl et al. (1982) reported the highest percentage (33 percent) based on a chart review. Interestingly, Kraepelin (1921) originally reported that 17 percent of his 900 manic-depressive patients were exclusively manic. Some feel that the longer or the more closely a patient is followed, the more likely it will be that depression is recognized.

RISK FACTORS

Bipolar illness is the disease of much earlier onset and much more limited risk. The onset is usually from the teens to the 50s, with the average age of onset being 30. More than one-third (Winokur et al., 1969) begin in the teenage years. Numerous studies have indicated that in the teenage years, bipolar illness can be mistakenly called schizophrenia, antisocial personality, or borderline personality disorder. Actually, there should be more adolescents diagnosed as bipolar (either manic or depressive) than as schizophrenic. Akiskal (1983) indicated that the clinical presentation of adolescents with bipolar disorders, in decreasing frequency, are "psychosis," alcohol and drug problems, "moodiness," suicidal ideation or attempt, academic failure, philosophic brooding, obsessional brooding, somatic complaints, school phobia, "hyperactivity," stupor, and flagrant antisocial behavior. Although the last was extremely uncommon, it can occur. The literature on late-onset bipolar illness is confusing because some of the patients discussed had episodes of depression before age 50 but did not become manic until after age 50. Reviews fail to take this into consideration, but still, there are onsets after 50 (Yassa et al., 1988; Rubin, 1988; Stone, 1989; Young and Klerman, 1992) that are not associated with organic pathology. Since this age group is increasing, we should see more.

In keeping with this young age of onset, Akiskal et al. (1983b) found that depression in a person under age 25 was highly correlated with a bipolar outcome in follow-up. A psychotic depression or any severe depression in a teenager should always be considered potentially the onset of a bipolar illness. The same is true of a schizoaffective illness (Joyce, 1984). This is important because of the implications for treatment in the acute episode and the willingness to consider maintenance therapy if such episodes recur.

The sex ratio shows only a slight preponderance of women over men. There are no racial differences in the incidence or prevalence of this illness. A fair amount of recent literature indicates that both Hispanics and blacks (Jones et al., 1981, 1983; Keisling, 1981) have high rates of bipolar affective disorder when inpatients are studied and that it is frequently misdiagnosed as schizophrenia. In the ECA study (Robins et al., 1984), there were no differences in the lifetime prevalence of mania by race, and in fact, in the St. Louis data there seemed to be an excess of mania in the blacks. In the same data set, mania was equally prevalent in urban or rural residents but was significantly more prevalent in non-college graduates than in college graduates. These race and education findings may be related.

Interestingly enough, there is little comment on the marital status of bipolar patients. In the collaborative study there were significantly more single bipolar patients than single unipolar patients, a fact also mentioned in the reports on race and bipolar illness. Young age of onset probably correlates with singleness.

A positive association between bipolar affective disorder and high socioeconomic status was noted previously (Clayton, 1981) but not confirmed in the ECA study. Coryell et al. (1989) reported significantly higher socioeconomic status in only the relatives of bipolar patients. The data on immigration status of bipolar patients are controversial.

A well-done study by Ambelas (1987) has confirmed what clinicians suspected: There is a strong correlation between stressful life events and first manic admissions, which lessen as the illness progresses. This is particularly true for younger bipolar patients and is significantly linked to mania and not depression. Studies of bereavement have shown that the most common somatic symptom following this stress is insomnia (Clayton, 1982b), and this, coupled with data from sleep-deprivation studies, has caused researchers (Wehr et al., 1987) to posit sleep reduction as a final common pathway to mania. Knowledge about the association between stressful life events and insomnia is essential in managing bipolar patients.

All studies have confirmed the postpartum period as a risk period for mania in known bipolar patients (Winokur et al., 1969), patients with serious previous depression (Akiskal, 1983b), and probably those with a bipolar diathesis (Kendell et al., 1987).

Periodicity of this illness is true for some patients, with fall/winter depression and spring/summer mania being most frequently described. The suicide rate is highest in April. Sayer et al. (1991) recently confirmed in the southern hemisphere what had been reported in the northern hemisphere (Carney et al., 1988), that hospital admissions for mania have a spring/summer peak. Onset of illness should be recorded for each episode in order to highlight patterns of illness. More recently, the seasonality of the mood disorders has been emphasized, leading to the classification of seasonal affective disorder (SAD) (Rosenthal et al., 1984; Rosenthal and Wehr, 1987). Large numbers of SAD patients are bipolar. Depending on the number of bipolar II patients included, percentages vary from 8 to 100 percent (Goodwin and Jamison, 1990), with most studies recording more than 50 percent as bipolar spectrum.

The personality traits of bipolar patients are not yet clarified. Akiskal et al. (1977) identified 46 outpatients (2.3 percent of the outpatient population) as cyclothymic and reported that 22 percent became bipolar in the follow-up period. Some researchers (Jamison et al., 1980; Targum et al., 1981; Bouman et al., 1992) indicated that even in remission, manics evaluate themselves in a positive way. Others (Akiskal et al., 1983a; Matussek and Feil, 1983) emphasized the achievement-oriented personality of the bipolar patients. Still others (MacVane et al., 1978; Lumry et al., 1982) have found that bipolar patients who are well or stabilized on lithium have personalities similar to those of controls. Bech et al. (1980) suggested that lithium mutes the cyclothymia and causes bipolar patients to test more like unipolar patients. Angst and Clayton (1986), comparing premorbid personality traits in young men who developed bipolar illness with those who remained well, found no differences. Unfortunately, the personality test did not measure obsessionality, the trait Klein and Depue (1985) reported may be associated with risk for bipolar disorder in the offspring of bipolar probands. Thus no personality trait or feature can be identified as a risk factor, and as yet, no childhood features are predictive of bipolarity. Cyclothymia is probably an early manifestation of the illness rather than a personality trait (Akiskal et al., 1983a; Pritz and Mitterauer 1984). It seems as likely that personality traits associated with early-onset recurrent depression will identify bipolar patients.

CLINICAL PICTURE

As previously emphasized, the typical bipolar patient starts with an episode of pure depression.

Angst (1978) reported that the ratio of depression to mania in the first episode was 3:1 for women and 3:2 for men.

Still, mania or a mixed manic and depressive state is the hallmark of this illness (Winokur et al., 1969). Pure and mixed states probably occur with equal frequency, although some reports combine mixed and cycling episodes, which elevates the percentage presenting as a mixed state (Keller et al., 1986; Secunda et al., 1987; Prien et al., 1988; Post et al., 1989; Bauer et al., 1991). Mania can begin suddenly with the development of a full-blown syndrome over hours (causing some to posit a substance in the bloodstream), or it may be a more gradual state, developing over days. It seldom takes weeks to develop. A history of a change in the patient's behavior is usual, although unless the onset is sudden, close relatives miss the first indications. Mania may begin with a short period of depression. Early in the course of illness, mania can be preceded by life events, including bereavement, but as the illness continues, there are fewer precipitants.

The picture can vary from an excited, talkative, loud, overreactive, somewhat amusing individual to a completely disorganized, intrusive psychotic. The mood is always elated, angry, or irritable. Many patients appear overly confident, bragging, self-aggrandizing, and happy but become irritable when their ideas are not enthusiastically endorsed. Frequently they become most angry at those who are closest to them, particularly their spouses. They interrupt conversations but dislike being interrupted themselves. They are distractible. Racing thoughts, pressured speech, circumstantiality, irrelevancies, and flight of ideas characterize thoughts and language. Decreased need for sleep or insomnia, an increase in sexual thoughts, and an increase in alcohol intake are all common in the manic patient. During the full-blown syndrome, there may be periods of depression lasting from minutes to hours. Grandiose ideas and delusions are common and are probably the basis for the symptoms of excessive telephone calls, extravagances, and excessive writing. One or two themes usually predominate. The themes may be religious, political, financial, sexual, or persecutory. All varieties of psychotic symptoms have been reported in the manic patient (Clayton et al., 1965; Abrams and Taylor, 1981). The best documentation of this is probably the Carlson and Goodwin (1973) study on the evolution of a manic episode. At the height of the manic episode, patients exhibited unusual psychomotor activities, incoherent thought processes, and delusions and hallucinations that were bizarre and idiosyncratic. They found that besides hyperactivity, extreme verbosity, pressure of speech, grandiosity, manipulativeness, irritability, euphoria, labile mood, hypersexuality, and flight of ideas, 75 percent had delusions that were either of control or sexual, persecutory, or religious; 75 percent had assaultive or threatening behavior; 70 percent had distractibility,

loose associations, and a fear of dying; 60 percent were intrusive; 55 percent had some delusions; 50 percent had religiosity; 45 percent used the telephone excessively; 45 percent had regressive behavior (urinating or defecating inappropriately and exposing themselves); 40 percent demonstrated symbolization or gesturing; 40 percent had auditory and visual hallucinations; and 35 percent were confused. Confusion is a well-documented symptom of acute mania. In a chart review, 58 percent of 31 manics (Clayton et al., 1965) were reported either to be disoriented or to have memory lapses. Kraepelin (1921) used the term delirious mania.

Andreasen (1979a, 1979b) and Andreasen and Powers (1974) looked at thought disorder in mania and found that besides being overinclusive, both behaviorally and conceptually, manics were tangential and had derailment, incoherence, and illogicality that was equally prominent as in schizophrenics. The manics were more likely to have pressured speech, distractibility, and circumstantiality. The schizophrenics more frequently had poverty of both speech and content of speech. Harrow et al. (1982) confirmed and extended this, indicating that at follow-up, in partial remission, almost half continued to have thought pathology. Brockington et al. (1983) reported similar follow-up findings. Catatonic features during a manic episode have been well documented by Abrams and Taylor (1976) and reconfirmed by Fein and McGrath (1990). Pope and Lipinski's (1978) comprehensive article emphasized that between 20 and 50 percent of well-validated bipolar patients have psychotic symptoms, including hallucinations, delusions, catatonia symptoms, and schneiderian first-rank symptoms.

Depression is well described in Chapter 5. Most, but not all, investigators report inconsistent and minimal differences in symptoms in bipolar and unipolar depressives (Mitchell et al., 1992). The one exception may be delusional depression, especially occurring in people under age 30. Delusional depression, by clinical course, outcome, treatment, and family studies, predicted bipolarity in the patient and family members. Weissman et al. (1988) even reported that children (ages 6 to 23 years) of delusional depressives compared with children of nondelusional depressives had a threefold increase in cyclothymia, were more often described by health professionals as hyperactive, and had increased school and social impairments. Although not confirmed, perhaps even older-onset delusional depressives should be considered part of the bipolar spectrum, especially in deciding treatment, maintenance, and genetic studies. Bipolar depressives have high anxiety scores similar to unipolar patients. They also make more serious suicide attempts during follow-up.

The following case illustrates a bipolar illness with an untreated, unrecognized first episode of depression and psychotic mania.

A 22-year-old single man was referred for consultation. He gave a clear history of episodes of psychosis beginning in May and June at age 17, after graduation from high school. He was going with a group to Israel, and in anticipation of this trip, he got excited and experienced insomnia. On the airplane he developed the idea that his peers were sending messages by some strange visual communication. He thought that their facial expressions told other stories and began to think that he could read their thoughts and minds. He also developed the idea that something was visibly wrong with him and that security guards in Israel noted this. In the midst of this he lost track of time and became convinced that they couldn't go to the Wailing Wall because it was Friday, when indeed it was Wednesday, so he refused to leave his room. After that he included the group leader in his scheme, thinking "they" were trying to fool him and retain him in Israel. He remembered that his thinking was loud and fast and that he was angry. He was hospitalized in Israel and returned to a hospital in the United States.

His second episode occurred in April, 2 years later. In this episode his psychotic symptoms were grounded in the grandiose delusion to save the world. He began to write a book. He also wrote clever but disjointed letters to the governor that pertained to fighting crime (this was probably originally based on some incident such as an attempted rape in his dorm). He developed the idea that one way to help crime and stabilize the financial market was to construct more jails, so he began to buy stock in construction companies. He believed that he would become famous for this plausible plan. Finally, because of his letter writing, the police decided that he might be dangerous, and he was committed. Again, he remembered being excited, needing no sleep, talking fast, and not eating.

His third episode occurred again in April of the next year and had a similar theme. Each time he was diagnosed as manic and was put on lithium and a major tranquilizer, but he objected to taking lithium continuously. When I saw him, he was on no medicine. He was depressed, with slowed thinking, difficulty concentrating, and difficulty making decisions. He had intermittently returned to a difficult college and had completed courses but had not completed his degree. He felt discouraged about that and thought that it was useless to go to school or work. He was thin and distraught looking. In retrospect, he stated that he probably was depressed in high school in the *spring* of his senior year, when his grades fell and he didn't do as well on the swimming team and developed a great deal of interpersonal difficulty with his father. His mother had recurrent bipolar affective disorder, but he has always blamed his father for his illness.

For several years he was stabilized on lithium and an antidepressant. He graduated from college but found no suitable long-term work. He was fired from a job as a postman before the probation period was up. He was far from well-adjusted. He complained that he never smiled. He remained single, lived at home, and was dependent on his family. His goal was to marry and have a reasonable job. He has had numerous long trials of psychotherapy. Because of side effects (alopecia, tremor) and no mania for 7 years, he stopped the lithium. We discussed the symptoms that we should anticipate if he got manic. He voluntarily listed the following symptoms: racing thoughts, distractibility, grandiosity, driving faster and in more of a hurry, talking faster, excessive buying and long-distance telephone calls, increased humorousness with free associations and punning, playing records louder, listening to music and bothering more people in the household, and becoming evangelistic. He did not think that his sexual interest changed (it was always high) or that he had weight loss or increased energy. After years of managing him on one antidepressant or another, he finally agreed to take a monoamine oxide (MAO) inhibitor. Previously, he had resisted because he maintained that the treatment might interfere with treatment for an acute asthma attack or at other times the drugs were dangerous and I was trying to kill him. Within days on an MAO inhibitor (he frequently escalated the dose without approval), he became irritable, humorous, argumentative. Mania was diagnosed. He stopped the MAO inhibitor but refused treatment. His family also would not intervene. He moved to a motel. He had some care, but not hospitalization. The illness essentially ran its course. He now takes lithium and antidepressants and sees another psychiatrist.

COURSE

Bipolar illness is definitely a recurring illness. Bratfos and Haug (1968) found in a 6-year follow-up of 42 patients that 7 percent recovered without relapse, 48 percent had one or more episodes, and 45 percent had chronic courses. On the other hand, Tohen et al. (1990a, 1990b), in a 4-year follow-up, reported that 46 percent ($n = 24$) of the first-episode manics and 28 percent ($n = 75$) of the total suffered no relapse. One assumes that there were none with chronic courses. Although 79 percent were taking medications (only 54 percent of the first-episode manics), this did not predict outcome. In this series, the short-term outcome (6 months) was worse than the 48-month outcome. Relapse occurred early. Harrow et al. (1990), with a shorter follow-up (1.7 years), reported less favorable results, although the number of first-episode patients was not given, and 78 percent were psychotic at index. Here again, a surprising number (40 percent) were medication-free at follow-up, and there was no relationship between somatic therapy and outcome. These data, however, start with patients with mania. Since more than 50 percent of patients have first episodes that are depressive, by the time they are identified as bipolar, they have already had two episodes. Grof et al. (1974) reported that virtually every patient had a recurrence. There are no comparable data from an outpatient clinic, although the lithium/placebo studies show high relapses when such patients are put on placebo and therefore complement these data.

The clearest data on the characterization of the illness come from the collaborative study of Grof et al. (1974; Angst et al., 1986; Angst, 1980). Patients were treated for their affective episodes and received no prophylactic treatment between episodes. The investigators were particularly interested in documenting numbers of episodes, lengths of episodes, and other details pertaining to episodes. The average manic episode lasted for about 3 months, and the average depressive episode lasted for about 4 months. The duration of episodes did not change remarkably with increasing numbers of episodes. Initially, with each episode, the interval between the episodes tended to decrease. However, once the patient had gone through a number of episodes, perhaps more than five, the duration of the cycle—defined as the time from the beginning of one episode to the beginning of the next—became stable. Thus the duration of the time between attacks had a tendency to decrease and the course deteriorated, but it ultimately bottomed out at a cycle every 6 to 9 months. The authors concluded that the most useful way to predict a patient's future course was by his or her past course; e.g., if a patient had three episodes in the past 2 years, the short-term future course would be similar.

Between 15 and 20 percent of bipolar patients who present for treatment exhibit rapid cycling. Coryell et al. (1992) applied prospectively the usual definition for rapid cyclers (four or more episodes of mania, hypomania, or depression in a single year) to the first 52 weeks of an intensive follow-up and compared these patients with non-rapid cycling bipolar patients. Rapid cyclers were far more likely to be female (75 percent), but in every other way, including thyroid status, family history, and long-term treatment outcome, as well as suicide and suicide attempts, they seemed similar to other bipolar patients. Rapid cyclers had less previous mania but more cycling, especially with hypomania. After the defined first year, they did less well for the second year, but by the third, fourth, and fifth years, their outcomes were as good as those of other bipolar patients, and there was no relationship between treatment with antidepressants and outcome. Whether or not there is an association between rapid cycling and low-grade hypothyroidism is controversial (Bauer et al., 1990; Bauer and Whybrow, 1990), although, since these are refractory patients, levothyroxine should be tried.

In summary, numerous studies have shown that if the presentation is mania (Keller et al., 1986; Prien et al., 1988; Secunda et al., 1987; Post et al., 1989; Coryell et al., 1990, 1992; Cohen et al., 1989; Tohen et al., 1990a, 1990b), then dysphoric mania, rapid cycling, and psychosis predict a less favorable 6- and 48-month outcome. If the presentation is depression (Coryell et al., 1987; Keller et al., 1986), rapid cycling predicts a poorer 2-year outcome. If the bipolar disorder is complicated by alcoholism or substance abuse (Black et al., 1988a, 1988b; Brady and Lydiard, 1992), the outcome is also less favorable. The longer-term outcome still seems more favorable.

This is consistent with the interesting and tentative finding from the work of Grof et al. (1974) that there may be an extinction of the pattern of episodes after a certain number. The authors found that although the total number of episodes in a lifetime varied from 2 to more than 30 (and 42 percent of them had more than 10 episodes), still, the median number was 9 whether the patient had been studied for 5 or 40 years. The authors interpreted this to mean that while the short-term prognosis of bipolar affective disorder may be poor, the long-term course may be better. Winokur (1975) suggested the same thing from a different data base. Here, however, the studies on lithium maintenance would speak against this, for they show that even patients up to age 65 who have recurring bipolar illness relapse if lithium is discontinued. Perhaps lithium blocks the extinction of the illness.

The occurrence of chronicity in bipolar disease is not a moot point. Grof and collaborators did not characterize the social disabilities of their patients. Without stating so specifically, they give the impression that between episodes the patients were relatively free of symptoms other than minor mood swings. Winokur et al. (1969) painted a picture more similar to that of Bratfos and Haug (1968). In a 2-year follow-up of 28 patients, 14 percent were well in every way, 46 percent had additional episodes but were well in between, 29 percent never achieved more than a partial remission of symptoms, and 11 percent were chronically ill. There were only four patients who were in the first episode of the illness, and in these four, one had a partial remission, two had complete remissions with subsequent episodes, and one remained entirely well. Welner et al. (1977) reviewed a large number of studies of bipolar illness and indicated that chronicity, if defined as presence of symptoms, social decline, or both, occurred in at least one-third of the bipolar patients. Chronic mania, however, is uncommon. The only more favorable outcome comes from Petterson's study (1977) of a group of patients treated in Sweden. She observed the clinical, social, and genetic aspects of 123 patients for approximately 5 years. At the end of the study, a large number of patients showed more satisfactory work capacity and better social adaptation. This was a group treated by a single investigator. It may be that in treating chronically ill patients who require maintenance therapy, psychological skills are an essential ingredient to a more favorable outcome.

Complications

The most serious consequence of this illness is suicide. Not dividing patients by polarity, a summary of the relationship between suicide and primary affective disorder showed that the suicide risk among patients with affective disorder was more than 30 times greater than that of the general population (Guze and Robins, 1970). Between 10 and 15 percent of all deaths of patients with affective disorder were accounted for by suicide (Tsuang, 1978). In bipolar disease, as in unipolar disease, there is a trend for the suicide to occur early in the illness and less frequently as the disease continues (Tsuang, 1978). Several recent studies have found lower suicide rates in unipolar and bipolar patients (Petterson, 1977; Khuri and Akiskal, 1983; Martin et al.,

1985). Morrison (1982) found lower rates in unipolar patients but not in bipolar patients. The follow-ups in these studies were sufficiently long to consider that this could be a positive result of lithium and of other acute and maintenance therapies. There appears to be an increase in mortality from other causes, especially in inadequately treated bipolars (Avery and Winokur, 1976; Tsuang and Woolson, 1977).

Suicide attempts have been reported to be higher in bipolar patients, especially men (Woodruff et al., 1972; Johnson and Hunt, 1979). And everyone reports an increased mortality among bipolar patients over and above that which is due to suicide. There also may be a link between bipolar disorder and excess cardiovascular mortality (Yates and Wallace, 1987; Weeke et al., 1987). One report (Lilliker, 1980) showed an increased prevalence of diabetes in hospitalized bipolar patients compared with *all* other hospitalized patients, such as schizophrenics, alcoholics, and the retarded. Both Bratfos and Haug (1968) and Angst (personal communication) reported that these patients develop dementia at a higher frequency than would be expected compared with appropriate age-matched controls, but without autopsy findings, it is unclear if this is Alzheimer's disease.

In addition, there may be an increased association between heavy drinking and acute mania and between alcoholism and bipolar disorder (Helzer and Prybeck, 1988) and substance abuse and bipolar disorder (Brady and Lydiard, 1992). There is also an association between pathologic gambling and a bipolar diagnosis (McCormick et al., 1984).

Some have indicated that bipolar patients' marriages ended in divorce more frequently than those of unipolar patients or appropriate controls (Brodie and Leff, 1971). Even in those not ending in divorce, 53 percent of well spouses compared with 5 percent of the bipolar patients indicated that they would not have married the spouse, and 47 percent of the well spouses compared with 5 percent of the patients would not have had children had they known about the bipolar illness before making these decisions (Targum et al., 1981). The illness has an impact on marriage, job, child rearing, and all aspects of life. Once more, Petterson (1977) reported better social and medical outcomes. In her data, the distribution of marital state and frequency of marriage was largely in agreement with the general population. In several cases there were divorces that occurred in connection with the patient's illness, but there also were reconciliations that were attributed to lithium treatment.

The bipolar patients she studied had fewer children and more childless marriages than the general Swedish population. The finding of decreased fertility also was reported by Baron et al. (1982).

With regard to criminality, Petterson's patients had fewer convictions than expected in comparison with the general population, a finding replicated in other studies. An interesting set of studies (London and Taylor, 1982), however, indicates that symptoms of mania are more common in forensic settings than was generally thought. In studying patients admitted to St. Elizabeth's Hospital in Washington, D.C., the authors found that 11 of the 13 attempted crimes against the president of the United States, so-called White House cases, were perpetrated by people diagnosed as having an affective disorder, and the majority of them were bipolar.

In summary, although numerous problems can be anticipated with the development of a bipolar affective disorder, there is some hope that maintenance therapy can significantly alter the course of the illness.

DIFFERENTIAL DIAGNOSIS

As indicated, there are other disorders that have similar symptoms, course, and outcome, including high chronicity and suicide, as well as similar age of onset, type of onset, and percentage single. Only family history can reliably distinguish the bipolar patient. Pritz and Mitterauer (1984) emphasize well the spectrum of mood phenomenon in bipolar disorder. Symptoms are not absorbed from the patient; they are elicited. Therefore, all symptoms, including mood, should be asked of the patient.

Schizophrenia

Schizophrenia and mania are alike in many ways. The symptoms of a current episode can be similar in mania and schizophrenia. There is not one symptom that is pathognomonic for either, although the mood of merriment, elation, ecstasy, or even irritability is much more likely to occur in the manic than in the schizophrenic, but there are some hypochondriacal or grandiose schizophrenics who maintain a haughty, elated affect. Studies of diagnostic criteria for mania (Young et al., 1983) indicated that the triad of symptoms—manic mood, rapid or pressured speech, and hyperactivity—is robust so that perhaps any patient with all three symptoms should be considered manic regardless of number or content of other symptoms. In patients partially treated with lithium or other antimanic drugs, these symptoms may be muted, and the prominent symptoms may only be psychotic symptoms.

Mania, for the most part, should have a relatively sudden onset, with the only extended prodromal being a depressive syndrome, and should be characterized as a change from the person's premorbid self. Schizophrenia should be more insidious, but it, too, can begin with depression *or* anxiety.

The course of the illnesses could be similar. At least one-third of bipolar patients have either social disabilities or symptoms that may be more than just low-grade depressive symptoms. Still, all studies show significantly better follow-up outcome in manics than in schizophrenics. Both have high suicide rates, with 10 to 15 percent dying by suicide.

The most reliable difference in these two illnesses is the family history. Although both are hereditary/familial, at least 50 percent of manic patients should have some family history of an affective disorder (mania or depression). Studies of schizophrenics show a significant but less striking increase in schizophrenia in their families but no increase in affective disorder over the population prevalence of about 6 to 8 percent.

Paranoid Schizophrenia

After the teenage years, many manics are misdiagnosed as paranoid schizophrenics. This seems to be particularly true with blacks and Hispanics. Again, the other indications of a manic syndrome, such as previous episodes, mode of onset, and family history, should help to differentiate patients.

Catatonic Schizophrenia

Since, when looking at catatonic symptoms, patients are more frequently bipolar or manic than any other diagnosis, all patients in whom the diagnosis of catatonic schizophrenia is entertained should be evaluated carefully for depressive and manic symptoms, previous episodes, and family history. Some manics become mute when their thoughts go so fast that they cannot speak. A "flat affect" is not uncommon or unusual in a bipolar patient treated with or maintained on phenothiazines. The amytal interview may still be useful in uncovering depressive delusions, disjointed manic thoughts, or disorientation (organicity).

Schizoaffective

Using the research diagnostic criteria (RDC) definition of schizoaffective, which splits patients into schizoaffective mania and schizoaffective depression, all studies show that the schizoaffective manics (Clayton, 1982a, 1987) are similar to manics, especially mood-incongruent mania, as defined in DSM-III. They all agree that the schizoaffective manic probably has an earlier age of onset and a more malignant course, but the biologic markers and the family history data indicate that they are in the bipolar spectrum. Joyce (1984) also concluded that patients with teenage onset have *more* schizophrenic symptoms. Because schizoaffective mania is so much like mania, it probably is wise not to use it for manic patients and to reserve it for schizoaffective depressives only.

On the other hand, schizoaffective depressives, who are usually a smaller group, seem to be a conglomerate of many different patients, such as schizophrenics, depressives, the spectrum of anxiety disorders with secondary depression, and alcoholics or drug abusers with secondary depression (Clayton,

1983). When schizoaffective manics are removed from schizoaffective depressives, there are almost no schizoaffective depressives who become bipolar at follow-up. It is a much more unstable diagnostic entity, but it should be retained to reflect uncertainty. Previous episodes of "pure" mania or depression and family history again help to discriminate.

Organic Mental Disorders

Because at least one-third of manics have either disorientation or some memory blanks during an episode, it might be easy to think of mania as a toxic state. Although certain drugs can precipitate manic episodes, usually even these syndromes are treated with neuroleptics or lithium, or both. In a first episode it may be impossible to distinguish or to make a definitive diagnosis. Previous history and family history should be useful in confirming a diagnosis. It is most difficult in a catatonic stupor. It is important not to be sidetracked by the confusion of mania and delay treatment for a long time (1 week) while completing extensive organic workups.

Personality Disorders (Antisocial, Borderline) and Alcohol and Drug Abuse

There are many presentations of bipolar disorder. In the teenage years, a change in behavior would be the key to distinguishing the manic from the typical sociopath. It is easy if the sociopathic behavior is manic—that is, stealing with some grandiose plan in mind—but less easy if it is typical of all adolescent antisocial acts. The same can be said of alcohol or drug problems, school phobia, and borderline personality diagnoses. Here again, the premorbid adjustment should be stable, and this should be a change in behavior that could not have been expected or anticipated. Depressive symptoms or, less commonly, manic symptoms should be present if inquired about. These things, coupled with a family history of affective disorder, should help in making the proper diagnosis.

Suicide Attempter

Because a suicide attempt may be trivial or serious in a bipolar depressive or manic (rarely), all suicide attempters should be considered potential unipolar or bipolar patients. Onset, symptoms, previous history, premorbid adjustment, and family history should help in making a diagnosis. Again, all suicidal or psychotic teenage depressives should be considered potential bipolar patients with all that this implies.

TREATMENT

No psychosocial management can be accomplished with a patient in the manic state. The patient is talkative, irritable, irritating, sexually aroused, confident, expansive, and completely lacking in insight or good judgment. Because of the uplifted mood, the patient feels no need of treatment and refuses with vehemence offers of assistance. Hospitalization is necessary and frequently entails commitment. The patient must be protected against the serious social and medical consequences of this state. In my opinion, because of the manic's intrusiveness and potential for creating conflict, it is almost always possible to think of that person as being dangerous to himself or herself. In the collaborative study of depression in St. Louis, the first death in the follow-up period was in a manic who was killed in a fight in a bar. If manics have other illnesses, such as hypertension, that are controlled by medication, those illnesses get out of control as the manic neglects medications, creating another reason for hospitalization.

When manics are hospitalized, their excessive energy is easy to handle if they are given space to roam and are not confined to a locked room. This does not mean that they can be on an unlocked unit, since they are capable of excessive spending even while in the hospital. Manic patients are also intrusive and speak in an uncensored way, so they can provoke arguments anywhere, including the hospital. In addition, enormous bills and bad feelings can develop in such patients if telephone use is not restricted. Hospitalization is also welcomed by the relatives, who are worn down and exasperated by the manic's behavior and relieved to know that he or she is being protected in the hospital. Such patients are also superalert; they hear and interpret every sound and see and interpret everything in their visual field. It is best to maintain them in an environment with as little stimulation as possible—groups, occupational therapy, and television should be minimized until the illness is remitting.

In treating manic patients, physicians should always remember that certain interpersonal traits are part of the manic illness. Janowsky et al. (1970, 1974) outlined a series of interpersonal behaviors that they had originally thought were part of the manic's premorbid personality but later discovered to be symptoms of the manic episode. In addition to the classic manic symptoms of hyperactivity, push of speech, flight of ideas, irritability, distractibility, poor judgment, and increased social contact, they found that manic behavior included such things as the testing of limits, flattery, shifting responsibility for their actions to others, exploiting other's soft spots, dividing the staff, and provoking anger. These traits led to marked interpersonal, marital, and ward conflict. Therefore, in treating the manic patient, one must take into consideration these symptoms and behaviors and respond to them as if they were part of the illness. This is best done by setting limits in an unambivalent, firm, and rather arbitrary way.

In acute mania, the efficacy of lithium is well accepted. With this in mind, the following choices are available, although the order may be debatable and may depend on the severity of the presenting symptoms: (1) lithium, (2) a neuroleptic or a benzodiazepine such as clonazepam or lorazepam plus lithium, (3) anticonvulsants such as carbamazepine or valproate alone or in addition, and (4) electroconvulsive therapy (ECT). Early studies comparing lithium with chlorpromazine or lithium, chlorpromazine, and haloperidol indicated that lithium was superior to the others in terms of earlier discharge. These studies, however, indicated that chlorpromazine, haloperidol, and other such neuroleptics control the hyperactivity/excitement of the acutely manic patient more quickly than does lithium. Some maintained that, clinically, the end result was superior with lithium alone, whereas others felt that haloperidol alone was sufficient for the acute illness. Because there have been a few isolated reports that the combination of haloperidol and lithium can produce adverse side effects (Garfinkel et al., 1980; Dunner, 1983), and because bipolars are at increased risk for tardive dyskinesia (Rosenbaum et al., 1977; Kane et al., 1980; Rush et al., 1982), more recent investigators have used lorazepam (1–2 mg q4–6h) or clonazepam (1 mg q4–6h) for sedation. In the most recent efficacy studies of valproate, lorazepam has been the supplemental drug allowed for insomnia or agitation (McElroy et al., 1992).

Before beginning treatment with lithium, the patient should have a complete medical workup, including a physical examination, tests for thyroid and renal function (blood urea nitrogen and creatinine), a white blood cell count, and electrocardiography. Other medications should be recorded, particularly the use of diuretics. Lithium is not contraindicated, however, in patients taking these drugs or with hypertension alone. Lithium should not be started in a pregnant woman. The issue of becoming pregnant while on lithium maintenance is discussed later. Patients should be monitored daily for symptoms of toxicity, such as tremor, nausea, vomiting, diarrhea, and confusion. Lithium levels should be monitored frequently. Symptoms of toxicity necessitate immediate change in the lithium dose. In general, however, if the dose is raised gradually, toxicity can be avoided. Skin rash is another potential problem.

The usual starting dose of lithium in acute manic attack is 300 mg three times a day, which is gradually raised until a blood level of 1.0 to 1.2 mEq/liter is achieved. Improvement typically occurs in 8 to 10 days. Since improvement occurs rapidly, patients may be discharged from the hospital long before the illness has run its course. The most common mistake in treating the acute manic attack is to discharge the patient too early, only to have him or her readmitted shortly after discharge. The manic should have a marked decrease in symptoms and an awareness about the illness and be thoroughly committed to continuing lithium before discharge

(Young et al., 1982). In addition, the patient's family should be educated and understanding about the illness.

Other Treatment Therapies

Carbamazepine is useful in the treatment of the acute mania (Ballenger and Post, 1980; Post, 1982; Post et al., 1983; Nolen, 1983; Kishimoto et al., 1983). Carbamazepine also has been used as a maintenance therapy for bipolar illness. Although the numbers are small in all studies, it seems to be a worthwhile second choice for select patients. The average daily dose varies across studies from 400 to 1000 mg, and the average blood level to be achieved varies between 6 and 12 μg/ml. Before beginning, a complete blood count and liver function tests are recommended.

Valproic acid also has been shown to be effective by double-blind, placebo-controlled studies in the treatment of acute mania and as a maintenance drug (McElroy et al., 1992; Prien and Gelenberg, 1989; Prien and Potter, 1990; Gerner and Stanton, 1992). This, too, is a second-line drug that should be used if lithium fails. Either carbamazepine or valproic can be added to lithium, and if the patient improves, the lithium can be discontinued. Depakote (enteric coated divalproex sodium) is a delayed-release tablet that causes less nausea. The usual starting dose is 750 mg per day in a divided dose, raised after 2 days to 1000 mg and after an additional 2 days to 1250 mg. This should achieve a blood level of somewhere between 50 and 120 μg/ml. In treatment with both carbamazepine or valproate, there may be sedation initially, which diminishes over time. Tremor can occur.

Both drugs can produce benign elevation of liver function tests. With valproate, hepatic failure has been reported, but the incidence is low, and it is rarely seen in patients above age 2. Carbamazepine reduces white blood and platelet counts in a dose-related manner, but this does not predict the most dangerous but rare complication of aplastic anemia or agranulocytosis.

These two drugs are pharmacologically different. Carbamazepine induces its own metabolism, causing the blood concentrations to drop so that an upward adjustment of medication is often necessary. Because it induces liver enzymes, it also may make blood levels of average doses of valproate lower if it is started. Reversely, blood levels need to be monitored closely if carbamazepine is discontinued. Other drugs also may have their concentrations reduced during treatment with carbamazepine, notably the neuroleptics and birth control pills.

It is necessary to monitor the blood levels of these antimanic drugs as they are being first administered. After reaching a stable dose, steady-state values can be expected for lithium in 4 days, for carbamazepine in 3 days, and for valproic acid in 2 days. Both drugs can be used together with lithium, neuroleptics, thyroid medication, and tricyclic antidepressants.

Although it is said that these anticonvulsants are particularly useful for mixed or dysphoric mania and for rapid cyclers, the one study that compared lithium to valproate did not sustain this claim (Clothier et al., 1992), and there have not been other double-blind studies to test this hypothesis. In addition, there have been no adequate tests of claims that these drugs are better in rapid cyclers, patients with organic mania, or patients with atypical or a schizoaffective bipolar disorder. These drugs should be used as second choices when a patient is nonresponsive to lithium or when the side effects of lithium are disturbing, particularly polyuria or acne. It is also said that if the patient has psoriasis, one of these drugs is preferable. Side effects will be further discussed later.

McCabe (1976) compared manics treated with ECT with untreated matched controls who were gathered before the introduction of ECT. In a second paper (McCabe and Norris, 1977), a third group of patients treated with chlorpromazine was added. McCabe found that both ECT and chlorpromazine were far superior to no treatment in acute mania when measured by duration of hospitalization, condition at discharge, and social recovery, but there were no significant differences between the two treatments. He did not, however, have a comparison group of patients treated with lithium. Black et al. (1987) retrospectively compared ECT and lithium and found that patients treated with ECT (unilateral or bilateral) had a significantly greater percentage who showed marked improvement, especially with schizoaffective disorder, manic type. Small et al. (1988) compared lithium and bilateral ECT in patients randomized to treatment and found ECT better in the first 8 weeks but no difference in longer outcomes. Finally, Mukherjee and Debsikdar (1992) reported a very favorable outcome in India in 30 manic patients treated with unmodified ECT. It seemed particularly good for dysphoric mania and severe cases. It also should be considered in those patients who have had such frequent episodes that lithium is not efficacious. Many authors have shown that the rapid cycler is a poor responder to most pharmacotherapy, and there have been no studies treating such patients with electrotherapy.

Treatment of the Depressive Episode

This is well covered in Chapter 5 and the last chapter on treatment (Chapter 33) and will not be replicated.

Maintenance Therapy

Everyone agrees (Prien, 1983) that lithium is an effective prophylactic agent. Not only does it significantly decrease the number of manic episodes, but it also decreases the number of depressive episodes. Many believe that this later finding is true because if lithium decreases the number of manic episodes—since it is frequently a biphasic or triphasic illness—it automatically decreases the potential for depressive episodes. Also, the quality of the episodes that do occur is changed (shorter, less severe), and hospitalization is avoided. Because mood swings still occur, however, patients on maintenance lithium need to be followed regularly so that the physician can add a phenothiazine, an antidepressant, or other drugs if necessary. Recent work (Gelenberg et al., 1989) has shown that lithium plasma levels need to be maintained between 0.8 and 1.0 mEq/liter. New data indicate that lithium can be given in a single bedtime dose that can be either lithium carbonate or a sustained-release lithium. Controversy reigns over whether this is better for the kidney; however, most agree that compliance is increased with a single daily dose. The association between relapse and plasma lithium levels is still unclear partially because the half-life of lithium is short and plasma levels fall quickly with missed doses and rise rapidly with extra doses, giving spurious impressions of compliance. Red blood cell lithium may be a better indicator than plasma lithium of brain lithium. However, red blood cell–plasma lithium studies still are inconclusive and should only be used as a research tool.

Carbamazepine and valproic acid are also good maintenance therapies, and here, too, the dose for maintenance is the same as that necessary to treat the acute attack.

Reanalysis of the NIMH collaborative study of bipolar patients (Shapiro et al., 1989) showed that if the patients presented with mania, lithium or lithium plus imipramine was efficacious, whereas if the patient presented with depression, the combination was the best treatment. This speaks against antidepressants causing rapid cycling, an area of unresolved controversy (Wehr and Goodwin, 1987). Others (Maj et al., 1989) also have shown that lithium alone is not the best maintenance for those who present with depression.

As mentioned earlier, all investigators have found that rapid cyclers (four episodes per year) have the poorest lithium response. They relapse quickly. Studies indicate that the more quickly the relapse occurs after beginning maintenance therapy, the more likely a second relapse will occur. The converse is also true; that is, the longer the patient is maintained without relapse, the better is his or her long-term prognosis. Early relapse is not correlated with anything else, such as sex, age, age of onset, or family history (Fleiss et al., 1978; Clayton, 1978). It should be noted that stereotactic tractotomy (Lovett, 1987; Poynton et al., 1988) is still being used for the most resistant cases.

The question of when to start maintenance therapy and how long to continue it is unanswered. Everyone would agree that a patient with two severe manic or depressive episodes within a certain period should be started on maintenance therapy. Some would automatically start every patient on maintenance therapy after the second manic or schizoaffective manic episode. Age, age of onset, severity of episodes, length of episodes, and many other factors must be considered in making a decision.

All recent data (Strober et al., 1990; Suppes et al., 1991) indicated that there is a tremendous risk of recurring episodes (even an increased risk) if lithium maintenance is discontinued, so it is not recommended. As might be expected, those who had been without episodes for the longest period before discontinuation were the least likely to experience relapse.

A 45-year-old successful businessman came for consultation about a decision to stop lithium. He had had several manic episodes in his 20s and finally became well stabilized on lithium. He had discontinued it at age 37 and done well for 3 years. He then developed a severe prolonged depression, during which time he shot himself in the chest in his psychiatrist's office. After his recovery from depression with ECT, he was stabilized on lithium and had done well. Again, he wanted to stop lithium because of weight gain and tremor. It was not encouraged. Now a different maintenance treatment would be recommended, but weight gain is a problem with all except maybe the addition of certain antidepressants.

On maintenance lithium, thyroid and renal functions need to be monitored. With carbamazepine and valproate, blood counts and liver function needs to be monitored. Blood levels should be done one to two times a year.

Jamison and Goodwin (1983) have outlined the therapeutic issue surrounding maintenance therapy with lithium, including patient and physician compliance. O'Connell et al. (1991) also discussed family and psychosocial factors in the outcome of lithium-maintained bipolar patients, as did Clarkin et al. (1990). This is an important point, because when the literature on maintenance therapy is reviewed, there are far more relapses in collaborative treatment studies of multiple impartial investigators than in studies reported by individual therapists treating a cohort of patients. It is definitely a disorder in which therapy and management make a difference.

Side Effects of Antimanic Drugs

The side effects of lithium are numerous and disturbing to the patient but seldom deleterious to his or her health. Many patients complain of tremor while on lithium. This can be treated with 10 mg propranolol, although it need not be given on a regular basis but can be taken by the patient before those situations which might prove embarrassing. Weight gain is a problem. Almost 50 percent of patients gain some weight, and weight gains of up to 30 kg have been reported. Weight gain, for the most part, is due to increased caloric intake and not water weight and needs to be treated with a low-carbohydrate diet. Patients should be warned not to treat an increased thirst with calorie-laden drinks. Some patients develop polyuria and polydipsia, and some patients cannot concentrate their urine. If this occurs, an adjustment in the dose of lithium should be made. Careful studies of long-range effects do not indicate permanent kidney damage (Povlsen et al., 1992). Memory problems, tiredness, and a dulling of senses have been reported to be present while the patient is on lithium, although these also could be symptoms of a low-grade depression. Certain antidepressants or psychostimulants may be helpful. Some patients report diarrhea. A few patients develop hypothyroidism while on lithium. If this occurs, thyroxine needs to be added to the drug regimen. A few develop leukocytosis. Finally, some patients develop alopecia.

Since there are reported prenatal deaths and congenital malformations in babies of women on lithium, lithium should be discontinued, if possible (Kallen and Tandberg, 1983), before pregnancy. Carbamazepine and valproate have associated teratogenic effects and should not be used in women who are trying to become pregnant. Many of the side effects described above are also reported with the anticonvulsants, although supposedly the cognitive dysfunctions are less with valproate. All acute and maintenance dose side effects should be discussed with the patient and the family.

Others (Ahlfors et al., 1981) have cautiously recommended the use of long-acting phenothiazines for maintenance in the patients whose illness is primarily manic.

Other untested drugs used in the acute or maintenance phase include acetazolamide and verapamil (Gerner and Stanton, 1992). Thyroid augmentation (T_3 or T_4) also has been recommended.

There is no doubt that bipolar illness is a devastating and difficult illness to treat, but the gratitude of patients who achieve remission justifies the concern, the patience, the tolerance, the persistence, the imagination, and the good judgment such treatment takes. And remembering the natural history, a certain number of patients will achieve long remissions.

REFERENCES

Abrams R, Taylor MA: Catatonia: A prospective clinical study. Arch Gen Psychiatry 33:579–581, 1976.

Abrams R, Taylor MA: Importance of schizophrenic symptoms in the diagnosis of mania. Am J Psychiatry 138:658–661, 1981.

Abrams R, Taylor MA, Hayman MA, Krishna NR: Unipolar mania revisited. J Affective Disord 1:59–68, 1979.

Ahlfors UG, Baastrup PC, Dencker SJ, et al: Flupenthixol decanoate in recurrent manic-depressive illness: A comparison with lithium. Acta Psychiatr Scand 64:226–237, 1981.

Akiskal HS: The bipolar spectrum: New concepts in classification and diagnosis. In Grinspoon L (ed): Psychiatry Update, vol. 2. Washington, American Psychiatric Press, 1983.

Akiskal HS, Djenderedjian AH, Rosenthal RH, Khani MK: Cyclothymic disorder: Validating criteria for inclusion in the bipolar affective group. Am J Psychiatry 134:1227–1233, 1977.

Akiskal HS, Hirschfeld RMA, Yerevanian BI: The relationship of personality to affective disorders: A critical review. Arch Gen Psychiatry 40:801–810, 1983a.

Akiskal HS, Walker P, Puzantian VR, et al: Bipolar outcome in the course of depressive illness: Phenomenologic, familial, and pharmacologic predictors. J Affective Disord 5:115–128, 1983b.

Akiskal HS, Cassano GB, Musetti L, et al: Psychopathology, temperament, and past course in primary major depressions: 1. Review of evidence for a bipolar spectrum. Psychopathology 22:268–277, 1989.

Ambelas A: Life events and mania: A special relationship? Br J Psychiatry 150:235–240, 1987.

Amsterdam JD, Winokur A, Lucki I, et al: A neuroendocrine test battery in bipolar patients and healthy subjects. Arch Gen Psychiatry 40:515–521, 1983.

Andreasen NC: Thought, language, and communication disorders: I. Clinical assessment, definition of terms, and evaluation of their reliability. Arch Gen Psychiatry 36:1315–1321, 1979a.

Andreasen NC: Thought, language, and communication disorders: II. Diagnostic significance. Arch Gen Psychiatry 36: 1325–1330, 1979b.

Andreasen NJC, Powers PS: Overinclusive thinking in mania and schizophrenia. Br J Psychiatry 125:452–456, 1974.

Angst J: Zur Atiologie und Nosologie endogener depressiver Psychosen. Mongraphien aus desm Gesamtgebiete der Neurologie und Psychiatrie. Berlin, Springer-Verlag, 1966.

Angst J: Discussion. In Angst J (ed): Classification and Prediction of Outcome of Depression. New York, Symposia Medica Hoechst 8, F. K. Schattauer Verlag, 1974.

Angst J: The course of affective disorders: II. Typology of bipolar manic-depressive illness. Arch Psychiatr Nervenkr 226:65–73, 1978.

Angst J: Course of unipolar, depressive, bipolar manic-depressive, and schizoaffective disorders: Results of a progressive longitudinal study. Fortschr Neurol Psychiatr 48:3–30, 1980.

Angst J: The course of affective disorders. Paper prepared for the Consensus Development Conference on Mood Disorders: Pharmacologic Prevention of Recurrences, National Institutes of Health, Bethesda, MD, April 1984.

Angst J. Clayton PJ: Premorbid personality of depressive, bipolar, and schizophrenic patients: With special reference to suicidal issues. Compr Psychiatry 27:511–532, 1986.

Angst J, Felder W, Frey R: The course of unipolar and bipolar affective disorders. In Schou M, Stromgren E (eds): Origin, Prevention and Treatment of Affective Disorders. New York, Academic Press, 1979.

Angst J, Felder W, Frey R, Stassen HH: The course of affective disorders: I. Change of diagnosis of monopolar, unipolar, and bipolar illness. Arch Psychiatr Nervenkr 226:57–64, 1978.

Arnold E, Rudd S, Kirshner H: Manic psychosis following rapid withdrawal from baclofen. Am J Psychiatry 137:1466–1467, 1980.

Arumainayagam M, Kumar A: Manic-depressive psychosis in a mentally handicapped person. Seasonality: A clue to a diagnostic problem. Br J Psychiatry 156:886–889, 1990.

Avery D, Winokur G: Mortality in depressed patients treated with electroconvulsive therapy and antidepressants. Arch Gen Psychiatry 33:1029–1037, 1976.

Avissar S, Schreiber G: The involvement of guanine nucleotide binding proteins in the pathogenesis and treatment of affective disorders. J Biol Psychiatry 31:435–459, 1992.

Ballenger JC, Post RM: Carbamazepine in manic-depressive illness: A new treatment. Am J Psychiatry 137:782–790, 1980.

Banks RE, Aiton JF, Cramb G, Naylor GJ: Incorporation of inositol into the phosphoinositides of lymphoblastoid cell lines established from bipolar manic-depressive patients. J Affective Disord 19:1–8, 1990.

Baron M, Risch N, Mendlewicz J: Differential fertility in bipolar affective illness. J Affective Disord 4:103–112 1982.

Bauer MS, Whybrow PC, Winokur A: Rapid cycling bipolar affective disorder: I. Association with grade I hypothyroidism. Arch Gen Psychiatry 47:427–432, 1990.

Bauer MS, Whybrow PC: Rapid cycling bipolar affective disorder: II. Treatment of refractory rapid cycling with high-dose levothyroxine: A preliminary study. Arch Gen Psychiatry 47: 435–440, 1990.

Bauer MS, Crits-Christoph P, Ball WA, et al: Independent assessment of manic and depressive symptoms by self-rating. Arch Gen Psychiatry 48:807–812, 1991.

Baxter LR, Schwartz JM, Phelps ME, et al: Reduction of prefrontal cortex glucose metabolism common to three types of depression. Arch Gen Psychiatry 46:243–250, 1989.

Bech P, Shapiro RW, Sihm F, et al: Personality in unipolar and bipolar manic-melancholic patients. Acta Psychiatr Scand 62:245–257, 1980.

Bertelsen A, Harvald B, Hauge M: A Danish twin study of manic-depressive disorders. Br J Psychiatry 130:330–351, 1977.

Black DW, Winokur G, Nasrallah A: Treatment of mania: A naturalistic study of electroconvulsive therapy versus lithium in 438 patients. J Clin Psychiatry 48:132–139, 1987.

Black DW, Winokur G, Hulbert J, Nasrallah A: Predictors of immediate response in the treatment of mania: The importance of comorbidity. Biol Psychiatry 24:191–198, 1988a.

Black DW, Winokur G, Bell S, et al: Complicated mania: Comorbidity and immediate outcome in the treatment of mania. Arch Gen Psychiatry 45:232–236, 1988b.

Blacker D, Tsuang MT: Unipolar relatives in bipolar pedigrees: Are they bipolar? Psychiatric Genetics 3:5–16, 1993.

Bouman TK, de Vries J, Koopmans IH: Lithium prophylaxis and interepisode mood: A prospective longitudinal comparison of euthymic bipolars and nonpatient controls. J Affective Disord 24:199–206, 1992.

Boyd JH, Weissman MM: Epidemiology of affective disorders: A reexamination and future directions. Arch Gen Psychiatry 38:1039–1046, 1981.

Brady KT, Lydiard B: Bipolar affective disorder and substance abuse. J Clin Psychopharmacol 12:17S–22S, 1992.

Bratfos O, Haug J: The course of manic-depressive psychosis. Acta Psychiatr Scand 44:89–112, 1968.

Brockington IF, Hillier VF, Francis AF, et al: Definitions of mania: Concordance and prediction of outcome. Am J Psychiatry 140:435–439, 1983.

Brodie HKH, Leff MJ: Bipolar depression—A comparative study of patient characteristics. Am J Psychiatry 127:1086–1090, 1971.

Carlson GA, Goodwin FK: The stages of mania: A longitudinal analysis of the manic episode. Arch Gen Psychiatry 28: 221–228, 1973.

Carney MWP, Chary TKN, Bottiglieri T: Switch mechanism in affective illness and oral S-adenosylmethionine (SAM). Br J Psychiatry 150:724–725, 1987.

Carney PA, Fitzgerald CT, Monaghan CE: Influence of climate on the prevalence of mania. Br J Psychiatry 152:820–823, 1988.

Carroll BJ, Feinberg M, Greden JF, et al: A specific laboratory test for the diagnosis of melancholia: Standardization, validation, and clinical utility. Arch Gen Psychiatry 38:15–22, 1981.

Cassano GB, Akiskal HS, Musetti L, et al: Psychopathology, temperament, and past course in primary major depressions: 2. Toward a redefinition of bipolarity with a new semistructured interview for depression. Psychopathology 22: 278–288, 1989.

Clark AF, Davison K: Mania following head injury: A report of two cases and a review of the literature. Br J Psychiatry 150: 841–844, 1987.

Clarkin JF, Glick ID, Haas GL, et al: A randomized clinical trial of inpatient family intervention: V. Results for affective disorders. J Affective Disord 18:17–28, 1990.

Clayton PJ: Bipolar affective disorder—Techniques and results of treatment. Am J Psychother 32:81–92, 1978.

Clayton PJ: The epidemiology of bipolar affective disorder. Compr Psychiatry 22:31–43, 1981.

Clayton PJ: Schizoaffective disorders. J Nerv Ment Dis 170: 646–650, 1982a.

Clayton PJ: Bereavement. In Paykel ES (ed): Handbook of Affective Disorders. Edinburgh, Churchill Livingstone, 1982b.

Clayton PJ: A further look at secondary depression. In Clayton PJ, Barrett JE (eds): Treatment of Depression: Old Controversies and New Approaches. New York, Raven Press, 1983.

Clayton PJ: Bipolar and schizoaffective disorders. In Tischler G (ed): Diagnosis and Classification in Psychiatry. Cambridge, England, Cambridge University Press, 1987.

Clayton PJ, Pitts FN Jr, Winokur G: Affective disorder: IV. Mania. Compr Psychiatry 6:313–322, 1965.

Clothier J, Swann AC, Freeman T: Dysphoric mania. J Clin Psychopharmacol 12:13S–16S, 1992.

Cohen S, Khan A, Cox G: Demographic and clinical features predictive of recovery in acute mania. J Nerv Ment Dis 177:638–642, 1989.

Cook BL, Shukla S, Hoff AL, Aronson TA: Mania with associated organic factors. Acta Psychiatr Scand 76:674–677, 1987.

Coryell W, Endicott J, Reich T, et al: A family study of bipolar II disorder. Br J Psychiatry 145:49–54, 1984.

Coryell W, Andreasen NC, Endicott J, Keller M: The significance of past mania or hypomania in the course and outcome of major depression. Am J Psychiatry 144:309–315, 1987.

Coryell W, Endicott J, Keller M, et al: Bipolar affective disorder and high achievement: A familial association. Am J Psychiatry 146:983–988, 1989.

Coryell W, Keller M, Lavori P, Endicott J: Affective syndromes, psychotic features, and prognosis: II. Mania. Arch Gen Psychiatry 47:658–662, 1990.

Coryell W, Endicott J, Keller M: Rapidly cycling affective disorder: Demographics, diagnosis, family history, and course. Arch Gen Psychiatry 49:126–131, 1992.

Dewan MJ, Haldipur CV, Lane EE, et al: Bipolar affective disorder: I. Comprehensive quantitative computed tomography. Acta Psychiatr Scand 77:670–676, 1988a.

Dewan MJ, Haldipur CV, Boucher MF, et al: Biopolar affective disorder: II. EEG, neuropsychological, and clinical correlates of CT abnormality. Acta Psychiatr Scand 77:677–682, 1988b.

Dunner DL: Drug treatment of the acute manic episode. In Grinspoon (ed): Psychiatry Update, vol 2. Washington, American Psychiatric Press, 1983.

Emrich HM, Zihl J, Raptis C, Wendl A: Reduced dark-adaptation: An indication of lithium's neuronal action in humans. Am J Psychiatry 147:629–631, 1990.

Extein I, Pottash ALC, Gold MS, Cowdry RW: Using the protirelin test to distinguish mania from schizophrenia. Arch Gen Psychiatry 39:77–81, 1982.

Fein S, McGrath MG: Problems in diagnosing bipolar disorder in catatonic patients. J Clin Psychiatry 51:203–205, 1990.

Fischer M: Twin studies and dual mating studies in defining mania. In Belmaker RH, van Praag, HM (eds): Mania: An Evolving Concept. New York, Spectrum, 1980.

Fleiss JL, Prien RF, Dunner DL, Fieve RR: Actuarial studies of the course of manic-depressive illness. Compr Psychiatry 19: 355–362, 1978.

Garfinkel PE, Stancer HC, Persad E: A comparison of haloperidol, lithium carbonate and their combination in the treatment of mania. J Affective Disord 2:279–288, 1980.

Gelenberg AJ, Kane JM, Keller MB, et al: Comparison of standard and low serum levels of lithium for maintenance treatment of bipolar disorder. N Engl J Med 321:1489–1493, 1989.

Gerner RH, Stanton A: Algorithm for patient management of acute manic states: Lithium, valproate, or carbamazepine? J Clin Psychopharmacol 12:57S–63S, 1992.

Gershon ES, Hamovit J, Guroff JJ, et al: A family study of schizoaffective, bipolar I, bipolar II, unipolar, and normal control probands. Arch Gen Psychiatry 39:1157–1167, 1982.

Gershon ES, Hamovit JH, Guroff JJ, Nurnberger JI: Birth-cohort changes in manic and depressive disorders in relatives of bipolar and schizoaffective patients. Arch Gen Psychiatry 44:314–319, 1987.

Gershon ES, McKnew D, Cytryn L, et al: Diagnoses in school-age children of bipolar affective disorder patients and normal controls. J Affective Disord 8:283–291, 1985.

Giles DE, Rush AJ, Roffwarg HP: Sleep parameters in bipolar I, bipolar II, and unipolar depressions. Biol Psychiatry 21: 1340–1343, 1986.

Glue P: Rapid cycling affective disorders in the mentally retarded. Biol Psychiatry 26:250–256, 1989.

Goodwin FK, Jamison KR: Manic-Depressive Illness. New York, Oxford University Press, 1990.

Gough SP, Cookson IB: Khat-induced schizophreniform psychosis in UK. Lancet 1:455, 1984.

Grof P, Angst J, Haines T: The clinical course of depression: Practical issues. In Angst J (ed): Classification and Prediction of Outcome of Depression. New York, Symposia Medica Hoeschst 8, F.K. Schattauer Verlag, 1974.

Guze SB, Robins E: Suicide and primary affective disorders. Br J Psychiatry 117:437–438, 1970.

Hammen C, Burge D, Burney E, Adrian C: Longitudinal study of diagnoses in children of women with unipolar and bipolar affective disorder. Arch Gen Psychiatry 47:1112–1117, 1990.

Harrow M, Grossman LS, Silverstein ML, Meltzer HY: Thought pathology in manic and schizophrenic patients: Its occurrence at hospital admission and seven weeks later. Arch Gen Psychiatry 39:665–671, 1982.

Harrow M, Goldberg JF, Grossman LS, Meltzer HY: Outcome in manic disorders: A naturalistic follow-up study. Arch Gen Psychiatry 47:665–671, 1990.

Helzer JE, Pryzbeck TR: The co-occurrence of alcoholism with other psychiatric disorders in the general population and its impact on treatment. J Stud Alcohol 49:219–224, 1988.

Hudson JI, Lipinski JF, Frankenburg FR, et al: Electroencephalographic sleep in mania. Arch Gen Psychiatry 45:267–273, 1988.

Jamison KR, Goodwin FK: Psychotherapeutic issues in bipolar illness. In Grinspoon L (ed): Psychiatry Update, vol 2. Washington, American Psychiatric Press, 1983.

Jamison KR, Gerner RH, Hammen C, Padesky C: Clouds and silver linings: Positive experiences associated with primary affective disorders. Am J Psychiatry 137:198–202, 1980.

Jampala VC, Abrams R: Mania secondary to left and right hemisphere damage. Am J Psychiatry 140:1197–1199, 1983.

Janowsky DS, El-Yousef MK, Davis JM: Interpersonal maneuvers of manic patients. Am J Psychiatry 131:250, 1974.

Janowsky, DS, Leff M, Epstein RS: Playing the manic game: Interpersonal maneuvers of the acutely manic patient. Arch Gen Psychiatry 22:252, 1970.

Janowsky DS, Risch SC, Judd LL, et al: Behavioral and neuroendocrine effects of physostigmine in affective disorder patients. In Clayton PJ, Barrett JE (eds): Treatment of Depression: Old Controversies and New Approaches. New York, Raven Press, 1983.

Johnson GF, Hunt G: Suicidal behavior in bipolar manic-depressive patients and their families. Compr Psychiatry 20:159–164, 1979.

Jones BE, Gray BA, Parson EB: Manic-depressive illness among poor urban blacks. Am J Psychiatry 138:654–657, 1981.

Jones BE, Gray BA, Parson EB: Manic-depressive illness among poor urban hispanics. Am J Psychiatry 140:1208–1210, 1983.

Joyce PR: Age of onset in bipolar affective disorder and misdiagnosis as schizophrenia. Psychol Med 14:145–149, 1984.

Joyce PR, Donald RA, Elder PA: Individual differences in plasma cortisol changes during mania and depression. J Affective Disord 12:1–5, 1987.

Joyce PR, Sellman JD, Donald RA, et al: The unipolar-bipolar depressive dichotomy and the relationship between afternoon prolactin and cortisol levels. J Affective Disord 14:189–193, 1988.

Kagan BL, Sultzer DL, Rosenlicht N, Gerner RH: Oral S-adenosylmethionine in depression: A randomized, double-blind, placebo-controlled trial. Am J Psychiatry 147:591–595, 1990.

Kahlbaum K: Die Katatonie oder das Spannugsirresein. Berlin, 1874.

Kallen B, Tandberg A: Lithium and pregnancy: A cohort study on manic-depressive women. Acta Psychiatr Scand 68:134–139, 1983.

Kane J, Struve FA, Weinhold P, Woerner M: Strategy for the study of patients at high risk for tardive dyskinesia. Am J Psychiatry 137:1265–1267, 1980.

Kato T, Shioiri T, Takahashi S, Inubushi T: Measurement of brain phosphoinositide metabolism in bipolar patients using in vivo ^{31}P-MRS. J Affective Disord 22:185–190, 1991.

Keisling R: Underdiagnosis of manic-depressive illness in a hospital unit. Am J Psychiatry 138:672–673, 1981.

Keller MB, Lavori PW, Coryell W, et al: Differential outcome of pure manic, mixed/cycling, and pure depressive episodes in patients with bipolar illness. JAMA 255:3138–3142, 1986.

Kendell RE, Chalmers JC, Platz C: Epidemiology of puerperal psychoses. Br J Psychiatry 150:662–673, 1987.

Khuri R, Akiskal HS: Suicide prevention: The necessity of treating contributory psychiatric disorders. Psychiatr Clin North Am 6:193–207, 1983.

Kishimoto A, Ogura C, Hazama H, Inoue K: Long-term prophylactic effects of carbamazepine in affective disorder. Br J Psychiatry 143:327–331, 1983.

Klein DN, Depue RA: Obsessional personality traits and risk for bipolar affective disorder: An offspring study. J Abnorm Psychol 94:291–297, 1985.

Kraepelin E: Manic-Depressive Insanity and Paranoia. Edinburgh, E&S Livingstone, 1921.

Krauthammer C, Klerman GL: Secondary mania: Manic syndromes associated with antecedent physical illness or drugs. Arch Gen Psychiatry 35:1333–1339, 1978.

Krauthammer C, Klerman GL: The epidemiology of mania. In Shopsin B (ed): Manic Illness. New York, Raven Press, 1979.

Kupfer DJ: Application of the sleep EEG in affective disorders. In Davis JM, Maas JW (eds): The Affective Disorders. Washington, American Psychiatric Press, 1983.

Lange C: Periodiske Depressioner. Copenhagen, 1895.

Larson EW, Richelson E: Organic causes of mania. Mayo Clin Proc 63:906–912, 1988.

Lasch K, Weissman M, Wickramaratne P, Bruce ML: Birth-cohort changes in the rates of mania. Psychiatry Res 33:31–37, 1990.

Leonhard K: Aufteilung der Endogenen Psychosen. Berlin, Akademie Verlag, 1957.

Lewis DA, McChesney C: Tritiated Imipramine Binding to Platelets in Manic Subjects. J Affective Disord 9:207–211, 1985.

Lewis DA, McChesney C: Tritiated imipramine binding distinguishes among subtypes of depression. Arch Gen Psychiatry 42:485–488, 1985.

Lilliker SL: Prevalence of diabetes in a manic-depressive population. Compr Psychiatry 21:270–275, 1980.

London WP, Taylor BM: Bipolar disorders in a forensic setting. Compr Psychiatry 23:33–37, 1982.

Lovett LM: Outcome in bipolar affective disorder after stereotactic tractotomy. Br J Psychiatry 151:113–116, 1987.

Lumry AE, Gottesman II, Tuason VB: MMPI state dependency during the course of bipolar psychosis. Psychiatry Res 7:59–67, 1982.

MacVane JR, Lange JD, Brown WA, Zayat M: Psychological functioning of bipolar manic-depressives in remission. Arch Gen Psychiatry 35:1351–1354, 1978.

Maj M, Pirozzi R, Starace F: Previous pattern of course of the illness as a predictor of response to lithium prophylaxis in bipolar patients. J Affective Disord 17:237–241, 1989.

Martin R, Cloninger C, Guze S, Clayton P: Mortality in a follow-up of 500 psychiatric outpatients: II. Cause-specific mortality. Arch Gen Psychiatry 42:58–66, 1985.

Matussek P, Feil WB: Personality attributes of depressive patients: Results of group comparisons. Arch Gen Psychiatry 40:783–790, 1983.

McCabe MS: ECT in the treatment of mania: A controlled study. Am J Psychiatry 133:688, 1976.

McCabe MS, Norris B: ECT versus chlorpromazine in mania. Biol Psychiatry 12:245, 1977.

McCormick RA, Russo AM, Ramirez LF, Taber JI: Affective disorders among pathological gamblers seeking treatment. Am J Psychiatry 141:215–218, 1984.

McElroy SL, Keck PE Jr, Pope HG Jr, Hudson JI: Valproate in the treatment of bipolar disorder: Literature review of clinical guidelines. J Clin Psychopharmacol 12:42S–52S, 1992.

McLaughlin M: Bipolar affective disorder in Down's syndrome. Br J Psychiatry 151:116–117, 1987.

Meltzer HY, Arora RC, Tricou BJ, Fang VS: Serotonin uptake in blood platelets and the dexamethasone suppression test in depressed patients. Psychiatry Res 8:41–47, 1983.

Mendlewicz J, Rainer JD: Adoption study supporting genetic transmission in manic-depressive illness. Nature 268:327–329, 1977.

Menninger K, Mayman M, Pruyser P: The Vital Balance: The Life Process in Mental Health and Illness. New York, Penguin Books, 1977.

Merikangas KR: Assortative mating for psychiatric disorders and psychological traits. Arch Gen Psychiatry 39:1173–1180, 1982.

Merikangas KR, Bromet EJ, Spiker DG: Assortative mating, social adjustment, and course of illness in primary affective disorder. Arch Gen Psychiatry 40:795–800, 1983.

Mitchell P, Parker G, Jamieson K, et al: Are there differences between bipolar and unipolar melancholia? J Affective Disord 25:97–106, 1992.

Morrison JR: Suicide in a psychiatric practice population. J Clin Psychiatry 43:348–352, 1982.

Mukherjee S, Debsikdar V: Unmodified electroconvulsive therapy of acute mania: A retrospective naturalistic study. Convulsive Ther 8:5–11, 1992.

Myers JK, Weissman MM, Tischler GL, et al: Six-month prevalence of psychiatric disorders in three communities: 1980–1982. Arch Gen Psychiatry 41:959–967, 1984.

Nolen WA: Carbamazepine, a possible adjunct or alternative to lithium in bipolar disorder. Acta Psychiatr Scand 67:218–225, 1983.

Nurnberger JI, Gershon ES: Genetics. In Paykel ES (ed): Handbook of Affective Disorders. Edinburgh, Churchill Livingstone, 1982.

Nurnberger J, Roose SP, Dunner DL, Fieve RR: Unipolar mania: A distinct clinical entity? Am J Psychiatry 136:1420–1423, 1979.

O'Connell RA, Mayo JA, Flatow L, et al: Outcome of bipolar disorder on long-term treatment with lithium. Br J Psychiatry 159:123–129, 1991.

Olfson M: An old treatment for mania. Lancet 2:221–222, 1987.

Pederson A, Poort R, Schou H: Periodical depression as an independent nosological entity. Acta Psychiatr Neurol 23:285–319, 1947.

Perris C: A study of bipolar (manic depressive) and unipolar recurrent depressive psychoses. Acta Psychiatr Scand 42:1–188, 1966 (suppl 194).

Perris C: The separation of bipolar (manic depressive) from unipolar recurrent depressive psychoses. Behav Neuropsychiatry 1:17–24, 1969.

Petterson U: Manic-depressive illness: A clinical, social and genetic study. Acta Psychiatr Scand (Suppl) 269, 1977.

Petty F, Sherman AD: Plasma GABA levels in psychiatric illness. J Affective Disord 6:131–138, 1984.

Pfohl B, Vasquez N, Nasrallah H: Unipolar vs. bipolar mania: A review of 247 patients. Br J Psychiatry 141:453–458, 1982.

Pope HG Jr, Lipinski JF Jr: Diagnosis in schizophrenia and manic depressive illness: A reassessment of the specificity of "schizophrenic" symptoms in the light of current research. Arch Gen Psychiatry 35:811–828, 1978.

Pope HG Jr, McElroy SL, Satlin A, et al: Head injury, bipolar disorder, and response to Valproate. Compr Psychiatry 29:34–38, 1988.

Post RM: Editorial. Use of the anticonvulsant carbamazepine in primary and secondary affective illness: Clinical and theoretical implications. Psychol Med 12:701–704, 1982.

Post RM, Uhde TW, Ballenger JC, Squillace KM: Prophylactic efficacy of carbamazepine in manic-depressive illness. Am J Psychiatry 140:1602–1604, 1983.

Post RM, Weiss SRB, Chuang D: Mechanisms of action of anticonvulsants in affective disorders: Comparisons with lithium. J Clin Psychopharmacol 12:23S–35S, 1992.

Post RM, Rubinow DR, Uhde TW, et al: Dysphoric mania: Clinical and biological correlates. Arch Gen Psychiatry 46:353–358, 1989.

Povlsen UJ, Hetmar O, Ladefoged J, Bolwig TG: Kidney functioning during lithium treatment: A prospective study of patients treated with lithium for up to ten years. Acta Psychiatr Scand 85:56–60, 1992.

Poynton A, Bridges PK, Bartlett JR: Resistant bipolar affective disorder treated by stereotactic subcaudate tractotomy. Br J Psychiatry 152:354–358, 1988.

Prien RF: Long-term prophylactic pharmacologic treatment of bipolar illness. In Grinspoon L (ed): Psychiatry Update, vol 2. Washington, American Psychiatric Press, 1983.

Prien RF, Gelenberg AJ: Alternatives to lithium for preventive treatment of bipolar disorder. Am J Psychiatry 146:840–848, 1989.

Prien RF, Potter WZ: NIMH workshop report on treatment of bipolar disorder. Psychopharmacol Bull 26:409–427, 1990.

Prien RF, Himmelhoch JM, Kupfer DJ: Treatment of mixed mania. J Affective Disord 15:9–15, 1988.

Pritz WF, Mitterauer BJ: Bipolar mood disorders: An affected sibling study: I. Genetic background and course of illness. Psychopathology 17:67–79, 1984.

Rice JP, McDonald-Scott P, Endicott J, et al: The stability of diagnosis with an application to bipolar II disorder. Psychiatry Res 19:285–296, 1986.

Rice J, Reich T, Andreasen NC, et al: The familial transmission of bipolar illness. Arch Gen Psychiatry 44:441–447, 1987.

Robbins TW, Sahakian BJ: Animal models of mania. In Belmaker RH, van Praag HM (eds): Mania: An Evolving Concept. New York, Spectrum, 1980.

Robins LN, Helzer JE, Weissman M, et al: Lifetime prevalence of specific psychiatric disorders in three sites. Arch Gen Psychiatry 41:949–958, 1984.

Rosenbaum KM, Niven RG, Hanson HP, Swanson DW: Tardive dyskinesia: Relationship with primary affective disorder. Dis Nerv Syst 38:423–426, 1977.

Rosenthal NE, Wehr TA: Chronobiology: Seasonal affective disorders. Psychiatr Ann 17:670–674, 1987.

Rosenthal NE, Sack DA, Gillin JC, et al: Seasonal affective disorder: A description of the syndrome and preliminary findings with light therapy. Arch Gen Psychiatry 41:72–80, 1984.

Rubin EH: Aging and mania. Psychiatr Dev 4:329–337, 1988.

Rush M, Diamond F, Alpert M: Depression as a risk factor in tardive dyskinesia. Biol Psychiatry 17:387–392, 1982.

Sayer HK, Marshall S, Mellsop GW: Mania and seasonality in the southern hemisphere. J Affective Disord 23:151–156, 1991.

Schou HI: La depression psychique. Acta Psychiatr Neurol 2:345–353, 1927.

Secunda SK, Swann A, Katz MM, et al: Diagnosis and treatment of mixed mania. Am J Psychiatry 144:96–98, 1987.

Sedler MJ: Falret's discovery: The origin of the concept of bipolar affective illness. Am J Psychiatry 140:1127–1133, 1983.

Shapiro DR, Quitkin FM, Fleiss JL: Response to maintenance therapy in bipolar illness: Effect of index episode. Arch Gen Psychiatry 46:401–405, 1989.

Shukla S, Cook BL, Mukherjee S, et al: Mania following head trauma. Am J Psychiatry 144:93–96, 1987.

Shulman K, Post F: Bipolar affective disorder in old age. Br J Psychiatry 136:26–32, 1980.

Silverskiöld P, Risberg J: Regional cerebral blood flow in depression and mania. Arch Gen Psychiatry 46:253–259, 1989.

Sitaram N: Faster cholinergic REM sleep induction as a possible trait marker of affective illness. In Davis JM, Maas JW (eds): The Affective Disorders. Washington, American Psychiatric Press, 1983.

Small JG, Klapper MH, Kellams JJ, et al: Electroconvulsive treatment compared with lithium in the management of manic states. Arch Gen Psychiatry 45:727–732, 1988.

Starkstein SE, Boston JD, Robinson RG: Mechanisms of mania after brain injury: 12 case reports and review of the literature. J Nerv Ment Dis 176:87–100, 1988.

Stokes PE, Stoll PM, Koslow SH, et al: Pretreatment DST and hypothalamic-pituitary-adrenocortical function in depressed patients and comparison groups: A multicenter study. Arch Gen Psychiatry 41:257–267, 1984.

Stone K: Mania in the elderly. Br J Psychiatry 155:220–224, 1989.

Strober M, Morrell W, Lampert C, Burroughs J: Relapse following discontinuation of lithium maintenance therapy in adolescents with bipolar illness: A naturalistic study. Am J Psychiatry 147:457–461, 1990.

Suppes T, Baldessarini RJ, Faedda GL, Tohen M: Risk of recurrence following discontinuation of lithium treatment in bipolar disorder. Arch Gen Psychiatry 48:1082–1088, 1991.

Swann AC, Secunda S, Davis JM, et al: CSF monoamine metabolites in mania. Am J Psychiatry 140:396–400, 1983.

Targum SD, Dibble ED, Davenport YB, Gershon ES: The family attitudes questionnaire: Patients' and spouses' views of bipolar illness. Arch Gen Psychiatry 38:562–568, 1981.

Tatetsu S: Methamphetamine psychosis. Folia Psychiatr Neurol Jpn 17 (suppl 7):377–380, 1963.

Tatetsu S: Methamphetamine psychosis. In Ellinwood EH, Cohen S (eds): Current Concepts on Amphetamine Abuse (DHEW publ no HSM 72-9085). Washington, 1972, pp 159–161.

Thompson C, Stinson D, Smith A: Seasonal affective disorder and season-dependent abnormalities of melatonin suppression by light. Lancet 336:703–706, 1990.

Tohen M, Waternaux CM, Tsuang MT: Outcome in mania. A 4-year prospective follow-up of 75 patients utilizing survival analysis. Arch Gen Psychiatry 47:1106–1111, 1990a.

Tohen M, Waternaux CM, Tsuang MT, Hunt AT: Four-year follow-up of twenty-four first episode manic patients. J Affective Disord 19:79–86, 1990b.

Tsuang MT: Suicide in schizophrenics, manics, depressives, and surgical controls. Arch Gen Psychiatry 35:153–155, 1978.

Tsuang MT, Woolson RF: Mortality in patients with schizophrenia, mania, depression and surgical conditions. Br J Psychiatry 130:162–166, 1977.

Waters B, Marchenko I, Abrams N, et al: Assortative mating for major affective disorder. J Affective Disord 5:9–17, 1983.

Weeke A, Juel K, Vaeth M: Cardiovascular death and manic-depressive psychosis. J Affective Disord 13:287–292, 1987.

Wehr TA, Goodwin FK: Can antidepressants cause mania and worsen the course of affective illness? Am J Psychiatry 144:1403–1411, 1987.

Wehr TA, Sack DA: Sleep disruption: A treatment for depression and a cause of mania. Psychiatr Ann 17:654–663, 1987.

Wehr TA, Sack DA, Rosenthal NE: Sleep reduction as a final common pathway in the genesis of mania. Am J Psychiatry 144:201–204, 1987.

Weissman MM, Warner V, John K, et al: Delusional depression and bipolar spectrum: Evidence for a possible association from a family study of children. Neuropsychopharmacology 1:257–264, 1988.

Welner A, Welner Z, Leonard MA: Bipolar manic-depressive disorder: A reassessment of course and outcome. Compr Psychiatry 18:327–332, 1977.

Winokur G: The Iowa 500: Heterogeneity and course in manic-depressive illness (bipolar). Compr Psychiatry 16:125–131, 1975.

Winokur G: Mania and depression: Family studies and genetics in relation to treatment. In Lipton MA, DiMascio A, Killam KF (eds): Psychopharmacology: A Generation of Progress. New York, Raven Press, 1978.

Winokur G, Wesner R: From unipolar depression to bipolar illness: 29 who changed. Acta Psychiatr Scand 76:59–63, 1987.

Winokur G, Clayton PJ, Reich T: Manic depressive illness. St. Louis, Mosby, 1969.

Woodruff RA Jr, Clayton PJ, Guze SB: Suicide attempts and psychiatric diagnosis. Dis Nerv Syst 33:617–621, 1972.

Wu JC, Bunney WE: The biological basis of an antidepressant response to sleep deprivation and relapse: Review and hypothesis. Am J Psychiatry 147:14–21, 1990.

Yassa R, Nair NPV, Iskandar H: Late-onset bipolar disorder. Psychiatr Clin North Am 11:117–131, 1988.

Yates WR, Wallace R: Cardiovascular risk factors in affective disorder. J Affective Disord 12:129–134, 1987.

Young MA, Abrams R, Taylor MA, Meltzer HY: Establishing diagnostic criteria for mania. J Nerv Ment Dis 171:676–682, 1983.

Young RC, Klerman GL: Mania in late life: Focus on age at onset. Am J Psychiatry 149:867–876, 1992.

Young RC, Nysewander RW, Schreiber MT: Mania ratings at discharge from hospital: A follow-up (brief communication). J Nerv Ment Dis 170:638–639, 1982.

Zetin M, Potkin S, Urbanchek M: Melatonin in depression. Psychiatr Ann 17:676–681, 1987.

CHAPTER 5

Unipolar Depression

GEORGE WINOKUR

DEFINITION

Unipolar depression is a depressive syndrome seen in patients who have never suffered a mania. A depressive syndrome is characterized by a low mood and such symptoms as loss of interest and energy, anorexia, weight change, sleep disturbance, psychomotor retardation, agitation, feelings of unworthiness, self-condemnation, trouble concentrating, and suicidal ideation. The DSM-IIIR classification includes major depression and dysthymic disorder as well as adjustment disorders with depressed mood. Other depressive disorder codes are organic mood disorder, depressed type, and uncomplicated bereavement. New classifications such as the *Diagnostic and Statistical Manual of Mental Disorders*, fourth edition (DSM-IV) and the *International Classification of Diseases* (ICD-10) follow this general guideline.

EPIDEMIOLOGY

Occasionally unpleasant circumstances exist in the lives of most people. A barely perceptible nod from a previously friendly boss or professor or an error-ridden game for a person who has previously been an extremely good athlete who may produce unhappiness or "depression." Usually this state of mind in these cases is transient and the person continues to function in a perfectly ordinary fashion. In unipolar depression, however, a person should be considered different from his or her usual self and have some degree of functional incapacity. It is possible for a person to have a depression and continue to function in an ordinary fashion, but this is unusual. Social incapacity and suicidal ideas often bring a person to seek help.

Unipolar depression is relatively common and occurs 8 times as frequently as bipolar illness and possibly 12 times as frequently as incapacitating schizophrenia. The epidemiology of depression has been studied throughout the world, and Table 5-1 lists three separate studies that present the lifetime expectancy for a depression in people selected from a population. Robins et al. (1984) have published data on lifetime prevalence, the proportion of persons in the population who have experienced a disorder up to the date of assessment. The lifetime prevalence for a major depressive episode varies between 3.7 and 6.7 percent over three catchment areas. The lifetime prevalence for dysthymia (minor depressive disorder) varies between 2.1 and 3.8 percent. This may be contrasted with the lifetime prevalence for a manic episode, which is between 0.6 and 1.1 percent, a considerably lower figure than what is seen for unipolar depression.

In Table 5-1, the proportions of the population that developed depression are dependent on the individual study. The reasons are explainable. The study in Iowa dealt with a population of relatives of psychiatrically well surgical patients (Tsuang et al., 1984). Thus the relatives presumably were not related to anybody who had a psychiatric illness. Even though this is true, however, it is notable that the 8.1 percent in this "purified" population is similar to the Robins et al. study when one adds major depressive episodes to the dysthymic diagnoses. The New Haven and Iceland population studies were done out in the community, and no effort was made to evaluate the people who came from psychiatrically well families (Weisman and Meyers, 1978; Helgason, 1979). Many studies show that psychiatric illnesses run in families; therefore, one would expect that the population from the Iowa study would contain less illness than the other two

TABLE 5-1. *Lifetime Illness in Control Populations*

| Study | Risk for depression (%) | | |
	MALES	FEMALES	TOTAL
Iowa	3.8	11.9	8.1
New Haven	12.3	25.8	18.0
Iceland	9.4	14.4	12.0

Source: Adapted from Winokur, 1991.

populations. The fact that the finding is comparable with the recent large study of Robins et al. suggests that the effect of attempting to "purify" a population may not be very successful. There are other differences in the epidemiologic studies. In the Iowa population, the person had to be ill for at least 4 weeks to qualify for a diagnosis, whereas a much shorter time constraint was used in the New Haven study. Also, different methods were used in obtaining populations.

All studies show that females are more likely to be affected with unipolar depression than are males. All these studies take into account both hospitalized and nonhospitalized patients in the population. In the Iceland study, about 48 percent of the males and 37 percent of the females with major affective disorders (bipolar plus unipolar) were never admitted to any hospital. Although some may have escaped medical notice, many were seen by family practitioners.

Annual incidence studies in unipolar depression are numerous; these vary between 247 and 7800 cases per 100,000 per year. In a series of incidence studies, between 82 and 201 men and between 320 and 500 women per 100,000 per year began receiving treatment for depression (Boyd and Weisman, 1981).

Studies in various cultures and in various countries suggest that unipolar depression is ubiquitous. There may be some changes in the symptom pictures between cultures, but the general overall syndrome exists and is recognized. Differences in frequency between various cultures suggest various etiologic factors, both environment and genetic.

The contributions of genetic epidemiology deserve mention. It is possible that some known genetic disorders are related to unipolar depression (Swift et al., 1991). As an example, Wolfram syndrome is an autosomal recessive neurodegenerative syndrome in which one-quarter of the affected homozygous people have psychiatric symptoms leading to suicide or psychiatric hospitalizations. Likewise, their relatives have an increased incidence of these kinds of findings. A depression was found in large degree in these relatives. Thus epidemiologic studies comparing relatives and patients with known genetic diseases on the variable of depression compared with controls might produce some interesting clues as to the pathophysiology and etiology of depression.

CLINICAL PICTURE

Although a depressive syndrome may be chronic, the person presenting himself to the hospital or clinic usually complains of an acute change. In a sense, the patient considers himself changed in some way from his usual state. A good question to ask a patient, then, would be whether he is different from what he is usually like.

A person may be diagnosed as depressed if he describes his state of mind as being dysphoric and uses such terms as *feeling depressed, sad, blue, despondent, hopeless, irritable, down in the dumps, fearful, worried, discouraged, and worthless.* Having described himself in this fashion, other symptoms are necessary. Common symptoms in depression include poor appetite or weight loss, difficulty in sleeping, energy loss or fatigability, agitation or retardation, loss of interest in usual activities, as well as loss of interest in sexual matters, feelings of worthlessness or guilt, and complaints of not being able to think or concentrate. Recurrent thoughts of death or suicidal ideas also are presented by depressive patients (Feighner et al., 1972). Such symptoms are, in part, seen in patients who have experienced personal tragedies. For example, bereavement may produce a syndrome that resembles depression (Clayton et al., 1974). This is, in a sense, a normal reactive depression. Such symptoms as suicidal thoughts, retardation, and feelings of worthlessness usually are not seen in a depression associated with grief. A person ordinarily gets over such a depression in a short period of time, but occasionally, it is prolonged. Other circumstances also may produce for a short period a mental state that fulfills a depressive syndrome. Thus a parent whose child suffered an injury might show depression, but this would not be considered a depressive illness. Also, such an episode would be short-lived. A time constraint is needed on the diagnosis of depression, and various amounts of time have been used. A conservative time constraint would be the presence of depressive symptoms for 1 month continuously.

Many studies have systematically evaluated the clinical status of depressed patients. Table 5-2 presents the common symptoms in 100 unipolar depressive patients. Although there were twice as many females in this group of 100 as males, there were no meaningful differences between the sexes regarding the frequency of symptoms (Baker et al., 1971).

Some of the symptoms deserve special comment. When a patient complains of impaired concentration, it is quite possible that his boss or spouse or close friends will not note any difficulty in his thinking. However, the patient himself believes that he is neither tracking nor concentrating as well as he did before he became depressed. The differences are subtle, and studies have shown that the difficulties in thinking are demonstrable on psychological tests (Stromgren, 1977).

TABLE 5-2. *Symptoms of Index Episode Occurring in More Than 50 Percent of Patients*

Symptoms	No. and percentage of patients (n = 100)
Reduced energy level	97
Impaired concentration	84
Anorexia	80
Initial insomnia	77
Loss of interest	77
Difficulty starting activities	76
Worry more than usual	69
Subjective agitation	67
Slowed thinking	67
Difficulty with decision making	67
Terminal insomnia	65
Suicide ideation or plans	63
Weight loss	61
Tearfulness	61
Movements slowed (subjective perception)	60
Increased irritability	60
Feels will never get well	56

Source: Adapted from Baker et al., 1971.

TABLE 5-3. *Symptoms of Index Episode Occurring in 10 to 50 Percent of Patients*

Symptoms	No. and percentage of patients (n = 100)
Diurnal variation	46
Difficulty finishing activities once started	46
Prominent self-pity	45
Inability to cry	44
Constipation	43
Impaired expression of emotions	42
Ruminations of worthlessness	38
Decreased libido	36
Anxiety attacks	36
Difficulty doing activities once started	35
Ruminations of guilt	32
Complains more than usual	28
Any type of delusion	27
Phobias during depression only	27
Multiple somatic symptoms during depression only	25
Communication of suicidal ideas, plans, or attempts	22
Place major blame for illness on others	19
At least one depressive delusion	16
Death wishes without suicidal ideation	16
Suicide attempts	15
Other delusions	14
Obsessions during depression only	14
Depersonalization and derealization	13
Ruminations of sinfulness	12

Decision making is often impaired in depressive patients. This creates some difficulty in dealing with such patients. As an example, a patient who had shot himself through the mouth and lived to tell the tale appeared with his wife in the office of a psychiatrist after medical treatment for the effects of the gunshot wound. This was a few months after the suicide attempt, and he was still as depressed as he had been before. When he was told that he would have to come into the hospital for treatment of his depressive illness, he was unable to make up his mind to do this. Instead, he vacillated back and forth over the idea of what would be best for him. This kind of uncertainty is fairly typical of patients who have unipolar depression, although usually the circumstances are not as dramatic as in the case described.

The sleep difficulties in unipolar depression are characteristic of the disorder. Although some patients complain of having trouble getting to sleep, the hallmark symptom is terminal insomnia. The individual says that he can fall asleep all right but wakes after a few hours and cannot get back to sleep, or he complains of getting up several hours earlier in the morning than is his usual habit and not being able to get back to sleep. This is *terminal insomnia* or *early-morning awakening*. This symptom is common also in bereavement as well as in depressed patients who are very anxious. Often, during these periods of wakefulness, the patient will ruminate over past guilt and difficulties in his life.

Table 5-3 shows symptoms that occur often during a depressive episode but not in the majority of patients. Most are seen equally in males and in females, but females are more than twice as likely to complain of inability to cry, and males are twice as likely to complain of multiple somatic symptoms during the depressive illness only. Some of the symptoms deserve special note. *Diurnal variation* describes mood change over the course of the day. A person who has this symptom awakens in the morning and feels quite depressed or agitated or inert. As the day wears on, he or she improves, sometimes almost to normality. There are probably no pathognomonic symptoms of depressive illness, but diurnal variation comes as close to being specific as any. *Anxiety attacks* occur frequently during a depressive episode. In unipolar depression these are associated only with the episode itself. Unlike in other illnesses (agoraphobia, panic disorder), the anxiety attack is not present on a long-term or chronic basis. Often a depressive patient is *delusional*. Delusions seen in depressives are of two types. The first comprises depressive delusions, which include delusions of guilt, sinfulness, worthlessness, and failure. A man who cheated on his income tax in 1927 entered the hospital in 1957. He was guilty about having cheated and believed that he was being persecuted by the government because of this. He thought that this was appropriate because he had been such a dishonest person. This type of depressive delusion is called a *mood-congruent delusion* because it is consistent with a state of mind of the depressed individual. Other types of delusions seen in depression are *mood-incongruent delusions*, which have nothing to do with feelings of guilt or worthlessness. It is important to recognize that even in the presence of mood-incongruent delusions and hallucinations, a diagnosis of unipolar depression may be made as long as the individual shows the appropriate symptom picture, a relatively acute onset, and no suggestion of another illness (e.g., schizophrenia, alcoholism, organic brain syndrome).

Table 5-4 shows mental status signs exhibited by patients being admitted to the hospital. What is notable is that almost half the patients show no clear signs of the illness. Formal thought disorder in the mental status consists of blocking or circumstantiality. No patient in this group shows tangentiality or loosening of associations. Again, males and females are not different from each other in showing these signs, although there is a slight increase in retardation of movements and speech in men.

Some differences in the clinical picture are related to other variables. Patients who are admitted after having had previous episodes are different from those who are admitted with a first episode. First-episode patients are more likely to complain of subjective agitation and tearfulness and less likely to complain of constipation, inability to cry, inability to express emotions, trouble making decisions, and slowed thinking. Perhaps some of the most striking clinical differences are seen in young (under 40) patients when they are compared with older depressive patients. Agitation is more common in the older group, and retardation is more common in the younger group (Winokur et al., 1973).

Finally, some statement should be made about the concept of the *endogenous* depression (synonymous with *melancholia*). Such a depression is considered to be physiologic, or somatic, or coming from within the body. It is ordinarily differentiated from *neurotic-reactive* depressions, which are presumed to be the result of difficult life stresses. Symptoms that are especially seen in endogenous depressions include diurnal variation, delusions, early-morning awakening, marked guilt, hopeless-

ness, and hallucinations. Symptoms that are seen in the neurotic-reactive type of unipolar depression include initial insomnia, emotional lability, blaming others, many somatic complaints, and a stormy lifestyle with difficulties in marriage, school, and job (Kay et al., 1971). At least one study (Parker et al., 1990) suggests that mental status signs are better than symptoms in separating melancholia from other depressions. Psychomotor retardation and agitation as expressed in face, posture, speech, and movement were found particularly effective in defining melancholia phenomenologically. In endogenous depression, the concept has to do with a specific definable illness; in neurotic-reactive depression, the concept is related to a set of symptoms that are either a response to life events or a lifestyle that remains unchanged over years. There is an overlap of symptoms between the endogenous and the neurotic-reactive (Kendell, 1968). Nevertheless, it is conceivable that these concepts do identify a certain group of patients at one or the other end of a continuum. The separation into two diagnoses, endogenous versus neurotic-reactive, may have some usefulness in predicting course as well as in prescribing treatment.

The clinical picture is composed of depressive affect and a number of related symptoms. Some patients, however, simply have the affect and relatively few or even none of the related symptoms. This clinical presentation suggests a depressive personality. Patients with a chronic depressive personality look on the dark side of life and view circumstances with extreme pessimism. Often such people are mistrustful and seem to have little capacity for pleasure. They are excessively critical and full of derogatory comments about themselves and their friends. Minor defeats lead them to conclude that their entire life has been a failure. An innocent or insignificant comment causes them to feel slighted. They have been described as being unaggressive, kindly people who are vulnerable or, alternatively, as ill-humored people who are surly, bitter, suspicious, and irritable. Because they have received what they consider to be the short end of the stick, they are often malicious and jealous of other people's success (Schneider, 1959). On occasion they will go from showing a depressive personality to being incapacitated with the full assortment of symptoms. The relationship of the depressive personality to the clear and unequivocal depressive syndrome with incapacitation is difficult to determine. Some believe that these depressive personalities are a minor form of a depressive illness; others believe that they exist independently of major depressive syndromes. A relationship of the depressive personality either with significant incapacitating depressive syndromes or with a presence of major depressive illness in the family would lead one to believe that the depressive personality is, in fact, a kind of *forme fruste* of unipolar depressive illness.

TABLE 5-4. *Mental Status Findings*

Findings	No. and percentage of patients ($n = 100$)
Mental status without evidence of agitation, retardation, or formal thought disorder	45
Agitation	30
Psychomotor retardation	19
Formal thought disorder	8
Both agitation and retardation	6

SOME ILLUSTRATIVE CASES

As is the case with other illnesses in medicine, certain behaviors are rather typical. Take the case of a man who found it unpleasant to stand in front of a classroom teaching because he felt "insignificant and unlearned." He had trouble making up his mind to get up in the morning or to eat breakfast or to go to his classes for his teaching chores. He couldn't decide whether he should sleep through the day. As time passed, he stayed in bed all the time, "lying rigidly in the fetal position facing the wall." He shut out the light from his room, spending his days in the blackened room "with the blankets pulled over his head." It was not possible to get him to move. In addition, he had anxiety attacks with "choking and suffocation." Over time, he showed some improvement and became more mobile. This is a typical picture of a severe and retarded depression, and it was a state suffered by Samuel Beckett, who went on to win the Nobel Prize for literature (Bair, 1990). Following are some cases of people less famous but not all that dissimilar.

Case History 1

Present Illness: Mrs. A., aged 40, was admitted in 1939. Her illness had begun 9 months earlier, when she expressed "queer ideas." She wrote letters to her minister and others stating that if anything happened to her, somebody should take care of her child. She worried about finances, started to sleep poorly, and lost her job taking care of children. She had ideas of reference and believed that people were talking about her. She became more irritable and complained of pain in the abdomen, which led her to the hospital.

At admission, her mental status was striking. She appeared weak and tired. Her facial expression was sad and downcast. On occasion she would moan and whimper to herself. She refused to eat or drink, saying that she was unable to swallow. At times she would become excited and squirm around in bed. Her stream of talk was such that she often would not answer questions, and if she did, she would answer them in a weak voice. She cried and at other times would become agitated. She expressed no delusions or hallucinations on questioning. Her sensorium was such that she fluctuated in and out of orientation.

Past History: In 1917, 22 years before, she had had a nervous breakdown similar to the present illness. At that time she was mute, restless, wept, picked at her clothing, and had to be cared for. This condition cleared up in 6 months, but she was left more irritable than before. In 1922 she married for economic reasons, and in 1924 her first child was stillborn after a difficult labor. In 1925 and 1929 she had normal pregnancies, and in 1931 she had a gastroenterostomy performed for a perforated gastric ulcer.

Mrs. A. was a nervous person, irritable, given to talking a lot about inconsequential things. She had few friends. She took disappointments hard. She worked conscientiously. Her heterosexual interest was minimal, and she married her husband only for economic advantages, which, unhappily, did not ensue.

As regards family history of psychiatric disease, her father was quite possibly a chronic alcoholic.

Course of Illness. Mrs. A. had a similar illness at age 18, from which she recovered. In 1939 (index admission) she was admitted to a psychiatric hospital because of weakness, emaciation, weight loss, and confused behavior. She was tube fed and gained 10 pounds. She then felt considerably stronger. However, she became more depressed and had poor contact with other people. With sedative medication, she improved to the point where she could eat by herself, and she talked more. She was not well, however, and was transferred to a state hospital.

Case History 2

Mrs. A.F. was admitted in June 1939 to a psychiatric hospital. Her illness started around February 1939, when she learned that a foster brother had absconded with money from a company for which he was working. She cried a great deal about this and stated that it was her own fault. She believed this because her foster brother had had behavior problems and she had not given him adequate support. She gave voice to a number of self-deprecatory ideas and self-accusations.

At admission to the hospital, her attitude and general behavior indicated profound depression, mostly associated with her guilt about her interaction with her foster brother. She was somewhat agitated and expressed suicidal ideas on occasion. She was uncomfortable with her attitude toward religion, and she inquired whether she was a bad person because of her failure to believe implicitly in the Bible and in God. She also wondered whether she had started her children off wrong and blamed herself for preventing her husband from attending theology school. Because of the persistence of these self-condemnatory symptoms, she was admitted to the hospital.

Her mental status was replete with many ideas of self-accusation and many self-deprecatory delusions. She protested vehemently that all her troubles were of her own making because she was constantly self-centered. She conceived of herself as a "congenital defective" who should expect no more than she was getting. Her outlook was dismal, and she stated that she would end her days in an "asylum with the most violent type of mental disease which I justly deserve because I am such a despicable character."

Past History: Mrs. A.F. was always considered a reactive kind of a person and might have had a previous depression 4 years earlier, when her husband lost his job. At this point she worried over the circumstances, was depressed, blamed herself for coming to the city in which she lived, and seemed absentminded and preoccupied. After several months, she stopped worrying and returned to normal.

She was talented. She graduated from college and was described as an energetic person who enjoyed social activities. As a young child, she was fearful of dogs and other animals, but this phobia did not persist.

Course of Illness: Mrs. A. F. remained in the hospital for about 2 months and continued profoundly depressed throughout her hospitalization. She was started on Metrazol convulsive therapy (the predecessor of electroconvulsive therapy) and showed dramatic improvement after the second treatment. Although she slipped back somewhat, she was discharged less depressed than on admission. After being out of the hospital for one day, she was readmitted. There was an exacerbation of depressive affect and self-deprecatory ideas. She believed that she would spend the rest of her days in a madhouse. She was given another series of Metrazol therapy treatments (this time seven; the first time five). There was a marked improvement in her mood after the first treatment, and this affective improvement was maintained. Interestingly, there was an attempt to determine whether there was any organic impairment from the Metrazol treatments, and it was noted that she did better on an IQ test (I.Q. 134) than she did at the time of her first hospital admission (I.Q. 124). She was discharged as well after 3 weeks in the hospital and was followed up in 1940, 1941, 1942, 1943, and 1944. She continued well and functional during all of those followups.

Case History 3
Present Illness: Mr. M.H., 47 years old, was admitted in August 1938. His illness had been noted for about 1 year. In February 1937 he had fallen from a bridge, and this was rumored to be a suicide attempt. He began to scratch all parts of his body and stated that he had lost his soul and had sinned. On several occasions he said that he wanted to die; once he was found with a gun, and another time he took a rope into a building but left it there. A month before admission he was found clinging to the inner edge of a cistern; he had intended to commit suicide but then thought better of it. He was restless and wandered. He refused food even when he stated that he was hungry.

His mental status showed retardation and perseveration in thinking. His general mood was one of depression, and ideas of guilt and unworthiness were expressed. On occasion he said that people made noises and did things to make him angry but that this was done to punish him. There was no evidence of hallucinations.

Past History. Mr. M.H. was born in Norway and moved to the United States as a young child. His wife died of tuberculosis 19 years before his illness. He was described as a congenial, well-liked person, interested in school activities, and an officer in church organizations.

Family History: A brother had had a nervous breakdown. He was not hospitalized, and he improved. The family was considered intelligent, stable, and successful in business. A nephew was admitted to the same hospital as a patient with a diagnosis of depression.

Course of Illness: At admission, Mr. M.H. was in a semistuporous state. He was tearful and agitated and said that his children would be better off without him, that he wanted to go away and live in a little shack. He said that he used to be goodhearted, but that he was currently bad. He talked of losing his soul and of committing crimes. He was transferred to a long-term state mental hospital after a couple of weeks of hospitalization. Seven years after his admission to the hospital, an attempt was made to follow him up. His daughter responded to the inquiry by saying, "I am answering your letter . . . regarding the health of my father, which has been real good these past years and does not show any signs of mental or physical complaints."

CLINICAL COURSE

The first episode of unipolar depression is usually, but not invariably, reported as occurring after puberty. Table 5-5 shows the cumulative proportion of patients for age of first episode. In this table, males and females are combined, as the ages of onset were not significantly different for the two sexes (Dorzab, et al., 1971).

A fifth of the patients first become ill in their teens, and by age 65, almost all of them who are going to fall ill have had an episode. Some people, however, do have their first episodes even after age 70. The median age of onset for unipolar depression is 37 years. If a depressive person has a family

TABLE 5-5. *Age of Onset in Unipolar Depression: Cumulative Proportion of Ill People*

Age	Proportion (%)
10–19	19
20–29	39
30–39	54
40–49	73
50–59	87
60–69	96
70–79	100

Mean age of onset 37.3 years.
Source: Adapted from Dorzab et al., 1971.

history of unipolar depression or a family history of alcoholism, the age of onset is usually earlier, probably around age 33. If there is no family history of either alcoholism or depression, the age of onset is later. These "sporadic" cases normally start in the late 30s or early 40s, or even at an older age.

Unipolar depressive illness shows multiple episodes. Single-episode cases are seen, but if one follows patients for more than 15 years, single-episode illnesses are rarely observed (Angst et al., 1973). In 20 years, the average number of episodes in unipolar depression is five or six.

EDITORS' COMMENT

In many patients there is a periodicity to the mood disorder. Epidemiologic evidence (Eastwood MR, Psychol Med 18:799–806, 1988) shows that major affective disorder depressed type peaks largely in the spring at different latitudes and in different countries. The term seasonal affective disorder, coined by Rosenthal et al. (Arch Gen Psychiatry 41:72–80, 1984) described a syndrome of recurrent depression that had its onset in fall–winter with specific symptoms of weight gain, carbohydrate craving, and hypersomnia. They suggest that light might be a useful treatment. It probably is not a specific, unique disorder (Pichot JT, et al., Jefferson J Psychiatry 7:41–50, 1989). At least 50 percent (Goodwin and Jamieson, Manic-Depressive Illness, 1990) of such patients are bipolar with spring and summer manias or hypomanias. Still, it is very important to record with the patient the daily, monthly, and yearly variations in the mood disorder.

Untreated episodes often last longer than treated episodes. Untreated episodes lasted 6 to 13 months. In current times, about 50 percent of patients with major depression recover by 1 year from onset. Speed of recovery with active treatment is more rapid, with 63 percent of patients recovered by 4 months (Keller et al., 1982). About 35 percent of depressives relapse within 40 weeks after recovery; patients with three or more prior episodes relapse even sooner (40 percent in 15 weeks) (Keller et al., 1983). The length of each episode of depression generally remains constant throughout the individual's lifetime, but *cycle length*—defined as the time from the beginning of one episode of depression to the beginning of the next—shortens from episode to episode.

Age seems to play a role in the clinical course. As women grow older, their episodes are likely to become longer. Thus women with age show a considerable amount of chronicity. As men grow older they seem to show an increasing number of episodes but not necessarily chronicity (Winokur and Morrison, 1973). There may be a limitation to the mean number of episodes in the unipolar depressive group. As noted earlier, unipolar depressives in follow-up have five to six episodes. This is true whether they are followed for 20 years or for 25, 30, or 35 years. This self-limitation in the mean number of episodes may indicate that after a certain number of episodes, the illness has run its course and the future will be good for the absence of occurrences.

Some unipolar depressives go on to show a mania (bipolar illness) some time in the future. This occurs in about 5 percent of unipolar depressive patients followed for a period of 3 to 5 years. Following the patients for up to 40 years shows that about 10 percent of unipolar patients convert to bipolarity in the course of time (Winokur et al., 1982).

In a group of untreated seriously ill depressives admitted to the hospital and followed for a period of 3 to 5 years, about 30 percent will remain chronically ill. This will be more common in females, about 36 percent, as compared with males, 26 percent. By about 5 years, 70 to 75 percent of depressives will have had a recovery. If one follows a group for 15 years, 85 percent will have recovered. One of the most interesting things about chronicity in depressed patients is that a group of patients may be chronically ill for a period of 10 years, but if one follows them for another 10 years, most will have recovered. ''Late-onset'' patients (i.e., after age 50), who have their first episode at that point, often remain ill for prolonged periods but ultimately recover spontaneously. Thus chronicity is a limited affair that may last for up to 10 years but does not continue indefinitely. It is important to emphasize that these observations refer only to the natural history of untreated unipolar depression; with treatment, chronicity is less of a problem (Winokur, 1974). Depressives who have been chronically ill for 2 years in modern times will show a recovery in the next 3 years in 80 percent of cases. At the end of a 5-year follow-up, those hitherto chronic depressives will have been well for at least 6 months in 41 percent of the cases (Coryell et al., 1990).

Some findings suggest that a family history of alcoholism in a unipolar depressive predicts an absence of chronicity. In other words, if alcoholism exists in a first-degree family member, a depressed patient is not likely to have an unremitting illness; rather, it will be an illness that is more variable.

In bipolar affective disorder, a short-term follow-up indicated that a high proportion of patients remained chronically ill but had superimposed exacerbations or episodes on this baseline state (Winokur et al., 1969). This course was termed *partial remission with episodes*. Such a finding also has been reported in unipolar illness. In a 2-year follow-up of unipolar depressives, a *subsyndromal* picture is reported as an underlying problem. This means that the full set of depressive symptoms is absent but may recur at any point; in fact, the patient may exhibit the full clinical picture of depression off and on during the follow-up but never be completely asymptomatic. This course is termed a *double depression* (Keller et al., 1983).

If one follows a group of unipolar depressives for a prolonged period (35 years) and compares them with a group of controls, it is clear that the controls will have fared better (see Table 5-6). Most of the controls will be considered to have no disability at the time of a 35-year follow-up, whereas slightly more than half the depressed patients will be considered severely or moderately disabled. In this case, the disability would take into account employment status, physical health, and the presence of psychiatric symptoms. Nonetheless, as may be noted from Table 5-6, 46 percent had no psychiatric disability of any sort.

In any discussion of the course of the illness, one must keep in mind some severe consequences. In unipolar depression these would be suicide and mortality from natural causes. A number of studies have shown a remarkably consistent finding. In groups of patients chosen for the diagnosis of affective disorder (usually unipolar depression plus bipolar illness), about 14 to 16 percent of the deceased patients will have died by suicide. In one study, a large group of unipolar depressives who were admitted to the hospital between 1935 and 1940 were chosen as subjects and followed for 35 to 40 years. These were compared with a group of controls who were followed for approximately the same length of time. Table 5-7 shows the suicide rates for the two groups. What is clear is that suicide risk for patients who have a unipolar depressive

TABLE 5-6. *Psychiatric Disability After a 35-Year Follow-up*

| | No. followed up | Disability (%) | | |
		SEVERE	MODERATE	NONE
Unipolar depressives	145	26	28	46
Controls	83	0	11	89

TABLE 5-7. *Incidence of Suicide Among Proband and Control Groups in a 30- to 40-Year Follow-up Study*

Item	Depressives	Controls
No. followed up	182	109
No. of suicides	14	0
Percentage of suicides	7.7	0.0
No. deceased at followup	132	37
Percentage of suicides among total deceased	10.6	0.0

Source: Adapted from Winokur and Tsuang, 1975.

illness is far greater than the risk that one would expect from the general population (Winokur and Tsuang, 1975).

The risk for suicide in patients with unipolar depression is highest shortly after discharge from hospital or treatment. The question of mortality is a more difficult one to answer. There have been a variety of studies of mortality in the affective disorders. One investigation showed that the survival rate in patients with unipolar depression is shortened. One of the causes of the increased mortality in such patients is unnatural deaths. These include suicides and accidents. It is possible, however, that other causes of death are implicated. For the first decade after admission to a hospital (in the years when relatively little treatment was available), the increased number of deaths in depressives, when compared with the general population and a control group, was about twofold (Tsuang et al., 1980).

Finally, it is important to assess whether or not patients with a diagnosis of unipolar depression change the character of their illness over time. When one deals with diagnoses that are made primarily on the basis of a clinical evaluation, some error is likely to be present. As noted earlier, in about 10 percent of the cases there is a change in diagnosis to bipolar illness. Changes to other diagnoses are considerably less common. About 5 percent of unipolar depressives in a 30- to 40-year follow-up will earn a diagnosis of schizophrenia. If one simply evaluates medical records, 84 percent of unipolar depressives, on readmission, will earn the same diagnosis (Tsuang et al., 1981). This kind of stability of psychiatric diagnosis in the case of the unipolar depressive group is reassuring. The lack of change to another diagnosis is evidence of a true illness.

ETIOLOGY

Both biologic and psychosocial factors have been implicated in the cause of unipolar depression. This seems quite rational because clinicians have separated unipolar depression into two types: *endogenous* (having origin within the organism), and neurotic-reactive. A reasonable definition of *neurotic-reactive depression* would be a depression seen in

a person who either has life events that provoke the syndrome or a history of multiple neurotic or personality difficulties (a stormy lifestyle) that culminate in a depressive episode (Klerman et al., 1979). In this definition, such people have symptoms of personality difficulties but do not meet criteria for a true diagnosis of a personality disorder. Thus they are people with problems in living.

A model for a reactive depression is seen in widows and widowers who develop a depressive syndrome after the death of their spouses. A third of the bereaved survivors meet criteria for depression. Women and men are equally likely to show a depression after bereavement, which is different from the sex ratio in a clinic or hospital. Such depressions may last for a considerable period, sometimes a year or longer. Some differences in clinical symptomatology exist between hospitalized depressives and patients who suffer depression after bereavement; suicidal thoughts, retardation, and feelings of hopelessness and worthlessness are far less common in bereavement depressions. Likewise, these patients are less likely than ordinary depressives to show loss of interest in personal relationships. Nevertheless, the bereaved depressive meets reasonable criteria for depression, indicating that depression can occur because of precipitating factors (Clayton et al., 1972).

The role of precipitating factors or life events in the depressed patient who is either hospitalized or seen in the clinic is more difficult to assess. Regardless of whether the patient is defined as endogenous or neurotic-reactive, some data suggest that life events are likely to occur around the onset of the illness (Paykel, 1982). Studies have shown that life events are more likely to occur in psychiatric patients who have a depressive syndrome when compared with people selected from the general population. More specifically, these kinds of life events are separations from important people in the individual's background. This appears to be consonant with the bereavement studies described previously. One of the problems in assessing the importance of life events is the difficulty in determining the onset of a depressive episode. Some of the things that might be particularly unpleasant to an individual could in fact be brought on as a consequence of the symptoms that are seen in the illness itself (e.g., losing a job or experiencing a marital problem). In other words, the depression may produce life events as well as be caused by them, and until a good method exists for evaluating the onset of depression, it may not be possible to determine the strength of the contribution of life events. The existence of a true reactive depression, however, is not in dispute. The occurrence of a depressive episode after bereavement, a natural disaster (e.g., Hurricane Andrew), economic recession, or in conjunction with a serious medical illness (e.g., myocardial infarction) is adequate evidence that a depression can be precipitated by life events (Winokur, 1991).

Other etiologic possibilities that are related to psychosocial events include the idea that early parental loss may lead to affective disorder later in life. Here the findings are mixed, with many studies showing that early parental loss is in fact related and other studies showing that early parental loss has no bearing on the subsequent development of a depression. Interestingly, most of the studies have not controlled for the possibility that early parental loss, either through death or disturbed family relationships, might be due to the presence of the illness itself in the parent. Therefore, a relationship of early parental loss and adult depression may indicate a familial (genetic) factor just as much as an environmental factor.

Genetic factors have been well studied in unipolar depression. After bipolar and unipolar illnesses were separated in the mid-1960s, it was possible to do genetic and family studies with an independent assessment of each of the illnesses. Before that time, most of the studies had been performed on mixed groups of unipolar depressives and bipolar patients. To suggest a genetic factor in an illness, one would need to demonstrate more illness in the families of unipolar depressives than in the families of a control population. It would be well to perform such a study blindly, with the investigator not knowing the diagnosis of the index case (the patient whose family is evaluated). Further, such a study should use valid and systematic criteria for the diagnosis of a family member.

Table 5-8 shows the results of a study in which bipolars, unipolar depressives, and controls were selected (Winokur et al., 1982). These cases were then followed up for 35 to 40 years, and a systematic family study was accomplished. This investigation was performed by researchers who were blind to the diagnosis of the index case. It is noteworthy that a far higher proportion of relatives of unipolar depressives also were ill with unipolar depression than

TABLE 5-8. *Unipolar Depression in First-Degree Relatives*

Index cases	No. of relatives	No. (%) blindly interviewed with unipolar depression
Unipolar (n = 203)	416	34 (8.2)
Control (n = 160)	541	25 (4.6)

	No. of deceased relatives	No. (%) with unipolar depression confirmed by charts
Unipolar (n = 203)	606	13 (2.1)
Control (n = 160)	322	1 (0.3)

Source: Adapted from Winokur et al., 1975.

is found in the relatives of the controls. The controls were surgical patients who were admitted at approximately the same time as the unipolar depressives. The ratio of ill family members in the unipolar depressives to the ill family members in the controls, when personally examined, is about 2:1. Deceased relatives also were evaluated. Psychiatric records were obtained on deceased relatives of unipolar depressives. There were 13 charts of relatives who were admitted with the same illness, a far higher number than was found in the deceased relatives of the control group. There the ratio is 7:1. The conclusion is that there is a much higher family history of unipolar depression in the family members of unipolar depressives than one would expect from studying the normal population. Another important type of genetic study is concerned with a comparison of concordance for depression in monozygotic versus dizygotic twins. Because monozygotic twins entertain all the same genes and dizygotic twins only 50 percent, one would expect a higher concordance rate in the monozygotic group. A study by Bertelson et al. (1977) in Scandinavia shows this to be true. In the monozygotic pairs of unipolar depressives, 43 percent were concordant. In the dizygotic pairs, only 19 percent were concordant. Other twin studies show similar findings. Notably when the family members of bipolar patients are compared with the family members of unipolar depressed patients, the former group contains significantly more people with mania. This is the major finding that suggests that bipolar and unipolar depressions are separate entities.

Such studies as those described do not prove a genetic factor beyond a shadow of doubt. The way to prove a genetic factor would be by conducting adoption, linkage, or association studies. In adoption studies, children of parents with affective disorder who were adopted away at an early age would be more likely to have the illness than would children who were adopted but born of normal biologic parents. Such a study has been reported by Cadoret (1978), in which a higher proportion of adopted children of parents with unipolar illness themselves had unipolar illness than did adopted children of parents who had no psychiatric illness. Nevertheless, more studies of unipolar depression using the adoption technique are needed. Linkage and association studies have been reported for bipolar illness. A linkage study would indicate that two genes, that of a genetic marker and that of a psychiatric illness, are next to each other on the same chromosome. Therefore, within a family (but not in the population) the marker and the illness would be found together more often than one would expect by chance alone. Association indicates that some seemingly unrelated genetic trait is more likely seen in persons who have a particular illness than in persons from the general population. To accomplish an association study, a group of depressives would be compared with an appropriate control population. Studies of linkage and association would be useful, and some have been attempted, but no unequivocal findings in unipolar depression have emerged as yet.

Another point should be made about the family or genetic studies. Depression can be classified on the basis of family background. Implicit in such a classification is that a specific type of family history of psychiatric illness has etiologic significance. Unipolar depressive illness can be divided into three groups. The first group is called *depression spectrum disease*, which is a depression in an individual who has a first-degree relative who has alcoholism or sociopathy. Such an individual may or may not have a relative with depression. A second group is that of *familial pure depressive disease*. This is a depression in an individual who has a family history of depression but not of alcoholism or sociopathy. The third group is *sporadic depressive disease*, which is a depression in an individual who has no family history of alcoholism, antisocial personality, or depression. None of these depressives should have a family history of mania. When one divides patients into these kinds of familial subtypes, there are some differences in the clinical picture. One of the most striking differences is that in many studies a clinical diagnosis of neurotic-reactive depression is related to a family history of alcoholism (depression spectrum disease). Alternatively, a family history of depression only (familial pure depressive disease) is related to a clinical diagnosis of endogenous depression. Thus, clinically and familially, some differences do exist in these groups. A patient with a depression spectrum disease is likely to have a stormy life history, with multiple marital and social problems. This is less likely in a patient with familial pure depressive disease. Sporadic depressive disease patients are differentiable from the other two groups on a later age of onset (Winokur, 1982).

The evidence for a genetic factor in unipolar depression is strong. In regard to etiology, this does not tell us anything about the proximal cause of the illness. It indicates that there are significant biologic factors that must, by definition, come into play in causing the illness. There are three sets of data that may shed some light on the proximal etiology of the illness.

One set concerns the biogenic amine hypotheses. These hypotheses were formulated because of the observation that a drug such as reserpine, which depletes the brain of amines, was associated with the development of a depressive syndrome. Biogenic amine hypotheses are best viewed as two hypotheses rather than as one. The first assumes that a decrease in catecholamines at important synapses in the central nervous system is associated with a depression. The other hypothesis is similar but considers the indole amines to be important factors. Such drugs as the monoamine oxidase inhibitors would decrease the breakdown of the monoamines and therefore be efficacious in the

treatment of depression. The tricyclic antidepressants would prevent reuptake of the monoamines and, therefore, likewise be associated with a remission from a depressive state. Various of the tricyclic antidepressants have differential effects in preventing reuptake of specific monoamines and therefore may be differentially efficacious in the treatment of certain depressions. Because some patients may respond to one antidepressant and not to another, this has given rise to the idea that certain kinds of depressive illnesses are associated with functional deficits of certain kinds of monoamines. The results of a large recent study reveal that some unipolar depressed patients show raised levels of 5-hydroxyindoleacetic acid, the metabolite of serotonin, in spinal fluid and that some show high levels of 3-methoxy-4-hydroxyphenyl-glycol (MHPG), a metabolite of the catecholamines (Koslow et al., 1983). The same study showed raised levels of vanillylmandelic acid, normetanephrine, metanephrine, norepinephrine, and epinephrine in urine in depressives. Such findings have not been invariable, and they have not been consistently related to specific kinds of affective disorder (e.g., bipolar versus unipolar). Nevertheless, the biogenic amine hypotheses are viable at the present time. They may well be involved in the etiology of all the affective disorders and even specifically in unipolar depression.

Recent findings have related receptor differences in the central nervous system to depressive illness. An example is that there may be reduced numbers of platelet imipramine binding sites in depression when compared with controls. Platelet binding sites may reflect those in the brain. Another reported finding is a decrease in serotonin uptake in platelets in depressed patients, even after recovery (Meltzer et al., 1983). In line with prior biogenic amine studies is a recent finding by Ågren et al. (1991), who reported a significantly lower uptake of radiolabeled L-5-hydroxytryptophane (the serotonin precursor) across the blood–brain barrier in major depressives as compared with controls. This was found irrespective of phase of illness, thus suggesting a trait finding that the transport of the serotonin precursor across the blood–brain barrier is compromised in major depression.

A second set of biologic findings relevant to depression is related to the endocrine system. Serious or endogenous depressions have been associated with an abnormal response to dexamethasone. Whereas a normal person has a marked reduction in circulating cortisol in response to a 1-mg challenge with dexamethasone, some depressed patients escape the effect of the dexamethasone and show high serum cortisol levels. This response is seen in about 50 percent of endogenous depressives. In some studies, patients with a family history of depression but not of alcoholism (familial pure depressive disease) are particularly noted to show abnormal nonsuppression. The finding of the abnormal dexamethasone test is paralleled by the finding that some depressive patients have high hourly plasma cortisol concentrations compared with controls (Sachar, 1975; Carroll et al., 1976; Schlesser et al., 1979). These findings suggest an abnormality in the hypothalamic–pituitary–adrenal axis, but the specific location of the "lesion" is unknown.

At one time an abnormal dexamethasone suppression test was considered specific for depression. However, reports have come out indicating that specificity is not quite as great as was previously thought and that some patients with obsessional neurosis, schizophrenia, anorexia nervosa, and Alzheimer's disease are abnormal suppressors. Nevertheless, the test is a good lead, since the response is commonly different in depressives as compared with controls.

Another abnormal endocrine response in depression is deficient thyroid-stimulating hormone (TSH) response to an infusion of thyrotropin-releasing hormone (TRH). This is not seen in all cases, and there is no reason to believe that the person with the abnormal cortisol response will have the abnormal TSH response to TRH. In other words, the two endocrine abnormalities may not be highly correlated. There is a possibility that the low TSH response to TRH continues after recovery, but this is not certain (Kirkegaard et al., 1975). A recent finding connects the biogenic amine theory to the endocrine abnormalities (O'Keane and Dinan, 1991). Prolactin and cortisol responses to D-fenfluramine were significantly impaired in depressives as compared with control subjects. Since D-fenfluramine is a selective serotonin challenge agent, this suggests a lowered serotonin responsivity in depression.

One problem with biologic studies is that there is no way to examine directly the organ that is considered responsible for the depression—the brain. One studies blood, urine, and spinal fluid, whereas it would be important to determine the pathophysiology of the brain during depression. At present, there is no satisfactory answer to the problem.

Another set of data is promising. Studies have shown that there is an abnormally short onset of rapid eye movement (REM) sleep in seriously ill depressives. REM sleep is associated with dreaming in a healthy individual. In patients with major depressions or endogenous depressions, the onset of REM sleep is far shorter than in the normal population. This shortened REM latency is not seen in patients who have secondary depressions to serious medical illnesses or other psychiatric illnesses. Also, it seems that patients who have a family history of alcoholism as well as a depression (depression spectrum disease) are less likely to have a shortened REM latency (Kupfer, 1976; Akiskal, 1983).

None of the findings has provided final answers to the etiology of unipolar depression, but they have stimulated a great deal of research and have considerable heuristic value.

DIFFERENTIAL DIAGNOSIS

The diagnosis of a unipolar depression is the diagnosis of a syndrome, not necessarily a disease. The simple finding of a depressive syndrome is not meaningful in terms of a diagnosis. Evaluating a depressive syndrome must be done in the context of a full medical and psychiatric workup. A true evaluation of a depression is an exercise in differential diagnosis; Figure 5–1 shows a system that may be used for this purpose (Winokur, 1991).

An *induced depressive syndrome* occurs from a variety of causes. Withdrawal from alcoholism is often, if not invariably, associated with a depressive syndrome that is relatively short-lived and usually lasts for no more than a couple of weeks. Patients treated with steroids may develop a depression. Other brain diseases or metabolic disturbances that may be associated with a depressive syndrome include left-sided stroke, Huntington's disease, Alzheimer's disease, and reserpine therapy for hypertension. It is the induced depressions particularly that make it necessary to obtain a full medical and psychiatric history.

The next group are the *neurotic depressions*. These are so named because they occur in the context of a stormy lifestyle, considerable conflict, and often other diagnoses. When they occur in the context of other diagnoses, they are called *secondary depressions* (Winokur, 1972). Thus an illness that occurs well after the onset of an anxiety disorder, somatization disorder, or alcoholism will have a high likelihood of developing a depression over time. These are secondary depressions. Patients with secondary depressions thus have a depressive syndrome which is superimposed on a preexisting illness such as panic disorder, agoraphobia, somatization disorder, substance-abuse disorder, or any other psychiatric condition.

Another group within the neurotic depressions are those patients who have a family history of alcoholism. These have been called *depression spectrum disease* (DSD) patients. They have a long history of difficult problems and stormy life events. These are, however, primary depressions, because the patients have never suffered any other psychiatric illness.

The third group that would fit the concept of neurotic depression is that of secondary depressions to personality disorders. The most obvious one is the secondary depression in an individual who has an antisocial personality. However, other less well defined personality disorders (e.g., borderline personality, histrionic personality) also show depressive episodes over time.

The reactive depressions are those which occur in the context of either a medical illness or a severe life stress. The medical illness in this case does not affect the brain, and consequently, the depression cannot be called induced. There is good evidence that bereavement is associated with a depression

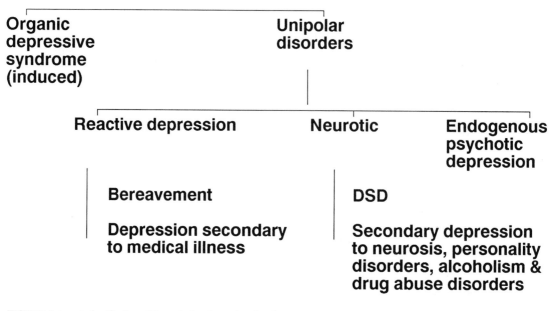

FIGURE 5-1. *A classification of the unipolar depressive disorders.*

that is reactive. Also, medical disease (Stewart et al., 1965) may precipitate a depression. Natural tragedies, such as earthquakes, radioactive spills, and volcanic eruptions, are often disruptive enough to be associated with an increase in depressive illness in the community. A reactive depression occurs in times of economic depression; that this becomes a problem is supported by the fact that the suicide rate goes up in times of economic depression and farm foreclosures.

Finally, the third type of illness that must be considered is *endogenous-psychotic depression.* These are primary depressions. Familially, these patients may be separated from the neurotic depressives of the depression spectrum disease type by virtue of the fact that they have only a family history of depression or no family history at all (sporadic). They are more likely to show psychotic symptomatology than the neurotic depressives, and they have fewer problems in living, e.g., sexual problems, problems in marriage, and personality difficulties.

The preceding classification has both treatment and etiologic meaning and may be useful in predicting the course of illness. In such a differential diagnosis, one thing should be kept in mind—the course of the illness. Most sets of criteria use a time constraint. A reasonable time constraint would be 1 month of continuous depression. This would remove such patients who had withdrawal syndromes as well as some of the patients who are simply experiencing unhappy life events that make

them acutely unhappy but do not necessarily provoke a long-standing depression.

LABORATORY FINDINGS

Some laboratory tests performed in unipolar depression have shown abnormal findings that are associated with a depressed state. Perhaps the best known is the 1-mg dexamethasone suppression test, discussed earlier under "Etiology." This test is accomplished in the following way. One milligram of dexamethasone is administered to a patient at 10:30 P.M. The next morning at 8:00 A.M. the patient's blood is drawn for a determination of serum cortisol. This determination is repeated at 4:00 P.M. A level of cortisol in the blood above 5 μg/dl at either 8:00 A.M. or 4:00 P.M. is considered an abnormal test. When dexamethasone is administered to nondepressives, their cortisol levels at those times the next day are usually quite low, well below 5 μg/dl and generally in the range of 1 to 2 μg/dl. Investigators have found some groups of patients with endogenous depression to have as high as 50 percent abnormal nonsuppressors. Patients who have familial pure depressive disease (a depression in a person with a family history of depression but no familial alcoholism) have been noted to be abnormal in some studies in 70 to 85 percent of cases. Neurotic-reactive depressives and secondary depressives are generally considered to be normal suppressors, as are patients with depression spectrum disease. Certainly not all studies are in agreement with these subtype findings, but most agree that patients with major depressions are more likely to be nonsuppressors than are normal controls or other psychiatric patients. The test may not be reliable in patients with recent weight loss, endocrine disturbances, pregnancy, and hepatic and renal disease or in those who are on such drugs as phenytoin (Dilantin). Nevertheless, most studies do support the finding that unipolar depressives whose illness is severe enough to get them admitted to the hospital have a high likelihood of abnormal nonsuppression. The test might be used as an aid in determining whether the patient has improved. Normalization of the dexamethasone test might indicate that the person is no longer suffering from the illness. Recent findings, however, have indicated that patients who have multiple episodes and admissions vary over time (Coryell and Schlesser, 1983). When depressed during one admission, they will be nonsuppressors; at other admissions, and with equal severity, they will be normal suppressors. This makes the use of the test as a monitor for improvement a dubious prospect. The test generally is considered important because it is an abnormal finding associated with psychiatric illness, and this abnormal finding may in fact provide a clue to the proximal etiology of the disease.

The dexamethasone suppression test (DST) has been subjected to extensive review (Coryell, 1984). One may conclude that due to modest sensitivity, the DST is not particularly effective for screening. However, the specificity is very high, and it is useful for confirmation if the suspicion of an endogenous depression is high. One must keep in mind, however, that the specificity may be somewhat compromised by the fact that schizophrenia with negative symptomatology and dementia now show a higher proportion of nonsuppressors. The DST may turn out to be particularly useful for differential diagnosis within the unipolar depression groups. Table 5-9 presents data regarding the performance of the test with varied subtypes of depression (Coryell, 1989).

Other endocrine tests have been reported to be abnormal besides the blunted TSH response to TRH. Growth hormone abnormalities have been noted. In one study, a decreased drop in blood glucose to insulin injection after recovery has been reported in familial pure depressives and bipolar depressives when compared with depression spectrum patients (Lewis et al., 1983). None of these findings is validated well enough for use in diagnosis or in monitoring progress in treatment, but they do indicate areas in which laboratory findings might be useful in the future.

One finding that may be clinically useful comes from the sleep laboratory (Kupfer, 1976). REM sleep shows a less-than-normal latency period in depressives. Other sleep disturbances also have been reported. Patients with secondary depression

TABLE 5-9. *The Dexamethasone Suppression Test in Subtypes of Major Depression*

	Nonsuppression (%)	Specificity (%)
Primary	41	90
Secondary	10	
Endogenous	32–59	76–84
Nonendogenous	16–24	
With melancholia	40	69
Without melancholia	31	

Source: Adapted from Coryell, 1984.

have been noted to have normal REM latency, as have patients with depression spectrum disease. Like the endocrine tests, the sleep laboratory tests show considerable promise in testing out pathophysiology of the illness that we call unipolar depression and in helping to make clinical evaluations.

Most depressed hospitalized patients have a medical workup of some sort. The finding of abnormal electrolyte tests or of abnormal levels of blood constituents is usually an indication that something else besides depression may be wrong with the patient. This does not mean that a patient cannot have two illnesses—a medical illness and a depression—but certainly no ordinary laboratory finding that is obtained on admission has been strongly associated with depression. Thus abnormal findings in plasma, serum, urine, or spinal fluid should be pursued, since they may indicate another illness that may be responsible for the depression or that may exist independent of the depression.

TREATMENT

For practical purposes, treatment may be divided into four major headings: general management, psychological therapy, pharmacologic therapy, and other somatic therapies.

General Management

General management is an important area. The person with unipolar depression is at some risk for suicide. Further, in the midst of his depression, he is likely to be irritable or hard to manage. Such a person has the potential of turning family relationships or social situations into disasters.

If a person is judged to be a suicidal risk, he or she must be protected. This can be done by having him enter a hospital. Often a patient with a depression is indecisive and will not make such a decision on his own. The physician should take the responsibility for such a decision by strongly advising the responsible people in the patient's life that they must have him in the hospital, even if he is opposed. This sounds easy, but often the family is reluctant to take the responsibility for committing the patient to the hospital against his will. Thus there is a standoff: the doctor reluctant to take care of the patient if he is not fully protected by being in a hospital and the family recognizing that the patient is at risk but unwilling to make the appropriate moves. On rare occasions the physician will go to the courts and recommend commitment. Most of the time, however, the physician is constrained to do the best he can with a patient who is not being optimally cared for. These kinds of ambiguities and uncertainties make the management of depressives difficult at times. There is no final answer; one must attempt to use good judgment.

Patients who are depressed have considerable difficulty with concentration and thinking. Consequently, it seems unreasonable to force them into situations where they have to be responsible for much intellectual work. Often depressed patients will vegetate unless they are pushed into some kind of activity, but the activity ought to be more physical than cerebral. Thus a physician is unlikely to suggest that the patient go to a book club while depressed and report on something he has read. Rather, the physician might suggest that the patient involve himself in such physical activity as might be reasonable. Insisting on intellectual activity may well make the patient more depressed.

In the midst of a depression the patient may want to make major decisions. Because of irritability, divorce may seem to be an appropriate response to a marital conflict. Quitting a job that the depressed patient believes he can no longer perform is hardly uncommon. Patients should be discouraged from making major changes in their lives during the period of depression. Once they are well, they will again become free agents and can make any decisions they want. But while they are depressed, it seems unreasonable to support their burning bridges or making foolish decisions that might come back to haunt them. One of the largest problems in managing the depressed patient is that he often finds reasons for his depression. Because depression is akin to being unhappy, it seems reasonable to him that something terrible may have caused the state. The patient who believes that his condition is due to disturbed life events may not be correct, and the physician should attempt to prevent him from acting on false premises.

It is well to deal with the depressed patient as if he were a collaborator, rather than as if he were a totally dependent individual. Thus it is often useful to discuss the illness with the patient and point out to him that although he is ill at the present time, all available evidence indicates that he will get well, that he will be as well as he ever was, and that he will not end up as a patient on the chronic ward of a state hospital. The patient often believes that he is going to lose his mind permanently. It is important to reassure him that this is not an end point of unipolar depression. In a sense, dealing with a depressive is similar to dealing with an intelligent

diabetic. The more he knows about his illness, the better off everybody is likely to be. It is interesting to note that a retarded depressed patient may lose a good bit of his retardation during a discussion with a physician. Giving the patient reassurance that he will get better may make for an acute improvement. The patient will feel better for a short period of time. This kind of reassurance, however, is no permanent treatment for the depression. The next day the patient will be back to where he was before the discussion.

One thing should be mentioned about the family. Often the wife or the parents or the children are prone to take blame themselves for the depressed relative. There are no data to support the idea that anybody's behavior causes a depression. The family should be reassured that the depression is best looked on as an illness, that they are not to blame, and that their sympathetic understanding will be useful. It will not cure the depression, but it may help with the management.

Intense exploration into personal problems during a depression may be contraindicated. Constant questioning of the person's behavior may make him feel more guilty and depressed.

During a depression the patient may need to visit the physician more frequently than usual. When he feels frightened or guiltier or more ashamed and in need of reassurance, the patient may ask to be seen more often. The physician should honor this request.

Psychological Therapy

Psychotherapy as a treatment for unipolar depression, after a time in the "yellow leaf," has once more become a viable concept. A variety of specific psychotherapies have been used recently to treat depressives (Rush, 1982). At this point in time, cognitive therapy has been extensively investigated. Cognitive therapy is based on the concept that a depressive regards himself in a negative fashion. The individual thinks of himself as being worthless and believes that life can never be worthwhile again. In cognitive therapy, the person offering the treatment attempts to use both verbal and behavioral techniques to help a patient recognize that these negative viewpoints (cognitions) are related to feeling states and behavior. The cognitive therapy is an effort to help the patient examine the circumstances and recognize that his ideas about himself are not consistent with reality. Self-condemnatory distortions may be expressed; when the patient realizes that they are inappropriate, the therapist suggests the substitution of a more reality-oriented concept. A high percentage of patients in cognitive therapy show marked improvement. That certain patients receive a great deal of benefit from cognitive therapy seems to be supported by the available evidence. Clarification of what specific kinds of patients with unipolar depressions might receive benefit is necessary at this point. Would they be patients who have had multiple somatic treatments with failure? Would they be patients who have mild depressions? Would they be patients who were reactive-neurotic, rather than endogenous? Answers to these questions are needed in order to determine the place of cognitive therapy in the treatment of unipolar depression.

Another kind of psychotherapy that has been reported to be useful is interpersonal psychotherapy. This kind of psychotherapy seems related to the idea that depression resembles unhappiness. Interpersonal psychotherapy is offered as a way to improve the patient's social functioning by increasing the ability to deal with stresses and by helping the patient to manage personal and social consequences of the depression. In interpersonal psychotherapy, special techniques have been developed for managing depressed patients who have experienced grief and loss, interpersonal deficits, and marital problems. Some studies of interpersonal psychotherapy in depressives suggest that it may be as effective as pharmacologic treatments. Antidepressant medication used in combination with interpersonal psychotherapy may be particularly effective. The patients in whom this technique has been used have generally been mildly depressed outpatients. Again, whether this technique would be useful in severely retarded or agitated inpatients is open to question.

A large multicenter collaborative study on the effectiveness in depression of cognitive-behavior therapy and interpersonal therapy as compared with pharmacotherapy and placebo (Elkin et al., 1989) helps put psychotherapy in a reasonable context. Generally, pharmacotherapy did best and placebo worst. The two psychotherapies were in between but closer to pharmacotherapy. For the least severe patients, all therapies did well. For the most severe patients, pharmacotherapy plus clinical management did the best, although there was some evidence of efficacy with psychotherapy.

Pharmacologic Therapy

For seriously ill depressives, specific antidepressant drug therapy is probably the most common treatment. These antidepressant drugs are related to the biogenic amine hypotheses, which have been previously discussed. Two classes are used. The first of these are the tricyclic antidepressants, which prevent reuptake of biogenic amines and thus increase the concentration of these amines at the synaptic junction. The other type of drug is the monoamine oxidase inhibitor, which prevents breakdown of the biogenic amines at the synaptic junction.

The tricyclic antidepressants are most frequently used. These drugs include amitriptyline, nortriptyline, which is a metabolic product of amitriptyline, imipramine, desipramine, which is a metabolic product of imipramine, and doxepine. These drugs differentially prevent reuptake of the different neurotransmitters. Desipramine prevents reuptake of norepinephrine very well, whereas amitriptyline prevents the reuptake of serotonin more effectively. Two of the drugs, amitriptyline and doxepin, are particularly sedative. Because of this, they are valuable in patients who might need a certain amount of sedation or who have sleep difficulties. A large proportion of the dose given at night might well be effective in producing a better sleep pattern. Imipramine or desipramine are less likely to be sedative. Thus a retarded patient might be considered a good candidate for these two drugs. Some of the tricyclics are associated with weight gain. The use of desipramine might be indicated if that becomes a problem, since less weight gain has been reported with this drug. Improvement is expected to occur in about 3 weeks, but the data indicate that it may occur within 1 week and continue thereafter.

The tricyclic drugs are given by starting the individual at about 50 to 75 mg in divided doses. In a few days the dose is raised to 150 mg a day. This is a reasonable dose for effectiveness. Some people metabolize tricyclics in aberrant ways; if this is suspected, blood levels may be obtainable for the drugs. After the individual has been built up to a dose of about 150 mg a day, it is possible to give a larger proportion at night, to help the patient fall asleep. If the person does not improve at this level after a period of time, the dose may be increased to 200 or 300 mg a day.

Side effects of these drugs have been noted. Lowered blood pressure and heart arrhythmias may be seen with some of the drugs, and this could be an adverse effect for a person with cardiac problems. Hypotension is an important effect, and often patients on the tricyclics will fall and suffer fractures. This can be a problem for elderly patients with fragile skeletal systems. On rare occasions confusional states and disorientation occur. Withdrawal of the medicine is usually accompanied by an improvement of these symptoms. Common side effects are dry mouth, inability to urinate, and constipation. Some drugs cause more potent side effects than others.

The monoamine oxidase inhibitors are not usually first-choice treatment for depression because of their possibly serious side effects. The drugs most commonly used are tranylcypromine sulfate, isocarboxazid, and phenelzine. Usually treatment is started by giving one 15-mg tablet of phenelzine on the first day, and the dose is increased over the next several days to 60 mg a day. In the case of tranylcypromine sulfate, over a period of a few days the dose is raised to about 30 mg in 10-mg doses. Side effects include lowered blood pressure and sometimes marked fatigue. A serious side effect is related to the presence of tyramine, which is found in some foods and beverages (e.g., aged cheese, red wine, pickled herring, and chocolate). If monoamine oxidase inhibitors are given and the tyramine is not inactivated, severe headaches and hypertension and death can result.

Monoamine oxidase inhibitors may be particularly useful for depressed patients who are somewhat atypical. These might be patients who show marked anxiety or do not show the classic symptoms described in depression. In other words, there is some reason to believe that the neurotic-reactive type of patient might be particularly responsive to monoamine oxidase inhibitors.

Two new antidepressants are now available, fluoxetine hydrochloride and bupropion hydrochloride. As a starting dose for fluoxetine, 20 mg per day is recommended. Serious side effects with this drug are uncommon, making it particularly useful, and acute overdoses with large amounts are unlikely to lead to death, making it a reasonable drug for depressives who may be suicidal. Bupropion also shows few adverse effects when used at doses of 450 mg per day or less. Higher doses have been associated with seizures. With adequate treatment of the primary condition, it has been noted that secondary depressions to such psychiatric illnesses as eating disorders and anxiety disorders improve, even without specific antidepressant therapy.

Electroconvulsive Therapy

For years, electroconvulsive therapy (ECT) was used as an effective treatment in depression. As originally given, electrodes were placed on each temple, and a current was passed between them. A grand mal seizure occurred, with the ordinary train of changes seen in any convulsion. Further, vertebral fractures occurred in the early days of ECT, as well as considerable confusion. Today ECT is far less traumatic to watch or to experience. It is usually administered three times a week. Before the treatment the patient is given nothing by mouth after supper until the treatment the next morning. About 30 minutes before the treatment, the patient is given atropine, which dries up secretions. At the time of treatment a rubber mouthpiece is inserted to ensure a good airway. Oxygen is given from a face mask. Electrodes are placed on the patient's temples and the physician injects a short-acting anesthesia, methohexital, until the patient is asleep. Through the same needle, a muscle relaxant is injected. After about 45 to 60 seconds, a current is administered and the patient has a modified convulsion. Often it is virtually impossible to tell that a convulsion has occurred because of the effectiveness of the muscle relaxant. After the convulsion, the face mask is placed over the patient's face and oxygen is given to the person. Within 50 to 80 seconds after the convulsion, breathing occurs. The patient then rests for a short while and eats breakfast. ECT is a safe treatment. The major side effect has to do with memory loss, which occurs for events around the period of time of the treatments. This occurs if the electrodes are placed bitemporally. Within several weeks, however, the patient has recalled most of the things

that he has forgotten. Certainly after a few weeks have passed the patient's ability to retain new memories is as good as it ever was. If the electrodes are placed unilaterally, less acute confusion results, but some clinicians believe that the efficacy is reduced as compared with the bilateral method. The average number of treatments administered is between 6 and 12. The patient is usually given treatments while hospitalized, but outpatient ECT has been used with success.

The effect of ECT is of considerable importance. When compared with antidepressant drug therapy, ECT tends to be equal in producing improvement (Homan et al., 1982; see Table 5-10). Of particular interest is that *marked* improvement is more likely to result with ECT than with antidepressant medication. Likewise, if one follows patients who have been treated with ECT and compares them with patients who have been followed after receiving adequate antidepressant therapy, a difference can be seen in the number of suicide attempts after treatment. Fewer patients with ECT (1 percent) than with antidepressant therapy (7 percent) are likely to attempt suicide during hospitalization and followup (Avery and Winokur, 1978), indicating that ECT may be more effective than antidepressant therapy. This possibility is relevant to the idea that perhaps there are certain kinds of patients in whom ECT should be the treatment of choice. These would be middle-aged men who have shown marked suicidal trends. Such men who were diagnosed as having unipolar depression are at particularly high risk for suicide; perhaps these patients should be given the most effective treatment for a marked recovery (i.e., ECT).

Prevention

A continuation of tricyclic medication has been associated with prevention of relapse in unipolar depression. An average dose of 200 mg imipramine daily and monthly interpersonal therapy have prophylactic value (Frank et al., 1990). Lithium also may be useful. It has been effective in preventing depressive episodes in patients with unipolar depression who have had multiple episodes in the past (Coppen et al., 1971). The individual may be kept on a dose that produces a serum level of about 0.6 to

TABLE 5-10. *Treatment Results in Hospitalized Unipolar Depressives*

	ECT (%) (n = 76)	Antidepressant medication (%) (n = 101)
No improvement	8	6
Moderate improvement	49	82
Marked improvement	43	12

Source: Adapted from Homan et al., 1982.

1.0 mEq/liter for a long period. Outpatient maintenance ECT also has been used to prevent the occurrence of depression.

REFERENCES

Ågren H, Reibring L, Hartvig P, et al: Low brain uptake of L-[^{11}C]5-hydroxytryptophane in major depression: A positron emission tomography study on patients and healthy volunteers. Acta Psychiatr Scand 83:449–455, 1991.

Akiskal H: Diagnosis and classification of affective disorders: New insights from clinical and laboratory approaches. Psychiatr Develop 2:123–160, 1983.

Angst J, Baastrup P, Grof P, et al: The course of monopolar depression in bipolar psychoses. Psychiatr Neurol Neurochir 76:489–500, 1973.

Avery D, Winokur G: Suicide, attempted suicide and relapse rates in depression. Arch Gen Psychiatry 35:749–753, 1978.

Bair D: Samuel Beckett: A Biography. New York, Simon and Schuster, 1990.

Baker M, Dorzab J, Winokur G, Cadoret R: Depressive disease: Classification and clinical characteristics. Compr Psychiatry 12:354–365, 1971.

Bertelson A, Harvald B, Haug A: Danish twin study of manic depressive disorders. Br J Psychiatry 130:330–351, 1977.

Boyd J, Weissman M: Epidemiology of affective disorders: A re-examination and future directions. Arch Gen Psychiatry 38:1039–1046, 1981.

Cadoret R: Evidence for genetic inheritance of primary affective disorder in adoptees. Am J Psychiatry 135:463–466, 1978.

Carroll B, Curtis G, Mendels J: Neuroendocrine regulation in depression. II. Discrimination of depressed from non-depressed patients. Arch Gen Psychiatry 33:1051–1058, 1976.

Clayton P, Halikas J, Maurice W: The depression of widowhood. Br J Psychiatry 120:71–77, 1972.

Clayton P, Herjanic M, Murphy G, Woodruff R: Mourning and depression: Their similarities and differences. Can Psychiatr Assoc J 19:309–312, 1974.

Coppen A, Noguera R, Bailey J, et al: Prophylactic lithium in affective disorders. Lancet 2:275–279, 1971.

Coryell W, Schlesser M: Dexamethasone suppression test response in major depression: Stability across hospitalizations. Psychiatry Res 8:179–189, 1983.

Coryell W, Endicott J, Keller M: Outcome of patients with chronic affective disorder: A five-year follow-up. Am J Psychiatry 147:1627–1633, 1990.

Coryell W: The use of laboratory tests in psychiatric diagnosis: The DST as an example. Psychiatr Dev 3:139–159, 1984.

Dorzab J, Baker M, Winokur G, Cadoret R: Depressive disease: Clinical course. Dis Nerv Syst 32:269–273, 1971.

Elkin I, Shea T, Watkins J, et al: National Institute of Mental Health Treatment of Depression Collaborative Research Program: General effectiveness of treatments. Arch Gen Psychiatry 46:971–982, 1989.

Feighner J, Robins E, Guze S, et al: Diagnostic criteria for use in psychiatric research. Arch Gen Psychiatry 26:57–63, 1972.

Frank E, Kupfer D, Perel J, et al: Three-year outcomes for maintenance therapies in recurrent depression. Arch Gen Psychiatry 47:1093–1099, 1990.

Helgason T: Epidemiological investigations concerning affective disorders, in Schou M, Stromgren E (eds): Origin, Prevention, and Treatment of Affective Disorders. New York, Academic Press, 1979.

Homan S, Lachenbruch P, Winokur G, Clayton P: An efficacy study of electroconvulsive therapy and antidepressants in the treatment of primary depression. Psychol Med 12:615–624, 1982.

Kay D, Garside R, Beamish P, Roy J: Endogenous and neurotic syndromes of depression: A factor analytic study of 104 cases. Clinical Features. Br J Psychiatry 115:377–388, 1971.

Keller M, Lavori P, Endicott J, et al: Double depression: Two year follow-up. Am J Psychiatry 140:689–694, 1983.

Keller M, Lavori P, Lewis C, Klerman G: Predictors of relapse in major depressive disorder. JAMA 250:3299–3304, 1983.

Keller M, Shapiro R, Lavori P, Wolfe N: Recovery in major depressive disorder. Arch Gen Psychiatry 39:905–910, 1982.

Kendell R: The Classification of Depressive Illness. London, Oxford University Press, 1968.

Kirkegaard C, Norlein N, Lauridsen U, et al: Protirelin stimulation test and thyroid function during treatment of depression. Arch Gen Psychiatry 32:1115–1118, 1975.

Klerman G, Endicott J, Spitzer R, Hirschfeld R: Neurotic depressions: A systematic analysis of multiple criteria and meanings. Am J Psychiatry 136:57–61, 1979.

Koslow S, Maas J, Bowden C, et al: CSF and urinary biogenic amines and metabolites in depression and mania. Arch Gen Psychiatry 40:999–1010, 1983.

Kupfer D: REM latency—A psychobiological marker for primary depressive disease. Biol Psychiatry 2:159–174, 1976.

Lewis D, Kathol R, Sherman B, et al: Differentiation of depressive subtypes by insulin insensitivity in the recovered stage. Arch Gen Psychiatry 40:167–170, 1983.

Meltzer H, Arora R, Tricou B, Fang V: Serotonin uptake in blood platelets and the dexamethasone suppression test in depressed patients. Psychiatry Res 8:41–47, 1983.

O'Keane V, Dinan T: Prolactin and cortisol responses to D-fenfluramine in major depression: Evidence for diminished responsivity of central serotonergic function. Am J Psychiatry 148:1009–1015, 1991.

Parker G, Hadzi-Pavlovic D, Boyce R, et al: Classifying depression by mental state signs. Br J Psychiatry 157:55–65, 1990.

Paykel ES: Life events and early environment, in Paykel ES (ed): Handbook of Affective Disorders. Edinburgh, Churchill Livingstone, 1982, pp 146–161.

Robins L, Helzer J, Weissman M, et al: Lifetime prevalence of specific psychiatric disorders in three sites. Arch Gen Psychiatry 41:949–958, 1984.

Rush J: Short-term Psychotherapies for Depression. New York, Guilford Press, 1982.

Sachar E: Neuroendocrine abnormalities in depressive illness, in Sachar E (ed): Topics in Psychoendocrinology. New York, Grune & Stratton, 1975, pp 135–156.

Schlesser M, Winokur G, Sherman B: Genetic subtypes of unipolar primary depressive illness distinguished by hypothalamic-pituitary-adrenal activity. Lancet 1:739–741, 1979.

Schneider K: Clinical Psychopathology. New York, Grune & Stratton, 1959.

Stewart M, Drake F, Winokur G: Depression among medically ill patients. Dis Nerv Syst 26:1–7, 1965.

Stromgren L: The influence of depression on memory. Acta Psychiatr Scand 56:109–128, 1977.

Swift R, Perkins D, Chase C, et al: Psychiatric disorders in 36 families with Wolfram syndrome. Am J Psychiatry 148:775–779, 1991.

Tsuang M, Winokur G, Crowe R: Psychiatric disorders among relatives of surgical controls. J Clin Psychiatry 45:420–422, 1984.

Tsuang M, Woolson R, Fleming J: Premature deaths in schizophrenia and affective disorders: An analysis of survival curves and variables affecting the shortened survival. Arch Gen Psychiatry 37:979–983, 1980.

Tsuang M, Woolson R, Winokur G, Crowe R: Stability of psychiatric diagnosis, schizophrenia and affective disorders followed up over a 30 to 40 year period. Arch Gen Psychiatry 38:535–539, 1981.

Weissman M, Meyers J: Affective disorders in a U.S. urban community: The use of research diagnostic criteria in an epidemiological survey. Arch Gen Psychiatry 35:1304–1311, 1978.

Winokur G: Family history studies. VIII. Secondary depression is alive and well and . . . Dis Nerv Syst 33:94–99, 1972.

Winokur G: Genetic and clinical factors associated with course and depression: Contributions to genetic aspects. Pharmacopsychiatr Neuropsychopharmacol 7:122–126, 1974.

Winokur G: The development and validity of familial subtypes in primary unipolar depression. Pharmacopsychiatria 15:142–146, 1982.

Winokur G: Mania and Depression: A Classification of Syndrome and Disease. Baltimore, Johns Hopkins University Press, 1991.

Winokur G, Clayton P, Reich T: Manic Depressive Illness. St. Louis, CV Mosby, 1969.

Winokur G, Morrison J: The Iowa 500: Follow-up of 225 depressives. Br J Psychiatry 123:543–548, 1973.

Winokur G, Morrison J, Clancy J, Crowe R: The Iowa 500: Familial and clinical findings favor two kinds of depressive illness. Compr Psychiatry 14:99–107, 1973.

Winokur G, Tsuang M: The Iowa 500: Suicide in mania, depression, and schizophrenia. Am J Psychiatry 132:650–651, 1975.

Winokur G, Tsuang M, Crowe R: The Iowa 500: Affective disorder in relatives of manic and depressed patients. Am J Psychiatry 139:209–212, 1982.

CHAPTER 6

Schizophrenia

MING T. TSUANG
STEPHEN V. FARAONE

To the clinician and researcher alike, schizophrenia is a most paradoxical disorder. It is a clinically heterogeneous illness, yet it defies subclassification. Patients with schizophrenia exhibit extreme dysfunctions in perception, thinking, behavior, and emotions; nevertheless, the cerebral source of these anomalies has remained elusive. For some time we have known that genes play a role in etiology, but the search for specific mutations has been frustrated by diagnostic dilemmas. We have studied the disorder for over 100 years with increasingly powerful neurodiagnostic technologies and criterion-keyed diagnostic systems; however, our diagnostic criteria still rely on observations of psychiatric phenomenology made by astute clinicians, as they did at the turn of the century.

Despite these paradoxes, the diagnosis and treatment of schizophrenia have taken great strides. The introduction of neuroleptic medication in the 1950s made it possible for many patients to live outside mental institutions. The recent introduction of clozapine promises to help the many patients who do not benefit from typical neuroleptic treatment. We are also hopeful that, in this "decade of the brain," that is, the 1990s, we are entering a new century of schizophrenia research that will lead us to the etiologic and pathophysiologic mechanisms underlying this bewildering illness.

DIAGNOSIS

Historical Background

In 1896, before Bleuler coined the term *schizophrenia* (Bleuler, 1911/1950), Kraepelin described an illness characterized by hallucinations, delusions, and thought disorder (Kraepelin, 1919/1971). He termed this disorder *dementia praecox* (after Morel), since it appeared to have an early onset (praecox) of an irrecoverable mental deterioration (dementia). He later modified this position when he found that a small percentage of these patients recovered fully.

With regard to symptomatology, Kraepelin felt that "one must on principle beware of attributing characteristic significance to a single morbid phenomenon" (Kraepelin, 1919/1971, p. 261). He also said, "Unfortunately, there is in the domain of psychic disorders no single morbid symptom which is thoroughly characteristic of a definite malady." Diagnosis must include the "total clinical picture, including development, course and issue" (p. 261).

Bleuler (1911/1950) thought that schizophrenia encompassed, but was not necessarily limited to, Kraepelin's "dementia praecox." He named four fundamental symptoms that came to be known as "Bleuler's four A's": autism, ambivalence, abnormal thought associations, and abnormal affect. Evidence of any of these was sufficient for the diagnosis of schizophrenia. Bleuler believed delusions and hallucinations to be accessory symptoms that were not essential to the diagnosis. He coined the term *schizophrenia*, which literally means "split mind"; he believed that his four A's indicated a splitting between thought, emotion, and behavior. Outside the mental health community, schizophrenia is commonly thought to mean "split" or multiple personality, but this is incorrect. We now know that multiple personality and schizophrenia are distinct disorders.

To Bleuler, symptoms of mood disturbance were not incompatible with schizophrenia, but schizophrenic symptoms were incompatible with mood disorder. He believed that schizophrenics never recovered fully; some residual evidence of the fundamental symptoms of the illness could always be found. Bleuler's four fundamental symptoms of schizophrenia became the basis of the American definition of schizophrenia and remained so for many years until the *Diagnostic and Statistical Manual of Mental Disorders*, third edition (DSM-III), was published (American Psychiatric Association, 1980). Because there were many interpretations of the meaning of these four symptoms, many clinical pictures seemed to fit within the definition of schizophrenia. Bleuler himself stated: "Dementia praecox comprises the majority of psychoses heretofore designated as functional" (Bleuler, 1911/1950 p. 271). And so in American psychiatry before DSM-III, schizophrenia was more often diagnosed than other psychoses.

Morton Kramer (1961), at the National Institute of Mental Health, noticed that the hospital incidence of schizophrenia in the United States significantly exceeded that of Great Britain (28.0 versus 17.9 per 100,000 population). Conversely, in the hospitals of Great Britain, mood disorders were diagnosed much more often than in U.S. hospitals (36 versus 7 per 100,000). Kramer questioned whether these differences were real or were simply artifacts of diagnostic definitions or practices. The U.S.–U.K. project was begun to determine the source of these differences (Cooper et al., 1972). To gather information from patients, psychiatrists used a structured interview, based on the Present State Examination (PSE). The glossary from the *International Classification of Diseases*, eighth edition, (ICD-8), served as a reference standard for making project diagnoses. In all, 250 hospital patients in Brooklyn, New York, and 250 hospital patients in London were examined. The rates of schizophrenia and manic-depressive illness were similar in the two cities when the ICD-8 project diagnoses were used: 32 percent of the New York group and 26 percent of the London group received a project diagnosis of schizophrenia. However, based on hospital diagnoses, the rates of these disorders were quite different: 65 percent of the New York group but only 34 percent of the London group received hospital diagnoses of schizophrenia. Thirty-eight percent of the New York patients with a hospital diagnosis of schizophrenia received a project diagnosis of affective disorder, including 20 patients with bipolar disorder.

The International Pilot Study of Schizophrenia, a larger international collaborative project, also considered the problem of classification (World Health Organization, 1973). In nine countries (five developed and four developing), 1202 patients were examined with the PSE. The diagnosis of schizophrenia was made in three ways—clinical judgment, computer assessment of PSE data (CATEGO), and cluster analysis. A total of 306 patients were diagnosed as being schizophrenic by all three methods. Restricted affect, poor insight, audible thoughts, widespread delusions, incoherent speech, unreliable information, bizarre delusions, and nihilistic delusions were characteristic of these 306 schizophrenics. Depressed facies, elation, and waking early (all symptoms of mood disorder) were negatively associated with the diagnosis of schizophrenia. Carpenter et al. (1973) incorporated these findings from the International Pilot Study into a system for diagnosing schizophrenia called the "flexible system."

At about the same time, researchers at Washington University in St. Louis were concerned with the need for operational definitions of psychiatric disorders. Based on the research literature, they developed the Washington University criteria for 15 disorders, including schizophrenia (Feighner et al., 1972). Subsequently, Spitzer's group in New York, in collaboration with the Washington University group, refined and elaborated on these diagnostic systems to create the research diagnostic criteria (RDC) (Spitzer et al., 1978). The RDC defined 25 diagnoses, several with multiple subclassifications.

Overview of Symptomatology

POSITIVE SYMPTOMS

Positive symptoms are particularly common in schizophrenia, although they may occur in other psychoses as well. These symptoms are called *positive* to denote the production of abnormal phenomena. This feature sets them apart from *negative* symptoms (discussed below), which reflect the absence or reduction of normal thoughts, feelings, and behaviors. Positive symptoms are often referred to in the general literature on schizophrenia, and several are referred to specifically in the current criteria for schizophrenia. Thus knowledge of these symptoms is necessary for understanding the clinical picture of schizophrenia.

Mellor's (1970) descriptions of positive symptoms are as follows: (1) *audible thoughts* (i.e., voices that speak the patient's thoughts out loud), (2) *voices arguing* (i.e., two or more voices argue or discuss, usually with the patient as the subject, who is often referred to in the third person), (3) *voices commenting* (i.e., a voice describes or comments on the patient's activities as he or she performs them), (4) *somatic passivity* (i.e., some outside agency imposes sensations on the patient, often by some extraordinary means, such as x-rays), (5) *thought withdrawal* (i.e., some outside agency withdraws the patient's thoughts; usually the patient feels for a time that his mind is empty), (6) *thought insertion* (i.e., some outside agency inserts thoughts into the patient's mind), (7) *thought broadcasting* (i.e., the patient feels that his thoughts escape into the environment and are overheard by other people; the patient may ascribe this to telepathy but usually distinguishes this from the belief that others can read his mind), (8) *made feelings* (i.e., some outside agency imposes on the patient feelings that are not his own), (9) *made impulses (drives)* (i.e., the patient experiences the drive or impulse to act as coming from some outside agency), (10) *made volitional acts* (i.e., the patient's actions are, he believes, completely controlled by an outside force; the patient may feel as if he were a robot or a zombie), and (11) *delusional perception* (i.e., the patient attributes a private meaning to a normal perception; the meaning is delusional and is not simply related to a previous personal experience).

Loose associations is the term applied to thought production in which there is no recognizable relationship between ideas. Thoughts appear unconnected or, at best, obliquely related to one another. *Tangentiality, derailment, word salad,* and *talking past the point* are related terms that apply to abnormal relationships between ideas. *Catatonic excitement* occurs when the patient becomes hyperactive. During the excited phase, the patient may be destructive or violent. This differs from the hyperactivity of mania in that other manic symptoms, such as euphoria, are not present and the patient does not meet criteria for mania (see DSM-III for the definition of mania).

The preceding discussion indicates how positive symptoms are all *active* symptoms that involve the production of perceptions, thoughts, and feelings. As this list of symptoms suggests, hallucinations and delusions constitute a core component of the schizophrenic picture. Hallucinations are false perceptions in the absence of real sensory stimuli. These differ from illusions, which are misperceptions of real external stimuli. A delusion is a fixed false belief that the believer maintains even in the face of considerable evidence or likelihood to the contrary. Delusions can be of many sorts. Paranoid delusions may include beliefs that one is being persecuted, harassed, spied on, poisoned, or in some other way plotted against. The patient may name family, friends, or some specific organization or may not know who the perpetrators are.

In ideas of reference, the patient believes that events that are of no obvious relevance to him refer personally to him. For example, the patient may believe that people are talking about him when they pass him on the street or that radio or television programs or newspaper articles are about him.

NEGATIVE SYMPTOMS

Although positive symptoms had, for some time, been considered the key characteristic of schizophrenia, negative symptoms are also common in schizophrenia, particularly in nonparanoid forms. Whereas positive symptoms involve the production of abnormal phenomena, the absence or reduction of normal phenomena is the shared feature of negative symptoms. Andreasen (1982) classified negative symptoms into five groups and described systematic procedures for their rating:

1. Affective flattening or blunting
   a. Unchanging facial expression
   b. Decreased spontaneous movements
   c. Paucity of expressive gestures
   d. Poor eye contact
   e. Affective nonresponsivity
   f. Inappropriate affect
   g. Lack of vocal inflections
2. Alogia
   a. Poverty of speech
   b. Poverty of content of speech
   c. Blocking
   d. Increased latency of response
3. Avolition-apathy
   a. Poor grooming and hygiene
   b. Impersistence at work or school
   c. Physical anergy
4. Anhedonia-asociality
   a. Decrease in or lack of recreational interests or pleasure from recreational activities.
   b. Lack of sexual interest or activity
   c. Decreased ability to feel intimacy or closeness
   d. Decrease in or lack of relationships with friends and peers
5. Attentional impairment
   a. Work inattentiveness
   b. Inattentiveness during mental status examination
   c. Subjective complaints of inattentiveness

Many of the symptoms are self-explanatory. Some require explanation. *Affect* refers to emotion expressed by the subject and observed by the examiner. *Blunted affect* is a marked reduction in the amount of affect. *Flat affect* refers to the absence of affect. *Inappropriate affect* is affect that is strikingly inconsistent with the thought content or environmental circumstances of the patient.

Poverty of speech means that speech is extremely reduced in amount; for example, the patient says very little in response to questions that, with an ordinary person, would elicit considerable talk. *Poverty of content of speech* refers to speech that is devoid of content. Despite normal verbal production, nothing is communicated. *Blocking* is when speech is interrupted before a thought has been completed, and the patient cannot recall what he or she was saying or had intended to say before the interruption of thought. *Increased latency of response* means there is an abnormally long delay before the patient speaks. *Physical anergy* refers to physical inactivity, such as sitting and doing nothing for long periods.

Catatonic negative symptoms, including negativism, mutism, waxy flexibility, posturing, and catatonic stupor, may be present. *Negativism,* loosely defined, refers to the refusal of the patient to comply with requests. More narrowly defined, it refers to the active resistance on the part of the patient to most or all demands made on him. *Mutism* is self-explanatory; the patient does not talk; it may be accompanied by *catatonic stupor*, in which the patient is unresponsive and immobile although conscious. *Waxy flexibility* may be elicited by first instructing the patient that he does not have to cooperate and then, while distracting with conversation or questions, placing a limb of the patient in some position. If waxy flexibility is present, the patient will hold the position for at least several minutes. *Posturing* refers to the holding of unusual positions for long periods. Schizophrenics also may display *mannerisms*, which are goal-directed movements that are stilted, bizarre, or out of context. *Stereotypies* are repetitive non-goal-directed movements that are more complex than a tic.

None of the positive or negative symptoms are pathognomonic of schizophrenia; they all may occur in other disorders. Kraepelin's original work (1919/1971) and *Fish's Schizophrenia* (Hamilton, 1984) are good sources for more detailed descriptions of the symptomatology of this disorder.

Current Diagnostic Criteria

The DSM-IIIR criteria for schizophrenia are given in Table 6-1 (American Psychiatric Association, 1987). Six major criteria must be present to diagnose the disorder. There are three types of major criteria: core symptoms, course criteria, and exclusion criteria. The core symptoms are listed in criterion A, which requires the presence of signs and symptoms indicative of massive disruptions in thought, perception, emotions, and motor behavior. These must occur for at least 1 week unless successfully treated. As the subcriteria that constitute criterion A indicate, nonbizarre delusions are not sufficient on their own. Neither are some types of hallucinations. To be diagnostic of schizophrenia,

these must occur in the presence of one another or with incoherence, marked loosening of associations, catatonic behavior, flat affect, or grossly inappropriate affect.

Two of the criteria are course criteria. That is, they require that the time course of the symptoms correspond to a specific pattern. Criterion B reflects the kraepelinian idea that schizophrenia is associated with a deteriorating course of social and occupational functioning. That is, schizophrenia cannot be diagnosed among individuals if the signs and symptoms of criterion A are not associated with impaired functioning in the patient's daily life. Criterion D is another course criterion. It requires "continuous signs of the illness" to be present for at least 6 months. These signs include both the core symptoms of criterion A and the prodromal or residual symptoms listed in Table 6-2. The symptoms are termed *prodromal* if they preceded the episode of core symptoms; they are otherwise termed *residual*.

The exclusion criteria (C, E, and F) indicate conditions under which the diagnosis of schizophrenia cannot be made, even if the core symptoms and course criteria are present. Criterion C requires the absence of a schizoaffective or mood disorder. As we discuss below, these are two of the most difficult of the differential diagnoses for schizophrenia. Schizophrenia is also excluded by criterion E if we establish that an organic factor initiated and maintained the disturbance. Note that the organic factor must both initiate and maintain the illness. For example, if the patient has a drug-induced psychosis that does not remit following cessation of drug use, the diagnosis of schizophrenia is still possible. Criterion F excludes the diagnosis of schizophrenia for autistic patients if prominent delusions or hallucinations are not present.

The DSM-IIIR criteria for schizophrenia are best seen as nosologic hypotheses rather than infallible indicators of a homogeneous disorder. Indeed, these criteria are currently being updated for DSM-IV, and additional revisions are likely until we have

---

TABLE 6-1.   *DSM-IIIR Criteria for Schizophrenia*

A. Presence of 1, 2, or 3 for at least 1 week (unless successfully treated)
  1. Two of the following
    a. Delusions
    b. Prominent hallucinations
    c. Incoherence or marked loosening of associations
    d. Catatonic behavior
    e. Flat or grossly inappropriate affect
  2. Bizarre delusions
  3. One of the following prominent hallucinations
    a. A voice with no relation to depression or elation
    b. A voice maintaining a running commentary on the patient
    c. Voices conversing with one another
B. Deterioration in functioning in such areas as work, social relations, and self-care
C. Schizoaffective disorder and psychotic mood disorder have been ruled out
D. Continuous signs of the disturbance for at least 6 months
E. Organic factors cannot account for the disturbance
F. If there is a history of autistic disorder, prominent hallucinations or delusions must be present

Adapted from American Psychiatric Association: Diagnostic and Statistical Manual of Mental Disorders, 3d ed revised. Washington, American Psychiatric Association, 1987.

TABLE 6-2.   *DSM-IIIR Prodromal and Residual Symptoms of Schizophrenia*

1. Marked social isolation or withdrawal
2. Marked impairment in role functioning
3. Markedly peculiar behavior (e.g., collecting garbage, talking to self)
4. Marked impairment in personal hygiene and grooming
5. Blunted or inappropriate affect
6. Digressive, vague, overelaborate, or circumstantial speech, poverty of speech, or poverty of content of speech
7. Odd beliefs or magical thinking influencing behavior and inconsistent with cultural norms
8. Unusual perceptual experiences (e.g., recurrent illusions)
9. Marked lack of initiative, interests or energy

Adapted from American Psychiatric Association: Diagnostic and Statistical Manual of Mental Disorders, 3d ed revised. Washington, American Psychiatric Association, 1987.

a comprehensive understanding of the etiology and pathophysiology of this illness. Nevertheless, the criterion-based diagnosis of schizophrenia that evolved into DSM-IV is much more reliable than the ill-defined entity that had preceeded it (Helzer et al., 1981; Stephens et al., 1982). By carefully excluding mood disorders and other "good prognosis" psychoses, such as schizophreniform disorder and brief reactive psychosis, the current diagnosis of schizophrenia creates a relatively homogeneous group for both treatment and research. In the absence of a classification system based on etiology, it is important that a diagnosis perform two basic functions: the prediction of outcome and the prediction of treatment. Both are essential aspects of practical day-to-day clinical medicine.

Subtypes of Schizophrenia

Schizophrenia is a clinically heterogeneous disorder and has traditionally been divided into a number of categories. Tsuang and Winokur (1974) developed criteria for paranoid and hebephrenic schizophrenia. These are displayed in Table 6-3. By their criteria, all the patients must first have fulfilled Washington University criteria for schizophrenia. Then, by application of subtyping criteria, they are divided into paranoid, hebephrenic, and undifferentiated subtypes. These criteria separate patients by outcome better than other criteria for these sub-

TABLE 6-3. *Tsuang-Winokur Criteria for Hebephrenic and Paranoid Schizophrenia*

I. Hebephrenic (A through D must be present)
  A. Age of onset and sociofamilial data (one of the following)
    1. Onset before age 25
    2. Unmarried or unemployed
    3. Family history of schizophrenia
  B. Disorganized thought
  C. Affect changes (either 1 or 2)
    1. Inappropriate affect
    2. Flat affect
  D. Behavioral symptoms (either 1 or 2)
    1. Bizarre behavior
    2. Motor symptoms (either a or b)
      a. Hebephrenic traits
      b. Catatonic traits (if present, subtype may be modified to hebephrenia with catatonic traits)
II. Paranoid (A through C must be present)
  A. Age of onset and sociofamilial data (one of the following)
    1. Onset after 25 years
    2. Married or employed
    3. Absence of family history of schizophrenia
  B. Exclusion criteria
    1. Disorganized thoughts must be absent or of mild degree, such that speech is intelligible.
    2. Affective and behavioral symptoms, as described in hebephrenia, must be absent or of mild degree.
  C. Preoccupations with extensive, well-organized delusions or hallucinations

---

Adapted from Tsuang MT, Winokur G: Criteria for subtyping schizophrenia: Clinical differentiation of hebephrenic and paranoid schizophrenia. Arch Gen Psychiatry 31:43–47, 1974.

groups (Kendler et al., 1984). In general, the paranoid group has a better outcome than the hebephrenic and undifferentiated groups and as good an outcome as that of a bipolar comparison group (Kendler et al., 1984). For example, 64 percent of the paranoid group at a 35- to 40-year follow-up were not occupationally disabled compared with 28 percent of the hebephrenic group and 40 percent of the undifferentiated group. By comparison, 76 percent of bipolar patients were not occupationally disabled. The DSM-IIIR criteria for paranoid, disorganized (hebephrenic), and undifferentiated schizophrenia are similar to the Tsuang-Winokur criteria. DSM-IIIR, however, does not include the age at onset and sociofamilial criteria used in the Tsuang-Winokur criteria. DSM-IIIR also includes a separate catatonic subtype that is not nested under the definition of hebephrenic schizophrenia.

A key problem in establishing the validity of subtype diagnoses has been that subtype diagnosis changes over time. Depue and Woodburn (1975) found that over a 10-year period, 50 percent of paranoid schizophrenic patients changed to a nonparanoid diagnosis. The shift in subtype diagnosis usually occurred about 6 years after the first admission with schizophrenia. Kendler et al. (1985) examined the stability of subtype diagnoses over a 30- to 40-year period. Using Tsuang-Winokur criteria, they found that 71 percent of the hebephrenics and 59 percent of the paranoids changed their subtype diagnosis at follow-up. Those patients who changed diagnosis were diagnosed as undifferentiated at follow-up. Thus, subtype diagnosis is not a consistent characteristic of the schizophrenic illness. This is important to consider when comparing research studies that may use different definitions of subtypes and may study patients at different times in the course of their illness. Indeed, as one might expect from the instability of the diagnosis, biologic studies comparing paranoid and nonparanoid subforms of schizophrenia have produced equivocal results (Farley et al., 1978; Bersani et al., 1989; Bornstein et al., 1989; Rosse et al., 1991).

Genetic studies of the distinction between paranoid and nonparanoid schizophrenia have tended to find that relatives of nonparanoid schizophrenics are at greater risk for schizophrenia compared with relatives of paranoid schizophrenics (Gottesman and Shields, 1972, 1982; Farmer et al., 1984; McGuffin et al., 1987). Furthermore, there is some evidence for subtype concordance among twin pairs (McGuffin et al., 1987) and family members (Gottesman and Shields, 1982). By *subtype concordance*, we mean that pairs of relatives with schizophrenia are more likely than chance to be of the same subtype. Not all studies find subtype concordance, and some of the studies finding subtype concordance have been criticized on methodologic grounds (Onstad et al., 1991). Nevertheless, given that measurement error and misclassification will tend to reduce evidence for subtype concordance (Kendler, 1987), the hypothesis that paranoid and nonparanoid subtypes breed true, at least to some extent, is viable. This hypothesis would suggest that the two subtypes are etiologically distinct. An alternative view is that paranoid and nonparanoid subforms lie on a continuum of severity, with the latter type being the more severe form (McGuffin et al., 1987). Much research is currently being devoted to testing these two viable hypotheses.

Differential Diagnosis

GENERAL PRINCIPLES

The making of a differential diagnosis presumes an understanding of certain basic principles of diagnosis. In general, psychiatric diagnoses cannot be based on a single dimension, such as cross-sectional symptomatology, course, family history, response to treatment, or laboratory findings. Usually, the more dimensions along which an illness has been defined, the more reliably it can be differentiated from other disorders.

Specific considerations in the differential diagnosis of schizophrenia are as follows:

1. Establish a clear sensorium, the absence of which precludes any immediate diagnosis of schizophrenia.
2. Use reliable, narrow definitions of symptoms.
3. Carefully determine the course of each symptom, including mode of onset, first occurrence, and course.
4. If possible, gather information on psychiatric illness in other family members.
5. Determine response to any treatment that may have been given in the past.
6. Specifically review symptoms of bipolar mood disorder and major depressive disorder, since the exclusion of these two disorders is required for the diagnosis of schizophrenia.
7. Be patient and observe until relevant diagnostic information can be gathered.
8. Carefully rate the presence or absence of features required for the diagnosis.
9. Remember that most symptoms of schizophrenia can occur in other disorders.

We are looking for characteristic patterns of course and symptoms. Remember, *pathognomonic features do not exist.* Usually, after these steps are carefully executed, application of the diagnostic criteria to the information gathered will clarify the diagnosis and help to avoid the ludicrous labeling of individuals as schizophrenic in the manner reported by Rosenhan (1973).

DISORDERS TO BE CONSIDERED IN THE DIFFERENTIAL DIAGNOSIS

The differential diagnosis of schizophrenia should include

- Organic mental disorder
- Bipolar disorder
- Major depression
- Schizophreniform disorder
- Psychotic disorder not otherwise specified (NOS)
- Induced psychotic disorder
- Schizoaffective disorder
- Brief reactive psychosis
- Schizotypal personality disorder
- Paranoid disorder
- Paranoid personality
- Borderline personality disorder

This list includes most of the disorders that are likely to share symptomatology with schizophrenia. Less commonly, the following may be confused with schizophrenia: somatization disorder, agoraphobia, obsessive-compulsive disorder, antisocial personality disorder, atypical anxiety disorder, and atypical depressive disorder.

Almost every major psychiatric disorder is included in the list. This is so because many disorders share symptoms with schizophrenia or have symptoms that may be confused with those of schizophrenia. For example, in a study of 116 consecutively admitted patients with hallucinations, Goodwin et al. (1971) found that only 32 (28 percent) had schizophrenia. Abrams and Taylor (1981) examined 111 manics who met Washington University criteria, research diagnostic criteria, and DSM-III criteria for mania. Only 42 (38 percent) had none of the following symptoms: formal thought disorder, catatonic symptoms, auditory hallucinations, persecutory delusions, and other positive symptoms. Andreasen (1979) found similar patterns of "thought-language-communication disorder" in 45 schizophrenics and 32 manics, including poverty of content of speech, tangentiality, derailment, incoherence, illogicality, loss of goal, and perseveration.

Research reviewed in this chapter suggests that the course and outcome of symptoms are the primary factors that differentiate schizophrenia from other psychoses. When based on symptoms alone, particularly isolated symptoms, the diagnosis of schizophrenia often has been erroneous (Pope and Lipinski, 1978). This was Kraepelin's basic position many years ago (Kraepelin, 1919/1971). The importance of establishing not only symptoms, but also their pattern and course, has been recognized by DSM-IIIR: In many cases it requires a specific course of symptoms for the diagnosis of a given disorder, particularly for schizophrenia.

SPECIFIC SOURCES OF CONFUSION IN THE DIFFERENTIAL DIAGNOSIS

There are many case reports of organic mental disorders being confused with schizophrenia or schizophreniform disorder. However, most reported cases of organic mental disorders confused with schizophrenia do not show a typically schizophrenic course of symptoms. For example, in an acute brain syndrome, symptoms begin much more abruptly and may include visual hallucinations or bizarre behavior resulting from a clouded consciousness; these are usually qualitatively different from the positive symptoms that are characteristic of schizophrenia. In a chronic brain syndrome, symptoms that might be confused with negative symptoms result from intellectual deterioration. The schizophrenic typically can describe the course of hallucinations and delusions over the duration of the illness. The patient with a brain syndrome recalls only vaguely what has occurred. The problems of differentiating organic illness from schizophrenia have been discussed in more detail by Hall (1980) and Lishman (1978).

The organic mental disorders most likely to be confused with schizophrenia are temporal lobe epilepsy and psychoses related to alcohol and drug abuse. In temporal lobe epilepsy (complex partial seizures), delusions and hallucinations may follow a course resembling that of schizophrenia. However, these symptoms usually occur after the onset of complex partial seizures (in one series an average of 14 years after the seizures began) (Slater and Beard, 1963). Thus a history of other seizure phenomena is useful in making this differential diagnosis.

Transient hallucinations and delusions occur frequently in alcoholics. Victor and Hope (1958) found that 15 of 76 patients had onset of hallucinations while still drinking. In the patients for whom the time of the last drink could be determined, 32 (60 percent) had onset of hallucinations within 12 to 48 hours of the last drink. In the 75 patients for whom the duration of hallucinations could be determined, 64 (85 percent) had a duration of hallucinations of 6 days or less. Only 8 of 75 (11 percent) had a duration of hallucinations of 6 weeks. Schuckit and Winokur (1971) found no increase in the incidence of schizophrenia in the relatives of alcoholics with hallucinosis. Also, the patients were no more likely than other alcoholics to have a history of schizophrenia. Thus alcoholic hallucinosis differs from schizophrenia in that it occurs after prolonged alcohol abuse, is usually of abrupt onset and short duration, and is not associated with a family history of schizophrenia.

Amphetamine abuse may produce a paranoid psychosis with visual, auditory, and tactile hallucinations. Unlike the insidious onset typical of true schizophrenia, the psychosis may begin relatively abruptly (e.g., during a several-day course of high intake of amphetamines) and resolve within a few days after cessation of drug use (Grinspoon and Bakalar, 1980; Ellison and Eison, 1983). It is more difficult to distinguish between individuals with preexisting psychiatric illness who may abuse drugs and drug abusers who may have prolonged psychoses (Tsuang et al., 1982). Tsuang et al. (1982)

defined *prolonged psychosis* as at least 6 months of symptoms without return to previous levels of functioning. They found that the risk for schizophrenia in the families of 45 drug abusers with prolonged psychosis was 6.5 percent. This was similar to the risk for families of 46 schizophrenics (6.8 percent). In addition, families of drug abusers with prolonged psychosis had increased risk for mood disorder, suggesting that this group of patients with psychosis was genetically heterogeneous. The psychoses of the patients, however, resembled schizophrenia in terms of course and symptomatology. Because chronic psychoses in drug abusers may begin at an earlier age than those in non-drug abusers, some authorities have suggested that drug abuse precipitates the illness in the genetically predisposed (Tsuang et al., 1982; Bowers and Swigar, 1983). In sum, a psychosis in a drug abuser that does not remit after prolonged cessation of drug use and that otherwise meets criteria for schizophrenia probably is schizophrenia.

Mood disorders, particularly mania, often were diagnosed as schizophrenia in the New York sample of the U.S.–U.K. study (Cooper et al., 1972). Abrupt onset and the predominance of affective symptoms usually distinguish bipolar mood disorder from schizophrenia (Pope and Lipinski, 1978). Manics may have many symptoms, such as paranoid delusions and thought disorder, that once were considered indicative of schizophrenia. Flight of ideas may be confused with loose associations, but these rarely occur without other symptoms of mania, such as euphoria, decreased sleep, and hyperactivity. Schizophrenics may sleep badly and have episodes of hyperactivity, but these symptoms are usually secondary to delusions and hallucinations or part of catatonic symptomatology; they usually are not accompanied by the typical euphoria, grandiosity, and social hyperactivity of the manic.

Major depression may involve paranoid delusions, usually mood-congruent. By *mood-congruent*, we mean that the delusion content is consistent with depressive themes (e.g., guilt, worthlessness, suicide). Sometimes *mood-incongruent* delusions occur, but more typical symptoms of depression usually precede them. Patients with depression may report hearing voices or having other hallucinations. These reports are typically fragmented; the experiences are not of many months' duration, and they occur within the context of a predominantly affective constellation of symptoms. Occasionally, at first examination, the clinician may have difficulty establishing the course of symptoms. In such cases, more information needs to be gathered before the final diagnosis is decided. The nosologic status of mood disorder with mood-incongruent features needs further clarification (Coryell et al., 1982; Kendler, 1991).

In schizophrenia, episodes of depression usually occur along with other schizophrenic symptoms and within the context of an otherwise typical schizophrenic illness (Guze et al., 1983). The social withdrawal, lack of interest, and psychomotor retardation of depression may resemble schizophrenic social deterioration and thought disorder. A careful history will reveal whether these symptoms occur in the context of a typical depressive illness, with other symptoms such as poor appetite, terminal insomnia, and self-reproach, or whether the onset of a depressed mood preceded the marked withdrawal, lack of interest, and psychomotor retardation.

Schizophreniform disorder has the same symptoms as schizophrenia, but they are of shorter duration. It thus appears to function as a residual category for those patients with schizophrenic symptoms who have an abrupt, rather than an insidious, onset. However, schizophreniform disorder historically has been used for individuals who do have some of the symptoms of schizophrenia but who differ from schizophrenics in ways other than mode of onset and duration (Tsuang and Loyd, 1985). For example, emotional turmoil and intellectual confusion or perplexity may be prominent; psychosocial stresses may play a larger role than in schizophrenia; premorbid adjustment is usually good. Nonetheless, the most important distinctions between the two disorders are mode of onset and duration of episode.

Psychosis NOS (not otherwise specified) is a residual diagnostic category. When diagnostic rules are carefully applied, many patients called schizophrenic in years past will fall into this category. The main identifying characteristic of these patients is that they have psychotic symptoms but do not fit into any more rigorously defined category. Using this category rather than forcing a choice between the more carefully defined categories is important. It reminds the clinician that more information needs to be gathered before deciding on course of treatment and counseling the patient and family as to future outcome. In many cases the psychosis NOS diagnosis serves as a temporary category for newly onset patients until the course of their symptoms reveals their diagnosis.

Schizoaffective disorder differs from schizophrenia in that both affective and schizophrenic features are equally prominent (Tsuang et al., 1976; Tsuang and Loyd, 1985). The affective symptoms do not occur in an otherwise typical schizophrenic course of illness, or vice versa. Rather, both categories of symptoms occur together. Schizoaffective patients also may have a relatively abrupt onset and fail to meet the duration criterion for schizophrenia. In DSM-IIIR, the diagnosis of schizoaffective disorder requires that the duration of all episodes of mood disturbance (mania or depression) has not been brief relative to the total duration of the psychotic disturbance (American Psychiatric Association, 1987, p. 210). Since the criteria do not define *brief*, this distinction is often very difficult to make.

Brief reactive psychosis (Tsuang and Loyd, 1985) should not be confused with schizophrenia, except in cases where a history cannot be obtained. Otherwise, a history of an abrupt-onset psychosis with rapid resolution of symptoms should distinguish the two. Brief reactive psychosis may be confused with schizophrenia when the patient has a preexisting personality disorder that bears some similarities to the prodromata of schizophrenia. However, since schizophrenics are usually psychotic for many months before coming to treatment, this is usually not a problem in most clinical settings. For new, acute-onset cases of schizophrenia, this differential diagnosis will be difficult until the course of the illness becomes clear.

Paranoid disorder is relatively rare (Winokur, 1977). It may be confused with paranoid schizophrenia and perhaps rightly so, since the boundaries between the two are unclear (Kendler and Tsuang, 1981). In paranoid disorder, only a single, well-encapsulated delusional system occurs. The delusions of paranoid disorder are plausible in the sense that they *could* occur. There are no hallucinations, bizarre or fantastic delusions, or negative symptoms, as in typical schizophrenia, and delusions are not fragmented.

Schizotypal personality disorder may be genetically related to schizophrenia. However, the symptoms never quite reach the stage of full-blown delusions or hallucinations. The patient may appear suspicious and superstitious. He or she may complain of vague ideas of reference and have few social contacts. But no symptoms such as those described under category A of schizophrenia are unequivocally present. Similarly, paranoid personality should not be confused with schizophrenia, since no delusions, hallucinations, changes in affect, thought disorder, or other schizophrenic symptoms are present. Initially, one might suspect that delusions lie behind the suspiciousness, guardedness, and hostility, but none can be found.

Borderline, histrionic, and other personality disorders have been confused with schizophrenia when broad criteria were applied. Strict application of the diagnostic criteria, using reliable and narrow definitions of features, obviates such errors. Although some of the symptoms of these disorders resemble the prodromal symptoms of schizophrenia, these patients do not develop the narrowly defined symptoms in criterion A of the diagnostic criteria for schizophrenia. However, since they may exhibit psychotic symptoms and be susceptible to brief reactive psychoses, the question of schizophrenia may arise.

In one group of patients, the mentally retarded, the diagnosis of schizophrenia may be difficult even if all the recommendations in this chapter are carefully followed. Many schizophrenic features are symptoms that only the patient can report. Patients with severe communication defects may not be able to communicate these symptoms to an observer. Less frequently, it may be difficult to differentiate misperceptions of events or fantasy from delusions or hallucinations (Wright, 1982).

The diagnosis of schizophrenia must be based on the presence of specific symptoms and a specific course of symptoms. DSM-IIIR specifies these symptoms and their course. Other disorders differ from schizophrenia if symptoms are narrowly defined and their course is taken into account. When the history and psychiatric examination of a psychotic patient do not reveal a pattern of symptoms and symptom duration that clearly corresponds to a well-defined disorder, it is prudent to use the category of psychosis NOS.

EPIDEMIOLOGY

Prevalence and Incidence

The three basic questions of psychiatric epidemiology are: How many people have a disorder at a given point or period in time (the *prevalence*)? How many new cases occur during a specified period of time (the *incidence*)? And what is the cumulative risk for the disorder over an entire lifetime (the *lifetime prevalence*)? Prevalence studies of schizophrenia are summarized in Table 6-4. The large majority of these studies find schizophrenia in less than 1 percent of the general population. Taken together, they suggest that schizophrenia will be found in approximately 1/2 of 1 percent of the general population at any point in time. The variability of rates in Table 6-4 do not clearly follow any simple categorizations of their countries of origin. Whether we consider East versus West, developed countries versus less developed countries, or other classifications, the prevalence of schizophrenia remains at approximately 0.5 percent. One notably large prevalence is the 1.7 percent rate reported by Böök et al. (1978). These investigators studied a northern Swedish population that is isolated from the rest of the country and located in a bleak environment. It may be that such environments are attractive for the many schizophrenics who prefer a socially withdrawn and isolated lifestyle.

We present incidence studies of schizophrenia in Table 6-5. These numbers indicate the *new* cases observed each year per 1000 persons in the population. The incidence rates range from a low of 0.10 to a high of 0.70. Consistent with the prevalence figures, the incidence of schizophrenia is not highly variable over time or across geographic areas. Table 6-6 displays the lifetime prevalence estimates for schizophrenia. Again, there is little evidence for cultural or temporal variation in these rates. They range from a low of 2.6 to a high of 37. The lifetime prevalence rates are more variable across studies than are the prevalence or incidence rates. This is probably due to methodologic differences in how the rates are computed. The differences in the magnitudes of the prevalence, incidence, and lifetime prevalence rates underscore the importance of using these terms correctly. As the tables clearly

TABLE 6-4. *Prevalence of Schizophrenia*

Study	Location	Prevalence per 1000
Brugger (1931)	Germany	2.4
Brugger (1933)	Germany	2.2
Klemperer (1933)	Germany	10.0
Strömgren (1935)	Denmark	3.3
Lemkao (1936)	U.S.A.	2.9
Roth and Luton (1938)	U.S.A.	1.7
Brugger (1938)	Germany	2.3
Lin (1946–1948)	China	2.1
Mayer-Gross (1948)	Scotland	4.2
Bremer (1951)	Norway	4.4
Böök (1953)	Sweden	9.5
Larson and Sjögren (1954)	Sweden	4.6
National Survey (1954)	Japan	2.3
Essen-Möller (1956)	Sweden	6.7
Yoo (1961)	Korea	3.8
Juel-Nielsen et al. (1962)	Denmark	1.5
Ivanys et al. (1963)	Czechoslovakia	1.7
Krasik (1965)	U.S.S.R.	3.1
Hagnell (1966)	Sweden	4.5
Wing et al. (1967)	England	4.4
	Scotland	2.5
	U.S.A.	7.0
Lin et al. (1969)	Taiwan	1.4
Jayasundera (1969)	Ceylon	3.2
Kato (1969)	Japan	2.3
Dube (1970)	India	3.7
Roy et al. (1970)	Canada	
	Indians	5.7
	Non-Indians	1.6
Crocetti et al. (1971)	Yugoslavia	
	Rijeka	7.3
	Zagreb	4.2
Kulcar et al. (1971)	Yugoslavia	
	Lubin	7.4
	Sinj-Trogir	2.9
Bash et al. (1972)	Iran	2.1
Zharikov (1972)	U.S.S.R.	5.1
Babigian (1975)	U.S.A.	4.7
Temkov et al. (1975)	Bulgaria	2.8
Rotstein (1977)	U.S.S.R.	3.8
Nielsen and Nielsen (1977)	Denmark	2.7
Ouspenskaya (1978)	U.S.S.R.	5.3
Böök et al. (1978)	Sweden	17.0
Lehtinen et al. (1978)	Finland	15.0
Wijesinghe et al. (1978)	Ceylon	5.6
Weissman (1980)	New Haven	4.0
Hafner and Klug (1980)	Germany	1.2
Walsh et al. (1980)	Ireland	8.3
Rin and Lin (1982)	Taiwan	0.9
Sikanartey et al. (1984)	Ghana	0.6
Meyers et al. (1984)	New Haven	11.0
	Baltimore	10.0
	St. Louis	6.0
Von Korff et al. (1985)	Baltimore	6.0
Hwu (1989)	Taiwan	2.4
Astrup (1989)	Norway	7.3
Hwu (1989)	Taiwan	2.4
Bøjholm (1989)	Denmark	3.3
Lee (1990)	Korea	3.1
Stefánsson (1991)	Iceland	3.0
Youssef (1991)	Ireland	3.3

indicate, the risk for developing schizophrenia over one's lifetime is much higher than either the incidence or prevalence of the disease.

Tables 6-4, 6-5, and 6-6 show that schizophrenia has been found in all cultures. In industrialized societies, schizophrenics usually belong to

TABLE 6-5. *Incidence of Schizophrenia*

Study	Country	Annual number of new cases per 1000
Ødegaard (1946)	Norway	0.24
Hollingshead and Redlich (1958)	U.S.A.	0.30
Norris (1959)	U.K.	0.17
Jaco (1960)	U.S.A.	0.35
Dunham (1965)	U.S.A.	0.52
Warthen (1967)	U.S.A.	0.70
Adelstein et al. (1968)	U.K.	0.26–0.35
Walsh (1969)	Ireland	0.46–0.57
Hafner and Reimann (1970)	Germany	0.54
Lieberman (1974)	U.S.S.R.	0.19–0.20
Hailey et al. (1974)	U.K.	0.10–0.14
Babigian (1975)	U.S.A.	0.69
Nielsen (1976)	Denmark	0.20
Helgason (1977)	Iceland	0.27
Krupinski (1983)	Australia	0.18
Folnegovic (1990)	Croatia	0.22
Youssef (1991)	Ireland	0.16

lower socioeconomic groups (Cooper, 1978). Dunham's (1965) work suggests that the excess of schizophrenics in the lowest socioeconomic group results either from downward drift or from the schizophrenic's failure to move into a higher class. Goldberg and Morrison (1963) found that the social class distribution of the fathers of schizophrenics did not differ from that of the general population. Male schizophrenics tended to have lower job achievement than did fathers, brothers, and other male relatives. Whereas fathers tended to rise in job status, schizophrenic sons tended to fall into jobs of lower and lower status or become disabled. Thus it appears that although low socioeconomic status is known to have deleterious effects, it is primarily an effect of schizophrenia rather than its cause.

ETIOLOGY AND PATHOPHYSIOLOGY

A variety of noxious psychological influences have been thought to cause schizophrenia. Society, social class, "schizophrenogenic" mothers, double binds, and other abnormal patterns of communication or behavior in the family have been implicated. At times it has even been suggested that schizophrenia is actually a healing process or a beneficial spiritual experience rather than an illness. However, after critically reviewing these theories, Wing (1978) and Leff (1978) concluded that advocates of these various explanations for schizophrenia had produced little evidence in their support.

In contrast, two domains have been robustly implicated in the etiology and pathophysiology of schizophrenia. First, family, twin, and adoption studies have unequivocally demonstrated that genetic factors play a substantial, albeit not exclusive, role in the etiology of the schizophrenic disorders (Gottesman and Shields, 1982). Second, although the details of schizophrenic pathophysiology have yet to be worked out, numerous studies have demonstrated both structural and functional abnormalities in the brains of schizophrenic patients. These abnormalities have been demonstrated both indirectly, as in neuropsychological assessment, and directly, as in computed tomography, magnetic resonance imaging, positron emission tomography, regional cerebral blood flow, and postmortem studies (Henn, 1982; Nasrallah and Weinberger, 1986). Indeed, along with indications of genetic factors, structural and functional brain abnormalities are among the most consistent findings in schizophrenia research (Wyatt et al., 1988).

Schizophrenia Is a Genetic Disorder

FAMILY STUDIES

A number of studies over the years have demonstrated a fourfold increase in the rate of functional psychosis in the families of patients with psychosis compared with the families of patients without psychosis. Most research suggests that the increased rate is illness-specific; that is, the increased risk in the families of patients is significant for the illness from which the patient suffers. Table 6-7 summarizes the risk for schizophrenia from the older literature (Tsuang and Vandermey, 1980). The figures clearly show that the more closely a person is related to a schizophrenic, the greater is that person's risk of having schizophrenia.

TABLE 6-6. *Lifetime Prevalence of Schizophrenia*

Study	Country	Lifetime prevalence per 1000
Hagnell (1966)	Sweden	14.0
Brugger (1931)	Germany	3.8
Brugger (1933)	Germany	4.1
Klemperer (1933)	Germany	14.0
Brugger (1938)	Germany	3.6
Strömgren (1938)	Denmark	5.8
Ødegaard (1946)	Norway	18.7
Fremming (1947)	Denmark	9.0
Böök (1953)	Sweden	26.6
Sjögren (1954)	Sweden	16.0
Helgason (1964)	Iceland	8.0
Helgason (1977)	Iceland	4.9
Böök (1978)	Sweden	24.8
Robins (1984)	New Haven, U.S.A.	19.0
	Baltimore, U.S.A.	16.0
	St. Louis, U.S.A.	10.0
Widerlov (1989)	Denmark	37.0
Lehtinen (1990)	Finland	13.0
Hwu (1989)	Taiwan	2.6
Youssef (1991)	Ireland	6.4

TABLE 6-7. *Risk to Relatives of Schizophrenic Patients*

Relation	Risk (%)
First-degree relatives	
Parents	4.4
Brothers and sisters	8.5
Neither parent schizophrenic	8.2
One parent schizophrenic	13.8
Fraternal twin	
Opposite sex	5.6
Same sex	12.0
Identical twin	57.7
Children	12.3
Both parents schizophrenic	36.6
Second-degree relatives	
Uncles and aunts	2.0
Nephews and nieces	2.2
Grandchildren	2.8
Half-siblings	3.2
General population	0.8

Adapted from Tsuang MT, Vandermey R: Genes and the Mind: Inheritance of Mental Illness. Oxford, Oxford University Press, 1980.

Contemporary studies using rigorous research methods and narrow, criterion-based definitions of schizophrenia are also consistent with the genetic hypothesis. However, they report risk figures that are somewhat lower than those seen in Table 6-7. Tsuang et al., (1980), for example, reported the risk of schizophrenia to first-degree relatives of schizophrenics to be 3.2 percent compared with 0.6 percent for relatives of nonpsychiatric controls. Guze et al. (1983) reported comparable figures of 3.6 and 0.56 percent, respectively. In both studies, the increased risk for schizophrenia among relatives of schizophrenics remained statistically significant despite the lower risk figures. As can be seen, contemporary studies report risk estimates approximately one-third the magnitude of those obtained by the earlier European studies, which employed a broader definition of schizophrenia. Diagnostic practices appear to play a strong role in these differences. For example, the figure of 3.2 percent obtained by Tsuang et al (1980) when using stringent Washington University criteria increases to 3.7 percent when DSM-III criteria are applied. It increases to 7.8 percent if the schizophrenia category is broadened to include atypical schizophrenics. Thus, as Kendler et al. (1985) noted, the risk figures for schizophrenia based on contemporary criteria are similar to the figures obtained by the earlier European studies when atypical cases are included. The exclusion of atypical schizophrenic patients from family studies also may explain why two recent family studies failed to find familial transmission in schizophrenia. Pope et al. (1978) found no cases of schizophrenia among first-degree relatives of their schizophrenic probands. Abrams and Taylor (1983) found the risk for schizophrenia to be only 1.6 percent among 128 first-degree relatives of schizophrenics. Nevertheless, contemporary figures as well as those reported in Table 6-7 suggest that the risk for schizophrenia among the first-degree relatives of schizophrenic patients exceeds the observed rate in the general population by 5 to 10 times. There would appear to be little doubt that schizophrenia is a familial disorder (Tsuang et al., 1991).

TWIN STUDIES

Monozygotic (MZ) twins are genetically identical, and dizygotic (DZ) twins share, on average, only one-half their genes. Therefore, a higher concordance rate for schizophrenia among MZ twins compared with DZ twins is strong evidence for the importance of genetic mechanisms in the etiology of a disorder. The logic of twin research requires the assumption that both MZ and DZ twins share a common environment but differ in the degree to which they share genes. Current evidence supports this assumption (Kendler, 1983). The twin study data for schizophrenia are unequivocal in implicating genetic factors. Gottesman and Shields (1972) studied a pooled sample of 550 MZ and 776 DZ twin pairs in a review of the literature. They reported concordance rates of 57.7 and 12.8 percent for MZ and DZ twins, respectively.

Kendler (1983) reviewed the evidence for environmental influences peculiar to MZ twins that might make their likelihood of developing schizophrenia greater than that of DZ twins. He concluded that there is little evidence of such a difference. He also summarized nine twin studies from eight countries involving 401 monozygotic twin pairs and 478 dizygotic twin pairs. Overall, 211 (53 percent) of the MZ twin pairs were concordant for schizophrenia, whereas only 74 (15 percent) of the DZ twin pairs were concordant. This significant difference between concordance rates for the two types of twin pairs strongly implicates genetic factors in the causation of schizophrenia.

Monozygotic twins raised apart provide a unique opportunity to separate genetic factors from environmental factors. Gottesman and Shields (1972) summarized eight such investigations. Eleven of 17 monozygotic twin pairs reared apart (65 percent) were concordant for schizophrenia.

ADOPTION STUDIES

Environmental factors can confound family and twin studies. They can be eliminated in part by studying children of schizophrenics who were not raised by their schizophrenic parent. Heston (1966) compared the rates of schizophrenia in 47 adopted-away children of schizophrenic mothers with 50 adopted-away children of nonschizophrenic mothers. Five of the children of schizophrenic mothers had schizophrenia at follow-up compared with none of the control children.

A series of studies known as the Danish-American Adoption Study of Schizophrenia demonstrated that 173 biologic relatives of adoptees with schizophrenia had significantly higher rates of schizophrenia (6.4 percent) than 174 biologic relatives of control adoptees without schizophrenia (1.7 percent) and 74 nonbiologic adoptive relatives of schizophrenics (1.4 percent) (Kety et al., 1978).

In utero influences may confound adoption studies. Because paternal half-siblings have different mothers, their comparison eliminates such an influence. Kety et al. (1978) found that 8 of 63 paternal half-siblings of schizophrenic adoptees (12.7 percent) had definite schizophrenia on interview compared with only 1 of 64 paternal half-siblings of control adoptees (1.6 percent).

In sum, family, twin, and adoption studies implicate a significant genetic component in the causation of schizophrenia. Genetic factors alone, however, cannot explain schizophrenia; otherwise, monozygotic twin pairs would be 100 percent concordant for schizophrenia. Thus environmental factors must play a critical role.

QUANTITATIVE MODELING OF GENETIC TRANSMISSION

Attempts to fit mathematical genetic models to schizophrenia family data have been contradictory. Single-gene models accurately predict the general population prevalence, the risk to offspring of schizophrenics, and the risk to siblings of schizophrenics. Collectively, however, segregation analyses do not support the single-gene model of inheritance for schizophrenia. All studies that provide statistical tests of model adequacy reject the model. Those which cannot rule out the model note that the risk to MZ twins and the offspring of two schizophrenics are underpredicted by the single-gene model (Faraone and Tsuang, 1985; Faraone et al., 1988; McGue and Gottesman, 1989a, 1989b; Gottesman and McGue, 1990).

The failure to find a single-gene model that accounts for the familial transmission of schizophrenia has led to the testing of polygenic models. Limited loci polygenic (LLP) models propose a relatively limited number of loci, whereas multifactorial polygenic (MFP) models propose a large, unspecified number of loci. Most segregation-analysis studies comparing the single-gene and LLP models agree that there are no dramatic differences between their abilities to account for the familial transmission of schizophrenia (Faraone and Tsuang, 1985). However, Risch (1990a, 1990b) finds that two- and three-locus models including gene interactions can account for the familial pattern of illness in schizophrenia, including the risks to MZ and DZ twins.

Multifactorial polygenic (MFP) models do not specify the number of loci involved in schizophrenia. Instead, they assume that there are many loci and that genes at these loci have small, additive effects on the predisposition for schizophrenia. This model assumes that all individuals have some unobservable liability or predisposition to develop schizophrenia. Compared with the single-gene model, the MFP model provides more accurate predictions of the risks observed to relatives in family studies. This is especially notable for the risk to MZ twins and the risk to offspring of two schizophrenics (McGue and Gottesman, 1989). However, these results cannot rule out the possibility of a mixed model in which a single-gene component and an MFP component both exist. However, attempts to fit mixed models have not been illuminating (Risch and Baron, 1984; Vogler et al., 1990).

Although these considerations suggest that the search for one or more etiologic genes may not be fruitful for schizophrenia, there are several reasons for pursuing hypotheses that one or several genes play a substantial etiologic role in schizophrenia. First, definitive evidence for or against the hypotheses will require results from linkage analysis (see discussion below). Second, as Gershon (1990) notes, the data on which the assertions of Risch (1990a, 1990b) and McGue and Gottesman (1989) are based were collected well before the development of modern family study and psychiatric diagnostic methodology. These studies also did not provide information about disorders such as schizotypal personality that are probably genetic variants of schizophrenia. Third, although the negative statistical results for the single-gene model seem compelling, the rejection of the model may indicate that some of the nongenetic assumptions of the model are wrong. In fact, Sham and McGuffin (1990) report that including reduced fertility, assortative mating, mutations, carrier advantage, and common twin environment in a single-gene model provides accurate risks to different classes of relatives.

LINKAGE ANALYSIS OF SCHIZOPHRENIA

The methodology for finding genes, known as *linkage analysis*, is now fairly routine. With the molecular genetic methodology currently available, there is no question that it is possible to find the genes responsible for many disorders. In fact, the list of disorders for which there is already an identified genetic locus grows every year. This list includes Huntington's disease, cystic fibrosis, Duchenne's muscular dystrophy, myotonic dystrophy, familial colon cancer, von Recklinhausen neurofibromatosis, and a form of mental retardation due to the fragile X syndrome. Linkage analysis offers the potential of a more powerful method of establishing genetic etiology for the psychiatric disorders than the statistical methods of segregation analysis.

Linkage analysis is based on the crossing over of homologous chromosomes during meiosis, the process whereby gametes are created. The occurrence of genetic transmission is due to an individual's inheriting one member of each pair of chromosomes from the mother and one from the father. However, these inherited haploid chromosomes are not identical to any of the original parental chromosomes. During meiosis, the original chromosomes in a pair cross over each other and exchange portions of their DNA. After multiple cross-overs, the resulting two chromosomes each consist of a new and unique combination of genes. After meiosis, each gamete will contain one chromosome from each of the newly formed pairs. Whether two genes on the same chromosome will remain together or will recombine during meiosis is a function of their physical proximity to each other. Linkage occurs when two loci on the same original chromosome are so close to each other that crossing over rarely or never occurs between them. Closely linked genes usually remain together on the same chromosome after meiosis is complete (Ott, 1985; Baron et al., 1990).

While comprehensive searches of all the chromosomes have yet to be completed in the linkage-study approach to schizophrenia, a few preliminary and isolated analyses have been reported. Interest in chromosome 5 followed the report of schizophrenia cosegregating with a partial trisomy of the chromosome in a family of Asian descent (Bassett et al., 1988). Two members of the pedigree shared a distinct chromosomal abnormality. Both met criteria for a narrowly defined schizophrenic syndrome and exhibited dysmorphic facial features and other structural anomalies. These findings led to speculation concerning the long arm region of chromosome 5 as a potential genetic locus for schizophrenia. Following this report, Sherrington et al. (1988) studied seven British and Icelandic families having schizophrenic members in at least three generations. Using two DNA markers to track the inheritance pattern of schizophrenia in these families, these investigators demonstrated genetic linkage to the same region of the long arm of chromosome 5. Their results, suggesting the existence of a dominant schizophrenia susceptibility allele in this region, are consistent with the deletion mapping of DNA markers to the region of chromosome 5 that cosegregates with schizophrenia in the Bassett et al. (1988) pedigree (Bassett, 1989; Gilliam et al., 1989; Kaufmann et al., 1989; McGillivray et al., 1990).

Unfortunately, subsequent linkage studies have not replicated this linkage finding. Using a detailed search of the suspected chromosome 5 region with the aid of seven DNA markers, Kennedy et al. (1988) found strong evidence *against* linkage of schizophrenia in a single large Swedish pedigree. Kennedy et al. suggested that the conflicting results might be due to the genetic heterogeneity of schizophrenia. That is, there could be different loci resulting in a "final common pathway" phenotype of schizophrenia in different families. However, St.

Claire et al. (1989) examined 15 Scottish pedigrees and also found no evidence for linkage regardless of how broadly the schizophrenic phenotype was defined. They found that linkage could be excluded to the region implicated by the Bassett et al. and Sherrington et al. findings. However, the pedigrees examined by these investigators demonstrated significant levels of mood disorder. Eight of the 15 pedigrees contained bipolar members, and 4 contained major depressives. Nevertheless, other investigators have excluded the chromosome 5 region (Detera-Wadleigh et al., 1989; Kaufmann et al., 1989; McGuffin et al., 1990; Crowe et al., 1991; Diehl et al., 1991).

Recent data have implicated a pseudoautosomal locus in the etiology of schizophrenia. The pseudoautosomal region is a small area at the tip of the Y chromosome that crosses over with the X chromosome. A pseudoautosomal locus was initially implicated by the finding of sex concordance between siblings affected with schizophrenia for families with a paternal, but not a maternal, history of schizophrenia (Crow et al., 1989). Support for this hypothesis was found by Collinge et al. (1991) using the linkage-analysis method of affected sibling pairs. They reported a significant linkage between schizophrenia and a pseudoautosomal telomeric locus among 83 sibships having two or more members with schizophrenia or schizoaffective disorder. Unfortunately, other investigators have excluded linkage to the pseudoautosomal region (Parfitt et al., 1991).

Some workers have noted that genetic heterogeneity may explain the conflicting linkage results (Kennedy et al., 1988). That is, there may be more than one gene that causes schizophrenia. In contrast, others have suggested that the initial positive linkage finding may have been wrong (Matthysse, 1990; McGuffin et al., 1990; Risch, 1990a). A reasonable, and conservative, guideline is that we should not conclude that a linkage exists until it has been confirmed independently by a second group of investigators. Also, we should not use genetic heterogeneity to explain discordant finding unless both findings have been replicated independently. It is notable that similar controversies have arisen for bipolar illness (Faraone et al., 1990; Tsuang and Faraone, 1990). These conflicting results for schizophrenia and bipolar disorder may indicate that although developments in molecular and statistical genetics have made it straightforward to find and replicate linkage for *simple* single-gene disorders, it will be more challenging to map etiologically complex disorders like schizophrenia (Risch, 1990).

Schizophrenia Is a Brain Disease

As we enter this "decade of the brain," it is timely to note that despite our ignorance of the details of etiology and pathophysiology, we can say that schizophrenia is, assuredly, a disease of the central nervous system. During the past century, as new neurodiagnostic technologies emerged, they were swiftly applied to the study of schizophrenia. Most of these measurements led to the same conclusion, namely, that the structure and function of the schizophrenic brain were not normal. In this section we provide a selective overview of this work.

STRUCTURAL BRAIN ABNORMALITIES

Weinberger et al. (1983), in a review of neuropathologic findings in schizophrenia, concluded that although abnormalities of the brain were common among schizophrenic patients, a lesion specific to the illness had not been found. More recent work continues to find evidence of abnormality, but again, a pathognomonic lesion has not yet been found. For example, atypical cell architecture and neuronal loss have been reported for a variety of structures, including the prefrontal cortex (Benes et al., 1986), the cingulate cortex (Benes et al., 1987), the entorhinal cortex (Falkai et al., 1988), and the hippocampus (Jakob and Beckmann, 1986).

In 1927, Jacobi and Winkler reported enlarged ventricles in 18 of 19 schizophrenics studied with pneumoencephalography (Weinberger and Wyatt, 1982). Subsequently, more than 30 studies reported similar results (Weinberger and Wyatt, 1982). These results were, by and large, ignored until recent work using computer tomography (CT) and magnetic resonance imaging (MRI) confirmed that, as a group, schizophrenics had larger ventricles than did controls.

For example, Johnstone et al. (1976) reported that 17 institutionalized schizophrenics had, on average, larger ventricles than 8 matched controls. Patients with the larger ventricles had more cognitive impairment, fewer positive symptoms of schizophrenia, and more negative symptoms. Subsequent work by several researchers suggests that, depending on the population studied, between 20 and 50 percent of schizophrenics may have enlarged ventricles (Luchins, 1982).

Patients with enlarged ventricles tend to have negative symptoms, cognitive impairment, more neurologic signs, less independent residential living, longer inpatient hospital stays, and a poor response to neuroleptic treatment (Johnstone et al., 1976; Golden et al., 1980; Weinberger et al., 1980; Andreasen et al., 1982; Weinberger, 1984; Zec and Weinberger, 1986; Raz and Raz, 1990; Seidman et al., 1992). After reviewing 10 studies, Lewis (1987) concluded that ventricular enlargement was more common among schizophrenic patients without a family history of schizophrenia. A subsequent review of additional studies also supported this conclusion (Lyons et al., 1989). These results initially suggested that ventricular enlargement may be a useful means for identifying subtypes of schizophrenia. However, researchers have not yet been able to isolate a homogeneous subtype with this feature (Daniel et al., 1991).

The weight of the evidence suggests that the ventricular enlargement associated with schizophrenia is present at the onset of the illness and is not due to progressive deterioration through the course of the illness (Weinberger, 1984; Seidman et al., 1992). However, ventricular enlargement is not confined to schizophrenia. It also has been reported in mania, schizoaffective disorder, and adolescent obsessive-compulsive disorder (Nasrallah et al., 1982; Rieder et al., 1983; Behar et al., 1984).

Although MRI is relatively new, it has been applied to the problem of schizophrenia with some success. In addition to confirming the finding of ventricular enlargement (Seidman et al., 1992), several MRI studies report reduced volume of temporal limbic structures on both sides of the brain (Barta et al., 1990; Bogerts et al., 1990; Suddath et al., 1990).

ABNORMALITIES OF BRAIN FUNCTIONING

Several lines of evidence suggest that schizophrenics have abnormalities of brain function. For example, total brain blood flow is reduced in schizophrenia (Mathew et al., 1982; Ariel et al., 1983), and regional blood flow measurements suggest a particular reduction in frontal blood flow (Buchsbaum and Ingvar, 1982; Ariel et al., 1983). Glucose metabolism, as measured by positron emission tomography, is a more direct indicator of regional metabolism than of regional blood flow. Such studies also have shown a relative reduction in metabolic activity in the frontal cortex of schizophrenics compared with controls, especially when the subject is required to perform a relevant cognitive task during the procedure (Farkas et al., 1984; Weinberger and Berman, 1988; Buchsbaum et al., 1990).

A number of investigators have postulated left hemisphere dysfunction in schizophrenia. Gur (1979) concluded from her own work and a review of the literature that schizophrenics had a dysfunctional left hemisphere, overactivation of the dysfunctional hemisphere, and failure to shift processing to the right hemisphere. Left hemisphere dysfunction may include an attentional deficit (Niwa et al., 1983).

In schizophrenics, Gur et al. (1983) found that the relative amount of blood flow to the left and right hemispheres differentiated schizophrenic patients from controls. For a verbal task, the patients showed no flow asymmetries, and controls showed an increase in left hemisphere flow. For a spatial task, the patients showed greater left hemisphere increases than right hemisphere increases; the controls showed a larger right hemisphere increase on the same task. Left temporal lobe epilepsy has been associated with an increased risk of a psychosis with schizophrenic symptomatology, and right temporal epilepsy, with an increased risk of affective symptoms (Flor-Henry, 1983).

The electroencephalogram (EEG) has a long history of use in schizophrenia studies. Between 20 and 40 percent of schizophrenics have EEG abnormalities, but their presence is not related to subtype, duration of illness, or severity of illness (Itil, 1977; Seidman, 1983). These abnormalities are usually diffuse or bilateral (Seidman, 1983). No EEG pattern is specific to schizophrenia, and epileptiform activity is rarely found among these patients (Itil, 1977).

Brain potential imaging (BPI) is a newer electrophysiologic technique that allows the electrical activity of several cortical areas to be measured at one time. The result is an electrophysiologic map of brain functioning that allows for subtle comparisons between brain regions. BPI studies of schizophrenic patients are consistent with regional blood flow studies in finding evidence of relatively lower levels of brain activity in the frontal cortex compared with other brain regions (Morihisa et al., 1983; Morstyn et al., 1983; Guenther and Breitling, 1985).

Positron emission tomography (PET) studies also have found evidence for physiologic dysfunction of the frontal cortex (Cohen et al., 1988; Buchsbaum et al., 1990). Like the regional blood flow studies, the finding of hypofrontality is more reproducible if the subject is performing a task mediated by the frontal lobes while being assessed.

ABNORMALITIES IN NEUROTRANSMITTER SYSTEMS

Neurotransmitter-based theories of the etiology of schizophrenia include the dopamine hypothesis (Snyder, 1976; Wyatt, 1985) and other hypotheses based on noradrenergic (Lake et al., 1987), serotonergic (Stahl and Wets, 1987), neuropeptide (Nemeroff and Bissette, 1987), and phospholipid and prostaglandin (Brody et al., 1987) pathways. The three monoamines are interrelated in their metabolism and share some of the enzymes for their synthesis and degradation. For example, norepinephrine (NE) is derived from dopamine (DA) by the action of dopamine-β-hydroxylase (DBH) and therefore shares the two preceding steps with the dopamine pathway. These two steps are catalyzed by the enzymes tyrosine hydroxylase (TH), which converts tyrosine to L-dopa, and L-dopa decarboxylase (DDC), which converts L-dopa to dopamine. DDC is also shared between the catecholamines (DA, NE, and epinephrine) and the 5-hydroxytryptophan pathways. Moreover, monoamine oxidase (MAO), particularly the type A isoenzyme, is a major enzyme in degradation pathways of all three of these monoamines.

A common theme of the neurotransmitter hypotheses of schizophrenia is that imbalances in the concentration of neurotransmitters or abnormal activities in the pathways cause symptoms of the syndrome. For example, in the DA hypothesis, the positive symptoms of schizophrenia are due to hyperactivity of the dopamine system. The opposite is postulated for negative symptoms. Cadet (1987)

postulated that during the degradation of DA or other catecholamines by MAO, peroxides and cytotoxic free radicals are formed. If these free radicals are in excess and cannot be removed quickly, destruction of neuronal pathways may ensue. In this model, the overproduction of DA leads to hyperactivity in dopaminergic neurons and the positive symptoms of schizophrenia. After a long exposure to the toxic effects of DA metabolites, destruction or "burnout" of DA pathways in some area of the brain may occur. This "burnout" may then cause negative symptoms. Neuronal pathways in the brain are highly interconnected; thus models involving other neurotransmitters such as GABA and acetylcholine also can be used to explain the development of the positive and negative symptoms. Although still very speculative, these models provide guidance for research.

The dopamine (DA) hypothesis emerged from several lines of evidence. First, drugs that increase brain DA activity, such as amphetamine (Snyder, 1972) and L-dopa (Davis, 1978), exacerbate schizophrenic symptoms. Also, amphetamine can cause schizophrenia-like symptoms that are clinically indistinguishable from schizophrenia and are reversible by neuroleptic drugs. Second, the effect of neuroleptic drugs has been shown to be due to their blockade of dopamine D_2 receptors (Carlsson and Lindqvist, 1963), since their therapeutic efficacy correlates with their blocking capacity (Creese et al., 1976; Wyatt, 1976). Also, DA receptor density is elevated in the postmortem brains of both medicated and unmedicated schizophrenic patients (Wong et al., 1986; Jaskiw and Kleinman, 1988; Wong, 1990). This increase is selective for type D_2 DA receptors (DRD_2); no changes have been detected in the D_1 or D_3 DA or other neurotransmitter receptors. Seeman et al. (1984) reported a bimodal distribution of DA receptor densities in the caudate nucleus, putamen, and nucleus accumbens of schizophrenic patients; both treated and untreated patients were present in both subgroups. In contrast, they found a uniformly distributed receptor density in control brains. The authors speculated that the high-density subgroup may represent a genetically distinct population. Wong et al. (1986), using PET scanning, demonstrated that the D_2 receptor density in the caudate nucleus was significantly higher in both 5 treated and 10 drug-naive schizophrenia patients compared with 11 normal volunteers. However, Farde et al. (1987) could not confirm this finding.

Significantly lower levels of DBH have been found in cerebrospinal fluid (CSF) of schizophrenics who were responsive to neuroleptic treatment compared with those who were not; these levels were constant over time in the same individual (Sternberg et al., 1982). Wise et al. (1973) reported reduced DBH activity in the postmortem brains of schizophrenic patients. However, others could not confirm this finding (Wyatt et al., 1978).

The potentiation effect of the TH inhibitor alpha-methyltyrosine in the treatment of chronic schizophrenics suggests a role of TH in schizophrenia (Walinder et al., 1976; Larsson et al., 1984). Moreover, significantly higher levels of postmortem TH and homovanillic acid, a dopamine metabolite, characterize the basal ganglia of schizophrenics, and a markedly high activity of TH was measured in a catatonic schizophrenic patient who had not taken antipsychotic drugs for 3 months before death (Toru et al., 1982). These results suggest that overactivity of TH may lead to higher DA concentrations in some regions of the brain for some subtypes of schizophrenia.

Norepinephrine (NE) is derived from dopamine (DA) through the action of the enzyme DBH. MAO degrades both NE and DA. Such a close metabolic relationship, plus the fact that some drugs show much overlap in their action on these catecholamines, suggests the logical possibility of some derangement of NE in schizophrenia. Further, some antipsychotics such as clozapine are more potent alpha-adrenergic antagonists and only weak DA blockers. Abnormal levels of NE have been reported in schizophrenic patients in the brain (Farley et al., 1978; Wyatt et al., 1981), in the CSF (Gomes et al., 1980; Kemali et al., 1982; Sternberg et al., 1982), and in the plasma (Castellani et al., 1982; Kemali et al., 1982).

The serotonin hypothesis emerged in the 1950s following observations of the striking similarities between serotonin and the hallucinogen LSD. Later, reports that serotonergic-depleting drugs such as reserpine can alleviate some symptoms of schizophrenia led to the theory that an increase in serotonin may be causally related to the disease (Stahl and Wets, 1987). While results from studies on the therapeutic potency of serotonin antagonists, brain and CSF levels of serotonin metabolites, and LSD binding to frontal cortex have been inconsistent, more recent results indicate that mean serotonin concentrations in schizophrenic patients with abnormal CT brain scans are higher than in patients with normal CT scans and in normal controls (DeLisi et al., 1981). This recent result is consistent with the serotonin hypothesis. Further, it points out the importance of subgrouping schizophrenic patients in testing biochemical and genetic hypotheses.

The Role of the Environment

Psychopathologists have long abandoned the nature—nurture controversy. The question is not, What causes schizophrenia—genes or environment? As Meehl (1973) observed some time ago, the appropriate question is much more complicated: What constellation of environmental factors interacts with what genetically determined factors to produce the disorder?

It is perhaps ironic that the most definitive evidence for the role of the environment in schizo-phrenia comes from a genetic paradigm, namely, the twin study. As we discussed earlier, the monozygotic twins of schizophrenic patients have only a 50 percent risk of developing the illness themselves. Thus it is likely that the schizophrenic genotype requires the action of environmental etiologic factors before the disorder emerges. For example, some neurobiologic studies of monozygotic twins discordant for schizophrenia find structural brain abnormalities in the affected twins only (Suddath et al., 1990).

FAMILY RELATIONSHIPS

It had been thought that family relationships caused schizophrenia. For example, some thought that certain personality traits of mothers caused schizophrenia in their children. Hence the term *schizophrenogenic mother*. Another hypothesis implicated abnormal communication between parent and child as etiologically relevant to schizophrenia. The *double-bind situation* was said to occur when the child was repeatedly exposed to contradictory messages. Such communication was believed to cause schizophrenia based on clinical observations of patients and their families. A third hypothesis suggested that an abnormal marital relationship between parents caused schizophrenia in their children. Two kinds of abnormal marital relationship were characterized. In the *skewed* relationship, one parent yielded to the abnormal parent, who then dominated the family. In *marital schism*, there was conflict between the parents, who competed for the child's support.

As the reader may suspect, these hypotheses about the etiology of schizophrenia have been rejected. Although the families of schizophrenic patients may have a variety of communication problems, none of these has been shown to cause the illness (Leff, 1978; Wing, 1978a, 1978b).

PREGNANCY AND DELIVERY COMPLICATIONS

Many studies have found increased rates of pregnancy and delivery complications (PDCs) in the births of children who eventually become schizophrenic. For example, schizophrenic patients are more likely to have been born prematurely and to have had relatively low birth weights (Lane and Albee, 1966; Woerner et al., 1971).

EDITORS' COMMENT

The low IQ (Angst and Clayton, 1986) repeatedly reported in good premorbid studies of schizophrenics also points to some intrauterine developmental abnormality.

It is possible that the effect of PDCs is to activate the genetic predisposition to schizophrenia. This is seen most dramatically in studies of children born to schizophrenic mothers. These "high-risk" children are not more likely than other children to have

PDCs (Mednick and Schulsinger, 1968). However, among the high-risk children, PDCs are predictive of subsequent psychiatric abnormality (Mednick, 1970). Subsequent work on the same sample (Parnas et al., 1982) reported a tendency for the children who became schizophrenic to have had more PDCs. They also found that those with the least complicated births had "borderline schizophrenia" (i.e., schizotypal personality disorder). They suggested that children with the schizophrenic genotype would not develop schizophrenia if they had unusually uncomplicated births.

The finding that PDCs are predictive of subsequent schizophrenia has been confirmed in other studies (McNeil and Kaij, 1978; Jacobsen and Kinney, 1980). Also, PDCs have been shown to predict ventricular enlargement in both schizophrenic and normal samples (Pearlson et al., 1985; Turner et al., 1986; Nimgaonkar et al., 1988). Some, but not all, family studies support the hypothesis that PDCs interact with a genetic predisposition to the illness. For example, in one study, schizophrenic patients had larger ventricles and more birth complications than their well siblings (DeLisi et al., 1986). Another possibility is that PDCs cause a nongenetic form of schizophrenia. In support of this, several studies have found more PDCs among patients without a family history of schizophrenia compared with patients with a family history (Kinney and Jacobsen, 1978; Lewis et al., 1987; Lyons et al., 1989; O'Callaghan et al., 1990). However, other studies find no difference (Pearlson et al., 1985; Reddy et al., 1990), and there is no straightforward way to interpret these inconsistencies (Lyons et al., 1989; Lyons et al., 1989; Kremen et al., 1992).

THE VIRAL HYPOTHESIS

The theory that schizophrenia is caused by a virus was articulated as early as 1845 (Torrey and Kaufmann, 1986). In its contemporary formulation, the viral hypothesis has been put forward to explain several epidemiologic and clinical observations. Foremost among these is the finding that the births of schizophrenic patients are more likely to occur during the late winter and spring months than during other parts of the year (Dalen, 1975). Since births during these months are at increased risk for exposure to viruses, the seasonality-of-birth effect has led some to conclude that a neurotoxic virus may be involved in the etiology of some cases of schizophrenia (Hare et al., 1974; Hare, 1976). Two studies find that the seasonality-of-birth effect is most pronounced among patients without a family history of schizophrenia (Shur, 1982; O'Callaghan et al., 1991). Thus it may be that viral cases of schizophrenia do not have a genetic origin or that genetic factors are of lesser importance in such cases.

Torrey and Kaufmann (1986) noted additional indirect evidence for the viral hypothesis as follows.

First, if a neurotoxic virus acting on the fetus leads to adult schizophrenia, we would expect to observe additional evidence of such effects. Two such effects have been observed in schizophrenia. First, schizophrenic patients have elevated rates of physical anomalies. Second, they also have abnormal dermatoglyphic patterns. Although both effects could be caused by PDCs or genetic abnormalities, their presence in schizophrenia is also consistent with the actions of a neurovirus.

Evidence supportive of the viral hypothesis also comes from studies of persons born during influenza epidemics. Mednick et al. (1988) studied a Finnish cohort who had been fetuses during a 1957 epidemic of influenza. They report that those exposed to the epidemic during their second trimester of development were at increased risk for subsequently being diagnosed with schizophrenia. However, this finding was not replicated in a Scottish study that failed to consistently find an increased risk for schizophrenia associated with influenza epidemics in 1918, 1919, or 1957; analyses limited to the city of Edinburgh in 1957 supported the viral hypothesis, but the nationwide data did not (Kendell and Kemp, 1989). Also, only limited evidence of an association between viral epidemics and schizophrenia was found in an American study (Torrey et al., 1988). Barr et al. (1990) criticized these studies on methodologic grounds. They also replicated the Finnish results in a Danish sample. Thus, although more research is needed, it seems reasonable to conclude that viral infection during fetal development may play a role in the etiology of schizophrenia.

COURSE AND OUTCOME

Both Kraepelin (1919/1971) and Bleuler (1911/1950) thought that recovery from schizophrenia was rare. Identifying criteria that might predict the course of illness has been difficult. However, narrow criteria, such as those in DSM-IIIR, have been more successful at separating good-prognosis patients from poor-prognosis patients than have broader criteria (Helzer et al., 1981; Stephens et al., 1982). For example, 35 to 40 years after admission, Tsuang et al. (1979) followed up 186 schizophrenics, 86 manics, and 212 depressives diagnosed by Washington University criteria (Feighner et al., 1972). Thirty-three of the schizophrenics met Tsuang-Winokur criteria for the paranoid subtype, and 40, for the hebephrenic subtype (Kendler et al., 1984). Table 6-8 summarizes their outcomes. Schizophrenics had significantly poorer outcomes in all three areas examined than did manics and depressives.

Manfred Bleuler (1978) personally followed 208 schizophrenic patients for more than 20 years. Fifty-six patients were excluded because they either were dead or had not reached a stable end state.

TABLE 6-8. *Comparative Outcome of Schizophrenics, Manics, and Depressives*

	Schizophrenia (n = 186)			Mood disorders (n = 298)	
	Paranoid (%) (n=33)	Hebephrenic (%) (n=40)	Total	Mania (%) (n=86)	Depression (%) (n=212)
Work-disabled from psychiatric illness	36	72	58	24	17
Severe psychiatric symptoms	36	62	54	29	22
Residence in county home or mental hospital	39	77	40	17	13

Twenty percent of the remaining 152 patients recovered fully. They were able to reassume former social and family roles, were regarded by their families as rational, and had no psychotic symptoms on examination. Thirty-three percent of the patients had mild end states. They could converse sensibly about topics other than their hallucinations and delusions. Overt behavior was normal, and they were usually able to work. However, they continued to have definite schizophrenic symptoms. Forty-seven percent had moderate to severe end states, characterized by marked psychiatric symptoms and marked impairment in most or all role functioning.

In Bleuler's series of patients, 62 percent had acute onsets of less than a 6-month duration. Acute onset and undulating course were both associated with a more favorable outcome than were insidious onset and chronic course. Bleuler described several combinations of course and outcome similar to those later described by Ciompi (1980), who followed up 289 surviving patients from an initial sample of 1642 schizophrenics. Follow-up was as much as 50 years after hospitalization. End states were defined with Bleuler's criteria (Bleuler, 1978). At follow-up, 27 percent of the patients had recovered fully, 22 percent had mild symptoms, 24 percent had moderately severe symptoms, 18 percent had severe symptoms, and 9 percent had uncertain outcome.

Of the 289 patients, mode of onset, course type, and end state (follow-up status) were known for 228 (79 percent). Onset was divided into two types: acute and chronic (insidious). Course was divided into two types: episodic and continuous. End state was defined as recovery/mild or moderate/severe. Table 6-9 summarizes the resulting eight course combinations.

Acute onset was associated with a better outcome than insidious onset, and episodic course was associated with a better outcome than continuous course. Of those patients who would probably receive the DSM-IIIR classification of schizophrenia early in the course of their illness (patients with insidious onset or acute onset with continuous course), 40 percent were recovered or had a mild end state at follow-up. Of the acute-onset group with episodic course, 68 percent were recovered or had a mild end state.

The onset of schizophrenia is usually insidious. Schizophrenics, particularly males, may have con-

TABLE 6-9. *Course of Schizophrenia*

Mode of onset	Course type	End state	Percent of 228 patients
Acute	Episodic	Recovery/mild	25.4
Acute	Episodic	Moderate/severe	11.9
Acute	Continuous	Moderate/severe	8.3
Acute	Continuous	Recovery/mild	5.3
Insidious	Continuous	Moderate/severe	24.1
Insidious	Continuous	Recovery/mild	10.1
Insidious	Episodic	Recovery/mild	9.6
Insidious	Episodic	Moderate/severe	5.3

Adapted from Ciompi L: Catamnestic long-term study on the course of life and aging in schizophrenics. Schizophr Bull 6:606–618, 1980.

duct disturbances as children, lower IQs, lower school grades, and completion of fewer grades (Robins, 1966; Offord, 1974). Between 50 and 70 percent of schizophrenics have had certain schizoid personality traits, such as aloofness, few close friends, and less involvement in social activities than their peers (Slater and Roth, 1969). Among children at high risk for schizophrenia, Fish (1977) has described a syndrome involving dysregulation of physical growth; motor, visual-motor, and cognitive development; proprioception; and vestibular responses. Several such children developed overt schizophrenia by early childhood. Other investigators have reported similar findings (Erlenmeyer-Kimling et al., 1982).

Usually, by the time the patient with schizophrenia consults a psychiatrist, deterioration from the previous level of functioning has been under way for months or years. In a group of 52 nonparanoid schizophrenics defined by Tsuang-Winokur criteria (see Table 6-3), positive or negative symptoms or both had been present for an average of 1 year before admission (Pfohl and Winokur, 1982). Nevertheless, a retrospective follow-up study from Vermont suggested that favorable outcome may be more common among schizophrenic patients than was previously believed (Harding et al., 1987). This study examined 82 DSM-III–defined schizophrenic patients 32 years after their index hospital admissions. At follow-up, most of these patients were free of schizophrenic symptomatology (68 percent), required little or no help to meet basic needs (81 percent), and led a moderate to very full life (73 percent).

Throughout the course of the illness, positive symptoms tend to be less persistent than negative symptoms (Pfohl and Winokur, 1982) and may serve to precipitate admission to a psychiatric hospital. Certain negative symptoms, such as avolition, may begin early in the course of the illness. In contrast to positive symptoms, however, negative symptoms may become more and more prominent as the illness progresses. In the Iowa 500 follow-up study, only 12 of 120 patients (10 percent) originally diagnosed as being nonparanoid schizophrenics received the diagnosis of paranoid schizophrenia at follow-up (Tsuang et al., 1981).

Depression is common in the course of schizophrenia. Over a 6- to 12-year span, Guze et al. (1983) reported that 25 of 44 schizophrenics (57 percent) had one or more depressive episode. Relatives of these schizophrenics were not at increased risk for mood disorder compared with relatives of schizophrenics without depressive episodes. It is important to note that these schizophrenics had an otherwise typical course of schizophrenic symptoms. Their illness did not appear to begin with affective symptoms and was not episodic.

One aspect of the course of an illness is the stability of the symptoms over time, as reflected in diagnostic stability. Personal interviews of 93 of 117 living patients who had been diagnosed schizophrenic 35 to 40 years earlier and who met Washington University criteria on chart review confirmed the diagnosis in 86 (93 percent). Only 4 of the 93 (4 percent) were found to have mood disorders at follow-up (Tsuang et al., 1981). Guze et al. (1983) have reported similar results in a prospective follow-up of 19 narrowly defined schizophrenics. None were rediagnosed with a mood disorder.

Mortality in schizophrenics is elevated compared with the general population (Tsuang and Woolson, 1977; Ciompi, 1980; Simpson, 1988). A good portion of this increased mortality is due to suicide (Simpson, 1988).

EDITORS' COMMENT

In a 6-year follow-up study (Knesevich et al., *Am J Psychiatry* 140:1507–1510, 1983) of carefully diagnosed good- and poor-prognosis schizophrenics, 3 of 25 (12 percent) committed suicide, and a significant number showed organic impairment (e.g., the dementia of dementia praecox).

Tsuang (1978) found that 10 percent of deceased schizophrenics died by suicide; this represents 4 percent of the total sample of 195 who could be traced to either death or present residence. Schizophrenics have an increased risk of death owing to physical illness as well. However, a reported decreased risk for cancer death appears to be an artifact of inappropriate statistical analysis (Tsuang et al., 1980).

We can summarize studies of course and outcome as follows: (1) Acute onset and episodic course are associated with better outcome than are insidious onset and chronic course. (2) Acute onset is more likely to be associated with an episodic course than is insidious onset. As a result, many patients with an acute onset of schizophrenic symptoms will not qualify for a DSM-IIIR diagnosis of schizophrenia. (3) Impaired role functioning is much more likely to occur in schizophrenia than in mood disorders. (4) Tsuang-Winokur criteria for paranoid and hebephrenic schizophrenia separate schizophrenia into three groups: paranoid, hebephrenic, and undifferentiated. The paranoid group has an outcome similar to that of the mood disorder group and significantly better than that of the other two schizophrenic subgroups. (5) Schizophrenics have increased rates of mortality, primarily by suicide. (6) Hebephrenic symptoms tend to be more enduring than paranoid symptoms.

The Family and Social Environments

Although in our discussion earlier we stated that the psychosocial environment does not play a role in the *etiology* of schizophrenia, some data suggest that it does affect the *course* of the illness. Specific types of family interactions may worsen the illness and result in increased rates of relapse (Leff, 1976). Also, stressful life events may predispose to an acute resurgence of symptoms (Leff et al., 1983), and low levels of social stimulation may increase social withdrawal and deterioration of self-care (Wing, 1978).

To investigate the relationship between emotional environment in the family and relapse in schizophrenia, researchers divided families into high-expressed-emotion (high-EE) and low-expressed-emotion (low-EE) groups. Expressed emotion was defined in terms of number of critical comments, amount of hostility, and degree of emotional overinvolvement of the family with the patient.

In a series of studies in which a total of 128 schizophrenic patients and their families were investigated, 13 percent (9 of 71) from low-EE families relapsed after 9 months. In the high-EE families, 51 percent (29 of 57) relapsed over a 9-month period. In the latter group, relapse rates were lower for those patients who had spent less than 35 hours per week in face-to-face contact with the family (28 percent) than for those who spent more than 35 hours per week in such contact (69 percent) (Leff, 1976). Two studies designed to reduce expressed emotion in families have demonstrated reduced relapse rates in the treated families (Falloon et al., 1982; Leff et al., 1982; Falloon and Liberman, 1983; Falloon et al., 1986).

Chronic institutionalization with little social stimulation also may increase schizophrenic deterioration. This deterioration may be reversed to some degree with increased social stimulation, but too much social stimulation may cause a relapse (Wing, 1978).

In sum, high amounts of expressed emotion in the families of schizophrenics and greater exposure to expressed emotion increase relapse rates in schizophrenics. Family treatment designed to reduce expressed emotion appears to reduce these relapse rates. Schizophrenics have increased social deterioration with low levels of social stimulation, but high levels of stimulation increase the chance of relapse.

TREATMENT

In the treatment of schizophrenia, the following modalities should be considered: hospitalization, administration of antipsychotics, and behavioral rehabilitation and family therapies.

Hospitalization

Hospitalization is used for four basic reasons: (1) diagnostic evaluation, as described in the section "Differential Diagnosis," (2) regulation of medication, (3) reduction of danger to the patient or others, and (4) other acute management problems. Rarely is the hospital used for chronic care, as in the past. Lengthy hospitalization has not been found to be more effective than brief hospitalization (Caton, 1982), although some authors have reported minor differences (Hargreaves et al., 1977).

Pharmacotherapy

Neuroleptic medication reduces relapse rates in schizophrenia. Davis's (1975) review of the older literature indicates that relapse rates are two to four times higher in placebo-treated groups than in drug-treated groups. For example, Hogarty et al. (1974) found that 80 percent of placebo-treated patients had relapsed by the end of 2 years compared with 48 percent of drug-treated patients. Hogarty and Ulrich (1977) report that the placebo-treated group was two to three times more likely to relapse over a 3-year period than was the treated group. Chronic schizophrenics may relapse if neuroleptics are discontinued, even after several years' remission (Cheung, 1981). After 2 to 3 years of treatment without relapse, 65 percent of 43 patients withdrawn from medication had an exacerbation of symptoms during the next year (Hogarty et al., 1976).

Neuroleptic side effects include sedation, dry mouth, hypotension, blurred vision, tachycardia, cardiac effects, galactorrhea, amenorrhea, loss of sexual interest, weight gain, hyperpyrexia, allergic reactions, pigmentary retinopathy, and seizures (Hollister, 1977). During the course of treatment with antipsychotics, acute extrapyramidal symptoms—dystonia, akathisia, and pseudoparkinson-ism—may occur in 40 to 60 percent of patients (Perry et al., 1981). *Dystonic reactions* are involuntary tonic muscle contractions of a striated muscle group and typically involve muscles of the head and face. *Akathisia* is a subjective feeling of restlessness. It may be expressed by pacing, rocking from foot to foot, or other motor activity and, at times, by insomnia. *Pseudoparkinsonism* is the production of an extrapyramidal syndrome that is virtually indistinguishable from Parkinson's disease, including tremor, rigidity, akinesia, and parkinsonian gait. These symptoms may be treated with anticholinergics (Perry et al., 1981).

Prolonged administration of antipsychotics may produce a late-onset dyskinetic syndrome known as *tardive dyskinesia*. This syndrome consists of involuntary dyskinetic movements, frequently involving the mouth, lips, and tongue. The prevalence of tardive dyskinesia among neuroleptic-treated patients has been highly variable across studies, ranging from 6 to 46 percent, with a mean of 18 percent (Jeste and Wyatt, 1982; Kane and Smith, 1982). These prevalences show a tendency to increase over time. Although the reasons for this increase are unknown, the resulting increase in malpractice suits has added an additional complication to the use of neuroleptic medication (Applebaum et al., 1985). Although withdrawal of antipsychotics may reverse the dyskinesia in about 37 percent of cases, the syndrome is frequently irreversible (Jeste and Wyatt, 1982).

Neuroleptic malignant syndrome is a rare but sometimes fatal reaction to neuroleptic medication. The clinical signs of the syndrome are fever, tachycardia, rigidity, altered consciousness, abnormal blood pressure, tachypnea, and diaphoresis (Levenson, 1985). These patients usually have high serum levels of creatinine phosphokinase and increased white blood cell counts. Levenson (1985) provides suggestions for the prevention and treatment of neuroleptic malignant syndrome.

Because of the high frequency and severity of neuroleptic side effects, clinical strategies have been developed to minimize the cumulative dose of neuroleptics that a patient receives during a lifetime. Excessive use of neuroleptics occurs when the dose required to manage acute psychotic symptoms is not reduced following clinical stabilization. The extended use of large doses of neuroleptics cannot be justified without evidence that lower doses are not effective.

During outpatient treatment, two strategies are available, low-dose treatment and intermittent treatment (Schooler, 1991). With a low-dose strategy, patients are maintained on a dose that is much lower than that initially required. In some cases, this is as much as 90 percent less. More intensive treatment is reserved for periods of symptom exacerbation. The maintenance dose of medication that will keep target symptoms reduced to a satisfactory level is highly individual and can be determined only by trial and error (Baldessarini and Davis, 1980). The intermittent-medication strategy withdraws all medication during periods of remission and uses neuroleptics only when the patient appears to be at risk for relapse.

Recent work in the psychopharmacology of schizophrenia has focused on the atypical neuroleptic clozapine (Bruhwyler et al., 1990). In addition to being an effective antipsychotic agent, clozapine has several distinct advantages over other neuroleptics. It has relatively few extrapyramidal side effects, and it is effective in many patients who are not helped by other neuroleptics (Safferman et al., 1991). It does not appear to cause tardive dyskinesia and may even suppress the syndrome when it is caused by other neuroleptics (Bruhwyler et al., 1990).

Common side effects of clozapine are sedation, hypersalivation, tachycardia, dizziness, constipation, nausea, and vomiting. Less common are hypotension, sweating, dry mouth, urinary problems, tremor, visual disturbances, fever, hypertension weight gain, seizures, akathisia, and rigidity. The most serious side effect is agranulocytosis, a life-threatening condition that occurs in 2 percent of patients after 1 year of clozapine therapy (Bruhwyler et al., 1990; Safferman et al., 1991). Hematologic monitoring of clozapine-treated patients reduces the mortality due to agranulocytosis. Thus systematic and frequent monitoring is necessary.

A number of other medications have been suggested for the treatment of schizophrenia. Lithium has been shown to be effective in as many as 50 percent of schizophrenic patients (Delva and Letemendia, 1982). Depression, sometimes termed *postpsychotic depression*, is common in schizophrenia (Guze et al., 1983). It usually responds to antipsychotics alone (Knights and Hirsch, 1981), but a role for antidepressants in the treatment of depression in schizophrenia has not been clearly established (British Medical Journal, 1980). Benzodiazepines have produced mixed results. Although they are helpful in some cases, they appear to be deleterious in others (Arana et al., 1986; Cott and Kurtz, 1987). Carbamazepine may be an effective treatment, especially for violent patients (Cott and Kurtz, 1987). However, it does not appear to be effective as a maintenance-treatment method (Carpenter et al., 1991). Electroconvulsive therapy has not proved to be effective in chronic schizophrenia (Kendell, 1981), but it may produce brief improvements in some patients (Wyatt et al., 1988).

The principles of psychopharmacology for schizophrenia are as follows (Klein et al., 1980; Perry et al., 1981; Bitter et al., 1991; Ruskin and Nyman, 1991; Van Putten et al., 1991):

- Define target symptoms.
- Choose an antipsychotic with the profile of side effects least likely to exacerbate other medical problems. If an antipsychotic has proven bene-

ficial in the past, it may be restarted or the dose increased. If an antipsychotic in adequate dose has not proved beneficial in the past or has particularly troublesome side effects, choose an antipsychotic from another class.

- Increase medication as tolerated, and observe target symptoms for several weeks. Evaluation of the effect of an antipsychotic may take up to several weeks of observation on a therapeutic dose of that antipsychotic. If there has been no change in target symptoms after this time, consider further increases in medication if side effects are tolerable, or change to a different class of antipsychotics. In either case, reevaluate target symptoms and appropriateness of diagnosis.
- After the patient has been stabilized clinically, consider reducing the dose to prevent future side effects.
- Avoid polypharmacy.
- If the patient is noncompliant and medication is clearly indicated, consider use of a long-acting (1 to 3 weeks) depot antipsychotic administered intramuscularly.
- If the patient does not respond to typical neuroleptics, consider clozapine and other medications.

Psychotherapy

After a review of the literature on psychotherapy for schizophrenia and other disorders, the American Psychiatric Association Commission on Psychotherapies (American Psychiatric Association, 1982) concluded

Psychotherapy as the sole therapeutic modality seems to be useful in such conditions as some psychoneuroses, personality disorders, and maladjustments. Psychotherapy alone has been shown to be less effective for the major affective disorders and much less so for schizophrenia. The prototypic relationship between psychotherapy and pharmacotherapy seems reciprocal, favoring psychotherapy for personality disorders and favoring pharmacotherapy for psychotic disorders. For many conditions the interrelationship seems to be additive [p. 227].

This conclusion does not rule out psychotherapy for schizophrenic patients, but it clearly indicates that it should not be used as a replacement for pharmacologic treatment. In clinical practice, the skills of the psychotherapist are useful in a variety of ways. The development of a productive patient–therapist relationship will foster compliance with drug therapy and motivation for behavioral and family treatments. Regular follow-up visits for monitoring symptoms, medication compliance, medication side effects, and social problems are advisable and can reduce hospitalization rates (Hogarty et al., 1974a, 1974b; American Psychiatric Association, 1982). Too vigorous an intervention, however, particularly in the symptomatic patient, may be worse than no intervention (Goldberg et al., 1977).

Behavioral Therapy

As a rule, schizophrenics have many social problems. Assistance in dealing with social agencies and such matters as finances and family stress is as important for the schizophrenic as it is for any handicapped individual. For example, marked social isolation appears to produce more schizophrenic deterioration. On the other hand, too much social stimulation may produce an increase in florid symptoms (Wing, 1978). If counselors and relatives do not understand the need for the schizophrenic to control social stimulation and the protective nature of some social withdrawal, they may place too much pressure on him or her to engage in social activities. In cases where the schizophrenic lives with his or her family, family therapy designed to reduce the level of expressed emotion may reduce relapse rates (Falloon et al., 1982; Leff et al., 1982).

The behavioral rehabilitative program for a patient with schizophrenia must be tailored to the particular handicaps of that patient. This may involve day care of a low intensity (Linn et al., 1979), sheltered employment, and sheltered housing (Bennett, 1978). To be effective, it must take into account not only the psychiatric phenomenology of the patient but also the cognitive impairments that are concomitants of structural and functional brain dysfunction (Seidman et al., 1992). In what follows, we briefly review three behavioral methods that have been effective in the treatment of schizophrenia: operant techniques, response acquisition methods, and behavioral family therapy.

OPERANT TECHNIQUES

The principles of operant conditioning describe how the systematic manipulation of rewards and punishments will modify behavior. These principles have been applied systematically to schizophrenic patients in a therapeutic program known as the "token economy" (Ayllon and Azrin, 1968; Kazdin and Bootzin, 1972; Kazdin, 1977). The token economy is useful for inpatient, day hospital, and group home settings where patients can be observed for long periods of time. The "token" is any object that is small and easily identified (e.g., a poker chip). The tokens are used to reward patients for appropriate behavior. It is best if they are individualized to avoid theft, gambling, and other exchanges of tokens among patients. Tokens are given freely to patients who are new to the program. They learn to use these tokens to buy rewards from the staff. These rewards can be specific items (e.g., valued foods) or access to privileges (e.g., use of television or game rooms). Rewards that are similar to those which may occur in the patient's posthospital circumstances are preferable because these will promote generalization.

The patient learns the reward value of tokens by buying rewards from the staff with the tokens given at the outset of the program. After this learning is established, the patient must earn tokens. Tokens are earned according to rules specified by staff in an individualized behavioral program. The program specifies the types and degree of behavior change required to earn a specified number of tokens. Initially, these requirements are relatively easy so that the patient can "learn to learn." Subsequently, they are made more difficult to encourage continued behavior change.

The modification of behavior with a token economy is relatively easy. It is, however, fairly difficult to program change so that it is maintained in the community (Kazdin and Bootzin, 1972). The generalization of behavior changes to situations where tokens are not available will not occur unless systematic procedures are applied. Ideally, one should increase behaviors that are rewarded in the community (e.g., job-related skills). We also suggest that the presentation of tokens be accompanied by social rewards such as praise and affection. If possible, tokens should be phased out and behavior should be maintained with social rewards alone.

A key problem with operant techniques is that to increase the likelihood of a behavior, it must already exist in the patient in some, albeit rudimentary, form. In many cases, the patient will not emit the desired behavior in any form. This is most relevant for social interactive behaviors. Indeed, many patients emit very little, if any, appropriate social behavior. Response acquisition procedures were created to deal with this problem. Since this work has focused mostly on social behaviors, these techniques are often referred to as *social skills training* (Curran and Monti, 1982).

RESPONSE ACQUISITION METHODS

Social skills training is usually performed with groups of patients to create a social context for learning. One program uses groups of three or four patients and two cotherapists (Curran et al., 1985). In a typical therapy session, the therapists do the following: (1) review previous session's material and homework; (2) present a summary of the session's lesson, (3) model the skills described in the lesson or present a videotape model, (4) answer questions and quiz patients on major points, (5) videotape the patients role playing the skills, (6) observe the videotape, provide feedback, and lead the discussion, (7) have patients master the skill with repeated practice, and (8) assign homework so that patients practice skills outside the group.

BEHAVIORAL FAMILY THERAPY

Behavioral family therapy assumes that family behaviors have an impact on the course of the illness but does not assume that the illness was directly or indirectly caused by deviant family interaction. Its goal is to reduce stress in the patient's life and to encourage the family to participate in the community treatment of the illness (Curran et al., 1986; Falloon et al., 1986). There are three major components of behavioral family therapy (Curran et al., 1986): education, communication, and problem-solving. The educational component attempts to reduce the family's self-blame for the illness. Once families learn about the biologic bases of the illness, they can throw off guilty feelings and more productively cooperate in the treatment of their schizophrenic relative. Understanding biologic bases also helps families accept the necessity of neuroleptic medication. Families are also taught that the manifestations of schizophrenia are outside the patient's control, and they are encouraged to avoid unrealistic expectations. Indeed, accusing the patient of being purposefully symptomatic or having high expectations for social or occupational performance is very stressful for the patient. Perhaps most important, the families are taught how to identify potential stresses for the patient in the home environment. This includes discussions of the concept of expressed emotion and findings in the research literature.

Many families do not have the communication skills needed to benefit fully from the educational component of treatment. Thus response acquisition methods are often used to teach these skills. The method of teaching is similar to that described for patients, although it emphasizes those communication skills which are most needed in the family environment (Curran et al., 1986; Falloon et al., 1986). Some families can identify relevant problems but do not have the skills to find and implement solutions. Thus problem-solving therapies have been applied to families with some success in reducing schizophrenia relapse rates to a clinically significant degree (Curran et al., 1986; Falloon et al., 1986).

Summary

In conclusion, the optimal treatment for schizophrenia should include

- Careful diagnostic evaluation.
- Hospitalization for acute management, if necessary, such as with the suicidal, homicidal, or assaultive patient, the patient who requires skilled nursing care and intensive medical management.
- Antipsychotics in an appropriate dose and dose form.
- Regular monitoring of symptoms, medication side effects, and compliance with medication
- Behavior therapy to teach patients socially appropriate behavior and to help families cope with patients and help in the management of their illnesses.

CASE HISTORIES

The case histories that follow illustrate many of the clinical features of schizophrenia that have been described in previous sections.

Case 1

M.C. is a 25-year-old male high school graduate who lives with his parents and receives Social Security disability income. His grades in high school were average but not as good as those of his siblings. He never dated and had few friends. After high school he worked at one job for about 2 years, but he has not been able to hold a job since then for more than a few months, although several of his father's friends have hired him as a favor.

His first psychiatric admission was at age 20. This followed a period of withdrawal, during which he refused to eat with his family and became hostile for no clear reason. His family brought him to the hospital after he became agitated. The records do not describe any clear hallucinations or delusions but do note that he had flat affect, talked little during his hospitalization, and laughed to himself. He was treated with neuroleptic medication and became quite agreeable, although he still was somewhat withdrawn. He returned home and attempted to return to his work. However, he was eventually fired for making too many mistakes.

His second hospitalization, at age 22, followed a similar episode of withdrawal, hostility, and agitation. At this time he complained of being God or the devil and of being influenced by spirits. His account was fragmented and vague. He again responded well to neuroleptic medication and was discharged in the care of his family.

One year later, his symptomatology reemerged while his antipsychotic dose was being reduced. He became withdrawn, refused again to eat with the family, refused to bathe, and over a period of several weeks took nearly every pill he could find in his parents' home. He could give no rational explanation for his behavior. In between his acute episodes of agitation and psychosis he had blunted affect, talking little during psychiatric evaluations; he often smiled peculiarly when answering questions with his usual one- or two-word answers, as if something funny had just happened and he were trying to suppress a giggle. His family reported that he seldom left the house and had no social life.

This patient meets Tsuang-Winokur criteria for hebephrenic schizophrenia (Tsuang and Winokur, 1974, Table 6-3). Onset of symptoms occurred before age 25; he is unmarried and unemployed. His thinking is disorganized during acute exacerbations; between episodes he shows poverty of speech and his affect is flat, except when he smiles inappropriately. He has behaved bizarrely, such as taking all the pills in the house and refusing to eat with his family without a rational explanation.

Case 2

R.F. is a 58-year-old male who lives with his parents and has never married. He lives on disability income, although he claims that he does not need it. He tore his last check into shreds in a fit of anger that terrified his aging parents. He has a 30-year history of believing that government agents have replaced most of his internal organs with artificial ones. He also believes that two teams of scientists continually experiment on him. At an examiner's first contact with this patient, he refused to answer most questions, replying, "You know, you know," with a hostile tone of voice and a sarcastic smile. He insisted that the examiner belonged to the "gold team" because his last name began with two I's and because he had asked some questions twice. When informed that the examiner's last name began with only one I, the patient still insisted that the examiner belonged to the "gold team." The patient would allow the examiner to talk with him only for 10 to 15 minutes at a time and then would become even more hostile and insist that the doctor leave the room. During these brief interviews the patient admitted that, at times, external forces would control his mind and body, causing him to think thoughts and perform actions against his will. He indignantly insisted that these were violations of his rights by the experimenting scientists.

The family reported that no other family members had ever had a similar illness. After 4 days in the hospital, the patient signed himself out against medical advice, despite the encouragement of his relatives to stay for treatment.

This patient meets Tsuang-Winokur criteria for the paranoid subtype (Table 6-3). No first-degree relative has had schizophrenia. He has no disorganized thoughts or hebephrenic symptoms, and he is preoccupied with a well-organized delusional system.

REFERENCES

Abrams R, Taylor MA: Importance of schizophrenic symptoms in the diagnosis of mania. Am J Psychiatry 138:658–661, 1981.

Abrams R, Taylor MA: The genetics of schizophrenia: A reassessment using modern criteria. Am J Psychiatry 140:171–175, 1983.

American Psychiatric Association: Diagnostic and Statistical Manual of Mental Disorders (DSM-III). Washington, American Psychiatric Association, 1980.

American Psychiatric Association: Commission on Psychotherapies: Psychotherapy Research: Methodological and Efficacy Issues. Washington, American Psychiatric Association, 1982.

American Psychiatric Association: Diagnostic and Statistical Manual of Mental Disorders, 3d ed, revised. Washington, American Psychiatric Association, 1987.

Andreasen NC: Thought, language, and communication disorders: II. Diagnostic significance. Arch Gen Psychiatry 36:1325–1330, 1979.

Andreasen NC: Negative symptoms in schizophrenia: Definition and reliability. Arch Gen Psychiatry 39:784–788, 1982.

Andreasen NC, Olsen SA, et al: Ventricular enlargement in schizophrenia: Relationship to positive and negative symptoms. Am J Psychiatry 139:297–302, 1982.

Applebaum PS, Schaffner K, et al: Responsibility and compensation for tardive dyskinesia. Am J Psychiatry 142:806–810, 1985.

Arana GW, Ornsteen ML, et al: The use of benzodiazepines for psychotic disorders: A literature review and preliminary clinical findings. Psychopharmacol Bull 22:77, 1986.

Ariel RN, Golden CJ, et al: Regional cerebral blood flow in schizophrenics: Tests using the xenon 133 inhalation method. Arch Gen Psychiatry 40:258–263, 1983.

Ayllon T, Azrin NH: The Token Economy: A Motivational System for Therapy and Rehabilitation. New York, Appleton-Century-Crofts, 1968.

Baldessarini RJ, Davis JM: What is the best maintenance dose of neuroleptics in schizophrenia? Psychiatry Res 3:115–122, 1980.

Baron M, Endicott J, et al: Genetic linkage in mental illness: Limitations and prospects. Br J Psychiatry 157:645–655, 1990.

Barr CE, Mednick SA, et al: Exposure to influenza epidemics during gestation and adult schizophrenia: A 40-year study. Arch Gen Psychiatry 47:869–874, 1990.

Barta PE, Pearlson GD, et al: Auditory hallucinations and smaller superior temporal gyral volume in schizophrenia. Am J Psychiatry 147:1457–1462, 1990.

Bassett AS: Chromosome 5 and schizophrenia: Implications for genetic linkage studies. Schizophr Bull 15(3):393–402, 1989.

Bassett AS, McGillivray BC, et al: Partial trisomy chromosome 5 cosegregating with schizophrenia. Lancet 1:799–801, 1988.

Behar D, Rapoport JL, et al: Computerized tomography and neuropsychological test measures in adolescents with obsessive-compulsive disorder. Am J Psychiatry 141:363–369, 1984.

Benes FM, Davidson J, et al: Quantitative cytoarchitectural studies of the cerebral cortex of schizophrenics. Arch Gen Psychiatry 43:31–35, 1986.

Benes FM, Majocha R, et al: Increased vertical axon numbers in cingulate cortex of schizophrenia. Arch Gen Psychiatry 44:1017–1021, 1987.

Bennett D: Social forms of psychiatric treatment. In Schizophrenia: Towards a New Synthesis. New York, Grune & Stratton, 1978.

Bersani G, Valeri M, et al: HLA antigens and neuroleptic response in clinical subtypes of schizophrenia. J Psychiatr Res 23 (3–4):213–220, 1989.

Bitter I, Volavka J, et al: The concept of the neuroleptic threshold: An update. J Clin Psychopharmacol 11(1):28–33, 1991.

Bleuler E: Dementia Praecox or the Group of Schizophrenias (1911). New York, International Universities Press, 1950.

Bleuler M: The Schizophrenic Disorders: Long-Term Patient and Family Studies. New Haven, Yale University Press, 1978.

Bogerts B, Ashtari M, et al: Reduced temporal limbic structure volumes on magnetic resonance images in first episode schizophrenia. Psychiatry Res Neuroimaging 35:1–13, 1990.

Book JA, Wetterberg L, et al: Schizophrenia in a North Swedish geographical isolate, 1900–1977: Epidemiology, genetics and biochemistry. Clin Genet 14:373–394, 1978.

Bornstein RA, Nasrallah HA, et al: Neuropsychological deficit in schizophrenic subtypes: Paranoid, nonparanoid, and schizoaffective subgroups. Psychiatry Res 31:15–24, 1989.

Bowers MB, Swigar ME: Vulnerability to psychosis associated with hallucinogen use. Psychiatry Res 9:91–97, 1983.

British Medical Journal: Use of antidepressants in schizophrenia. Br Med J 1:1037–1038, 1980.

Brody D, Wolkin A, et al: Phospholipids and prostaglandins in schizophrenia. In Neurochemistry and Neuropharmacology of Schizophrenia. Amsterdam, Elsevier Science Publishers, 1987, pp 319–336.

Bruhwyler J, Chleide E, et al: Clozapine: An atypical neuroleptic. Neurosci Behav Rev 14:357–363, 1990.

Buchsbaum MS, Ingvar DH: New visions of the schizophrenic brain: Regional differences in electrophysiology, blood flow, and cerebral glucose use. In Schizophrenia as a Brain Disease. New York, Oxford University Press, 1990.

Buchsbaum MS, Nuechterlein KH, et al: Glucose metabolic rate in normals and schizophrenics during the continuous performance test assessed by positron emission tomography. Br J Psychiatry 156:216–227, 1990.

Cadet JL, Lohr JB, et al: Tardive dyskinesia and schizophrenic burnout: The possible involvement of cytotoxic free radicals. In Neurochemistry and Neuropharmacology of Schizophrenia. Amsterdam, Elsevier Science Publishers, 1987, pp 425–438.

Carlsson A, Lindqvist M: Effect of chlorpromazine and haloperidol on formation of 3-methoxytyramine and normetanephrine in mouse brain. Acta Pharmacol Toxicol 20:140–144, 1963.

Carpenter WT Jr, Kirkpatrick B, et al: Carbamazepine maintenance treatment in outpatient schizophrenics. Arch Gen Psychiatry 48:69–72, 1991.

Carpenter WT, Strauss JS, et al: Flexible system for the diagnosis of schizophrenia: Report from the WHO international pilot study of schizophrenia. Science 182:1275–1278, 1973.

Castellani S, Ziegler MG, et al: Plasma norepinephrine and dopamine-beta-hydroxylase activity in schizophrenia. Arch Gen Psychiatry 39:1145–1149, 1982.

Caton CLM: Effect of length of inpatient treatment for chronic schizophrenia. Am J Psychiatry 139:856–861, 1982.

Cheung HK: Schizophrenics fully remitted on neuroleptics for 3–5 years—To stop or continue drugs? Br J Psychiatry 138: 490–494, 1981.

Ciompi L: Catamnestic long-term study on the course of life and aging in schizophrenics. Schizophr Bull 6:606–618, 1980.

Cohen RM, Semple WE, et al: From syndrome to illness: Delineating the pathophysiology of schizophrenia with PET. Schizophr Bull 14:169–176, 1988.

Collinge J, DeLisi LE, et al: Evidence for a pseudo-autosomal locus for schizophrenia using the method of affected sibling pairs. Br J Psychiatry 158:624–629, 1991.

Cooper B: Epidemiology. In Schizophrenia: Towards a New Synthesis. New York, Grune & Stratton, 1978.

Cooper JE, Kendell RE, et al: Psychiatric Diagnosis in New York and London: A Comparative Study of Mental Hospital Admissions. London, Oxford University Press (Institute of Psychiatry, Maudsley Monographs, No. 20), 1972.

Coryell W, Tsuang MT, et al: Psychotic features in major depression: Is mood congruence important? J Affective Disord 4:227–237, 1982.

Cott JM, Kurtz NM: New pharmacological treatments for schizophrenia. In Neurochemistry and Neuropharmacology of Schizophrenia. Amsterdam, Elsevier Science Publishers, 1987, pp 203–226.

Creese I, Burt DR, et al: Dopamine receptor binding predicts clinical and pharmacological potencies of antischizophrenic drugs. Science 192:481–482, 1976.

Crow TJ, DeLisi LE, et al: Concordance by sex in sibling pairs with schizophrenia is paternally inherited: Evidence for a pseudoautosomal locus. Br J Psychiatry 155:92–97, 1989.

Crowe RR, Black DW, et al: Lack of linkage to chromosome 5q11–q13 markers in six schizophrenia pedigrees. Arch Gen Psychiatry 48:357–361, 1991.

Curran JP, Monti PM: Social Skills Training: A Practical Handbook for Assessment and Treatment. New York, Guilford, 1982.

Curran JP, Faraone SV, et al: Inpatient treatment of schizophrenia and other psychotic disorders. In Practice of Inpatient Behavior Therapy: A Clinical Guide. New York, Grune & Stratton, 1985.

Curran JR, Faraone SV, et al: Behavioral family therapy in an acute inpatient setting. In Handbook of Behavioral Family Therapy. New York, Guilford, 1986.

Dalen P: Season of Birth: A Study of Schizophrenia and Other Mental Disorders. Amsterdam, Elsevier, 1975.

Daniel DG, Goldberg TE, et al: Lack of a bimodal distribution of ventricular size in schizophrenia: A Gaussian mixture analysis of 1056 cases and controls. Biol Psychiatry 30:887–903, 1991.

Davis JM: Maintenance therapy in psychiatry: I. Schizophrenia. Am J Psychiatry 132:1237–1245, 1975.

Davis JM: Dopamine theory of schizophrenia: A two-factor theory. In The Nature of Schizophrenia. New York, Wiley, 1978.

DeLisi LE, Goldin LR, et al: A family study of the association of increased ventricular size in schizophrenia. Arch Gen Psychiatry 43:48, 1986.

DeLisi LE, Neckers LM, et al: Increased whole blood serotonin concentrations in chronic schizophrenic patients. Arch Gen Psychiatry 38:647–650, 1981.

Delva NJ, Letemendia FJJ: Review article: Lithium treatment in schizophrenia and schizoaffective disorders. Br J Psychiatry 141:387, 1982.

Depue RA, Woodburn L: Disappearance of paranoid symptoms with chronicity. J Abnorm Psychol 84:84–86, 1975.

Detera-Wadleigh SD, Goldin LR, et al: Exclusion of linkage to 5q11–13 in families with schizophrenia and other psychiatric disorders. Nature 340:391–393, 1989.

Diehl S, Su Y, et al: Linkage studies of schizophrenia: Exclusion of candidate regions on chromosomes 5q and 11q (abstract). Psychiatr Gene 2(1):14–15, 1991.

Dunham HW: Community and Schizophrenia: An Epidemiological Analysis. Detroit, Wayne State University Press, 1965.

Ellison GD, Eison MS: Continuous amphetamine intoxication: An animal model of the acute psychotic episode. Psychol Med 13:751–761, 1983.

Erlenmeyer-Kimling L, Cornblatt B, et al: Neurological, electrophysiological, and attentional deviations in children at risk for schizophrenia. In Schizophrenia as a Brain Disease. New York, Oxford University Press, 1982.

Falkai P, Bogerts B, et al: Limbic pathology in schizophrenia: The entorhinal region—A morphometric study. Biol Psychiatry 24:515–521, 1988.

Falloon IRH, Liberman RP: Behavioral family intervention in the management of chronic schizophrenia. In Family Therapy in Schizophrenia. New York, Guilford, 1983.

Falloon IRH, Boyd JL, et al: Family management in the prevention of exacerbations of schizophrenia: A controlled study. N Engl J Med 306:1437–1440, 1982.

Falloon IRH, Boyd, JL, et al: Family management in the prevention of morbidity of schizophrenia: Clinical outcome of a two-year controlled study. Arch Gen Psychiatry 42:887–896, 1986.

Faraone SV, Tsuang MT: Quantitative models of the genetic transmission of schizophrenia. Psychol Bull 98(1):41–66, 1985.

Faraone SV, Kremen WS, et al: Genetic transmission of major affective disorders: Quantitative models and linkage analyses. Psychol Bull 108(1):109–127, 1990.

Faraone SV, Lyons MJ, et al: Schizophrenia: Mathematical models of genetic transmission. In Nosology, Epidemiology and Genetics. Amsterdam, Elsevier Science Publishers, 1988, pp 501–530.

Farde L, Wiesel F-A, et al: No D_2 receptor increase in PET study of schizophrenia. Arch Gen Psychiatry 44:671–672, 1987.

Farkas T, Wolf AP, et al: Regional brain glucose metabolism in chronic schizophrenia: A positron emission transaxial tomographic study. Arch Gen Psychiatry 41:293–300, 1984.

Farley IJ, Price KS, et al: Norepinephrine in chronic paranoid schizophrenia: Above normal levels in limbic forebrain. Science 200:465–468, 1978.

Farmer AE, McGuffin P, et al: Searching for the split in schizophrenia: A twin study perspective. Psychiatry Res 13: 109–118, 1984.

Feighner JP, Robins E, et al: Diagnostic criteria for use in psychiatric research. Arch Gen Psychiatry 26:57–63, 1972.

Fish B: Neurobiologic antecedents of schizophrenia in children: Evidence for an inherited, congenital neurointegrative defect. Arch Gen Psychiatry 34:1297–1313, 1977.

Flor-Henry P: Determinants of psychosis in epilepsy: Laterality and forced normalization. Biol Psychiatry 18:1045–1057, 1983.

Gershon ES: Genetic linkage and complex diseases: A comment. Genet Epidemiol 7:21–23, 1990.

Gilliam TC, Freimer NB, et al: Deletion mapping of DNA markers to a region of chromosome 5 that cosegregates with schizophrenia. Genomics 5:940–944, 1989.

Goldberg EM, Morrison SL: Schizophrenia and social class. Br J Psychiatry 109:785–802, 1963.

Goldberg SC, Schooler NR, et al: Prediction of relapse in schizophrenic outpatients treated by drug and sociotherapy. Arch Gen Psychiatry 44:171–184, 1977.

Golden CJ, Moses JA, et al: Cerebral ventricular size and neuropsychological impairment in young chronic schizophrenics: Measurement by the standardized Luria-Nebraska neuropsychological battery. Arch Gen Psychiatry 37:619–623, 1980.

Gomes UCR, Shanley BC, et al: Noradrenergic overactivity in chronic schizophrenia: Evidence based on cerebrospinal fluid noradrenaline and cyclic nucleotide concentrations. Br J Psychiatry 137:346–351, 1980.

Goodwin DW, Alderson P, et al: Clinical significance of hallucinations in psychiatric disorders: A study of 116 hallucinatory patients. Arch Gen Psychiatry 24:76–80, 1971.

Gottesman II, McGue M: Mixed and mixed-up models for the transmission of schizophrenia. In Thinking Clearly About Psychology: Essays in Honor of Paul E. Meehl. St. Paul, University of Minnesota Press, 1990.

Gottesman II, Shields J: Schizophrenia and Genetics: A Twin Study Vantage Point. New York, Academic Press, 1972.

Gottesman II, Shields J: Schizophrenia: The Epigenetic Puzzle. Cambridge, Cambridge University Press, 1982.

Grinspoon L, Bakalar JD: Drug dependence: Nonnarcotic agents. In Comprehensive Textbook of Psychiatry, 3d ed. Baltimore, Williams & Wilkins, 1980.

Guenther W, Breitling D: Predominant sensorimotor area left hemisphere dysfunction in schizophrenia measured by brain electrical activity mapping. Biol Psychiatry 20:515–532, 1985.

Gur RE: Cognitive concomitants of hemispheric dysfunction in schizophrenia. Arch Gen Psychiatry 36:269–274, 1979.

Gur RE, Skolnick BE, et al: Brain function in schizophrenic disorders: I. Regional blood flow in medicated schizophrenics. Arch Gen Psychiatry 40:1250–1254, 1983.

Guze SB, Cloninger R, et al: A follow-up and family study of schizophrenia. Arch Gen Psychiatry 40:1273–1276, 1983.

Hall CW: Psychiatric Presentations of Medical Illness: Somatopsychic Disorders. New York, SP Medical and Scientific Books, 1980.

Hamilton M: Fish's Schizophrenia. Bristol, John Wright & Sons, 1984.

Harding CM, Brooks GW, et al: The Vermont longitudinal study of persons with severe mental illness: I. Methodology, study sample, and overall status 32 years later. Am J Psychiatry 144:718–726, 1987.

Hare E: The season of birth of siblings of psychiatric patients. Br J Psychiatry 129:49, 1976.

Hare E, Price J, et al: Mental disorder and season of birth. Br J Psychiatry 124:81, 1974.

Hargreaves WA, Glick ID, et al: Short vs. long hospitalization: A prospective controlled study: VI. Two-year follow-up results for schizophrenics. Arch Gen Psychiatry 34:305–311, 1977.

Helzer JE, Brockington IF, et al: Predictive validity of DSM-III and Feighner definitions of schizophrenia: A comparison with research diagnostic criteria and CATEGO. Arch Gen Psychiatry 38:791–797, 1981.

Henn FA: A role in psychosis or schizophrenia. In Schizophrenia as a Brain Disease. New York, Oxford University Press, 1982.

Heston LL: Psychiatric disorders in foster home-reared children of schizophrenic mothers. Br J Psychiatry 112:819–825, 1966.

Hogarty GE, Ulrich RF: Temporal effects of drug and placebo in delaying relapse in schizophrenic outpatients. Arch Gen Psychiatry 34:297–301, 1977.

Hogarty GE, Goldberg SC, et al: Drug and sociotherapy in the aftercare of schizophrenic patients: II. Two year relapse rates. Arch Gen Psychiatry 31:603–608, 1974a.

Hogarty GE, Goldberg SC, et al: Drug and sociotherapy in the aftercare of schizophrenic patients: III. Adjustment of nonrelapsed patients. Arch Gen Psychiatry 31:609–618, 1974b.

Hogarty GE, Ulrich RF, et al: Drug discontinuation among longterm, successfully maintained schizophrenic outpatients. Disord Nerv Syst 37:494–500, 1976.

Hollister LE: Antipsychotic medications and the treatment of schizophrenia. In Psychopharmacology: From Theory to Practice. New York, Oxford University Press, 1977.

Itil TM: Qualitative and quantitative EEG findings in schizophrenia. Schizophr Bull 3:61–79, 1977.

Jacobsen B, Kinney DK: Perinatal complications in adopted and non-adopted schizophrenics and their controls: Preliminary results. Acta Psychiatr Scand Suppl 285(62):337, 1980.

Jakob H, Beckmann H: Prenatal developmental disturbances in the limbic allocortex in schizophrenics. J Neural Transm 65:303–326, 1986.

Jaskiw G, Kleinman J: Postmortem Neurochemistry Studies in Schizophrenia. New York, Oxford University Press, 1988.

Jeste DV, Wyatt RJ: Therapeutic strategies against tardive dyskinesia. Arch Gen Psychiatry 39:803–816, 1982.

Johnstone EC, Crow TJ, et al: Cerebral ventricular size and cognitive impairment in chronic schizophrenia. Lancet 2: 924–926, 1976.

Kane JM, Smith JM: Tardive dyskinesia: Prevalence and risk factors, 1959 to 1979. Arch Gen Psychiatry 39:473–481, 1982.

Kaufmann CA, DeLisi LE, et al: Physical mapping, linkage analysis of a putative schizophrenia locus on chromosome 5q. Schizophr Bull 15(3):441–452, 1989.

Kazdin AE: The Token Economy: A Review and Evaluation. New York, Plenum, 1977.

Kazdin AE, Bootzin RR: The token economy: An evaluative review. J Appl Behav Anal 5:343–372, 1972.

Kemali D, Del Vecchio M, et al: Increased noradrenaline levels in CSF and plasma of schizophrenic patients. Biol Psychiatry 17:711–717, 1982.

Kendell RE: The present status of electroconvulsive therapy. Br J Psychiatry 139:265–283, 1981.

Kendell RE, Kemp JW: Maternal influenza in the etiology of schizophrenia. Arch Gen Psychiatry 46:878–882, 1989.

Kendler KS: Overview: A current perspective on twin studies of schizophrenia. Am J Psychiatry 140:1413–1425, 1983.

Kendler KS: The impact of diagnostic misclassification on the pattern of familial aggregation and coaggregation of psychiatric illness. J Psychiatr Res 21(1): 55–91, 1987.

Kendler KS: Mood-incongruent psychotic affective illness: A historical and empirical review. Arch Gen Psychiatry 48: 362–369, 1991.

Kendler KS, Tsuang MT: Nosology of paranoid, schizophrenic, and other paranoid psychoses. Schizophr Bull 7:594–610, 1981.

Kendler KS, Gruenberg AM, et al: Outcome of schizophrenia subtypes defined by four diagnostic systems. Arch Gen Psychiatry 41:149–154, 1984.

Kendler KS, Gruenberg AM, et al: Psychiatric illness in first-degree relatives of schizophrenic and surgical control patients: A family study using DSM-III criteria. Arch Gen Psychiatry 42:770–779, 1985.

Kendler KS, Gruenberg AM, et al: Subtype stability in schizophrenia. Am J Psychiatry 142(7):827–832, 1985.

Kennedy JL, Giuffra LA, et al: Evidence against linkage of schizophrenia to markers on chromosome 5 in a northern Swedish pedigree. Nature 336:167–170, 1988.

Kety SS, Rosenthal D, et al: The biologic and adoptive families of adopted individuals who became schizophrenic: Prevalence of mental illness and other characteristics. In The Nature of Schizophrenia: New Approaches to Research and Treatment. New York, Wiley, 1978.

Kinney DK, Jacobsen S: Environmental factors in schizophrenia: New adoption evidence. In The Nature of Schizophrenia: New Approaches to Research and Treatment. New York, Wiley, 1978, pp. 38–51.

Klein DF, Gittelman R, et al: Diagnosis and Drug Treatment of Psychiatric Disorders: Adults and Children. Baltimore, Williams & Wilkins, 1980.

Knights A, Hirsch SR: "Revealed" depression and drug treatment of schizophrenia. Arch Gen Psychiatry 38:806–811, 1981.

Kraepelin E: Dementia Praecox and Paraphrenia (1919). Huntington, NY, Robert Krieger, 1971.

Kramer M: Some problems for international research suggested by observations on differences in first admission rates to the mental hospitals of England and Wales and of the United States. In Proceedings of the Third World Congress of Psychiatry, 1961.

Kremen WS, Tsuang MT, et al: Using vulnerability indicators to compare conceptual models of genetic heterogeneity in schizophrenia. J Nerv Ment Dis 180:141–152, 1992.

Lake CR, Kleinman JE, et al: Norepinephrine metabolism in schizophrenia. In Neurochemistry and Neuropharmacology of Schizophrenia. Amsterdam, Elsevier, 1987, pp 227–256.

Lane EA, Albee GW: Comparative birthweights of schizophrenics and their siblings. J Psychol 64:227, 1966.

Larsson M, Ohman R, et al: Antipsychotic treatment with alpha-methyltyrosine in combination with thioridazine: Prolactin response and interaction with dopaminergic precursor pools. J Neural Transm 60(2):115–132, 1984.

Leff J: Schizophrenia and sensitivity to the family environment. Schizophr Bull 2:566–574, 1976.

Leff J: Social and psychological causes of the acute attack. In Schizophrenia: Towards a New Synthesis. New York, Grune & Stratton, 1978.

Leff J, Kuipers L, et al: A controlled trial of social intervention in the families of schizophrenic patients. Br J Psychiatry 141:121–134, 1982.

Leff J, Kuipers L, et al: Life events, relatives' expressed emotion and maintenance neuroleptics in schizophrenic relapse. Psychol Med 13:799–806, 1983.

Levenson JL: Neuroleptic malignant syndrome. Am J Psychiatry 142:1137–1145, 1985.

Lewis SW, Reveley AM, et al: The familial/sporadic distinction as a strategy in schizophrenia research. Br J Psychiatry 151: 306–313, 1987.

Linn MW, Caffey EM, et al: Day treatment and psychotropic drugs in the aftercare of schizophrenic patients. Arch Gen Psychiatry 36:1055–1066, 1979.

Lishman WA: Organic Psychiatry: The Psychological Consequences of Cerebral Disorder. Oxford, Blackwell Scientific, 1978.

Luchins DJ: Computed tomography in schizophrenia: Disparities in the prevalence of abnormalities." Arch Gen Psychiatry 39:859–860, 1982.

Lyons MJ, Faraone SV, et al: Familial and sporadic schizophrenia: A simulation study of statistical power. Schizophr Res 2: 345–353, 1989.

Lyons MJ, Kremen WS, et al: Investigating putative genetic and environmental forms of schizophrenia: Methods and findings. Int Rev Psychiatry 1:259–276, 1989.

Mathew RJ, Duncan GC, et al: Regional cerebral blood flow in schizophrenia. Arch Gen Psychiatry 39:1121–1124, 1982.

Matthysse S: Genetic linkage and complex diseases: A comment. Genet Epidemiol 7:29–31, 1990.

McGillivray BC, Bassett AS, et al: Familial 5q11.2–q13.3 segmental duplication cosegregating with multiple anomalies, including schizophrenia. Am J Med Gen 35:10–13, 1990.

McGue M, Gottesman II: Genetic linkage in schizophrenia: Perspectives from genetic epidemiology. Schizophr Bull 15 (3):453–464, 1989a.

McGue M, Gottesman II: A single dominant gene still cannot account for the transmission of schizophrenia. Arch Gen Psychiatry 46:478–479, 1989b.

McGuffin P, Farmer A, et al: Is there really a split in schizophrenia? The genetic evidence. Br J Psychiatry 150:581–592, 1987.

McGuffin P, Sargeant M, et al: Exclusion of a schizophrenia susceptibility gene from the chromosome 5q11–q13 region: New data and a reanalysis of previous reports. Am J Hum Genet 47:524–535, 1990.

McNeil TF, Kaij L: Obstetric factors in the development of schizophrenia: Complications in the births of preschizophrenics and in reproduction by schizophrenic parents. In The Nature of Schizophrenia: New Approaches to Research and Treatment. New York, Wiley, 1978, pp 401–429.

Mednick SA: Breakdown in individuals at high risk for schizophrenia: Possible predispositional perinatal factors. Ment Hyg 54:50, 1970.

Mednick SA, Schulsinger F: Some premorbid characteristics related to breakdown in children with schizophrenic mothers. In The Transmission of Schizophrenia. Oxford, Pergamon Press. 1968, pp 267–291.

Mednick SA, Machon RA, et al: Adult schizophrenia following prenatal exposure to an influenza epidemic. Arch Gen Psychiatry 45:189–192, 1988.

Meehl PE: Specific genetic etiology, psychodynamics, and therapeutic nihilism. In Psychodiagnosis: Selected Papers. New York, WW Norton, 1973, pp 182–199.

Mellor CS: First rank symptoms of schizophrenia. Br J Psychiatry 117:15–23, 1970.

Morihisa JM: Duffy FH, et al: Brain electrical activity mapping (BEAM) in schizophrenic patients. Arch Gen Psychiatry 40:719–728, 1983.

Morstyn R, Duffy FH, et al: Altered topography of EEG spectral content in schizophrenia. Electroencephalogr Clin Neurophysiol 56:263–271, 1983.

Nasrallah HA, McCalley-Whitters M, et al: Cerebral ventricular enlargement in young manic males: A controlled CT study. J Affective Disord 4:15–19, 1982.

Nasrallah HA, Weinberger DR (eds): The Neurology of Schizophrenia: Handbook of Schizophrenia. Amsterdam, Elsevier Science Publishers, 1986.

Nemeroff CB, Bissette G: The role of neuropeptides in schizophrenia. In Neurochemistry and Neuropharmacology of Schizophrenia. Amsterdam, Elsevier Science Publishers, 1987, pp 297–317.

Nimgaonkar VL, Wessely S, et al: Response to drugs in schizophrenia: The influence of family history, obstetric complications and ventricular enlargement. Psychol Med 18:583–592, 1988.

Niwa SI, Hiramatsu KI, et al: Left hemisphere's inability to sustain attention over extended time periods in schizophrenics. Br J Psychiatry 142:477–481, 1983.

O'Callaghan E, Gibson T, et al: Season of birth in schizophrenia: Evidence for confinement of an excess of winter births to patients without a family history of mental disorder. Br J Psychiatry 158:764–769, 1991.

O'Callaghan E, Larkin C, et al: Obstetric complications, the putative familial-sporadic distinction, and tardive dyskinesia in schizophrenia. Br J Psychiatry 157:578–584, 1990.

Offord DR: School performance of adult schizophrenics, their siblings and age mates. Br J Psychiatry 125:12–19, 1974.

Onstad S, Skre I, et al: Subtypes of schizophrenia: Evidence from a twin–family study. Acta Psychiatr Scand 84:203–206, 1991.

Ott J: Analysis of Human Genetic Linkage. Baltimore, Johns Hopkins University Press, 1985.

Parfitt E, Asherson P, et al: A linkage study of the pseudoautosomal region in schizophrenia (abstract). Psychiatr Genet 2(1):92–93, 1991.

Parnas J, Schulsinger F, et al: Perinatal complications and clinical outcome within the schizophrenia spectrum. Br J Psychiatry 140:416, 1982.

Pearlson GD, Garbacz DJ, et al: Symptomatic, familial, perinatal and social correlates of CAT changes in schizophrenics and bipolars. J Nerv Ment Dis 173:42, 1985.

Perry PJ, Alexander B, et al: Psychotropic Drug Handbook. Cincinnati, Harvey Whitney Books, 1981.

Pfohl B, Winokur G: Schizophrenia: Course and outcome. In Schizophrenia as a Brain Disease. New York, Oxford University Press, 1982.

Pope HG, Lipinski JF: Diagnosis in schizophrenia and manic-depressive illness: A reassessment of the specificity of "schizophrenic" symptoms in the light of current research. Arch Gen Psychiatry 35:811–828, 1978.

Raz S, Raz N: Structural brain abnormalities in the major psychoses: A quantitative review of the evidence from computerized imaging. Psychol Bull 108:93–108, 1990.

Reddy R, Mukherjee S, et al: History of obstetric complications, family history, and CT scan findings in schizophrenic patients. Schizophr Res 3:311–314, 1990.

Rieder RO, Mann LS, et al: Computed tomographic scans in patients with schizophrenia, schizoaffective, and bipolar affective disorder. Arch Gen Psychiatry 40:735–739, 1983.

Risch N: Genetic linkage and complex diseases, with special reference to psychiatric disorders. Genet Epidemiol 7:3–7, 1990a.

Risch N: Linkage strategies for genetically complex traits: I. Multilocus models. Am J Hum Genet 46:222–228, 1990b.

Risch N, Baron M: Segregation analysis of schizophrenia and related disorders. Am J Hum Genet 36:1039–1059, 1984.

Robins L: Deviant Children Grown Up. Baltimore, Williams & Wilkins, 1966.

Rosenhan DL: On being sane in insane places. Science 179: 250–258, 1973.

Rosse RB, Schwartz BL, et al: Subtype diagnosis in schizophrenia and its relation to neuropsychological and computerized tomography measures. Biol Psychiatry 30:63–72, 1991.

Ruskin PE, Nyman G: Discontinuation of neuroleptic medication in older, outpatient schizophrenics: A placebo-controlled, double-blind trial. J Nerv Ment Dis 179(4):212–214, 1991.

Safferman A, Lieberman JA, et al: Update on the clinical efficacy and side effects of clozapine. Schizophr Bull 17(2):247–261, 1991.

Schooler NR: Maintenance medication for schizophrenia: Strategies for dose reduction. Schizophr Bull 17(2):311–324, 1991.

Schuckit MA, Winokur G: Alcoholic hallucinosis and schizophrenia: A negative study. Br J Psychiatry 119:549–550, 1971.

Seeman P, Ulpian C, et al: Bimodal distribution of dopamine receptor densities in brains of schizophrenics. Science 225:728–731, 1984.

Seidman LJ: Schizophrenia and brain dysfunction: An integration of recent neurodiagnostic findings. Psychol Bull 94: 195–238, 1983.

Seidman LJ, Cassens G, et al: The neuropsychology of schizophrenia. In Clinical Syndromes in Adult Neuropsychology: The Practitioner's Handbook. Amsterdam, Elsevier Science Publishers, 1992, pp. 381–499.

Sham PC, McGuffin P: A monogenic model of schizophrenia. Behavior Genetics Association, 20th Annual Meeting, Aussois, France, 1990.

Sherrington R, Brynjolfsson J, et al: Localization of a susceptibility locus for schizophrenia on chromosome 5. Nature 336: 164–167, 1988.

Shur E: Season of birth in high and low genetic risk schizophrenics. Br J Psychiatry 140:410–415, 1982.

Simpson J: Mortality studies in schizophrenia. In Nosology, Epidemiology and Genetics of Schizophrenia. Amsterdam, Elsevier Science Publishers, 1988, pp 245–273.

Slater E, Beard AW: The schizophrenia-like psychoses of epilepsy: I. Psychiatric aspects. Br J Psychiatry 109:95–150, 1963.

Slater E, Roth M: Clinical Psychiatry. Baltimore, Williams & Wilkins, 1969.

Snyder S: The dopamine hypothesis of schizophrenia: Focus on the dopamine receptor. Am J Psychiatry 133:197–202, 1976.

Snyder SH: Catecholamines in the brain as mediators of amphetamine psychosis. Arch Gen Psychiatry 27:169–179, 1972.

Spitzer RL, Endicott J, et al: Research diagnostic criteria: Rationale and reliability. Arch Gen Psychiatry 35:773–782, 1978.

St. Clair D, Blackwood D, et al: No linkage of chromosome 5q11–q13 markers to schizophrenia in Scottish families. Nature 339:305–309, 1989.

Stahl SM, Wets K: Indoleamines and schizophrenia. In Neurochemistry and Neuropharmacology of Schizophrenia. Amsterdam, Elsevier Science Publishers, 1987, pp 257–296.

Stephens JH, Astrup C, et al: A comparison of nine systems to diagnose schizophrenia. Psychiatry Res 6:127–143, 1982.

Sternberg DE, VanKammen DP, et al: Schizophrenia: Dopamine beta-hydroxylase activity and treatment response. Science 216(4553):1423–1425, 1982.

Suddath RL, Christison GW, et al: Anatomical abnormalities in the brains of monozygotic twins discordant for schizophrenia. N Engl J Med 322:789–794, 1990.

Torrey EF, Kaufmann CA: Schizophrenia and neuroviruses. In The Neurology of Schizophrenia. Amsterdam, Elsevier Science Publishers, 1986, pp 361–376.

Torrey EF, Rawlings R, et al: Schizophrenic births and viral diseases in two states. Schizophr Res 1:73–77, 1988.

Toru M, Nishikawa T, et al: Dopamine metabolism increases in postmortem schizophrenic basal ganglia. J Neural Transm 54:181–191, 1982.

Tsuang MT: Suicide in schizophrenics, manics, depressives, and surgical controls: A comparison with general population suicide mortality. Arch Gen Psychiatry 35:153–155, 1978.

Tsuang MT, Faraone SV: The Genetics of Mood Disorders. Baltimore, Johns Hopkins University Press, 1990.

Tsuang MT, Loyd DW: Other psychotic disorders. In Psychiatry. Philadelphia, Lippincott, 1985, pp 1–17.

Tsuang MT, Vandermey R: Genes and the Mind: Inheritance of Mental Illness. London, Oxford University Press, 1980.

Tsuang MT, Winokur G: Criteria for subtyping schizophrenia: Clinical differentiation of hebephrenic and paranoid schizophrenia. Arch Gen Psychiatry 31:43–47, 1974.

Tsuang MT, Woolson RF: Mortality in patients with schizophrenia, mania, depression, and surgical conditions. Br J Psychiatry 130:162–166, 1977.

Tsuang MT, Dempsey M, et al: A study of "atypical schizophrenia": Comparison with schizophrenia and affective disorder by sex, age of admission, precipitant, outcome, and family history. Arch Gen Psychiatry 33:1157–1160, 1976.

Tsuang MT, Gilbertson MW, et al: The genetics of schizophrenia: Current knowledge and future directions. Schizophr Res 4:157–171, 1991.

Tsuang MT, Simpson JC, et al: Subtypes of drug abuse with psychosis: Demographic characteristics, clinical features, and family history. Arch Gen Psychiatry 39:141–147, 1982.

Tsuang MT, Winokur G, et al: Morbidity risks of schizophrenia and affective disorders among first-degree relatives of patients with schizophrenia, mania, depression, and surgical conditions. Br J Psychiatry 137:497–504, 1980.

Tsuang MT, Woolson RF, et al: Long-term outcome of major psychoses: I. Schizophrenia and affective disorders compared with psychiatrically symptom-free surgical conditions. Arch Gen Psychiatry 36:1295–1301, 1979.

Tsuang MT, Woolson RF, et al: Premature deaths in schizophrenia and affective disorders: An analysis of survival curves and variables affecting the shortened survival. Arch Gen Psychiatry 37:979–983, 1980.

Tsuang MT, Woolson RF, et al: Stability of psychiatric diagnosis: Schizophrenia and affective disorders followed up over a 30- to 40-year period. Arch Gen Psychiatry 38:535–539, 1981.

Turner SW, Toone BK, et al: Computerised tomographic scan changes in early schizophrenia. Psychol Med 16:219, 1986.

Van Putten T, Marder SR, et al: Neuroleptic plasma levels. Schizophr Bull 17(2):197–216, 1991.

Victor M, Hope JM: The phenomenon of auditory hallucinations in chronic alcoholism: A critical evaluation of the status of alcoholic hallucinosis. J Nerv Ment Dis 126:451–481, 1958.

Vogler GP, Gottesman II, et al: Mixed model segregation analysis of schizophrenia in the Lindelius Swedish pedigrees. Behav Genet 1990, 20:461–472.

Walinder J, Skott A, et al: Potentiation by metyrosine of thioridazine effects in chronic schizophrenics: A long-term trial using double-blind crossover technique. Arch Gen Psychiatry 33(4):501–505, 1976.

Weinberger DR: CAT scan findings in schizophrenia: Speculation on the meaning of it all. J Psychiatr Res 18:477–490, 1984.

Weinberger DR, Berman KF: Speculation on the meaning of cerebral metabolic hypofrontality in schizophrenia. Schizophr Bull 14:157–168, 1988.

Weinberger DR, Wyatt RJ: Brain morphology in schizophrenia: In vivo studies. In Schizophrenia as a Brain Disease. New York, Oxford University Press, 1982.

Weinberger DR, Llewellyn BB, et al: Cerebral ventricular enlargement in chronic schizophrenia: An association with poor response to treatment. Arch Gen Psychiatry 37:11–13, 1980.

Weinberger DR, Wagner RI, et al: Neuropathological studies of schizophrenia: A selective review. Schizophr Bull 9: 193–212, 1983.

Wing JK: The management of schizophrenia. In Schizophrenia: Towards a New Synthesis. New York, Grune & Stratton, 1978a.

Wing JK: Reasoning About Madness. London, Oxford University Press, 1978b.

Wing JK: Social influences on the course of schizophrenia. In The Nature of Schizophrenia: New Approaches to Research and Treatment. New York, Wiley, 1978c.

Winokur G: Delusional disorder (paranoia). Compr Psychiatry 18:511–521, 1977.

Wise CD, Stein L: Dopamine-beta-hydroxylase deficits in the brains of schizophrenic patients. Science 181(97):344–347, 1973.

Woerner MG, Pollack M, et al: Birthweight and length in schizophrenics, personality disorders and their siblings. Br J Psychiatry 118:461, 1971.

Wong DF: Elevated dopamine receptors in psychosis. Annual Meeting of the American Psychiatric Association, New York, 1990.

Wong HN, Tune LE, et al: Positron emission tomography reveals elevated D_2 dopamine receptors in drug-naive schizophrenics. Science 234:1558–1563, 1986.

World Health Organization: The International Pilot Study of Schizophrenia. Geneva, World Health Organization, 1973.

Wright EC: The presentation of mental illness in mentally retarded adults. Br J Psychiatry 141:496–502, 1982.

Wyatt RJ: Biochemistry and schizophrenia: IV. The neuroleptics—Their mechanism of action: A review of the biochemical literature. Psychopharmacol Bull 12:5–50, 1976.

Wyatt RJ: The dopamine hypothesis: variations on a theme. In Research in the Schizophrenic Disorders: The Stanley R. Dean Award lectures. Jamaica, NY, Spectrum, 1985, pp 225–247.

Wyatt RJ, Erdelyi E, et al: Difficulties in comparing catecholamine-related enzymes from the brains of schizophrenics and controls. Biol Psychiatry 13(3):317–334, 1978.

Wyatt RJ, Alexander RC, et al: Schizophrenia, just the facts: What do we know, how well do we know it? Schizophr Res 1:3–18, 1988.

Wyatt RJ, Potkin SG, et al: The schizophrenia syndrome: Examples of biological tools for subclassification. J Nerv Ment Dis 169:100–112, 1981.

Zec RF, Weinberger DR: Relationship between CT scan findings and neuropsychological performance in chronic schizophrenia. Psychiatr Clin North Am 9:49–61, 1986.

CHAPTER 7

Schizoaffective and Schizophreniform Disorders

WILLIAM CORYELL

DEFINITION

Ambiguous terminology has impeded the accumulation of knowledge in psychiatry. Particularly affected have been efforts to clarify the boundary between schizophrenia and affective disorders. The number of terms proposed to label such patients reflects the failure of any one definition to meet with wide acceptance. Moreover, differing definitions have attached to certain of these terms, definitions that, until recently, were purely descriptive; they provided no clear rules for inclusion and exclusion and therefore did not lend themselves to use by other researchers. The advent of operational diagnostic systems 20 years ago remedied this situation somewhat, and for the first time, researchers have attempted to replicate one another using the same definitions.

Nevertheless, confusion surrounding the term *schizoaffective disorder* persists, owing in part to the conceptual difficulties inherent in any intermediate or boundary category and in part to a series of profound shifts in term's definition. The Research Diagnostic Criteria (RDC) (Spitzer et al., 1976) provided the first definition that was both widely used and operational. These relatively inclusive criteria differed according to whether a manic or depressive syndrome was present but, in essence, required a full affective syndrome accompanied either by schneiderian first-rank symptoms or by history of mood-incongruent psychotic features ''in the absence of'' or ''to the relative exclusion of'' affective symptoms. The RDC definitions have been used in more studies of schizoaffective disorder than any other single, operational definition. Yet they were supplanted, at least in the official American nomenclature, by the DSM-III definition. In contrast to the RDC, the DSM-III assigned this term to a residual category for those who did not meet criteria for

schizophrenia or affective disorder but who appeared to have features of both. Moreover, the boundaries for major affective disorders were expanded so that many patients with RDC schizoaffective disorder met criteria in the DSM-III for major depression or mania with mood-incongruent psychotic features (Coryell et al., 1985). The DSM-IIIR reoperationalized the term and applied it only to patients who had had delusions or hallucinations without ''prominent mood symptoms'' for at least 2 weeks in the index episode. Very little work has appeared to characterize either the DSM-III or the DSM-IIIR definition of schizoaffective disorder, yet the deliberations published at the time of this writing (American Psychiatric Association, 1991) promise that DSM-IV will again substantially redefine *schizoaffective disorder*.

The circumstances recommend a generic use of the term *schizoaffective disorder* in any broad overview of the topic. Thus the following will apply the term to any condition in which there is a coincidence of schizophrenic and affective symptoms or in which there is the occurrence of an affective syndrome at one point and a schizophrenic syndrome at another. At the same time, the full interpretation of any particular study requires attention to the definition of schizoaffective disorder used in that study.

ETIOLOGY

Many demonstrable organic insults can produce symptoms suggesting schizoaffective disorder. Identification of a cause, however, precludes the diagnosis, and in DSM-IIIR, the diagnosis becomes one of an organic delusional syndrome, organic hallucinosis, or an organic mood syndrome. The etiology of schizoaffective disorder is, by definition, unknown.

The question then becomes, does schizoaffective disorder share its unknown etiology with schizophrenia, with affective disorder, with both, or with neither? Or does schizoaffective disorder simply label a genotypically mixed group made up partly of affective disorder patients and partly of schizophrenic patients? Because both schizophrenia and affective disorder are heritable, family studies offer one approach to weighing these alternatives. The relevant hypotheses can be tested in the following ways: (1) if schizoaffective disorder is simply a variant of affective disorder (Clayton et al., 1968; Pope et al., 1980), then schizoaffective probands should have no more familial loading for schizophrenia than do affective disorder probands; (2) if schizoaffective probands have simply a variant of schizophrenia, as implied in the formerly used DSM-II (American Psychiatric Association, 1968), their families should contain no more affective disorder than the families of schizophrenic probands; (3) if schizophrenia, schizoaffective disorder, and affective disorder all share a common etiology and form a spectrum, patients in any of these three categories should have relatives at increased risk for disorders in the other two categories; and (4) if schizoaffective disorder is a separate disorder, the first and second predictions listed above should obtain and the families of schizoaffective probands should be loaded for schizoaffective disorder, provided this condition is, likewise, familial.

Table 7-1 summarizes the informative studies published in English over the past 20 years. Because schizophrenia-like symptoms may have different implications when they coexist with depressive syndromes than when they coexist with manic ones (Clayton, 1982), this review summarizes studies in three groups: those which isolated schizoaffective manics, those which isolated schizoaffective depressives, and those which did neither. The intent of this display is to reveal overall patterns in group relationships. Many pairwise comparisons were statistically significant, but this information was omitted because statistical significance depends heavily on sample sizes and these varied greatly across studies. For studies using DSM-III and DSM-IIIR systems, the schizoaffective proband group is comprised of patients who met the corresponding criteria for major depression or mania with mood-incongruent psychotic features or, more rarely, for schizoaffective disorder. The affective disorder proband groups are comprised of those with affective disorder with or without mood-congruent psychotic features.

Those studies which did not separate schizoaffective manic patients from schizoaffective depressed patients consistently failed to support the first hypothesis. In seven of seven studies, relatives of schizoaffective probands were more likely to have schizophrenia than were relatives of affective disorder probands. The same was true in six of the seven studies that considered schizoaffective depression apart. Earlier studies of schizoaffective mania failed to follow this trend (Abrams and Taylor, 1976; Pope et al., 1980; Rosenthal et al., 1980), but more recent studies (Gershon et al., 1988; Bocchetta et al., 1990) show patterns more consistent with those found in studies of schizoaffective depression.

Although fewer studies included schizophrenia cohorts for a comparison, they are consistent in finding higher rates of affective disorder in the families of schizoaffective probands than in the families of schizophrenics. Thus the second of the hypotheses—that schizoaffective disorder is altogether a variant of schizophrenia—can be rejected.

The consistency with which schizophrenia was overrepresented in the families of schizophrenia probands, as well as the regular predominance of affective disorder in the families of affective disorder probands, argues against a spectrum hypothesis. Moreover, those few studies which have included normal control probands have generally shown no increase in affective disorder within families of schizophrenic probands (Kendler et al., 1985; Coryell and Zimmerman, 1988; Maj et al., 1991) nor any increase in schizophrenia within the families of affective disorder probands (Coryell and Zimmerman, 1988; Maj et al., 1991).

EDITORS' COMMENT

In a 30- to 40-year follow-up study and a blind psychiatric evaluation of relatives of schizophrenics, manics, unipolar depressives, and controls, the morbid risk for schizophrenia in first-degree relatives was 3.2 percent for schizophrenic probands, 1.0 percent for manic probands, 0.9 percent for depressive probands, and 0.6 percent for controls. All the relatives were personally interviewed. The increase in the relatives of schizophrenic probands was significantly higher than in any of the other groups (Tsuang M, et al, *Br. J. Psychiatry* 137:497–504, 1980).

Attempts to address the fourth hypothesis—that there is a "third psychosis"—presents special problems. Most relatives are, by necessity, diagnosed in retrospect, particularly if their lifetime diagnosis involves an episodic condition. Although past depressive episodes can be reliably assessed (Andreasen et al., 1981), the existence and nature of psychotic symptoms apparently cannot (Orvaschel et al., 1982; Rosenthal et al., 1979). Unless a researcher evaluates the relative during a psychotic episode, or unless records taken during that episode are available, the distinction between mood-congruent and mood-incongruent psychotic features, and thus the precise diagnosis, will be elusive. Indeed, the eight studies that made this diagnosis in relatives yielded mixed results (see Table 7-1).

Other approaches to familial psychopathology may be more germane to this fourth hypothesis. Cohen et al. (1972) described a large series of

TABLE 7-1. *Rates of Illness Among Relatives of Probands with Schizoaffective, Mood-Incongruent, or Atypical Psychoses: Comparisons to Probands with Affective Disorder or Schizophrenia*

	Proband diagnosis		
	Affective disorder	Schizoaffective or equivalent	Schizophrenia
Schizoaffective probands not divided by polarity			
Reference (definition of schizoaffective disorder used in study)			
Angst J, 1973 (author's def.)			
No. of probands	254	73	—
MR% schizophrenia*	1.4	5.9	
MR% affective disorder	13.3	7.1	
MR% schizoaffective	0.7	3.8	
Tsuang et al., 1976 (author's def.)			
No. of probands	325	85	200
% FH + for schizophrenia†	0.5	1.3	1.3
% FH + for affective disorder	8.3	7.6	3.1
Suslak et al., 1976 (author's def.)			
No. of probands	37	10	—
MR% schizophrenia	0.9	4.0	
MR% affective disorder	12.5	6.5	
Tsuang et al., 1977 (author's def.)			
No. of probands	289	52	183
MR% schizophrenia	0.5	0.9	1.3
MR% affective disorder	8.3	11.8	3.2
Mendlewicz et al., 1980 (author's def.)			
No. of probands	110	55	55
MR% schizophrenia	2.5	10.8	16.9
MR% affective disorder	34.0	34.6	8.6
Scharfetter, 1981 (author's def.)			
No. of probands	89	40	102
MR% schizophrenia	3.3	13.5	~7.4
MR% affective disorder	11.4	4.4	~1.0
MR% schizoaffective	3.4	2.5	—
Baron et al., 1982 (RDC)			
No. of probands	85	50	50
MR% schizophrenia	0.3	2.2	7.9
MR% affective disorder	25.2	18.9	5.1
Schizoaffective mania vs. mania (vs. schizophrenia)			
Abrams and Taylor, 1976 (RDC)			
No. of probands	78	10	—
% FH + for schizophrenia	0	0	—
% FH + for affective disorder	14.1	13.9	—
Pope et al., 1980 (RDC)			
No. of probands	34	52	41
% FH + for schizophrenia	0	0	9.8
% FH + for affective disorder	32.4	40.4	9.8
Rosenthal et al., 1980 (RDC)			
No. of probands	28	25	—
MR% schizophrenia	0	0	—
MR% affective disorder	24.8	24.6	—
Gershon et al., 1988 (RDC)			
No. of probands	130	12	24
MR% schizophrenia	0.3	3.3	3.1
MR% affective disorder	22.1	16.6	16.0
MR% schizoaffective	5.0	1.7	0.6
Bocchetta et al., 1990 (RDC)			
No. of probands	65	56	—
MR% schizophrenia	0.20	0.80	—
MR% affective disorder	9.1	4.2	—
MR% schizoaffective	1.3	3.4	—
Schizoaffective depression vs. depression (vs. schizophrenia)			
Coryell et al., 1982 (DSM-III)			
No. of probands	221	95	235
MR% schizophrenia	0.5	1.6	2.8
MR% affective disorder	13.0	8.2	5.8
Abrams and Taylor, 1983 (DSM-III)			
No. of probands	14	17	31
MR% schizophrenia	0	0	1.6
MR% affective disorder	12.9	19.3	6.8

Table continued on following page

TABLE 7-1. *Rates of Illness Among Relatives of Probands with Schizoaffective, Mood-Incongruent, or Atypical Psychoses: Comparisons to Probands with Affective Disorder or Schizophrenia Continued*

	Proband diagnosis		
	Affective disorder	Schizoaffective or equivalent	Schizophrenia
Endicott et al., 1986 (RDC)			
No. of probands	275	23	—
MR% schizophrenia	0	3.0	—
MR% affective disorder	35.9	25.2	—
MR% schizoaffective	0.3	1.0	—
Gershon et al., 1988 (RDC)			
No. of probands	31	12	24
MR% schizophrenia	0	1.7	3.1
MR% affective disorder	19.6	19.5	16.0
MR% schizoaffective	0.7	3.4	0.6
Coryell and Zimmerman, 1988 (RDC)			
No. of probands	29	47	21
MR% schizophrenia	0	2.3	1.4
MR% affective disorder	27.5	24.7	13.1
MR% schizoaffective	1.0	2.5	0
Bochetta et al., 1990 (RDC)			
No. of probands	29	26	—
MR% schizophrenia	0	0.5	—
MR% affective disorder	3.3	3.7	—
MR% schizoaffective	0.4	0.5	—
Maj et al, 1991 (DSM-III-R)			
No. of probands	46	43	28
MR% schizophrenia	0.9	6.1	8.8
MR% affective disorder	15.0	3.4	1.7

*Morbid risk % $= \dfrac{\text{no. of relatives with a disorder}}{\text{no. of relatives at risk for that disorder}}$

[†]% Family history positive $= \dfrac{\text{no. of probands with a family history of a disorder}}{\text{total no. of probands}}$

monozygotic twin pairs and found a higher concordance rate for schizoaffective disorder than for manic depressive disorder or schizophrenia. Moreover, among pairs concordant for any psychosis, there was 100 percent concordance for this specific diagnosis. This would argue powerfully for a third psychosis, except that the medical records of each twin were assessed to gather information about cotwins, and this allowed substantial rater bias. Although there are no blindly rated twin studies with which to gauge this effect, Tsuang (1975) did describe a series of blindly diagnosed sibling pairs, and the results led to very different conclusions. Of the 35 pairs concordant for any psychosis, only 4 (11.4 percent) were concordant for schizoaffective disorder. Of 17 siblings with schizoaffective disorder, 5 (29.4 percent) had a cosibling with schizophrenia, 8 (47.1 percent) had a cosibling with affective disorder, and only 4 (23.5 percent) had a cosibling with schizoaffective disorder. Moreover, those schizoaffective siblings with affective disorder cosiblings were significantly older at onset than were the schizoaffective siblings with schizophrenic cosiblings. These findings are quite consistent with a final hypothesis, that some schizoaffective patients are genotypically schizophrenic while others are genotypes for affective disorder.

Indeed, the morbid risk patterns common to almost all family studies (see Table 7-1) clearly favor this hypothesis over the others. It is essentially a "heterogeneity" or "diagnostic uncertainty" hypothesis. Patients with this label may, for practical purposes, be viewed in terms of the likelihood that they suffer from either schizophrenia or affective disorder. There are undoubtedly also patients with this label who are suffering from both illnesses. The prevalence figures for psychotic affective disorder and for schizophrenia indicate that such coincidences are rare and would account for only a small proportion of patients with schizoaffective disorder. This rarity, and the lack of any clear means with which to identify such a subgroup, gives its existence very little practical significance.

On the other hand, the likelihood that most schizoaffective patients have schizophrenia or affective disorder gives considerable importance to subdivisions within schizoaffective disorder. Within the affective disorders, the bipolar/unipolar distinction is well supported by family and outcome studies and is widely accepted. Its application to a group that is substantially comprised of individuals with affective disorder thus seems reasonable. Another intuitively compelling subdivision is based on the relative predominance of schizophrenic or affective features. In the RDC, schizoaffective patients who exhibit mood-incongruent psychotic features for at least 1 week without manic or depressive symptoms or who have premorbid features suggesting schizophrenia have the "mainly schizophrenic" subtype. Two family studies clearly support this distinction (Table 7-2).

EDITORS' COMMENT

A third study is also in favor of the large proportion of the schizoaffective manics with an acute onset having a relationship to ordinary affective disorder (Winokur G, et al, *Schizoaffective Psychoses*, edited by Marneros and Tsuang. Heidelberg, Springer-Verlag, 1986). A group of 66 schizoaffective manics who had either mood-incongruent delusions and hallucinations or catatonic symptoms were compared with bipolar patients who lacked these symptoms. Family history for affective disorder in primary relatives was 12 and 11 percent, respectively. In this study, there was an increase in schizophrenia when parents, grandparents, and third-degree relatives were all taken into account. There were 2.1 percent of such relatives having schizophrenia in the schizoaffective bipolar patients as opposed to 0.7 percent in the ordinary bipolar patients. This would be consistent with a small amount of misdiagnosis in the probands, a few of them having schizophrenia rather than bipolar disorder as a true diagnosis. Of importance is the fact that there were no course or follow-up differences between the schizoaffective bipolar and other bipolar patients in this study.

The DSM-IIIR concept of schizoaffective disorder closely resembles the RDC mainly schizophrenic subtype in that it requires a period of delusions or hallucinations without prominent mood symptoms. DSM-IIIR major affective disorder with mood-incongruent psychotic features, in turn, closely approximates the RDC mainly affective subtype. Not surprisingly, the only family study of DSM-IIIR schizoaffective disorder available as of this writing (Maj et al., 1991) replicates the patterns displayed in Table 7-2. The relatives of schizoaffective probands had twice the rate of schizophrenia as the relatives of probands with major depression and mood-incongruent psychotic features (morbid risk was 8.7 and 3.8 percent, respectively) and one-half the rate of major affective disorders (morbid risk was 2.4 and 6.5 percent, respectively). Notably, both Kendler et al. (1986) and Maj et al. (1991)

TABLE 7-2. *Rates of Illness Among Relatives of Probands with RDC Schizoaffective Disorder Divided by Subtype*

	Proband diagnosis	
	Mainly schizophrenic	Mainly affective or other
Baron et al., 1982		
No. of probands	28	22
MR% schizophrenia	4.1	0
MR% affective disorder	10.9	28.1
Kendler et al., 1986		
No. of probands	19	28
MR% schizophrenia	8.2	3.8
MR% affective disorder	7.3	14.5

provided values for normal controls. In comparison with those controls, RDC mainly schizophrenic probands (Kendler et al., 1986) and DSM-IIIR schizoaffective probands (Maj et al., 1991) had no increase in familial loading for affective disorder. Pending further replications of these patterns, we may conclude that the large majority of patients who meet these narrow definitions of schizoaffective disorder in fact have schizophrenia. Groups with RDC mainly affective schizoaffective disorder or with DSM-IIIR major depression and mood-incongruent psychotic features apparently retain substantial heterogeneity; familial rates of schizophrenia were substantially higher in both studies (Kendler et al., 1986; Maj et al., 1991), though not significantly so, than the rates for normal controls.

EPIDEMIOLOGY

Most community surveys have not described rates of schizoaffective disorder. Given the many definitions in use and the low concordance across these definitions (Brockington and Leff, 1979), such rates would have been widely disparate. The National Institute of Mental Health (NIMH) epidemiologic catchment program (Regier et al., 1984) encompassed a very broad base, but published results have used DSM-III, and as noted above, this system leaves schizoaffective disorder as a residual nonoperationalized category. Two community surveys have appeared using the RDC. Weissman and Myers (1978) found a 0.4 percent lifetime prevalence for RDC schizoaffective disorder, whereas Vernon and Roberts (1982) found 0.8 percent. These figures were based on only three and four cases, respectively, however, and none of these were ill when interviewed.

Brockington and Leff (1979) found 10 patients who met at least three of eight definitions for schizoaffective disorder from approximately 222 consecutive admissions; 6 (2.7 percent) met RDC criteria for schizoaffective disorder (1 manic and 5 depressed). These figures are similar to those derived from all consecutive admissions seen over a several-year period; of 388 patients, 11 (2.8 percent) met RDC criteria for schizoaffective disorder (Coryell, unpublished data). In a subsequent series of 97 consecutively admitted nonmanic psychotics, 48.4 percent had RDC schizoaffective disorder, depressed type (Coryell and Zimmerman, 1986). In the same series, only 21 met RDC criteria for schizophrenia. Thus, while conditions meeting one or more definitions for schizoaffective disorder may be rare in the community, they comprise a large portion of psychotic patients who come to treatment.

Some have used prevalence data to address an additional epidemiologic hypothesis—that schizoaffective disorder represents the chance coexistence of schizophrenia and affective disorder. According to Brockington and Leff (1979), this chance coexistence should occur only once in a year in Great Britain, yet they found 10 in 1 year in only three hospitals.

CLINICAL PICTURE

A description of the clinical picture seen in schizoaffective disorder is necessarily circular. Most definitions of schizoaffective disorder depend entirely on the clinical picture, and since these definitions vary so markedly (Brockington and Leff, 1979), the associated clinical picture also will vary depending on the label. By definition, then, patients with RDC schizoaffective disorder, with DSM-III or DSM-IIIR affective disorder and mood-incongruent psychotic features, or with DSM-IIIR schizoaffective disorder, can exhibit in cross section any symptom characteristic of schizophrenia and any symptom characteristic of affective disorder. Such a patient may report low mood, anorexia, insomnia, fatigue, and thoughts of suicide, as well as thought broadcasting, delusions of passivity, and hallucinations in any sphere. He or she may exhibit euphoria, hyperactivity, recklessness, and grandiosity, as well as blunted affect, bizarre behavior, catatonia, and loose associations.

Also by definition, schizoaffective disorder differs from, or is atypical of, affective disorder because of the presence of schizophrenic features. In turn, the presence of affective symptoms distinguishes schizoaffective disorder from schizophrenia.

EDITORS' COMMENT

Unfortunately, follow-up studies describing the course of schizophrenics (Guze S et al., *Arch Gen Psychiatry* 40: 1273–1276, 1983) indicated that more than 50 percent have superimposed episodes of major depression (also called *secondary depression*).

Phenomenologic differences may extend further, however. In one study, patients with RDC schizophrenia had delusions that were significantly more bizarre than those reported by schizoaffective patients. Schizophrenic patients also were more likely to exhibit loosening of associations and a blunted or inappropriate affect (Coryell and Zimmerman, 1986). Moreover, when compared with patients with psychotic major depression, schizoaffective patients reported greater severity of 12 depressive symptoms, among which the endogenous rather than the nonendogenous depressive symptoms were overrepresented. This pattern emerged in another sample as well (Coryell et al., 1985). Thus, broadly defined, *schizoaffective depression* designates patients who, on average, have depressive syndromes that are less typical than those of patients with psychotic depression and schizophrenic symptoms that are less typical than those of schizophrenic patients. These patterns also support a "heterogeneity" hypothesis.

Because these patients suffer from psychosis, an associated loss of insight, and often, severe psychomotor disturbance, many are poor historians. This feature deserves special emphasis. At the time of admission, affective symptoms may be altogether overshadowed by the patient's delusional preoccupation, hallucinations, or bizarre behavior. Indeed, at this point such patients often deny affective symptoms that they later recall and that other informants describe when questioned carefully. The distinction between affective, schizoaffective, and schizophrenic psychosis, therefore, must not depend on the patient interview alone. In all cases the clinician must seek knowledgeable informants to learn whether affective symptoms preceded the psychotic ones. Serial interviews of the patient are also more useful than is generally appreciated (Dysken et al., 1979).

CLINICAL COURSE

The prognosis for schizoaffective disorder appears to be worse than that for affective disorder (Table 7-3), although a small minority of studies have yielded results to the contrary.

EDITORS' COMMENT

In a large study of unipolar depressives and manics divided into three groups—those nonpsychotic, those with congruent psychotic symptoms, and those with incongruent psychotic symptoms—these acute-onset unipolar patients appear very similar as regards marked improvement at discharge, marked improvement with electroconvulsive therapy (ECT), lack of relapse in follow-up of 2 years, and suicide attempts and completed suicides in follow-up. Similar findings were true of the acute-onset manics. Thus the definition of schizoaffective disorder in the RDC, which depends on the presence of mood-incongruent symptomatology, did not alter the course from the more classically diagnosed depressives or manics (Winokur et al., *Affective and Schizoaffective Disorders*, edited by Marneros and Tsuang. Heidelberg, Springer-Verlag, 1990). Acute onset in schizoaffectives separates those related to the affective disorders from those related to schizophrenia.

At one point, the schizoaffective designation seemed prognostically less important for manic syndromes than for depressive syndromes, but studies done in the past 5 years have not supported this conclusion. Proportions with good outcomes vary widely across studies, and this reflects such methodologic particulars as the length of follow-up and the definitions of good outcome. The prognostic differences between schizoaffective and affective disorders also vary and appear to reflect important differences in how schizoaffective disorder was defined. Specifically, schizoaffective patients so identified because of the persistence of schizophrenia-like symptoms between affective episodes may constitute a different group from those defined solely by

TABLE 7-3. *Course of Illness Among Patients with Schizoaffective, Mood-Incongruent, or Atypical Psychoses: Comparisons to Probands with Affective Disorder or Schizophrenia*

	Affective disorder	Schizoaffective or equivalent	Schizophrenia
Schizoaffective disorder not divided by polarity			
Reference (definition of schizoaffective disorder used in study)			
Tsuang et al., 1976 (author's def.)			
No. of patients	325	85	200
% recovered	58	44	8
Angst, 1980 (author's def.)			
No. of patients	254	150	—
% with "full remission"	39	27	—
Himmelhoch et al., 1981 (author's def.)			
No. of patients	409	34	—
"Improved within 2 months"	39.7	5.9	—
Moller et al., 1988 (ICD)			
No. of patients	36	27	34
% with "favorable outcome"	84	78	65
Grossman et al., 1991 (RDC)			
No. of patients	40	41	20
% with outcomes better than			
"very poor"	85	57	45
Schizoaffective mania vs. mania (vs. schizophrenia)			
Brockington, Wainwright, and Kendell, 1980b (author's def.)			
No. of patients	66	30	53
% recovered	94	77	34.0
Abrams and Taylor, 1976 (RDC)			
No. of patients	78	10	—
Mean treatment response (4 = full remission)	3.2	3.5	—
Pope et al., 1980 (RDC)			
No. of patients	18	35	27
% with "marked improvement" after treatment	79	73	7.3
% with "excellent" globally assessed outcome	44	26	0
Rosenthal et al., 1980 (RDC)			
No. of patients	28	25	—
Probability of remaining well at 16 weeks	70	86	—
van Praag and Nijo, 1984 (RDC)			
No. of patients	21	10	19
% with "good" treatment responses after 6 weeks	62	40	5
Grossman et al., 1984 (RDC)			
No. of patients	33	15	47
% with "good" overall functioning	33	13	9
Maj, 1985 (RDC)			
No. of patients	16	17	—
Mean score (SD) on Strauss-Carpenter Outcome Scale (16 = optimal score)	13.7 (2.6)	12.6 (1.7)	—
Coryell et al., 1990b (RDC)			
No. of patients	56	14	—
% recovered from index episode	95	79	—
Marneros et al. 1990a (author's def.)			
No. of patients	30	56	
% with "no difficulties"	66.7	46.4	
Schizoaffective depression vs. depression (vs. schizophrenia)			
Brockington, Kendell, and Wainwright, 1980a (author's def.)			
No. of patients	66	75	53
% recovered	94.0	69.3	34.0
Coryell et al., 1982 (DSM-III)			
No. of patients	149	43	171
% recovered during follow-up	57.1	32.6	7.0

Table continued on following page

TABLE 7-3.   *Course of Illness Among Patients with Schizoaffective, Mood-Incongruent, or Atypical Psychoses: Comparisons to Probands with Affective Disorder or Schizophrenia Continued*

	Affective disorder	Schizoaffective or equivalent	Schizophrenia
Abrams et al., 1983 (DSM-III)			
No. of patients	29	12	19
% with "good" treatment			
van Praag and Nijo, 1984 (RDC)			
No. of patients	29	12	19
% with "good" treatment response			
after 6 weeks	69.0	50.0	5.3
Grossman et al., 1984 (RDC)			
No. of patients	330	24	—
% with "good" overall			
functioning	38	8	9
Maj, 1985 (RDC)			
No. of patients	23	19	
Mean score (SD) on Strauss-			
Carpenter Outcome Scale			
(16 = optimal score)	13.3 (2.5)	11.6 (3.6)	
Coryell and Zimmerman, 1986 (RDC)			
No. of patients	29	46	20
% recovered during follow-up	58.6	39.1	10.0
Opjordsmoen, 1989 (DSM-III)			
No. of patients	50	33	94
% "healthy" at follow-up	66	42	10
Coryell et al., 1990a (RDC)			
No. of patients	73	30	
% recovered from			
index episode	89	73	
Marneros et al., 1990b (author's def.)			
No. of patients	76	45	
% with "no difficulties			
at follow-up"	63.2	55.6	

the presence of first-rank symptoms in the midst of an affective syndrome. The studies finding the largest outcome differences between affective disorder and schizoaffective disorder were those which defined the latter disorder by the persistence of schizophrenia-like symptoms between affective episodes (Angst et al., 1970; Himmelhoch et al., 1981; Johnson, 1970; Zall and Therman, 1968). In contrast, one of the few studies finding a superior outcome for schizoaffective disorder explicitly excluded subjects with psychotic symptoms persisting between episodes (Rosenthal et al., 1980).

Because lithium is generally thought to be effective in mania and much less so in schizophrenia, acute and prophylactic response to this drug affords another view of schizoaffective disorder. With one exception, lithium studies describing five or more schizoaffective patients report poorer responses in that group than in more typically manic groups (Table 7-4). Subdivisions within schizoaffective groups are probably very meaningful to response prediction, but few studies have considered them. Maj (1988) did find that the RDC subtyping strongly predicted prophylactic response to lithium. Those with the mainly affective subtype, but not those with the mainly schizophrenic subtype, showed a significant reduction in number of episodes with lithium therapy.

Such comparisons serve to summarize the literature, but their simplicity can be misleading, since there are many shades of "response," "improved," and "recovered." In light of the most tenable hypothesis on etiology, some schizoaffective patients should have a course typical of psychotic affective disorder; the psychosis may be profound, but eventual recovery is complete. Others may display a waxing and waning of symptoms, which might be perceived initially as recovery and relapse but which eventually evolve into chronicity and avolition characteristic of narrowly defined schizophrenia. Patients, as well as families and physicians, need to know which course to expect.

Recent findings from the National Institute of Mental Health Collaborative Program on the Psychobiology of Depression bear directly on this issue (Coryell et al., 1990a, 1990b). These analyses sought to predict the presence or absence of a persistent psychosis 5 years in the future for patients who presented with psychotic affective or schizoaffective disorders. Overall, such outcomes emerged in 24 individuals, or 14 percent of the sample. For patients who were depressed at intake, only a history of mood-incongruent psychotic features to the relative exclusion of depressive symptoms significantly and independently predicted persistent psychosis (Coryell et al., 1990a). Among those who were

TABLE 7-4. *Outcome with Lithium Therapy in Patients with Schizoaffective (or Equivalent) Mania: Comparisons to Patients with Manic Disorder*

	Manic disorder	Schizoaffective mania
Reference (definition of schizoaffective disorder used in study)		
Schou et al., 1954 (author's def.)		
No. of patients	30	8
% with "+ effect" acutely or prophylactically	40.0	25.0
Baastrup and Schou, 1967 (author's def.)		
No. of patients	51	15
% reduction of no. of episodes with lithium	95.2	71.3
Zall et al., 1968 (author's def.)		
No. of patients	33	10
% with "complete recovery"	78.8	10.0
Angst et al., 1970 (WHO criteria)		
No. of patients	114	72
% with improvement in frequency of episodes with lithium	67	49
Aranoff and Epstein, 1970 (author's def.)		
No. of patients	7	6
% with "unequivocal" acute response	71.4	33.3
Johnson, 1970 (author's def.)		
No. of patients	19	11
% in "remission"	79.0	9.1
Prien et al., 1974 (author's def.)		
No. of patients	86	5
% without episodes during 1 yr of prophylaxis	60.5	40.0
Pope et al., 1980 (RDC)		
No. of patients	13	20
% with "marked" improvement	92.3	80.0
Rosenthal et al., 1980 (RDC)		
No. of patients	27	15
Probability of remaining well after 16 wk	0.70	0.86

manic at intake, significant and independent predictors consisted of a history of any formal thought disorder in the absence of prominent manic symptoms, loosening of associations at intake, and greater global severity at intake. When manic and depressed patients were pooled (Coryell et al., 1990b), a stepwise regression analysis revealed the following independent predictors of a sustained psychotic outcome (in order of robustness): longer duration of index episode, history of psychotic features without (or to the exclusion of) affective symptoms, poor adolescent friendship patterns, never married, and never manic. Very few other studies have attempted to predict schizophrenia-like outcomes in such a sample. The most important of these yielded very similar results, however. Brockington et al. (1980a) selected as the single most valuable predictor of such an outcome "the presence of schizophrenic symptoms in the absence of affective symptoms."

LABORATORY FINDINGS

As yet there are no generally accepted roles for laboratory tests in the clinical distinction between schizophrenia and depression, and the laboratory, therefore, has little to offer in subdividing schizoaffective disorders. Some tests may eventually prove useful in this way, however. Among these are the thyroid-releasing hormone stimulation test (Kirkegaard et al., 1978) and the dexamethasone suppression test (DST) (Carroll et al., 1981). So far the latter shows the most promise as a diagnostic aid and has received by far the most attention. As used in psychiatry, it is modification of a test long used to screen for Cushing's disease. One milligram of dexamethasone is given at 11:00 P.M., and blood samples for cortisol assay are drawn the next day at 8:00 A.M., 4:00 P.M., and 11:00 P.M. Postdexamethasone cortisol values over 4 or 5 μg/dl generally indicate an abnormal resistance of the hypothalamic-pituitary-adrenal axis to suppression by exogenous steroid (nonsuppression).

Early work with this test suggested a high level of specificity for psychotic depression, and it appeared to hold promise as a clinically useful diagnostic tool. Subsequent work has shown that nonsuppression rates among schizophrenics, while consistently lower than those for patients with psychotic depression, are nevertheless higher than those for normal controls (Sharma et al., 1988). It now appears that nonsuppression among individuals with narrowly defined schizophrenia has a different meaning from nonsuppression among patients with psychotic depression or mania. In particular, nonsuppression among schizophrenic patients appears to be associated with relatively prominent negative features (Newcomer et al., 1991; Altamura et al., 1989; Saffer et al., 1985; Tanden et al., 1991). Nonsuppression may nevertheless have prognostic significance among other patients with depression and psychotic features, i.e., those with psychotic major depression or schizoaffective depression. Two studies (Coryell and Zimmerman, 1989; Coryell and Tsuang, 1992) have found that among such patients, nonsuppressors are substantially more likely to have recovered at the end of follow-up (1 and 8 years, respectively). However, the DST was not predictive in two other follow-up studies of schizoaffective disorder (Maj et al., 1987; Tandon et al., 1989). Thus, although it holds promise, the DST does not yet qualify as a prognostic tool for schizo-affective patients.

DIFFERENTIAL DIAGNOSIS

As with other conditions seen by psychiatrists, the differential diagnosis when affective and psychotic symptoms coexist should begin with the distinction between conditions that arise from demonstrable lesions (organic illness) and those which do not (functional illness). Depressive, manic, and schizo-phrenic syndromes can be produced by a variety of identifiable insults, and the differential diagnosis for each of these conditions is provided in more detail in the corresponding chapters. With those other possi-bilities in mind, there are several general features that should increase the suspicion that psychiatric symptoms are arising from an organic condition. "Depression" with only two or three of the possible eight criteria symptoms should raise such suspi-cions, as should the appearance of affective or psy-chotic symptoms in an elderly individual with no prior psychiatric history. Confusion that is out of proportion to the depressive symptoms and that features approximate answers rather than refusal or reluctance to answer also increases the possibility of medical illness as etiology. Likewise, "catatonia" in an individual with no recent or remote history of affective disorder or schizophrenia should be con-sidered undiagnosed until a full syndrome can be identified.

Several conditions are of particular note in the differential diagnosis of schizoaffective syndromes. High doses of exogenous steroids may produce con-ditions in which symptoms of affective disorder, schizophrenia, and delirium alternate rapidly. Lia-bility to this condition is dose-related, and symp-toms typically resolve within 3 weeks, rarely lasting longer than 6 weeks (Lewis and Smith, 1983). The crucial feature here is the history of high doses of steroids preceding the onset of the symptoms. Be-cause this history is almost always apparent, diag-nosis is usually not a problem. Patients with per-sistent symptoms, particularly those with a prior history of similar symptoms not preceded by steroid ingestion, may, however, have a purely functional condition (Lewis and Smith, 1983).

Amphetamines and other sympathomimetics may produce hyperactivity, euphoria, racing thoughts, and pressured speech typical of mania shortly after ingestion. A "crash" may occur after several days of continuous amphetamine ingestion and often features dysphoria, hyperphagia, hyper-somnia, and extreme irritability—a picture that may resemble depression. These conditions rarely, of themselves, lead individuals to seek psychiatric help. Between these two phases of amphetamine intoxication, however, a psychosis may emerge that is indistinguishable from paranoid schizophrenia in cross section. Delusions typically resolve within several days to 1 or 2 weeks, and simple observation for this period usually clarifies the diagnosis.

Phencyclidine (PCP) intoxication may be more difficult to recognize. The diagnosis is frequently missed, even by those who are familiar with its presentation (Yago et al., 1981). This may be due in part to the protean nature of the symptoms; para-noid delusions in a clear sensorium may alternate with marked depressive symptoms, or these syn-dromes may coexist with or without evidence of delirium. In one Los Angeles emergency room, 78.5 percent of involuntary psychiatric admissions had detectable PCP in the admission blood sample. In only 21 percent of these cases was there an initial diagnosis of PCP psychosis; a diagnosis of schizo-phrenia was given to more than a third of these cases and primary affective disorder to another third (Yago et al., 1981). Drug screening available to most clinicians is probably inadequate for the detection of clinically significant PCP levels (Analine et al., 1980), since the drug is highly lipophilic and is secreted in only minute quantities over an extended period. However, this condition often involves cer-tain physical symptoms that may help to distinguish it from functional psychosis—slurred speech, ataxia and nystagmus, ptosis, hypertension, analgesia, and hyperreflexia. The level of suspicion also should depend in large part on the patient's demographic features and the pattern of drug use in the patient's subculture.

Temporal lobe epilepsy also may produce affec-tive psychosis, schizophrenia-like psychosis, or a mixture of the two (Flor-Henry, 1969), and the syndromes can closely resemble their functional counterparts (Slater and Beard, 1963). In only 3 of the 69 cases described by Slater and Beard (1963) did the psychosis and epilepsy begin in the same year; in all other cases the psychosis followed the epilepsy, usually by many years. Thus the likelihood that epilepsy lies at the base of a new case of psy-chosis is greatly reduced when there is no history of clinically manifest seizures.

TREATMENT

Clinicians should consider the hypotheses de-scribed previously when selecting treatment. The most efficient approach, the one most consistent with follow-up and family history data, assumes that schizoaffective patients have either schizophrenia or affective disorder. The clinician must weigh the probability of one of these illnesses over the other using all available data—demographics, both present and past psychopathology, premorbid or prodromal features, and family history.

Emphasis should be given to the affective disorder alternative, particularly in treatment-naive patients, since treatment of affective disorder is generally more specific than treatment of schizophrenia. For instance, ECT is much more effective for psychotic depression than for schizophrenia, and the prophylactic value of lithium in affective disorder is clearly established, while there is relatively little support for its use in schizophrenia. In contrast, neuroleptics ameliorate psychotic symptoms regardless of the underlying disorder. Because of the risk of tardive dyskinesia with chronic neuroleptic treatment, other potentially more specific approaches—lithium, tricyclic antidepressants, monoamine oxidase inhibitors, and ECT—should be given preference unless indications for chronic neuroleptic treatment are clear.

Nevertheless, acute treatment usually requires antipsychotics unless ECT is given (Glassman et al., 1975). In the absence of clear indications for long-term use of neuroleptics, these drugs should be discontinued gradually when delusions remit. The clinicians should then determine whether lithium or a tricyclic antidepressant will provide adequate protection against relapse. This will require careful surveillance, particularly in the first 6 months, when the risk of relapse is the highest (Keller et al., 1982). Because relapse is likely to involve a loss of insight, the family's help will be important in this effort. After one or more episodes, they will learn the early warning signs and help the patient to seek early intervention.

More judgments are necessary when relapse does occur. Was the relapse preceded by poor compliance? If so, does the patient find the side effects peculiar to that drug intolerable, or does he or she simply require more time to develop the acceptance and habits necessary for adequate compliance? Because the options for effective prophylaxis are limited, it is important not to abandon a given drug prematurely. Also, it must be remembered that prophylactic efficacy may require time to develop. In fact, maintenance therapy may take several years to show clear effects for depression or hypomania (Dunner et al., 1982).

If, with these cautions in mind, tricyclic antidepressants and lithium appear ineffective, carbamazepine might be considered before chronic neuroleptics. Several controlled trials have found this agent effective in patients with affective disorders resistant to more conventional treatment (Ballenger and Post, 1980; Okuma et al., 1979; Post and Uhde, 1985; Post et al., 1990). Likewise, sodium

valproate apparently has efficacy in bipolar illness (McElroy et al., 1988). However, open trials strongly suggest that schizoaffective patients have poorer outcomes with these agents than do patients with typical bipolar affective disorder (Emrich et al., 1985; McElroy et al., 1988; Elphick, 1985).

EDITORS' COMMENT

Because these patients may be flagrantly psychotic and poorly responsive to treatment, Clozapine should be considered.

SCHIZOPHRENIFORM DISORDER

Langfeldt coined the word *schizophreniform* in 1939 (Langfeldt, 1939) to describe schizophrenia-like psychoses with relatively good prognoses. He intended this to be a heterogeneous group that would include "exogenically precipitated psychosis" (Langfeldt, 1982). Indeed, the words *schizophreniform* and *schizoaffective* have been used interchangeably through much of the subsequent literature. The definitions found in DSM-III and DSM-IIIR are original, however; they separate schizophreniform disorder from schizophrenia solely on the basis of a duration of less than 6 months, including the prodromal phase. DSM-III and DSM-IIIR thus set schizophreniform disorder apart both from affective disorder with mood-incongruent psychotic features and from schizoaffective disorder. This departure from convention must be borne in mind in any review of recent literature on atypical schizophrenia. The preceding section under schizoaffective disorder describes schizophreniform disorder equally well, according to common usage before DSM-III. This section is therefore restricted to studies using the DSM-III/DSM-IIIR definitions.

Table 7-5 summarizes all such studies. Five of seven studies suggest that, like schizoaffective disorder, schizophreniform disorder defines an intermediate or heterogeneous group (Coryell and Tsuang, 1986; Helzer et al., 1981; Targum, 1983; Beiser et al., 1988; Guldberg et al., 1990). However, one found no difference between schizophrenia and schizophreniform disorder (Weiberger et al., 1982), while another concluded that schizophreniform disorder simply represented "atypical affective disorder" (Fogelson et al., 1982).

Consensus may not be forthcoming for several reasons. First, the distinction between schizophrenia and schizophreniform disorder often hinges on the presence of a prodromal syndrome, and many of the components of this syndrome (i.e., social isolation, blunted affect, and digressive speech) shade gradually into the normal spectrum of behavior. Many acutely psychotic patients are unable to give valid accounts of such features in retrospect. Affective syndromes are also difficult to assess in patients who are delusional or halluci-

TABLE 7-5. DSM-III/DSM-IIIR Schizophreniform Disorder: Studies of Validity*

Study	No. with SF	Comparison groups	Design	Results
Helzer et al., 1981	7 (of 134 admissions with psychosis: 5.2%)	19 with schizophrenia	Systematic follow-up averaging 6.5 years	SF patients had significantly better "combined social status score" and "outcome regression score"; less percentage of time in hospital; more manic symptoms
Coryell and Tsuang, 1982	93 (of 810 admissions studied: 11.5%)	86 bipolar AD; 203 unipolar AD; 214 schizophrenia	Chart follow-up averaging 3.1 years; family history study	16% of SF patients recovered vs. 8% of S patients and 58% of AD patients; SF resembled S patients more than AD patients in terms of MR for S and AD
Fogelson et al., 1982	6 (of 50 consecutive admissions: 12%)	None	Individual case reports	Outcome, response to treatment, family and DST results (5/6 abnormal) lead to conclusion that SF is atypical AD
Weinberger et al., 1982	35 (of 128 with CT scans: 27.3%)	17 schizophrenia; 23 affective disorder; 27 other disorders; 26 neurologic controls	Computed tomographic study (CTs routinely obtained)	SF group had distribution of ventricular to brain ratio indistinguishable from those for S group, significantly less than controls, less (but not significantly) than other psychiatric illnesses
Targum, 1983	21 (of 145 admissions: 14.5%)	76 unipolar AD; 10 bipolar AD; 24 other disorders; 14 schizophrenia	Neuroendocrine evaluation (DST and TRH-ST) with 6-month follow-up of only SF patients	% with: +DST† Blunted TRH-ST† AD 44 32 SF 24 29 S 7 7 Neuroendocrine test results predicted outcome among SF patients
Coryell and Tsuang, 1986	93	298 affective disorder; 219 schizophrenia	Systematic follow-up of 40 years	SF patients were significantly more likely than AD patients, but only slightly less likely than schizophrenic patients, to be symptomatic at follow-up
Beiser et al., 1988	29 (of 575 patients with nonorganic psychosis: 4.5%)	60 with schizophrenia; 73 with affective disorder	Systematic follow-up of 18 months	18 (62.1%) rediagnosed as schizophrenic on follow-up: 8 others (27.6% of the sample) had recovered
Guldberg et al., 1990	16	None	Systematic follow-up of 4 to 12 years	6 (37.5%) recovered; "confusion" and "perplexity" were associated with good outcomes

*AD, affective disorder; SF, schizophreniform disorder; S, schizophrenia; DST, dexamethazone suppression test; TRH-ST, thyroid-releasing hormone stimulation test.

†With certain exceptions, a positive DST and a blunted TRH-ST may be specific to major depression.

nating. Even when such patients report typical depressive symptoms, these are often attributed to understandable effects of acute psychosis. A careful history taken from knowledgeable informants will remedy these problems to some extent. Unfortunately, few studies describe the availability of such informants or the thoroughness with which they were interviewed. Reasons for discordance across these studies are, therefore, hard to trace.

In light of this, the clinician must maintain doubtfulness about the true nature of schizophreniform disorder in a given case. As with schizoaffective disorder, the clinician should use all the clinical data available to weight the likelihood of schizophrenia over an affective disorder, giving at least initial weight to the presumption that the overall course and treatment response will ultimately suggest affective disorder.

REFERENCES

Abrams R, Taylor MA: Mania and schizoaffective disorder, manic type: A comparison. Am J Psychiatry 133:12, 1976.

Abrams R, Taylor MA: The importance of mood-incongruent psychotic symptoms in melancholia. J Affective Disord 5: 179–181, 1983.

Altamura C, Guercetti G, Percudani M: Dexamethasone suppression test in positive and negative schizophrenia. Psychiatry Res 30:69–75, 1989.

American Psychiatric Association, Committee on Nomenclature and Statistics: Diagnostic and Statistical Manual of Mental Disorders, 3d ed. Washington, American Psychiatric Association, 1980.

American Psychiatric Association: Diagnostic and Statistical Manual of Mental Disorder, 2d ed. Washington, American Psychiatric Association, 1968.

American Psychiatric Association: DSM-IV Options Book: Work in Progress—9/1/91. Washington, American Psychiatric Association, 1991, pp f15–f16.

Analine O, Allen RE, Pitts FN, et al: The urban epidemic of phencyclidine use: Laboratory evidence from a public psychiatric hospital inpatient service. Biol Psychiatry 15:813–816, 1980.

Andreasen NC, Grove WM, Shapiro RW, et al: Reliability of lifetime diagnosis. Arch Gen Psychiatry 38:400–405, 1981.

Angst J, Weis P, Grof P, Baastrup PC, Schou M: Lithium prophylaxis in recurrent affective disorder. Br J Psychiatry 116:604–614, 1970.

Angst J: Course of unipolar depressive, bipolar manic depressive and schizoaffective disorder: Results of a prospective longitudinal study. Fortschr Neurol Psychiatr 48:3–30, 1980.

Angst J: The etiology and nosology of endogenous depressive psychoses. Foreign Psychiatry 2:1–108, 1973.

Aronoff MS, Epstein RS: Factors associated with poor response to lithium carbonate: A clinical study. Am J Psychiatry 127:4, 1970.

Baastrup PC, Schou M: Lithium as a prophylactic agent. Arch Gen Psychiatry 16:162–172, 1967.

Ballenger JC, Post RM: Carbamazepine in manic-depressive illness: A new treatment. Am J Psychiatry 137:782–790, 1980.

Baron M, Gruen R, Asnis L, Kane J: Schizoaffective illness, schizophrenia and affective disorders: Morbidity risk and genetic transmission. Acta Psychiatr Scand 65:253–262, 1982.

Beiser M, Fleming AE, Iacono DG, Lin T: Refining the diagnosis of schizophreniform disorder. Am J Psychiatry 145:695–700, 1988.

Bocchetta A, Bernardi F, Garau L, et al: Familial rates of affective illness in Sardinia with special reference to schizoaffective disorder. Eur Arch Psychiatr Clin Neurosci 240:16–20, 1990.

Brockington IF, Leff JP: Schizoaffective psychosis: Definitions and incidence. Psychol Med 9:91–99, 1979.

Brockington IF, Kendell RE, Wainwright S: Depressed patients with schizophrenic or paranoid symptoms. Psychol Med 10:665–675, 1980a.

Brockington IF, Wainwright S, Kendell RE: Manic patients with schizophrenic or paranoid symptoms. Psychol Med 10: 73–83, 1980b.

Carroll BJ, Feinberg M, Greden JF, et al: A specific laboratory test for the diagnosis of melancholia. Arch Gen Psychiatry 38: 15–22, 1981.

Clayton PJ: Schizoaffective disorders. J Nerv Ment Dis 170: 646–650, 1982.

Clayton PJ, Rodin L, Winokur G: Family history studies: III. Schizoaffective disorder, clinical and genetic factors including a one to two year follow-up. Comp Psychiatry 9:31, 1968.

Cohen SM, Allen M, Pollin W, Hrubec Z: Relationship of schizoaffective psychosis to manic depressive psychosis and schizophrenia. Arch Gen Psychiatry 26:539–546, 1972.

Coryell W: The use of laboratory tests in psychiatric diagnosis: The DST as an example. Psychiatr Dev 3:139–159, 1984.

Coryell W, Tsuang D: HPA-axis hyperactivity and psychosis: Recovery during an eight-year follow-up. Am J Psychiatry 149:1033–1039, 1992.

Coryell W, Tsuang MT: Outcome after forty years in DSM-III schizophreniform disorder. Arch Gen Psychiatry 43:324–328, 1986.

Coryell W, Zimmerman M: Outcome following ECT in primary unipolar depression: A test of newly proposed response predictors. Am J Psychiatry 141:862–867, 1984.

Coryell W, Zimmerman M: Demographic, historical and symptomatic features of the nonmanic psychoses. J Nerv Ment Dis 174:585–592, 1986.

Coryell W, Zimmerman M: The heritability of schizophrenia and schizo-affective disorders: A family study. Arch Gen Psychiatry 45:323–327, 1988.

Coryell W, Zimmerman M: HPA-axis hyperactivity and recovery from functional psychoses. Am J Psychiatry 146:473–477, 1989.

Coryell WH, Tsuang MT: DSM-III schizophreniform disorder: Comparisons with schizophrenia and affective disorder. Arch Gen Psychiatry 39:66–69, 1982.

Coryell W, Tsuang MT, McDaniel J: Psychotic features in major depression: Is mood congruence important? J Affective Disord 4:227–236, 1982.

Coryell W, Endicott J, Keller M, Andreasen NA: Phenomenology and family history in DSM-III psychotic depression. J Affective Disord 9:13–18, 1985.

Coryell W, Keller M, Lavori P, Endicott J: Affective syndromes, psychotic features and prognosis: I. Depression. Arch Gen Psychiatry 47:651–657, 1990a.

Coryell W, Keller M, Lavori P, Endicott J: Affective syndromes, psychotic features and prognosis: II. Mania. Arch Gen Psychiatry 47:658–664, 1990b.

Dunner DL, Stallone F, Fieve RR: Prophylaxis with lithium carbonate: An update. Arch Gen Psychiatry 39:1344–1345, 1982.

Dyksen MW, Kooser JA, Havaszti JJ, Davis JM: Clinical usefulness of sodium amobarbital interviewing. Arch Gen Psychiatry 36:789–794, 1979.

Elphick M: An open clinical trial of carbamazepine in treatment resistant bipolar and schizoaffective psychotics. Br J Psychiatry 147:198–200, 1985.

Emrich HM, Dose M, Von Zerssen D: The use of sodium valproate, carbamazepine and oxcarbamazepine in patients with affective disorders. J Affective Disord 8:243–250, 1985.

Endicott J, Nee J, Coryell W, et al: Schizoaffective, psychotic and nonpsychotic depression: Differential familial association. Compr Psychiatry 27:1–13, 1986.

Flor-Henry P: Psychosis and temporal lobe epilepsy. Epilepsia 10:363–395, 1969.

Fogelson DL, Cohen BM, Pope HG: A study of DSM-III schizophreniform disorder. Am J Psychiatry 139:1281–1285, 1982.

Gershon E, DeLisi L, Hamovit J, et al: A controlled family study of chronic psychoses. Arch Gen Psychiatry 45:328–336, 1988.

Gershon ES, Hamovit J, Guroff JJ, et al: A family study of schizoaffective, bipolar I, bipolar II, unipolar and normal control probands. Arch Gen Psychiatry 132:716–718, 1975.

Glassman AH, Kantor SJ, Shostak M: Depression, delusions and drug response. Am J Psychiatry 132:716–718, 1975.

Griffith JD, Cavanaugh T, Held J, Oates JA: Experimental psychosis induced by the administration *d*-amphetamine. In Costa E, Gavattini S (eds): Amphetamine and Related Compounds. New York, Raven Press, 1970.

Grossman LS, Harrow M, Fudala JL, Meltzer HY: The longitudinal course of schizoaffective disorder. J Nerv Ment Dis 172:140–149, 1984.

Grossman LS, Harrow M, Goldberg JF, Fichtner CG: Outcome of schizoaffective disorder at two long term follow-ups: Comparisons with outcome of schizophrenia and affective disorders. Am J Psychiatry 148:1359–1365, 1991.

Guldberg CA, Dahl AA, Hansen H, Bergem M: Predictive value of the four good prognostic features in DSM-III-R schizophreniform disorder. Acta Psychiatr Scand 82:23–25, 1990.

Helzer JE, Brockington IF, Kendell RE: The predictive validity of DSM-III and Feighner definitions of schizophrenia: A comparison with RDC and CATEGO. Arch Gen Psychiatry 38:791–797, 1981.

Himmelhoch JM, Fuchs CZ, May SJ, et al: When a schizoaffective diagnosis has meaning. J Nerv Ment Dis 169:277–282, 1981.

Johnson G: Differential response to lithium carbonate in manic-depressive and schizoaffective disorders. Dis Nerv Syst 9:613–615, 1970.

Keller MB, Shapiro RW, Lavori TW, Wolfe N: Relapse and major depressive disorder. Arch Gen Psychiatry 39:911–915, 1982.

Kendler KS, Gruenberg AM, Tsuang MT: Psychiatric illness in first-degree relatives of schizophrenic and surgical control patients. Arch Gen Psychiatry 42:770–779, 1985.

Kendler KS, Gurenberg AM, Tsuang MT: A DSM-III family study of the nonschizophrenic psychotic disorders. Am J Psychiatry 143:1098–1105, 1986.

Kirkegaard C, Bjorum N, Cohn D, Lauvidsen UG: Thyrotrophin-releasing hormone (TRH) stimulation test in manic depressive illness. Arch Gen Psychiatry 35:1017–1021, 1978.

Langfeldt G: Definition of "schizophreniform psychoses" (letter). Am J Psychiatry 139:703, 1982.

Langfeldt G: The Schizophreniform States. London, Oxford University Press, 1939.

Lewis DA, Smith RE: Steroid-induced psychiatric syndromes. J Affective Disord 5:319–332, 1983.

Maj M: Lithium prophylaxis of schizoaffective disorders: A prospective study. J Affective Disord 14:129–135, 1988.

Maj M, Starace F, Demali D: Prediction of outcome by historical, clinical and biological variables in schizoaffective disorder, depressed type. J Psychiatr Res 21:289–295, 1987.

Maj M, Starace F, Pirozzi R: A family study of DSM-III-R schizoaffective disorder, depressive type, compared with schizophrenia and psychotic and nonpsychotic major depression. Am J Psychiatry 148:612–616, 1991.

Marneros A, Deister A, Rohde A: The concept of distinct but voluminous groups of bipolar and unipolar diseases: I. Bipolar diseases. Eur Arch Psychiatr Clin Neurosci 240:77–84, 1990a.

Marneros A, Rohde A, Deister A: The concept of distinct but voluminous groups of bipolar and unipolar diseases: II. Unipolar diseases. Eur Arch Psychiatr Clin Neurosci 240:85–89, 1990b.

McElroy SL, Keck PE, Pope HG, Hudson JI: Valproate in primary psychiatric disorders: Literature review and clinical experience in a private psychiatric hospital. In McElroy SL, Pope HG (eds): Use of Anticonvulsants in Psychiatry. Clifton, NJ, Oxford Health Care, Inc., 1988, pp 25–41.

Meltzer HY, Fang BS, Tricou BJ, et al: Effect of dexamethasone on plasma prolactin and cortisol levels in psychiatric patients. Am J Psychiatry 139:763–768, 1982.

Mendlewicz J, Linkowski P, Wilmotte J: Relationship between schizoaffective illness and affective disorders or schizophrenia. J Affective Disord 2:289–302, 1980.

Moller HJ, Schmid-Bode W, Cording-Tommel C, et al: Psychopathological and social outcome in schizophrenia vs. affective/schizoaffective psychoses and prediction of poor outcome in schizophrenia. Acta Psychiatr Scand 77:379–389, 1988.

Newcome JW, Faustman WO, Whitefored HA, et al: Symptomatology and cognitive impairment associate independently with post-dexamethasone cortisol concentrations in unmedicated schizophrenic patients. Biol Psychiatry 29:855–864, 1991.

Okuma T, Inanaga K, Otsuki S, et al: Comparison of the antimanic efficacy of carbamazepine and chlorpromazine: A double-blind control study. Psychopharmacology 66:211–217, 1979.

Orvaschel H, Thompson WD, Belanger A, et al: Comparison of the family history method of direct interview. J Affective Disord 4:49–59, 1982.

Opjordsmoen S: Long-term course and outcome in unipolar affective and schizoaffective psychoses. Acta Psychiatr Scand 79:317–326, 1989.

Pope HG, Lipinski JF, Cohen BM, Axelrod DT: "Schizoaffective disorder": An invalid diagnosis? A comparison of schizoaffective disorder, schizophrenia and affective disorder. Am J Psychiatry 137:921–927, 1980.

Post RM, Uhde TW: Carbamazepine in bipolar illness. Psychopharmacol Bull 21:10–17, 1985.

Post RM, Leverich GS, Rosoff AS, Altshuler LL: Carbamazepine prophylaxis in refractory affective disorders: A focus on long-term follow-up. J Clin Psychopharmacol 10:318–327, 1990.

Prien RF, Caffey Em, Klett J: Factors associated with treatment success on lithium carbonate prophylaxis. Arch Gen Psychiatry 31:189–192, 1974.

Regier DA, Myers JK, Kramer M, et al: The NIMH catchment program. Arch Gen Psychiatry 41:934–941, 1984.

Rosenthal NE, Rosenthal LN, Stallone F, et al: The validation of RDC schizoaffective disorder. Arch Gen Psychiatry 37:804–810, 1980.

Rosenthal NE, Rosenthal LN, Stallone F, et al: Psychosis as a predictor of response to lithium maintenance treatment in bipolar affective disorder. J Affective Disord 1:237–245, 1979.

Rzewuska M, Angst J: Prognosis of periodic bipolar manic depressive and schizoaffective psychosis. Arch Psychiatr Nervenkr 231:471–486, 1982.

Saffer D, Metcalfe M, Coppen A: Abnormal dexamethasone suppression test in type II schizophrenia. Br J Psychiatry 147:721–723, 1985.

Scharfetter C: Subdividing defunctional psychosis: A family hereditary approach. Psychol Med 11:637–640, 1981.

Schou M, Juel-Nielsen N, Stromgren E, Voldby H: The treatment of manic psychoses by the administration of lithium salts. J Neurol Neurosurg Psychiatry 17:250, 1954.

Sharma RP, Pandey GN, Janicak PG, et al: The effect of diagnosis and age on the DST: A meta-analytic approach. Biol Psychiatry 24:555–568, 1988.

Slater E, Beard AW: The schizophrenia-like psychoses of epilepsy: Psychiatric aspects. Br J Psychiatry 109:95–150, 1963.

Spitzer RL, Endicott J, Robins E: Research diagnostic criteria: Rationale and reliability. Arch Gen Psychiatry 35:773–786, 1978.

Suslak L, Shopsin B, Silbey E, et al: Genetics of affective disorders: I. Familial instance study of bipolar, unipolar and schizoaffective illness. Neuropsychobiology 2:18–27, 1976.

Tandon R, Mazzara C, DeCuardo J, et al: Dexamethasone suppression test in schizophrenia: Relationship to symptomatology, ventricular enlargement, and outcome. Biol Psychiatry 29:953–964, 1991.

Tandon R, Mazzara C, Dequardo JR: The DST and outcome in schizophrenia. Am J Psychiatry 146:1648–1649, 1989.

Targum SD: Neuroendocrine dysfunction in schizophreniform disorder: Correlation with 6 month clinical outcome. Am J Psychiatry 140:309–313, 1983.

Taylor MA: Schneiderian first-rank symptoms and clinical prognostic features in schizophrenia. Arch Gen Psychiatry 26:64–67, 1972.

Tsuang MT, Dempsey GM, Dvoredsky A, Struss A: A family history study of schizoaffective disorder. Biol Psychiatry 12:331–338, 1977.

Tsuang MT, Dempsey M, Ranscher F: A study of "atypical schizo-phrenia." Arch Gen Psychiatry 33:1157–1160, 1976.

Tsuang MT: Genetics of affective disorder. In Mendels J (ed): The Psychobiology of Depression. New York, Spectrum, 1975, pp 85–100.

van Praag H, Nijo L: About the course of schizo-affective psy-choses. Compr Psychiatry 25:9–22, 1984.

Vernon SW, Roberts RE: Use of the SADS-RDC in a triethnic community survey. Arch Gen Psychiatry 39:47–52, 1982.

Weinberger DR, DeLisi LE, Perman GP, et al: Computed tomogra-phy and schizophreniform disorder and other acute psychi-atric disorders. Arch Gen Psychiatry 39:778–783, 1982.

Weissman MM, Myers J: The affective disorders in a U.S. urban community. Arch Gen Psychiatry 35:1304–1311, 1978.

Yago KB, Pitts FM, Burgoyne RW, et al: The urban epidemic of phencyclidine (PCP) use: Clinical and laboratory evidence from the Public Hospital Emergency Service. J Clin Psychia-try 42:193–196, 1981.

Zall H, Therman PG: Lithium carbonate: A clinical study. Am J Psychiatry 125:549–555, 1968.

CHAPTER 8

Delusional (Paranoid) Disorders

RAYMOND R. CROWE
MARC-ANDRÉ ROY

DEFINITION

If any psychiatric illness with delusions is considered to be a paranoid disorder, then these disorders are among the most common conditions in psychiatry (Freedman and Schwab, 1978). For example, 48 percent of manic and 33 percent of bipolar depressives are delusional (Winokur et al., 1969), and practically all schizophrenics experience delusions at some time during the course of their illness. Therefore, if the concept of a paranoid disorder is to have any validity as a diagnostically pure group of patients, it must be defined by paranoid delusions in the absence of other psychiatric illness that might account for the delusional thinking.

Although the term *paranoia* dates from the time of Hippocrates, Kahlbaum (1863) was the first to use it to designate a diagnostically separate group of disorders that remained so over their course (Lewis, 1970; Tanna, 1974). Kraepelin (1921) further developed the concept of paranoia as a chronic and unremitting system of delusions that was distinguished from schizophrenia by the absence of hallucinations and other psychotic features. These ideas were incorporated into the first diagnostic manual (DSM-I) of the American Psychiatric Association (1952), and paranoid reactions were defined as illnesses with persistent persecutory or grandiose delusions, ordinarily without hallucinations, and with emotional responses and behavior consistent with the ideas held. Subtypes included paranoia, a chronic disorder characterized by an intricate and complex delusional system, and paranoid state, usually of shorter duration and lacking the systematization of paranoia. These concepts of paranoid disorders and their subtypes have been preserved in all their essential features by DSM-II (1968) and DSM-III (1980).

In DSM-IIIR, paranoid disorders have been renamed *delusional disorders*, because of the confusion that arose from the use of paranoia in its narrow meaning, e.g., persecutory delusion (American Psychiatric Association, 1987). Moreover, the category has been expanded to include patients presenting with erotomanic, grandiose, somatic, or other delusions, as long as they fulfill the other criteria. Another departure from DSM-III has been the removal of the distinction between acute and chronic subtypes. In DSM-IIIR, induced psychotic disorder (i.e., folie à deux) has been removed from the delusional disorders and classified under psychotic disorders not otherwise specified. This fascinating topic is reviewed by Sacks (1988) and will not be considered further here.

International Classification of Diseases (ICD)-9 classifies most paranoid disorders under "paranoid states" and includes four types. Simple paranoid states are those in which "delusions, especially of being influenced, persecuted, or treated in some special way, are the main symptom." They may be acute or chronic. Paranoia is a "chronic psychosis in which logically constructed systematized delusions have developed gradually without concomitant hallucinations." When hallucinations are prominent, the disorder is classified as a paraphrenia, the third subtype. The diagnostic classification of patients who share all the clinical characteristics of the delusional disorders but also present prominent hallucinations remains controversial; while there is a general consensus, some authorities (Winokur, 1985; Munroe, 1988) propose to keep them in the separate and distinct category of psychosis not otherwise specified. Some authors propose to call hallucinatory delusional disorder *paraphrenia* (Munroe, 1988), a term often used to designate a late-onset schizophrenia-like psychosis.

EPIDEMIOLOGY

Delusional disorders have always been considered uncommon illnesses, but until recently, little was known of their epidemiology. Demographic reports from the United States and other countries have now provided a reasonably complete picture of the epidemiology of these conditions (Table 8-1) (Kendler, 1982).

The annual incidence ranges from 0.7 to 3.0 new cases per 100,000 population per year. This rate accounts for 1.3 percent of all first admissions to mental hospitals and 3.9 percent of first admissions for nonorganic psychoses. Moreover, the incidence appears to have been stable from 1932 to 1952, with a small decrease since 1952 owing to an increase in the number of first admissions for other illnesses. Thus there seems to have been little change recently in the incidence of new cases.

Prevalence refers to the number of active and inactive cases in the population at any given time. For the delusional disorders, it is approximately 24 to 30 cases per 100,000 population, which substantiates clinical impressions that these are indeed uncommon conditions. Thus, for every case of delusional disorder, there are approximately 30 cases of schizophrenia and 150 of affective disorder (assuming a prevalence of 1 percent for schizophrenia and 5 percent for affective disorder; Goodwin and Guze, 1979). These figures show how much more likely a delusional patient is to have one of the more common psychoses than a delusional disorder.

This relative rarity of delusional disorder may well be secondary to the reluctance of these patients to visit mental health professionals. For example, there are clear indications that delusions of parasitosis are not a rare condition within dermatology clinics.

Delusional disorders are most likely to appear in mid life. The peak age of onset and the age at first admission both occur in the fourth to fifth decade and range from the teens into senescence (Winokur, 1977; Kendler, 1982). The sexes are nearly equally affected, although most studies have found a small excess of females, about 55 percent of first admissions being women.

ETIOLOGY

Because delusional disorders are uncommon, and because schizophrenia and depression can both present with paranoid delusions, the question arises whether delusional disorders represent a separate group of illnesses or simply atypical forms of these more common ones. This question is important because of the obvious treatment implications, and several lines of evidence converge to provide a reasonably consistent answer.

Epidemiologic findings suggest that delusional disorders are unrelated to either affective disorder or schizophrenia (Kendler, 1980). Delusional disorders are far less prevalent than either of the other two. They begin at a later time in life than schizophrenia, and the sex ratio is closer to unity than that of the affective disorders, with their prominent excess of females. Although these findings are suggestive, they by no means prove the case for a diagnostically separate condition.

The familial findings are more convincing. If delusional disorders were a form of either schizophrenia or affective disorder, the incidence of these latter conditions should be increased in the families of delusional disorders, but this has not been found (Kolle, 1931; Debray, 1985; Winokur, 1977; Kendler and Hays, 1981). Familial rates of schizophrenia range from 0.6 to 1.7 percent, and those of affective disorder, from 1.1 to 5.0 percent. Both are within the population expectation for their respective prevalences. Moreover, reanalysis of data from a large adoption study of schizophrenia did not find a higher rate of delusional disorders in the biologic relatives of schizophrenic adoptees than in other groups of relatives (adoptive relatives of the same adoptees and biologic and adoptive relatives of control adoptees) (Kendler and Hays, 1981).

While it is relatively clear that delusional disorders do not breed true with either affective or schizophrenic disorders, a few recent studies have shown a family history of paranoid personality disorders or traits in the relatives of delusional disorder patients (Winokur, 1985; Kendler et al., 1985). These findings suggest that these two conditions may be genetically related to each other.

Our own unpublished data (Table 8-2) confirm these findings. We reviewed the medical records of 257 patients with either simple delusional disor-

TABLE 8-1. *Epidemiology of Delusional Disorders*

Incidence*	0.7–1.3
Prevalence*	24–30
Percent of first admissions*	1.3
Mean age of onset†	39
Sex ratio (F/M)	1.18

The figures for incidence, prevalence, and sex ratio represent cases per 100,000 population.
* From Kendler, 1982.
† From Retterstol, 1966.

TABLE 8-2. *Family History in Delusional Disorder*

	Simple delusional	Hallucinatory delusional	Paranoid schizophrenia
Number of cases	101	38	118
Number of relatives	643	285	653
Affect disorder (%)	1.6	1.8	2.1
Schizophrenia (%)	0.5	1.8	1.5
Paranoid traits (%)	2.3	1.1	0.6

ders, hallucinatory delusional disorders, or paranoid schizophrenia. We reviewed all available information on relatives and assigned them blind diagnoses. As can be shown, the relatives of patients with simple delusional disorders were characterized by a higher prevalence of paranoid traits and a lower frequency of schizophrenia compared with the relatives of schizophrenic subjects, while the relatives of hallucinatory patients were between those two groups. However, only the rates of paranoid traits reached statistical significance.

Follow-up studies of delusional disorders range in length of follow-up from a few months to 20 years and indicate that the diagnosis of delusional disorder tends to remain stable over time (Kendler, 1980). If it were a form of affective disorder or schizophrenia, this length of observation should allow sufficient time for the correct diagnosis to declare itself. However, 78 to 93 percent of delusional disorder patients retained the same diagnosis, only 3 to 22 percent developing schizophrenia and less than 6 percent developing affective disorder.

These observations indicate that Kahlbaum's original concept of paranoid disorders as uncommon but distinct entities was correct. They appear to form a chronologically stable group of disorders that are biologically distinct from the other psychoses.

CLINICAL PICTURE

The hallmark of the delusional disorders is the delusional system. This consists of a unique set of false ideas that are rigidly adhered to despite all contradictory evidence. The uniqueness of the delusion distinguishes these patients from persons with idiosyncratic ideas shared by a larger social group, such as a religious cult. The fixed quality of the delusion also separates them from nondelusional persons with unusual ideas. A third feature of delusions is that facts are reinterpreted to fit the delusion, rather than the delusion being modified to fit the facts. The delusion is thus characteristically fed by constant misinterpretations of the facts. It is thus important to emphasize that the chronic delusional patient does not base his or her delusional beliefs on hallucinations. For example, the paranoid patient on seeing persons laughing will think they are laughing at him or her. The perception of persons laughing is correct; it is the interpretation of the perception that is abnormal.

The delusions of delusional disorders are usually systematized and encapsulated to varying degrees. *Systematized* refers to the ramifications of the delusional system being connected by a common theme. *Encapsulation* refers to thought processes outside the delusional system remaining unaffected. As the French psychiatric tradition has emphasized, delusions can vary quite a lot in their degree of *extension*. This term refers to the extent of ramification. For example, an *unextended* delusion would be limited to a relatively small sphere of the person's life, while an *extended* delusional system might infiltrate most of the person's activities. However, even in these extreme cases, thought processes outside the delusional system remain unaffected.

DSM-IIIR emphasizes that the quality of the delusions be nonbizarre. Winokur (1977) has proposed that the delusion be possible even though implausible, as opposed to impossible, as a test criterion for being nonbizarre.

Many delusional disorders are accompanied by hallucinations that are not sufficiently prominent to justify a diagnosis of schizophrenia. Some would exclude any patient with hallucinations (Winokur, 1977), whereas others would include them as long as the hallucinations are not prominent (Kendler, 1980). At the present time, it seems reasonable to consider infrequent hallucinations to be a symptom of delusional disorders.

When a thought disorder is present, it is not prominent and does not affect communication as the thought disorder of schizophrenia does. Winokur (1977) found loquacity and circumstantiality in 30 percent of his cases. When this occurs, it usually accompanies descriptions of the delusional system.

Another hallmark of the delusional disorders is the relative preservation of the personality. Outside the areas of life involved in the delusional system, patients should not show major impairments in areas such as housework, occupational performance, and social relationships. However, the impairments of delusional patients can be severe, particularly if their delusions are extended to involve many areas of their life. Their behavior will seem normal when their delusions are not discussed or acted on, and they will show neither blunted nor discordant affect. When present, these impairments should be easily explained by the delusions. For example, a person could have problems at work because of a conviction of being persecuted; other than that, his or her performance should remain relatively unimpaired. This impairment is often further aggravated by the characteristic tendency of these patients to act on their delusions. For example, the person who feels persecuted may complain to the police or attempt revenge; the erotomanic, convinced he is loved, may write or otherwise attempt to contact or stalk the object of his delusion. This is an area that the clinician should always inquire about given the potential consequences of these acts.

DSM-IIIR has outlined five subtypes that closely parallel those proposed by Monro (1988). These are erotomanic, grandiose, jealous, persecutory, and somatic types. However, other delusional themes are consistent with a diagnosis of delusional disorder as long as they meet the major defining criteria.

Persecutory delusions may develop insidiously from a situation in which some degree of suspicion is justified. As the illness develops, the bounds of reason are exceeded, and simple suspiciousness is replaced by a delusional system. In time, the system becomes increasingly elaborate as more details are incorporated into it. The following case illustrates this development, as well as the preservation of affect leading the patient to act on the delusion.

SOME ILLUSTRATIVE CASES

Case History 1: Persecutory Delusional Disorder
A 22-year-old single man, who lived on a farm with his parents, was brought to the hospital because of increasing suspiciousness of a neighbor. There had been long-standing friction between the patient's family and the neighbor, but over the preceding 3 weeks the patient had become convinced that the neighbor was involved in a grain and beef theft ring (which was indeed operating in the area) and informed the Federal Bureau of Investigation of his suspicions. He became convinced that his house was bugged and that some apples his father bought were poison because they had been purchased from a friend of the neighbor. He was hospitalized when he began sleeping with a gun for self-protection. On interview he was cooperative, although suspicious at times. The affect was appropriate to the delusional system. The speech was circumstantial and, at times, tangential when discussing the delusion. Over a 1-month hospitalization, the delusion cleared rapidly, and at discharge he had gained complete insight into the irrationality of his former beliefs. However, his suspiciousness toward the neighbor remained.

A. Meyer suggested the following stages in the development of paranoid symptomatology (Muncie, 1939). Meyer's stages started with (1) "a rigid makeup with a tendency to pride and self-contained haughtiness, mistrust and disdain," (2) "appearance of affectively charged dominant notions, as autochthonous ideas or revelation which illuminates all the brooding questioning in a manner to leave no need for further check," (3) "an irresistible need for working over the material for evidence to support the dominant notion. That it will support it is a foregone conclusion." (4) "Systematization of a sort that is so tightly knit that it remains logically correct if the original dominant notion be admitted." (5) "When the present has been ransacked for proofs and systematized, the attention is turned to the past with a re-examination of the past experiences in the light of newer certainty. There result misinterpretations of past events and retrospective falsification. . . . " No psychiatrist has ever done a better job describing the march of circumstances in delusional disorder.

Case History 2: Jealous Delusional Disorder
Delusional disorder with jealous delusions is referred to as *conjugal paranoia*. Such patients become convinced that their spouses are unfaithful, and they become preoccupied with proving the infidelity and extracting a confession. Of all the paranoid disorders, these patients spend the greatest amount of time attempting to verify their suspicions (Shepherd, 1961).

A 22-year-old college student was brought to the hospital for threatening his wife with a hammer. She first became aware of his jealousy on their honeymoon, 3 years earlier, when he accused her of infidelity because she was not home on one occasion when he returned. Over the ensuing 3 years he often nagged her for confessions of past affairs. His bullying led to frequent arguments of such intensity that the police were once called. During the year before his admission, his suspicions had intensified to the point that he accused her of having affairs after work whenever she was not home as promptly as he expected. He called her at work to check on her, set traps around the house, inspected her underwear, and even examined a vaginal smear under a microscope. He often kept her awake all night attempting to extract a confession of infidelity. His deteriorating school performance was blamed on his wife for the anguish she was causing him. He was hospitalized after the incident with the hammer and viewed the admission as an attempt by his wife and the doctors to "railroad" him and threatened to "even the score." On admission he was antagonistic and threatening, with a superior attitude. Although the speech was pressured, it was coherent. The affect was intense but appropriate to his suspicions. After his admission he became calmer, but the delusion remained unchanged during a 1-month hospitalization. He was discharged to another hospital, and his wife separated from him and obtained a divorce.

EDITORS' COMMENT

Clinicians have noted that patients with delusional jealousy will lose most of the pressure and need to add interpretations and delusions when they are divorced. They will get along in the community in a satisfactory manner and appear ordinary, though they will continue to be delusional about the past. On remarriage they will have a recrudescence of their jealous delusions, this time attached to the new spouse.

Erotic delusional patients have delusions of secret suitors, and they interpret ordinary comments and gestures from the delusional suitor as concealed messages proclaiming their love. The "suitor" is often a prominent person with whom the patient has had some dealings. When their overtures are not reciprocated, such patients only become more convinced of the other's love for them, which, for various reasons, cannot be returned openly. Eventually, they may feel jilted and attempt to avenge themselves against their former "lover." This type of paranoid disorder is also known as *erotomania* and as *DeClerambault's syndrome* (Hollender and Callahan, 1975; Seeman, 1978; Segal, 1989).

Case History 3: Erotic Delusional Disorder
A 46-year-old farm wife, who had been unhappily married for 15 years, fell in love with an itinerant evangelist conducting tent meetings in her town. Convinced that her love was secretly reciprocated, she neglected her housework to spend hours writing him unanswered letters. In her letters she asked him not to reply if he loved her, as it would cause a scandal in the community. She then interpreted his lack of response as proof of his love. The only abnormality noted on admission to the hospital was the erotic delusion, which failed to clear over a 3-week hospitalization. She was discharged home unimproved.

Grandiose paranoids believe themselves to be persons of special importance. Common delusions of this genre include those of inventions and discoveries, as well as delusions of being an important part of an organization such as the Central Intelligence Agency. They can describe their delusions with such enthusiasm and loquatiousness that they may initially appear manic.

Case History 4: Grandiose Delusional Disorder
A 56-year-old businessman developed diabetes 4 years before admission. Shortly thereafter, he developed his own treatment for the disease, which consisted of replacing sugar lost in the urine with a diet rich in sugar. He began publishing materials on his new treatment and advertised courses in it over the radio. Because he charged a nominal fee for these, he was arrested on charges of mail fraud and hospitalized for a court-ordered psychiatric examination. On admission he was cooperative and discussed his ideas with considerable loquatiousness and circumstantiality. His affect was appropriate to the ideas discussed. The delusional system remained fixed over a 3-week hospitalization, and he was discharged unimproved.

Patients with somatic delusional disorders are preoccupied with the appearance, odor, or function of their body (Munro, 1980). Common examples are delusions of body odor or halitosis. These patients are convinced of having a bad smell. Typically, they do not perceive the odor themselves, but they interpret benign remarks or nonverbal reactions as signs of disgust over the imagined odor. If the patient indeed smells an odor, this is a hallucination, and another disorder such as schizophrenia or an organic disorder should be suspected. With delusions of infestation or parasitosis, the patient believes that he or she is infested with insects or other foreign bodies under the skin. With dysmorphic delusions, the patient is convinced that he or she has a disfiguring anatomic feature, such as a distorted chin or nose. With delusional hypochondriasis, the patient believes that he or she is affected by a serious illness and characteristically visits multiple physicians as well as other healers.

COURSE

The data on outcome of delusional disorders are scarce. However, Retterstol (1966) published an interesting description of his personal follow-up of delusional patients. He reported his results using the distinction between acute and chronic delusional disorders, and we thus will summarize them using this distinction, which seems relevant with regard to prognosis (Table 8-3). He compared these two subtypes on different variables. First, the chronic subtype has a slightly later onset (44 versus 37 years, on average). Second, an acute onset was more frequent in the acute subgroup (93 versus 67 percent). Third, 53 percent of the chronic subtype and 90 percent of

TABLE 8-3.   *Course of Delusional Disorders*

	Paranoia	Acute paranoid disorder
Mean age of onset	44	37
Acute onset (%)	67	93
Six-month duration (%)	88	54
Predominant delusion	Jealous	Persecutory
Remission (%)	54	90
Relapse (%) (of those remitting)	7	41

Data from Retterstol, 1966. Paranoia is used instead of paranoiac, and acute paranoid disorder, instead of paranoid in the reference.

the acute subtype were free from any delusions on follow-up. Fourth, in both subgroups, about 80 percent were self-supporting at follow-up, and 80 percent were at most only briefly incapacited from work. Thus the overall picture provides the basis for some optimism about the prognosis of delusional disorders. Another long-term (mean 25 years) retrospective follow-up of 88 patients with delusional disorders identified through hospital records arrived at results quite different from Retterstol's; among the delusional patients, only 36 percent were completely recovered, 54 percent were still delusional, and 29 percent were living in institutions (Crowe et al., 1988). Therefore, it is probable that the outcome of delusional disorders is quite variable, ranging from complete recovery to severe incapacitation.

DIFFERENTIAL DIAGNOSIS

Because delusional disorders are so uncommon, the possibility that a delusional illness is caused by some other condition must always be kept in mind. A large number of causes are possible; these include organic brain syndromes, affective disorders, schizophrenia, and schizophreniform disorder (Manschreck and Petri, 1978).

Three organic brain syndromes can present with delusions. Delirium is characterized by a fluctuating state of consciousness, and the delusions are likewise evanescent and rapidly changing, while those of delusional disorders remain relatively fixed for the duration of the illness. In addition, the cognitive symptoms of delirium (e.g., disorientation and memory impairment) are absent in delusional disorders.

Dementia may be accompanied by delusions and should be suspected in an elderly paranoid patient. Suspiciousness and delusional thinking can be more prominent than the cognitive impairment of the dementia, but the latter can usually be uncovered by a careful mental status examination. In questionable cases, psychometric testing for organicity may lead to the correct diagnosis. Organic delusional syndromes present a greater diagnostic problem because of the absence of the cognitive impairment of delirium and dementia. For this reason, a careful medical history, with particular attention to the drug history, should be obtained. These organic delusions can result from a variety of medical illnesses and drugs (see Cummings, 1986, for a comprehensive review). Pathology of the basal ganglia, such as Huntington's and Wilson's disease, or of the limbic system, such as temporal lobe epilepsy, is the most likely etiology, but other etiologies also should be considered. These include presenile dementia and metabolic (systemic lupus erythematosus, porphyria, pernicious anemia), endocrine (Addison's disease, hypoparathyroidism), and infectious etiologies. Delusions are associated with a variety of commonly abused drugs, such as amphetamines and cocaine. Among prescription drugs, delusions can occur with steroids and L-dopa.

Delusions are often the initial psychotic symptoms of schizophrenia. This diagnosis should be suspected whenever the delusions tend toward the bizarre, when the affect is blunted or inappropriate, or when a thought disorder is prominent. If the correct diagnosis is schizophrenia, this will usually become apparent with the passage of time.

Affective disorder should be suspected whenever the delusional content is depressive or expansive, when a preexisting affective illness is present, or when the family history is positive for one. Chronology of the delusions versus that of the depressive symptoms should help. Often the depressed patient will view the persecution as deserved and just punishment. With grandiose and erotomanic delusional disorders, the delusions may be so expansive as to be confused with manic depressive illness; however, in these subtypes, the psychomotor and vegetative symptoms of mania will be absent.

Hypochondriasis differs from somatic delusional disorder in that in the former the patient suspects the presence of an illness, whereas in the latter he or she is convinced of it.

Paranoid personality disorder presents a diagnostic problem when the suspiciousness becomes so pronounced that it resembles a delusion. However, these disorders never become truly delusional and are distinguished in this way from delusional disorders.

LABORATORY EXAMINATIONS

Several laboratory examinations are useful in ruling out other diseases that can present as a delusional disorder. Neuropsychological tests demonstrating organic brain damage raise the possibility of a dementia or an organic delusional syndrome. A positive drug screen for amphetamine or other substances known to cause delusions raises the possibility of a drug-induced organic delusional syndrome.

TREATMENT

Given the relative rarity of these disorders and the reluctance of these patients to be treated, it is not surprising that the treatment literature consists mainly of case series and reports. While there is no controlled trial on their effectiveness with these patients, a trial of neuroleptics seems to be warranted, given numerous anecdotal reports of substantial improvement with their use, particularly with patients suffering from delusional parasitosis. Among the neuroleptics, pimozide has been used more often; while some investigators claim its superiority over the other neuroleptics, this remains an open question (Munro, 1988). The use of antidepressants should be considered, given some case reports describing a good response to these agents, particularly for patients who show obsessive-compulsive or phobic features or have a family history of affective disorders or a previous personal history of affective disorders, even in the absence of a full depressive picture (Akiskal, 1983).

Some general guidelines are useful in the relationship with these sometimes difficult patients. It is particularly important to be honest, flexible, and noncontrolling in order to avoid being viewed as unsympathetic or even as another persecutor. It is thus important to identify how the patient suffers as a consequence of the delusions and to be empathic to this suffering.

An important issue concerns the confrontation of the delusional system. Most often it is better not to attack the delusional conviction directly. The therapist may help the patient more by questioning the consequences of the psychotic behavior and showing him or her how counterproductive acting on the delusional conviction can be. Sometimes, the therapist can help in further encapsulating the delusion by encouraging the patient to discuss it only within therapy sessions.

REFERENCES

Akiskal HS, Arana GW, Baldessarini RJ, Barreira BJ: A clinical report of thymoleptic-responsive atypical paranoid psychoses. Am J Psychiatr 140:1187–1190, 1983.

American Psychiatric Association: Diagnostic and Statistical Manual of Mental Disorders. Washington, American Psychiatric Association, 1952.

American Psychiatric Association: Diagnostic and Statistical Manual of Mental Disorders, 2d ed (DSM-II). Washington, American Psychiatric Association, 1968.

American Psychiatric Association: Diagnostic and Statistical Manual of Mental Disorders, 3d ed (DSM-III). Washington, American Psychiatric Association, 1980.

American Psychiatric Association: Diagnostic and Statistical Manual of Mental Disorders, 3d ed revised (DSM-III). Washington, American Psychiatric Association, 1987.

Crowe RR, Clarkson C, Tsai M, Wilson R: Delusional disorder: Jealous and nonjealous types. Eur Arch Psychiatr Neurol Sci 237:179–183, 1988.

Cummings JL: Organic psychoses: Delusional disorders and secondary mania. Psychiatr Clin North Am 9:293–311, 1086.

Debray Q: A genetic study of chronic delusions. Neuropsychobiology 1:313–321, 1985.

Freedman R, Schwab PJ: Paranoid symptoms in patients on a general hospital psychiatric unit: Implications for diagnosis and treatment. Arch Gen Psychiatry 35:387–390, 1978.

Goodwin DW, Guze SB: Psychiatric Diagnosis. New York, Oxford University Press, 1979.

Hollender MH, Callahan AS: Erotomania or deClerambault syndrome. Arch Gen Psychiatry 32:1574–1576, 1975.

Kahlbaum K: Die Gruppirung der Psychischen Krankheiten. Danzig, Kafemann, 1863.

Kendler KS: The nosologic validity of paranoia (simple delusional disorder): A review. Arch Gen Psychiatry 37:699–707, 1980.

Kendler KS: Demography of paranoid psychosis (delusional disorder): A review and comparison with schizophrenia and affective illness. Arch Gen Psychiatry 39:890–902, 1982.

Kendler KS, Hays P: Paranoid psychosis (delusional disorder) and schizophrenia: A family history study. Arch Gen Psychiatry 38:547–551, 1981.

Kendler KS, Gruenberg AM, Strauss JS: An independent analysis of the Copenhagen sample of the Danish adoption study of schizophrenia. Arch Gen Psychiatry 38:985–987, 1981.

Kendler KS, Masterson CC, Davis KL: Psychiatric illness in first-degree relatives of patients with paranoid psychosis, schizophrenia and medical illness. Br J Psychiatry 147:524–531, 1985.

Kolle K: Die Primare Verruckheit (Primary Paranoia). Leipzig, East Germany, Thieme, 1931.

Kraepelin E: Manic-Depressive Insanity and Paranoia, trans by Barclay RM. Edinburgh, E&S Livingstone, 1921.

Lewis A: Paranoia and paranoid: A historical perspective. Psychol Med 1:2–12, 1970.

Manschreck TC, Petri M: The paranoid syndrome. Lancet 2:251–253, 1978.

Mooney HB: Pathologic jealousy and psychochemotherapy. Br J Psychiatry 111:1023–1042, 1965.

Muncie W: Psychobiology in Psychiatry. St. Louis, CV Mosby, 1939.

Munro A: Monosymptomatic hypochondriacal psychosis. Br J Hosp Med 24:34–38, 1980.

Munro A: Delusional (paranoid) disorders: Etiologic and taxonomic considerations: II. A possible relationship between delusional and affective disorders. Can J Psychiatry 33:175–178, 1988.

Retterstol N: Paranoid and Paranoiac Psychoses. Springfield, IL, Charles C Thomas, 1966.

Retterstol N: Jealousy-paranoiac psychoses: A personal follow-up study. Acta Psychiatr Scand 43:75–107, 1967.

Sacks MH: Folie á Deux. Compr Psychiatry 29:270–277, 1988.

Seeman MV: Delusional loving. Arch Gen Psychiatry 35:1265–1267, 1978.

Segal JH: Erotomania revisited: From Kraepelin to DSM-IIIR. Am J Psychiatry 146:1261–1266, 1989.

Shepherd M: Morbid jealousy: Some clinical and social aspects of a psychiatric syndrome. J Ment Sci 197:687–753, 1961.

Tanna VL: Paranoid states: A selected review. Compr Psychiatry 15:453–470, 1974.

US Department of Health and Human Services: The International Classification of Diseases, 9th rev Clinical Modification (ICD-9 CM). DHHS publ. No. (PHS) 80–1260. Washington, Government Printing Office, 1980.

Winokur G: Familial psychopathology in delusional disorder. Compr Psychiatry 26:241–248, 1985.

Winokur G: Delusional disorder (paranoia). Compr Psychiatry 18:511–521, 1977.

Winokur G, Clayton PJ, Reich T: Manic-depressive Illness. St Louis, CV Mosby, 1969.

CHAPTER 9

Anxiety Disorders

RUSSELL NOYES, JR.
CRAIG S. HOLT

Anxiety is a prominent clinical feature of the disturbances grouped together under the heading of anxiety disorders in DSM-IIIR (American Psychiatric Association, 1987). These disorders include panic disorder, agoraphobia, generalized anxiety disorder, simple phobia, social phobia, obsessive-compulsive disorder, and posttraumatic stress disorder. The focus of anxiety in panic disorder is on panic attacks, whereas in generalized anxiety disorder it is on apprehensive expectation or worry about many threatening life circumstances. The anxiety in social and simple phobias is centered on objects or situations that evoke unreasonable fear. Finally, the anxiety of posttraumatic stress disorder is linked to reminders of a traumatic event and is focused on perceived environmental threats.

Together these disorders have a lifetime prevalence in the general population of 10 to 20 percent; thus they are among the most prevalent of all mental disorders. They, along with the mood and substance use disorders, make up the three largest groups in terms of their occurrence. Although most anxiety disorders are mild in comparison with the major psychiatric illnesses (e.g., usually treated as outpatients), they tend to be chronic and to cause substantial morbidity. Even so, the majority of anxiety disorders go untreated. This is unfortunate, because available drug and behavioral therapies are quite effective (Noyes, 1991a). In fact, much of the renewed interest in these disorders in the past decade and a half has resulted from the discovery of effective treatments.

In addition to effective treatment, the new classification of psychiatric disorders has stimulated research and clinical interest in the anxiety disorders (American Psychiatric Association, 1980). However, a number of issues remain unsettled with regard to the DSM-IIIR classification. One of these has to do with whether certain categories should be separated from one another. The separation of generalized anxiety disorder from panic disorder and panic disorder from agoraphobia remains controversial (Noyes, 1988). Another issue concerns the relationship between coexisting disorders. Most patients with anxiety disorders have coexisting conditions, and the functional relationships between them are often unclear. Still another issue has to do with where the threshold for various disorders should be established. For example, many people experience panic attacks, but at what frequency do they constitute a disorder?

PANIC DISORDER AND AGORAPHOBIA

Definition

Panic disorder is named for its essential feature, recurrent panic attacks. These attacks are characterized by sudden intense anxiety, together with autonomic nervous system arousal. Typically, panic attacks last minutes and, at least initially, are unexpected; that is, they occur without exposure to phobic objects or situations. Other manifestations of the illness include anticipatory anxiety and agoraphobic symptoms.

Classification

Diagnostic criteria for panic disorder are as follows:

A. At some time during the disturbance, one or more panic attacks (discrete periods of intense fear or discomfort) have occurred that were (1) unexpected (i.e., did not occur immediately before or on exposure to a situation that almost always caused anxiety) and (2) not triggered by situations in which the person was the focus of others' attention.

B. Either four attacks, as defined in criterion A, have occurred within a 4-week period, or one or more attacks have been followed by a period of at least a month of persistent fear of having another attack.

C. At least four of the following symptoms developed during at least one of the attacks:
   1. Shortness of breath (dyspnea) or smothering sensations
   2. Dizziness, unsteady feelings, or faintness
   3. Palpitations or accelerated heart rate (tachycardia)
   4. Trembling or shaking
   5. Sweating
   6. Choking
   7. Nausea or abdominal distress
   8. Depersonalization or derealization
   9. Numbness or tingling sensations (paresthesias)
   10. Flushes (hot flashes) or chills
   11. Chest pain or discomfort
   12. Fear of dying
   13. Fear of going crazy or of doing something uncontrolled

D. During at least some of the attacks, at least four of the criteria C symptoms developed suddenly and increased in intensity within 10 minutes of the beginning of the first symptom of the attack.

E. It cannot be established that an organic factor initiated and maintained the disturbance (e.g., amphetamine or caffeine intoxication, hyperthyroidism).

In the majority of cases, persons with panic disorder develop symptoms of agoraphobia. Agoraphobia consists of fear of places or situations from which escape might be difficult (or embarrassing) or in which help might not be available in the event of a panic attack. As a result of this fear, persons find they are unable to travel or need to have a companion in order to do so. Common agoraphobic situations include being away from home alone, being in crowded places, or, standing in a line, or traveling in a car, bus, or plane.

Etiology

GENETIC FACTORS

Although the cause of panic disorder, is unknown, genetic factors appear to be important. Family studies have found the same disorder in 18 percent of first-degree relatives compared with 2 percent of control relatives. Sixty percent of panic disorder patients have at least one similarly affected family member compared with 15 percent of controls (Crowe, 1990). Female relatives are at greater risk than males, but male relatives more often develop

alcoholism. Twin studies provide further evidence for the importance of hereditary factors. Monozygotic twins have a higher concordance rate (45 percent) than dizygotic twins (15 percent) (Torgersen, 1983). The mode of inheritance has not been determined, but a single autosomal locus predisposing to the disease has not been ruled out.

BIOLOGIC FACTORS

Studies of autonomic function in panic disorder patients show physiologic activation. Baseline measures of heart rate, blood pressure, and skin conductance usually show elevations (Nesse et al., 1984). However, these elevations are correlated with the level of anxiety, and no changes have been observed during sleep or nonanxious parts of the day. Autonomic activation also occurs in response to psychological stimuli such as exposure to phobic situations. Thus, autonomic arousal accompanies anxiety, but whether it is a cause or an effect of panic or panic vulnerability is unclear.

The early observation of elevations in blood lactate after exercise in patients with anxiety neurosis prompted investigators to infuse this metabolic by-product in an attempt to reproduce anxiety symptoms (Pitts and McClure, 1967). Sodium lactate consistently causes panic attacks in most panic disorder patients but not normal controls. However, the mechanism remains unknown; while hypocalcemia and alkalosis have been proposed, neither has received strong support. Also, a phobic response to perceived internal change has been offered as an alternative explanation.

Hyperventilation may play a role in the pathogenesis of panic. Studies have found evidence for chronic hyperventilation in panic patients, and forced overbreathing produces panic symptoms. The finding that carbon dioxide inhalation provokes panic also has suggested that respiratory dysfunction may be involved. The mechanism, like that of lactate-induced panic, is not understood. Hypotheses include CO_2-induced firing of the locus ceruleus, hypersensitivity of the suffocation alarm mechanism, and stimulation of brainstem chemoreceptors (Gorman et al., 1988a). However, cognitive factors also may play a role.

A variety of physical illnesses are associated with panic-like symptoms, and the possibility that panic disorder may be a manifestation of underlying organ system pathology has been considered. Abnormalities in the cardiovascular, vestibular, and gastrointestinal systems have received attention. Mitral valve prolapse has been found in a high proportion of patients with panic disorder, but the meaning of the relationship remains unclear. The lack of an association between panic and mitral prolapse in family and community studies suggests that ascertainment bias may explain the relationship observed in clinical samples (Gorman et al., 1988b). Preliminary studies of vestibular function have shown abnormalities in panic patients. The finding of irritable bowel syndrome in 40 percent of patients with panic disorder suggests that there may be a relationship between these disorders.

Neurochemical Abnormalities
There is strong evidence for the involvement of the noradrenergic system in panic disorder (Charney et al., 1990). This neurotransmitter system mediates arousal, and increased noradrenergic activity causes hyperarousal and anxiety. The noradrenergic hypothesis was originally based on studies showing that activation of the locus ceruleus produced fear in monkeys (Redmond, 1979). Evidence supporting the hypothesis comes from several sources, including the demonstration of increased norepinephrine and its metabolite, MHPG, in the cerebrospinal fluid and plasma of anxious patients. Also, drugs that increase the synaptic availability of norepinephrine, such as yohimbine, can induce anxiety. In addition, a number of challenge tests have demonstrated increased sensitivity to norepinephrine uptake blockers and postsynaptic adrenoceptor down-regulation. These abnormalities point to excessive reactivity of the adrenergic system rather than excessive tone.

DEVELOPMENTAL FACTORS

Developmental factors are thought to play a role in the occurrence of panic disorder and agoraphobia. In some studies, agoraphobics viewed their parents as having been more overprotective. Epidemiologic studies have found relationships between parental death or divorce during childhood and the occurrence of panic disorder or agoraphobia in the general population (Tweed et al., 1989). Such findings fit with the hypothesized role of separation anxiety in the development of this disorder (Gittleman and Klein, 1985). Stressful life events of various kinds are commonly associated with the onset of panic disorder, although the importance of such events is unknown.

PERSONALITY FACTORS

Recently, behavioral inhibition has been identified in the young children of agoraphobic parents and in children with anxiety disorders (Biederman et al., 1990). This disturbance of social interaction may be a temperamental antecedent of adult panic disorder. Patients with panic disorder have more dependent, avoidant, and histrionic personality traits compared with nonanxious controls. Such traits improve with treatment, but whether they represent a premorbid disturbance or the influence of anxiety on personality functioning is difficult to determine.

COGNITIVE FACTORS

Cognitive disturbances appear to contribute to panic vulnerability. These abnormalities include preoccupation with and sensitivity to bodily sensations and vigilance toward environmental threats, anticipation of harm, catastrophic thoughts, and perceived lack of safety. However, the origin of the cognitive disturbances remains unclear; they may be the cause or the result of panic anxiety. Peripheral physiologic change may trigger panic by way of conditioned emotional responses or learned perceptual associations (Barlow, 1988). Studies have shown that panic disorder patients misinterpret bodily sensations and have catastrophic thoughts related to them (e.g., "I must be having a heart attack") at the start of attacks.

Epidemiology

Recent epidemiologic studies have found lifetime rates for panic disorder ranging between 0.1 and 2.2 percent and for agoraphobia between 3.8 and 4.3 percent (Oakley-Browne and Joyce, in press). These figures are consistent with earlier estimates of 2 to 5 percent for anxiety neurosis (DSM-II). According to the epidemiologic catchment area (ECA) study, nearly 10 percent of the population have experienced at least one panic attack, and a smaller proportion have had recurrent attacks (Regier et al., 1984). Only a small proportion of those who have recurrent attacks qualify for the diagnosis of panic disorder. However, the level of impairment associated with recurrent attacks suggests that the threshold for the disorder is too conservative in DSM-IIIR.

Data from the ECA study have shown morbidity associated with panic disorder comparable with that associated with major depression (Markowitz et al., 1989). Poor marital adjustment, financial dependency, alcohol abuse, and suicide attempts were all reported by similar proportions of subjects with panic disorder and major depression. In addition, data from this study showed that health care utilization by persons with panic disorder is three times that of persons with no disorder. Most seek treatment from primary-care physicians, to whom they typically present somatic symptoms referable to the cardiovascular, neurologic, or gastrointestinal systems (Katon, 1991). As many as 13 percent of primary-care patients meet criteria for panic disorder with or without major depression.

Community surveys have found that the prevalence of panic disorder is highest in the 25 to 44 age group and that it declines thereafter (Eaton et al., 1991). This is consistent with the age of onset from clinic populations of about 25, with a range of 15 to 35 years. Women are affected twice or three times as often as men, but the reason for this female preponderance is unknown. The occurrence of panic and agoraphobia in the general population is associated with divorced marital status and low social class. Such environmental factors may contribute to the development of the disorder but also may reflect the influence of the disorder on social functioning.

Clinical Picture

PANIC ATTACKS

Panic or anxiety attacks are characterized by the sudden onset of extreme anxiety and autonomic arousal like that caused by life-threatening danger. Most attacks occur spontaneously and may even awaken a person from sleep, although they may be provoked by strong emotion, excitement, or even physical exertion. Persons having panic attacks report that they feel suddenly frightened for no reason. They may feel as though electricity is passing through their body. Their heart may pound, and they may feel as though blood is rushing to their face. Some report that their legs feel wobbly and that their sense of imbalance is impaired.

Anxiety of panic proportions is accompanied by a feeling of impending doom or the thought that something terrible is about to happen. Patients feel that they may lose control of themselves (e.g., faint, urinate, or cry out) or experience serious illness (e.g., a heart attack or stroke). At the height of their anxiety, many feel that they are about to die.

During attacks, patients are visibly distressed and show obvious physiologic signs of anxiety. They are often pale, with a fearful expression and pleading manner. Many have a rapid pulse and labored breathing; others are diaphoretic and tremulous. Their behavior is motivated by an overpowering urge to escape from circumstances that are perceived as being dangerous. This takes many to emergency rooms in search of lifesaving interventions.

Between attacks, most patients experience some degree of generalized anxiety. They find themselves worried, anxious, and fearful. Many ruminate about future attacks and what might be done to avoid them.

AGORAPHOBIA

The majority of patients develop agoraphobic symptoms. Agoraphobia consists of fear related to situations from which escape might be difficult or help might not be readily available. Commonly feared situations include crowds, travel, and being alone. Agoraphobic patients avoid such situations or enter them only when accompanied by a trusted companion. Phobic situations often provoke panic attacks accompanied by a strong impulse to escape from immediate surroundings. The agoraphobic person is distressed not only by phobic situations but also by the anticipation of having to confront them. Such persons become preoccupied with arranging activities so as to minimize their discomfort, but as activities are given up, their lives become increasingly restricted.

Course and Complications

COURSE

Commonly, a spontaneous panic attack is the abrupt, initial manifestation of panic disorder, although many patients report a period of increasing generalized anxiety. Regardless of its timing, the first attack often leaves a lasting and painful impression. As mentioned, precipitating events or circumstances are often associated with the onset of symptoms. These include emotionally disturbing events, such as the death of a family member, divorce, and financial loss. Physical illness, surgical procedures, and events associated with hormonal change, such as pregnancy, childbirth, and menopause, also may be associated with initial symptoms.

Typically, panic disorder follows a chronic, fluctuating course, although remissions and exacerbations are experienced by some patients. Most patients report that their symptoms are reactive to life circumstances and are most severe during periods of environmental stress. A favorable outcome is found in half of psychiatric patients and two-thirds of general medical patients (Noyes et al., 1990). Agoraphobic symptoms impose restrictions on the activities of many patients. As a consequence, some are unable to work or engage in social activities, and a few, with severe agoraphobic symptoms, become housebound.

A number of predictors of poor long-term outcome have emerged from follow-up studies (Noyes, 1992). Several of these, including more severe anxiety symptoms, greater phobic avoidance, and longer duration of illness, reflect greater severity and chronicity of illness. Others, such as the presence of a personality disorder or major depression, involve coexisting disturbances. Demographic factors predictive of poor outcome include female gender and low socioeconomic status.

COMPLICATIONS

The most common complications of panic disorder are depression and alcohol abuse. Secondary depression (i.e., depression that begins after the primary disorder) develops in about half patients (Lesser, 1990). Such depression is usually mild and reactive to environmental circumstances. In some it is precipitated by distressing events; in others it is associated with worsening symptoms. Depression may explain the increased risk of suicide in patients with panic disorder (Noyes, 1991b).

Alcohol abuse complicates panic disorder in about 20 percent of patients (Kushner et al., 1990). Patients who use alcohol in an effort to control their symptoms may become dependent on the substance. Likewise, a small proportion of patients who use benzodiazepines find themselves increasing the dose to achieve the same effect; others have difficulty discontinuing their use. Dependence on these drugs occasionally results from overzealous prescribing by physicians.

Whether physical illness is a complication of anxiety disorders remains an unanswered question. Long-standing increases in sympathetic arousal have been hypothesized to explain high rates of peptic ulcer and hypertension observed in some panic subjects (Katon, 1991). The finding of excess mortality in panic disorder patients followed for 35 years suggests this possibility (Coryell et al., 1982). A portion of the excess appeared to have been due to cardiovascular disease in men.

Differential Diagnosis

PHYSICAL ILLNESS

The differential diagnosis of panic disorder includes a variety of physical as well as psychiatric illnesses. A number of cardiac, neurologic, and endocrine disorders are commonly associated with episodic symptoms that resemble panic attacks (Raj and Sheehan, 1987).

The most common cardiac conditions associated with recurrent attacks are angina pectoris and cardiac arrhythmias. Angina is characterized by episodes of chest pain, dyspnea, and palpitations that are precipitated by exercise or emotional stress. The diagnosis may depend on coronary arteriography when symptoms are atypical. Recent studies have shown that a high proportion of patients with chest pain and negative angiography or treadmill tests have panic disorder (Beitman et al., 1987). Cardiac arrhythmias may cause palpitation, chest discomfort, dyspnea, and faintness. The diagnosis of an arrhythmia is made by identifying the abnormal rhythm during an attack. Portable monitoring may facilitate this.

Hypoglycemia is seldom associated with anxiety symptoms. A low blood glucose level is accompanied by sweating, weakness, hunger, tremor, and headache and may be confirmed by measurement of blood glucose levels during an acute episode. Reactive hypoglycemia is identified by an oral glucose tolerance test during which the glucose level falls below 45 mg/dl.

Hypoparathyroidism is associated with anxiety symptoms in a minority of patients. Symptoms include muscle cramps and paresthesias of the hands, feet, and mouth. Carpopedal spasm is a diagnostic sign. Useful diagnostic tests include serum calcium and phosphorous levels.

Partial complex seizures may be accompanied by fear or anxiety either as part of the aura or as part of the seizure itself. An electroencephalogram, using nasopharyngeal leads or continuous monitoring, is used to establish the diagnosis.

PSYCHIATRIC ILLNESS

Panic attacks may accompany almost any psychiatric illness. Most commonly they are associated with mood disorders and other anxiety disorders such as phobic disorders, obsessive-compulsive disorder, and posttraumatic stress disorder. Such attacks occur in 20 percent of patients with major depression, making the differential diagnosis difficult. Panic disorder has an earlier onset, and when panic attacks appear for the first time after age 40, they are commonly part of a depressive syndrome. Because panic disorder is chronic, a history of discrete episodes suggests depression. A family history of depression also suggests an affective disorder diagnosis.

Panic symptoms are also shared by phobic disorders. Both simple and social phobias may have panic-like attacks, but they are confined to phobic situations. Panic-like symptoms also may occur in patients with generalized anxiety disorder on exposure to stressful situations or excessive worry, but the attacks in panic disorder patients often occur without worry.

Anxiety symptoms are also prominent in patients with posttraumatic stress disorder. Emotionally traumatic events are associated with the onset of this disorder and form its mental content. The diagnosis depends on establishing a connection between a traumatic event and the ensuing disturbance.

Treatment

Effective treatment of panic disorder rests on establishing and communicating the diagnosis. Of course, examination and reassurance are important initial steps when patients present with acute symptoms. These measures not only rule out more serious illness but also have an important anxiety-relieving function. In the face of persisting symptoms, education becomes important. Discussion of the diagnosis and prognosis forms a basis for understanding and accepting the condition.

DRUG THERAPY

Except in the mildest cases, drug treatment should be considered for patients with panic disorder. It may provide temporary control of acute symptoms and long-term reduction of chronic ones. The goal is control rather than permanent relief of symptoms, because relapse after stopping effective drug therapy is common. The most useful drugs belong to four classes: tricyclic antidepressants, monoamine oxidase inhibitors, benzodiazepines, and serotonin uptake blockers (Noyes, 1991a).

The tricyclic compound imipramine is the treatment of choice for panic disorder. Imipramine blocks panic attacks and may relieve generalized anxiety as well. Of those who tolerate the drug, nearly 70 percent report at least moderate improvement, and most become free of panic attacks. A few patients respond to less than 100 mg daily, but others require 200 mg or more. Anxiety symptoms are relieved gradually, and improvement may not be maximal for 6 weeks. Because some patients are sensitive to its side effects, the drug is often started at a dose of 25 mg and increased by 25 mg every 3 days.

Once a patient has responded to imipramine, the dose may be reduced gradually to a maintenance level where improvement is sustained. After 6 to 12 months, it should be discontinued gradually to assess continuing need. Other tricyclic compounds also may be effective, and drugs such as nortriptyline and desipramine may be better tolerated. Clomipramine may be effective in low dose (i.e., 25 to 100 mg daily). Imipramine is a relatively safe drug for long-term administration; still, about a third of patients gain weight on the drug, and an overdose may be life-threatening.

Patients who fail to respond to imipramine should be switched to phenelzine. This monoamine oxidase inhibitor is very effective, but because of the need for a tyramine-free diet and the risk of hypertensive crises, it is usually reserved for patients who have failed to respond to other drugs. Postural hypotension and initial insomnia are sometimes troublesome side effects, and weight gain may occur later on. Tranylcypromine is less likely to produce postural hypotension and weight gain. The serotonin uptake–blocking drug, fluoxetine, has been shown recently to be an effective antipanic agent.

In controlled studies, alprazolam has been shown to be effective and well tolerated for panic disorder (Ballenger et al., 1988). In doses of up to 6 mg daily, the drug frees the majority of patients from panic attacks. Sedation, when it occurs, usually subsides in a few days or responds to a reduction of dose. The drug should not be given to patients who have a history of alcohol or drug abuse, nor should it be given without warning patients of its habit-forming potential (Noyes et al., 1988). Because response to the drug is rapid, it is useful for achieving prompt control of symptoms. Other benzodiazepines, such as clonazepam, also appear to be effective.

COGNITIVE AND BEHAVIORAL THERAPY

Patients with panic disorder who have phobic avoidance should receive exposure in vivo regardless of whether they are given a drug to control panic attacks (Marks, 1987). Studies have shown that this is the most effective behavioral intervention and that it significantly reduces agoraphobia in about 70 percent of patients. In its simplest form, exposure consists of therapist instructions for patients to challenge themselves in phobic situations. Some patients respond to this approach alone; the remainder require therapist supervision of practice sessions in which they expose themselves to progressively more difficult situations. Because behavior and drug therapies interact positively, they should usually be administered together.

Cognitive behavioral treatment also may be effective for panic disorder without agoraphobia (Barlow, 1988). With use of this approach, panic attacks can be eliminated by exposure to bodily sensations that trigger attacks. These sensations (e.g., palpitations, light-headedness) often prompt catastrophic interpretations which lead to panic.

Patients are taught to elicit these sensations by spinning, running in place, hyperventilating, and so on to produce habituation. In addition, patients are informed about the origin of panic symptoms and the role of fearful cognitions in maintaining them. Cognitive restructuring is used to correct catastrophic misinterpretations of symptoms and stimulate more adaptive thinking. Symptom-management techniques, such as breathing retraining and relaxation training, are also effective in reducing symptoms (Barlow and Craske, 1989).

GENERALIZED ANXIETY DISORDER

Definition

The essential feature of generalized anxiety disorder (GAD) is unrealistic or excessive worry (apprehensive expectation) about life circumstances. Common sources of such worry include health, finances, social acceptance, job performance, and marital adjustment. When anxious, individuals with this disorder experience symptoms of central nervous system arousal (vigilance and scanning), motor tension, and autonomic hyperactivity. DSM-IIIR allows the diagnosis of GAD to be made in the presence of other anxiety disorders, providing the focus of worry is not a manifestation of the other disorder (American Psychiatric Association, 1987). That is, worry must not be centered on panic attacks, as in panic disorder.

Classification

Diagnostic criteria for generalized anxiety disorder are as follows:

A. Unrealistic or excessive anxiety and worry (apprehensive expectation) about two or more life circumstances for a period of 6 months or longer, during which the person has been bothered more days than not by these concerns.
B. If another disorder is present, the focus of the anxiety and worry is unrelated to it.
C. The disturbance does not occur only during the course of a mood disorder or a psychotic disorder.
D. At least 6 of the following 18 symptoms are often present when anxious (does not include symptoms present only during panic attacks):

Motor tension
  1. Trembling, twitching, or feeling shaky
  2. Muscle tension, aches, or soreness
  3. Restlessness
  4. Easy fatigability

Autonomic hyperactivity
  5. Shortness of breath or smothering sensations
  6. Palpitations or accelerated heart rate (tachycardia)

7. Sweating or cold, clammy hands
8. Dry mouth
9. Dizziness or light-headedness
10. Nausea, diarrhea, or other abdominal distress
11. Flushes (hot flashes) or chills
12. Frequent urination
13. Trouble swallowing, or "lump in throat"

Vigilance and scanning
14. Feeling keyed up or on edge
15. Exaggerated startle response
16. Difficulty concentrating or "mind going blank" because of anxiety
17. Trouble falling or staying asleep
18. Irritability

E. It cannot be established that an organic factor initiated and maintained the disturbance (e.g., hyperthyroidism, caffeine intoxication).

Generalized anxiety disorder (GAD) was originally a residual category created in DSM-III by removing panic disorder from anxiety neurosis (American Psychiatric Association, 1980). Although it is more precisely defined and given equal status in DSM-IIIR, the diagnosis remains controversial (American Psychiatric Association, 1987). Phenomenologically, GAD resembles normal anxiety or the reaction to stressful circumstances. Generalized anxiety symptoms accompany many other anxiety and mood disorders and often represent a prodrome or residual of such disorders. GAD is perhaps the most common coexisting disorder among patients with other anxiety disorders, and the distinction between them is not always clear (Di Nardo and Barlow, 1990).

Etiology

Little can be said about the etiology of GAD because few studies have been done and findings have been inconsistent. Epidemiologic data suggest that environmental stressors play an important role in the occurrence of generalized anxiety symptoms, supporting earlier studies in which a variety of stressors appeared to be responsible for the emergence and persistence of anxiety symptoms (Blazer et al., 1991).

A preliminary family study showed that while relatives of persons with GAD were more likely to have the same disorder, life events were important in the development of the illness in relatives (Noyes et al., 1987). One twin study showed no difference in concordance for generalized anxiety disorder among monozygotic compared with dizygotic twins (Torgersen, 1983). However, the results of a large twin registry study showed that genetic factors accounted for most of the variance in the occurrence of GAD among twin pairs.

EDITORS' COMMENT

The definition of the illness requires that a GAD diagnosis not be made in the presence of a major depression. In addition, *worry* is one of the 10 most common symptoms elicited in patients with primary unipolar depression (Clayton et al., *Am J Psychiatry* 148:1512–1517, 1991). Kendler et al. (*Arch Gen Psychiatry* 49:716–722, 1992) recently reported that in female twins the liability to major depression and GAD is influenced by the same genetic factors. It may well be that if we absorbed some patients with GAD into major depression and others into adjustment disorder with anxious mood, we would not need the category of GAD.

PHYSIOLOGIC ABNORMALITIES

The hyperarousal reported by patients with GAD is evident in electroencephalographic and sleep recordings. Anxious patients typically have reduced alpha activity, poor alpha organization, and increased beta activity (Koella, 1981). With respect to sleep pattern, GAD patients, unlike those with depression, have reduced stage I sleep and reduced rapid eye movement (REM) sleep. Patient reports of muscle tension are also supported by physiologic measures.

The increased arousal that manifests itself in heightened alertness and increased muscle tension appears to be associated with inhibition of the autonomic nervous system. Studies have shown that compared with normal persons, anxious subjects show few differences in heart rate, skin conductance, and catecholamine levels. In response to stimulation, however, these subjects show a less reactive skin conductance response that is slower to return to resting levels. Hoehn-Saric and McLeod (1988) have referred to this phenomenon as *reduced autonomic flexibility*.

Endocrine function in GAD patients differs little from that in normal controls. Few differences in catecholamines, cortisol, and thyroid levels have been found.

NEUROCHEMICAL ABNORMALITIES

Understanding of the neurobiology of anxiety has come from study of the action of pharmacologic agents that reduce anxiety. The benzodiazepines have been the most widely used drugs, and the discovery of benzodiazepine receptors in the brain has been of major importance in this regard (Insel et al., 1984). Benzodiazepines facilitate synaptic transmission within the gamma-aminobutyric acid (GABA) neurotransmitter system and act on benzodiazepine receptors to produce their modulatory action. These receptors are unique in mediating not only the effects of benzodiazepine agonists, which reduce anxiety, but also the effects of inverse agonists, such as beta-carbolines, which generate anxiety in animals and humans. A search for compounds synthesized in the central nervous system that are endogenous ligands continues.

Studies of the locus ceruleus in monkeys have yielded evidence for involvement of the noradrenergic neurotransmitter system in anxiety (Redmond, 1979). Electrical and pharmacologic activation of this nucleus produces behaviors like those observed in monkeys exposed to threats in the wild. In contrast, electrical lesions and pharmacologic inhibition of this nucleus abolish these behaviors. Also, drugs that increase locus ceruleus activity, such as yohimbine and piperoxane, or that decrease locus activity, such as clonidine and benzodiazepines, have anxiogenic and anxiolytic properties in humans.

The serotonergic neurotransmitter system is also regarded as having an important role in the neurochemistry of anxiety. The discovery of antagonists that inhibit serotonin activity in the brain and that reduce the psychological and somatic symptoms of anxiety suggests involvement of this system.

Epidemiology

Data from the ECA study, using DSM-III criteria, show that GAD is one of the most common anxiety disorders (Blazer et al., 1991). The 1-year prevalence was estimated at 2.0 to 3.6 percent and the lifetime prevalence at 4.1 to 6.6 percent of the population. Rates were higher in women, blacks, and persons under age 30. The disorder was associated with low occupational status and low income. Also, unmarried persons had a higher prevalence than married persons. The data showed that most persons with GAD had had at least one other psychiatric disorder, the most common being panic disorder and major depression.

Persons with the disorder made increased use of mental health services, but use of general health services was not affected. Most patients with GAD are treated by primary-care physicians. The prevalence in one medical clinic was found to be 4.6 percent (Von Korff et al., 1987). The disorder is common among persons with chronic physical conditions but the relationship to these conditions is not known.

Clinical Picture

The symptoms of GAD involve both psychological and somatic spheres. Psychological symptoms fall under the headings of apprehensive expectation and vigilance and scanning, whereas somatic symptoms are grouped under muscle tension and autonomic hyperactivity. Apprehensive expectation is the hallmark of GAD. Patients find themselves worried, anxious, or fearful. Many ruminate about unfortunate events that might happen, such as the death of a family member, financial disaster, social rejection, serious illness, or job termination. Anxious preoccupation about such events persists despite recognition that the concern is unrealistic. Some patients focus on stressful circumstances or uncertainties about which they worry excessively.

Vigilance and scanning typically accompany such anxious cognitions. Many patients feel tense, keyed up, or restless and find it difficult to relax. Persons with GAD have a tendency to startle and find themselves irritable and impatient. Their concentration is often poor, and some experience memory difficulty. At night their minds remain active so that they have difficulty in falling asleep, and later, they sleep in a fitful and interrupted manner. Dreams of an anxiety-provoking character are frequent.

Muscular tension is also a typical feature. Patients experience aching and tightness in their muscles, especially across the shoulders and back of the neck, and frequently have tension headaches. Muscle tension is often accompanied by restlessness, trembling, and easy fatigability.

Autonomic hyperactivity often involves both the sympathetic and parasympathetic nervous systems. Many patients report palpitations, sweating, and symptoms associated with hyperventilation, such as tightness in the chest, light-headedness, numbness, and tingling. Others report dry mouth, abdominal distress, nausea, diarrhea, or urinary frequency, all parasympathetic symptoms. Some patients eat to relieve tension and gain weight as a consequence, although weight loss also may occur.

Associated features include symptoms of other anxiety disorders and avoidant behavior. Some patients experience infrequent panic attacks, but such patients probably have subsyndromal panic disorder. Simple and social phobic features also may be present. At times the anxious ruminations of patients with GAD take on an obsessional quality and may be difficult to distinguish from obsessive-compulsive symptoms. Also, patients tend to avoid activities that increase their symptoms, such as risk taking, exposure to criticism, and confronting stressful life circumstances.

Course and Complications

The average age of onset for GAD is 21 years, although the range covers the lifespan (Thyer et al., 1985). Many patients report that they have been nervous all their lives but that symptoms were made worse by life stressors. Stressful events are often associated with the onset, and the severity of the disorder often depends on the number and severity of perceived external stressors. As currently defined, GAD is a chronic disorder lasting at least 6 months. The illness has a prolonged course with symptoms that fluctuate in severity over time (Anderson et al., 1984; Barlow et al., 1986).

GAD is, compared with panic disorder and major depression, a relatively mild disturbance. Persons with the illness make up only about 10 percent of the anxious patients seen by psychiatrists. Nevertheless, work efficiency is often reduced by poor concentration or fatigue, and interpersonal relations are strained by irritability and impatience.

Patients also tend to become overly conscientious or excitable and disorganized under stress.

The most common complications are depression or substance abuse. Mild depressive symptoms commonly coexist with GAD, and many patients experience one or more episodes of major depression over the course of the illness (Breslau and Davis, 1985). Some patients use alcohol or drugs to control symptoms but, in the course of so doing, develop problems related to substance abuse.

Differential Diagnosis

The differential diagnosis of GAD includes a variety of physical as well as psychiatric illnesses. However, most of these are uncommon and cause few diagnostic problems. Hyperthyroidism is the most common endocrine disturbance associated with a generalized anxiety syndrome. Symptoms include palpitations, insomnia, sweating, heat intolerance, increased appetite, and diarrhea. Signs include tachycardia, tremor, weight loss, and warm, moist skin. A diffuse goiter and exophthalmos are often present. The diagnosis is established by tests of thyroid function.

Pheochromocytoma is a rare, catecholamine-secreting tumor of the adrenal medulla. Flushing and headache are prominent, and sustained hypertension is present in most patients who have this tumor. A urine metanephrine assay is usually diagnostic.

Certain medications may be associated with generalized anxiety symptoms. Caffeine may produce symptoms when the daily intake exceeds 250 mg. The diagnosis is confirmed when symptoms disappear after discontinuation of the drug. Other substances that may produce anxiety symptoms include nicotine, cocaine, and alcohol. Medications that may cause anxiety include ephedrine, aminophylline, amphetamines, methylphenidate, phenmetrazine, levodopa, antihistamines, indomethacin, and thyroid preparations.

Discontinuation of alcohol and various other substances is often associated with a withdrawal syndrome that includes generalized anxiety symptoms. Withdrawal symptoms include anxiety, insomnia, tremor, restlessness, ataxia, nausea, loss of appetite, and so on. This syndrome is perhaps the most common cause of a missed diagnosis in patients whose substance abuse is not suspected. Signs of autonomic hyperarousal include tachycardia, diaphoresis, flushing, tremor, and nausea. Abnormal liver function tests are often present. Other drugs that may be associated with anxious withdrawal syndromes are benzodiazepines, barbiturates, sedatives, hypnotics, and opiates. Short-acting drugs, such as alprazolam, are especially prone to withdrawal reactions.

Generalized anxiety symptoms may accompany almost any psychiatric disorder. The most common of these are mood and other anxiety disorders. Anxiety symptoms are often prominent in patients with depression (e.g., anxious or agitated depression), making the differential diagnosis difficult.

Treatment

When patients present mild symptoms in association with psychosocial stressors, nonpharmacologic treatment may be satisfactory. With more severe or persistent symptoms, some combination of drug and nondrug therapies may be considered. Psychological treatments include supportive psychotherapy, self-regulatory therapies, and behavior therapies. Pharmacologic treatments include the benzodiazepines, azaspirones (buspirone), and tricyclic antidepressants.

Patients will often benefit from an explanation of their symptoms and what affects them. Symptoms that are described as part of the "fight or flight" response or as a surge of adrenalin may seem less alarming. Also, muscle tension may lead to aching and hyperventilation to light-headedness and paresthesias. Patients should be aware that caffeine, nicotine, and alcohol may increase symptoms as well as fatigue and loss of sleep. Environmental stress usually increases symptoms even when it is not the cause of them.

PSYCHOLOGICAL TREATMENT

Patients seeking help for GAD often feel overwhelmed and demoralized (Frank, 1984). They feel that they are losing control and do not know where to turn. Supportive counseling or therapy can reverse these trends. The physician should give the patient an opportunity to talk about work or family problems and help him or her see connections between these and recent symptoms. Ways to modify circumstances to reduce distress may then be explored. Brief sessions on a weekly basis may provide considerable relief.

Self-regulatory treatments include relaxation, biofeedback, and meditation (Goldberg, 1982). These produce a relaxation response that can lessen anxiety and reduce the feeling of loss of control. The method of progressive relaxation involves systematic tensing and relaxing of muscle groups. Electromyographic and electrodermal feedback and transcendental meditation also may be useful where they are available and appeal to patients. However, like relaxation, they take effect gradually and must be practiced regularly.

Relaxation is often combined with one or more cognitive or behavioral techniques to achieve greater benefit. These techniques aim at modifying avoidant behavior or anxious cognitions that accompany generalized anxiety. One behavioral strategy, known as *anxiety symptom management*, has several components designed to reduce anxious cognitions. These include an explanation of anxiety symptoms, training in distraction, and practice in counterbalancing anxious thoughts with reassuring, rational ones.

PHARMACOLOGIC TREATMENT

Drug treatment is indicated for patients with more severe or persistent symptoms. Such treatment should usually be administered for short periods of time along with nondrug interventions (Hollister, 1979). This approach is consistent with the natural, fluctuating course of generalized anxiety. Of course, patients who are likely to abuse medications should not receive agents with dependence potential. These include patients who have previously abused alcohol or drugs or patients with unstable personalities. Benzodiazepines continue to be the most widely prescribed drugs for generalized anxiety.

Diazepam remains the standard among benzodiazepines, although some newer high-potency agents, such as alprazolam, may be less sedating in equivalent dosage. Ten milligrams of diazepam at bedtime may be effective in promoting sleep as well as reducing daytime anxiety. However, dose adjustment within the range of 5 to 30 mg daily is important to achieve maximum benefit and minimize side effects. If necessary, one-third of the daily dose may be taken at noon. The range for alprazolam is 0.5 to 3.0 mg daily, and this should be given in divided doses. Sedation is dose-related and tends to subside with a reduction in dose or continued use.

Benzodiazepines should be taken on a regular basis for a few days to a few weeks to give patients a respite from anxiety. During this period, factors contributing to anxiety may subside, or action may be taken to modify them. Patients may then be encouraged to reduce the dose, take the drug on an "as necessary" basis, and finally discontinue it. Long-acting drugs such as diazepam or prazepam have the advantage of a built-in tapering effect when stopped (Hollister, 1979). They also may be given once daily, at bedtime, thus eliminating the daytime titration of dose that can lead to dependence. Even after stopping the drug, many patients are comforted by the knowledge that relief is available should they need it.

Tricyclic antidepressants are also useful in the treatment of patients with generalized anxiety, particularly when depressive symptoms are prominent. Sedating tricyclics such as doxepin and amitriptyline act rapidly and may be effective in low dose (e.g., 25–100 mg at bedtime) (Gorman, 1987). Tolerance to the sedative effects develops rapidly, but patients need to be aware that the drugs may be very sedating initially. Nonsedating tricyclics, such as imipramine or desipramine, may be effective in the usual antidepressant doses (100 to 200 mg daily). However, because anxious patients are sensitive to the side effects of these drugs, dosing should begin with 25 mg daily and be increased in 25-mg increments. Buspirone is a nonbenzo-diazepine anxiolytic that appears to have no abuse potential and that causes little sedation.

SIMPLE PHOBIA

Definition

A simple phobia is excessive fear of an object or situation, the *phobic stimulus*. Contact with the phobic stimulus almost always provokes a fear response. This produces a persistent fear of the phobic object, which is either avoided or endured with intense discomfort. Anticipatory anxiety and avoidant behavior may generalize to diverse situations associated with phobic stimuli, leading to interference in activities and, in severe cases, to a restricted lifestyle. In other instances, individuals suffering from simple phobia can establish a routine that excludes phobic stimuli, and it is only when some life change disrupts this routine that the phobic person seeks treatment.

Classification

Diagnostic criteria for simple phobia are as follows:

A. A persistent fear of a circumscribed stimulus (object or situation) other than fear of having a panic attack (as in panic disorder) or of humiliation or embarrassment in certain social situations (as in social phobia).
B. During some phase of the disturbance, exposure to the specific phobic stimulus (or stimuli) almost invariably provokes an immediate anxiety response.
C. The object or situation is avoided or endured with intense anxiety.
D. The fear or the avoidant behavior significantly interferes with the person's normal routine or with usual social activities or relationships with others, or there is marked distress about having the fear.
E. The person recognizes that his or her fear is excessive or unreasonable.
F. The phobic stimulus is unrelated to the content of the obsessions of obsessive-compulsive disorder or the trauma of posttraumatic stress disorder.

The current classification of simple phobia used in the DSM-IIIR dates back to Marks (1970), who distinguished between phobias of external objects and internal circumstances. Maser (1985) provided a listing of different phobias that spans several pages. In practice, however, the most common phobic objects or situations fall within a limited number of categories, such as animals, blood or injury, heights, enclosed places, storms, dental procedures, driving, and air travel. Although most simple phobias are of external objects or situations, illness phobia has been gaining greater attention (Noyes et al., 1992). Illness phobia is a fear of specific medical conditions, such as heart disease, HIV infection, or malignant tumors, and is atypical in its focus on internal sensations as the source of potential threat.

Simple phobias can be diagnosed independently of other disorders, but this category is sometimes conceptualized as a residual diagnosis. Fears that are part of a more specific or pervasive anxiety disorder, such as agoraphobia, social phobia, or obsessive-compulsive disorder, should not receive a diagnosis of simple phobia.

Etiology

The etiology of simple phobia in the individual patient appears to be quite varied. In general, most etiologic factors that have been investigated have been either genetic or learning-based. Most research in this area is unclear, however, because studies of phobic disorders often grouped patients with agoraphobia and social phobia together with simple phobics. Also, among simple phobias, there may be etiologic factors associated with certain subtypes of phobias, such as blood phobia with distinctive changes in blood pressure.

GENETICS

In a study of family transmission among patients who sought treatment for simple phobias, Fyer et al. (1990) found that first-degree family members of patients were more likely to have a simple phobia and, to a lesser degree, other anxiety disorders than first-degree relatives of control subjects. However, simple phobics seeking treatment may have a more severe disorder than those who do not. Other studies using agoraphobic probands also have shown that phobias of various types aggregated in families but were not specific to type of fears. Ost (1992) noted that 61 percent of blood phobics had at least one first-degree relative with the same phobia, and that these relatives were likely to feel faint in the presence of blood, indicative of a similar vasovagal response. Vasovagal response in other phobics is uncommon.

Similarly, twin studies examining concordance rates of "fears" have consistently shown increased concordance in monozygotic twins compared with dizygotic twins. Torgeson (1979) suggested that increased concordance may be due as much to psychosocial factors as it is to genetic factors. In addition, the relation of fears to more severe phobias is unclear, so no proof of purely genetic transmission of phobias is available.

LEARNING FACTORS

The behavioral acquisition of various phobias has been the focus of several retrospective studies in which patients were asked to recall the origin of their fear (e.g., McNally and Steketee, 1985; Mun-

jack, 1984; Ost and Hugdahl, 1983). Many phobic patients *attribute* the origin of their fears either to direct conditioning (often recalling one or more traumatic events) or vicarious learning (e.g., modeling or information). A sizable proportion of phobics could not recall any salient origin to their fears.

Noting that phobias are likely to occur in response to a restricted set of objects or situations, Seligman (1971) hypothesized that humans are "prepared" to learn fears that have survival value in an evolutionary sense. Indeed, most phobic objects and situations are threatening in nature, but the phobic reaction is extreme and enduring. Positive or nonthreatening objects rarely become phobic stimuli. Seligman proposed that specific phobias originate from *prepared classic conditioning*, a type of conditioning that would be highly selective and resistant to extinction. His preparedness hypothesis, however, has not generated much clinical research. Also, conceptual shortcomings remain after several revisions of the theory, and it has not been proven in humans (McNally, 1987).

Epidemiology

From the ECA study, Myers et al. (1984) reported 6-month prevalence rates ranging from 4.5 to 11.8 percent for simple phobia. These rates were consistent with a much earlier study (Agras et al., 1969) that found the prevalence of phobias in the general population to be 7.7 percent. Agras et al. reported that only 9 per 1000 sufferers had seen a mental health professional for treatment. Simple phobia is uncommon in clinic populations because of the limited life disruption it causes relative to other psychiatric disorders (Barlow, 1988). Therefore, relatively few individuals with this common anxiety disorder seek professional treatment; those who do are likely to have a more severe disorder, face direct or frequent confrontation with phobic stimuli (e.g., being required to fly to meetings or ride in elevators), or present with other, more troublesome psychiatric disorders.

Overall, a greater proportion of women than men develop simple phobias. However, Agras et al. (1969) reported that males and females were equally likely to develop intense fears of illness, injury, or medical procedures. Simple phobics who present for treatment are predominantly female.

Clinical Picture

The simple phobic usually fears a single object or situation. Confronting the phobic stimulus results in a strong sense of dread and often a desire to flee. In addition, autonomic arousal may result in panic-like symptoms, such as trembling, shortness of breath, sweating, or tachycardia. Unlike other phobic patients, blood phobics are likely to have a sharp fall in blood pressure leading to dizziness and possible fainting. The focus of the fear for illness phobics is internal, such that avoidance is impossible, and episodic escalation of arousal to panic proportions, typical of other phobias, is rare.

Physiologically, the symptoms of simple phobia may become themselves so extreme as to be indistinguishable from panic attacks. However, unlike the uncued and unexpected anxiety attacks of panic disorder, anxiety attacks that occur in patients with simple phobia are elicited by phobic stimuli and are otherwise absent.

Even a simple phobia can cause significant interference with everyday life as a result of repeated encounters with the phobic object. For example, a claustrophobic who lives in a high-rise apartment serviced by an elevator or a driving phobic who commutes may experience considerable distress or remain constantly vigilant to avoid encounters with phobic stimuli. Simple phobics may develop superstitious or ritualistic behaviors that momentarily reduce ruminative anxiety. For example, an illness phobic may continually monitor vital signs, or a dental phobic may require a set and predictable routine for dental visits. Typically, simple phobics are able to organize their daily lives to avoid phobic stimuli. However, disruptions in this routine, such as taking a new job or moving to a new community, may result in renewed contact and a return of phobic anxiety.

Course

Most simple phobics report an age of onset prior to adulthood. Ost (1987) reported that animal phobics had the earliest average age of onset (7 years), followed by blood phobics (9 years), and dental phobics (12 years). Claustrophobics (20 years) had a mean age of onset closer to that of agoraphobics (28 years). Although studies show great variability in age of onset within diagnostic categories, a consistent pattern of average ages suggests that developmental factors may be involved in the acquisition of anxiety disorders. One hypothesis, based on ethologic studies of imprinting, is that of a critical developmental period during which an individual may be predisposed to acquire specific fears. Other developmental hypotheses address changes in individual capacities or environmental demands related to normative cognitive, affective, or social development. To date, no empirical support is available for any of these hypotheses.

Little is known about the course of untreated simple phobias. In most cases of a circumscribed phobia, daily routines can be established to minimize contact with phobic stimuli. With age, experience, and exposure to phobic stimuli, simple phobias may remit spontaneously, but extreme phobic reactions may continue unabated without treatment. Phobias with childhood onset are more likely to resolve over time than those with onset in adulthood (Agras et al., 1972).

Differential Diagnosis

The differential diagnosis mostly concerns the overlap of simple phobia with other anxiety disorders. Simple phobias can cause extreme autonomic arousal similar to panic disorder. In panic disorder, however, attention is focused on internal sensations and arousal sometimes occurs without a phobic stimulus; at other times, specific situations may become associated with fear and arousal in a phobic manner. In contrast, simple phobia is always elicited by the phobic stimulus. Agoraphobia is often difficult to distinguish from simple phobias, such as travel, but simple phobia arises from the possibility of a catastrophe rather than from fear of internal sensations, as it does in agoraphobia. As mentioned previously, illness phobia, with anxiety focused on a single symptom or illness, is difficult to distinguish from hypochondriasis, which is a more diffuse preoccupation with symptoms and possible illness.

EDITORS' COMMENT

Hypochondriasis is considered by many to be an anxiety disorder because its primary feature is preoccupation with a belief in or fear of having a serious illness (Warwick and Salkovskis, *Behav Res Ther* 28:105–117, 1990; Kellner et al., *J Nerv Ment Dis* 175:20–25, 1987). (Whether it belongs in simple phobia, panic disorder, or obsessive-compulsive disorder is still a matter of debate.)

Phobic presentations may be evident in persons with schizophrenia, obsessive-compulsive disorder, or posttraumatic stress disorder, but they do not constitute simple phobia if they are consistent with the presentation of the other disorder.

Treatment

One of the most effective treatments for a simple phobia is systematic desensitization, a behavior therapy in which the patient confronts increasingly anxiety-producing presentations of the phobic stimulus. Patients first learn a muscle-relaxation technique such as that developed by Benson (1975). Next, phobic situations are listed in order of the amount of anxiety that is elicited, from neutral to terrifying. Patients begin with the least anxiety-provoking situation and attempt to relax while confronted with that imagery. The incompatible response of relaxation and the natural habituation of the anxiety reaction reduce phobic responding with repeated exposures. As patients are able to relax in one situation, they move on to increasingly intense imagery until they are able to confront the entire hierarchy of situations. Imaginal exposure to phobic stimuli is assumed to generalize to actual encounters, but direct exposure (in vivo desensitization) is preferable when possible. This technique can be practiced in the home between sessions and has been found to be effective for motivated patients with uncomplicated phobias. Very brief treatment—sometimes a single prolonged in vivo exposure session—has been reported to be effective in the treatment of diverse phobias, such as animals, spiders, injections, or blood and injury.

Although there seems to be no substitute for exposure, cognitive therapy may be a useful adjunct in addressing exaggerated or irrational fears of threat and vulnerability that often accompany phobic anxiety. Cognitive therapy is also useful for reducing anticipatory anxiety and hypervigilence related to possible confrontations.

Medication has not proven useful in the treatment of simple phobias beyond symptom relief. It may be helpful in decreasing symptom intensity, thus allowing individuals to pursue activities outside the range of their normal daily routine, such as air travel necessary for a vacation. No research has demonstrated that phobic responding has been eliminated following a trial of medication by itself, and there is little to recommend anxiolytic medication as a separate treatment. As an adjunct to the initiation of behavior therapy, benzodiazepines may help reduce severe or pervasive phobic anxiety. However, concurrent use of medication for symptom relief interferes with systematic desensitization; the experience of tolerable levels of anxiety is viewed as a necessary component of this treatment.

Illness phobics, because of their focus on inescapable internal sensations and anxious rumination, may respond differently to treatment than other simple phobics. Graduated exposure to these sensations is not possible, and illness phobics often develop ritualized behavior (e.g., asking for reassurance, touching the area of concern, reading related information). Thus medication such as imipramine (Wesner and Noyes, 1991) may prove useful. Response prevention and distraction techniques common in the treatment of obsessive-compulsive disorder, also may be helpful, but there have been no reports of their use to date.

SOCIAL PHOBIA

Definition

Social phobia is an excessive fear of situations in which a person might do something embarrassing or be evaluated negatively by others. As with other phobias, involvement in phobic situations will almost always provoke a fear response; consequently, these situations are either avoided or endured with intense discomfort.

Classification

Diagnostic criteria for social phobia are as follows:

A. A persistent fear of one or more situations (the social phobic situations) in which the person is exposed to possible scrutiny by others and fears that he or she may do something or act in a way that will be humiliating or embarrassing.

B. If an Axis III or another Axis I disorder is present, the fear in criterion A is unrelated to it; e.g., the fear is not of having a panic attack (panic disorder), stuttering, trembling (Parkinson's disease), or exhibiting abnormal eating behavior (anorexia nervosa or bulimia nervosa).

C. During some phase of the disturbance, exposure to the specific phobic stimulus (or stimuli) almost invariably provokes an immediate anxiety response.

D. The phobic situation(s) is avoided or is endured with intense anxiety.

E. The avoidant behavior interferes with occupational functioning or with usual social activities or relationships with others, or there is marked distress about having the fear.

F. The person recognizes that his or her fear is excessive or unreasonable.

Social phobia became a separate diagnosis in DSM-III, which assumed that it, like simple phobia, focused on a single situation (Marks, 1970). Patients with fear across a broader range of social situations were to be considered for an exclusionary diagnosis of avoidant personality disorder (APD). DSM-IIIR recognizes that many social phobic patients fear more than one type of social situation. If a patient fears most social situations, a diagnosis of generalized subtype is given and an additional diagnosis of APD may be considered. Distinguishing the generalized subtype from other social phobics appears clinically useful. However, the criteria for this distinction need to be clarified, and their reliability needs to be established (Heimberg et al., in press).

Etiology

Little is known about the etiology of social phobia, but several differences between social phobics and comparison groups have suggested possibilities. The generalized subtype of social phobia may have a different etiology than more focal forms of the disorder that are more similar to simple phobias in clinical presentation and life interference.

DEVELOPMENTAL FACTORS

A review of studies of familial transmission of anxiety disorders concluded that subjects with phobic disorders (including agoraphobia, simple phobia, and social phobia) were more likely to report an early parenting environment with less affection and greater parental control (i.e., overprotection) than control subjects or other psychiatric patients (Gerlsma et al., 1990). Comparing perceptions of childhood and parental relations in social phobic and agoraphobic (with panic disorder) patients, social phobics perceived their mothers as more socially avoidant, more isolating, and overemphasizing of others' opinions (Bruch et al., 1989). Thus, there may be an increased risk of familial transmission of social phobia, but the relative contribution of genetic and environmental factors has not been determined.

BIOLOGIC FACTORS

No biologic abnormalities of etiologic significance have been found for social phobia. Social phobic patients, compared with panic disorder patients, were less likely to experience panic during lactate infusion (Liebowitz et al., 1985) or caffeine challenge (Tancer et al., 1990) and had normal sleep architecture and behavior (Uhde et al., 1991). Public speaking phobics have shown greater heart rate reactivity than generalized social phobics during an individualized behavioral challenge (Heimberg et al., 1990). One explanation for reduced reactivity would be consistent with the behavioral inhibition hypothesis mentioned below, i.e., that generalized social phobics experience autonomic arousal as more aversive. Consequently, their inhibited behavior serves to minimize arousal through social withdrawal and inattention (e.g., reduced eye contact, lack of initiation in conversation).

PERSONALITY FACTORS

Social phobics tend to be shy or self-conscious, but the etiologic significance of this is unclear. In one study, a substantial minority of social phobics likely met criteria for personality disorders, the most common being either avoidant (22 percent) or obsessive-compulsive personality (13 percent) disorder (Turner et al., 1991). When personality traits (i.e., subthreshold diagnoses) also were considered, 88 percent of the sample had significant personality disturbance. Histrionic or paranoid features also were observed in over 20 percent of the sample. Separation anxiety in childhood may be associated with adult social phobia, but it is also associated with adult agoraphobia.

Social phobia may develop from a general behavioral inhibition in unfamiliar situations that may be seen in early childhood and transmitted in families (see Rosenbaum et al., 1991). Behavioral inhibition may be manifest as social withdrawal or inactivity due to increased physiologic arousal in novel or challenging situations. This temperamental factor may be genetically transmitted, and it is more evident in children of anxiety disorder patients compared with children of community controls or depressed patients. Family reactions are also seen as important determinants of an inhibited pattern of responding. This hypothesis seems most applicable to generalized social phobia and APD, but methodologic limitations in developmental research are problematic.

LEARNING FACTORS

Behavioral and cognitive theories may provide important clues to etiology, particularly for phasic responding that occurs in some social situations but not others. These theories focus on cued physiologic arousal, anticipatory anxiety, and avoidance behavior. The primary assumption is that the phobic response (i.e., increased arousal and dread) is learned and subsequently triggered by environmental or somatic cues. Learning theorists believe phobias are learned alarm responses that may be acquired by direct, vicarious, or instructional means (Rachman, 1977).

Cognitive models of social phobia also have been considered. Specific cognitive schemata may be used to interpret an event as dangerous and beyond one's ability to neutralize the threat (Barlow, 1988; Beck and Emery, 1985). This evaluation of situations as threatening or dangerous activates affective, physiologic, and motor responses. Causal attributions allow the event to be viewed as uncontrollable but from an identifiable source (e.g., social evaluation, unfriendly others). Constructs in cognitive models (e.g., cognitive schemata of vulnerability, self-focused attention) have been identified in anxiety patients, but the etiologic significance of these constructs has not been proven.

Epidemiology

Social phobia has a prevalence of 1.2 to 2.2 percent, according to the ECA study (Myers et al., 1984), which used DSM-III criteria. Pollard and Henderson (1988) found that approximately 20 percent of a community sample reported extreme fears of public speaking, eating or writing in public, or using a public restroom, but only 2 percent of the sample met the severity and impairment criteria for a social phobia diagnosis. The diagnosis in DSM-IIIR includes more generalized presentations and, therefore, may increase the prevalence of the disorder. Females had a greater prevalence than males in the general population (Bourdon et al., 1988) but present in equal proportions for treatment. The age of onset for social phobia is typically in adolescence, around 16 years of age (Ost, 1987).

Clinical Picture

Anxiety upon exposure to the phobic situation partially defines the diagnosis. The social phobic stimulus may be a single or circumscribed set of situations (akin to a simple phobia). However, most cases of social phobia involve more than one social situation. Common situations feared by social phobics include public speaking, assertive interactions, group or didactic conversations, dating interactions, or even noninteractional behavior that may be observed by others (e.g., writing or eating in public) (Holt et al., 1992).

Social situations may be categorized as those of performance (in which the patient is center of attention) or social interaction (in which the patient engages others). More circumscribed social phobias tend to be performance-related, with public speaking phobia being by far the most common. A specific dating phobia is also common, having both a performance and interactional component. More generalized social phobias have social interactional and performance anxiety. For these patients, the performance anxiety is of minor importance compared with interactional distress.

Social phobics experience physiologic arousal in phobic situations, have a desire to avoid or withdraw from such situations, and have anxiety in anticipation of them. In addition, more generalized phobics worry excessively, similar to patients with generalized anxiety disorder, except that the focus is specific to social evaluation or embarrassment. A number of studies (Herbert et al., 1992; Holt et al., 1992; Schneier et al., 1991; Turner et al., 1992) have shown the generalized subtype to be more severe not only in the number of social situations feared but also with an early age of onset, longer duration of disorder, greater comorbidity with other psychiatric disorders, and greater life interference.

Course and Complications

The untreated course of social phobia is not known, but it is thought to be chronic and unremitting. For specific social phobics, life changes may eliminate the feared situation. Thus a dating phobic may become involved in a long-term relationship or a public speaking phobic may obtain a job in which speaking in front of others is not required. In most instances, however, patterns of avoidance or reduced participation serve both to reduce phobic distress and to perpetuate it by making phobic situations less rehearsed and, therefore, more uncomfortable when encountered.

Life interference varies by the types and number of feared situations. For generalized social phobics, and particularly those with APD, most social contacts are aversive and not well tolerated. This leads to interference with most social activities and, in severe cases, to a very restricted lifestyle. Persons who fear only public speaking or dating can sometimes avoid these situations without harm to employment or other social contacts. Such patients can establish a normal routine that excludes phobic situations, and it is often only during some life change that the person seeks treatment.

Alcohol and drug use, suicide attempts, and depression are prominent in patients with social phobia (Amies et al., 1983). Treatment for substance abuse may be hampered if it is administered in a group format or requires public speaking and being the center of attention. Additional mood and anxiety disorders frequently occur along with social

phobia. Simple phobia, dysthymia, and panic disorder with agoraphobia are common secondary diagnoses, and GAD, simple phobia, and panic disorder with agoraphobia are also likely to have a secondary social phobia (Sanderson et al., 1990). Social anxiety and fears are common among anxiety disorders other than social phobia (Rapee et al., 1988), but social phobic patients can be distinguished from those with panic disorder or GAD by the lack of autonomic hyperactivity away from phobic situations (Reich et al., 1988).

As noted earlier, personality disorders are common in social phobia, and APD occurs frequently with more severe social phobia. However, the proportion of social phobics who receive the APD diagnosis ranges from 22.1 to 70 percent in clinic samples (Herbert et al., 1992; Holt et al., 1992; Schneier et al., 1991; Turner et al., 1992), suggesting that diagnostic reliability is a problem and that sampling biases influence prevalence.

Treatment

Social phobia appears to respond favorably to both pharmacologic and psychotherapeutic interventions (for a review of treatment research, see Hope et al., in press). Unlike simple phobias, several different classes of medication appear to be effective, especially monoamine oxidase (MAO) inhibitors and benzodiazepines. The effectiveness of cognitive behavioral therapy is also well established. Evidence for efficacy of supportive or interpretive psychotherapy is notably absent.

PHARMACOTHERAPY

The role of pharmacotherapy in the treatment of social phobia is just now being understood (Liebowitz et al., 1991, Uhde et al., 1991). There are three main classes of drugs that are frequently prescribed: benzodiazepines, beta-adrenergic blockers, and MAO inhibitors. There is no consistent evidence that tricyclic antidepressants are effective for social phobia.

Only alprazolam, a benzodiazepine, and phenelzine, an MAO inhibitor, have been shown to be superior to placebo in controlled trials with social phobic samples. In direct comparison, both medications were equally effective over 12 weeks of treatment, but treatment gains were maintained over an additional 4-week period for phenelzine but not for alprazolam (Gelernter et al., 1991). Phenelzine also has been shown to be more effective than atenolol, a beta blocker, over 8 weeks of treatment (Liebowitz et al., 1991). Clonazepam, a benzodiazepine, produced favorable results over 11 months of treatment in an open trial (Davidson et al., 1991). Several clinical reports suggest that buspirone and fluoxetine may be effective but with less potency of response than with phenelzine (Liebowitz et al., 1991). However, with the side-effect profile and dietary restrictions of phenelzine and the dependence and withdrawal problems with benzodiazepines, further examination of alternative medications is warranted.

Beta-adrenergic blockers, such as propranolol or atenolol, may be effective when somatic manifestations of anxiety (e.g., sweating, palpitations, trembling, and blushing) are prominent or when more circumscribed social phobias are involved. Evidence for the effectiveness of beta-blocker treatment of social phobia consists mostly of acute single-dosage studies in analogue populations such as musicians with "stage fright" or athletes with performance anxiety (see reviews by R. J. Noyes, Jr., 1988; Schneier et al., 1990). In general, most studies report a superior subjective response to beta-blockers compared with placebo but equivocal effect for objective ratings of performance (i.e., quality of recital or speech or test or sports score). Atenolol was no better than placebo in the only controlled study to date (Liebowitz et al., 1991), although the effectiveness of beta blockers for more discrete performance-oriented social phobia has not been investigated. As with simple phobia, MAO inhibitor and benzodiazepine treatment may be less effective for more circumscribed social phobias than they are for more generalized phobias.

SOCIAL SKILLS TRAINING

Awkward behavior is common among social phobics in phobic situations and may be due to lack of social skills or to anxiety causing disruption of adequate skills. Therefore, determination of the source of behavioral impairment is recommended before selecting a psychological intervention (Hope et al., in press). Social skills training for social phobia assumes that the impairment is due to deficient social behavior, and emphasis is placed on identifying target social behaviors. Target behaviors are then modeled and rehearsed with specific feedback and reinforcement for adequate performance. Although this approach appears to be at least moderately effective in reducing social anxiety, the mechanism may be similar to that for treatments using graduated exposure that do not identify target behaviors.

COGNITIVE BEHAVIORAL THERAPIES

In patients whose social awkwardness is due more to anxiety disruption than to lack of social skills, exposure to the feared situation is an effective intervention. Exposure may be most efficient if there are few feared situations and the focus is on performance rather than on interactional anxiety. However, Butler (1985) suggests that exposure to interactional situations may be more difficult than exposure to other phobic objects or situations. The nature of social interaction is inherently more complex and variable than, say, the presentation of a spider, a trip to the mall, or even speaking to an audience. Adequate social behavior is difficult to define, and feedback is often either ambiguous or unavailable. The nature of the behavioral disruption in social interactions is complex and open to interpretation and is determined in part by the reaction of the others involved in that interaction.

The addition of cognitive techniques in the treatment of *social* phobia is useful because the phobic stimulus involves personal perspective, and access to the patient's perceptions is necessary for setting treatment goals and delivering useful feedback. Cognitive interventions are particularly effective when they are combined with in-session exposure and structured, between-session assignments. These cognitive interventions are based on identification of negatively biased observations, evaluations or self-statements, and replacement with more positive and productive evaluations of social interaction. Patients are typically challenged in role-play interactions to examine assumptions arising from unrealistic performance standards, overreliance on misleading arousal cues, or ambiguous reactions of others that occur during the interaction. This analysis is then used to set more realistic and objective performance goals to improve subsequent social encounters.

POSTTRAUMATIC STRESS DISORDER

Definition

Posttraumatic stress disorder (PTSD) is a disturbance resulting from an extreme and emotionally traumatic event. Traumatic events most often include combat, torture, violent crime and sexual assault, and natural disasters. Characteristic postevent features include hypervigilence and hyperarousal, avoidance of stimuli associated with the event, and reexperiencing of the trauma. PTSD can develop immediately following the event or after some delay, usually with avoidance of reminders of the trauma.

Classification

PTSD first appeared in the diagnostic nomenclature in the third edition of the *Diagnostic and Statistical Manual of Mental Disorders* (DSM-III; American Psychiatric Association, 1980). It was classified among the anxiety disorders, and its description emphasized autonomic arousal, avoidance, and reexperiencing of a "stressor that would evoke significant distress in almost anyone." In the revision of DSM-III (DSM-IIIR; American Psychiatric Association, 1987), the diagnostic criteria were more precisely defined and increased in number, allowing for greater patient heterogeneity within the category. Because most changes were clarifications, the diagnosis was made more reliable without greatly affecting prevalence rates established under DSM-III criteria.

Diagnostic criteria for posttraumatic stress disorder are as follows:

A. The person has experienced an event that is outside the range of usual human experience and that would be markedly distressing to almost anyone (e.g., a serious threat to one's life or physical integrity; a serious threat or harm to one's children, spouse, or other close relatives and friends; sudden destruction of one's home or community; or seeing another person who has recently been or is being seriously injured or killed as the result of an accident or physical violence).

B. The traumatic event is persistently reexperienced in at least one of the following ways:
    1. Recurrent and intrusive distressing recollections of the event (in young children, repetitive play in which themes or aspects of the trauma are expressed)
    2. Recurrent distressing dreams of the event
    3. Sudden acting or feeling as if the traumatic event were recurring [includes a sense of reliving the experience, illusions, hallucinations, and dissociative (flashback) episodes, even those which occur upon awakening or when intoxicated]
    4. Intense psychological distress at exposure to events that symbolize or resemble an aspect of the traumatic event, including anniversaries of the trauma

C. Persistent avoidance of stimuli associated with the trauma or numbing of general responsiveness (not present before the trauma), as indicated by at least three of the following:
    1. Efforts to avoid thoughts or feelings associated with the trauma
    2. Efforts to avoid activities or situations that arouse recollections of the trauma
    3. Inability to recall an important aspect of the trauma (psychogenic amnesia)
    4. Markedly diminished interest in significant activities (in young children, loss or recently acquired developmental skills such as toilet training or language skills)
    5. Feeling of detachment or estrangement from others
    6. Restricted range of affect (e.g., unable to have loving feelings)
    7. Sense of a foreshortened future (e.g., does not expect to have a career, marriage, or children or a long life)

D. Persistent symptoms of increased arousal (not present before the trauma), as indicated by at least two of the following:
    1. Difficulty falling or staying asleep
    2. Irritability or outbursts of anger
    3. Difficulty concentrating
    4. Hypervigilance
    5. Exaggerated startle response
    6. Physiologic reactivity upon exposure to events that symbolize or resemble an aspect of the traumatic event

E. Duration of the disturbance (symptoms in criteria B, C, and D) of at least 1 month

Etiology

The diagnostic criteria specify that PTSD must occur after an event outside the range of normal experience. However, this stressor is, by itself, insufficient to cause PTSD. That is, not everyone exposed to the same stressor (e.g., combat, rape) will develop the disorder, and even relatively common stressful events, such as divorce or death of a significant other, can produce PTSD phenomenology. Nevertheless, for combat PTSD, the number of exposures and the severity of each contribute to the development of PTSD (Foy et al., 1984; Kulka et al., 1990).

Apart from characteristics of the traumatic event, little is known about the etiology of PTSD. Much of what is known about premorbid functioning of PTSD patients was determined retrospectively and is more likely to reflect current functioning than etiologic factors. Prior psychopathology has been discussed as a predisposing factor. However, when other disorders are present, establishment of an independent and subsequent PTSD diagnosis is problematic (Barlow, 1988).

Reviews of preservice records of combat veterans with PTSD found that basal physiologic data, such as blood pressure and heart rate, did not differ from those of combat veterans without PTSD. Thus differences in physiologic arousal between PTSD patients and controls are probably not etiologic but occur subsequent to the stressful event. Heightened physiologic reactivity (i.e., accelerated change from tonic levels due to stressors) and longer latency in return to tonic levels have been demonstrated in PTSD veterans and have been named as possible etiologic factors.

An animal model of response to inescapable shock has been shown to produce autonomic hyperactivity and depletion of the norepinepherine system. According to this model, PTSD patients are thought to have lowered thresholds for responding to stimuli. This phenomenon, termed *kindling*, has been demonstrated in animal research to explain epileptiform reactivity. The effectiveness of antikindling medications (e.g., tegretol or valproate) for a subset of chronic PTSD patients has been offered as support for this hypothesis.

A learned helplessness model has been used to explain avoidance and social withdrawal, which are common negative symptoms of PTSD. This model, originally formulated to explain depressive disorders, describes a learned response to repeated and inescapable shock, in which animals exhibit autonomic arousal but also inactivity rather than escape. Cognitive self-statements consistent with this model (e.g., "Nothing I do will make a difference") are common in posttrauma patients.

Similarly, cognitive and learning explanations for positive symptoms of hypervigilence and arousal have shown biased attentional focus and memory processes (encoding and recall) for threatening rather than nonthreatening stimuli. Biased attention and processing, however, describe existing differences between PTSD patients and other comparison groups.

The occurrence of PTSD is lower in victims of group disasters compared with combat veterans or individual victims of crime. This suggests that public acknowledgment of the trauma, availability of social support, or opportunities to talk about the traumatic event may reduce the incidence of PTSD and lessen the severity and duration of the disorder once it occurs. Thus, social isolation and the inability to process the impact of the trauma may be important etiologic factors.

Epidemiology

The prevalence of PTSD in the general population is about 1 percent using DSM-III criteria (Helzer et al., 1987). Incidence rates following specific stressors may be a more meaningful indication of PTSD occurrence. The most common stressor events are combat, sexual assault or other violent crimes, and natural disasters. As stated previously, PTSD reactions can either be immediate or delayed, further complicating the assessment of prevalence.

Among male Vietnam veterans, Kulka et al. (1990) estimated that 15.2 percent currently suffer from PTSD. Among female Vietnam veterans, current prevalence was placed at 8.5 percent. Lifetime prevalence was estimated at 30.9 percent for males and 26.9 percent for females. These prevalence rates include all personnel assigned to the Vietnam theater of operations regardless of the types of duty. Prevalence rates increased for both genders with amount, intensity, and duration of combat exposure. Helzer et al. (1987) reported that 20 percent of Vietnam veterans met DSM-III criteria for PTSD and 60 percent of veterans report some PTSD symptomatology.

In a community sample of 2000 women, Kilpatrick et al. (1985) found that almost 500 had been victims of crime and that, of these, 100 reported having been raped. In addition to PTSD, robbery, aggravated assault, and rape experiences increased the likelihood of reporting "nervous breakdowns" (7.8 to 16.3 percent of victims compared with 3.3 percent of noncrime controls), suicidal ideation (14.9 to 44.0 percent of victims compared with 6.8 percent of controls), or suicide attempts (8.1 to 19.1 percent of victims compared with 2.2 percent of controls).

Rates of emotional difficulties following civilian disasters or other trauma are relatively low compared with combat or individual trauma. Generally, survivors of civilian disasters (e.g., a high-casualty fire, Three Mile Island radiation release, Lebanese students and civilians) experience stress reactions, but these do not cause significant life interference or require substantial clinical intervention.

GENDER AND AGE DISTRIBUTION

Among Vietnam veterans, younger persons (who entered between the ages of 17 and 19 years of age) were more likely to develop PTSD. This may reflect the type of combat duty assigned. No such age differential was found for female veterans. For PTSD secondary to other traumatic events, there have been no reports of differential incidence according to age or gender. Higher prevalence rates for rape-related PTSD in women reflect the nature of the crime.

Clinical Picture

As noted earlier, the most common traumatic events are combat, sexual assault or other violent crimes, and natural disasters. Such events usually involve the immediate threat of death or injury and engender a profound sense of vulnerability.

Individuals with PTSD may present with heterogeneous symptomatology. As Davidson and Foa (1991) note, these patients share features not only with other anxiety disorders but also with depressive and dissociative disorders. Anxiety is considered the predominant affective response, as described in the diagnostic criteria, but anger and dysphoria are also common responses. Emotional blunting or numbing is often present, as is emotional lability.

Reliving, flashbacks, nightmares, or intrusive thoughts of the traumatic event are necessary for the diagnosis, but psychogenic amnesia for important aspects of the event also may occur. Other sleep disturbances (insomnia and parasomnias) also have been reported. Cognitive functioning is also impaired, with decreased concentration and memory.

PTSD patients tend to avoid contact with situations that are similar to or that may symbolize the traumatic event. Fear-based avoidance of stimuli associated with the traumatic event may result in a presentation that is similar to other phobias. Hypervigilance to threat is common with other anxiety disorders.

In general, PTSD patients exhibit increased tonic arousal, but they also have shown physiologic reactivity specific to auditory and visual stimuli that represent the traumatic event (e.g., gunfire, screams, loud crashes). However, they may not be more reactive to other negative stimuli when compared with other psychiatric or community groups. The exaggerated startle response appears to be nonspecific.

Course and Complications

The nature of the traumatic event directly affects the course of the disorder. For example, a natural disaster may mobilize community-wide social support and resources that assist in amelioration of emotional responses. Alternatively, a rape victim may not perceive commonalties with other such victims and may not be aware of community resources to cope with the trauma. In this instance, the isolated individual may not have an opportunity to deal openly with the trauma and receive available support.

PTSD usually begins soon after the traumatic event with an acute phase, in which extreme distress, disorientation, or dissociation may be common, followed by a chronic course. Onset of PTSD symptomatology may be delayed for months or even years, but the determining factors for an acute versus delayed onset are still unknown. Emotional numbing and dissociation may contribute to such delay and appear to be characteristic responses to *repeated* traumatic events. Repeated traumas (e.g., combat, familial sexual abuse) that are similar in nature make PTSD symptomatology more severe, more likely to occur along with other disorders, and thus less likely to subside with out intervention.

Depression and other anxiety disorders, with onset prior or subsequent to the development of PTSD, are also common complications. Substance abuse is also a complication. It is not uncommon for PTSD symptomatology to go undetected for years in Vietnam combat veterans until substance abuse has been treated, at which time the veteran recognizes continuing problems related to unresolved combat experiences.

Treatment

Treatment options for PTSD include crisis management, outpatient psychotherapy, antidepressant and anxiolytic medications, and multidisciplinary intensive inpatient protocols. As Barlow (1988) notes, however, there is less evidence for the effectiveness of either psychotherapy or pharmacotherapy for PTSD than there is for any other emotional disorder. The effectiveness of most interventions is still under investigation, and many of the parameters for treatment outcome are poorly understood. The type of precipitating event, the type of response exhibited, and the time before initiation of treatment all appear to be important. However, an overall review of treatment outcome is also confounded because various patient populations are more likely to receive one type of treatment or another. For example, most research concerning pharmacotherapy for PTSD have studied combat-related etiologies of long-standing duration. By contrast, behavior therapy for combat-related PTSD is almost nonexistent but somewhat better developed for victims of crime and sexual assault. Chronic PTSD in Vietnam veterans is complicated by at least 20 years in which substance abuse and other problems with living may have greatly compounded the clinical picture. Often an intensive and multimodal course of treatment is required to address not only current distress and incapacitation but also disruption in home and work environments.

CRISIS INTERVENTION

Early crisis intervention is one of the most useful treatments for PTSD. Ideally, secondary prevention efforts involving community resource mobilization have been shown to minimize the overall incidence of stress disorders following natural disasters. Even before full PTSD symptomatology has emerged, an individual may be assisted in talking through the traumatic event and employing coping skills. It also may be useful to normalize short-term adjustment problems and educate the patient on the natural course of coping with trauma. Such minimal therapeutic efforts may help the patient at risk for PTSD to recognize emotional disturbance as a necessary process of coping with trauma.

BEHAVIOR AND COGNITIVE THERAPY

For uncomplicated cases, systematic desensitization (SD) with imaginal exposure and relaxation therapy have been useful in reducing arousal and avoidance associated with PTSD. SD, as mentioned previously, uses increasingly intense exposure to anxiety-provoking imagery while the patient attempts to remain relaxed. Though effective, it is unclear whether SD is more effective than relaxation therapy, which also instructs patients to confront avoidance in daily routines.

Cognitive therapy also may help patients by exploring the nature of the traumatic event and the patient's continuing reactions to it. The primary goal of cognitive therapy is to reduce the patient's sense of threat and vulnerability. Recognizing and reinterpreting hypervigilance and arousal may decrease the threatening nature of the reactions and reduce a patient's avoidance of potentially arousing and uncomfortable situations.

PHARMACOTHERAPY

The magnitude of medication response and the percentage of responding patients remain modest, although Vietnam veterans (many of whom had previous medication or therapy trials and were at least 10 years posttrauma) have been the most commonly studied patient population. Tricyclic antidepressants and MAO inhibitors have been the most widely investigated medications. Both may be useful for long-term control of positive symptoms. Lithium carbonate, alprazolam, clonidine, and propranolol also have been useful for some patients in open trials. Antikindling drugs, such as carbamazepine and valproate, appear to be potentially effective treatments for anger outbursts, flashbacks, and sleep disturbances. For PTSD cases complicated by other Axis I or Axis II disorders, Silver et al. (1990) recommend medications that are appropriate for the other disorder, such as benzodiazepines or buspirone for anxiety disorders and tricyclic antidepressants or MAO inhibitors for depressive disorders. For uncomplicated PTSD, they recommend an initial trial of antidepressant medication, and for persistent symptoms of autonomic arousal, they advise medications that inhibit adrenergic tone, such as propranolol or clonidine.

REFERENCES

Agras SW, Chapin HN, Oliveau DC: The natural history of phobia: Course and prognosis. Arch Gen Psychiatry 26:315–317, 1972.

Agras, SW, Sylvester D, Oliveau D: The epidemiology of common fears and phobia. Compr Psychiatry 10:151–156, 1969.

American Psychiatric Association: Diagnostic and Statistical Manual of Mental Disorders, 3d ed revised. Washington, APA, 1987.

American Psychiatric Association: Diagnostic and Statistical Manual of Mental Disorders, 3d ed. Washington, APA, 1980.

Amies BL, Gelder MG, Shaw PM: Social phobia: A comparative clinical study. Br J Psychiatry 142:174–179, 1983.

Anderson DJ, Noyes R Jr, Crowe RR: Panic disorder and generalized anxiety disorder: A comparison. Am J Psychiatry 141:572–575, 1984.

Ballenger JC, Burrows G, DuPont RL, et al: Alprazolam in panic disorder and agoraphobia: Results of a multicenter trial: I. Efficacy in short-term treatment. Arch Gen Psychiatry 45:413–422, 1988.

Barlow DH: Anxiety and Its Disorders: The Nature and Treatment of Anxiety and Panic. New York, Guilford, 1988.

Barlow DH, Craske M: Mastery of Your Anxiety and Panic. State University of New York at Albany, Center for Stress and Anxiety Disorders, 1989.

Barlow DH, Blanchard EB, Vermilyea JA, et al: Generalized anxiety and generalized anxiety disorder: Description and reconceptualization. Am J Psychiatry 143:40, 1986.

Beck AT, Emery G: Anxiety Disorders and Phobias: A Cognitive Perspective. New York, Basic Books, 1985.

Beitman BD, Basha I, Flaer G, et al: Atypical or nonanginal chest pain: Panic disorder or coronary artery disease. Arch Intern Med 147:1548–1552, 1987.

Benson H: The Relaxation Response. New York: Wm Morrow and Company, 1975.

Biederman J, Rosenbaum JF, Hirshfeld DR, et al: Psychiatric correlates of behavioral inhibition in young children of parents with and without psychiatric disorders. Arch Gen Psychiatry 47:21–26, 1990.

Blazer DG, Hughes D, George LK, et al: Generalized anxiety disorder. In Robins LN (ed): Psychiatric Disorders in America: The Epidemiologic Catchment Area Study. New York, Free Press, 1991, pp 180–203.

Bourdon KH, Boyd JH, Rae DS, et al: Gender differences in phobias: Results of the ECA community survey. J Anxiety Disord 2:227–241, 1988.

Breslau N, Davis GC: Further evidence on the doubtful validity of generalized anxiety disorder. Psychiatry Res 16:177–179, 1985.

Bruch M, Heimberg RG, Berger P, Collins TM: Social phobia and perceptions of early parental and personal characteristics. Anxiety Res 2:57–65, 1989.

Butler G: Issues in the application of cognitive and behavioral strategies to the treatment of social phobia. Clin Psychol Rev 9:91–186, 1989.

Charney DS, Woods SW, Nagg LM, et al: Noradrenergic function in panic disorder. J Clin Psychiatry 51(suppl):5–11, 1990.

Clayton PJ, Grove WM, Coryell W, et al: Follow-up and family study of anxious depression. Am J Phychiatry 148:1512–1517, 1991.

Coryell W, Noyes R, Clancy J: Excess mortality in panic disorder. Arch Gen Psychiatry 39:701–703, 1982.

Crowe RR: Panic disorder: Genetic considerations. J Psychiatr Res 24:129–134, 1990.

Davidson JRT, Foa EB: Diagnostic issues in posttraumatic stress disorder. J Abnorm Psychol 100:346–355, 1991.

Davidson JRT, Ford SM, Smith RD, Potts NLS: Long-term treatment of social phobia with clonazepam. J Clin Psychiatry 52(11, suppl):16–20, 1991.

Di Nardo PA, Barlow DH: Syndrome and symptom co-occurrence in the anxiety disorders. In Maser JD, Cloninger CR (eds): Comorbidity of Mood and Anxiety Disorders. Washington, American Psychiatric Press, 1990, pp 205–230.

Eaton WW, Dryman A, Weissman MM: Panic and phobic. In Robins LN, Regier DA (eds): Psychiatric Disorders in America: The Epidermiologic Catchment Area Study. New York, Free Press, 1991, p 155.

Foy DW, Sipprelle RC, Rueger DB, Carroll EM: Etiology of posttraumatic stress disorder in Vietnam veterans: Analysis of premilitary, military, and combat exposure influences. J Consult Clin Psychol 52:79–87, 1984.

Frank JD: The psychotherapy of anxiety. In Grinspoon L (ed): Psychiatry Update, vol 3. Washington, American Psychiatric Press, 1984, pp 418–425.

Fyer AJ, Mannuzza S, Gallops MS, et al: Familial transmission of simple phobias and fears. Arch Gen Psychiatry 47:252–256, 1990.

Gerlernter CS, Uhde TW, Cimbolic P, et al: Cognitive-behavioral and pharmacological treatment of social phobia. Arch Gen Psychiatry 48:938–945, 1991.

Gerslma C, Emmelkamp PMG, Arrindell WA: Anxiety, depression and perception of early parenting: A meta-analysis. Clin Psychol Rev 10:251–277, 1990.

Gittleman R, Klein DF: Childhood separation anxiety and adult agoraphobia. In Tuma AH, Maser J (eds): Anxiety and Anxiety Disorders. Hillsdale, NJ, Erlbaum, 1985.

Goldberg RJ: Anxiety reduction by self-regulation: Theory, practice, and evaluation. Ann Intern Med 96:483–487, 1982.

Gorman JM: Generalized anxiety disorder. Mod Probl Pharmacopsychiatry 22:127–140, 1987.

Gorman JM, Fyer MR, Goetz R, et al: Ventilation physiology of patients with panic disorder. Arch Gen Psychiatry 45:31–39, 1988a.

Gorman JM, Goetz RR, Fyer M, et al: The mitral valve prolapse-panic disorder connection. Psychosom Med 50:114–122, 1988b.

Heimberg RG, Hope DA, Dodge CS, Becker RE: DSM-III-R subtypes of social phobia: Comparison of generalized social phobics and public speaking phobics. J Nerv Ment Dis 178:172–179, 1990.

Heimberg RG, Holt CS, Schneier F, et al: The issue of subtypes in the diagnosis of social phobia. J Anxiety Disord (in press).

Helzer JE, Robins LN, McEvoy L: Posttraumatic stress disorder in the general population: Findings from the Epidemiologic Catchment Area survey. N Engl J Med 317:1630–1634, 1987.

Herbert JD, Hope DA, Bellack AS: Validity of the distinction between generalized social phobia and avoidant personality disorder. J Abnorm Psychol 102:332–339, 1992.

Hoehn-Saric R, McLeod DR: The peripheral sympathetic nervous system: Its role in normal and pathological anxiety. Psychiatr Clin North Am 11(2):375–386, 1988.

Hollister LE: Prudent use of antianxiety drugs in medical practice. In Brown BS (ed): Clinical Anxiety/Tension in Primary Care Medicine. Amsterdam. Excerpta Medica, 1979, pp 51–65.

Holt CS, Heimberg RG, Hope DA. Avoidant personality disorder and the generalized subtype of social phobia, J Abnorm Psychol 101:318–325, 1992.

Holt CS, Heimberg RG, Hope DA, Liebowitz ML: Situational domains of social phobia. J Anxiety Disord 6:63–77, 1992.

Hope DA, Holt CS, Heimberg RG: Social Phobia. In T. Giles (ed): Handbook of Effective Psychotherapy. New York: Plenum, in press.

Insel TR, Ninan PT, Aloi J, et al: Benzodiazepine receptors and anxiety in non-human primates. Arch Gen Psychiatry 41: 741–750, 1984.

Katon W: Panic Disorder in the Medical Setting. Washington, American Psychiatric Press, 1991.

Katon W: Panic Disorder: Epidemiology, diagnosis and treatment. J Clin Psychiatry 47:21–27, 1986.

Kilpatrick DG, Best CL, Veronen LJ, et al: Mental health correlates of criminal victimization: A random community survey. J Consult Clin Psychol 53:866–873, 1985.

Koella WP: Electroencephalographic signs of anxiety. Prog Neuropsycopharmacol Biol Psychiatry 5:187–192, 1981.

Kulka R, Schlenger WE, Fairbank JA, et al: Trauma and the Vietnam War Generation: Report of the Findings from the National Vietnam Veterans Readjustment Study. New York, Brunner/Mazel, 1990.

Kushner MG, Sher KJ, Beitman BD: The relation between alcohol problems and the anxiety disorders. Am J Psychiatry 147: 685–695, 1990.

Lesser IM: Panic disorder and depression: Co-occurrence and treatment. In Ballenger J (ed): Clinical Aspects of Panic Disorder. New York, Wiley, 1990, pp 181–194.

Liebowitz MR, Fyer AJ, Gorman JM, et al: Specificity of lactate in social phobia versus panic disorder. Am J Psychiatry 142: 947–950, 1985.

Liebowitz MR, Schneier FR, Hollander E, et al: Treatment of social phobia with drugs other than benzodiazepines. J Clin Psychiatry 52:(11, suppl):10–15, 1991.

Markowitz JS, Weissman MM, Ouellette R, et al: Quality of life in panic disorder. Arch Gen Psychiatry 46:984–992, 1989.

Marks IM: Fears, Phobias, and Rituals: Panic, Anxiety, and Their Disorders. New York, Oxford University Press, 1987.

Marks IM: The classification of phobic disorders. Br J Psychiatry 116:377–386. 1970.

Maser JD: List of phobias. In Tuma AH, Maser JD (eds): Anxiety and the Anxiety Disorders. Hillsdale, NJ: Erlbaum, 1985.

McNally RJ: Preparedness and phobias: A review. Psychol Bull 101:283–303, 1987.

McNally RJ, Steketee GS: The etiology and maintenance of severe animal phobias. Behav Res Ther 23:431–435, 1985.

Munjack DJ: The onset of driving phobias. J Behav Ther Exp Psychiatry 15:305–308, 1984.

Myers JD, Weissman MM, Tischler GL, et al: Six-month prevalence of psychiatric disorders in three communities. Arch Gen Psychiatry 41:959–967, 1984.

Nesse ZM, Cameron OG, Curtis GC, et al: Adrenergic function in patients with panic anxiety. Arch Gen Psychiatry 41: 771–776, 1984.

Noyes R: Treatments of choice for anxiety disorders. In Coryell W, Winokur G (eds): The Clinical Management of Anxiety Disorder. New York, Oxford University Press, 1991a, pp 140–153.

Noyes R: Suicide in panic disorder: A review. J Affective Disord 22:1–11, 1991b.

Noyes R: The outcome of panic disorder as influenced by illness variables and coexisting syndromes. In Burrows GD, Roth M, Noyes R (eds): Handbook of Anxiety, vol 5. Amsterdam, Elsevier, pp 137–160, 1992.

Noyes R: Revision of the DSM-III classification of anxiety disorders. In Noyes R, Roth M, Burrows GD (eds): Handbook of Anxiety, vol 2. Amsterdam, Elsevier, 1988, pp 81–108.

Noyes R, Garvey MJ, Cook BL, et al: Benzodiazepine withdrawal: A review of the evidence. J Clin Psychiatry 49:382–389, 1988.

Noyes RJ Jr: Beta-adrenergic blockers. In Last C, Hersen M (eds): Handbook of Anxiety Disorders New York: Pergamon, 1988, pp 445–459.

Noyes RJ Jr, Wesner RB, Fisher MA: A comparison of patients with illness phobia and panic disorder. Psychosomatics 33:92–99, 1992.

Noyes RJ Jr, Clarkson D, Crowe RR, et al: Generalized anxiety disorder: A family study. Am J Psychiatry 144:1019–1024, 1987.

Noyes RJ Jr, Reich JH, Christiansen J, et al: Outcome of panic disorder: Relationship to diagnostic subtypes and comorbidity. Arch Gen Psychiatry 47:809–818, 1990.

Oakley-Browne MA, Joyce PR: New perspectives for the epidemiology of anxiety disorders. In Burrows GD, Roth M, Noyes R (eds): Handbook of Anxiety, vol 5. Amsterdam, Elsevier, pp 57–78, 1992.

Ost LG: Blood and injection phobia: Background and cognitive, physiological and behavioral variables. J Abnorm Psychol 101:68–74, 1992.

Ost LG: Age at onset in different phobias. J Abnorm Psychol 96:223–229, 1987.

Ost LG, Hugdahl K: Acquisition of phobias and anxiety response pattens in clinical patients. Behav Res Ther 19:439–447, 1981.

Pitts FN, McClure JN: Lactate metabolism in anxiety neurosis. N Engl J Med 277:1329–1336, 1967.

Pollard CA, Henderson JG: Four types of social phobia in a community sample. J Nerv Ment Disord 176:440–445, 1988.

Rachman SJ: The conditioning theory of fear acquisition: A critical examination. Behav Res Ther 15:375–387, 1977.

Raj A, Sheehan DV: Medical evaluation of panic attack. J Clin Psychiatry 48:309–313, 1987.

Rapee RM, Sanderson WC, Barlow DH: Social phobia features across the DSM-III anxiety disorders. J Psychopathol Behav Assess 10:287–299, 1988.

Redmond DE Jr: New and old evidence for the involvement of a brain norepinephrine system in anxiety. In Fann WE, Karachan I, Porkorny AD (eds): Phenomenology and Treatment of Anxiety. New York, Spectrum, 1979, pp 153–203.

Regier DA, Myers JK, Kramer M, et al: The NIMH Epidemiologic Catchment Area Program: Historical context, major objectives, and study population characteristics. Arch Gen Psychiatry 41:934–941, 1984.

Reich J, Noyes R Jr, Yates W: Anxiety symptoms distinguishing social phobia from panic and generalized anxiety disorders. J Nerv Ment Disord 176:510–513, 1988.

Rosenbaum JR, Biederman J, Hirshfeld DR, et al: Behavioral inhibition in children: A possible precursor to panic disorder or social phobia. J Clin Psychiatry 52:(11, suppl):5–9, 1991.

Sanderson WC, Di Nardo PA, Rapee RM, Barlow DH: Syndrome comorbidity in patients diagnosed with a DSM-IIIR anxiety disorder. J Abnorm Psychol 99:308–312, 1990.

Schneier FR, Levin AP, Liebowitz MR: Pharmacotherapy of Social Phobia. In Bellack AS, Hersen M (eds): Handbook of Comparative Treatments of Adult Disorders. New York, Wiley, 1990, pp 219–239.

Schneier FR, Spitzer RL, Gibbon M, et al: The relationship of social phobia subtypes and avoidant personality disorders. Compr Psychiatry 32:496–502, 1991.

Seligman MEP: Phobias and preparedness. Behav Ther 2:307–320, 1971.

Silver JM, Sandberg DP, Hales RE: New approaches in the pharmacotherapy of posttraumatic stress disorder. J Clin Psychiatry 51:33–38, 1990.

Tancer ME, Stein MB, Uhde TW: Anxiogenic effects of caffeine in patients with social phobia: Comparison with panic disorder patients and normal controls. Presented at the 10th annual meeting of the Anxiety Disorders Association of America, Bethesda, MD, 1990.

Thyer BA, Parrish RT, Curtis GC, et al: Ages of onset of DSM-III anxiety disorders. Compr Psychiatry 26:113, 1985.

Torgersen S: Genetic factors in anxiety disorders. Arch Gen Psychiatry 40:1085–1089, 1983.

Torgersen S: The nature and origin of common phobic fears. Br J Psychiatry 134:343–351, 1979.

Turner SM, Beidel DC, Townsley RM: Social phobia: A comparison of specific and generalized subtypes and avoidant personality disorder. J Abnorm Psychol 102:326–331, 1992.

Tweed LG, Schoenbach JJ, George LK, Blazer DG: The effects of childhood parental death and divorce on six-month history of anxiety disorders. Br J Psychiatry 154:823–828, 1989.

Uhde TW, Tancer ME, Black B, Brown TM: Phenomenology and neurobiology of social phobia: Comparison With Panic Disorder. J Clin Psychiatry 52:(11, suppl):31–40, 1991.

Von Korff M, Shapiro S, Burke JD, et al: Anxiety and depression in a primary care clinic: Comparison of diagnostic interview schedule, general health questionnaire, and practitioner assessments. Arch Gen Psychiatry 44:152–156, 1987.

Watson J, Raynor R: Conditioned emotional reactions. J Genet Psychol 37:394–419, 1920.

Wesner RB, Noyes R Jr: Imipramine: An effective treatment for illness phobia. J Affective Disord 22:43–48, 1991.

CHAPTER 10

Obsessive-Compulsive Neurosis

THOMAS B. MACKENZIE

DEFINITION

Obsessive-compulsive neurosis, commonly referred to as *obsessive-compulsive disorder* (OCD), is a chronic mental disorder dominated by obsessions and compulsions. An *obsession* is a recurrent, intrusive mental experience recognized by the subject as originating in his or her mind and as being unreasonable or improbable. It may take the form of a thought, a fear, a doubt, an image, an impulse, or a feeling. The experience is distressing, and attempts to resist the content or form of the mental experience are not successful. A *compulsion*, also referred to as a *ritual*, is a cognition or behavior such as praying, counting, checking, or washing that is recurrent, stereotypic, purposeful, and recognized by the patient as originating from within himself or herself. Great importance may be assigned to conducting the ritual in a fixed manner, and any interruption or deviation may force repetition of the entire sequence. Performing the compulsion is variably accompanied by a reduction in anxiety.

The *Diagnostic and Statistical Manual of Mental Disorders*, third edition revised (American Psychiatric Association, 1987), classifies OCD among the anxiety disorders and specifies that the presence of either obsessions or compulsions is sufficient to make the diagnosis. This chapter takes the position that compulsions are invariably preceded by a mental state, albeit as simple as a feeling of tension, that corresponds to an obsessional component. For example, a periodic need to touch the right-hand wall for no apparent reason is preceded by a feeling of tension that can only be reduced by that activity.

ETIOLOGY

Research has implicated specific neuroanatomic regions and neurotransmitter systems in the pa-

thophysiology of OCD. Functional neuroimaging techniques have shown abnormal metabolic rates in the basal ganglia and orbitalfrontal cortex of OCD patients (Insel, 1992). The finding of reduced caudate volume measured by quantitative x-ray computed tomography (Luxenberg et al., 1988) and the increased prevalence of OCD in Tourette's disorder (Hollander et al., 1989) and in patients with Sydenham's chorea (Swedo et al., 1989a) also point to the basal ganglia region. Neuropsychological and electroencephalographic disturbances indicative of frontal lobe dysfunction also have been demonstrated in OCD (Flor-Henry et al., 1979). Nonlocalizing signs of neurologic dysfunction also have been observed more frequently in OCD patients (Hollender et al., 1990b).

Several hypotheses have been advanced to explain these findings (Modell et al., 1989; Baxter et al., 1990; Rapoport, 1990). In general, they propose dysfunction of the basal ganglia, which compromises the integration of routine sensations and actions. This, in turn, leads to compensatory activity in the orbitalfrontal cortex and the neural circuits connecting these regions. Complex interactions with thalamic nuclei and the cingulum are also proposed. These theories parallel the cybernetic model advanced by Pitman (1987), which postulates a persistent mismatch between what is perceived and what is expected. Unable to reduce the error signal associated with this mismatch and obtain an "all clear" signal, the OCD patient feels anxious and engages in rituals in an attempt to align the external and internal signals.

The response of OCD to psychotropic agents which block the presynaptic uptake of serotonin has implicated this neurotransmitter in the pathophysiology of OCD (Murphy and Pigott, 1990). The results of manipulating the serotonergic system using agonists such as *m*-chlorophenylpiperazine (*m*-CPP) (Zohar et al., 1987) and antagonists such as metergoline (Benkelfat et al., 1989) also suggest an important role for this neurotransmitter. Approaches using neuroimaging techniques to explore treatment effects in OCD suggest that serotonin uptake blockers not only improve OCD but concomitantly reduce the "hyperfrontality" characteristic of cerebral metabolism in OCD (Hoehn-Saric et al., 1991). Baxter et al. (1992) have extended this finding to behavioral treatment, demonstrating similar reductions in the metabolic rate in the right caudate in patients who responded to either behavioral or drug treatment.

Cocaine abuse (Satel and McDougle, 1991), isoniazid administration (Bhatia, 1990), multiple sclerosis (George et al., 1989), head injury (Drummond and Gravestock, 1988), frontal lobe lesions (Ward, 1988), focal striatal abnormalities (Weilburg et al., 1989), benzodiazepine withdrawal (Drummond and Matthews, 1988), and the onset of epilepsy (Kettl and Marks, 1986) have been associated with the onset of OCD.

EPIDEMIOLOGY

Once thought to be an uncommon disorder (Woodruff and Pitts, 1964), recent estimates of the lifetime prevalence of OCD derived from careful epidemiologic studies of the general population are in the 1 to 2 percent range (Karno et al., 1988). This corresponds to a staggering fifty-fold increase in the recognized prevalence of OCD.

Family history studies strongly suggest a genetic contribution to the development of OCD. Studies of both children and adults with OCD indicate a higher rate of psychopathology in first-degree relatives. McKeon and Murray (1987) found that the first-degree relatives of OCD patients had a significantly greater lifetime prevalence of mental illness than controls (36 versus 17 percent), the difference being due to an excess of depressive and anxiety disorders. However, they found only one case of OCD in 149 first-degree relatives. Likewise, Insel et al. (1983b) failed to find any OCD among the parents of 27 patients with the disorder. On the other hand, Lenane et al. (1990) found that 25 percent of fathers and 9 percent of mothers of 46 children and adolescents with severe OCD had this disorder. It is therefore possible that childhood-onset OCD represents a subtype associated with a stronger genetic component.

CLINICAL PICTURE

The essential feature of OCD is the presence of obsessions. Obsessions generally involve themes of dirt contamination (excreta, germs, semen, blood, illness), aggression (physical or verbal assault, accidents, calamities, wars), inanimate-impersonal objects (locks, leaking substances, mathematical figures and their totals), sex (sexual advances, incestuous impulses, competence), or religion (the existence of God, violation of religious canons, blasphemous thoughts), in decreasing order of frequency (Akhtar et al., 1975). They are often accompanied by a dysphoric mood (Goodwin et al., 1969). At least half of patients have more than one obsession (Akhtar et al., 1975), and the content of these changes over time (Goodwin et al., 1969). Women are more likely to show fears of contamination than are men (Dowson, 1977), and persons of low intelligence tend to have less structured and less abstract ideation (Ingram, 1961).

Three-quarters of OCD patients experience compulsions (Akhtar et al., 1975). These involve cleaning (51 percent), avoiding (51 percent), repeating (40 percent), checking (38 percent), completeness (11 percent), and meticulousness (9 percent) (Stern and Cobb, 1978). To this list should be added slowness in which the components of an action must be performed perfectly and in the correct sequence, leading at times to complete cessation of activity and hoarding, which involves the accumulation of ordinary materials such as food containers, newspapers, and mail accompanied by an inability to discard anything least it prove important.

There is no agreement on whether avoidance of situations which elicit obsessions should be considered a compulsion. Avoidance is not practiced in a stereotypic fashion and is driven by fear of obsessive-compulsive symptoms rather than by their actual occurrence. The degree of impairment caused by avoidance can be massive even in the absence of obsessions. For example, a patient may altogether avoid leaving home for years to avoid airborne contaminants.

Stern and Cobb (1978) found that 40 percent of patients had little resistance to carrying out their ritual but that 80 percent felt that the ritual was silly or absurd. They reported that reassurance from others had no effect on the ritual in 50 percent of patients and that 88 percent of rituals occurred in more than one place. Only 8 of 45 patients had a single type of ritual.

Compulsions may be classified according to whether they involve yielding to an obsession, such as hand washing in response to a fear of contamination, or controlling an obsession, such as counting in the face of urges to harm others. A worse prognosis was noted for yielding compulsions in the era prior to specific psychopharmacologic treatments for OCD (Akhtar et al., 1975). Compulsions also may be divided into rituals that resemble everyday activities or involve bizarre/magical components. According to Capstick and Seldrup (1977), patients with the latter more frequently give a history of abnormal birth, raising the possibility of an association between bizarre content and cerebral damage.

Obsessions and the rituals that accompany them can last for hours and be so exhausting that patients will go to great lengths to avoid stimuli that elicit them. A patient may avoid a shower knowing its completion may take several hours.

Obsessive compulsives appear to have a higher than average intelligence. Whether this reflects their intrinsic endowment or the overrepresentation of upper- and middle-class patients among obsessionals is not clear (Black, 1974).

Premorbid obsessional traits, such as indecisiveness, orderliness, rigidity, punctuality, scrupulosity, and conscientiousness, are by no means ubiquitous among obsessive compulsives. Using a structured interview, Baer et al (1990) found that while 52 percent of OCD patients had at least one personality disorder, only 6 percent had obsessive-compulsive personality disorder. The most frequently diagnosed personality disorders were mixed, dependent, and histrionic.

Obsessional patients are consistently reported to have an unusually high celibacy rate, ranging from 40 to 50 percent (Black, 1974). Men show a higher rate of celibacy than do women (Ingram, 1961). Further, Kringlen (1965) observed that among those who married, the relationship was bad or extremely bad in 25 of 90 cases.

The average age of onset for OCD in men and women is in the early twenties (Black, 1974). Men and women are equally affected. Men have an earlier onset, and patients with checking have an earlier onset than those with washing (Noshirrani et al., 1991). The disorder commonly has a childhood onset, and Kringlen (1965) noted that half of his adult patients had become ill before age 20 and one-fifth of them before puberty. Although the symptoms and clinical picture of the childhood disorder are virtually identical to those of adult patients (Rapoport et al., 1981), it has been suggested that in children the onset is more likely to be sudden (Elkins et al., 1980).

Ingram (1961) noted a significant precipitating factor in 70 percent of his obsessional patients, as opposed to 50 percent of his anxiety neurotics. He found that the most common precipitants in women were pregnancy and childbirth. In each case, similar symptoms were noted: fears of harming the child with consequent washing and avoidance rituals. Black (1974) cited sexual experiences, marital difficulties, and bereavement as additional precipitants in both sexes.

According to Pollitt (1975), the most common initial symptoms are fears and rituals. The same author described the intrusion of the first symptom as sudden and dramatic. Kringlen (1970) described an acute onset in 65 percent of women and 40 percent of men. Symptoms are frequently disguised by the patient to avoid ridicule. The disguise can be maintained for long periods if the behavior involves an activity such as checking or avoidance. Cleaning, however, is usually readily evident, especially in family settings, where the bathroom may be occupied for hours at a time (Stern and Cobb, 1978).

The interval between onset of symptoms and psychiatric treatment is typically lengthy, the average duration between onset and consultation being 7.5 years (Pollitt, 1975). If hospitalization is necessary, it tends to take place in the midthirties (Kringlen, 1965) and is often related to the emergence of depression (Marks et al., 1980).

The Maudsley Inventory (Hodgson and Rachman, 1977) and the Leyton Inventory (Cooper, 1970) are widely used self-report scales that quantitate obsessive-compulsive symptoms and, in the case of the Leyton, rate their severity. The Yale-Brown Obsessive Compulsive Scale (Y-BOCS) (Goodman et al., 1989b), completed by a trained rater, combines measures of time spent, interference, distress, resistance, and control for all obsessions and compulsions into a total score that can be used to monitor treatment effects.

CLINICAL COURSE

Black (1974) reviewed outcome studies completed before the development of effective behavioral and pharmacologic therapies. Among outpatients, 114 of 190 (60 percent) followed up for 1 to 14 years were asymptomatic, much improved, or improved. Forty percent showed slight or no improvement or were worse. Patients who had been hospitalized showed a slightly worse symptomatic outcome; 142 of 309 (46 percent), when followed for 1 to 20 years, were asymptomatic, much improved, or improved.

Pollitt (1957) reported that among his cohort of inpatients and outpatients, 50 percent had showed a phasic course, with episodes lasting for approximately 1 year. He noted that most of this group had three or fewer attacks. In contrast, Ingram (1961) reported that at follow-up, only 13 percent of his inpatients had a phasic course marked by periods of recovery.

Grimshaw (1965) pointed out that there may be a dissociation of symptomatic outcome and social and occupational adjustment. Thirteen percent of his socially recovered outpatients remained unchanged or were worse as far as symptoms. He concluded that many patients maintained social adaptation in the face of severe symptoms.

According to Ingram (1961), factors associated with a negative prognosis include childhood symptoms, compulsions, and a lengthy interval between onset and treatment. An episodic course, mild or atypical symptoms, and precipitating factors are favorable prognostic signs (Black, 1974; Goodwin et al., 1969). Evidence on the contribution of personality to outcome is mixed. On the one hand, Kringlen (1965) concludes that obsessive premorbid personality is associated with a poor prognosis. On the other hand, Pollitt (1957) assigns a positive prognostic significance to the presence of moderate obsessional traits. Schizotypal personality disorder confers a poor prognosis (Jenike et al., 1986). The content and form of obsessional phenomena appear to be irrelevant to prognosis (Akhtar et al., 1975).

The most common complication of OCD is depression (Goodwin et al., 1969). Nearly one-third of obsessive-compulsive inpatients develop depression in the course of their illness (Rosenberg, 1968). Marks et al. (1980) reported that 38 of 40 chronic obsessive-compulsive ritualizers accepted for a clinical study were depressed. According to Insel (1982), mood change correlates weakly with obsessive-compulsive symptoms. This agrees with Marks et al. (1980), who noted that even after substantial and sustained improvement in rituals and social adjustment, their patients had a strong tendency to have depressive episodes. Despite the high incidence of depression in obsessive compulsives, the risk of suicide is lower than that observed in other neurotics (Rosenberg, 1968; Coryell, 1981).

The development of schizophrenia at follow-up in obsessive compulsives has been described in anywhere from 0.0 to 12.3 percent of patients (Black, 1974). The reported incidence of schizophrenia in OCD has steadily fallen since the 1960s (Black, 1974), suggesting that the earlier reported association of OCD and schizophrenia was substantially a reflection of diagnostic practices.

According to Kringlen (1970), misuse of alcohol and drugs frequently occurs, but typical patterns of substance abuse rarely emerge.

LABORATORY FINDINGS

No laboratory determination is diagnostic of OCD. However, a number of abnormalities have been described. Compared with normal controls, OCD patients had less total sleep, more awakenings, a decreased percentage of delta sleep, and a 50 percent reduction in rapid eye movement (REM) latency (Insel et al., 1982a). On the latter measure, they resembled depressed subjects (Insel et al., 1982a). The same investigators noted that 6 of 16 patients with chronic, severe OCD showed nonsuppression on the dexamethasone suppression test (Insel et al., 1982b). Four of the six nonsuppressors showed significant depression. In a related study, a number of the same patients showed a diminished growth hormone response to intravenous clonidine similar to that observed in depressed patients (Siever et al., 1983). Thoren et al. (1980a) noted normal cerebrospinal fluid (CSF) concentrations of 5-hydroxyindoleacetic acid, homovanillic acid, and 3-methoxy-4-hydroxyphenylglycol in patients participating in a clomipramine treatment study. Elevated levels of arginine vasopressin in CSF and increased release into plasma of the same substance with hypertonic saline challenge in OCD patients have been reported (Altemus et al., 1992). Plasma levels of immunoreactive beta-endorphin were 36 percent lower in OCD patients than normal controls (Weizman et al., 1990).

Neuropsychological testing of OCD patients has yielded inconsistent results. Flor-Henry et al. (1979) reported neuropsychological deficits indicative of left frontal dysfunction in 11 adults. Children with severe obsessive-compulsive disorder exhibited disturbances in spatial orientation and maze-solving abilities (Behar et al., 1984). In contrast, Insel et al. (1983a) found no significant abnormalities in adult patients using standard neuropsychological instruments.

Contemporary EEG studies using strict diagnostic criteria have produced variable results. Mild nonspecific abnormalities were observed in 10 percent of patients by Insel et al. (1983a) and Rapoport et al. (1981). On the other hand, Jenike and Brotman (1984) discovered abnormalities consistent with partial complex seizures in 4 of 12 patients. Because patients with organic mental disorders had been excluded in all three studies, it is not clear what accounts for this difference.

Computed tomography and magnetic resonance imaging of the head have yielded mixed results. Abnormalities in the orbital frontal cortex (Garber et al., 1989), reduced caudate volume (Luxenberg et al., 1988), and ventricular enlargement (Behar et al., 1984) contrast with normal studies (Insel et al., 1983a; Rapoport et al., 1981; Kellner et al., 1991).

An association of blood group A and OCD has been observed (Rinieris et al., 1978). Other investigators (McKeon and McColl, 1982) have not been able to confirm this finding, and its reliability and meaning remain unestablished.

DIFFERENTIAL DIAGNOSIS

Obsessions must be distinguished from two related phenomena: phobias and delusions. A *phobia* is a persistent, unreasonable fear of an object, activity, or situation that generates avoidance behavior. Anxiety is usually in proportion to the probability of encountering the phobic stimulus and can be virtually eliminated by avoidance. The act of avoiding need not conform to fixed rules. The imagined consequences of encountering the stimulus are overwhelming anxiety and personal danger. In contrast, the distress associated with obsessions is not directly related to the probability of encounter or occurrence. Unlike phobias, virtually any situation can serve to enhance the intrusion of obsessions. Compulsive behaviors, such as checking, avoiding, and washing, are rarely executed once but must be repeated in exactly the same way many times. The imagined consequences of an encounter often exceed feeling frightened or being hurt, extending to catastrophic, even absurd, consequences, such as killing someone, getting tetanus, or transmitting leukemia to someone hundreds of miles away.

Ordinarily, obsessive-compulsive experiences are distinct from *delusions* in that their irrationality and self-origin are recognized by the patient. However, some obsessions are held with such tenacity and so little insight that they merge with psychosis. An argument for an obsessive-compulsive psychosis has recently been advanced (Insel and Akiskal, 1986). The presence of hallucinations or disturbance in progression of thought cannot be attributed to OCD.

It may be difficult to distinguish the obsessions of OCD from the worries of generalized anxiety disorder (Mackenzie et al., 1990). The latter are not experienced as alien or intrusive, and efforts to resist them are not undertaken.

While only a small percentage of OCD patients have Tourette's disorder, as many as 50 to 75 percent of persons with the disorder may have OCD (Pauls et al., 1986). By convention, both diagnoses are made when both tics and obsessive-compulsive symptoms coexist.

Distinguishing OCD from depression is complicated by the fact that at least 33 percent of obsessives become depressed (Rosenberg, 1968) and as many as 25 percent of depressives develop state-dependent obsessional symptoms (Gittleson, 1966). Further, OCD shows sleep and endocrine abnormalities resembling those seen in depression (Insel et al. 1982a, 1982b; Siever et al., 1983). According to Black (1974), obsessional illness is heralded by anxiety, fears, and rituals and the onset is often sudden. In contrast, depression usually has an insidious onset (Black, 1974). If obsessions appear during a depression, they often show a diurnal variation in intensity and frequently involve such themes as suicide and homicide (Gittleson, 1966). Depressive symptoms in obsessionals appear in relationship to the dysfunction created by the core symptoms. Signs of melancholia are rarely present unless a major depression has set in as a complication. The observation that eight times as many primary depressives have a family history positive for depression as do obsessive compulsives (Coryell, 1981) may be of assistance in ambiguous cases.

It can be difficult to distinguish between OCD and body dysmorphic disorder, hypochondriasis, and illness phobias. Some patients with eating disorders have intrusive concerns about gaining weight and rituals such as weighing themselves several times a day which resemble obsessive-compulsive symptoms. These disorders have been referred to as *OCD variants* (Tynes et al., 1990).

By convention, trichotillomania is considered an impulse-control disorder, but phenomenologically it overlaps with OCD and appears to respond to some serotonin uptake–blocking agents effective in OCD (Swedo et al., 1989b).

Activities such as gambling, paraphilias, kleptomania, pathologic shopping, and substance abuse, which have a compulsive quality, are generally considered distinct from OCD because the behaviors were at one time pleasurable and resisted only because of negative consequences.

TREATMENT

Since the 1960s, behavioral therapy has emerged as the treatment of choice for OCD with rituals. In vivo exposure with response prevention has been effective in 60 to 75 percent of patients followed up at 2 years (Cobb, 1983). The treatment involves immersing the patient in a situation that provokes obsessional experiences and then preventing ritualization. Substantial improvement can be observed after 20 daily sessions lasting for 1 hour (Marks et al., 1975). This technique showed greater success in patients with overt ritualistic behavior, in vivo exposure being most effective in reducing anxiety, and response prevention, in reducing rituals (Steketee et al. 1982). Relaxation techniques are ineffective in the treatment of OCD (Marks et al., 1975). One-quarter of patients may reject exposure–response prevention therapy, and 20 percent may need retreatment at follow-up (Steketee et al., 1982). Disturbances in mood are poorly responsive to behavioral therapy (Marks, 1981), and treatment failure or early relapse has been correlated with severe depression and conviction that fears were realistic (Foa, 1979). Inpatient hospitalization may be necessary in selected cases to implement behavioral treatments (Megens and Vandereycken, 1989).

To date, the most effective psychotropic agent in the treatment of OCD is the potent serotonin uptake blocker clomipramine hydrochloride. In at least four double-blind, placebo-controlled trials, clomipramine has been shown to produce significant symptomatic improvement (Marks, 1983). No correlation between pretreatment characteristics and therapeutic outcome was noted among 260 patients treated with clomipramine for 10 weeks (DeVeaugh-Geiss et al., 1990). A therapeutic window for the parent compound and its primary metabolite, desmethyl clomipramine, itself a norepinephrine uptake blocker, has been reported (Stern et al., 1980). The drug appears to exert a maximum effect at 10 to 18 weeks (Marks et al., 1980), and discontinuation of the drug may be followed rapidly by relapse (Pato et al., 1988; Thoren et al., 1980b). However, dosage reductions over time of up to 50 percent may not result in loss of benefit (Pato et al., 1990). Recent reports suggest that intravenous clomipramine may be more effective than the oral form in cases which are refractory or have severe side effects (Warneke, 1989). Fluoxetine (Pigott et al., 1990), fluvoxamine (Goodman et al., 1989), and sertraline (Chouinard et al., 1990) have all been shown to be superior to placebo in controlled trials. A combination of clomipramine and fluoxetine has been used (Simeon et al., 1990) but has not been shown to be more effective than either agent alone in controlled trials. Buspar has been reported to augment the benefits of fluoxetine (Jenike et al., 1991a) and in one study was shown to have effect by itself (Pato et al., 1991). Lithium

(Howland, 1991) and fenfluramine (Hollander et al., 1990a) have both been used to augment the effects of serotonin uptake blockers. Clonazepam (Hewlett et al., 1990) and trazodone (Hermesh et al., 1990) are effective in selected cases. Monoamine oxidase inhibitors have been recommended for patients with associated phobic anxiety or panic attacks (Jenike et al., 1983). Loxitane was found to be effective in a case where paranoid ideation was prominent (Bulkeley and Hollender, 1982). Carbamazepine was associated with modest improvement in one of four patients with electroencephalograms suggestive of temporal lobe epilepsy (Jenike and Brotman, 1984).

The combination of a serotonin uptake blocker and pimozide, a neuroleptic, may be useful in the treatment of patients with both Tourette's and OCD (Delgado et al., 1990). The use of electroconvulsive therapy has yielded unimpressive results. However, in selected cases, it may be successful (Mellman and Gorman, 1984).

For patients with OCD refractory to other therapies, psychosurgery may be considered. Four different procedures have been used in the last three decades. These include (1) lesions in the orbitomedial quadrant of the frontal lobe (subcaudate tractotomy), (2) addition to the preceding procedure of lesions to the cingulum (limbic leukotomy), (3) lesions in the anterior cingulum (cingulotomy), and (4) interruption of the anterior limb of the internal capsule (capsulotomy). The latter two procedures are the most well known in North America. Follow-up of 35 patients with severe, treatment-refractory OCD who had undergone bilateral cingulotomy during the previous 25 years revealed that 30 percent had benefited substantially from the procedure (Jenike et al., 1991b). Nine percent had easily controlled seizures. A review of capsulotomy in 172 OCD patients drawn from seven centers concluded that 67 percent were free of symptoms or much improved and that 8 percent were unchanged or worse (Mindus, 1991). Until recently, the standard psychosurgical technique involved radiofrequency heat lesions produced by a stereotactically placed probe. This method is being replaced by the so-called gamma knife, which eliminates craniotomy by focusing hundreds of external gamma emitters on a selected brain area, creating a radiosurgical lesion (Mindus, 1991).

It is generally conceded that the response of OCD to intensive, dynamically oriented psychotherapy has been disappointing (Salzman and Thaler, 1981). Nonetheless, certain guidelines have been advanced with respect to interacting with obsessive-compulsive patients. The patient should be apprised that he or she has a well-known illness that may improve spontaneously, that he or she is not losing his or her mind, and that impulses to act destructively will almost certainly not be carried out (Goodwin et al., 1969).

REFERENCES

Akhtar S, Wig NN, Varma NN, et al: A phenomenological analysis of symptoms in obsessive-compulsive neurosis. Br J Psychiatry 127:342–348, 1975.

Altemus MA, Pigott T, Kalogeras KT, et al: Abnormalities in the regulation of vasopressin and corticotropin-releasing factor secretion in obsessive-compulsive disorder. Arch Gen Psychiatry 49:9–20, 1992.

American Psychiatric Association, Committee on Nomenclature and Statistics: Diagnostic and Statistical Manual of Mental Disorders, 3d ed revised. Washington, American Psychiatric Association, 1987.

Baer L, Jenike MA, Ricciardi JN, et al: Standardized assessment of personality disorders in obsessive-compulsive disorder. Arch Gen Psychiatry 47:826–830, 1990.

Baxter LR, Schwartz JM, Bergman KS, et al: Caudate glucose metabolic rate changes with both drug and behavior therapy for obsessive-compulsive disorder. Arch Gen Psychiatry 49:681–689, 1992.

Baxter LR, Schwartz JM, Guze GH, et al: PET imaging in obsessive compulsive disorder with and without depression. J Clin Psychiatry 51:61–69, 1990.

Behar D, Rapoport JL, Berg CJ, et al: Computed tomography and neuropsychological test measures in adolescents with obsessive-compulsive disorder. Am J Psychiatry 141:363–368, 1984.

Benkelfat C, Murphy DL, Zohar J, et al: Clomipramine in obsessive-compulsive disorder: Further evidence for a serotonergic mechanism of action. Arch Gen Psychiatry 46:23–28, 1989.

Bhatia MS: Isoniazid-induced obsessive compulsive neurosis (letter). J Clin Psychiatry 51:387, 1990.

Black A: The natural history of obsessional neurosis in obsessional states. In Beech HR (ed): Obsessional States. London, Methuen, 1974, pp 19–54.

Bulkeley NR, Hollender MH: Successful treatment of obsessive-compulsive disorder with loxitane. Am J Psychiatry 139:1345–1346, 1982.

Capstick N, Seldrup J: Obsessional states: A study in the relationship between abnormalities occurring at the time of birth and the subsequent development of obsessional symptoms. Acta Psychiatr Scand 56:427–431, 1977.

Chouinard G, Goodman W, Greist J, et al: Results of a double-blind, placebo-controlled trial of new serotonin uptake inhibitor, sertraline, in the treatment of obsessive-compulsive disorder. Psychopharmacol Bull 26:279–284, 1990.

Cobb J: Behavior therapy in phobic and obsessional disorders. Psychiatr Dev 4:351–365, 1983.

Cooper J: The Leyton Obsessional Inventory. Psychol Med 1:48–64, 1970.

Coryell W: Obsessive-compulsive disorder and primary unipolar depression. J Nerv Ment Dis 169:220–224, 1981.

Delgado PL, Goodman WK, Price LH, et al: Fluvoxamine/pimozide treatment of concurrent Tourette's and obsessive-compulsive disorder. Br J Psychiatry 157:762–765, 1990.

DeVeaugh-Geiss J, Katz R, Landau P, et al: Clinical predictors of treatment response in obsessive compulsive disorder: Exploratory analyses from multicenter trials of clomipramine. Psychopharmacol Bull 26:54–59, 1990.

Dowson JH: The phenomenology of severe obsessive-compulsive neurosis. Br J Psychiatry 131:75–78, 1977.

Drummond LM, Gravestock S: Delayed emergence of obsessive-compulsive neurosis following head injury: Case report and review of its theoretical implications. Br J Psychiatry 153:839–842, 1988.

Drummond LM, Matthews HP: Obsessive-compulsive disorder occurring as a complication in benzodiazepine withdrawal. J Nerv Ment Dis 176:688–691, 1988.

Elkins R, Rapoport J, Lipsky A: Obsessive-compulsive disorder of childhood and adolescence. J Am Acad Child Psychiatry 19:511–524, 1980.

Flor-Henry P, Yendall LT, Koles ZJ, Howarth BG: Neuropsychological and powerspectral EEG investigations of the obsessive compulsive syndrome. Biol Psychiatry 14:119–130, 1979.

Foa EB: Failure in treating obsessive-compulsives. Behav Res Ther 17:169–176, 1979.

Garber HJ, Ananth JV, Chiu LC, et al: Nuclear magnetic resonance study of obsessive-compulsive disorder. Am J Psychiatry 146:100–1005, 1989.

George MS, Kellner CH, Fossey MD: Obsessive-compulsive symptoms in a patient with multiple sclerosis. J Nerv Ment Dis 177:304–305, 1989.

Gittleson NL: The phenomenology of obsessions in depressive psychosis. Br J Psychiatry 112:261–264, 1966.

Goodman WK, Price LH, Rasmussen SA, et al: Efficacy of fluvoxamine in obsessive-compulsive disorder: A double-blind comparison with placebo. Arch Gen Psychiatry 46:36–44, 1989a.

Goodman WK, Price LH, Rasmussen SA, et al: The Yale-Brown Obsessive Compulsive Scale. Arch Gen Psychiatry 46: 1006–1011, 1989b.

Goodwin DW, Guze SB, Robins E: Follow-up studies in obsessional neurosis. Arch Gen Psychiatry 20:182–187, 1969.

Grimshaw L: The outcome of obsessional disorder: A follow-up study of 100 cases. Br J Psychiatry 111:1051–1056, 1965.

Hermesh H, Aizenberg D, Munitz H: Trazodone treatment in clomipramine-resistant obsessive-compulsive disorder. Clin Neuropharmacol 13:322–328, 1990.

Hewlett WA, Vinogradov S, Agras WS: Clonazepam treatment of obsessions and compulsions. J Clin Psychiatry 51:158–161, 1990.

Hodgson RJ, Rachman S: Obsessional-compulsive complaints. Behav Res Ther 15:389–395, 1977.

Hoehn-Saric R, Pearlson GD, Harris GJ, et al: Effects of fluoxetine on regional cerebral blood flow in obsessive-compulsive patients. Am J Psychiatry 148:1243–1245, 1991.

Hollander E, Liebowitz MR, DeCaria CM: Conceptual and methodological issues in studies of obsessive-compulsive and Tourette's disorders. Psychiatr Dev 7:267–296, 1989.

Hollander E, DeCaria CM, Schneier FR, et al: Fenfluramine augmentation of serotonin reuptake blockade antiobsessional treatment. J Clin Psychiatry 51:119–123, 1990a.

Hollander E, Schiffman E, Cohen B, et al: Signs of central nervous system dysfunction in obsessive-compulsive disorder. Arch Gen Psychiatry 47:27–32, 1990b.

Howland RH: Lithium augmentation of fluoxetine in the treatment of OCD and major depression: A case report (letter). Can J Psychiatry 36:154–155, 1991.

Ingram IM: Obsessional illness in mental hospital patients. Br J Psychiatry 107:382–402, 1961.

Insel TR: Toward a neuroanatomy of obsessive-compulsive disorder. Arch Gen Psychiatry 49:739–744, 1992.

Insel TR: Obsessive-compulsive disorder: Five clinical questions and a suggested approach. Compr Psychiatry 23:241–251, 1982.

Insel TR, Akiskal HS: Obsessive-compulsive disorder with psychotic features: A phenomenologic analysis. Am J Psychiatry 143:1527–1533, 1986.

Insel TR, Hoover C, Murphy DL: Parents of patients with obsessive-compulsive disorder. Psychol Med 13:807–811, 1983b.

Insel TR, Donnelly EF, Lalakea ML, et al: Neurological and neuropsychological studies of patients with obsessive-compulsive disorder. Biol Psychiatry 18:741–751, 1983a.

Insel TR, Gillin C, Moore A, et al: The sleep of patients with obsessive-compulsive disorder. Arch Gen Psychiatry 39: 1372–1377, 1982a.

Insel TR, Kalin NH, Guttmacher LB, et al: The dexamethasone suppression test in patients with primary obsessive-compulsive disorder. Psychiatry Res 6:153–160, 1982b.

Jenike MA, Brotman AW: The EEG in obsessive-compulsive disorder. J Clin Psychiatry 45:122–124, 1984.

Jenike MA, Baer L, Buttolph L: Buspirone augmentation of fluoxetine in patients with obsessive compulsive disorder. J Clin Psychiatry 52:13–14, 1991a.

Jenike MA, Baer L, Ballantine T, et al: Cingulotomy for refractory obsessive-compulsive disorder: A long-term follow-up of 33 patients. Arch Gen Psychiatry 48:548–555, 1991b.

Jenike MA, Baer L, Minichiello WE, et al: Concomitant obsessive-compulsive disorder and schizotypal personality disorder. Am J Psychiatry 143:530–532, 1986.

Jenike MA, Surman OS, Cassem NH, et al: Monoamine oxidase inhibitors in obsessive-compulsive disorder. J Clin Psychiatry 44:131–132, 1983.

Karno M, Golding JM, Sorenson SB, Burnam MA: The epidemiology of obsessive-compulsive disorder in five U.S. communities. Arch Gen Psychiatry 45:1094–1099, 1988.

Kellner CH, Jolley RR, Holgate RC, et al: Brain MRI in obsessive-compulsive disorder. Psychiatry Res 36:45–49, 1991.

Kettl PA, Marks IM: Neurological factors in obsessive compulsive disorder: Two case reports and a review of the literature. Br J Psychiatry 149:315–319, 1986.

Kringlen E: Natural history of obsessional neurosis. Semin Psychiatry 2:403–419, 1970.

Kringlen E: Obsessional neurosis: A long term follow-up. Br J Psychiatry 111:709–722, 1965.

Lenane MC, Swedo SE, Leonard H, et al: Psychiatric disorders in first-degree relatives of children and adolescents with obsessive compulsive disorder. J Am Acad Child Adolesc Psychiatry 29:407–412, 1990.

Luxenberg JS, Swedo SE, Flament MF, et al: Neuroanatomical abnormalities in obsessive-compulsive disorder detected with quantitative x-ray computed tomography. Am J Psychiatry 145:1089–1093, 1988.

Mackenzie TB, Christenson G, Kroll J: Obsession or worry? Am J Psychiatry 147:1573, 1990.

Marks IM: Are there anti-compulsive or anti-phobic drugs? Review of the evidence. Br J Psychiatry 143:338–347, 1983.

Marks IM: Review of behavioral psychotherapy: I. Obsessive-compulsive disorders. Am J Psychiatry 138:584–592, 1981.

Marks IM, Hodgson R, Rachman S: Treatment of chronic obsessive-compulsive neurosis by in vivo exposure: A two-year follow-up and issues in treatment. Br J Psychiatry 127: 349–364, 1975.

Marks IM, Stern RS, Mawson D, et al: Clomipramine and exposure for obsessive-compulsive rituals, part I. Br J Psychiatry 136:1–25, 1980.

McKeon JP, McColl D: ABO blood groups in obsessional illness: State and trait. Acta Psychiatr Scand 65:74–78, 1982.

McKeon P, Murray R: Familial aspects of obsessive-compulsive neurosis. Br J Psychiatry 151:528–534, 1987.

Megens J, Vandereycken W: Hospitalization of obsessive-compulsive patients: The "forgotten" factor in the behavior therapy literature. Compr Psychiatry 30:161–169, 1989.

Mellman LA, Gorman JM: Successful treatment of obsessive-compulsive disorder with ECT. Am J Psychiatry 141:596–597, 1984.

Mindus P: Capsulotomy in Anxiety Disorders: A Multidisciplinary Study. Stockholm, Karolinska Institute, 1991.

Modell JG, Mountz JM, Curtis GC, Greden JF: Neurophysiologic dysfunction in basal ganglia/limbic striatal and thalamocortical circuits as a pathogenetic mechanism of obsessive compulsive disorder. J Neurol Psychiatry 1:27–36, 1989.

Murphy DL, Pigott TA: A comparative examination of a role for serotonin in obsessive compulsive disorder, panic disorder, and anxiety. J Clin Psychiatry 51:53–58, 1990.

Noshirvani HF, Kasvikis Y, Marks IM, et al: Gender-divergent etiological factors in obsessive-compulsive disorder. Br J Psychiatry 158:260–263, 1991.

Pato MT, Hill JL, Murphy DL: A clomipramine dosage reduction study in the course of long-term treatment of obsessive-compulsive disorder patients. Psychopharmacol Bull 26: 211–214, 1990.

Pato MT, Pigott TA, Hill JL, et al: Controlled comparisons of buspirone and clomipramine in obsessive-compulsive disorder. Am J Psychiatry 148:127–129, 1991.

Pato MT, Zohar-Kadouch R, Zohar J, Murphy DL: Return of symptoms after discontinuation of clomipramine in patients with obsessive-compulsive disorder. Am J Psychiatry 145:1521–1525, 1988.

Pauls DL, Towbin KE, Leckman JF, et al: Gilles de la Tourette's syndrome and obsessive-compulsive disorder. Arch Gen Psychiatry 43:1180–1182, 1986.

Pigott TA, Pato MT, Bernstein SE, et al: Controlled comparisons of clomipramine and fluoxetine in the treatment of obsessive-compulsive disorder: Behavioral and biological results. Arch Gen Psychiatry 47:926–932, 1990.

Pitman RK: A cybernetic model of obsessive-compulsive psychopathology. Compr Psychiatry 28:334–343, 1987.

Pollitt J: Obsessional states. Br J Psychiatry 9:133–140, 1975.

Pollitt J: Natural history of obsessional states. Br Med J 1:194–198, 1957.

Rapoport J: Obsessive compulsive disorder and basal ganglia dysfunction. Psychol Med 20:465–469, 1990.

Rapoport J, Elkins R, Lancer DH, et al: Childhood obsessive-compulsive disorder. Am J Psychiatry 138:1545–1554, 1981.

Rinieris PM, Stefanis CN, Rabavilas AD, Vaidakis NM: Obsessive-compulsive neurosis, anancastic symptomatology and ABO blood types. Acta Psychiatr Scand 57:377–381, 1978.

Rosenberg CM: Complications of obsessional neurosis. Br J Psychiatry 114:477–478, 1968.

Salzman L, Thaler FH: Obsessive-compulsive disorders: A review of the literature. Am J Psychiatry 138:286–296, 1981.

Satel SL, McDougle CJ: Obsessions and compulsions associated with cocaine abuse (letter). Am J Psychiatry 148:947, 1991.

Siever LJ, Insel TR, Jimerson DC, et al: Growth hormone response to clonidine in obsessive-compulsive patients. Br J Psychiatry 142:184–187, 1983.

Simeon JG, Thatte S, Wiggins D: Treatment of adolescent obsessive-compulsive disorder with a clomipramine-fluoxetine combination. Psychopharmacol Bull 26:285–290, 1990.

Steketee G, Foa EB, Grayson JB: Recent advances in the behavioral treatment of obsessive-compulsives. Arch Gen Psychiatry 39:1365–1371, 1982.

Stern RS, Cobb JP: Phenomenology of obsessive-compulsive neurosis. Br J. Psychiatry 132:233–239, 1978.

Stern RS, Marks IM, Mawson D, Luscombe DK: Clomipramine and exposure for compulsive rituals: II. Plasma levels, side effects and outcomes. Br J Psychiatry 136:161–166, 1980.

Swedo SE, Rapoport JL, Cheslow DL, et al: High prevalence of obsessive-compulsive symptoms in patients with Sydenham's chorea. Am J Psychiatry 146:246–249, 1989a.

Swedo SE, Leonard HL, Rapoport JL, et al: A double-blind comparison of clomipramine and desipramine in the treatment of trichotillomania. N Engl J Med 321:497–501, 1989b.

Thoren P, Asberg M, Bertilsson L, et al: Clomipramine treatment of obsessive-compulsive disorder: II. Biochemical aspects. Arch Gen Psychiatry 37:1289–1294, 1980a.

Thoren P, Asberg M, Cronholm B, et al: Clomipramine treatment of obsessive-compulsive disorder: I. A controlled clinical trial. Arch Gen Psychiatry 37:1281–1285, 1980b.

Tynes LL, White K, Steketee GS: Toward a new nosology of obsessive compulsive disorder. Compr Psychiatry 31:465–480, 1990.

Ward CD: Transient feelings of compulsion caused by hemispheric lesions: Three cases. J Neurol Neurosurg Psychiatry 51:266–268, 1988.

Warneke L: Intravenous chlorimipramine therapy in obsessive-compulsive disorder. Can J Psychiatry 34:853–859, 1989.

Weilburg JB, Mesulam MM, Weintraub S, Buonanno F: Focal striatal abnormalities in a patient with obsessive compulsive disorder. Arch Neurol 46:233–235, 1989.

Weizman R, Gil-Ad I, Hermesh H, et al: Immunoreactive beta-endorphin, cortisol, and growth hormone plasma levels in obsessive-compulsive disorder. Clin Neuropharmacol 13:297–302, 1990.

Woodruff R, Pitts FN: Monozygotic twins with obsessional illness. Am J Psychiatry 120:1075–1080, 1964.

Zohar J, Mueller EA, Insel TR, Zohar-Kadouch RC, Murphy DL: Serotonergic responsivity in obsessive-compulsive disorder: Comparison of patients and healthy controls. Arch Gen Psychiatry 44:946–951, 1987.

CHAPTER 11

Somatoform and Dissociative Disorders

C. ROBERT CLONINGER

The most prominent features of some psychiatric disorders are physical complaints that cannot be explained by known pathophysiologic mechanisms. Such unexplained physical complaints are common in all medical practices, so physicians must learn to recognize psychiatric disorders that mimic physical disorders. Such psychiatric disorders cannot be reliably recognized simply by excluding physical disorders or by treatment trials. Physical disorders may fail to respond to routine treatments or may go unrecognized because of atypical presentation or limitations of available assessment procedures. In addition, patients often present with combinations of physical and psychiatric symptoms that challenge the diagnostic and therapeutic skills of the most astute and patient physician.

One of the major innovations of the third edition of the American Psychiatric Association's *Diagnostic and Statistical Manual of Mental Disorders* (DSM-III) was its classification of psychiatric disorders associated with prominent physical complaints. DSM-III distinguishes five groups of disorders according to the role of known pathophysiologic mechanisms, psychological conflict, and voluntary control over symptoms (Table 11-1). The *somatoform disorders* refer to illnesses in which there is no known physical disorder or pathophysiologic mechanism to explain symptoms and in which psychological conflicts are currently assumed to lead to involuntary formation of physical signs and symptoms. These somatoform disorders include several explicitly described syndromes or discrete clinical disorders: *Briquet's syndrome* (also called *somatization disorder* or *chronic hysterical neurosis*), conversion disorder (or *acute hysterical neurosis, conversion type*), *psychogenic pain disorder, hypochondriasis* (or *hypochondriacal neurosis*), and other atypical somatoform disorders. In this chapter, each

of these categories of somatoform disorder is considered. Conversion disorders and dissociative disorders are often referred to collectively as *acute hysterical neurosis* because of similarities in their clinical course and in theories about their etiology. Accordingly, dissociative disorders are described here along with conversion disorders.

BRIQUET'S SYNDROME (SOMATIZATION DISORDER OR CHRONIC HYSTERIA)

Definition

Briquet's syndrome has been described by Guze and his associates (Perley and Guze, 1962; Guze, 1967; Woodruff, 1967) as a chronic syndrome of recurrent symptoms in many organ systems that begins before age 30 and is associated with psychological distress but no physical disorder. It is associated with excessive surgery and medical attention for a wide variety of medically unexplained complaints. Characteristic symptoms include frequent pains, gastrointestinal symptoms, sensorimotor conversion symptoms and dissociative reactions, sexual and menstrual problems, and a belief that the patient has been sickly most of his or her life. Anxiety and depressive symptoms are frequently associated with the recurrent physical complaints. Personal and social problems are also commonly observed in such patients. In 1962, Perley and Guze described 59 symptoms in 10 groups as characteristic of Briquet's syndrome and required at least 20 medically unexplained symptoms in 9 groups for diagnosis (Table 11-2). These patients were initially labeled as having hysteria or hysterical neurosis, but later the name *Briquet's syndrome* was suggested in order to distinguish this chronic polysymptomatic disorder

TABLE 11-1.   *DSM-II Criteria Used in the Differential Diagnosis of Symptom(s) Suggesting Physical Illness*

Classification	Physical mechanism explains the symptoms	Symptoms are linked to psychological factors	Symptoms initiation is under voluntary control	Obvious recognizable environmental goal
Somatoform and dissociative disorders	No	Yes	No	Variable
Factitious disorders	Variable	Yes	Yes	No
Malingering	Variable	Variable	Yes	No
Psychological factors affecting physical condition	Yes	Yes	No	Yes
Undiagnosed physical illness	Variable	Variable	No	No

Based on Hyler and Spitzer, 1978.

from acute conversion and dissociative reactions. The name recognizes the early work of the French physician Briquet, who described a similar syndrome in 1859 (Purtell et al., 1951; Guze, 1967; Mai and Merskey, 1980).

In order to facilitate clinical applications, an attempt was made in DSM-III (American Psychiatric Association, 1980) to simplify the original criteria of Perley and Guze. DSM-III also suggested the alternative name of *somatization disorder*. Depressive

TABLE 11-2.   *Symptom Items for Guze's Criteria for Briquet's Syndrome*

Group 1	Group 6
Headaches Sickly most of life	Abdominal pain Vomiting

Group 2	Group 7
Blindness Paralysis Anesthesia Aphonia Fits or convulsions Unconsciousness Amnesia Deafness Hallucinations Urinary retention Ataxia Other conversion symptoms	Dysmenorrhea Menstrual irregularity Amenorrhea Excessive bleeding

Group 8
Sexual indifference Frigidity Dyspareunia Other sexual difficulties Vomiting nine months pregnancy or hospitalized for hyperemesis gravidarum

Group 3
Fatigue Lump in throat Fainting spells Visual blurring Weakness Dysuria

Group 9
Back pain Joint pain Extremity pain Burning pains of the sexual organs, mouth, or rectum Other bodily pains

Group 4
Breathing difficulty Palpitation Anxiety attacks Chest pain Dizziness

Group 10
Nervousness Fears Depressed feelings Need to quit working or inability to carry on regular duties because of feeling sick Crying easily Feeling life was hopeless Thinking a good deal about dying Wanting to die Thinking of suicide Suicide attempts

Group 5
Anorexia Weight loss Marked fluctuations in weight Nausea Abdominal bloating Food intolerances Diarrhea Constipation

symptoms and panic attacks were omitted from the criteria to avoid overlap with depressive and anxiety disorders. The remaining 37 symptoms that best discriminated persons with Briquet's syndrome from others were retained. Requirements about the number of groups were dropped because this was found to add little information: the total number of somatization symptoms is highly correlated with the number of somatization groups. Finally, to reduce possible sex bias owing to the impossibility of menstrual and pregnancy symptoms in men, men were diagnosed who had 12 unexplained symptoms compared with the criterion number of 14 in women.

The DSM-III criteria for somatization disorder require a history of medically unexplained physical symptoms of several years' duration, beginning before age 30. These include at least 14 complaints in women and 12 in men of the following 37 symptoms: sickly, difficulty swallowing, loss of voice, deafness, double vision, blurred vision, blindness, fainting, unconsciousness, amnesia, seizures, trouble walking, paralysis or weakness, urinary retention, abdominal pain, nausea, vomiting, abdominal bloating, food intolerance, diarrhea, dysmenorrhea, menstrual irregularity, menorrhagia, hyperemesis gravidarum, sexual indifference, frigidity, painful intercourse, back pain, joint pain, extremity pain, genital pain, dysuria, other pain except headaches, shortness of breath, palpitations, chest pain, and dizziness.

The criteria for Briquet's syndrome consider 21 other symptoms besides those included in somatization disorder: headaches, anesthesia, hallucinations, fatigue, panic attacks, anorexia, weight loss, marked fluctuations in weight, constipation, amenorrhea, other sexual difficulties, nervousness, fears, depressed feelings, inability to carry on regular duties because of feeling sick, crying easily, hopelessness, thinking a good deal about dying, wanting to die, thinking of suicide, and suicide attempts. These 21 symptoms occur in 8 of the 10 groups delineated by Perley and Guze.

It is possible to satisfy the criteria for Briquet's syndrome and not somatization disorder as defined in DSM-III because the criteria for Briquet's syndrome include more than 20 symptoms that do not contribute to a diagnosis of somatization disorder. It is also possible to satisfy the criteria for somatization disorder and not Briquet's syndrome because the 14 symptoms required for somatization disorder are insufficient to satisfy the requirement of at least 20 for Briquet's syndrome. In clinical practice, discordance between the diagnosis of Briquet's syndrome and somatization disorder can be substantial. Among 123 women who received either diagnosis in a follow-up and family study of somatization disorder, only 63 percent received both diagnoses, 21 percent had somatization disorder only, and 16 percent had Briquet's syndrome only (Cloninger et al., 1986). Men and women with somatization

disorder only had a variety of heterogeneous disorders, particularly anxiety and personality disorders. There was familial aggregation for Briquet's syndrome but not for somatization disorder alone. Thus the agreement of the simplified DSM-III criteria, and other briefer screening criteria (Reveley et al., 1977), with the full criteria is too low for definitive diagnosis. The diagnosis of Briquet's syndrome may influence clinical decisions about treatment and risk for suicide, so clinicians are encouraged to use the full Briquet's syndrome criteria rather than any briefer criteria. Actually, the criteria for Briquet's syndrome are not substantially more time-consuming to administer than the DSM-III criteria because nearly all the additional items should be routinely elicited in psychiatric assessments.

DSM-IV Criteria

The full criteria for Briquet's syndrome are lengthy and difficult to remember. This complexity has limited their use in both clinical practice and research. Recently, an efficient set of criteria were developed for the American Psychiatric Association for DSM-IV (Cloninger, 1993). These criteria were validated by showing their close concordance with the original criteria for Briquet's syndrome and the criteria for somatization disorder in DSM-III.

Cloninger observed that there is an essential pattern and specific number of complaints that permit efficient screening for somatization disorder in clinical practice, as well as its diagnosis (Cloninger, 1993). First, the clinician should inquire about a history of pain in various parts of the body. Unless there is a lifetime history of pain in at least four different parts of the body, the diagnosis can be excluded without asking further questions. If there are four or more bodily pains, then these also must be medically unexplained and associated with treatment or functional impairment in order to permit the diagnosis.

Second, the clinician should inquire about a history of gastrointestinal symptoms other than pain, such as nausea, vomiting, diarrhea, and food intolerance. Unless there are two or more gastrointestinal symptoms other than pain, the diagnosis can be excluded without further questions. These symptoms can be compatible with a diagnosis of irritable bowel syndrome, which is frequent in somatization disorder.

Third, the clinician should inquire about any history of sexual or reproductive symptoms other than pain, such as sexual indifference in men or women. Sexual impotence is another common example of sexual dysfunction in men. Other examples of such symptoms in women are irregular menses, menorrhagia, or hyperemesis gravidarum. At least one sexual or reproductive symptom is required for diagnosis.

Fourth, patients who meet the earlier three requirements also must have a history of at least one conversion or dissociative symptom in order to receive a diagnosis of somatization. Finally, the onset of somatic complaints must begin before the age of 30 years and occur over a period of several years.

These criteria allow efficient stepwise screening using symptom clusters that are easy to remember. Since no questions about anxiety or depression are required, discrimination from anxiety and mood disorders is enhanced. Fortunately, patients who meet these criteria for somatization disorder also satisfy the full Briquet's syndrome criteria in 98 percent of cases. Also, the DSM-IV criteria identify about 90 percent of patients with the full Briquet's syndrome. The small number of discrepant cases are primarily individuals with more anxiety and depressive symptoms than other physical complaints, suggesting that the DSM-IV somatization disorder may be even more homogeneous than the original Briquet's syndrome. More crucially, the availability of easy and efficient screening and diagnostic procedures should facilitate both future research and routine clinical practice.

Etiology

Briquet's syndrome is familial: it is observed in 10 to 20 percent of the female first-degree relatives of probands with Briquet's syndrome, a fivefold to tenfold increase over the lifetime risk of the disorder in women in the general population (Woerner and Guze, 1968; Cloninger et al., 1975; Coryell, 1980; Cloninger et al., 1986). The male relatives of women with Briquet's syndrome also show an increased risk of antisocial personality and alcoholism (Woerner and Guze, 1968; Cloninger et al., 1975). A blind family interview study in St. Louis has confirmed the familial nature of Briquet's syndrome in women and the association with antisocial personality in male and female relatives. In contrast, men with many somatic complaints were found to be clinically heterogeneous and did not aggregate in families with either male or female somatizers (Cloninger et al., 1986). This suggests that somatization in women often has a common etiology with antisocial personality, but not somatization in men.

This familial aggregation could be caused by genetic factors, environmental influences, or both. An adoption study of somatoform disorders in Sweden has shown that the contributions of both genetic and environmental influences are substantial (Bohman et al., 1984). Two discrete types of somatoform disorders were distinguished in Swedish women using comprehensive lifetime medical records (Cloninger et al., 1984). One of these disorders, high-frequency somatization, was characterized by frequent headaches, backaches, and gastrointestinal and gynecologic complaints associated with psychiatric disability (Fig. 11-1). Extensive overlap with Briquet's syndrome was suggested by available psychiatric evaluations. Women who were adopted away at an early age had a fivefold

increase in high-frequency somatization disorder if their biologic parents were antisocial or alcoholic. Low social status of the adoptive parents also increased the risk of somatoform disorders in the adopted children. This indicates that both biologic and psychosocial influences contribute to the development of this disorder. The interaction of these genetic and environmental contributions was studied in a cross-fostering analysis (Fig. 11-2), which considers the possible combinations of genetic background (high or low risk) and of postnatal background (high or low risk). The analysis showed that both genetic and environmental background contribute to the risk of somatization regardless of the other.

Studies of the biologic and adoptive parents of hyperactive children also have provided evidence for genetic factors that are shared by Briquet's syndrome and attention-deficit disorder with hyperactivity in children. Briquet's syndrome and antisocial personality are increased in the biologic parents of hyperactive children in intact families, but not in the adoptive parents of other hyperactive children (Cantwell, 1972; Morrison and Stewart, 1973).

Objective experimental tests indicate that individuals with Briquet's syndrome have low pain thresholds (Bianchi, 1973) and an information-processing pattern characterized by distractibility, difficulty distinguishing target and nontarget stimuli, and impaired verbal communication (Ludwig, 1972; Bendefeldt et al., 1976; Almgren et al., 1978; Flor-Henry et al., 1981). This attentional deficit is associated with their failure to habituate to repetitive stimuli (Mears and Horvath, 1972). Flor-Henry et al. (1981) compared the neuropsychological function of patients with Briquet's syndrome with that of normal controls, psychotic depressives, and schizophrenics who were matched to the Briquet's patients for age, sex, handedness, and full-scale intelligence. Compared with the normal controls, the Briquet's patients had a bilateral and symmetrical pattern of frontal lobe impairment. This anterior cerebral impairment was substantially greater than posterior cerebral impairment, but the Briquet's patients exhibited some bilateral, but principally nondominant (right-sided), posterior temporal deficits in most cases also. The patients with Briquet's syndrome had greater dominant hemisphere impairment than did the psychotic depressives, as expected from their relationship to antisocial personality, and they had less nondominant hemisphere disorganization than did the schizophrenics. This characteristic pattern of neuropsychological impairment allowed patients with Briquet's syndrome to be distinguished from each of the other contrast groups.

Shapiro (1965) and Horowitz (1977) have suggested that this "hysterical" information-processing pattern explains many of their clinical features. Their "global deployment of attention" leads to

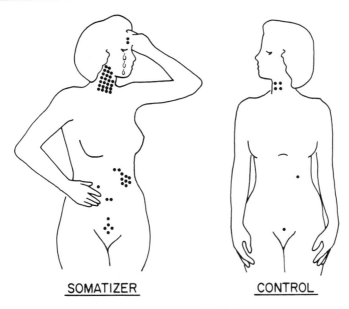

SOMATIZER   CONTROL

• I Somatic sick leave/IO person years
♭ I Psychiatric sick leave/IO person years

FIGURE 11-1.   *Distribution and number of sick leave occasions in Swedish high-frequency somatizers and control non-somatizers.*

CLASSIFICATION OF PREDISPOSITION   OBSERVED FEMALE ADOPTEES
TO TYPE I (High Frequency) SOMATIZATION

Congenital	Postnatal	Row Total (N)	Row% of Type I Somatizers
Low	Low	379	2.1%
Low	High	359	4.7%
High	Low	68	7.4%
High	High	53	13.2%

FIGURE 11-2.   *Cross-fostering analysis of type 1 (high frequency) somatization in Swedish adopted women (Bohman et al., 1984). "Congenital" refers to variables about biologic parents, whereas "postnatal" refers to variables about rearing experiences and adoptive placement. Classification of predisposition depended on whether the set of background variables were more like the average characteristics of adoptees with type 1 somatization (classified as high) or with type 2 or no somatization (classified as low).*

vague, nonspecific labels for experience; their "impressionistic grouping of constructs" leads to unclear and incomplete statement of ideas and feelings, circumstantial or partial patterns of association, and distortion of new information to fit earlier preconceptions. Their tendency to respond quickly and impulsively to external stimuli without sustained critical examination leads to suggestibility, shallowness, lability, and diminished reflective self-awareness. Schalling (1978) and her associates (1973) have shown that monotony avoidance and impulsivity are positively associated with somatization or somatic anxiety but not with obsessional traits or anticipatory anxiety. Thus somatization, impulsivity, and the hysterical information-processing pattern tend to occur in the same individual, as is observed in patients with Briquet's syndrome and their biologic relatives.

The hysterical information-processing deficit may underlie the frequent somatic complaints, mental status findings of vagueness and circumstantiality, as well as many social and personal problems that are prominent in patients with Briquet's syndrome and their biologic relatives (Horowitz, 1977; Cloninger, 1978; Flor-Henry et al., 1981). This pattern of information processing is associated with the use of what psychoanalysts describe as the defense mechanisms of repression and denial. Shapiro (1965) describes repression as "the loss not of affect but of ideational contents from consciousness, the failure of once-perceived contents to achieve the status of conscious memories." Schafer (1948) suggested that excessive reliance on repression and denial hampers the development of broad intellectual and cultural interests, impairs the ability for independent and creative thinking, and leads to emotional lability, immature interpersonal attachments, and a crisis-oriented lifestyle. In contrast, Shapiro suggested that the appearance of repression and the associated clinical problems are a consequence of the information-processing pattern. It is likely that the same neurobiologic phenomena are simply being described at different levels of observation so that arguments about whether the egg or the chicken came first are moot.

The perception of somatic sensations can be increased by selective attention and improves with practice or conditioning. Adam (1967) showed that individuals could be taught to perceive gastrointestinal movements that they were unaware of previously. Autonomic activity can be conditioned to signals that can occur below the level of awareness. For example, heart rate can be conditioned to vary with signals that subjects are not aware of consciously (Lacey et al., 1955). Transient physiologic disturbances associated with autonomic hyperactivity, muscle tension, or hyperventilation are associated with somatic symptoms and occur frequently in the general population (Mayou, 1976; Kellner and Sheffield, 1973). Examples of such somatic symptoms include tension headaches, irritable

bowel syndrome, and sensory changes, such as paresthesias (Weintraub, 1983). Presumably, the frequency of such physiologic disturbances or symptoms can be modified by selective attention and conditioning. Patients with Briquet's syndrome show rapid and marked responses to suggested shifts of their attention (Scallet et al., 1976) and frequently experience symptoms associated with such physiologic disturbances.

Social modeling and operant conditioning of sick role behavior can influence the frequency and intensity of somatization and are discussed later in relation to conversion symptoms and chronic pain states.

Epidemiology

AGE

The full Briquet's syndrome develops gradually. It is rarely diagnosable before age 14 (Robins and O'Neal, 1953). In the majority of cases, characteristic symptoms begin during adolescence, and full criteria are satisfied by age 25 (Purtell et al., 1951; Guze and Perley, 1963). The hysterical information-processing pattern and histrionic personality traits are usually recognizable during adolescence in those cases (about 70 percent) in whom they are ever prominent (Cloninger and Guze, 1970). Kimble et al. (1975) found histrionic personality and Briquet's syndrome highly correlated in adult women but noted that teenage girls with histrionic personality rarely fulfilled the criteria for Briquet's syndrome. Guze et al. (1973) found that among psychiatric clinic patients, the number of symptoms characteristic of Briquet's syndrome was unimodally distributed in women and peaked during the 20s, followed by a gradual decline. In men, on the other hand, there was a gradual increase in the number of symptoms with age, reaching a peak in the 50s and then declining. There was a significant sex difference under age 40 but not thereafter. Similar findings have been observed in different age cohorts of psychiatric outpatients in Sweden also (Lindberg and Lindegard, 1963), but in the absence of prospective studies, it remains uncertain whether such patterns reflect differences between various birth cohorts or actual clinical changes with age within birth cohorts. In any case, in patients who develop Briquet's syndrome, the characteristic symptoms are recurrent and lead to chronic disability.

LIFETIME RISK IN WOMEN

Several studies now suggest that the lifetime risk for Briquet's syndrome or somatization disorder is about 2 percent in women when age of onset and method of assessment are taken into account. Cloninger et al. (1975) found that 3 of 153 white women who had just experienced normal child deliveries had Briquet's syndrome. By counting the 59 unaffected women younger than age 25 as being, on average, only half through their lifetime risk period, the lifetime risk was estimated as 2.4 percent plus or minus 1.4 percent.

The prevalence of Briquet's syndrome or somatization disorder is underestimated in studies relying on interviews by nonphysicians. The diagnostic criteria require a judgment of whether or not the symptoms are medically explained. This judgment requires medical training to develop the skill to assess critically the description of the symptoms, diagnostic evaluations, and putative physical diagnoses. Psychiatrists and other physicians can do this reliably even in patients with multiple chronic medical illnesses (Woodruff, 1967; Reveley et al., 1977). Patients with Briquet's syndrome, however, often attribute symptoms to a variety of physical disorders, and nonphysicians are unable to critically evaluate such assertions adequately. As a result, when nonphysicians accept medical explanations offered by patients without properly judging their plausibility, Briquet's syndrome is underdiagnosed. In addition, people may be less motivated to describe somatic complaints to nonphysicians. The sensitivity (proportion of true cases recognized) of nonphysicians compared with psychiatrists is 55 percent for Briquet's syndrome and 41 percent for DSM-III somatization disorder (Robins et al., 1981). Specificity (proportion of noncases properly diagnosed) remains high (97 to 99 percent) for nonphysicians for both Briquet's syndrome and somatization disorder.

This underestimation of prevalence by nonphysicians may account for the low prevalence estimates of Briquet's in large-scale population surveys that use nonphysician interviewers. Weissman et al. (1978) obtained follow-up interviews on 511 adults in 1975–1976 (all over age 25) out of an original sample of 1095 adults identified in 1967. The follow-up sample differed significantly from the original population in that there were fewer nonwhite and low socioeconomic subjects. They found only two women with definite Briquet's syndrome. However, this is an underestimate owing to the biased attrition and the fact that interviews were done by nonphysicians. Correcting for sensitivity and specificity of nonphysician interviewers, the lifetime risk for Briquet's syndrome is about 1.6 percent in women. Similarly, in a more recent epidemiologic study using nonphysician interviewers, the lifetime risk of somatization disorder was reported as only 0.2 to 0.3 percent of women, but this does not correct for underdiagnosis by nonphysicians.

Comprehensive medical records are the most sensitive method for recognizing Briquet's syndrome or somatization disorder because they are unaffected by inconsistent self-reports (Martin et al., 1979). Using complete lifetime medical records in Sweden, high-frequency somatization disorder was observed in about 3 percent of 859 women in the general population. This is only slightly higher than estimates of Briquet's syndrome based on

comprehensive assessments by psychiatrists using personal interviews supplemented by selected medical records.

SEX DIFFERENCES

Briquet's syndrome is diagnosed predominantly in women, but infrequent cases do occur in men. In a recent study in St. Louis, 4 percent of 74 psychiatric outpatients with Briquet's syndrome were men. Some clinicians have suggested that this sex difference is artifactual. Warner (1978) found that male and female professionals tend to label men as antisocial and women as hysterical even when they have identical clinical features. Others have noted that the criteria for Briquet's syndrome were biased against diagnosis of men because some of its characteristic symptoms are inapplicable to men (e.g., pregnancy and menstrual complaints). Also, men generally report fewer symptoms than do women, and it has been suggested that there should be compensation for this response bias in the number of reported symptoms required for diagnosis in men (Temoshok and Attkisson, 1977).

DSM-III reduced the number of symptoms required to diagnose somatization disorder from 14 in women to 12 in men. This compensates for the inapplicable gynecologic symptoms but not for the general response bias in number of somatic complaints. Somatization disorder is much rarer in men than in women unless the number of somatic complaints required for diagnosis in men is reduced to half the number required in women (14 to 7). The symptoms characteristic of somatization disorder were counted in a study of psychiatric outpatients and their relatives (Cloninger et al., 1986). The cumulative frequency distributions of these counts are shown in Table 11-3 for probands at follow-

TABLE 11-3. *Frequency of Somatization Disorder Symptoms*

| Symptoms count | Probands of follow-up | | Relatives of nonsomatizers | |
	Men (n = 129) cum. col. (%)	Women (n = 277) cum. col. (%)	Men (n = 375) cum. col. (%)	Women (n = 479) cum. col. (%)
20 +	—	2.5	—	0.2
16–19	3.1	12.3	—	1.5
14–15	3.1	22.0*	—	2.9*
12–13	6.2	25.6	0.3	4.0
8–11	17.8*	48.4	2.7*	11.7
4–7	40.3	76.5	12.5	35.5
2–3	47.3	85.9	13.6	38.2
0–1	100.0	100.0	100.0	100.0

Relatives were excluded if the proband had 14 (women) or 8 (men) symptoms, whether the symptoms were judged medically explained or not, in order to best approximate a general population sample by excluding probands with medical and somatoform disorders.

*Percentages of subjects in each sex with somatization disorder if the criterion was taken as 14 and 8 medically unexplained symptoms in women and men, respectively.

up and for the relatives of definite nonsomatizers. Using the DSM-III criterion of 14 unexplained symptoms in women, the prevalence of somatization disorder was 22 percent in outpatient women compared with 2.9 percent in the female relatives of nonsomatizers. Using the DSM-III criterion of 12 unexplained symptoms in men, the prevalence of somatization disorder in the relatives of nonsomatizers was only 0.3 percent, making the disorder more than 10 times as prevalent in women as in men. If the required minimum symptom count for men was reduced to 7 or 8, the prevalences in men and women were about the same. However, these men with 7 to 11 somatic complaints had a wide variety of anxiety and personality disorders and did not aggregate in families with female somatizers. This suggests that the sex difference in somatization in the United States has practical clinical significance.

It is interesting that a study of 75 subjects with Briquet's syndrome in Greece included 21 men and 54 women (Rinieris et al., 1978). Further cross-cultural studies are needed to evaluate the importance of cultural influences on sex role stereotypes about the expression of somatization.

SOCIOECONOMIC ASSOCIATIONS

Briquet's syndrome is more common in individuals who have low socioeconomic, occupational, and educational status (Robins, 1966; Cloninger and Guze, 1970; Guze et al., 1971a). Low occupational status of either biologic or adoptive parents increased the risk of high-frequency somatization disorder in adopted Swedish women (Bohman et al., 1984).

Pathology

By definition, patients with Briquet's syndrome have no known pathologic abnormalities to explain their symptoms. The disorder often leads to surgery. Pathologic reports of surgically removed tissues are typically characterized as normal or describe coincidental abnormalities.

Clinical Picture

The most discriminating clinical feature is a medical history complicated by recurrent unexplained problems and the subjective complaint of sickliness. However, the chief complaint at a particular time need not be a physical complaint. Often the chief complaint involves social problems, a suicide attempt, or a nonpsychotic agitated depression. Frequently, patients with Briquet's syndrome are unable to specify a single chief complaint and instead describe many problems that are, at best, vaguely related (Purtell et al., 1951). In order to avoid misdiagnosis and inappropriate treatment, it is necessary to review the history of hospitalizations and

outpatient medical care as well as conduct a careful review of systems in all patients, regardless of their most prominent presenting symptoms, because of the variability and vagueness of chief complaints in Briquet's syndrome.

No one symptom or sign is pathognomonic of Briquet's syndrome; the cardinal feature is the chronic polysymptomatic pattern of physical complaints. Nevertheless, some symptoms are highly characteristic and discriminate Briquet's disorder from other psychiatric disorders. These include the complaint of sickliness for most of a patient's life, or a history of voluntary sterilization before age 30, or repeated surgery for unexplained pain. Individual symptoms or behaviors such as these suggest the possibility of Briquet's disorder but are an inaccurate basis for diagnosis because they are not frequent enough in Briquet's disorder and too common in other conditions. It is necessary to consider combinations of two or more symptoms in evaluating the possibility of Briquet's disorder.

Three symptom clusters have been identified that distinguish patients with Briquet's syndrome from patients with other psychiatric or medical disorders (Reveley et al., 1977). One syndrome, occurring in 30 percent of outpatients with Briquet's disorder, is the combination of onset of a complex illness before age 26, back pain, abdominal pain, and suicidal thoughts. This syndrome is similar to the symptom pattern that is characteristic of high-frequency somatizers in Sweden, as noted earlier. The second syndrome, occurring in another 28 percent of outpatients with Briquet's disorder, was the combination of recurrent vomiting and the conversion symptom ataxia. The third syndrome, occurring in most other patients with Briquet's syndrome, is the onset of a complex illness before age 26, back pain, painful menstrual periods, and either sexual indifference or conversion reactions. The presence of one of these symptom clusters should lead to especially careful consideration of the possibility of Briquet's syndrome, including detailed review of past medical records.

Recurrent somatic complaints lead to repeated hospitalizations for observation, laboratory tests, x-rays, and surgery. A wide variety of specialists may be consulted because of the range of unexplained complaints. Abdominal, pelvic, and back pain often lead to frequent gynecologic surgery: dilatation and curettage, uterine suspension, and hysterectomy. Gastrointestinal complaints lead to frequent x-rays and laparotomies. Complaints of headaches, fits, and other sensorimotor problems lead to neurologic evaluations. Psychiatrists are often consulted because of agitated depressions, suicide attempts, and interpersonal problems.

On mental status examination, histrionic personality traits and the hysterical information-processing deficit described earlier are prominent in most cases. Such patients are circumstantial, imprecise, and inconsistent historians. They recall their current situation and past history as a series of separate elements mixed together or mingled without sorting, discrimination, or apprehension of functional relationship and temporal order. As a result, it is useful to obtain collateral information from other observers and from records.

Social maladjustment is prominent in most cases also. This may include juvenile delinquency, frequent divorce or marital separations, child neglect and inconsistent parenting, and low job productivity. Interpersonal relations are often shallow and chaotic.

Clinical Course

The course of illness in Briquet's syndrome or somatization disorder is chronic, with fluctuation in the frequency and diversity of symptoms but without complete remission (Guze and Perley, 1963; Guze et al., 1986). The most floridly symptomatic phase is usually early adulthood, but aging does not lead to remission. Prospective longitudinal studies have confirmed that 80 to 90 percent of patients have a similar clinical picture and the same diagnosis over many years (Perley and Guze, 1962; Guze et al., 1986). This stability of clinical picture and consistency of diagnosis is observed for both Briquet's syndrome and DSM-III somatization disorder (Cloninger et al., 1986). Some clinicians have questioned whether this is a consequence of the requirement of many years of past sickliness. However, the course of somatoform disorders in the relatives of chronic somatizers is also chronic; there is no excess of individuals with acute or episodic disorders (Woerner and Guze, 1968). Also, chronic somatizers show qualitatively different neurophysiologic responses than do acute somatizers (Mears and Horvath, 1972). Although individual symptoms may wax and wane, these clinical, familial, and neurophysiologic observations indicate that the underlying disorder is a stable trait with a chronic course.

Laboratory Findings

Patients with Briquet's syndrome are not immune to other medical illnesses, so laboratory tests are useful to document concurrent illnesses objectively. However, no specific laboratory tests are available for diagnosis of Briquet's syndrome itself. Some nonspecific laboratory tests include low pain thresholds (Bianchi, 1973) and failure to habituate to repetitive stimuli (Mears and Horvath, 1972), but these are not sufficiently discriminating for use in routine clinical practice.

Differential Diagnosis from Physical Disorders

The individual symptoms encountered in Briquet's syndrome and somatization disorder are non-specific. In other words, they occur in many different medical disorders so that the differential diagnosis of the individual symptoms encompasses all of clinical medicine. Three features help to distinguish Briquet's syndrome from physical disorders: (1) involvement of multiple organ systems, (2) early onset and chronic course without development of physical signs of structural abnormalities, and (3) absence of characteristic laboratory abnormalities of other physical disorders. Medical disorders that begin with nonspecific functional and sensory abnormalities with transient or equivocal physical signs may present diagnostic problems. Multiple sclerosis and systemic lupus erythematosus are classic examples of conditions that are often misdiagnosed early in their course. However, they seldom satisfy the multisystem requirements for diagnosis of Briquet's syndrome; only about 14 percent of female medical inpatients have the range of symptoms characteristic of Briquet's syndrome even when symptoms are counted that may be medically explained (Reveley et al., 1977). Even patients with multiple coincident disorders can be distinguished by attention to the onset, course, and associated physical and laboratory findings of individual complaints (Woodruff, 1967). Two conditions that are associated with metabolic disturbances affecting multiple organ systems—porphyria and hypercalcemia—present clinical pictures that are most likely to be confused with the full Briquet's syndrome.

Acute intermittent porphyria (AIP) and other hepatic porphyrias may resemble Briquet's syndrome with a history of recurrent pains and neurologic disturbances. AIP is due to a hereditary partial deficiency of porphobilinogen (PBG) deaminase, which leads to the accumulation of PBG and its precursor, delta-aminolevulinic acid, in blood and their excretion in urine. Like Briquet's syndrome, AIP is familial. Carrier status, demonstrated by assay of erythrocyte PBG deaminase, is inherited as an autosomal dominant disorder. Carriers may complain of mood swings and pains even when their urine PBG levels are within the normal range (Bissell, 1982; Stein and Tschudy, 1970). Factors that increase the demand for heme synthesis lead to overproduction of heme precursors and clinical symptoms. Drugs such as alcohol and barbiturates that induce the microsomal cytochromes in liver often precipitate acute attacks. Other drugs that precipitate attacks include chlordiazepoxide, imipramine, and estrogens. Recurrent painful premenstrual exacerbations occur in some women and resolve with onset of menstruation. As in Briquet's syndrome, clinical symptoms are uncommon before puberty and carrier status is more often expressed in women than in men. PBG can be converted to a dark compound called porphobilin in the bladder; this is accelerated by exposure of voided urine to light, so some patients may notice that their urine darkens after voiding. PBG and its precursor appear to have neurotoxic effects. Neuropathic changes are variable, with patchy demyelination of peripheral nerves and focal degeneration of autonomic nerves. Acute attacks usually include complaints of abdominal, back, or extremity pain. Tachycardia, anorexia, nausea, and vomiting are also frequent. Constipation is often a chronic problem in carriers and may be exacerbated during acute attacks. In such cases, x-rays often reveal a paralytic ileus. Neuropsychiatric symptoms include seizures, paralysis, confusion, and psychotic behavior. Routine laboratory tests are usually normal except for slight elevation of serum transaminase activity, even during acute attacks. Urine PBG levels are elevated during attacks, and this may be documented by rapid qualitative methods (Schwartz-Watson or Hoesch tests). In 20 to 30 percent of carriers, however, urine PBG levels are within normal limits when they are not in acute distress. In these cases, only assay of erythrocyte PBG will identify carriers (Bissell, 1982). Other types of hepatic porphyrias are associated with elevated levels of serum porphyrins that lead to skin abnormalities not seen in Briquet's syndrome or in acute intermittent porphyria.

Various causes of hypercalcemia may present with symptoms that cross-sectionally suggest Briquet's syndrome. These include a large number of nonspecific symptoms in many organ systems: (1) central nervous system—lethargy, depression, emotional lability, confusion, and drowsiness; (2) neuromuscular system—easy fatigability, weakness (especially of the proximal muscles), joint pains, pruritus; (3) gastrointestinal system—anorexia, nausea, vomiting, constipation, dyspepsia; (4) cardiovascular system—hypertension, arrhythmias; and (5) renal system—polyuria, stone diathesis. Early onset and course of illness in Briquet's disorder distinguishes it from most causes of hypercalcemia, such as hyperparathyroidism, vitamin D or A toxicity, diuretic therapy, and cancer. Also, serum calcium is routinely tested by most physicians, so hypercalcemia is seldom mistaken for Briquet's syndrome.

Chronic systemic infections, such as brucellosis and trypanosomiasis, may present a picture suggestive of chronic somatization disorders. Although they are uncommon in general, they should be considered in patients who live in endemic areas or who have a history of relevant exposures, such as brucellosis in slaughterhouse workers. After returning from his voyage on the Beagle in 1836, at age 27, Charles Darwin was described as sickly and hypochondriacal by his friends, family, and physicians of the time, who could find no physical explanation for his chronic complaints of fatigue, recurrent abdominal pain, vomiting, abdominal bloating, palpitations, dizziness, chest pain, and insomnia. Darwin withdrew socially and remained a semi-invalid attentively ministered by his wife at home until his death of heart disease at age 73. Some psychiatrists have suggested that Darwin had hysterical or hypochondriacal neurosis, and his social withdrawal and acceptance of his wife's careful attention to his needs have been offered as evidence of his neurosis. It is known, however, that in 1835 in South America he had extensive bites from the insect *Triatoma infestans*, the most frequent carrier of the trypanosome of Chagas' disease (De Beer, 1980). This American trypanosome was not discovered until 1909, and the disease was not described by Chagas until 1916. The acute phase of this infestation is seldom recognized, and in the chronic phase there may be effects in multiple organ systems, with the cardiovascular and gastrointestinal systems most prominent clinically, as in Darwin's case (Macedo, 1982). With more sophisticated diagnostic methods and chemotherapy, such chronic infections have become uncommon in industrial societies.

Neurologic and other medical disorders that must be differentiated from conversion and dissociative reactions are discussed later because they seldom present with symptoms in multiple organ systems.

Differential Diagnosis from Psychiatric Disorders

The psychiatric disorders that must be considered in the differential diagnosis of Briquet's syndrome include the anxiety disorders, the affective disorders, and the schizophrenic disorders. The most difficult distinction is between anxiety disorders and Briquet's syndrome. Patients with Briquet's syndrome present with recurrent panic attacks in most cases. Similarly, features of generalized anxiety disorder (motor tension, autonomic hyperactivity, apprehensive expectation, and vigilance and scanning phenomena) are common in Briquet's syndrome. Age of onset and course are of little help in differentiating anxiety disorders from Briquet's disorder. Patients with anxiety disorders also often have disease fears and hypochondriacal disease convictions. Conversion and dissociative symptoms, sexual and menstrual problems, social maladjustment, and histrionic personality traits are the major distinguishing features. Men are more likely to have anxiety disorders than somatoform disorders also. The distinction may be difficult in individual cases, but it is clinically important because the family history and clinical management of Briquet's syndrome are different from that of anxiety disorders (Guze et al., 1971b).

Patients with unipolar and bipolar affective disorder may present with multiple somatic complaints associated with depressive syndromes. In fact, the chief complaint in depressive disorders is often a physical complaint like headache, gastrointestinal distress, or other pain. These complaints are transient, however, and resolve with the treatment of the depression, whereas in Briquet's syndrome the physical complaints persist regardless of the mood state.

Patients with schizophrenia sometimes present initially with somatic complaints. Only later are they found to have systematized delusions and hallucinations in addition to their somatic complaints. Some of their somatic complaints may be due to somatic hallucinations and delusions, but this is often difficult to resolve. There is no familial aggregation of schizophrenia and Briquet's syndrome so the somatic complaints appear to be symptomatic of schizophrenia.

Patients with antisocial and histrionic personality disorders often have associated Briquet's syndrome or somatization disorder. These disorders aggregate both within individuals and within families (Cloninger et al., 1970, 1975) and may have a common pathogenesis in many cases. Such personality disorders do not preclude an additional diagnosis of Briquet's syndrome or somatization disorder.

Occasional patients with Briquet's syndrome or somatization disorder may be found to produce some of their symptoms factitiously or to malinger. Even when this is documented for some occasions, the patient may insist that the symptom occurs spontaneously on other occasions. Such claims are difficult or impossible to resolve, and the distinction often has little or no practical consequence in clinical management.

Treatment and Clinical Management

The optimal treatment of Briquet's syndrome or somatization disorder is unknown. Claims of superiority of particular methods of management have often varied with the vogue of the times. A review of treatment studies (Scallet et al., 1976) shows that psychotherapeutic approaches, including psychoanalysis, dynamically oriented psychotherapy, behavior therapy, and group therapy, have no superiority over eclectic psychotherapy that mainly involves education about their illness, reassurance, and redirection of their attention from somatic complaints to work on improving social skills. Somatic therapies such as use of anxiolytics, electrosleep therapy, and electroconvulsive therapy have limited and transient benefits (Scallet et al., 1976). Patients with Briquet's syndrome or somatization disorder have a high rate of utilization of health care services so it is essential that all physicians understand the principles involved in their clinical management.

The first phase of clinical management must be the establishment of the diagnosis and of a therapeutic alliance. Patients with Briquet's syndrome or somatization disorder often change doctors after a short time or may go to several doctors at the same time. They quickly reject the conclusion that there is nothing wrong with them physically and seek another evaluation and more tests from another physician. They also quickly reject the suggestion that their symptoms are due to psychological distress or psychiatric disorder if this is equated with the absence of a physical basis to their complaints. There-

fore, it is useful to inform a patient who is suspected of having somatization that you recognize that they are ill and uncomfortable, but before beginning treatment, it will be necessary to see them at least a few times to know them more fully, to review their medical history carefully, and to obtain records of prior diagnostic evaluations and treatments. This communicates your empathy and willingness to evaluate their complaints seriously and is essential to establishing their confidence in your subsequent diagnosis and treatment plan. It also provides the time needed to properly evaluate alternative diagnoses; if neglected initially, the patient is likely to reject any reassurance that they are not physically ill because you do not really know enough about them. Thorough evaluations can be carried out in most cases without additional invasive tests. The time taken to carefully review and document the patient's history initially will pay long-term benefits in accuracy of diagnosis and effectiveness of compliance with follow-up and treatment. Considering the frequency and cost of the use of health care services by these patients, the time required is easily justified.

The second step is to explain to patients that they have Briquet's syndrome or somatization disorder and what this means. It is essential to communicate to patients that they have a real disorder that leads to their experiencing characteristic symptoms that distinguish their disorder from other disorders that leads to progressive physical deterioration and from other psychiatric disorders that do not have such prominent physical complaints. Many patients are reassured that their disorder has been recognized by physicians as a valid entity, that it has a name, that it is heritable, and that it does not lead to progressive physical deterioration. However, they will not be much reassured by this information alone because they are uncomfortable, disabled, and seeking relief of their discomfort and help to reduce their disability. It is important to communicate a realistic treatment plan and goals for the sake of both the patient and yourself.

The goal of treatment in Briquet's syndrome is to educate the patient to manage his or her own life more effectively, not for the physician to cure and relieve all symptoms passively. If a passive cure is promised or expected, both the patient and the physician will be frustrated and disappointed. Realistic goals include reduced frequency and severity of physical complaints, improved social adjustment, and reduced cost and frequency of medical treatment.

These goals can usually be achieved by adherence to a few treatment principles. First, it is essential to limit the number of doctors the patient is seeing. Often a primary-care physician alone can effectively manage a patient with Briquet's syndrome. Alternatively, patients with prominent psychosocial problems do best when seen by both a psychiatrist and a primary-care physician on different occasions but with close consultation. An important behavioral management principle is to schedule regular visits that are neither increased nor decreased in frequency in response to somatic complaints.

Second, it is essential that invasive or costly diagnostic evaluations and treatments only be undertaken in response to objective evidence, and not in response to subjective complaints alone. Of course, patients with Briquet's syndrome or somatization disorder are not immune to physical disorders. A physician who is responsible for all the health care needs of a patient over many years has much more knowledge of his or her usual status in order to recognize the emergence of another disorder. Sometimes a patient may be frustrated with the physician for not doing more tests or not prescribing a desired medication and threaten to change physicians. This should be met with an empathetic but firm response that such a change would be unfortunate because the physician knows his or her history well and this knowledge permits the physician to be most effective in carrying out his or her commitment to providing the best possible care of the patient in the long run. A thorough annual physical examination and routine tests provide reassurance.

Third, it is essential to recognize that patients with Briquet's syndrome or somatization disorder usually have much discomfort from anxiety or depressive symptoms that are often associated with many personal and social problems. They often have limited social skills and methods for dealing with stressful or difficult interpersonal problems. Often their physical complaints are precipitated or exacerbated coincident with increasing stress. They often have information-processing deficits that make it difficult for them to recognize the relationship between their physical complaints and social problems. When the information-processing deficit is not too great, it may be possible for them to improve their skill at recognizing what is upsetting them when they experience an exacerbation of somatic symptoms. Even if this is not accomplished, it is possible to modify the patient's behavior by simple behavioral management techniques. The physician should show little interest and attention in physical complaints and great interest in personal and social problems (Morrison, 1978). Alternative ways of dealing with social and personal problems can be concretely discussed by reviewing the advantages and disadvantages of each of several possible courses of action and inaction. The goal is to improve the patient's problem-solving skills by concrete, nondirective discussion to practical problems of immediate interest. It may be helpful for patients to keep a diary of their activities, symptoms, and associated circumstances in order to identify recurrent factors that precipitate symptoms or reinforce sick role behavior. Operant conditioning of sick role behavior is discussed in detail in relation to chronic pain later. Actual direction and advice must be avoided; direct advice fosters dependence rather

than increased self-esteem and facilitates manipulation of the therapist by the patient. In addition to teaching problem-solving techniques, the patient can be taught that regular brief periods of rest and relaxation may reduce tension and that this will indirectly reduce sensitivity to pain, muscle spasms, and other factors associated with somatic discomfort. A wide variety of relaxation techniques are available at little or no cost (Scallet et al., 1976). The combination of instruction in relaxation techniques and training in problem-solving and social skills may help the patient to deal with psychosocial stress with less disability from physical discomfort.

Fourth, the prescription of medication should be kept to a minimum and carefully monitored. Wheatley (1962, 1964, 1965) has shown that low doses of anxiolytic drugs provide some symptomatic improvement in these patients in a series of double-blind clinical trials with general practitioners. Chlordiazepoxide, phenobarbital, amobarbital, and the phenothiazine pericyazine were compared in various trials. Chlordiazepoxide was recommended because of safety, patient preference, and equivalent effectiveness in symptom relief (Wheatley, 1965). The best results were obtained by optimistic doctors using low doses of medication regardless of which anxiolytic drug was used. The preferred regimen was chlordiazepoxide, 5 mg three times daily. The response to placebo tablets was uniformly poor, and it was concluded that the use of placebo tablets is of little value in the treatment of somatizers. Other drugs besides anxiolytics may be preferable in some cases. Some patients with Briquet's syndrome as adults have a history of attention-deficit disorder with hyperactivity as children; these adult hyperkinetics often are dramatically improved on stimulants, such as methylphenidate, amphetamine, and the noneuphoriant pemoline (Wender et al., 1981). Other patients without childhood inattention, hyperactivity, and impulsivity do not tolerate such stimulants. More patients show improvement on antidepressants, but the effective doses are often lower than usually required in primary major depressive disorders: Mann and Greenspan (1976) reported rapid improvement on 25 to 50 mg imipramine. However, patients with Briquet's syndrome or somatization disorder are often erratic about taking medication; develop drug dependence on sedatives, analgesics, and euphoriant drugs; and may attempt suicide by overdosing. Accordingly, it is important to teach relaxation techniques in order to minimize the need for medication. Medication should be selectively prescribed in the lowest effective dosage schedule and discontinuation trials undertaken regularly.

Fifth, it is useful to maintain contact with family members. Patients with Briquet's disorder are such poor observers and historians that information from others involved in their lives on a daily basis is often needed for the physician to know what is really happening. Family members can assist the physician to maintain compliance with therapy and alert the physician to emerging social problems, doctor shopping, medication abuse, or forms of noncompliance with therapy.

Finally, it is essential that the physician place firm limits on excessive or manipulative demands by the patient (Murphy and Guze, 1960; Murphy, 1982). These limits should be guided by the preceding principles with an attitude of optimism and confidence that such patients can eventually reduce their disability and discomfort, learn to cope more effectively with their problems, and avoid unnecessary medical and social complications.

CONVERSION AND DISSOCIATIVE REACTIONS (ACUTE HYSTERIA)

Definition

A *conversion reaction* is a sudden, temporary loss or alteration in sensorimotor function or some other physical functions in response to psychological conflict. The classic examples of conversion reactions are sensorimotor abnormalities that suggest neurologic disorders. These include sensory losses, such as blindness, deafness, anosmia, anesthesia, and analgesia, or sensory alterations, such as diplopia and dysesthesias. Other classic examples often involve motor abnormalities alone, such as paralysis, ataxia, dysphagia, and aphonia, or in combination with disturbances of consciousness or sensation, such as pseudoseizures and unconsciousness. Thus the classic conversion reactions involve the special senses or voluntary nervous system, but DSM-III also includes some disturbances of the autonomic nervous system or endocrine system when these disturbances appear to be direct symbolic expressions of psychological conflict. For example, disgust or rejection of particular situations or activities may be symbolized by recurrent psychogenic vomiting; or the wish for pregnancy may be symbolized by pseudocyesis (false pregnancy). Many clinicians prefer to reserve the term *conversion reaction* for the classic sensorimotor disturbances because autonomic and endocrine disturbances more often have a chronic course (Cloninger, 1987). Conversion disorder is not diagnosed in DSM-III when symptoms are limited to pain (see psychogenic pain disorders later) or sexual dysfunction.

Conversion symptoms are not diagnosed simply by the exclusion of neurologic or other physical disorders. An essential element of the diagnosis is that there is a close temporal relationship between the onset of the symptom and an environmental precipitant that appears to involve a psychological conflict or need of the patient. Judgments about such precipitation are often uncertain unless the chain of events is repeated, so the diagnosis of a conversion reaction is unreliable unless the symptom is recurrent. DSM-III (1980) also permitted diagnosis of conversion disorder when there was no identifiable environmental precipitant, but the symptom enabled the individual to obtain "secondary gain." *Secondary gain* refers to the patient obtaining additional support or avoiding undesired activities because of the symptom. This has little diagnostic value, however, because many patients with medical illnesses obtain such secondary gain from their illness. Accordingly, the 1980 DSM-III criteria are being revised to exclude diagnosis based on secondary gain and to distinguish between isolated and recurrent conversions.

A *dissociative reaction* is a sudden, temporary, psychogenic loss of memory, alteration in consciousness, or alteration in identity. When there is an alteration in consciousness, important personal events cannot be recalled, and the patient may be disoriented, perplexed, and wander aimlessly. When there is an alteration in identity, the person may forget his or her usual identity, travel to a new location, and assume a new identity temporarily; this is called a *fugue*. An uncommon example of a dissociative disorder is the phenomenon of multiple personality: the existence of two or more fully integrated personalities within an individual, each of which is dominant at different times and with unique memories, complex social activities, and behavior patterns. Transition between personalities or the onset of amnesic or fugue states is usually precipitated by psychosocial stress, such as marital quarrels, personal rejection, or events associated with a high risk of injury or death. Thus both conversion and dissociative states are typically precipitated by severe psychosocial stress, but it is often difficult to elicit the relevant history before treatment without collateral informants. Both conversion and dissociative states suggest the possibility of neurologic disorders and are characterized by abrupt onset and resolution. Accordingly, they are sometimes grouped together as acute hysteria or hysterical neurosis.

Etiology

Dissociative and conversion reactions appear to depend, in at least some cases, on descending or corticofugal inhibitory brain mechanisms. This was initially suggested in 1963 by Hernandez-Peon, Chavez-Ibarra, and Aguilar-Figueroa based in part on a study of a patient with hysterical hemianesthesia, using averaged electroencephalographic (EEG) responses evoked by painful stimuli. No somatosensory responses were evoked by stimulation of the anesthetized side, but stimulation of the healthy side evoked normal responses. The inhibition was relative, operating only up to a certain level of stimulus intensity. Active inhibition was indicated by responses returning to normal with anesthesia. Similar findings have been obtained with visually evoked responses in 14 patients with hysterical blindness (Behrman and Levy, 1970). A longitudinal study of a patient with depersonalization revealed little or no fluctuation in skin conductance during the dissociative state (Lader, 1969), but she reverted to a state of marked agitation with frequent spontaneous fluctuations in skin conductance when the depersonalization state remitted.

These observations all support the hypothesis that conversion and dissociative reactions may be precipitated by excessive cortical arousal, which in turn triggers reactive inhibition of signals at synapses in sensorimotor pathways by way of negative feedback relationships between the cerebral cortex and the brainstem reticular formation (Berlyne, 1967; Hernandez-Peon, 1961). This accounts for the consistent temporal relationship between stressful events and the onset of acute hysteria (Raskin et al., 1966), the reduction in anxiety and autonomic activity during conversion and dissociative states (Lader, 1969), and the effectiveness of sodium amobarbital infusions—and other methods of sedation that are discussed later—in relieving the symptoms (Frumkin et al., 1981).

Before these modern physiologic studies were possible, detailed clinical studies of patients with conversion and dissociative reactions were a major impetus to the development of many psychodynamic concepts by Janet (1907) and Freud (1964). Both men thought that the development of hysterical symptoms was the result of disturbing mental associations becoming unavailable to consciousness by voluntary recall. Janet proposed that hysterical symptoms could arise when forces that normally serve to integrate mental function fail and some functions escape from active central control. This theoretical process was referred to by Janet as *dissociation*. In contrast, Freud suggested that there was an active process by which disturbing mental associations were removed from conscious awareness. This active process of removal from availability to voluntary recall was called *repression* and was conceived as a mechanism to protect the patient from emotional pain arising from either disturbing external circumstances or anxiety-provoking internal urges and feelings. The theoretical formulation of Freud is remarkably analogous to contemporary theories based on more refined neurophysiologic data.

Current psychodynamic theory suggests that conversion symptoms are a direct symbolic expression of the underlying psychological conflict rather than an undifferentiated reaction to stress. Primary gain is defined in terms of the effectiveness of a conversion symptom in reducing anxiety by symbolic expression of the repressed wish. In practice, however, the evaluation of symbolism is usually difficult or impossible in brief consultations (Raskin et al., 1966). Social learning, mimicry, and suggestion also appear to influence at least the form of conversion phenomena: patients with conversions often have been exposed to a model for their symptom (Raskin et al., 1966). The model may have been the illness of another person, a previous illness, or even concurrent physical disease. For example, individuals with epilepsy also may develop pseudoseizures that simulate their usual fits or a seizure by one person in a school or factory may herald "mass hysteria" in which conversion symptoms spread like contagion (Temoshok and Attkisson, 1977).

Individuals differ in their susceptibility to conversion and dissociative reactions. Individuals with histrionic, antisocial, or dependent personality disorders or with Briquet's syndrome are more likely to develop acute hysterical symptoms than others (Guze et al., 1971a; American Psychiatric Association, 1980). Increased susceptibility to conversion and dissociative reactions is found in individuals with low sedation thresholds, frontal lobe trauma or impairment, or dominant cerebral hemisphere dysfunction (Shagass and Jones, 1958; Slater, 1948; Flor-Henry et al., 1981). However, conversions may occur in individuals with no associated psychopathology or neuropsychological deficits.

Most studies have not distinguished between individuals with single and recurrent conversions, and these groups may be qualitatively distinct but overlapping populations. Acute hysterics habituate normally to repetitive sound stimuli whereas chronic hysterics do not (Mears and Horvath, 1972).

Most patients with conversion reactions have bilateral symptoms, but left-sided symptoms predominate when the symptoms are unilateral (Stern, 1977; Galin et al., 1977). The left-sided predominance is more pronounced in women than in men (Flor-Henry et al., 1981). Flor-Henry et al. (1981) suggest that this asymmetrical distribution of unilateral conversion reactions and of psychogenic pain (Merskey and Watson, 1979) is a direct consequence of brain neural organization. Wyke (1967) studied the effects of brain lesions on the rapidity of upper limb movement and found that left hemisphere lesions produced both ipsilateral and contralateral abnormalities, whereas right brain lesions had only contralateral effects. Similarly, in studies of discriminative touch sensibility, Semmes (1968) found ipsilateral deficits with left hemispheric lesions but contralateral deficits with right hemispheric lesions. Thus brain dysfunction is likely to be associated with either bilateral or left-sided sensorimotor symptoms.

Epidemiology

Estimates of the incidence and prevalence of conversion and dissociative reactions depend greatly on whether they are based on treated cases or on self-report of past symptoms regardless of treatment. A past history of one or more classic conversion or dissociative reactions was found in 27 percent of 100 normal postpartum women (Farley et al., 1968) and in 30 percent of 50 medically ill women (Woodruff, 1967). Most of these symptoms remitted quickly without treatment but were clearly recalled because of the dramatic and severe nature of the symptom. When the same interview was given to psychiatric outpatients, about 25 percent had a past history of conversions (Guze et al., 1971a), which is similar to the risk in the general population. This suggests that the association of conversion and dissociative reactions with psychopathology may be greatly influenced by treatment-seeking behavior.

In contrast, treated cases of conversion or dissociative reaction are uncommon. The incidence of treatment for conversion reactions over a 10-year period was 22 per 100,000 in New York and 11 per 100,000 in Iceland (Stefansson et al., 1976). The hospital incidence in New York during the same period was 4.5 percent for conversions. Dissociative reactions appear to be even more uncommon than conversions: only 1.3 percent of all admissions to an Air Force medical center were for dissociative reactions (Kirshner, 1973). Even in treated samples, however, a high proportion of patients in some settings have some conversion symptoms observed when assessment is systematic: about 25 percent of all men in a Veterans Administration neuropsychiatric hospital in Appalachia had one or more conversions at some time during their hospitalization (Weinstein et al., 1969).

Although it is often said that conversion and dissociative reactions are becoming less common, available data suggest no actual change (Stephens and Kamp, 1962). Some psychiatrists may now see fewer patients with acute hysteria than in the past because they are now often referred to neurologists or internists (Chodoff, 1974). Among patients referred for psychiatric consultation in medical centers, about 14 percent are referred because of conversion symptoms (Ziegler et al., 1960; McKegney, 1967).

Patients with acute hysteria are most often adolescents or young adults (Ziegler et al., 1960; Guze et al., 1971a), but patients of all ages may present with conversions (Temoshok and Attkisson, 1977). Women outnumber men by a factor of 2:1 (Stefansson et al., 1976) to 5:1 (Ziegler et al., 1960). Acute hysteria is more common in lower socioeconomic groups (Hollingshead and Redlich, 1958; Stefansson et al., 1976). Fewer patients with 1 or more years of college report a history of conversion or dissociative reactions than those with less education (Guze et al., 1971a). The incidence of treatment for acute hysteria may be higher in rural areas than in urban areas (Temoshok and Attkisson, 1977). Interpreting these differences is difficult because they are based on series of treated cases, and the vast majority of all conversion and dissociative reactions appear to remit spontaneously without treatment.

Pathology

By definition, there are no pathologic findings that account for the symptoms.

Clinical Picture

Conversion and dissociative reactions are not syndromes or discrete disorders with their own characteristic clinical picture. They are individual symptoms occurring in response to stress in a wide variety of psychiatric or medical disorders. Nevertheless, the diagnosis may be useful to distinguish individual psychogenic symptoms from individual symptoms of physical disorders. The fundamental clinical issue is to identify the associated clinical features that permit an accurate distinction from symptoms of physical disorders.

Investigators who have followed patients for several years after a diagnosis of conversion or dissociative reaction have identified those features that permit a reliable distinction from physical disorders. Several studies have found that a previous history of conversion or other unexplained physical complaints is the most reliable predictor that the patient will not later be proven to have a physical disorder (Gatfield and Guze, 1962; Slater, 1965; Perley and Guze, 1962; Raskin et al., 1966; Purtell et al., 1951; Guze et al., 1971a; Bishop and Torch, 1979). The diagnosis of conversion or dissociative reactions is unreliable in the absence of a definite history of Briquet's syndrome or a past history of transient unexplained symptoms that recur in association with well-defined precipitants.

Patients with Briquet's syndrome or a past history of conversion or dissociative reactions are not immune to physical disorders. Thus the presence of prior hysterical symptoms is not a sufficient basis for diagnosis. The evaluation of emotional stress is a difficult but necessary part of the clinical assessment. Events that are obviously stressful often precede the onset or exacerbation of physical disorders as well as various psychiatric disorders and do not distinguish true conversions from initially undiagnosed physical disorders (Raskin et al., 1966; Watson and Buranen, 1979). However, Raskin et al. (1966) reported success in distinguishing conversion symptoms from physical disorders by judgments about whether the symptoms appeared to solve a psychological conflict brought about by a precipitating stress. Their judgment was highly dependent on the patient's report of prior conversion symptoms or transient somatic complaints: that is, an event that would be trivial for an average individual was judged to be significant because it was reportedly associated with somatic symptoms in the past. Thus clinical judgments about psychogenic stress seem to be reliable only when the sequence of events has been repeated.

The *complete* resolution of symptoms by suggestion, hypnosis, or intravenous infusion of sedatives like amobarbital is useful in distinguishing conversion and dissociative reactions from physical disorders. For example, psychogenic amnesia often clears, whereas organic amnesia is often worsened with amobarbital infusions (Ward et al., 1978;

Frumkin et al., 1981). Physical disorders may be exacerbated by associated anxiety, and *partial* improvement with reassurance or sedation often occurs in such cases. Such concurrent anxiety or partial improvement with reduction of anxiety may lead to misdiagnosis of physical disorders (Gatfield and Guze, 1962; Watson and Buranen, 1979). For example, Gatfield and Guze (1962) found that 21 percent of 24 patients diagnosed as conversion reactions on a neurology service had definite neurologic diseases 3 to 10 years later to explain the original symptoms. All these diagnostic errors were due to temporary partial improvement with medical evaluation or sedation that had falsely suggested psychiatric illness.

Signs and symptoms that appear inconsistent with known anatomic distributions or that vary from one examination to another are frequent in patients with conversion reactions (Weintraub, 1983). Such judgments are notoriously unreliable because of limitations in knowledge of pathophysiology, marked variation in the presentation of physical disorders, and limited methods for objective assessment. Patients with undiagnosed physical disorders are often in distress and may exaggerate or misrepresent their symptoms. Consequently, patients with both physical disorders and somatoform disorders may be difficult to evaluate.

The diagnosis of conversion disorder is often suspected if patients are dramatic or suggestible. Such findings are associated with conversions but, like inconsistent signs and symptoms, are not a reliable basis for diagnosis in the absence of past history of recurrent psychogenic symptoms.

Clinical Course

The course of conversion and dissociative reactions depends on the organ system that is affected. Classic pseudoneurologic symptoms, including sensorimotor conversions and psychogenic amnesia or fugue states, are characterized by their abrupt onset and resolution. The duration of the individual attack is usually short and self-limited. Occasionally, pseudoneurologic symptoms may become chronic or recurrent, especially when the precipitating stress is chronic or recurrent, when there is associated chronic psychopathology, or when persistence of the symptom is reinforced by secondary gain. Patients with pseudoseizures are more likely to have recurrences than are patients with paralysis or aphonia (Hafeiz, 1980; Weintraub, 1983). The overall course of illness is dominated by the course of any underlying physical or psychiatric disease. For example, multiple personality disorder is often associated with chronic psychopathology, but the individual transitions usually are brief.

Endocrine disturbances are often chronic and misdiagnosed physical disorders. For example, most patients with symptoms suggestive of pseudocyesis can be shown to have an objective endocrine disturbance, most often a prolactinoma, with radioimmunoassays of serum prolactin (Cohen, 1982).

In contrast, patients with psychogenic vomiting, like psychogenic pain patients, usually have a chronic course. Psychogenic vomiting is seldom debilitating, despite its chronicity (Rosenthal et al., 1980; Wruble et al., 1982), whereas psychogenic pain is often disabling (Blumer and Heilbronn, 1982).

Laboratory Findings

Acute hysteria is not associated with abnormal laboratory findings. The results of neurophysiologic tests and other laboratory findings largely depend on any associated psychopathology or physical disease.

Differential Diagnosis

General aspects of the clinical picture that aid in differential diagnosis were noted earlier (also see Table 11-4) but differential diagnosis in individual cases depends on the particular symptoms. Marked weakness in the presence of normal deep tendon reflexes may suggest the possibility of a conversion reaction, but myasthenia gravis, periodic paralysis, myoglobinuric myopathy, polymyositis, and other acquired myopathies must be considered. In myasthenia gravis, weakness may come and go, but typical attacks last for weeks rather than for hours or days. Myopathies are usually associated with prominent myalgia, and muscle enzymes assays and electromyography permit differentiation. Also, discolored urine is observed with myoglobinuria.

TABLE 11-4. *Utility of Psychiatric Criteria for Distinguishing Conversion and Dissociative Reactions from Physical Disorders*

Putative diagnostic criteria	Predicts no physical disorder
Briquet's syndrome	Yes
Prior history of conversions	Yes
Prior history of recurrent somatic complaints	Yes
Current anxiety or dysphoria	No
Emotional stress before onset	
Any	No
Previous history of conversions with conflict resolution	Yes
With symbolism	No
Secondary gain	No
Partial improvement with suggestion or sedation	No
MMPI profile type*	No
Histrionic personality	
With prior history of conversions	Yes
No prior history of conversion	No
La belle indifference	No

*MMPI, Minnesota Multiphasic Personality Inventory.

Attacks of weakness in periodic paralysis are usually precipitated by exercise or by eating a large meal but also may be precipitated by frightening experiences or injections of epinephrine. Potassium metabolism is altered in periodic paralysis, and many cases are inherited as a mendelian dominant. Weakness of arms and legs is seen early in acute idiopathic polyneuritis of the Guillain-Barré type.

Sudden unilateral blindness owing to optic neuritis may be confused with a conversion reaction, since the funduscopic examination is normal in both conditions. Diminished direct light reflex usually permits a differentiation, and many patients with optic neuritis later develop other signs of multiple sclerosis.

Apparent dissociative phenomena, including amnesia, fugue, and multiple personality, may either result from complex partial seizures owing to a temporal lobe focus or be secondarily generalized from another brain region (Mayeux et al., 1979; Schenk and Bear, 1981). Prolonged or repetitive complex partial seizures with continuous interictal confusion have been documented in episodes lasting for as long as 3 days. Depression and anxiety may herald the onset of fugue caused by such complex partial seizures, and apparently, psychogenic behavior responds to anticonvulsant therapy (Mayeux et al., 1979).

A detailed, practical guide to the differential diagnosis of a wide variety of specific conversion, dissociative, and pain symptoms has been presented by Weintraub (1983).

Treatment

The diagnosis and treatment of conversion and dissociative reactions must be approached with caution and respect for the patient for two major reasons. The differentiation of physical and psychogenic symptoms is unreliable early in the course of illness, so the physician must observe carefully and avoid premature conclusions based on inadequate data. If the symptom is truly psychogenic, the patient is in distress and the symptom has an adaptive role. Relief of the symptom and treatment of associated psychosocial problems may have a major impact on later adjustment. If patients are told that there is nothing "real" wrong with them, they will often deteriorate rather than improve. If the symptom is relieved but the associated psychosocial problems that precipitated the symptom are not recognized and managed, the symptoms may recur. Improper management can have serious consequences, leading to chronic disability. In contrast, proper management can be rewarding because of the rapid and complete resolution of the symptoms.

As soon as possible after conversion and dissociative reactions are suspected, it is important to obtain collateral information about the circumstances associated with the onset of symptoms. The patient's own account is often incomplete or inaccurate before treatment, and this information can expedite treatment.

Once a presumptive diagnosis of conversion or dissociative reaction is made, the first phase of treatment is the reassurance and relaxation of the patient. Many patients are reassured by a calm and thorough history and physical examination. Some patients who remain overtly agitated may benefit from mild sedation. It is nearly always countertherapeutic to tell the patient initially that the symptom is psychogenic. It is more helpful to suggest to the patient that from your examination, you are confident that the symptom will disappear quickly and completely. It is also useful to suggest that the symptom may already be beginning to disappear. As long as the patient does not become more agitated, recent events and feelings may be discussed without drawing any specific causal connection with the symptom. If the patient becomes more agitated, he or she should be reassured and encouraged to relax quietly for a short while before continuing with further discussion.

If this conservative approach of reassurance and relaxation does not result in remission of the symptom, then an amobarbital (Amytal) interview has both diagnostic and therapeutic value. A 10% solution of Amytal is slowly injected intravenously; 500 mg of Amytal diluted in sterile water to 5 ml is injected at a maximum rate of 1 ml/min. Before the infusion begins the patient should be informed that you expect the conversion or dissociative symptom to disappear with this treatment. During the infusion, the physician should suggest that the symptom is beginning to disappear. The patient can be asked to try to recall the circumstances preceding the onset of the symptom, and it can be suggested that the medication being infused will help this recall. When the patient's words begin to slur, administration should be stopped and the patient observed. Often the removal of the symptom is accompanied by recall of the precipitating stress, which is expressed with much crying and sighing. The patient can be reassured that he or she will be able to discuss what was upsetting him or her without so much distress later and that the symptom will not recur.

Suggestion, hypnosis, Amytal, and other relaxation treatments are all effective in the first, acute phase of treatment (Weintraub, 1983; Hafeiz, 1980; Frumkin et al., 1981). Although some have suggested that amobarbital is more effective than other approaches (Frumkin et al., 1981), Hafeiz (1980) found that other relaxation techniques as well as 10 mg methylamphetamine injected intravenously were more effective than a 5% solution of amobarbital. Regardless of the particular technique used, the emphasis in this phase is on rapid relief of the symptom to prevent reinforcement of its persistence by secondary gain, to identify and recall precipitating psychosocial stressors, and to establish a therapeutic alliance. The treatment of acute hysteria is a psychiatric emergency requiring both empathy and a push for rapid resolution because the risk of recurrence and chronic disability are strongly associated with the prior duration of symptoms before treatment (Hafeiz, 1980).

The second phase of treatment is to support the patient and help him or her to recognize and cope with the psychosocial stress that initially precipitated the symptom. If the precipitating stress is unlikely to recur and the patient has no major underlying psychopathology, then this phase of treatment is likely to be brief, with little risk of recurrence. On the other hand, persistent stress or associated psychopathology may require long-term psychiatric treatment. The duration and type of treatment at this phase must be individualized according to these associated factors.

PSYCHOGENIC PAIN (CHRONIC IDIOPATHIC PAIN)

Definition

Pain is one of the most frequent and difficult symptoms that a physician must evaluate. It is a subjective experience, and a patient's pain threshold varies with his or her attention, mood, fatigue, and suggestion. In other words, there is always an interaction between physical stimuli and psychological state in the perception of pain, so the distinction between physical (pathogenic) and psychogenic pain is moot. Even when clinicians attempt to rate the etiology of chronic pain on an organic–nonorganic continuum based on comprehensive diagnostic data, the agreement among different raters is, at best, moderate; in a study of 100 consecutive patients referred to a pain clinic, Fordyce et al. (1978) found the interjudge correlation for such ratings was only 0.57, even though the raters had access to the same data. In a follow-up study of patients diagnosed as having psychogenic pain, Slater (1965) found that acute pain proved to result, in most cases, from physical disorders. When the pain remains unexplained despite repeated observation over 6 months, psychological factors that lead to persistence or exacerbation of the pain often develop. Nevertheless, obscure organic pathology may remain unrecognized. For example, Hendler et al. (1982) used thermography to evaluate 224 consecutive patients with no radiologic, neurologic, orthopedic, or laboratory abnormalities to explain their chronic pain. Abnormal results of thermography in 19 percent led to revised diagnoses of reflex sympathetic dystrophy, nerve root irritation, and thoracic outlet syndrome. Other series have found up to 54 percent abnormal thermograms (Weintraub, 1983). Thus attempts to evaluate the causes of pain according to the cartesian mind/body dichotomy are doubtful in principle and unreliable in practice.

DSM-III criteria for psychogenic pain are identical to those for conversion disorder except that the symptoms are limited to pain. The required judgments about psychogenicity have proved to be impossible in most patients, and it is now recommended that the pathogenic/psychogenic distinction not be attempted (Williams and Spitzer, 1982). Patients with chronic (6 months') preoccupation with pain are recognized as having idiopathic pain disorder if the pain is unexplained after extensive evaluation or if the functional impairment or complaints are grossly in excess of what would be expected from the physical findings. Such patients are clinically heterogeneous in terms of their prepain psychopathology, but most have a characteristic pattern of psychiatric symptoms and pain-related behaviors that appears to be learned or conditioned by the consequences of their recurrent complaints about pain.

Etiology

Pain-related behavior may be learned by either operant or classical conditioning. Operant conditioning occurs when certain behaviors are reinforced (increased in frequency or strength) through contingent rewards or when particular behaviors are decreased in frequency or strength by punishment or inhibition. For example, the frequency and intensity of pain-related complaints may be reinforced by increased attention from friends and relatives, relief from carrying out undesirable activities such as hard physical labor or undesired sexual obligations, the pleasurable effects of analgesics given as needed for pain, the possibility of monetary gain from litigation or disability compensation. At the same time, health-related behaviors may be inhibited by instruction by physicians, lawyers, and well-meaning associates not to work and to assume an invalid role or by the need to remain sick in order to collect compensation. Classical conditioning also can occur with chronic pain patients so that ordinary neutral objects begin to evoke pain-related behavior. A pain patient's bedroom or work area may evoke an increase in pain if earlier experience with these settings has been associated with pain. Such learned behavior cannot be eliminated by relief or correction of the original source of pain, so separation from such conditioned stimuli and behavioral modification in pain centers may be necessary.

Demoralization and learned helplessness, as described by Seligman (1975), may account for the prominence of depressive symptoms in many patients with chronic pain. Such patients appear anergic, anhedonic, dependent, and helpless after prolonged periods in which they are unable to achieve rewards for initiating health-related behavior (Morse, 1983).

There is some evidence that prior social models and cultural attitudes may predispose some individuals to developing chronic pain-related behavior.

Apley (1975) studied 1100 British school children and found that half of those with chronic unexplained abdominal pain had a close relative with chronic pain compared with such a family history in only one eighth of children with a clear physical explanation for their abdominal pain. It is believed that the Irish and Anglo-Saxons have greater pain tolerance than southern Mediterranean ethnic groups, suggesting substantial ethnic differences. Some empirical studies confirm these cultural and ethnic stereotypes about pain tolerance (Woodrow et al., 1972), but others do not. Flannery et al. (1981) found no significant difference in episiotomy pain among five ethnic groups (blacks, Italians, Jewish, Irish, and Anglo-Saxon Protestants). Zborowski (1969) found that ethnic differences are more prominent in first-generation immigrants than in later generations.

Neurons in the cerebral cortex and medulla can inhibit the firing of trigeminal and spinal pain transmission neurons. The activity of this descending pain inhibition system is mediated, at least in part, by endorphins, which are endogenous opiate-like compounds. Serotonin has an inhibiting effect on pain perception and is probably the neurotransmitter of the descending inhibitory pathways that arise in the raphe nucleus of the medulla (Posner, 1982). Accordingly, it is interesting that endorphins and serotonin metabolites are decreased in the cerebrospinal fluid of chronic pain patients (von Knorring et al., 1979). The extent of the reduction in endorphins correlates with the tendency to augment the intensity of incoming sensory stimuli as measured by the slope of the amplitude of averaged evoked EEG potentials in response to increasing stimulus intensities. Thus what appears to be an overdramatized description of pain in relation to physical abnormalities is associated with an objective neurophysiologic tendency to augment sensory input. It is unclear whether the amplification or abnormally decreased inhibition of pain in such patients is a cause or an effect of the observed clinical state. Regardless of the original direction of effects, there are objective neurophysiologic and biochemical differences between patients with chronic pain and patients with other psychiatric and medical conditions.

Epidemiology

Few epidemiologic data are available about chronic pain patients, but the number of pain-control facilities indicates that such patients are not uncommon. In 1979 the Pain Clinic Directory, published by the American Society of Anesthesiologists, listed 285 pain-control facilities in the United States. Most of the patients in such facilities have maladaptive pain-related behavior conditioned by the consequences of their chronic complaints (Brena and Chapman, 1983).

Pathology

Many postural and gait abnormalities can be caused by chronic misuse of braces, collars, and ambulatory devices by pain patients. Low activity and poor postural habits may lead to contractures and myofibrositis. Prolonged inactivity also can lead to osteoporosis, overweight, and circulatory and respiratory disorders. Abuse of aspirin and phenacetin can lead to gastric, renal, or hepatic damage. Thus pain-related behavior may, in turn, cause added nociceptive stimulation, creating a vicious cycle of progressive deterioration.

Clinical Picture

Patients with chronic pain-related behaviors manifest a lifestyle that has been characterized as the "disease of the *D*'s" (Brena and Chapman, 1983): (1) dramatic display in describing the painful experience: vague, diffuse complaints that are often inconsistent with documented organic pathology or known pathophysiologic mechanisms; (2) disuse and degeneration of various body functions as consequences of the pain-related behavior; (3) drug misuse and doctor shopping; (4) dependency: passivity and learned helplessness, which lead to demoralization and depression; (5) disability: pain-contingent financial compensation or desire for compensation through litigation and disability claims.

Blumer and Heilbronn (1982) evaluated a consecutive series of 129 patients with chronic unexplained pain and compared them with 36 patients with chronic rheumatoid arthritis who were receiving gold therapy. They noted that the chronic idiopathic pain patients had many more of the *D*'s than did the patients with chronic rheumatoid arthritis (Table 11-5). They also noted that such patients seemed unable to appreciate and verbalize their feelings. This inability to read one's own emotions has been called alexithymia (Nemiah, 1978). Although nearly all the patients showed depression and dependency after the onset of pain, only 12 percent had a history of depression before the onset of pain. The most prominent depressive symptoms are anergia, insomnia, and anhedonia, which are typically attributed to the pain; diurnal variation, loss of weight, and psychomotor retardation are unusual. Patients with chronic idiopathic pain had a history of more chronic overtime at work before onset of pain compared with those with rheumatoid arthritis (50 versus 28 percent) and more often took no annual vacation (48 versus 22 percent). A careful history from the patient and family members often reveals that the symptoms are almost identical with pain learned from a previous experience or observation. Patients often seek passive cures by physicians without accepting their own responsibility for modifying pain-related behavior, setting up what Berne (1964) called the

TABLE 11-5. *Clinical Features of Chronic Pain Patients*

Somatic complaints
Continuous pain of obscure origin Hypochondriacal preoccupation Desire for surgery and passive medical cures
Solid citizen
Denial of conflicts Idealization of self and of family relations Ergomania (prepain): "workaholism," relentless activity
Depression
Anergia (postpain): lack of initiative, inactivity, fatigue Anhedonia: inability to enjoy social life, leisure, and sex Insomnia Depressive mood and despair
History
Family (and personal) history of depression and alcoholism Past abuse by spouse Crippled relative Relative with chronic pain

Based on Blumer and Heilbronn, 1982.

"pain game," in which the doctor inevitably fails and feels guilty if he accepts the patient's premise that the doctor is responsible for the pain and its consequences.

Women tend to complain of pain in the face, abdomen, or genital region, whereas men usually complain of pain in the back or chest (Weintraub, 1983). Prepain psychopathology, if any, is highly variable: major affective disorders, alcoholism, Briquet's syndrome, and various anxiety states and personality disorders are the most common associated diagnoses.

Course

The course of illness depends on associated psychopathology, prior duration of pain, and extent of external reinforcement. Patients with lifelong adjustment problems, as in Briquet's syndrome, or pending or continuing monetary compensation are unlikely to improve regardless of treatment (Brena and Chapman, 1983). If there are many operantly conditioned pain-related behaviors, remission is unlikely without treatment in which the patient is removed from her usual environment and these contingencies are modified before the patient's return.

Laboratory Findings

Infrared thermography is useful in identifying changes in vascular flow associated with some cases of chronic pain. According to available studies, there is reduced vascular flow and lower temperature in the anatomical region of pain that is unde-

tected by other tests (Hendler et al., 1982). There is a low correlation between thermographic findings and clinical symptoms (Weintraub, 1983). Also, changes in vascular flow may be psychologically induced or learned, as in autogenic training or biofeedback, so that the question of original psychogenicity remains moot.

Differential Diagnosis

Several medical syndromes are characterized by chronic pain that cannot be diagnosed by routine evaluations, including electromyography, myelography, and tomography of affected regions. These include sympathetic reflex dystrophies and myofascial pain syndromes, such as tension headaches (Posner, 1982). Thermography is abnormal in these disorders.

Treatment

All physicians need to be knowledgeable about the first phase of pain management—the prevention of learned illness behavior associated with pain. Often chronic pain-related behaviors are, in part, iatrogenic and preventable. Prevention involves attention to behavioral management principles in prescription of medication, providing disability statements to employers and others, and educating the patient and his or her family about illness behavior.

Brena (1983) has summarized the following guidelines for use of drugs in chronic pain patients: (1) The use of any sedative or antianxiety drug has no lasting benefit and is a potential iatrogenic problem because of frequent misuse and complications. The patient and family should be informed that such drugs can cause depression and foster dependency. (2) The use of opiates should be limited to nonambulatory patients in cases of clear pathogenic pain. When the decision to use opiates is made, the drug must be given in doses high enough to provide effective analgesia. (3) In cases of chronic pain associated with a nonprogressive, noninvasive pathologic process of long duration, the drug of first choice is a tricyclic antidepressant, such as amitriptyline or doxepin, not sedatives or antianxiety medication. Depression, whether endogenous or reactive, should be treated with tricyclic antidepressants. If a rheumatic-type inflammatory process is documented, a nonsteroidal anti-inflammatory drug may be added. This permits encouragement of activity rather than inactivity. (4) No drug for chronic pain should be prescribed on an as-needed basis. Time-contingent prescriptions are less likely to lead to drug misuse through conditioning. Demands from the patient should be resisted, and drugs should never be prescribed, even temporarily, without proper assessment and follow-up. (5) Patients should be informed about possible drug reactions and complications in order to increase the likelihood that they will comply with prescribed limits. (6) Alternative treatment approaches, such as relaxation therapies, should be provided. Many patients requesting drugs for sleep and muscle spasms will have no further need for drugs after they have learned relaxation skills.

It is important for the physician to encourage appropriate activity rather than inactivity in order to avoid fostering sick role developments. The physician should explain the importance of normal activities of daily living in preserving physical and mental adjustment and should return the patient to activity that is appropriate for his or her physical status. This requires accurate assessment of physical limitations because premature or excessive activity can cause later avoidance of activity. Any statement of disability from the physician, whether to the patient, the family, employers, lawyers, or others, should be objectively documented, not based on subjective complaints alone, and should always be time-limited rather than indefinite. Most often operantly conditioned pain behavior is promoted by the patient's medical ignorance or misunderstanding, which the physician can correct. The patient and family should be informed when pain is not a symptom of a progressive disease and when physical activity can be increased without risk of harm. The meager rewards of chronic pain behavior are ultimately self-defeating and should be contrasted with those of effective well behavior. Disability benefits are generally adequate only for subsistence; depression and dependency accompany relief from responsibility; sympathy from others is usually brief and gives way to avoidance; and pain behaviors are not effective ways to communicate needs and feelings accurately to others.

In patients with chronic pain who have already developed conditioned pain-related behavior, it is important for the doctor and the patient to realize that the benefits of somatic treatment of any underlying physical disease will be independent of the benefits of psychiatric treatment of the learned sick role behaviors. Elimination of the original cause of the pain will not extinguish the conditioned sick role behavior and subjective complaints may actually intensify.

The goals of psychiatric treatment of chronic pain are to replace pain-related behavior with normal activity and to counteract the *D*'s by detoxifying patients misusing medication, decreasing subjective pain intensity, increasing activities of daily living, teaching competent coping skills to deal with impairment and suffering, and providing vocational evaluation and rehabilitation. It is often useful to have patients keep a diary of their daily activity, pain, and associated circumstances in order to identify any patterns suggesting conditioned behavior. This can be supplemented by interviewing family members. A wide variety of treatment strategies may be useful, including relaxation and biofeed-

back, cognitive therapy, behavior modification, and structured milieu-group therapy programs (Brena and Chapman, 1983). When conditioned pain behaviors are extensive, individual outpatient treatment is often unsuccessful, and it may be necessary to remove patients from their usual settings, evaluate and treat them in a pain clinic or comprehensive pain-control facility, educate their families, and restructure their environments before returning them home. Pain centers are medical facilities for diagnosis and treatment that are staffed by a team of physicians, psychologists, physical and occupational therapists, and consulting medical specialists. About 70 percent of patients who go through such pain-control programs are improved (Brena and Chapman, 1983). Many of the refractory patients have continuing disability compensation or associated chronic psychopathology, such as personality disorders, drug dependence, or Briquet's syndrome.

HYPOCHONDRIASIS AND OTHER SOMATOFORM DISORDERS

Hypochondriasis has been conceptualized in four ways that are supported by data (Barsky and Klerman, 1983). First, hypochondriasis is conceptualized as a psychiatric syndrome composed of "functional" somatic complaints, fear of disease, body preoccupation, and the persistent pursuit of medical care despite reassurance. Second, according to psychodynamic theory, the patient is disturbed by problems of anger and hostility, orality and dependency, low self-esteem, guilt, and masochism. Third, the cognitive set the patient uses to assess body sensations tends to amplify and augment normal body sensations so that the patient has a low threshold and tolerance of physical sensations, often misinterpreting normal sensations as an indication of disease. Fourth, hypochondriasis is socially learned sick role behavior and indirect interpersonal communication that is reinforced by success in eliciting caretaking and other secondary gains from the sick role. These features are all characteristic of the somatoform disorders in general, and serious doubt exists about whether there is a discrete disease entity corresponding to hypochondriacal neurosis.

The DSM-III criteria for hypochondriasis or hypochondriacal neurosis require preoccupation with an unrealistic fear or belief of having a serious disease and impaired social or occupational function despite medical evaluation and reassurance. The concept that such patients have an augmenting perceptual style and often misinterpret normal sensations is mentioned in the DSM-III description, but it is not part of the criteria.

Until the late nineteenth century, hypochondriasis was associated specifically with complaints involving the hypochondriac region of the abdomen—that is, below the costal cartilages—rather than with regionally nonspecific morbid disease preoccupation (Cloninger et al., 1984). The DSM-III criteria are essentially the same as proposed by Gillespie in 1928, who believed that hypochondriasis was an independent, discrete disease entity. Kenyon (1976) concluded from an extensive literature review and a controlled study of 512 psychiatric patients with hypochondriacal symptoms that hypochondriasis was always a secondary part of another syndrome, usually a depressive illness. In addition, Bianchi (1973) carried out a principal-components analysis of 235 psychiatric patients and identified one component that corresponded to a distinct group of female patients who had a syndrome of multiple somatic complaints, unnecessary surgery, and psychogenic pain associated with a low pain threshold. Bianchi concluded that these women had Briquet's syndrome and that other aspects of hypochondriasis were ancillary symptoms of other primary psychiatric disorders. For example, those scoring high on his disease conviction component usually had endogenous depressions and those with disease phobias usually had an anxiety neurosis.

It is important to note that most studies of hypochondriasis have been done in psychiatric patients rather than in the general population except for the recent Stockholm Adoption Study of somatoform disorders (Sigvardsson et al., 1984; Cloninger et al., 1984; Bohman et al., 1984). It may well be that few patients with hypochondriasis ever see psychiatrists because they believe that the symptoms of psychiatric patients are imaginary, not real, whereas they know that their own suffering is real. More studies with general or primary-care populations are needed before any conclusions about other somatoform disorders can be drawn.

REFERENCES

Adam G: Interception and Behavior. Budapest, Akademiai Kiado, 1967.

Almgren PE, Nordgren L, Skantze H: A retrospective study of operationally defined hysterics. Br J Psychiatry 132:670–673, 1978.

American Psychiatric Association Task Force on Nomenclature and Statistics: Diagnostic and Statistical Manual of Mental Disorders, 3d ed. Washington, American Psychiatric Association, 1980.

Apley J: The Child with Abdominal Pains. Oxford, Blackwell, 1975.

Barsky A, Klerman G: Overview: Hypochondriasis, bodily complaints, and somatic styles. Am. J. Psychiatry 140:273–283, 1983.

Behrman J, Levy R: Neurophysiological studies on patients with hysterical disturbances of vision. J Psychosom Res 14:187–194, 1970.

Bendefeldt F, Miller LL, Ludwig AM: Cognitive hysteria. Arch Gen Psychiatry 33:1250–1254, 1976.

Berlyne DE: Arousal and reinforcement. In Divine D (ed): Nebraska Symposium on Motivation. Lincoln, University of Nebraska Press, 1967, pp 1–110.

Berne E: Games People Play. New York, Grove Press, 1964.

Bianchi GN: Patterns of hypochondriasis. A principal components analysis. Br J Psychiatry 122:541–548, 1973.

Bishop ER Jr, Torch EM: Dividing "Hysteria": A preliminary investigation of conversion disorder and psychalgia. J Nerv Ment Dis 167:348–357, 1979.

Bissell DM: Porphyria, in Wyngaarden JB, Smith LH Jr (eds): Cecil's Textbook of Medicine, 16th ed. Philadelphia, WB Saunders Co, 1982, pp 1121–1126.

Blumer D, Heilbronn M: Chronic pain as a variant of depression disease: The pain-prone disorder. J Nerv Ment Dis 170:381–406, 1982.

Bohman M, Cloninger CR, von Knorring A-L, Sigvardsson S: An adoption study of somatoform disorders: III. Cross-fostering analysis and genetic relationship to alcoholism and criminality. Arch Gen Psychiatry 41:872–878, 1984.

Brena SF: Drugs and pain: Use and misuse. In Brena SF, Chapman SL (eds): Management of Patients with Chronic Pain. New York, Spectrum, 1983, pp 121–130.

Brena SF, Chapman SL (eds): Management of Patients with Chronic Pain. New York, Spectrum, 1983.

Briquet P: Traite clinique et therapeutique a l'hysterie. Paris, J-B Balliere & Fils, 1859.

Cantwell D: Psychiatric illness in the families of hyperactive children. Arch Gen Psychiatry 27:414–417, 1972.

Chodoff P: The diagnosis of hysteria: An overview. Am J Psychiatry 131:1073–1078, 1974.

Cloninger CR: Somatization disorder. In DSM-IV Sourcebook. Washington, American Psychiatric Press, 1993.

Cloninger CR: Diagnosis of somatoform disorders: A critique of DSM-III. In Tischler GL (ed): Diagnosis and Classification in Psychiatry. New York, Cambridge University Press, 1987.

Cloninger CR: The link between hysteria and sociopathy: An intergrative model of pathogenesis based on clinical, genetic, and neurophysiological observations. In Akiskal HS, Webb WL (eds): Psychiatric Diagnosis: Explorations of Biological Predictors. New York, Spectrum, 1978, pp 189–218.

Cloninger CR, Guze SB: Psychiatric illness and female criminality: The role of sociopathy and hysteria in the antisocial woman. Am J Psychiatry 127:303–311, 1970.

Cloninger CR, Reich T, Guze SB: The multifactorial model of disease transmission: III. Familial relationship between sociopathy and hysteria (Briquet's syndrome). Br J Psychiatry 127:11–22, 1975.

Cloninger CR, Martin RL, Guze SB, Clayton PJ: A prospective follow-up and family study of somatization in men and women. Am J Psychiatry 143:873–878, 1986.

Cloninger CR, Sigvardsson S, von Knorring A-L, Bohman M: An adoption study of somatoform disorders: II. Identification of two discrete somatoform disorders. Arch Gen Psychiatry 41:863–871, 1984.

Cohen LM: A current perspective of pseudocyesis. Am J Psychiatry 139:1140–1144, 1982.

Coryell W: A blind family history study of Briquet's syndrome: Further validation of the diagnosis. Arch Gen Psychiatry 37:1266–1269, 1980.

De Beer G: Charles Darwin. In Encyclopedia Britannica Macropedia, vol 5. Chicago, Encyclopedia Brittanica, Inc, 1980, pp 492–496.

Farley J, Woodruff RA Jr, Guze SB: The prevalence of hysteria and conversion symptoms. Br J Psychiatry 114:1121–1125, 1968.

Flannery RB, Sos J, McGovern P: Ethnicity as a factor in the expression of pain. Psychosomatics 22:39–50, 1981.

Flor-Henry P, Fromm-Auch D, Tapper M, Schopflocher D: A neuropsychological study of the stable syndrome of hysteria. Biol Psychiatry 16:601–626, 1981.

Fordyce WE, Brana SF, Holcomb RJ: Relationship of patient semantic pain descriptions to physician diagnostic judgments, activity level measures, and MMPI. Pain 5:293–303, 1978.

Freud S: Standard Edition of the Complete Psychological Works of Sigmund Freud. London, Hogarth Press, 1964.

Frumkin LB, Ward NG, Grim PS: A possible cerebral mechanism for the clearing of psychogenic symptoms with amobarbital. Biol Psychiatry 16:687–692, 1981.

Galin D, Diamond R, Braff D: Lateralization of conversion symptoms: More frequent on the left. Am J Psychiatry 134:578–580, 1977.

Gatfield PD, Guze SB: Prognosis and differential diagnosis of conversion reactions (A follow-up study). Dis Nerv Sys 23:1–8, 1962.

Gillespie R: Hypochondria: Its definition, nosology, and psychopathology. Guys Hosp Rep 78:408–460, 1928.

Guze SB: The diagnosis of hysteria: What are we trying to do? Am J Psychiatry 124:491–498, 1967.

Guze SB, Cloninger CR, Martin RL, Clayton PJ: A follow-up and family study of Briquet's syndrome. Br J Psychiatry, 149:17–23, 1986.

Guze SB, Perley MJ: Observations on the natural history of hysteria. Am J Psychiatry 119:960–965, 1963.

Guze SB, Woodruff RA Jr, Clayton PJ: A study of conversion symptoms in psychiatric outpatients. Am J Psychiatry 128:643–646, 1971a.

Guze SB, Woodruff RA Jr, Clayton PJ: Hysteria and antisocial behavior: Further evidence of an association. Am J Psychiatry 127:957–960, 1971b.

Guze SB, Woodruff RA Jr, Clayton PJ: Sex, age, and the diagnosis of hysteria (Briquet's syndrome). Am J Psychiatry 129:745–748, 1973.

Hafeiz HB: Hysterical conversion: A prognostic study. Br J Psychiatry 136:548–551, 1980.

Hendler N, Uematesu S, Long D: Thermographic validation of physical complaints in "psychogenic pain" patients. Psychosomatics 23:283–287, 1982.

Hernandez-Peon R: Reticular mechanisms in sensory control. In Rosenblith WA (ed): Sensory Communication. New York, Wiley, 1961.

Hernandez-Peon R, Chavez-Ibarra G, Aguilar-Figueroa E: Somatic evoked potentials in one case of hysterical anesthesia. EEG Clin Neurophysiol 15:889–892, 1963.

Hollingshead AB, Redlich FC: Social class and mental illness. New York, Wiley, 1958.

Horowitz MJ (ed): Hysterical Personality. New York, Jason Aronson, 1977.

Hyler S, Spitzer R: Hysteria split asunder. Am J Psychiatry 135:1500–1504, 1978.

Janet P: The Major Symptoms of Hysteria. New York, Macmillan, 1907.

Kellner R, Sheffield BF: The one week prevalence of symptoms in neurotic patients and normals. Am J Psychiatry 130:102–105, 1973.

Kenyon F: Hypochondriacal states. Br J Psychiatry, 129:1–14, 1976.

Kimble R, Williams JG, Agras S: A comparison of two methods of diagnosing hysteria. Am J Psychiatry 132:1197–1199, 1975.

Kirshner LA: Dissociative reactions: An historical review and clinical study. Acta Psychiatr Scand 49:698–711, 1973.

Lacey JI, Smith RL, Green A: Use of conditioned autonomic responses in study of anxiety. Psychosom Med 17:208–217, 1955.

Lader MH: Psychophysiology of anxiety, in Lader M (ed): Studies of Anxiety. Br J Psychiatry Special Pub No 3, 1969.

Lindberg BJ, Lindegard B: Studies of the hysteroid personality attitude. Acta Psychiatr Scand 39:170–180, 1963.

Ludwig AM: Hysteria: A Neurobiological theory. Arch Gen Psychiatry 27:771–786, 1972.

Macedo V: Chagas' disease (American trypanosomiasis). In Wyngaarden JB, Smith LH Jr (eds): Cecil's Textbook of Medicine, 16th ed. Philadelphia, WB Saunders Co, 1982, pp 1728–1731.

Mai FM, Merskey H: Briquet's treatise on hysteria. A synopsis and commentary. Arch Gen Psychiatry 37:1401–1405, 1980.

Mann HB, Greenspan SI: The identification and treatment of adult brain dysfunction. Am J Psychiatry 113:1013, 1976.

Martin RL, Cloninger CR, Guze SB: The evaluation of diagnostic concordance in follow-up studies: II. A blind follow-up of female criminals. J Psychiatr Res 15:107–125, 1979.

Mayeux R, Alexander MP, Benson DF, et al: Poriomania. Neurology 29:1616–1619, 1979.

Mayou R: The nature of bodily symptoms. Br J Psychiatry 129:55–60, 1976.

McKegney FP: The incidence and characteristics of patients with conversion reactions: I. A general hospital consultation service sample. Am J Psychiatry 124:542–545, 1967.

Mears R, Horvath TB: "Acute" and "chronic" hysteria. Br J Psychiatry 121:653–657, 1972.

Merskey H, Watson GD: The lateralization of pain. Pain 7:271–280, 1979.

Morrison JR: Management of Briquet's syndrome (hysteria). West J Med 128:482–487, 1978.

Morrison JR, Stewart MA: The psychiatric status of the legal families of adopted hyperactive children. Arch Gen Psychiatry 28:888–891, 1973.

Morse RH: Pain and emotions. In Brena SF, Chapman SL (eds): Management of Patients with Chronic Pain. New York, Spectrum, 1983, pp 47–54.

Murphy GE: The clinical management of hysteria. JAMA 247:2559–2564, 1982.

Murphy GE, Guze SB: Setting limits. Am J Psychother 14:30–47, 1960.

Nemiah JC: Alexithymia and psychosomatic illness. J Clin Exp Psychiatry 25–37, 1978.

Perley MJ, Guze SB: Hysteria—The stability and usefulness of clinical criteria. N Engl J Med 266:421–426, 1962.

Posner JB: Pain. In Wyngaarden JB, Smith LH (eds): Cecil's Textbook of Medicine, 16th ed. Philadelphia, WB Saunders Co, 1982, pp 1940–1948.

Purtell JJ, Robins E, Cohen ME: Observations on clinical aspects of hysteria. JAMA 146:901–909, 1951.

Raskin M, Talbott JA, Meyerson AT: Diagnosis of conversion reactions: Predictive value of psychiatric criteria. JAMA 197:102–106, 1966.

Reveley MA, Woodruff RA Jr, Robins LN, Taibleson M, et al: Evaluation of a screening interview for Briquet Syndrome (Hysteria) by the study of medically ill women. Arch Gen Psychiatry 34:145–149, 1977.

Rinieris PM, Stefanis CN, Lykouras EP, Varsou EK: Hysteria and ABO blood types. Am J Psychiatry 135:1106–1107, 1978.

Robins E, O'Neal P: Clinical features of hysteria in children. Nerv Child 10:246–271, 1953.

Robins LN: Deviant Children Grown Up. Baltimore, Williams & Wilkins, 1966.

Robins LN, Helzer JE, Croughan J, Ratcliff KS: National Institute of Mental Health Diagnostic Interview Schedule: Its history, characteristics, and validity. Arch Gen Psychiatry 38:381–389, 1981.

Rosenthal RH, Webb WI, Wruble LD: Diagnosis and management of persistent psychogenic vomiting. Psychosomatics 21:722–730, 1980.

Scallet A, Cloninger CR, Othmer E: The management of chronic hysteria: A review and double-blind trial of electrosleep and other relaxation methods. Dis Nerv Sys 37:347–353, 1976.

Schafer R: Clinical Application of Psychological Tests. New York, International Universities Press, 1948.

Schalling D: Psychopathy-related personality variables and the psychophysiology of socialization. In Hare RD, Schallings D (eds): Psychopathic Behavior: Approaches to Research. New York, Wiley, 1978, pp 85–106.

Schalling D, Cronholm B, Åsberg M, Espmark S: Ratings of psychic and somatic anxiety indicants—Interrater reliability and relations to personality variables. Acta Psychiatr Scand 49:353–368, 1973.

Schenk L, Bear D: Multiple personality and related dissociative phenomena in patients with temporal lobe epilepsy. Am J Psychiatry 138:1311–1316, 1981.

Seligman MEP: Helplessness. San Francisco, WH Freeman, 1975.

Semmes J: Hemispheric specialization: A possible clue to mechanism. Neuropsychologia 6:11–16, 1968.

Shagass C, Jones AL: A neurophysiological test for psychiatric diagnosis: Results in 750 patients. Am J Psychiatry 114:1002–1009, 1958.

Shapiro D: Neurotic Styles. New York, Basic Books, 1965.

Sigvardsson S, von Knorring A-L, Bohman M, Cloninger C: An adoption study of somatoform disorders: I. The relationship of somatization to psychiatric disability: Arch Gen Psychiatry 41:853–859, 1984.

Slater ETO: Psychopathic personality as a genetical concept. Br J Psychiatry 94:277–282, 1948.

Slater ETO: Diagnosis of hysteria. Br Med J 1:1395–1399, 1965.

Stefansson JG, Messina JA, Meyerowitz S: Hysterical neurosis, conversion type: Clinical and epidemiological considerations. Acta Psychiatr Scand 53:110–138, 1976.

Stein JA, Tschudy DP: Acute intermittent porphyria. A clinical and biochemical study of 46 patients. Medicine 49:1, 1970.

Stephens JH, Kamp M: On some aspects of hysteria: A clinical study. J Nerv Ment Dis 134:305, 1962.

Stern DB: Handedness and the lateral distribution of conversion reactions. J Nerv Ment Dis 164:122–128, 1977.

Temoshok L, Attkisson CC: Epidemiology of hysterical phenomena: Evidence for a psychosocial theory. In Horowitz MJ (ed): Hysterical Personality. New York, Jason Aronson, 1977, pp 145–222.

von Knorring L, Almay BGL, Johansson F, Terenius L: Endorphins in CSF of chronic pain patients, in relation to augmenting-reducing response in visual averaged evoked response. Neuropsychobiology 5:322–326, 1979.

Ward N, Rowlett D, Burke P: Sodium amylobarbitone in the differential diagnosis of confusion. Am J Psychiatry 135:75–78, 1978.

Warner R: The diagnosis of antisocial and hysterical personality: An example of sex bias. J Nerv Ment Dis 166:839–845, 1978.

Watson CG, Buranen C: The frequency and identification of false positive conversion reactions. J Nerv Ment Dis 167:243–247, 1979.

Weinstein EA, Eck RA, Lyerly OG: Conversion hysteria in Appalachia. Psychiatry 32:334–341, 1969.

Weintraub MI: Hysterical Conversion Reactions: A Clinical Guide to Diagnosis and Treatment. New York, Spectrum, 1983.

Weissman MM, Myers JK, Harding PS: Psychiatric disorders in a U.S. urban community: 1975–76. Am J Psychiatry 135:459–462, 1978.

Wender PH, Reimherr FW, Wood DR: Attention deficit disorder ("Minimal Brain Dysfunction") in adults: A replication study of diagnosis and drug treatment. Arch Gen Psychiatry 38:449, 1981.

Wheatley D: Evaluation of psychotherapeutic drugs in general practice. Psychopharmacol Bull 2:25–32, 1962.

Wheatley D: General practitioner clinical trials: Phenobarbitone compared with an inactive placebo in anxiety states. Practitioner 192:147–151, 1964.

Wheatley D: General practitioner clinical trials: Chlordiazepoxide in anxiety states: II. Long-term study. Practitioner 195:692–695, 1965.

Williams JBW, Spitzer RL: Idiopathic pain disorder: A critique to pain-prone disorder and a proposal for a revision of the DSM-III category psychogenic pain disorder. J Nerv Ment Dis 170:410–419, 1982.

Woerner PI, Guze SB: A family and marital study of hysteria. Br J Psychiatry 114:161–168, 1968.

Woodrow KM, Friedman GD, Siegelaub AB, Cohen MF: Pain tolerance according to age, sex and race. Psychosom Med 34:548–556, 1972.

Woodruff RA Jr: Hysteria: An evaluation of objective diagnostic criteria by the study of women with chronic medical illnesses. Br J Psychiatry 114:1115–1120, 1967.

Wruble LD, Rosenthal RH, Webb WL: Psychogenic vomiting: A review. Am J Gastroenterol 77:318–321, 1982.

Wyke M: Effect of brain lesions on the rapidity of arm movement. Neurology 17:113–120, 1967.

Zborowski M: People in Pain. San Francisco, Jossey-Bass, 1969.

Ziegler FF, Imboden JB, Meyer E: Contemporary conversion reactions: A clinical study. Am J Psychiatry 116:901–910, 1960.

CHAPTER 12

Anorexia Nervosa and Bulimia Nervosa

ELKE D. ECKERT
JAMES E. MITCHELL

Anorexia nervosa and bulimia nervosa are common, potentially serious disorders that primarily affect young females. Both disorders are characterized by peculiar attitudes and behaviors directed toward eating and weight accompanied by intense fear of weight gain. Anorexia nervosa is further characterized by obsessive pursuit of extreme thinness leading to emaciation, disturbance of body image, and, in females, amenorrhea.

The cardinal feature of bulimia nervosa is eating binges: powerful and intractable urges to consume large amounts of food over a short time. Usually, this is followed by either self-induced vomiting or ingestion of laxatives in an attempt to prevent weight gain. However, bulimia nervosa does not produce the emaciation, which accompanies anorexia nervosa.

Although anorexia nervosa and bulimia nervosa are described separately in this chapter, there are no clear boundaries between the two conditions. Not only can the one frequently develop from the other, but characteristics of both disorders are frequently present together in the same individual. Also, there are similarities in many of the important characteristics of the disorders (Table 12-1).

ANOREXIA NERVOSA

Etiology and Pathogenesis

The etiology of anorexia nervosa is unknown, although hypotheses abound that involve various psychological, sociocultural, neuroendocrine, and hypothalamic factors. Psychological theories have centered mostly on phobias and psychodynamic interpretations. One view is that anorexia nervosa can be seen as an eating or weight phobia; regardless of the initial stimulus for dieting, eating or weight gain begins to generate severe anxiety, while failure to eat or weight loss serves to avoid anxiety (Brady and Rieger, 1972). Crisp (1970) has postulated that a weight phobia springs from an avoidance response to the sexual and social demands of puberty. Bruch (1962) described early false learning experiences as causing disturbance in body image, disturbance in perception, and, in turn, lack of recognition of hunger, fatigue, and weakness. Sociocultural theories have pointed to a shift in cultural standards for feminine beauty toward thinness (Garner et al., 1980). This cultural ideal may indirectly contribute to the development of anorexia nervosa, particularly among vulnerable adolescents, who equate weight control and thinness with beauty and success. Some investigators have described family interactional patterns that they regard as related to the development and maintenance of the disorder. For example, Minuchin et al. (1975) identified dysfunctional characteristics in families of anorectics (enmeshment, overprotection, lack of conflict resolution, and rigidity) that they saw as supporting the anorectic symptoms.

Other theories have been biologic. Based on the observation that amenorrhea and disturbed hypothalamic thermoregulation are independent of emaciation in anorexia nervosa, Russell (1965) proposed that hypothalamic dysfunction contributes to the disorder. Barry and Klawans (1976) proposed that increased dopaminergic activity may account for major signs and symptoms of anorexia nervosa, specifically, anorexia, hyperactivity, decreased libido, and a morbid fear of becoming fat.

TABLE 12-1. *Comparison of Important Clinical Features of Anorexia Nervosa and Bulimia Nervosa*

Important features for anorexia nervosa	Important features for bulimia nervosa
Significant weight loss below normal range or refusal to maintain at a minimal normal weight for age and height*	Weight maintenance in normal range†
Intense fear of weight gain*	Intense fear of weight gain
Peculiar food handling (*may* include recurrent binge eating)‡	Peculiar food handling (*must* include recurrent binge eating*)
Severe self-inflicted behaviors directed toward weight loss (*may* include vomiting, laxative or diuretic abuse)	Severe self-inflicted behaviors directed toward weight loss (e.g., vomiting, laxative or diuretic abuse, or excessive exercise or fasting)*
Disturbance of body image or overconcern with body shape and weight*§	Overconcern with body shape and weight*
Amenorrhea in women*	Menstrual irregularities

*Required for the diagnosis according to DSM-IIIR.
†A minority of bulimics are above normal and some are below normal weight range.
‡In the proposed DSM-IV, anorexia nervosa is subtyped into bulimic and nonbulimic subtypes.
§In the proposed DSM-IV, denial of the seriousness of the low weight may substitute for this criterion.
Adapted from American Psychiatric Association: Diagnostic and Statistical Manual of Mental Disorders, 3d ed revised (DSM-3R), Washington, APA, 1987.

Evidence suggests that anorexia nervosa may be an atypical affective disorder occurring in an adolescent female at a time in her life when body image issues are important. Several findings support this view. Controlled family studies have shown an increased incidence of primary affective disorder in the families of anorectics compared with families of controls (Winokur et al., 1980; Gershon et al., 1983 Halmi et al., 1991). Also, follow-up of anorectics suggests an increased risk for affective disorder (Halmi et al., 1991; Cantwell et al., 1977). Biologic markers associated with primary affective disorders, such as elevated plasma cortisol levels, dexamethasone nonsuppression, low urine 3-methoxy-4-hydroxyphenylglycol levels, impaired growth hormone response to provocative stimuli, and an abnormal thyroid-stimulating hormone (TSH) response to thyrotropin-releasing hormone (TRH), also are found in anorectics, although the abnormalities appear reversible with weight gain (Halmi et al., 1978; Gross et al., 1979; Gerner and Gwirtsman, 1981; Sherman and Halmi, 1977; Casper and Frohman, 1982; Brown, 1983; Brown, Koslow, and Reichlin, 1984).

Newer evidence suggests anorexia nervosa is related to obsessive-compulsive disorders. During the acute illness, anorectics suffer from obsessions about food, weight, and body image, and they often have compulsions concerning dieting, exercising, food preparation, and weighing. A recent 10-year follow-up study indicated that 26 percent of the anorectics were given a lifetime diagnosis of obsessive-compulsive disorder even excluding obsessions and compulsions concerning the eating disorder symptoms (Halmi et al., 1991). There may be a common biologic substrate between at least some anorectics and obsessive-compulsive patients. For example, evidence is emerging that *m*-chlorophenylpiperazine (*m*-CPP), which increases obsessive-compulsive behavior in obsessive-compulsive patients, also increases obsessive-compulsive symptoms in anorectics (Buttinger et al., 1990).

EDITORS' COMMENT

Neuroendocrine alterations in anorexia nervosa are common [Brown GM, Koslow SH, and Reichlin S (eds): Neuroendocrinology and Psychiatric Disorder, Raven Press, New York, 1984; Brown GM: Endocrine alterations in anorexia nervosa. In Darby PL, Garfinkel PE, Garner DM, and Coscine DV (eds): Anorexia Nervosa: Recent Developments in Research. New York, Alan R. Liss, Inc., 1983] and controversy on the pathogenesis of these changes continues. Many of these changes relate directly to weight loss. These include alterations in TSH response to TRH, in resting gonadotropin levels and luteinizing hormone (LH) responses to provocative stimuli. Other hypothalamic disturbances, such as plasma growth hormone, T_3, and reverse T_3, directly relate to caloric restriction, since they respond rapidly to food (carbohydrate) intake before significant weight changes can occur. Some changes appear to be independent of body weight and diet intake. These include an increased cortisol production rate, an immature pattern of LH, and possibly a decrease in norepinephrine in the cerebrospinal fluid (Kaye WH, Ebert MH, Raligh M, Lake R: Abnormalities in CNS monoamine metabolism in anorexia nervosa. Arch Gen Psychiatry 41:350–354, 1984). Factors such as amount of exercise [relating to a high incidence of amenorrhea in runners and ballet dancers (Frisch RE, Wyshak G, Vincet L: Delayed menarche and amenorrhea in ballet dancers. N Engl J Med 303:17–19, 1980; Warren MP: The effects of exercise on pubertal progression and reproductive function in girls. J Clin Endocrinol Metab 51:1150–1157, 1980)] and emotional distress (perhaps relating to the elevated cortisol production rate) probably play a role. The possibility of an underlying hypothalamic abnormality remains.

The role of heredity in anorexia nervosa also is unclear. Increased rates of eating disorders among female family members of anorectic patients has been reported in several large series (Theander, 1970; Gershon et al., 1983). For example, Theander (1970) found a morbidity risk of anorexia nervosa among sisters of anorectic probands to be 6.6 percent. Twin studies have been largely limited to case reports. About 50 percent of monozygotic twin sets reported have been concordant for anorexia nervosa, but biased selection and the small numbers reported do not permit conclusions. A recent study of twins with anorexia nervosa, the largest to date, involved 34 twin pairs and one set of triplets (Holland et al., 1984). In this study, anorexia nervosa was more likely to affect both members of the twin pair if they were monozygotic. In discordant pairs, the affected twin had a higher rate of perinatal complications. The affected twin in the discordant pairs also was more likely to have reached menarche later and to be the less dominant twin.

In the absence of sufficient controlled studies, the etiologic factors are speculative. It is likely that a complex chain of events interact to precipitate the disorder.

EDITORS' COMMENT

It may be that genetic family studies would be enhanced if anorexia nervosa were considered as part of a spectrum, and obsessive-compulsive disorder or traits and obligatory runners or other extreme exercisers were included (Yates A, Leehy K, Shisslack CM: Running—An analogue of anorexia? N Engl J Med 308:251–255, 1983). Major depression is too nonspecific to include.

Epidemiology

Anorexia nervosa historically has seemed an uncommon illness. The incidence and prevalence in the general population have not been determined. In 1973, however, three separate psychiatric case registers in Scotland, England, and northeastern United States supported a low annual incidence of about 1 case per 100,000 population (Kendall et al., 1973). Recent evidence suggests that the incidence of anorexia nervosa is increasing. One study indicates that the incidence nearly doubled from 1960 to 1976 (Jones et al., 1980). The most recent study, which identified all anorectics in one midwestern community between 1935 and 1984, indicated that the incidence has increased among females 15 to 24 years of age but not among older women or among males. The overall age-adjusted incidence rate per 100,000 person-years was 14.6 for females (Lucas et al., 1991).

Recent prevalence studies indicate anorexia nervosa to be a common disorder in the age group at risk: 12 to 30 years. In 1976, Crisp et al. surveyed nine populations of high school girls in England. The prevalence was 1 severe case in 200 girls, and in those age 16 or older, the prevalence was even higher—1 severe case in every 100 girls. In the midwestern community study described above, the prevalence also was 1 case per 200 girls 15 to 19 years of age. Crisp et al. (1976) and other authors have reported anorexia nervosa to be more prevalent in the higher socioeconomic classes, but no controlled studies support this hypothesis.

Anorexia nervosa occurs predominantly in females. Only 4 to 10 percent of cases are males (Crisp and Burns, 1983; Lucas et al., 1991). Clini-

cally, except for amenorrhea, male anorectics are remarkably similar to the females. Anorexia nervosa appears to be uncommon in poorly developed countries, and it is seldom seen among blacks in the United States. It is overrepresented in females in certain occupations, such as models and ballerinas, who must rigorously control their body shape (Frisch et al., 1980; Garner et al., 1980).

Clinical Picture

The essential clinical features of anorexia nervosa and a comparison with the features of bulimia nervosa are listed in Table 12-1. Anorexia nervosa typically begins with a simple diet adopted in response to concern about real or imagined overweight. At first, high-calorie foods are eliminated. Then other foods are systematically curtailed as negative attitudes toward food develop. As weight loss progresses, disgust about eating and intense fear about being obese begin to outweigh hunger. The term *anorexia* is a misnomer because true loss of appetite is uncommon until late in the illness. Weight loss progresses until the patient becomes emaciated. The anorectic is typically unaware of her extreme thinness; instead, she continues to feel fat and loses more weight.

Attempts to assess body image disturbance, or the anorectic's failure to recognize her starved body as being too thin or to regard herself as normal, or even overweight, in the face of increasing cachexia, have relied on visual size estimation devices. Using these devices, various investigators have confirmed that anorectics overestimate the width of body parts, but there are wide individual variations among anorectics in their body size estimates (Casper et al., 1979; Button et al., 1977; Slade and Russell, 1973). Compared with anorectics who more accurately estimate the size of body parts, those who are relatively inaccurate have been found to be more likely to fail to acknowledge their illness, to vomit, to be more severely malnourished, to gain less weight during treatment, and to have failed to gain weight during previous hospitalizations (Casper et al., 1979; Button et al., 1977). Although body size overestimation is significant in a subgroup of anorexia nervosa, it cannot be considered unique to this population, since some studies have found no significant mean differences between anorectics and control groups (Casper et al., 1979; Button et al., 1977).

Anorectics exhibit odd behavior around food. They hide food all over the house. During mealtimes they deviously dispose of food. They cut food into tiny pieces or spend much time arranging food on their plates. Confrontation about these behaviors is often met with denial. Yet anorectics think constantly about food, often collect recipes, and engage in elaborate food preparation for others. Approximately 50 percent begin to gorge themselves with food (binge eating, or bulimia), up to 40 percent induce vomiting, and may begin using laxatives and diuretics in an attempt to reduce weight (Casper et al., 1980; Garfinkel et al., 1980). They also may become hyperactive and engage in strenuous ritualistic exercises to control weight.

Attempts to delineate subgroups have focused on clinical differences between anorectics who binge eat and those who do not. In two large surveys, bulimic anorectic patients were characterized by self-induced vomiting and by abuse of laxatives and diuretics (Casper et al., 1980; Garfinkel et al., 1980). They displayed impulsive behaviors, e.g., alcohol abuse, stealing, and suicide attempts. They were more extroverted but manifested greater anxiety, guilt, depression, and interpersonal sensitivity and had more somatic complaints than did anorectics who exclusively dieted to lose weight. In one study, a high frequency of obesity was found in mothers of the bulimic anorectics (Garfinkel et al., 1980). The delineation of these subgroups extends to the families. The incidence of alcoholism and drug abuse disorders is higher in families of bulimic anorectics than in families of nonbulimic anorectics (Eckert et al., 1979a; Strober et al., 1982). The bulimic subgroup of anorexia nervosa remarkably shares characteristics with bulimia nervosa described later. Possibly these two populations form a single group within the eating disorders. Anorexia nervosa patients who purge but who do not objectively binge eat also are encountered.

Anorexia nervosa patients have a high comorbidity with affective and anxiety disorders. In a recent study, 68 percent had a lifetime psychiatric diagnosis of major depression and 65 percent an anxiety disorder (26 percent obsessive-compulsive, 15 percent agoraphobia, 34 percent social phobia) (Halmi et al., 1991).

Clinical Course

Onset of anorexia nervosa occurs from prepuberty to young adulthood, generally between the ages 10 and 30. Most commonly, the disorder begins between the ages 13 and 20, and the mean age onset is age 16 (Theander, 1970; Halmi, 1974). Although rare cases outside this range are described, they must be scrutinized to rule out other psychiatric or organic disorders simulating anorexia nervosa.

Some investigators find no distinct premorbid personality, whereas others describe a typical case as well behaved, perfectionistic, obsessional, introverted, and shy.

Onset of dieting has been associated with precipitating events, such as moving to a new school, or a traumatic event involving dating or peer relations, but often no specific reason is apparent.

Anorexia nervosa has a variable course and outcome. The course varies from spontaneous recovery without treatment to gradual or rapid deterioration, resulting in death. There may be lasting recovery after one episode of weight loss or a fluctuating pattern of illness marked by remissions and exacerbations over many years. Although the short-term response of anorectics to well-organized hospital treatment programs is good, there are no consistent data concerning the effect of treatment on long-term outcome.

No follow-up study done has been free of methodological problems involving, primarily, sampling biases, inconsistent follow-up intervals, and different outcome measurement (Hsu, 1980; Cantwell et al., 1977; Dally, 1969; Morgan and Russell, 1975; Theander, 1970; Kay and Schapira, 1965; Schwartz and Thompson, 1981; Halmi et al., 1975, 1991). Full recovery occurs in half the anorectics, usually within 5 years. Others have persistent difficulties in maintaining weight, eating patterns, menses, and social, sexual, and psychological adjustment. A significant number remain amenorrheic despite a return to normal weight. Body weight remains persistently below 75 percent of normal in up to 25 percent. Obesity develops in less than 8 percent. Although weight may be normal at follow-up, abnormal eating behavior may persist; one-half still practice dietary restriction and avoid high-calorie foods, and binge eating or compulsive overeating, vomiting, and laxative abuse are common. Up to half the anorectics have unipolar affective disorder at follow-up (Cantwell et al., 1977; Halmi et al., 1991). Other common psychiatric problems at follow-up are obsessive-compulsive symptoms, social phobias, drug dependency, and stealing. Several studies indicate that psychiatric symptoms are more common and severe in anorectics who at follow-up have low weight and abnormal eating behavior or are preoccupied with food and weight (Halmi et al., 1991).

The most consistent favorable prognostic feature is early age of onset, and the most consistent unfavorable ones are late age of onset and more previous hospitalizations (Theander, 1970; Halmi et al., 1975; Morgan and Russell, 1975). Poorer outcome also has been associated with greater length of illness, the presence of bulimia, vomiting and laxative abuse, overestimation of body size, disturbed family relationships, more physical complaints, and symptoms of neuroticism, depression, and obsessionality.

The illness carries a considerable mortality (Halmi et al., 1991). The usual causes of death are starvation and electrolyte disturbance, but suicide is also a contributor. Although most studies report a death rate of less than 10 percent, several report a rate greater than 15 percent. Two studies with the longest period of follow-up report the highest death rates (Halmi et al., 1975; Theander, 1983). The most notable of these, a Scandinavian study conducted over 22 years, found an 18 percent mortality (Theander, 1983). The suicide rate was 5 percent. Most studies report suicide rates of around 1 percent.

Medical Findings

Amenorrhea is invariably present and may begin before, concurrently with, or after the onset of dieting (Falk and Halmi, 1982). Other common physical findings are hypotension, hypothermia, bradycardia, dry skin, and lanugo. Less common features are hair loss, petechiae, peripheral edema, carotenemic skin, and swollen salivary glands.

Medical abnormalities and complications noted in anorexia nervosa and a comparison with those noted in bulimia nervosa are given in Table 12-2. Most investigators believe that starvation and associated disordered eating behaviors produce most, if not all, of the abnormalities, but the data, especially in the neuroendocrine area, are still inconclusive. One notable finding in emaciated anorectics is the "immaturity" in the pattern of luteinizing hormone (LH) functioning, resembling that of prepubertal girls. After weight gain, the LH pattern usually returns to normal, but some anorectics continue to have an immature pattern. In one study those patients who continued to have abnormal eating patterns also continued to have an immature LH secretory pattern (Katz et al., 1977).

EDITORS' COMMENT

A follow-up of 140 hospitalized women with a diagnosis of anorexia nervosa (Brinch M, Isager T, Tolstrup K: Anorexia nervosa and motherhood: Reproduction pattern and mothering behavior of 50 women. Acta Psychiatr Scand 77:611–617, 1988) reported that 50 of them gave birth to 86 children, approximately one-third the expected fertility. Involuntary childlessness was similar to the comparison population, so this seemed to be due to the fact that the probands did not want to have children. More women in the group of mothers than in the group of nonmothers had better scores of all-around functioning at follow-up.

Other serious sequelae of the malnutrition associated with anorexia nervosa include skeletal abnormalities. Prepubertal patients may experience growth arrest and may not grow to anticipated heights. Prolonged amenorrhea with low weight is associated with potentially irreversible osteopenia and an increased rate of pathologic fractures (Rigotti et al., 1991).

The consequence of some medical findings is not clear. For example, abnormal CT scans of the brain may be found in more than half of anorectic patients (Krieg et al., 1988). Other complications such as sudden death (Schocken et al., 1989) may

TABLE 12-2. *Medical Abnormalities and Complications of Anorexia Nervosa and Bulimia Nervosa*

System	Anorexia nervosa	Bulimia nervosa
Hematologic	Leukopenia; thrombocytopenia; bone marrow hypocellularity; granulocyte killing rate decreased	
Renal	Elevated BUN (dehydration); decreased glomerular filtration rate; partial diabetes insipidus	Elevated BUN (dehydration)
Metabolism	Hypercholesterolemia; elevated carotene levels; low plasma zinc levels; abnormal liver function tests	Reduced energy expenditure
Gastrointestinal	Altered gastric emptying; low gastric secretion; salivary gland swelling; elevated amylase levels; superior mesenteric artery syndrome	Salivary gland swelling; elevated amylase levels; esophageal rupture
Cardiovascular	ECG abnormalities; arrhythmias, bradycardia; altered circulatory dynamics; hypotension; edema	
Dental	Caries; perimyolysis	Caries; perimyolysis
Fluid and electrolyte	Dehydration; alkalosis; hypochloremia; hypokalemia	Dehydration; alkalosis; hypochloremia; hypokalemia
Central nervous system	EEG abnormality; CAT scan abnormality	EEG abnormality
Gonadal steroids	Low LH, FSH; impaired response to LHRH; immature LH pattern; low urinary gonadotropins; low urinary estrogens; abnormal estrogen metabolism; low testosterone (in males)	
Thyroid	Low T_3, high rT_3; impaired TRH responsiveness	Impaired TRH responsiveness
Growth hormone	Elevated basal; pathologic responsiveness to provocative stimuli	Pathologic responsiveness to provocative stimuli
Glucose	Abnormal glucose tolerance test; fasting hypoglycemia	
Adrenal	Elevated cortisol levels; change in cortisol metabolism, secretion; Dexamethasone nonsuppression positive	Dexamethasone nonsuppression positive
Skeletal	Osteoporosis; growth (height) arrest; pathologic fractures	

These abnormalities are not necessarily seen in every patient, and many are seen in only a minority (Mitchell, 1984).

occur in patients who feel deceptively well and who have normal electrocardiograms.

Differential Diagnosis

The major confounding diagnosis is bulimia nervosa. The unclear boundaries between anorexia nervosa and bulimia nervosa are indicated by the fact that one frequently develops from the other and by the overlap in their essential features (see Table 12-1). Although binge eating occurs in both bulimia nervosa and anorexia nervosa, bulimic patients generally maintain weight within a normal range and do not show extreme pursuit of thinness. Body image disturbance has not yet been systematically assessed in bulimics. Amenorrhea is a variable feature of bulimia nervosa.

Anorexia nervosa must be differentiated from peculiar eating behavior and weight loss, which can occur in several other disorders. In general, the differentiation can readily be made on the basis of positive criteria of anorexia nervosa, such as fear of becoming obese and pursuit of thinness, which are absent in the other disorders.

Weight loss is common in depressive disorders but is generally severer in anorexia nervosa. Whereas depressed patients are aware of a loss of appetite, anorectics generally have a normal appetite, which they may deny. Anorectics, in contrast to depressives, are preoccupied with food. Agitation can be seen in depressive disorders, but it differs from the ritualistic activity of an anorectic.

Weight loss and peculiar eating behavior are sometimes seen in schizophrenics, usually on the basis of delusions. However, the delusions of schizophrenics differ in content and are not concerned with caloric content or fear of weight gain.

It is important to ascertain medical conditions that accompany or simulate anorexia nervosa. Lesions of the pituitary or the hypothalamus may be accompanied by appetite disturbance and weight loss. In general, starvation, resulting from causes other than anorexia nervosa, is associated with inactivity and apathy and not with the intense fear of weight gain, body image distortion, alertness, and hyperactivity seen in anorectics (Casper and Davis, 1977).

Treatment

There is no agreement about the best treatment. Treatment currently involves a combination of medical management, nutritional rehabilitation often using behavioral techniques, reeducative personal therapy, family therapy, and, sometimes, pharmacotherapy. The immediate aim of treatment during the acute anorectic phase is to correct dehydration and electrolyte imbalance and restore the nutritional state to normal. Starvation itself can lead to many problems, including depression, sleep disturbance, preoccupation with food, and irritability,

and improvement in the patient's psychological state will occur with nutritional rehabilitation (Morgan and Russell, 1975; Eckert et al., 1982). Treatment is done most efficiently in a structured hospital treatment program. Because many anorectic patients do not acknowledge that a problem exists, it is essential to obtain the family's support so that firm treatments can be effected. Those patients who are less severely ill, are not vomiting or using laxatives, and have family that will cooperate with prescribed treatment may respond to outpatient treatment.

It is advisable to prescribe a structured diet, gradually increasing calories to avoid stomach dilatation and circulation overload. Close observation during and after meals will minimize surreptitious mealtime behavior, such as hiding food and vomiting.

Behavioral contingencies after an operant conditioning paradigm probably increase the rate of weight gain (Agras and Kraemer, 1983). A typical positive reinforcement dependent on weight gain is opportunity for increased physical and social activity, including visitors, while negative reinforcements for failure to gain weight are bed rest, isolation, and tube feeding. However, a randomized, controlled treatment study did not demonstrate a clear advantage, expressed as weight gain, for behavior therapy (Eckert et al., 1979b).

Although there is no proven pharmacologic treatment for anorexia nervosa, drugs may be useful adjuncts. Antidepressant drugs may be useful because of the presence of depressive symptoms, although insufficient data are available in this area. One controlled, double-blind study of hospitalized anorectics did not find amitriptyline to decrease depression, although it had a marginal effect on increasing the rate of weight gain (Halmi et al., 1986). In the same controlled study, cyproheptadine, an antihistamine and serotonin antagonist, was found to decrease depression and increase the rate of weight gain in the nonbulimic subgroup of anorexia nervosa. Uncontrolled trials have suggested that fluoxetine may help some patients with weight restoration (Gwirtsman et al., 1990) and weight maintenance phases (Kaye et al., 1991). The usefulness of drugs such as metoclopramide to enhance gastric emptying and improve the gastrointestinal symptoms of patients with anorexia nervosa is unclear (Saleh and Lebwohl, 1980). Lithium is contraindicated for patients who vomit or abuse laxatives or diuretics because of the potential for lithium toxicity. The usefulness of antipsychotic medication is unproven.

No information is available about drugs affecting the long-term course of the disorder. However, anorectics who remain depressed after nutritional rehabilitation may benefit from antidepressants.

Psychoanalytically oriented therapy is not effective in treating anorexia nervosa (Bruch, 1970). Individual psychotherapy should aim at correcting cognitive errors of thinking, promoting independence, accepting responsibilities, improving psychosocial skill deficits, and promoting a positive self-concept.

Counseling of family members is a necessary component of an effective treatment program. This involves educating the family about the disorder, assessing the family's impact on maintaining the disorder, and assisting in methods to promote normal functioning of the patient.

BULIMIA NERVOSA

Definition

Bulimia nervosa is a disorder characterized by binge eating coupled with some other behavior designed to eliminate the ingested food or to promote weight loss (Russell, 1979). In DSM-IIIR, purging behavior such as self-induced vomiting or laxative abuse is not required, and less well studied accompanying behaviors, such as excessive exercise or fasting, can be used (American Psychiatric Association, 1987). However, the proposed diagnostic criteria for DSM-IV break bulimia nervosa into purging and nonpurging subtypes. The nonpurging subtype would include people who binge eat but also exhibit inappropriate compensatory behavior for binge eating, such as excessive exercise or fasting. These proposed changes reflect the growing awareness that the vast majority of patients presenting for treatment with bulimia nervosa engage in some purging behavior and that many of the medical complications attributed to the disorder probably result from the purging behavior rather than from the binging episodes per se. Also, nonpurging bulimics have been little studied, although there is a growing interest in this group (Marcus et al., 1985).

Etiology and Pathogenesis

Little is known concerning the causes of bulimia nervosa. As with anorexia nervosa, sociocultural preoccupation with thinness is commonly implicated. A relationship between obesity, dietary restraint, and binge eating has been suggested (Wardle and Beinart, 1981). This suggestion is supported by evidence showing that many patients who develop bulimia nervosa are overweight during adolescence, before the onset of the disorder, and that binges frequently begin during a period of dieting (Fairburn and Cooper, 1982; Pyle et al., 1981). Some patients also retrospectively link the onset of bulimia nervosa with traumatic events, particularly experience of separation or loss (Pyle et al., 1981).

A relationship between affective disorder and bulimia nervosa has been suggested. Several findings support this view. Many bulimic patients are depressed, improve with antidepressants, show dexamethasone nonsuppression, and have strong family histories of affective disorder (Hudson et al., 1982; Gwirtsman et al., 1983; Walsh et al., 1982). However, bulimia nervosa can occur in individuals without concomitant affective disorder and without a history of affective disorder, and it is unlikely that the disorder can be regarded simply as a variant of an affective disorder.

A predisposition to chemical abuse has been described (Pyle et al., 1981; Hatsukami et al., 1982). Bulimic patients and their families have been described as being at high risk for abuse of alcohol and other drugs. Also, studies which have examined the prevalence of bulimia nervosa in patients with alcohol or drug abuse indicate a higher than expected rate of bulimia nervosa. This is particularly interesting when one considers that there are many behavioral similarities between drug abuse and bulimia nervosa, including preoccupation with the substance, loss of control over the use of the substance, the secretive nature of the behavior, and the social isolation that accompanies and results from the behavior.

There is considerable variability as to what actually constitutes an eating binge. However, monitored eating binges in various laboratory paradigms have found that the majority of patients with bulimia nervosa have binge-eating episodes in excess of 1000 kilocalories and that the binge-eating episodes can be many times larger than this (Mitchell et al., 1985b). Binge eating may be used to alleviate a dysphoric state or a sense of boredom, but a variety of cues have been shown to trigger bulimic behavior in different individuals, and for many individuals binge eating becomes habitual.

Epidemiology

Most of the research studies looking at the prevalence of bulimia nervosa have focused on college and high school age women (Fairburn and Beglin, 1990). We know little about the prevalence of bulimia nervosa in the general population. The results in the available studies suggest that approximately 1 percent of young women will develop the full-blown symptoms of bulimia nervosa, although higher percentages will engage in binge-eating behavior and/or will experiment with self-induced vomiting or laxative abuse (Halmi et al., 1981; Pyle et al., 1983; Pope et al., 1984; Cooper and Fairburn, 1983). What little cross-cultural research is available suggests that bulimia nervosa occurs primarily in industrialized society where emphasis is placed on slimness as a model of attractiveness for women and where an abundance of food is available. Available data also suggest that bulimia nervosa can be seen in all socioeconomic groups. It can be present in minorities, particularly when they are of higher socioeconomic standing (Anderson and May, 1985).

Clinical Picture

In clinic populations 9 of 10 bulimic patients are female. At presentation they average several years older than anorexia nervosa patients, the majority being between 20 and 30 years old (Pyle et al., 1981; Fairburn and Cooper, 1984; Russell, 1979; Mitchell et al., 1985a).

The essential clinical features of bulimia nervosa are given in Table 12-1. Most bulimics are of normal weight but are very concerned about weight, are afraid of gaining weight, and desire a lower body weight. Unlike the typical patient with anorexia nervosa, bulimic patients complain of loss of control over their eating.

Binge eating, which usually occurs in isolation, is considered the hallmark of bulimia nervosa. Most binge eating is done in the afternoon and evening. Patients may eat 5000 or more calories within a few hours (Mitchell et al., 1981). Binge foods usually consist of high-calorie carbohydrate or fat-containing foods that the patients usually exclude from their regular diets because they are perceived as being "fattening." Bulimic patients have grossly disturbed eating habits in which regular meals are seldom eaten, and attempts at dietary restriction are interspersed with episodes of binge eating, followed usually by self-induced vomiting or laxative abuse. Early in the course of the illness, vomiting is usually induced by stimulating the gag reflex with the fingers or an object such as a toothbrush. Many patients eventually learn to vomit by reflex.

About two-thirds of patients with bulimia nervosa will use laxatives as a weight-control technique during the course of the illness (Mitchell et al., 1988). This usually involves the ingestion of large amounts of over-the-counter stimulant-type laxatives, which result in abrupt, watery diarrhea after several hours (Bo-linn et al., 1983). This engenders a sense of weight loss which is reinforcing to the patients. In reality, however, most of what is lost is fluid and electrolytes from the colon, and most of the ingested food is still in the upper gastrointestinal tract. However, this results in dehydration, in rebound hyperreninemia, and in subsequent fluid retention, which tends to predispose the patient to repeat laxative usage the next day. Between 15 and 20 percent of these patients will abuse diuretics, with basically the same sequelae as of laxative abuse. Twenty-eight percent will experiment with ipecac as a means to induce vomiting (Pope et al., 1986). This is a particularly dangerous behavior in that it may result in the development of myopathy or cardiomyopathy. A small percentage of patients engage in other behaviors such as rumination or misuse of enemas. Some chew and spit out food without swallowing as an alterative to binge eating and vomiting.

Anxiety and depression, with prominent expressions of guilt, worthlessness, and, sometimes, suicidal thoughts, are frequent. Mood tends to parallel control over eating; the less the control, the lower the mood (Russell, 1979). Some have diffuse difficulty controlling their impulses; they may abuse alcohol or drugs or they may steal (Pyle et al., 1981; Russell, 1979). Stealing often consists of shoplifting food (Krahn et al., 1991).

Clinical Course

Onset of bulimia generally occurs during adolescence or the young adult years, with a mean age onset for binge eating of 18 years (Pyle et al., 1981; Fairburn and Cooper, 1982; Mitchell and Eckert, 1987). The onset of vomiting occurs, on average, 1 year after onset of binge eating (Fairburn and Cooper, 1982).

Premorbid characteristics vary, but in general, a subgroup of patients with bulimia nervosa appears to have generalized impulse-control problems, not just around food. On the whole, bulimic patients are more outgoing, socially competent, and sexually experienced than anorexia nervosa patients.

Little is known about the longitudinal course of bulimia nervosa. A history suggesting episodes of anorexia nervosa before bulimia nervosa becomes manifest is found in a significant minority (Pyle et al., 1981; Fairburn and Cooper, 1984). The typical bulimic has been symptomatic for 3 to 6 years before seeking treatment, and the usual pattern is that the frequency of abnormal behaviors has increased over that period of time (Fairburn and Cooper, 1984; Pyle et al., 1981). Many patients lose weight when they first become bulimic; however, as the disorder progresses, they tend to gain weight, possibly because of increasing intensity and frequency of binge-eating episodes (Russell, 1979). Follow-up studies suggest that the illness may have a relapsing course. The exact influence of treatment on the long-term outcome is unclear. However, the available studies do suggest that this disorder has a much lower morbidity and mortality than that associated with anorexia nervosa (Herzog et al., 1988).

Medical Findings

Most bulimics menstruate regularly, but some menstruate irregularly or are amenorrheic (Fairburn and Cooper, 1984; Pirke et al., 1987). Medical abnormalities and complications noted in bulimia and a comparison with those noted in anorexia nervosa are given in Table 12-2. The most common problem is fluid and electrolyte abnormalities, which are found in approximately 50 percent of patients. Such abnormalities result from variable combinations of vomiting and laxative or diuretic abuse (Mitchell et al., 1984, 1991). The most common picture is one of alkalosis manifested by elevated serum bicarbonate level, sometimes accompanied by hypokalemia and hypochloremia. Metabolic acidosis, on the other hand, suggests recent laxative abuse, in that ingestion of large amounts of stimulant laxatives results in loss of large amounts of bicarbonate in the stool. A medical complication of particular concern is gastric dilatation after binge eating, which can result in gastric perforation and death (Abdu et al., 1987). Fortunately, this occurs infrequently. The pathogenesis of salivary gland swelling, usually involving the parotid glands, is unclear. Elevated serum amylase levels are presumably related to the parotid gland changes (Walsh et al., 1990). However, there also appears to be an association between bulimia nervosa and pancreatitis, and for this reason, an elevated amylase level should be fractionated. It is very common for these patients to develop problems of dentition, in that the highly acid gastric contents tend to erode the surface dental enamel (Roberts and Li, 1987). The changes are usually maximal on the posterior surface of the upper teeth, where the acidic contents hit as they are projected from the back of the mouth. Esophageal rupture also has been reported. Recent research suggests that reductions in energy expenditure relative to controls may occur, a finding that may predispose to weight gain (Devlin et al., 1990). These patients also demonstrate metabolic changes suggestive of starvation, despite an apparently normal body weight (Pirke et al., 1985).

Differential Diagnosis

The differential diagnosis includes organic disorders that produce binge eating, such as, Kleine-Levine syndrome, Prader-Willi syndrome, and Klüver-Bucy–like syndromes. However, overeating in these conditions is usually nonspecific, in that patients are hyperphagic constantly, which clearly differentiates them from bulimia nervosa.

There is currently a plan to include a separate diagnostic category, binge-eating disorder, in the Appendix of DSM-IV. This would target patients who do not engage in purging behavior or other significant inappropriate compensatory behavior for binge eating such as fasting or excessive exercise. This would include many overweight people who binge eat on a regular basis.

Treatment

There is still considerable controversy regarding the treatment of bulimia nervosa, although the controlled treatment literature for this condition has grown enormously over the last 10 years. Two general approaches have been used experimentally: pharmacotherapy approaches, primarily using antidepressant drugs, and psychotherapy approaches, primarily using cognitive behavioral techniques (Mitchell et al., 1989; Mitchell, 1991; Mitchell and Eckert, 1987). The pharmacologic treatment literature has focused on the use of heterocyclic compounds, and a dozen treatment studies have shown that in most cases mood (as well as eating behavior)

does improve substantially on these drugs. The decrements in the frequency of binge-eating and vomiting behavior are usually dramatic; however, one problem with the pharmacotherapy studies is that many of the patients remain symptomatic at the end of treatment, regardless of the degree of reductions in target eating behaviors. This raises questions about the adequacy of this form of treatment. The single drug studied most intensively has been fluoxetine hydrochloride, which in two large, multicentered trials has been shown to be superior to placebo. Interestingly, the drug appears to work best in this condition at 60 mg per day, as opposed to the 20-mg dose that is usually used in depression (Fluoxetine Bulemia Nervosa Collaborative Study Group, 1992). Available studies suggest that antidepressants may exert their therapeutic effect through a mechanism other than improving mood, since patients without affective disorders also benefit.

Psychotherapeutic approaches also have been tried in more than a dozen studies. Much of this literature has focused on the use of cognitive behavioral techniques, adapted from cognitive behavior therapy (CBT) for depression. These studies show quite clearly that CBT techniques are effective in suppressing bulimic behaviors, although in the majority of studies the number of subjects completely free of symptoms at the end of treatment is still low. More recent research has suggested that other psychotherapies not directly addressing eating behaviors such as interpersonal psychotherapy (IPT) also may be useful in the treatment of bulimia nervosa. The relative efficacy of IPT and CBT were recently tested in a controlled study: IPT and CBT achieved equivalent effects on the frequency of binge eating and purging as well as in other areas of symptoms, although there was a clear temporal difference in the pattern of response, with IPT taking longer to achieve its effect (Fairburn et al., 1993). In general, treatments specifically designed for bulimia nervosa include an emphasis on meal planning and nutritional education, self-monitoring techniques to increase patients' awareness of their eating patterns, goal setting to change eating behavior, manipulation of the behavioral antecedents and consequences of bulimic behavior, the use of problem-solving and adaptive skills techniques, and cognitive restructuring.

Three studies have examined the possible efficacy of adding antidepressants to cognitive behavioral psychotherapy, and all find that the addition of active drug to group or individual therapy may improve outcome on certain variables such as anxiety and depression and/or may help prevent relapse (Mitchell et al. 1990; Fichter et al. 1991; Agras et al. 1992). Overall, the available studies strongly suggest that outpatient treatment can be effective for bulimia nervosa and that inpatient care is rarely indicated.

REFERENCES

Abdu RA, Garritano D, Culver O: Acute gastric necrosis in anorexia nervosa and bulimia. Arch Surg 122:830–832, 1987.

Agras WS, Kraemer HC: The treatment of anorexia nervosa: Do different treatments have different outcomes? Psychiatric Ann 13:928, 1983.

Agras WS, Rossiter EM, Arnow B, et al: Pharmacologic and cognitive-behavioral treatment for bulimia nervosa: A controlled comparison. Am J Psychiatry 149:82–87, 1992.

American Psychiatric Association: Diagnostic and Statistical Manual of Mental Disorders. Washington, American Psychiatric Association, 1987.

Anderson AE, May A: Racial and socioeconomic influences in anorexia nervosa and bulimia. Int J Eat Disord 4:479–487, 1985.

Barry BC, Klawans HL: On the role of dopamine in the pathophysiology of anorexia nervosa. J Neural Transm 38:107, 1976.

Bo-linn G, Santa Ana C, Moranshi S, et al: Purging and calorie absorption in bulimic patients and normal women. Ann Intern Med 99:14–17, 1983.

Brady JP, Rieger W: Behavioral treatment of anorexia nervosa. In Proceedings of the International Symposium on Behavior Modification. New York, Appleton-Century-Crofts, 1972.

Brown GM: Endocrine alterations in anorexia nervosa. In Darby PL, Garfinkel PE, Garner DM, and Coscine DV (eds): Anorexia Nervosa: Recent Developments in Research. New York, Alan R. Liss, 1983.

Brown GM, Koslow SH, and Reichlin S (eds): Neuroendocrinology and Psychiatric Disorder. New York, Raven Press, 1984.

Bruch H: Perceptual and conceptual disturbances in anorexia nervosa. Psychosom Med 24:187, 1962.

Bruch H: Psychotherapy in primary anorexia nervosa. J Nerv Ment Dis 150:51, 1970.

Buttinger C, Hollander E, Walsh BT: m-CPP challenges in anorexia nervosa. Presented at the American Psychiatric Association Annual Meeting, New York, 1990.

Button EJ, Fransella F, Slade PD: A reappraisal of body perception disturbance in anorexia nervosa. Psychol Med 7:235, 1977.

Cantwell DP, Sturzenberger S, Burroughs J, et al: Anorexia nervosa—An affective disorder? Arch Gen Psychiatry 34:1087, 1977.

Casper RC, Davis JM: On the course of anorexia nervosa. Am J Psychiatry 134:974, 1977.

Casper RC, Eckert ED, Halmi KA, et al: Bulimia: its incidence and clinical significance in patients with anorexia nervosa. Arch Gen Psychiatry 37:1030–1035, 1980.

Casper RC, Frohman LA: Delayed TSH response in anorexia nervosa following injection of thyrotropin-releasing hormone (TRH). Psychoneuroendocrinology 7:59, 1982.

Casper RC, Halmi KA, Goldberg SC, et al: Disturbances in body image estimation as related to other characteristics and outcome in anorexia nervosa. Br J Psychiatry 134:60, 1979.

Cooper PJ, Fairburn CG: Binge eating and self-induced vomiting in the community: A preliminary study. Br J Psychiatry 142:139, 1983.

Crisp AH: Anorexia nervosa: "Feeding disorder," "nervous malnutrition," or "weight phobia"? World Rev Nutr Diet 12:452, 1970.

Crisp AH, Burns T: The clinical presentation of anorexia nervosa in males. Int J Eat Disord 2:5, 1983.

Crisp AH, Palmer RL, Kalucy RS: How common is anorexia nervosa? A prevalence study. Br J Psychiatry 128:549, 1976.

Dally PJ: Anorexia Nervosa. New York, Grune & Stratton, 1969.

Devlin MJ, Walsh MT, Kral JG, et al: Metabolic abnormalities in bulimia nervosa. Arch Gen Psychiatry 47:144–148, 1990.

Eckert ED, Goldberg SC, Halmi KA, et al: Alcoholism in anorexia nervosa. In Pickens RW, Heston LL (eds): Psychiatric Factors in Drug Abuse. New York, Grune & Stratton, 1979a.

Eckert ED, Goldberg SC, Halmi KA, et al: Behavior therapy in anorexia nervosa. Br J Psychiatry 134:55, 1979b.

Eckert ED, Goldberg SC, Halmi KA, et al: Depression in anorexia nervosa. Psychol Med 12:115, 1982.

Fairburn CG, Beglin SJ: Studies of the epidemiology of bulimia nervosa. Am J Psychiatry 147:401–408, 1990.

Fairburn CG, Cooper PJ: The clinical features of bulimia nervosa. Br J Psychiatry 144:238, 1984.

Fairburn CG, Jones R, Peveler RC et at: Psychotherapy and bulimia nervosa: longer-term effects of interpersonal psychotherapy, behavior therapy, and cognitive behavior therapy. Arch Gen Psychiatry 50:419–428, 1993.

Falk JR, Halmi KA: Amenorrhea in anorexia nervosa: Examination of the critical body weight hypothesis. Biol Psychiatry 17:799, 1982.

Fichter MM, Leibl K, Rief W, et al: Fluoxetine versus placebo: A double-blind study with bulimic inpatients undergoing intensive psychotherapy. Pharmacopsychiatry 24:1–7, 1991.

Fluoxetine Bulimia Nervosa Study Group: Fluoxetine in the treatment of bulemia nervosa: a multi-center, placebo-controlled, double-blind trial. Arch Gen Psychiatry 49:139–147, 1992.

Frisch RE, Wyshak G, Vincent L: Delayed menarche and amenorrhea in ballet dancers. N Engl J Med 303:17, 1980.

Garfinkel PE, Moldofsky H, Garner DM: The heterogeneity of anorexia nervosa: Bulimia as a distinct subgroup. Arch Gen Psychiatry 37:1036, 1980.

Garner DM, Garfinkel PE, Schwartz D, Thompson M: Cultural expectation of thinness in women. Psychol Rep 47:483, 1980.

Gerner, RH, Gwirtsman HE: Abnormalities of dexamethasone suppression test and urinary MHPG in anorexia nervosa. Am J Psychiatry 138:650, 1981.

Gershon ES, Hamovit JR, Schreiber JL, et al: Anorexia nervosa and major affective disorders associated in families: A preliminary report. In Guze SB, Earls FJ, Barrett JE (eds): Childhood Psychopathology and Development. New York, Raven Press, 1983.

Gross HA, Lake CR, Ebert MH, et al: Catecholamine metabolism in primary anorexia nervosa. J Clin Endocrinol Metab 49:805, 1979.

Gwirtsman HE, Guze BH, Yager J, Gainsley B: Fluoxetine treatment of anorexia nervosa: An open clinical trial. J Clin Psychiatry 51:378–382, 1990.

Gwirtsman HE, Roy-Byrne P, Yager J, Gerner RH: Neuroendocrine abnormalities in bulimia. Am J Psychiatry 140:559, 1983.

Halmi KA: Anorexia nervosa: Demographic and clinical features in 94 cases. Psychosom Med 36:18, 1974.

Halmi KA, Brodland G, Rigas C: A follow-up study of 79 patients with anorexia nervosa: An evaluation of prognostic factors and diagnostic criteria. Life Hist Rev Psychopathol 4:2990, 1975.

Halmi KA, Falk JR, Schwartz E: Binge eating and vomiting: A survey of a college population. Psychol Med 22:697, 1981.

Halmi KA, Eckert ED, La Du TJ, Cohen J: Anorexia nervosa: Treatment efficacy of cyproheptadine and amitriptyline. Arch Gen Psychiatry 43:177, 1986.

Halmi KA, Dekirmenjian H, Davis JM, et al: Catecholamine metabolism in anorexia nervosa. Arch Gen Psychiatry 35:458, 1978.

Halmi KA, Eckert E, Marchi P, et al: Comorbidity of psychiatric diagnoses in anorexia nervosa. Arch Gen Psychiatry 48:712–718, 1991.

Hatsukami D, Owen P, Pyle R, et al: Similarities and differences on the MMPI between women with bulimia and women with alcohol or drug abuse problems. Addict Behav 7:435, 1982.

Herzog DB, Keller MB, Lavori PW: Outcome in anorexia nervosa and bulimia nervosa: A review of the literature. J Nerv Ment Dis 176:131–143, 1988.

Holland AJ, Hall A, Murray RM, et al: Anorexia nervosa: A study of 34 twin pairs and one set of triplets. Br J Psychiatry 14:414, 1984.

Hsu LKG: Outcome of anorexia nervosa. Arch Gen Psychiatry 37:1041, 1980.

Hudson JI, Laffer PS, Pope HG Jr: Bulimia related to affective disorder by family history and response to dexamethasone suppression test. Am J Psychiatry 139:685, 1982.

Jones DJ, Fox MM, Babigian HM, Hutton HE: Epidemiology of anorexia nervosa in Monroe County, New York: 1960–1976. Psychosom Med 42:551, 1980.

Katz JL, Boyar RM, Roffway H, et al: LHRH responsiveness in anorexia nervosa: Intactness despite prepubertal circadian LH pattern. Psychosom Med 39:241, 1977.

Kay DWK, Schapira K: The prognosis in anorexia nervosa. In Meyer JE, Feldman H (eds): Symposium on Anorexia Nervosa. Stuttgart, Thieme-Verlag, 1965.

Kaye WH, Ebert MH, Raligh M, Lake R: Abnormalities in CNS monoamine metabolism in anorexia nervosa. Arch Gen Psychiatry 41:350–354, 1984.

Kaye WH, Weltzin TW, Hsu LKG, Bulik C: An open trial of fluoxetine in patients with anorexia nervosa. J Clin Psychiatry 52:464–471, 1991.

Kendall RE, Hall DJ, Hailey A, Babigian HM: The epidemiology of anorexia nervosa. Psychol Med 3:200, 1973.

Krahn DD, Nairn K, Goswell BA, Drewnowska A: Stealing in eating disordered patients. J Clin Psychiatry 52:112–115, 1991.

Krieg JC, Pirke KM, Lauer C, Barkmund H: Endocrine, metabolic, and cranial computed tomographic findings in anorexia nervosa. Biol Psychiatry 23(4):377–387, 1988.

Lucas AR, Beard CM, O'Fallon WM, and Kurland LT: 50-year trends in the incidence of anorexia nervosa in Rochester, Minnesota: A population-based study. Am J Psychiatry 148:917–922, 1991.

Marcus MD, Wing RR, Lamparski DM: Binge eating and dietary restraint in obese patients. Addict Behav 10:163–168, 1985.

Minuchin S, Baker L, Rosman BL, et al: A conceptual model of psychosomatic illness in children. Arch Gen Psychiatry 32:1031, 1975.

Mitchell JE: Medical complications of anorexia nervosa and bulimia. Psychiatr Med 1:229, 1984.

Mitchell JE: A review of the controlled trials of psychotherapy for bulimia nervosa. J Psychosomat Res 35:23–31, 1991.

Mitchell JE, Eckert ED: Scope and significance of eating disorders. J Consult Clin Psychol 55:628–634, 1987.

Mitchell JE, Haberman H, Pyle RL: An overview of the treatment of bulimia nervosa. Psychiatr Med 7:317–332, 1989.

Mitchell JE, Pomeroy C, Huber M: A clinicians guide to the eating disorders medicine cabinet. Int J Eat Disord 2:211–223, 1988.

Mitchell JE, Pyle RL, Eckert ED: Frequency and duration of binge-eating episodes in patients with bulimia. Am J Psychiatry 138:835, 1981.

Mitchell JE, Pyle RL, Eckert ED, et al: A comparison study of antidepressants and structured intensive group psychotherapy in the treatment of bulimia nervosa. Arch Gen Psychiatry 47:149–157, 1990.

Mitchell JE, Specker S, de Zwaan M: Comorbidity and medical complications of bulimia nervosa. J Clin Psychiatry 52: 13–20, 1991.

Mitchell JE, Hatsukami D, Eckert ED, Pyle RL: Characteristics of 275 patients with bulimia. Am J Psychiatry 142:482–485, 1985a.

Mitchell JE, Laine DC, Morley JE, et al: Naloxone but not CCK-8 may attenuate binge-eating behavior in patients with bulimia. Int J Eat Disord 4:177–183, 1985b.

Mitchell JE, Pyle RL, Eckert ED, et al: Electrolyte and other physiological abnormalities in patients with bulimia. Psychol Med 13:273, 1983.

Morgan HG, Russell GF: Value of family background in clinical

features as predictors of long-term outcome in anorexia nervosa. Psychol Med 5:355, 1975.

Pirke KM, Pohl J, Schweiger U, Wainkoff M: Metabolic and endocrine indices of starvation in bulimia: A comparison with anorexia nervosa. Psych Res 15:33–39, 1985.

Pirke KM, Fickter MM, Chlond C, et al: Disturbances of the menstrual cycle in bulimia nervosa. Clin Endocrinol 27: 245–251, 1987.

Pope HG Jr, Hudson JI, Yurgelon-Todd D: Anorexia nervosa and bulimia among 300 suburban women shoppers. Am J Psychiatry 141:292, 1984.

Pope HG, Hudson JJ, Nixon RA, et al: The epidemiology of ipecac abuse. N Engl J Med 314:245, 1986.

Pyle RL, Mitchell JE, Eckert ED: Bulimia: A report of 34 cases. J Clin Psychiatry 42:60, 1981.

Pyle RL, Mitchell JE, Eckert ED, et al: The incidence of bulimia in freshman college students. Int J Eat Disord 2:75, 1983.

Rigotti NA, Neer RM, Skates JJ, et al: The clinical course of osteoporosis in anorexia nervosa: A longitudinal study of cortical bone mass. JAMA 265:1133–1138, 1991.

Roberts MW, Li SH: Oral findings in anorexia nervosa and bulimia nervosa: A study of 47 cases. J Am Dent Assoc 115:407–410, 1987.

Russell G: Bulimia nervosa: An ominous variant of anorexia nervosa. Psychol Med 9:429, 1979.

Russell GFM: Metabolic aspects of anorexia nervosa. Proc R Soc Med 58:811, 1965.

Saleh JW, Lebwohl P: Metoclopromide-induced gastric emptying in patients with anorexia nervosa. Am J Gastroenterol 74:127, 1980.

Schocken DD, Holloway JD, Powers PS: Weight loss and the heart. Arch Intern Med 149:877–881, 1989.

Schwartz DM, Thompson MG: Do anorectics get well? Current research and future needs. Am J Psychiatry 138:319, 1981.

Sherman BM, Halmi KA: The effect of nutritional rehabilitation on hypothalamic-pituitary function in anorexia nervosa. In Vigersky RA (ed): Anorexia Nervosa. New York, Raven Press, 1977.

Slade PD, Russell GFM: Experimental investigations of bodily perception in anorexia nervosa and obesity. Psychother Psychosom 22:259, 1973.

Strober M, Salkin B, Burroughs J, Morrell W: Validity of the bulimic-restricter distinction in anorexia nervosa. J Nerv Ment Dis 170:345, 1982.

Theander S: Anorexia nervosa. Acta Psychiatr Scand Suppl 214:1–194, 1970.

Theander S: Research on outcome and prognosis of anorexia nervosa and results from a Swedish long-term study. Int J Eat Disord 12:167, 1983.

Walsh BT, Stewart JW, Wright L, et al: Treatment of bulimia with monoamine oxidase inhibitors. Am J Psychiatry 139:1629, 1982.

Walsh BT, Wong LM, Pesce MA, et al: Hyperamylasemia in bulimia nervosa. J Clin Psychiatry 51:373–377, 1990.

Wardle J, Beinart H: Binge eating: A theoretical review. Br J Clin Psychol 20:97, 1981.

Winokur A, March V, Mendels J: Primary affective disorder in relatives of patients with anorexia nervosa. Am J Psychiatry 130:695, 1980.

CHAPTER 13

Antisocial Personality

REMI CADORET

DEFINITION

Antisocial personality (sociopathy or sociopathic personality) is a chronic condition that manifests before age 15 and continues throughout adult life. It is characterized by repeated disturbances in interpersonal and social relations, such as aggressivity, various derelictions of social responsibility, and criminal activity.

ETIOLOGY

Sociopathy, like many psychiatric conditions, runs in families. Studies of families of convicted felons (most of whom have antisocial personalities) show higher numbers of relatives with antisocial personality or alcoholism than are found in the general population (Guze et al., 1967; Cloninger and Guze, 1973; Robins, 1966). As with other familial conditions, hereditary factors are usually confounded with environmental factors so that the relative importance of each factor is difficult to assess. Adoption studies offer a way of studying separately the effects of heredity and environment. Adoptees, separated at birth from biologic parents and placed with nonrelatives, bring to their adoptive environments a set of unrelated genes. In addition, the adoptive environments provide a varied spectrum of different conditions. Despite careful screening, many adoptive families have family members with psychiatric problems, such as depression, alcoholism, or antisocial behavior, so that the effect of these conditions can be assessed on adoptees from a variety of biologic backgrounds. A number of adoption studies have shown that children of convicted felons, of parents with antisocial types of behavior, are more likely to be diagnosed as antisocial person-

ality even though separated at birth from biologic parents (Cadoret, 1978; Crowe, 1972, 1974; Schulsinger, 1972). Adoption studies of criminal behavior also have shown that adopted-away offspring of convicted criminals are more likely themselves to be convicted of crimes (Bohman et al., 1982; Cloninger et al., 1982; Mednick et al., 1984). These studies are consistent with a genetic factor in criminal behavior and indirectly suggest that antisocial behavior traits may be the common transmitted features.

As noted earlier, family studies of antisocials have found relationships to alcoholism. Adoption studies have helped to elucidate this important relationship. Figure 13-1 shows, for an adoption sample, the relationship of biologic backgrounds of alcohol problems and antisocial behavior and adult adoptee alcohol abuse and antisocial personality. There appears to be some specificity of inheritance, with the biologic parent's alcohol problem predicting alcohol abuse in adult offspring (but not antisocial personality), while the biologic parent's antisocial behavior predicts antisocial personality in their separated-at-birth offspring (but not alcohol abuse). The environmental factor of having an individual in the adoptive family with alcohol problems increases the chance of adoptee alcoholism as well. Environmental factors such as psychiatric disturbance in adoptive family members have proved important in predicting *adolescent* antisocial behavior (Cadoret, 1985; Cadoret, et al., 1983). Recent adoption studies have shown that alcohol problems in both biologic and adoptive parents can separately and independently increase the number of adolescent antisocial behaviors, such as truancy, school suspensions and expulsions, running away from home, early substance use, and fighting (Cadoret et al., 1990). The diagram (Fig. 13-1) shows the strong

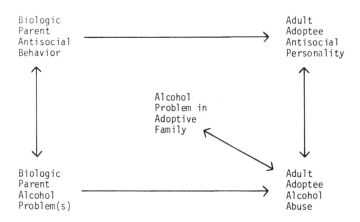

Key: Arrows indicate significant correlations of factors. If factors are not connected by arrows, their correlations are not significant.

FIGURE 13-1   *Inter-relationship of biologic and environmental factors in adult antisocial personality and alcohol abuse in males.*

correlation usually found between antisocial personality and alcohol abuse in adults (right-hand vertical arrow). The left-hand vertical arrow shows the correlation found in this particular sample of biologic parents and represents both a combination of selective mating (tendency for individuals with alcohol problems to mate with antisocials) and the simultaneous occurrence of antisocial behavior and alcohol abuse in one biologic parent. The independent genetic transmission of alcoholism and antisocial personality shown in Figure 13-1 is confirmed by family and population studies (Vaillant, 1983; Cloninger and Reich, 1983).

In a further study of adoptees, Cadoret et al. (1987) reported that antisocial behavior in an adoptive family member (usually another adopted sibling) significantly increased the probability of an antisocial personality diagnosis in the adoptee (odds ratio 16.6). Other environmental factors predicting increased antisocial personality in the adult adoptee were divorced adoptive parents and the socioeconomic level of the adoptive family. The latter relationship depended on the genetic background of the adoptee; adoptees from a criminal or delinquent biologic parent developed significantly more antisocial personalities in lower socioeconomic adoptive homes (odds ratio 12.02), and adoptees from biologic parents who were not criminal or delinquent did not appear to be influenced by the adoptive home socioeconomic level to develop antisocial personality (Cadoret et al., 1990).

EPIDEMIOLOGY

The incidence of antisocial personality is difficult to determine, since most population studies have used other definitions than those in the *Diagnostic and Statistical Manual of Mental Disorders,* third edition (DSM-III; American Psychiatric Association, 1980), for personality disorder. Depending on the study, anywhere from 0.1 to 10 percent of civilian populations have personality disorders (Ekblad, 1950; Hagnell, 1966; Sjogren, 1948). Figures from the United States suggest a value of about 3 percent for antisocial personality (Cloninger and Reich, 1983). The Environmental Catchment Area (ECA) Study done at five different sites in the continental United States estimated that lifetime prevalence of antisocial personality could be as high as 7.3 percent for men and 1.0 percent for women (Robins et al., 1991). As with alcoholism, many more men than women are affected, and family studies generally show a sex ratio of male–female antisocials from 3:1 to 8:1 (Guze et al., 1968, 1970; Winokur et al., 1970).

Antisocials often come from families with marked social disturbances, such as parental desertion, separation and divorce, alcohol and drug abuse, and criminality; families of antisocials are more likely to be of low socioeconomic status (Robins, 1966; Cowie et al., 1968; Guze et al., 1967).

CLINICAL PICTURE

The description of antisocial personality is organized around the DSM-III criteria, which are presented in Table 13-1. The clinical picture of antisocial personality varies to a certain degree, depending on the age at which the person is seen, since the quality of problems that adolescents or young adults can get into is sometimes different

TABLE 13-1. *DSM-III Diagnostic Criteria for Antisocial Personality Disorder*

A. Current age at least 18.

B. Onset before age 15 as indicated by a history of three or more of the following before that age:
1. Truancy (positive if it amounted to at least 5 days per year for at least 2 years, not including the last year of school)
2. Expulsion or suspension from school for misbehavior
3. Delinquency (arrested or referred to juvenile court because of behavior)
4. Running away from home overnight at least twice while living in parental or parental surrogate home
5. Persistent lying
6. Repeated sexual intercourse in a casual relationship
7. Repeated drunkenness or substance abuse
8. Thefts
9. Vandalism
10. School grades below expectations in relation to estimated or known IQ (may have resulted in repeating a year)
11. Chronic violations of rules at home and/or at school (other than truancy)
12. Initiation of fights

C. At least four of the following manifestations of the disorder since age 18:
1. Inability to sustain consistent work behavior, as indicated by any of the following: (a) too frequent job changes (e.g., three or more jobs in 5 years not accounted for by nature of job or economic or seasonal fluctuation); (b) significant unemployment (e.g., 6 months or more in 5 years when expected to work); (c) serious absenteeism from work (e.g., average 3 or more days of lateness or absence per month); (d) walking off several jobs without other jobs in sight. (*Note:* Similar behavior in an academic setting during the last few years of school may substitute for this criterion in individuals who by reason of their age or circumstances have not had an opportunity to demonstrate occupational adjustment.)
2. Lack of ability to function as a responsible parent as evidenced by one or more of the following: (a) child's malnutrition; (b) child's illness resulting from lack of minimal hygiene standards; (c) failure to obtain medical care for a seriously ill child; (d) child's dependence on neighbors or nonresident relatives for food or shelter; (e) failure to arrange for a caretaker for a child under 6 when parent is away from home; (f) repeated squandering, on personal items, of money required for household necessities
3. Failure to accept social norms with respect to lawful behavior, as indicated by any of the following: repeated thefts, illegal occupation (pimping, prostitution, fencing, selling drugs), multiple arrests, a felony conviction
4. Inability to maintain enduring attachment to a sexual partner as indicated by two or more divorces and/or separations (whether legally married or not), desertion of spouse, promiscuity (10 or more sexual partners within 1 year)
5. Irritability and aggressiveness as indicated by repeated physical fights or assault (not required by one's job or to defend someone or oneself), including spouse or child beating
6. Failure to honor financial obligations, as indicated by repeated defaulting on debts, failure to provide child support, failure to support other dependents on a regular basis
7. Failure to plan ahead, or impulsivity, as indicated by traveling from place to place without a prearranged job or clear goal for the period of travel or clear idea about when the travel would terminate, or lack of a fixed address for a month or more
8. Disregard for the truth as indicated by repeated lying, use of aliases, "conning" others for personal profit
9. Recklessness, as indicated by driving while intoxicated or recurrent speeding

D. A pattern of continuous antisocial behavior in which the rights of others are violated, with no intervening period of at least 5 years without antisocial behavior between age 15 and the present time (except when the individual was bedridden or confined in a hospital or penal institution)

E. Antisocial behavior is not due to either severe mental retardation, schizophrenia, or manic episodes.

From American Psychiatric Association: Diagnostic and Statistical Manual of Mental Disorders, 3d ed. Washington, American Psychiatric Association, 1980.

from those seen in older individuals. However, all the problems may be characterized by repeated disturbances in interpersonal and social relationships. The disturbance characteristically starts before age 15, and types of behavioral problems met with in this life period are shown in Table 13-2. As might be expected, since minors spend most of their waking time in school situations, a good deal of antisocial behaviors occurs in school. Truancy and consequences of truancy, such as school suspension and expulsion and poor school performance, are common, as can be seen from Table 13-2. Aggressiveness toward other individuals, especially toward authority figures, such as teachers, also can figure into school difficulties. School problems often lead to dropping out, and it is an unusual antisocial who has finished high school. Antisocials who do graduate high school usually are indifferent scholars who do not achieve their academic potential. Many young antisocials while truant from school will seek the company of others of similar interests, espe-

cially older adolescents, and engage with them in alcohol and other substance abuse, casual sex, thefts, and vandalism. If these behaviors are blatant enough and the individuals are detected in them, the adolescents will come to the attention of the police and be charged with delinquency. Misbehaviors are not confined to the school or the outside world but occur in the home as well, where antisocials are often aggressive toward parents and get into much difficulty by chronically violating rules, such as staying out when they are supposed to be home, not doing chores, stealing money and other items from the home to support such activities as drug habits, and frequent lying. Lying is done sometimes to escape the consequences of misbehavior or to cover up their tracks, or again, lying sometimes occurs as a form of self-aggrandizement, as, for example, when an adolescent boasts about having had contact with famous people. The young antisocial causes further problems at home and at school by his association with other children of bad

TABLE 13-2.   *Disturbed Behavior Before Age 15 in Antisocial Personality*

Behavior	Persons with adult diagnosis of antisocial personality who demonstrated this behavior (%)
Truancy	33
School expulsion	—
Delinquency	—
Running away	34
Persistent lying	45
Casual sex (premarital)	45
Alcohol or other substance abuse	50
Thefts	30
Vandalism	—
Poor school work	—
Chronic violation of home or school rules (stay out late)	32
Initiation of fights	
Aggressive toward relatives	32
Aggressive toward authority figures	28

Data from Robins LN: Deviant Children Grown Up. Baltimore, Williams & Wilkins, 1966. Reprinted with permission from Cadoret RJ, King LJ: Psychiatry in Primary Care, 2d ed. St. Louis, Mosby, 1983.

reputation and by his or her impulsive and reckless behavior. Many antisocials also have difficulty getting along with peers and are frequently disliked, especially because of their aggressivity, their thieving, their bullying, and their bad language. One of the early behaviors in adolescent antisocial girls is casual sex, with its concomitant increased risk of illegitimate pregnancy and venereal diseases. Alcohol and drug abuse also lead to early medical complications in some cases, such as accidents, so that antisocials are more often seen in an emergency department than in an office for counseling. Investigators, such as Lee Robins, have shown that there is a strong correlation between the total number of these early adolescent behaviors and the later diagnosis in adult life of antisocial personality. For example, she has shown that if an individual has 10 or more of the types of behavior shown in Table 13-2, then there is a 43 percent chance that the individual will receive a diagnosis of antisocial personality as an adult. If two or less of these behaviors are present, then there is only a 4 percent chance of such an adult diagnosis.

DSM-III diagnostic criteria for antisocial personality require that after age 18, a number of antisocial behaviors shown in Table 13-1 be present. The frequency of these behaviors in adult antisocials is compared with that in normal controls in Table 13-3. Some type of difficulty with work occurs in a high percentage of antisocial individuals, and such problems can be brought out by a carefully obtained job history, with attention to a careful chronological order of jobs held so that hiatuses in the job record can be detected. Reasons for leaving work also

should be routinely sought as part of the job history. Typical antisocial job histories are characterized by frequent changes of job, punctuated by episodes of unemployment. Reasons for leaving jobs are, characteristically, impulsive quitting because of fights or disagreements with people in authority, being fired for incompetency, fighting on the job, or coming in late or being absent without sufficient reason. Because of these types of job difficulties, antisocials frequently cross the white-collar–blue-collar line in a downward direction. As can be seen in Table 13-3, a high percentage of antisocials show frequent job changes, significant unemployment, and longer periods of unemployment. Job difficulty contributes to financial instability and increasing dependency of such individuals on state and federal funds. One important clinical feature of antisocial job performance was pointed out a number of years ago by Lee Robins, who showed that the length of time a job could be held appeared to be related to the amount of supervision. Solo jobs (such as a truck driver or a service person working alone) were associated with longer periods of employment. In contrast, highly supervised positions (such as clerks in stores or factory workers) were not held as long.

Inability to function as a responsible parent leads to such problems as child neglect and children being removed from the home for abuse or neglect. In part, this difficulty in parenting is probably associated with other behaviors of antisocials that occur in clinically significant numbers of patients. These behaviors are not specifically cited in the DSM-III criteria and are presented separately in Table 13-4. Antisocials often marry spouses with behavior difficulties, such as unfaithfulness, excessive drinking, or child neglect, and as a consequence, the home of the antisocial is more likely to show a chaotic environment. The chaotic home environment also may contribute to the high rate of behavior problems in children (item 3 in Table 13-4), and more children of antisocials are held back in school and themselves show antisocial behaviors, such as truancy, running away from home, and stealing. All these factors, then—poor choice of spouses and difficulty with children—are associated with inability to function responsibly as a parent.

Illegal behavior is an extremely common feature of antisocial adult behavior, as can be seen from Table 13-3, where the number of arrests for major crime is quite high, as well as high conviction rates for nontraffic offenses. In convicted felons, antisocial personality is probably the most common psychiatric diagnosis. Brushes with the law and the consequences, such as incarceration, lead to further disturbance of the antisocial's family and increased financial dependency of all concerned.

Inability to maintain an enduring attachment to a sexual partner, as manifested by a high divorce rate, unfaithfulness, and promiscuity, is prominent in antisocial behavior, as indicated in Table 13-3.

TABLE 13-3. *Diagnostic Disturbed Behavior in Adult Antisocials*

Area of behavior	Antisocials with this behavior (%)	Controls (%)
1. Poor work record		
Too frequent job changes (longest job held less than 2 years)	26	1
Median number of employers in 10-year period	6.4	2.6
Significant unemployment (ever unemployed in past 10 years)	78	23
Median duration of unemployment in months	19	3
Serious work absenteeism	—	—
Leaving job without another job to go to	—	—
2. Lack of ability to function responsibly as a parent		
Cited for child neglect	7	0
Placed children	20	0
3. Serious breaking of law		
Nontraffic arrests	94	17
Arrest for major crime of those ever arrested	73	13
Conviction rate for nontraffic offenses	80	0
4. Inability to maintain enduring attachment to sexual partner		
Unfaithful	28	4
Two or more divorces in those who remarry	54	12
Ever divorced	78	20
Promiscuity	56	12
Desertion	22	4
5. Aggressiveness		
Physical cruelty to spouse or children	12	5
Combative behavior reason for hospitalization if ever in hospital	5	0
6. Failure to honor financial obligations		
Derogatory credit report of those with credit record	57	13
Current debt	14	2
Nonsupport	22	10
7. Failure to plan ahead—impulsivity	67	—
8. Disregard for truth		
Pathologic lying	17	—
Use of alias	8	—
9. Recklessness	—	—

Data from Robins LN: Deviant Children Grown Up. Baltimore, Williams & Wilkins, 1966. Reprinted with permission from Cadoret RJ, King LJ: Psychiatry in Primary Care, 2d ed. St. Louis, Mosby, 1983.

Other antisocial characteristics also contribute to the high divorce rate, such as interpersonal aggressiveness, as shown in physical fighting. Impulsivity, which is present in adolescence and persists through adulthood, also plays a significant role in marital and family problems. In the Robins study, 67 percent of antisocials showed sudden, poorly thought out moves from one city to another, elopements from hospital, and unprovoked desertion of their spouses and children. Such behaviors can contribute significantly to social disruption and lead to divorces.

Irritability and aggressiveness are frequent features of the antisocial. Physical cruelty to spouse and children and physical fighting are two of the biggest reasons for placing the antisocial in the hospital. This increasing combativeness manifests in many situations. For example, antisocials who are alcoholic are much more likely to be arrested for disturbing the peace or for fighting in public than primary alcoholics (Cadoret et al., 1984).

Failure to honor financial obligations is part of the picture of social dereliction of duties and manifests by poor credit ratings, many debts, and, in those who are separated or divorced, failure to provide child support.

Failure to plan ahead, or impulsivity, occurs in a high proportion of antisocials and leads to vagrancy and wanderlust. In Robins's study of antisocials at least 60 percent had spent a period of several months hitchhiking around the country with no financial support or employment in prospect. Such individuals occasionally will sell drugs or take temporary jobs requiring little skills to support their wanderlust. Marked impulsivity seems to have a poor prognosis for antisocials, since Robins reported that individuals with this characteristic early in life seemed to have severer problems later with their antisocial behavior.

Disregard for the truth, such as pathologic lying or using an alias, occurs in a significant number of individuals. Many times the lies serve a useful purpose of "conning" someone else, and individuals who are extremely verbal can sometimes put up convincing arguments or rationalizations for their behavior. Frequently, conning procedures are used by antisocials in getting drugs from physicians by either reporting nonexistent physical symptoms or exaggerating ones that might be present. Hence the importance of knowing one's patients and realizing that antisocial individuals are likely to indulge in this type of activity should lead a physician to ques-

TABLE 13-4. *Nondiagnostic Areas of Behavioral Disturbance in Antisocials*

Area of behavior	Antisocials (%)	Controls (%)
1. Financial dependency		
Received welfare funds	45	2
Financial or work assistance	63	8
2. Behavior problems in spouse		
Desertion or unfaithfulness	28	6
Drinking to excess	28	5
Neglect of home or child	23	7
Arrests	21	7
Solution to problem spouse		
Divorce and remarry another		
problem spouse	42	13
Divorce	84	36
3. High rate of behavior problems in children		
Held back in school	30	15
Truant	16	0
Runaway	14	0
Stealing	11	0
High school graduations of		
sons 18 and older	9	69
4. Difficulties in armed forces (men)		
Reason for rejection		
Criminal record	41	0
Physical incapacity	37	24
Problems in service (of those who served)		
Dishonorable discharge	23	0
AWOL	40	3
Punishments	37	3
Court-martial	23	0
5. Alcohol and drug use		
Social and medical problems associated with alcohol abuse		
Any ever	62	7
Arrests	42	3
Fired from job	13	1
Drug addition ever	10	0
6. Poor socialization		
No contact with living siblings or parents	27	0
No contact with neighbors	75	33
Lack of planned social contacts	51	7
No organizational memberships	69	31
7. Increased psychiatric treatment and hospitalization		
Mental hospital	21	1
Any psychiatric attention	50	20
Reason for hospitalization*		
Alcohol	18	0
Drugs	14	0
Depressed or suicidal	18	100†
Dangerous to others	14	0
Prostitution (women only)	25	0
8. Suicidal behavior—suicide attempts	11	—
9. Unusual emotional response—lack of guilt at interview	40	—

*Reason for hospitalization (for those hospitalized).
†Reflects depression of the one control subject that had been hospitalized.
Data from Robins LN: Deviant Children Grown Up. Baltimore, Williams & Wilkins, 1966. Reprinted with permission from Cadoret RJ, King LJ: Psychiatry in Primary Care, 2d ed. St. Louis, Mosby, 1983.

tion requests for tranquilizers, narcotics, and other such medications from antisocials.

Recklessness is also a large feature of antisocial life, especially in late adolescence, and leads to arrests for speeding and public intoxication and involves the antisocial in accidents where they are likely to come in contact with physicians or other health care professionals.

All these behaviors may be detected by taking good histories from the patient or, better still, from reliable informants. It is necessary in obtaining the history to obtain a chronological accounting of behaviors in all these different areas so that important hiatuses can be noted and periods of time when embarrassing situations occurred that the patient does not wish to report can be detected (e.g., time done in prison).

As noted earlier, many other behaviors occur in antisocials more frequently than in individuals without these characteristics that may bring the individual in contact with physicians. These "nondiagnostic" behaviors appear in Table 13-4 and include financial dependency, marrying a spouse with significant behavior problems, and having chaotic families with high rates of behavior problems in children. Table 13-4 presents a number of additional behaviors that are important because they cause the antisocial to have contact with physicians. The first of these is difficulties in the armed forces. Many antisocials are rejected from service for a criminal record. Those who do serve have a disproportionate number of problems both in the service and when they are discharged. A high proportion during service get into difficulty with absent-without-leaves and other punishments, including court martial. A significant proportion eventually receive a less than honorable discharge. In the service, antisocials are likely to come in contact with physicians in trying to get drugs or in trying to get out of their service obligations by playing the sick role. Once these individuals are discharged from active duty, they request more veteran's benefits, such as treatment or pensions, than do non-antisocial individuals. Thus VA hospitals are more likely to contain individuals with this type of history and personality.

An important part of antisocial behavior that frequently brings antisocials in contact with health care professionals is their abuse of alcohol and drugs. Antisocials characteristically start such drug abuse much earlier in life than individuals who are primary alcoholics. It is not unusual to find alcoholic antisocials using alcohol regularly in grade school and early high school. In addition to alcohol, a large part of substance abuse is the use of illicit street drugs. One study of alcoholic antisocials who had been admitted for detoxification found that such individuals were much more likely to have significant illicit street drug abuse than were primary alcoholics admitted to the same unit (Cadoret et al., 1984). High amounts of alcohol and drug use are associated with many and early complications so that, in general, antisocial alcoholics are usually admitted to detoxification centers at an earlier age than primary alcoholics. Alcohol and drug use also contributes significantly to difficulty in holding jobs and to performing criminal acts to supply the money necessary for heavy drug and alcohol use. In Robins's study of antisocials, alcohol accounted for most of the hospitalizations, largely because of the aggressive behavior that was associated with drinking. In the Guze and Cantwell study (1965) of convicted felons, alcoholic antisocials showed a much higher rate of recidivism than those who were not alcoholic. Thus the use of drugs and alcohol is an important complication of antisocial personality. Adoption studies have shown a very significant relationship between the antisocial personality and drug abuse (Cadoret et al., 1986) and have implicated a genetic factor (alcoholic biologic parents) in promoting the move from drug user to drug abuser in a study of 28 male adoptee abusers, of whom 75 percent had antisocial personality (Cadoret, 1992).

Antisocial individuals show higher rates of psychiatric treatment and hospitalization, as indicated in Table 13-4. The reasons for hospitalization are frequently associated with alcohol and drugs. Depression and suicidal behavior are also important features of antisocial behavior that result in hospitalization. In general, suicide attempts far outweigh completed suicide, as evidenced in the Robins study. Other studies agree in suggesting that completed suicide in antisocials is probably relatively low (Pokorny, 1960; Robins et al., 1950; Tuckman and Youngman, 1965). A number of studies have shown that there is a high incidence of antisocial personality among individuals who come to hospital emergency departments with attempted suicide. These studies (Batchelor, 1954; James et al., 1963) indicate that between 20 and 25 percent of suicide attempters seen in hospital emergency departments are antisocial personalities. Suicide attempts in antisocials were more likely to be medically nonserious, in contrast to primary depressives, whose attempts were more likely to be medically serious. As one might expect, a high proportion of antisocials' attempts were regarded as impulsive and were often closely associated in time with a socially upsetting situation, such as a personal fight with a spouse or lover or the threat of being arrested and put in prison or a mental hospital. One study suggested that the most common motive for the suicide attempt was bad feelings for a person about whom there was considerable ambivalence so that the suicide attempt often represented a way of revenge to the antisocial individual. In only a few cases were the suicidal motives manipulative, in the sense that they were designed to change others' behavior. Many antisocials do suffer from feelings of guilt, especially in the presence of a depressive syndrome, although a goodly proportion of antisocials are reported as being cold and affectionless and not feeling guilt. For example, a recent study of 35 antisocial persons treated in an outpatient clinic showed that 22 of them had a secondary depression with marked self-deprecatory and guilt feelings. Indeed, secondary depression is probably one of the principal reasons for antisocials coming to physicians for treatment. Such individuals also can make suicide attempts.

One other area of disturbance brings antisocial individuals in contact with physicians. A high proportion of antisocial individuals show a large number of neurotic or somatic symptoms. These symptoms are shown in Table 13-5, where it can be seen that anxiety and gastrointestinal symptoms are rather high in frequency. Likewise, "neurologic" symptoms, such as blurred vision or even episodes of blindness and paralysis, including trances and amnesia, occur with significantly greater frequency in antisocial individuals. In the Robins series, 5 percent of hospitalizations were for amnesia. The presence of large numbers of such somatic or neurotic symptoms in some antisocials but not in others has raised the question of heterogeneity in antisocial personality. The ECA study showed that male and female antisocials were both much more likely to have increased rates of other psychiatric condi-

TABLE 13-5. *Somatic "Nonsociopathic" Symptoms in Adult Antisocials*

	Antisocials (%)	Controls with no disease (%)
1. Average number of symptoms	7.8	2.6
2. High level of neurotic or somatic symptoms (>9 symptoms and/or disabling symptoms)	37	—
3. Neurologic symptoms		
Blurred vision	17	3
Episode of blindness	8	0
Paralysis	7	1
Trouble walking	7	1
Trances	7	0
Amnesia	7	0
4. Anxiety symptoms		
Anxiety attacks	22	0
Dizzy spells	30	5
Dyspnea	30	12
Palpitations	30	10
"Nervous"	47	15
Chest pain	29	7
Anxiety in crowds	15	0
5. Other somatic symptoms		
Weakness	20	4
Nausea	32	9
Vomiting	22	8
Abdominal pain	28	8
Bowel trouble	28	8
Insomnia	30	12
Fatigue	22	10
Anorexia	12	5
Back pain	45	31

Data from Robins LN: Deviant Children Grown Up. Baltimore, Williams & Wilkins, 1966. Reprinted with permission from Cadoret RJ, King LJ: Psychiatry in Primary Care, 2d ed. St. Louis, Mosby, 1983.

tions such as drug abuse, obsessive-compulsive syndrome, alcohol abuse, depression, dysthymia, and panic and phobic states (Robins et al., 1991). In addition, diagnosis of mania and schizophrenia were more common.

Heterogeneity has long been described in sociopathy. Karpman (1947) distinguished primary and secondary psychopaths. *Secondary psychopaths* "act out" in antisocial and aggressive ways as a result of inner conflict and, as part of the clinical picture, often show guilt, anxiety, depression, remorse, paranoia, or other psychoneurotic symptoms. In contrast to this, *primary psychopaths* usually show a low level of anxiety, with little evidence of guilt. Primary psychopaths have been shown to be impulsive, undersocialized, aggressive, and lacking anxiety or other forms of subjective distress (Jenkins, 1966; Quay, 1964a, 1964b; Peterson et al., 1961). Prison populations that are high in proportion of sociopaths as defined in this chapter have shown evidence of these two types of antisocials (Blackburn, 1971; Hare, 1975). One study of primary and secondary sociopaths used scales derived from the Minnesota Multiphasic Personality Inventory and showed that secondary psychopaths had high levels for depression, tension, body symptoms, autistic thinking, and anxiety, in contrast to primary psychopaths, who had high levels of extraversion, impulsivity, aggression, suspicion, and psychopathic deviation (Blackburn, 1973). Evidence for two such groupings of sociopathics also was described in a study where alcoholic sociopaths were divided on the basis of low and high numbers of depressive symptoms (Whitters et al., 1984). Those with high numbers of depressive symptoms had larger numbers of manic, panic, schizophrenic, and somatic symptoms. These differences are shown in Table 13-6. One additional clinical difference of

practical importance was the high rate of drug abuse in those antisocials with a high number of depressive symptoms. Although heterogeneity as described above for primary and secondary neuropathy may be present, it is not recognized by DSM-III.

However, recent developments in nosology of antisocials describes a different type of heterogeneity. Two correlated factors have been described in prison populations which when present in different degrees could lead to differing clinical presentations (Harper et al., 1989). Factor 1 measures a selfish, callous, and exploitative use of others, and factor 2 measures an unstable lifestyle characterized by socially deviant behavior. The latter factor correlates very highly with criminal behavior; the first correlates only marginally with criminality and a diagnosis of antisocial personality as made by current diagnostic criteria (which emphasize socially deviant behavior). Factor 1 is characterized by traits of superficial charm and glibness, grandiose sense of self-worth, deception, conning and lack of sincerity, lack of remorse or guilt, and failure to accept responsibility for one's own actions. The applicability of factor 1 traits to clinical diagnosis of antisocial personality is currently under investigation in DSM-IV field trials.

PATHOLOGY

There is no known basic pathology process causing antisocial personality such as is found in a disease like Huntington's chorea. While, for example, abnormalities of electroencephalography or autonomic nervous system reactivity have been described more frequently in antisocial populations, many antisocials still do not show such abnormalities. Any basic structural, biochemical, or functional abnormality eludes us at present.

TABLE 13-6. *Clinical Differences Between Antisocial Alcoholics with High and Low Number of Depressive Symptoms*

	Low depressive symptoms (%), $n = 46$	High depressive symptoms (%), $n = 48$
Any drug abuse/ dependence diagnosis	37.0	70.0*
Average number of manic symptoms	.83	3.9†
Average number of panic symptoms	1.7	3.8*
Average number of schizophrenic symptoms	1.2	2.9†
Average number of somatic symptoms	1.0	2.1‡

*Significant 1.0% level.
†Significant 0.1% level.
‡Significant 5.0% level.
Data from Whitters A, Troughton E, Cadoret RJ, et al.: Evidence for clinical heterogeneity in antisocial alcoholics. Compr Psychiatry 25:158–164, 1984.

CLINICAL COURSE

In general, antisocial behavior seems to decrease as individuals grow older, although the condition is a chronic one, with one or more disturbed areas of behavior usually present. In the Robins series, approximately 40 percent improved later in life, with the median age of improvement being 35 years. The best predictor for remission in the series was the diagnosis of the father: 3 percent of children from antisocial fathers remitted, contrasted with 26 percent of children who improved whose fathers were not diagnosed antisocial. Other series (Maddocks, 1970) also report chronicity with a tendency for improvement later in life. In this latter series, those who had *not* improved were more likely to be alcoholic and to exhibit marked hypochondriacal symptoms. Although a certain amount of improvement seems to occur, especially regarding brushes with the law, many of these individuals are pathetically socially isolated. Some idea of this social isolation, which is little appreciated, can be seen in Table 13-4. Antisocials tend to stay by themselves, to have little contact with neighbors, to have few friends, and to be isolated, even from blood relatives and in-laws. When improvement later in life does occur, it is difficult to know how much can be attributed to treatment.

Vaillant's longitudinal study of alcoholics has shown that by the fifth decade of life, individuals diagnosed as sociopaths were *more* likely to be abstinent than were primary alcoholics (Vaillant, 1983). This suggests that improvement in psychopathology may be more likely to occur with older antisocials, since sociopathy is generally considered an unfavorable prognostic sign in the treatment of alcoholism (Gibbs and Flanagan, 1977).

DIFFERENTIAL DIAGNOSIS

Differentiation of antisocial personality from other psychiatric conditions is based mostly on long-term history rather than on a cross-sectional view of symptoms. Difficulty beginning in childhood or adolescence and continuing through adult life is the rule for antisocial personality, whereas most other psychiatric conditions have a more episodic course and a later onset. Psychiatric conditions that must be distinguished from the antisocial are as follows:

1. *Major depression.* Depressed individuals may act in self-destructive ways. Some of these self-destructive ways may involve criminal activity and resemble the kinds of behaviors done by antisocials, such as drug or alcohol abuse, sexual promiscuity, difficulties with discipline, recklessness (including reckless driving), neglect of work, and other derelictions of social responsibilities. As with other psychiatric conditions, the major feature distinguishing antisocial from primary depression is the time course, with antisocial behavior starting before age 15, as well as being more chronic. Depression generally starts later than age 15 and is more likely to be episodic with intervals of relatively good functioning. An antisocial individual also may suffer from major depression during his or her lifetime; if this is the case, then the diagnosis of antisocial personality with secondary depression can be made.

2. *Manic illness.* The distinguishing feature of manic illness, like that in depression, is the periodicity of mania and its onset usually in the late teens or early 20s, with relatively good functioning up to the point of onset. During manic episodes, behavior of antisocial flavor can occur, such as overspending, misusing credit cards, recklessness, financial irresponsibility, sexual promiscuity, and argumentativeness.

3. *Schizophrenia.* A number of children with conduct disorder or antisocial behavior turn out later in life to be schizophrenic (Robins, 1966). As shown in Table 13-6, antisocial individuals tend to complain more of psychiatric symptoms, including schizophrenic-type symptoms. This makes a differential diagnosis rather difficult at times. If symptoms and a course diagnostic of schizophrenia are present, then this condition should be diagnosed and treated. It should be kept in mind, however, that antisocial individuals frequently indulge in drug abuse and that this may be presenting as a schizophrenic-like picture in an antisocial individual. Hospital admission to a controlled environment in which drugs are not available might help to differentiate the situation from schizophrenia.

4. *Neuroses.* Classic obsessions and compulsions seem to be uncommon in antisocial individuals, although, as indicated in Table 13-5, a number of anxiety symptoms do occur and may raise the question of generalized anxiety, phobic disorder, or panic disorder. Again, phobic, panic, or generalized anxiety disorders usually do not have a preexisting antisocial history. If an antisocial history is present along with anxiety attacks, then it is reasonable to assume that the anxiety is part of the antisocial picture and treat it accordingly. Similar considerations should hold for symptoms of hysteria that, as indicated in Table 13-5, occur in antisocial individuals and raise the question of somatoform disorder, conversion disorder, or other dissociative disorders.

5. *Mental retardation.* Most definitions of antisocial personality, including that in DSM-III, eliminate individuals who are severely mentally retarded (see exclusion E in DSM-III diagnostic criteria, Table 13-1). However, a number of individuals with mild, or even moderate, retardation show considerable antisocial behavior. If these meet criteria for antisocial personality, then this condition may be diagnosed.

6. *Other personality diagnoses.* Sometimes differentiation of antisocial personality from other personality diagnoses may be difficult. This is especially true when distinguishing between passive-aggressive personality disorder and antisocials. Many individuals with passive-aggressive personality disorder manifest derelictions of social responsibility as part of their resistance, expressed through such mechanisms as procrastination, stubbornness, dawdling, intentional inefficiency, or "forgetfulness." The dependency of these individuals, including financial dependency, also smacks of antisocial personality. If features of antisocial and passive-aggressive personality disorder are clearly present, then the diagnosis of mixed personality disorder can be made.

The DSM-III borderline personality can also be confused with the antisocial. Impulsivity, self-destructive behaviors, such as gambling and substance abuse, temper outbursts, suicidal attempts, and gestures are characteristics that borderlines share with antisocials. The early onset in antisocials and their more criminal activity should help to make the distinction.

7. *Alcohol and drug abuse/dependency*. Diagnosis of these conditions should arouse suspicion of an underlying antisocial personality.

8. *Miscellaneous conditions*, such as factitious disorders or malingering, should raise the question of whether an underlying antisocial personality is present.

TREATMENT

Treatment of antisocial personalities is generally difficult owing to a number of factors. First, antisocial behaviors are embedded in a social matrix of bad company and other adverse environmental factors, which tends to enmesh the antisocial and encourage socially deviant behavior. Second, the length of time that these antisocial behaviors have been practiced and reinforced makes change difficult. Third, antisocial individuals seldom volunteer for treatment; hence their motivation for change is usually low. Physicians probably find that their major contact with antisocials is in such areas as emergency departments, where antisocials appear with impulsive suicide attempts, for treatment of injuries received in fights, or for treatment of drinking or drug-related problems, such as medical complications of their substance abuse. Many antisocials are brought to the attention of a physician when they are expelled from school and are creating a great deal of difficulty at home with discipline problems. No matter where the contact is made, the treating professional is impressed with the magnitude of the problems that beset antisocials and wonder where to begin management.

In dealing with antisocials, three questions must be raised: (1) What behaviors are involved in the present problems that bring the person to attention? (2) What is the patient's insight into his or her responsibility to affect changes in this area? (3) Most important, how motivated is the patient to try to make changes? Motivation to change is especially important, since most antisocials appear at professionals' doorsteps only under considerable social pressure from spouse, family, friends, or the police. Superficially, some appear to be motivated and elect treatment rather than some alternative, such as going to jail. Sometimes it is possible to arrange that social pressure be continued on the antisocial, thus ensuring a certain amount of motivation, e.g., by putting the individual on probation and requiring her or him to report for treatment regularly or go to jail for failure to comply. In the case of marital problems, separation from a spouse could be maintained as a means of applying pressure on the antisocial to change his or her behavior, with the reward for efforts to change being living again with the spouse. With a specific problem behavior in mind, then, and some motivation on the patient's part to change, some approach to treatment of antisocial behavior is possible. This rather

limited problem-oriented approach does not deal with all difficulties, but at least it allows, in many cases, more realistic goals to be set. It also may be less likely to lead therapists to expect too much and result in the often-quoted conclusion that response to treatment aimed at antisocial behavior is so bad that any treatment is an exercise in futility.

In describing treatment, discrete areas of disturbed behavior in antisocials, as shown in Tables 13-3 and 13-4, are considered, and some therapeutic approaches that might be tried for each of these areas are indicated. Some treatments may require elaborate settings, such as in an institution where such measures as token economies might be used. Other treatment methods, such as medication, group psychotherapy, family or marital counseling, could be used in outpatient settings.

Antisocial behavior that leads to trouble with the law (Table 13-3, area 3) has long been a prime target for treatment. Most of the studies that describe effects of treatment on criminals have dealt with incarcerated individuals so that some cooperation with treatment was enforced. The treatments used in such settings include individual or group psychotherapy, therapeutic communities, and behavioral psychotherapies, such as token economies. The use of these techniques has been detailed in some reports (LeVine and Bornstein, 1972). The past decade has seen an increased interest in application of principles of cognitive therapy to criminal thinking. This approach was suggested and pioneered by Yochelson and Samenow (1976, 1977), working with hospitalized criminals at St. Elizabeth's Hospital in Washington, D.C. The basic premise of this treatment is that antisocial behavior is a product of faulty and erroneous thinking. Individuals are taught to identify erroneous thinking and correct it. Thinking errors include such alterations of reality as the antisocial portraying himself or herself as always a victim (even in the commission of a crime), or as always questing power, or as espousing the view that injustice means getting caught for your crime. The maneuvers used by the criminal to get out of accountability are also identified: his or her feeling of uniqueness, failure to assume obligation, and blocking of communication. A large number of such thinking errors have been identified and used in treatment programs.

This treatment approach has been tested in a number of correctional settings, and a meta-analysis of published results from such settings has shown that the cognitive approach is generally superior to comparison treatments in leading to lower recidivism rates (Gendreau and Ross, 1987; Ross et al., 1988). Whether a cognitive approach could be used in a noncorrectional setting with individuals who are not prisoners is yet to be determined, but the positive results reported belie the generally accepted belief that "nothing helps" antisocials.

In treating antisocials, the physician faces the problem of finding an institution or treatment for a particular individual, since many public institutions may require a court commitment, thus limiting those admitted to antisocials with usually severe behavior problems. In some instances, patients and their families are also required to go the route of contact with a juvenile court. Many institutions limit intake to certain age groups, and there are few facilities, other than jails or hospitals, for adult antisocial individuals. In many communities, group homes or halfway houses are available for younger adolescents. Such facilities are usually organized along therapeutic community lines and are characterized by the setting of behavioral limits. In some communities, hospitals maintain live-in, long-term facilities where antisocial individuals may be exposed to controlled environments. Halfway houses, group homes, and long-term hospitalizations in therapeutic community situations can be useful not only for types of behavior leading to crime but also in situations where individuals come from chaotic homes in which discipline was absent or, at best, inconsistent.

One important factor in the therapy for antisocial behavior is the setting of behavioral limits. Institutionalization of some type is often the best way to achieve this. Outpatient management can be attempted, however, when parents or guardians are willing and able to try to set limits and carry out consistent discipline. Discipline appears to be an important ingredient of treatment. Robins's studies have shown that antisocial individuals often come from homes in which discipline is poor, inconsistent, or nonexistent. Craft (1965) has reported that in institutional settings, rigid discipline seems to result in greater improvements in incarcerated antisocials. Providing a disciplined environment can be done in family conferences, where the antisocial and the parents or guardians meet together and set up agreements or contracts as to which behaviors are to be changed, which behaviors are to be expected, and what rewards are to be obtained if change occurs and is maintained.

Aggressivity (Table 13-3, area 5), a cardinal manifestation of antisocial behavior, may be dealt with in a number of ways. Medications such as phenytoin (Dilantin) and major tranquilizers have been recommended, but there are no studies that show their efficacy. One study, however, has shown that maintenance lithium carbonate reduced the number of physical assaults in incarcerated individuals with severe personality disorders (Sheard et al., 1976). Thus a trial on lithium might be attempted for some individuals. Propranolol has recently been used with some success in children and adolescents who show rage and aggressive outbursts (Williams et al., 1982). Most of these individuals also have some significant organic brain dysfunction, such as cerebral palsy, moderate to severe mental retardation, or a seizure disorder. The value of propranolol for aggressive outbursts in antisocials is unknown. In behavior problems where impulsivity is a factor,

some type of individual psychotherapy might encourage the antisocial person to consider and try other responses to situations that might otherwise end with violence. For example, an antisocial and his spouse may receive marital counseling to help guide them around the situations that would ordinarily call forth aggression. Because alcohol or other drug abuse is often associated with aggressivity, it is important to assess this factor. Having the individual stop drinking may be sufficient to ameliorate significant aggression. Treatment of the alcohol problem in antisocials can involve administration of drugs, such as disulfiram, and antisocial individuals can certainly be referred to alcoholism treatment units for treatment and management of their alcohol problems if they see this as a contributing factor to their difficulties in life.

At one time, as a means of treatment or punishment, many antisocials were required to enlist in the armed forces (Table 13-4, area 4). Recent law now specifies that "antisocial attitudes and behavior" are reason for psychiatric rejection. Although some antisocial individuals may benefit from the discipline of the armed forces, the rate of significant behavior problems in the armed forces and subsequent problems after discharge would make armed forces service a poor general method of treatment.

Somatic symptoms (Table 13-5) frequently bring an antisocial in contact with a physician. Selecting the appropriate medication for specific conditions that might be causing such symptoms is important. Thus, for crippling anxiety attacks, usual medical methods of approach might include the use of propranolol, tricyclic antidepressants, or even monoamine oxidase inhibitors. There is no evidence that antisocials fail to respond to psychotropic drugs, so when somatic symptoms of depression, such as fatigue or sleeplessness, occur, antidepressants may be prescribed, perhaps with a bit more caution, realizing that antisocials may be more likely to abuse medication or mix it with other substances, such as illicit drugs or alcohol. Medications directed against specific somatic problems may be helpful to the individual antisocial and enable him or her to make a better general adjustment.

Suicide attempts (Table 13-4, area 8) are fairly common in antisocial individuals and are one of the main reasons for antisocials being seen by physicians in emergency departments. The suicidal motive is often a wish to take revenge on some significant other person. In some cases, marital or family therapy may help to uncover frictions and teach the patient to deal with frustration and anger in ways other than suicide attempts. One-to-one psychotherapy could be attempted with such individuals in order to point out alternative behaviors to suicide attempts, and training aimed at postponing impulsive activity, which is frequently associated with suicide attempts, could be given.

A poor work record (Table 13-3, area 1) and consequent financial dependency (Table 13-4, area

1), hallmarks of antisocial history, can be attacked in a number of ways. In properly motivated individuals, job training might be offered through such agencies as vocational rehabilitation. Intelligent sociopaths could be sent back to complete the schooling necessary for higher-level jobs. Job training should take into account the antisocial's interest and abilities. Job training could make the antisocial more competitive in the job market and help to reduce financial dependency.

Lack of ability to function responsibly as a parent (Table 13-3, area 2) and concomitant problems, such as inability to maintain enduring attachment to a sexual partner (Table 13-3, area 4), behavior problems in one's spouse (Table 13-4, area 2), and high rate of behavior problems in children (Table 13-4, area 3) might be handled in marriage and family counseling that deals with specific problems arising in the marriage or family relationships.

In many antisocials' lives one of the most important factors affecting their social behavior is alcohol (and other substance) abuse (Table 13-4, area 5). Substance abuse enters into all kinds of problems: family, job, and crime. One of the most positive changes that can be made in the antisocial lifestyle is to stop substance abuse. Antisocials can benefit from programs aimed at alcohol and drug abuse and should be encouraged to try such approaches to sobriety as Alcoholics Anonymous or Narcotics Anonymous.

Treatment goals are often limited. Whatever the goals, the chance of achieving success will be greater if they are agreed on in advance by all parties concerned. Sometimes changes in one target area (e.g., stopping substance abuse) will be reflected by large gains in other areas (e.g., acting more responsibly as a parent).

REFERENCES

American Psychiatric Association: Diagnostic and Statistical Manual of Mental Disorders, 3d ed. Washington, American Psychiatric Association, 1980.

Batchelor IRC: Psychopathic states and attempted suicide. Br Med J 1:1342–1347, 1954.

Blackburn R: Personality types among abnormal homicides. Br J Criminol 11:14–31, 1971.

Blackburn R: An empirical classification of psychopathic personality. Br J Psychol 127:456–460, 1973.

Bohman M, Cloninger CR, Sigvardsson S, et al: Predisposition to petty criminality in Swedish adoptees: I. Genetic and environmental heterogeneity. Arch Gen Psychiatry 39:1233–1241, 1982.

Cadoret RJ: Psychopathology in adopted-away offspring of biologic parents with antisocial behavior. Arch Gen Psychiatry 35:176–184, 1978.

Cadoret RJ: Genes, environment and their interaction in the development of psychopathology, in Sakai T, Tsuboi T (eds): Genetic Aspects of Human Behavior. Tokyo, Igaku-Shoin Ltd, 1985.

Cadoret RJ: Genetic and environmental factors in initiation of drug use and the transition to abuse. In Glanz M, Pickens R (eds): Vulnerability to Drug Abuse. Washington, American Psychological Association, 1992.

Cadoret RJ, Cain CA, Crowe RR: Evidence for gene-environment interaction in development of adolescent antisocial behavior. Behav Genet 13:301–310, 1983.

Cadoret RJ, Troughton E, O'Gorman TW: Genetic and environmental factors in alcohol abuse and antisocial personality. J Stud Alcohol 48:1–8, 1987.

Cadoret RJ, Troughton E, Widmer R: Clinical differences between antisocial and primary alcoholics. Compr Psychiatry 25:1–8, 1984.

Cadoret RJ, Troughton E, Bagford J, Woodworth G: Genetic and environmental factors in adoptee antisocial personality. Eur Arch Psychiatr Neurol Sci 239:231–240, 1990.

Cadoret RJ, Troughton E, O'Gorman TW, Heywood E: An adoption study of genetic and environmental factors in drug abuse. Arch Gen Psychiatry 43:1131–1136, 1986.

Cloninger CR, Guze SB: Psychiatric illness in the families of female criminals: A study of 288 first-degree relatives. Br J Psychol 122:697–703, 1973.

Cloninger CR, Reich T: Genetic heterogeneity in alcoholism and sociopathy. In Kety SS, Rowland LP, Sidman RL, Matthysse SW (eds): Genetics of Neurological and Psychiatric Disorders. New York, Raven Press, 1983, pp 145–166.

Cloninger CR, Sigvardsson S, Bohman M, et al: Predisposition to petty criminality in Swedish adoptees: II. Cross-fostering analysis of gene-environment interaction. Arch Gen Psychiatry 39:1242–1247, 1982.

Cowie J, Cowie V, Slater E: Delinquency in Girls. London, Humanities Press, 1968.

Craft M: Ten Studies into Psychopathic Personality. Bristol, England, J Wright & Sons, 1965.

Crowe RR: The adopted offspring of women criminal offenders. Arch Gen Psychiatry 27:600–603, 1972.

Crowe RR: An adoption study of antisocial personality. Arch Gen Psychiatry 31:785–791, 1974.

Ekblad M: A psychiatric and sociological study of a series of Swedish naval conscripts, in Stromgren E (ed): Statistical and Genetical Population Studies Within Psychiatry: Methods and Principal Results. Paris, Congres Internationale de Psychiatrie, 1950.

Gendreau P, Ross RR: Revivification of rehabilitation: Evidence from the 1980s. Justice Q 4:349–407, 1987.

Gibbs SE, Flanagan J: Prognostic indicators of alcoholism treatment outcome. Int J Addict 12:1097–1141, 1977.

Guze SB, Cantwell DP: Alcoholism and criminal recidivism: A study of 116 parolees. Am J Psychiatry 122:436–439, 1965.

Guze SB, Wolfgram ED, McKinney JK, et al: Psychiatric illness in the families of convicted criminals. A study of 519 first-degree relatives. Dis Nerv Syst 28:651–659, 1967.

Guze SB, Wolfgram ED, McKinney JK: Delinquency, social maladjustment and crime: The role of alcoholism (a study of first-degree relatives of convicted criminals). Dis Nerv Syst 29:238–243, 1968.

Guze SB, Goodwin DW, Crane JB: Criminal recidivism and psychiatric illness. Am J Psychiatry 127:832–835, 1970.

Hagnell O: A Prospective Study of the Incidence of Mental Disorder. Stockholm, Svenska Boknorloget Norstedts-Bonnias, 1966.

Hare RD: Psychophysiological studies of psychopathy. In Fowles DC (ed): Clinical Applications of Psychophysiology. New York, Columbia University Press, 1975, pp 1–105.

James IP, Derham SP, Scott-Orr DV: Attempted suicide: A study of 100 patients referred to a general hospital. Med J Aust 6:375–380, 1963.

Jenkins RL: Psychiatric syndromes in children and their relation to family background. Am J Orthopsychiatry 36:450–457, 1966.

Karpman B: Passive parasitic psychopathy: Toward the personality structure and psychogenesis of idiopathic psychopathy. Psychoanal Rev 34:102–118, 198–222, 1947.

LeVine WR, Bornstein PE: Is the sociopath treatable? The contribution of psychiatry to a legal dilemma. Wash Univ Law Q 693–711, 1972.

Maddocks PD: A five-year follow-up of untreated psychopaths. Br J Psychol 116:511–515, 1970.

Mednick SA, Gabrielli WF, Hutchings B: Genetic influences in criminal convictions: Evidence from an adoption cohort. Science 224:891–894, 1984.

Peterson DR, Quay HC, Tiffany TL: Personality factors related to juvenile delinquency. Child Dev 32:355–372, 1961.

Pokorny AD: Characteristics of 44 patients who subsequently committed suicide. Arch Gen Psychiatry 2:314–323, 1960.

Quay HC: Dimensions of personality in delinquent boys as inferred from the factor analysis of case history data. Child Dev 35:479–484, 1964a.

Quay HC: Personality dimensions in delinquent males as inferred from the factor analysis of behavior rating. J Res Crime Delinquency 1:33–37, 1964b.

Robins E, Murphy G, Wilkinson R Jr: Some clinical considerations in the prevention of suicide based on a study of 134 successful suicides. Am J Public Health 49:888–899, 1950.

Robins LN: Deviant Children Grown Up. Baltimore, Williams & Wilkins, 1966.

Robins LN, Tipp J, Przybeck T: Antisocial personality. In Robins LN, Regier DA (eds): Psychiatric Disorders in America. New York, Free Press, 1991.

Ross RR, Fabiano EA, Diemer-Ewles C: Reasoning and rehabilitation. Int J Offend Ther Compar Criminol 32:29–35, 1988.

Schulsinger F: Psychopathy, heredity, and environment. Int J Ment Health 1:190–206, 1972.

Sheard MH, Marini JL, Bridges CI, et al: The effect of lithium on impulsive aggressive behavior in man. Am J Psychiatry 133:1409–1413, 1976.

Sjogren T: Genetic, statistical and psychiatric investigations of a West Swedish population. Acta Psychiatr Neurol Scand 1948 Munksgaard, Copenhagen pp 102. [Suppl 52].

Tuckman J, Youngman W: Suicide and criminality. J Forens Sci 10:104–107, 1965.

Vaillant GE: The Natural History of Alcoholism. Cambridge, Harvard University Press, 1983.

Whitters A, Troughton E, Cadoret RJ, et al: Evidence for clinical heterogeneity in antisocial alcoholics. Compr Psychiatry 25:158–164, 1984.

Williams DT, Mehl R, Yudofsky S, et al: The effect of propranolol on uncontrolled rage outbursts in children and adolescents with organic brain dysfunction. J Am Acad Child Psychiatry 21:129–135, 1982.

Winokur G, Reich T, Rimmer J: Alcoholism. III. Diagnosis and familial psychiatric illness in 259 alcoholic probands. Arch Gen Psychiatry 23:104–111, 1970.

Yochelson S, Samenow SE: The Criminal Personality, vol 1: A Profile for Change. New York, Jason Aronson, 1976.

Yochelson S, Samenow SE: The Criminal Personality, vol 2: The Change Process. New York, Jason Aronson, 1977.

CHAPTER 14

ALCOHOLISM

BARRY LISKOW
DONALD W. GOODWIN

DEFINITION

The definition of *alcoholism* continues to be controversial. The three editions of the American Psychiatric Association's *Diagnostic and Statistical Manual of Disorders* since 1980 reflect changing opinions about what elements in the definition should be emphasized. The 1980 DSM-III (American Psychiatric Association, 1980) emphasized problems from drinking (called *substance abuse*) and specified that the term *alcohol dependence* (the officially preferred term for alcoholism) required evidence of physiologic tolerance and/or withdrawal. These criteria for abuse and dependence drew considerable criticism, and in 1987, the criteria were revised in DSM-IIIR with greater emphasis on patterns of compulsive use and less emphasis on dependence and withdrawal. Proposed criteria for alcohol dependence in DSM-IV resembled those in DSM-IIIR in not making physiologic dependence essential to the definition of the disorder, but the order of the criteria was changed so that items related to dependence were listed at the outset (American Psychiatric Association, Option 1, 1991).

The criteria for alcohol dependence presented here are modified from proposed criteria for DSM-IV.

A. A maladaptive pattern of alcohol use leading to clinically significant impairment or distress, as manifested by the following:
    1. Tolerance, as defined by any of the following:
       a. Need for markedly increased amounts of alcohol to achieve intoxication or desired effect.
       b. Markedly diminished effect with continued use of the same amount of alcohol.

       c. Has functioned adequately at doses or blood levels of alcohol that would produce significant impairment in a casual user.
    2. The characteristic withdrawal syndrome from excessive drinking.
    3. Alcohol is often taken to relieve or avoid withdrawal symptoms.
    4. Alcohol is often taken in larger amounts or over a longer period than intended.
    5. Any unsuccessful effort or persistent desire to cut down or control alcohol use.
    6. A great deal of time is spent in activities necessary to obtain alcohol (e.g., driving long distances), use alcohol, or recover from its effects.
    7. Recurrent alcohol use resulting in inability to fulfill major role obligations at work, school, or home (e.g., repeated absences or poor work performance related to alcohol use; alcohol-related absences, suspensions, or expulsions from school; neglect of children or household).
    8. Recurrent alcohol use in situations in which it is physically hazardous (e.g., driving an automobile or operating a machine when impaired by alcohol).
    9. Important social, occupational, or recreational activities given up or reduced because of alcohol.
    10. Recurrent alcohol-related legal or interpersonal problems (e.g., alcohol-related arrests and traffic accidents, physical fights related to alcohol use).
    11. Continued alcohol use despite knowledge of a persistent or recurrent problem(s) caused or exacerbated by the use of alcohol (e.g., drinks despite family arguments about it,

continued drinking despite recognition that an ulcer was made worse by alcohol).

DSM-IV retained the approach of DSM-IIIR in subdividing alcohol dependence into *mild, moderate*, and *severe* and specifying whether the dependence was in *partial* or *full remission*.

In DSM-III, the term *substance abuse* referred to a pattern of pathologic and compulsive use accompanied by impairment in social and occupational functioning. DSM-IIIR shifted items describing manifestations of compulsive use from alcohol abuse to alcohol dependence. As a consequence, in DSM-IIIR alcohol abuse was conceived of as no more than a residual category for those individuals whose pattern of alcohol use was not severe enough to warrant a diagnosis of dependence (Grob, 1991). The framers of DSM-IV proposed the following operational criteria for alcohol abuse:

A. A maladaptive pattern of alcohol use leading to clinically significant impairment or distress, as manifested by one or two of the following items:
  1. Recurrent alcohol use resulting in inability to fulfill major role obligations at work, school, or home (e.g., repeated absences or poor work performance as related to alcohol abuse; alcohol-rated absences, suspensions, or expulsions from school; neglect of children or household).
  2. Recurrent alcohol-related legal or interpersonal problems (e.g., arrests and traffic accidents and physical fights related to alcohol abuse).
  3. Important social, occupational, or recreational activities given up or reduced because of alcohol abuse.
  4. Recurrent alcohol use in situations in which it is physically hazardous (e.g., driving an automobile or operating a machine when impaired by alcohol use).

Other groups from time to time formulate different definitions for alcoholism. Toward this goal, a 23-member multidisciplinary committee of the National Council on Alcoholism and Drug Dependence and the American Society of Addiction Medicine conducted a 2-year study of the definition of alcoholism in the "light of recent research" (ASAM News, 1990). The goals of the group were to create by consensus a revised definition that was (1) scientifically valid, (2) clinically useful, and (3) understandable by the general public. The following definition emerged from this work:

Alcoholism is a chronic, progressive and potentially fatal disease. It is characterized by tolerance and physical dependence or pathological organ changes, or both—all the direct or indirect consequences of the alcohol ingested.

It was not clear how this definition was any more scientifically valid or clinically useful than the operational definition of DSM-IV. For research purposes, the DSM-IV criteria will probably prevail.

For a simple definition of alcoholism that embraces most of the elements of the above, the following might be recommended:

Alcoholism is a condition that involves compulsive drinking, causing harm to the person and others.

EPIDEMIOLOGY

Epidemiologic studies of alcohol use and abuse are bedeviled by the uncertainties of what to measure and how to measure it. The terms *alcoholism, alcohol dependence, alcohol abuse, problem drinking,* and *drinking problems* continue to be used by different researchers in different ways. To further complicate matters, such categories as abstainers and light, medium, and heavy drinkers, referring to quantity and frequency of alcohol use, are defined differently by various investigators. Finally, there is disagreement regarding which effects of alcohol use on a given population should be studied and over what period of time. It is therefore surprising that there is as much agreement regarding the scope of alcohol problems as there is.

Three distinct methods of epidemiologic investigation have been used in assessing the extent and effects of alcohol use. These are the estimation of apparent alcohol consumption, collection of data relating to morbidity and mortality from alcohol, and surveys of alcohol use and problems in the general population.

Apparent Consumption

Apparent per capita consumption of alcohol is calculated by adding up the amount of alcohol sold based on sales and tax data and dividing it by the adult population under consideration. Sales and tax data of various quality exist for the United States back to at least 1850. After being approximately level in the 1940s and 1950s, per capita consumption of alcohol for adults age 14 or over began rising, at first rapidly and then more slowly, from 2.07 gal of absolute alcohol per year in 1960 until peaking at 2.75 gal in 1980 and 1981, after which per capita consumption has progressively fallen to 2.54 gal in 1987 (NIAAA, 1989a). This current amount represents about 1 oz of absolute alcohol per day for every person age 14 or older in the United States, or about 1.5 oz for every drinking person. Such figures are misleading because it is estimated that 11 percent of adults drink 50 percent of the alcohol sold (Malin et al., 1982). The figure also may be misleading because it does not consider the amount of illicit (untaxed) alcohol made and consumed each year. Of the alcohol consumed, approximately 50 percent is from beer, 10 percent from wine, and 40 percent from liquor.

In the United States, apparent consumption is highest in the West and lowest in the South, highest in Nevada (where many drinking tourists evidently increase per capita consumption for this state) and lowest in Utah (USDHHS, 1990). Internationally, the highest per capita consumption occurs in France, Portugal, Italy, and Spain (Brenner, 1982). However, although international per capita consumption rose beginning in 1950, it leveled off in the mid-1970s and began declining in two-thirds of 25 countries surveyed between 1979 and 1984. The greatest declines occurred in Poland, Spain, Sweden, and Ireland. Increases, however, occurred in Denmark, Portugal and the former Soviet Union (Horgan et al., 1986). Decreases in consumption were generally accompanied by decreases in reported alcohol problems such as cirrhosis and death (Mann and Smart, 1990).

Morbidity and Mortality Attributable to Alcohol

Cirrhosis mortality historically has been used to assess the prevalence of alcoholism. Jellinek developed a formula for calculating the prevalence of alcoholism in a population by extrapolation from the number of deaths caused by cirrhosis in a given year (Jellinek and Keller, 1952). This method was chosen in the belief that population surveys would be futile because people (in the United States at least) would be unwilling to report accurately on their use of alcohol (Keller, 1975). The Jellinek formula was useful because it at least gave an estimate of the prevalence of alcoholism. It was hence widely used, with occasional modification, in the 1950s, despite numerous critics, including Jellinek himself (Keller and Effron, 1955; Jellinek, 1959). Currently, cirrhosis rates are considered important not because of what they reveal about the prevalence of alcoholism, but because of what they reveal about morbidity and mortality related to alcohol.

Cirrhosis death rates rose steadily in the United States from 1950 to 1973, when they peaked at 15.0 deaths per 100,000 population. Between 1973 and 1986 the rate fell steadily to 9.3 per 100,000, the lowest rate since 1955 (USDHHS, 1990). Schmidt and Popham (1975/76) and Brenner (1975) have hypothesized that cirrhosis death rates, as well as other complications of alcohol abuse, rise when per capita alcohol consumption increases, with a lag of 1 to 2 years. However, the recent fall in cirrhosis mortality has occurred earlier and perhaps faster than can be accounted for by decreases in per capita consumption, raising the possibility that improvements in medical and/or alcohol treatment methods may be partly responsible for these trends (Mann and Smart, 1990). Although cirrhosis mortality has been dropping among all groups, it remains highest for young urban nonwhite males, whose cirrhosis mortality is considerably higher than that of comparable white male groups (NIAAA, 1989).

Cirrhosis is not the only cause of alcohol-related mortality. Alcohol is involved in approximately 50 percent of fatal motor vehicle crashes, 17 to 53 percent of fatal falls, 37 to 64 percent of fatal burns, and 38 percent of fatal drownings (USDHHS, 1990; Hingson and Howland, 1987; Howland and Hingson, 1987, 1988). It is likely that alcohol's relationship to these traumatic deaths is significantly underreported. In addition, alcohol-related medical conditions that are contributory causes of death, such as cardiomyopathy, gastrointestinal hemorrhage, and pancreatitis, are often underreported on death certificates. All these factors make it difficult to estimate precisely alcohol's effect on mortality, but there is little doubt that it is substantial (USDHHS, 1990).

EDITORS' COMMENT

As discussed on page 6, there is increasing recognition of the strong association between increased alcohol consumption and hypertension and stroke. Even when hypertension is treated, heavier drinking compared with light drinking significantly increases blood pressure. Unfortunately, the reported higher age-specific mean blood pressure and higher prevalence of hypertension in blacks (Comstock GW, Am J Hygiene 65:271–315, 1957) fail to acknowledge this as a risk factor. As indicated on page 4, lifetime rates of alcoholism are similar in blacks, whites, and hispanic males, although in older age groups (above age 30) black males have the highest lifetime prevalence.

Morbidity associated with alcohol is also considerable. In the mid-1970s, hospital discharges for alcohol-related disorders ranged from 2.5 percent for short-stay hospitals to 17 percent for VA hospitals. Although precise figures are difficult to gather and studies are hampered by methodological problems, it has been estimated that alcohol is involved in 45 percent of violent crimes, 45 percent of episodes of marital violence, 40 percent of suicide attempts, 20 percent of nonfatal industrial accidents, and 15 percent of nonfatal traffic accidents. The cost of alcohol-related mortality and morbidity in the United States is estimated at $136 billion per year (Malin et al., 1982; Roizen, 1982; USDHHS, 1990). Although such morbidity and mortality data gathered from various agencies indicate the scope of the alcohol problem, they do not represent the full spectrum of such problems. Many people who drink and have problems from alcohol do not appear in such agency data. Population surveys are needed for a more complete picture of alcohol problems.

Population Surveys

General population surveys of drinking practices and problems began in earnest in the United States in the 1960s (Cahalan, 1970) and have been conducted regularly since the early 1970s by the National Institute of Alcohol Abuse and Alcoholism (NIAAA) and the National Institute on Drug Abuse

(NIDA) either separately or jointly. The most recent survey, the National Household Survey on Drug Abuse (NHSDA) was conducted in 1988 with funding from NIDA and NIAAA and the Department of Education and was conducted by the Research Triangle Institute in North Carolina. The survey, which covered alcohol and drugs, was able to use data from seven prior NHSDA surveys dating back to 1972 to ascertain trends in usage. It should be noted that these surveys probably seriously underestimate alcohol consumption. Apparent consumption data, based on sales and tax data, consistently have indicated that 50 to 75 percent of the alcohol consumed in the United States is unaccounted for when consumption is extrapolated from nationwide general population surveys (Malin et al., 1982). This may be due to a number of factors, including (1) alcohol use may be consciously, or unconsciously, underreported by those surveyed, (2) heavy drinkers may not be easily available for surveys that are generally done in households, (3) questionnaires and interview techniques may be inadequate, and (4) population groups, such as hospitalized patients, prisoners, and military personnel, that may contain large numbers of heavy drinkers are often excluded from population surveys. Despite these problems, these surveys allow an assessment of the trends in alcohol consumption and alcohol problems across time and in different segments of the U.S. population. Selective findings of the most recent survey (NIDA, 1990) include the following:

1. Use of alcohol peaked in the late 1970s and has since declined. However, the use rate remains high, with 85 percent of the population over the age of 11 having used alcohol in their lifetime, 68 percent in the past year, and 58 percent in the past month.

2. In all age groups assessed (12 to 17 years old, 18 to 25, 26 to 34, and greater than 35), males were more likely than females to have drunk in their lifetime, in the past year, and in the past month. In the year prior to the survey, 27 percent of men and 37 percent of women were abstainers. Daily use of alcohol (defined as 20 to 30 days of use in the past month) occurred in 11 percent of men and 4 percent of women. Heavy use (defined as 5 or more drinks per occasion on 5 or more days in the past 30 days) occurred in 8 percent of men and 2 percent of women. Heavy use peaked in the age group 18 to 25 for both men (17 percent) and women (4 percent).

3. Whites used alcohol at higher lifetime, last year, and last month rates than Hispanics, who were higher in these categories than blacks. The black abstention rate was 44 percent and the Hispanic abstention rate was 33 percent in the year prior to the survey. Daily use was most common in whites and slightly more common in blacks than in Hispanics (8.2 versus 4.7 versus 4.2 percent), and heavy drinking was most common in Hispanics, followed by whites and then blacks (5.6 versus 4.9 versus 3.9 percent).

4. Residents of large cities, outside the South, with more education, and employed were more likely to use alcohol in their lifetimes, the past year, and the past month than residents of small towns or rural areas, those in the South, with less education, and unemployed.

5. When asked if they experienced any of 11 problems in the past year which they attributed to alcohol, 10.5 percent of those who used alcohol in the past year reported such problems. Problems acknowledged included arguments or fights with family or friends (5.2 percent), finding it difficult to think clearly (4.6 percent), feeling irritable or upset (3.8 percent), and becoming depressed or losing interest in things (3.3 percent).

6. When asked if they experienced any of 18 negative experiences (e.g., lost or nearly lost a job, partner told me I should cut down, unable to remember what happened) with their drinking in the past year, 33 percent of those who drank in the past year reported one or more such experiences, and 17 percent reported three or more. These percentages were highest in the 12 to 17 and 18- to 25-year old age groups, with approximately 50 percent of these two age groups reporting one or more negative experiences and approximately 30 percent reporting three or more. In all age groups, there was a relationship between problems and frequency of being drunk in the past year, with 14 percent of those who had not been drunk reporting no problems, 59 percent of those who were drunk twice a month or less often reporting a problem, and 88 percent of those who were drunk more than twice a month reporting a problem.

This latest survey, like the ones before it, indicates that alcohol use is almost universal and that a substantial number of people have problems related to their alcohol use. However, until recently, there was no nationwide epidemiologic survey that began from the premise that alcoholism is a specific illness, separable from abusive drinking or problem drinking. There were surveys conducted on a more limited population (Hagnell and Tunving, 1972; Winokur and Tsuang, 1978; Weissman et al., 1980; Boyd et al., 1983) and having in common a definition of alcohol dependence requiring social impairment due to alcohol use, pathologic use of alcohol, and/or symptoms of tolerance or withdrawal because of alcohol. These studies, although differing in the population surveyed, year conducted, and operational definitions of alcoholism agreed that the lifetime prevalence of alcoholism in men was between 5 and 10 percent and in women was between 0.4 and 4 percent.

Recently, data from the Epidemiological Catchment Area (ECA) study as it relates to alcoholism have become available. This study was conducted in 1980 and surveyed 20,000 individuals in five geographic areas (New Haven, Conn., Baltimore, Md., St. Louis, Mo., Durham, N.C., and Los Angeles,

Calif.) using state-of-the-art epidemiologic techniques to obtain a population representative of these five areas and by extension to the country. An instrument, the Diagnostic Interview Schedule (DIS) was developed to allow lay interviewers to collect information by personal interview which resulted in DSM-III diagnoses. Follow-up interviews 1 year later also were conducted, but reports on alcoholism thus far relate only to the initial interviews.

Selective results from the ECA study (Helzer et al., 1991) include the following:

1. Lifetime prevalence of alcoholism (alcohol dependence and/or alcohol abuse) was 14 percent, which included 24 percent for men and 5 percent for women. These percentages, especially for men, are large. This may have been related to the fact that in order to qualify for a diagnosis, a minimum of two symptoms were required which did not have to occur at the same time. Also, 12 percent of men and 2 percent of women had one or more symptoms in the past year, and 6 percent of men and 1 percent of women had one or more symptoms in the past month.

2. Prevalence rates for alcoholism did not significantly differ for lifetime, 1-year, or 1-month time periods among whites, blacks, and Hispanics.

3. In young men (18 to 29 years old), lifetime prevalence of alcoholism in whites was double that in blacks (28 versus 13 percent), but in the 30 to 44 year old age range, black male lifetime prevalence exceeded white male rates (31 versus 27 percent), and the gap grew in succeeding age ranges. Hispanic male prevalence exceeded white male prevalence in all age ranges but was overtaken by black lifetime prevalence rates for ages older than 45. These differences were maintained for 1-year and 1-month prevalence rates for most age categories up to age 65, after which black males, although having a high lifetime prevalence for alcoholism, had a low 1-year and 1-month prevalence of alcoholism even compared with white males.

4. The male-to-female lifetime, 1-year, and 1-month prevalence ratios (3.9, 4.1, and 3.5) were lowest in the youngest age group (18 to 29), and this was true for all ethnic groups. This would seem to indicate that the male and female prevalence rates for alcoholism are converging in the younger age groups.

5. Higher educational attainment and a stable marriage were related to a lower lifetime prevalence of alcoholism. Being a professional or manager and being employed full time were related to a lower 1-year prevalence of alcoholism.

6. Forty-seven percent of alcoholics had a diagnosis of one or more additional psychiatric disorders compared with 35 percent of the total ECA sample. Comorbidity was more common in women alcoholics (65 percent) than in men (44 percent). The diagnoses with which alcoholism were most strongly associated included antisocial personality, mania, drug abuse/dependence, and schizophrenia.

In summary, although epidemiologic studies disagree about what should be measured and how to measure it, there is good agreement that the majority of adults in the United States drink, that a large minority of these drinkers have trouble at some time because of their drinking, and that those who do have trouble tend to be young males who drink a lot but who drink less as they grow older. The percentages of those who abstain, those who drink without problems, and those who drink with problems have remained relatively stable in the United States since the 1970s. However, per capita consumption and use rates are decreasing, allowing for optimism that improvement may occur in problem rates in the future. However, problem rates in all ages and ethnic groups, and especially in the young, remain uncomfortably high, and there is evidence that the percentage of young women with alcohol problems is approaching the percentage of young men with such problems. Although cirrhosis mortality rates have declined since the mid-1970s, the overall morbidity and mortality of alcoholism continue to be a tremendous drain on the human and financial resources of the United States. This morbidity and mortality are greatest among the men and women who are diagnosable as alcohol-dependent at some time in their lives, but it is not exclusive to them.

CLINICAL PICTURE

The clinical presentation of the alcohol-dependent patient is contingent on when in the course of the illness he or she presents. There are no pathognomonic signs or symptoms of alcohol abuse or dependence. Although medical symptoms may bring an alcoholic into his or her first contact with a possibility for therapy, early in the course of the illness there may be no physical or laboratory signs of this condition. Additionally, physician discomfort, judgmental attitudes, or inadequate training and patient denial raise additional barriers to effective diagnosis (Benzer, 1991). Often, indications of an alcohol problem can be gained only through a careful social and medical history. Specific inquiry regarding marital conflict, absenteeism from work or school, job losses, accidents, and legal difficulties should be made; such problems occur more commonly in alcoholics than in nonalcoholics. Patients who indicate that they have such problems should be asked about the relationship of alcohol to the problems and about specific drinking practices. Not infrequently, the alcoholic will deny or rationalize the relationship of alcohol to his or her problems and will underreport the quantity of alcohol consumed. If willing to admit to problem drinking, the early alcoholic may report sneaking drinks, hiding alcohol, feeling comfortable only with other drinkers, experiencing guilt associated with drinking, and attempting to control drinking by using alcohol only at specified times (Goodwin, 1984).

Medical complaints early in the course of alcoholism include anorexia, morning nausea and vomiting, gastroesophageal reflux, diarrhea, palpitations, insomnia, amenorrhea, impotence, and polyuria. Psychiatric and neurologic complaints may include depressed mood, anhedonia, anxiety, irritability, nervousness, blackouts (memory lapses), and subjectively poor memory (Holt et al., 1981; Helzer and Pryzbeck, 1988; Benzer, 1991).

Early in the course of alcohol use, hypertension can occur with as few as three drinks per day, with higher consumption associated with higher blood pressures (Klatsky, 1987; Benzer, 1991). An estimated 5 to 24 percent of hypertension is associated with alcoholism (Klatsky, 1987); thus internists should screen all hypertensives for possible alcoholism, and psychiatrists should measure blood pressures regularly and consider an alcoholism diagnosis in hypertensive patients. The physician should be aware that blood pressures decline and rise in tandem with active drinking (Benzer, 1991).

As alcoholism progresses, physical signs may begin to appear, such as an alcohol odor on the breath, careless grooming and hygiene, signs of intoxication (ataxia, slurred speech), multiple traumas, hepatomegaly (Holt et al., 1981), and certain facial features, including rhinophyma and persistent erythema, with or without telangiectasias. Later in the course, signs of chronic liver disease may appear, including jaundice, ascites, palmar erythema, spider angiomata, purpura, abdominal varices, testicular atrophy, gynecomastia, and Dupuytren's contractures. Associated symptoms of liver, pancreatic, and other chronic gastrointestinal disturbances may be reported, including abdominal pain, food intolerance, hematemesis, melena, weight loss, weakness, and fatigue. Specific diseases occurring more frequently in alcoholics than in controls include head, neck, and oral cancers (especially in conjunction with cigarette smoking), pneumonia (including tuberculosis), and hemorrhagic stroke unrelated to the hypertensive status of the patient (Benzer, 1991).

Neurologic and psychiatric signs and symptoms may occur in later-stage alcoholism and include seizures (unrelated to active drinking or withdrawal), withdrawal syndromes (seizures, hallucinations, delusions, delirium), psychotic syndromes (paranoia, hallucinations, and delusions in a clear sensorium), peripheral neuropathy (usually in the lower extremities, bilateral, symmetrical, and sensorimotor in type), and cognitive deficits (ranging from minor memory problems to dementia and the amnestic syndrome) (Sellers and Kalant, 1976; Mardsden, 1977; Goodwin and Hill, 1975; Schuckit, 1989; Geller, 1991; Ng et al., 1988).

Uncommonly, myopathy may occur acutely with muscle pain and swelling or chronically with progressive weakness and atrophy. Also, rarely, cardiomyopathy may occur with signs and symptoms of congestive heart failure (Benzer, 1991).

Another type of disorder described by Jones and colleagues in 1973 is the fetal alcohol syndrome, diagnosed by specific developmental abnormalities, including dysmorphic facial features and central nervous system abnormalities, occurring in infants born to alcoholic mothers. Longitudinally, such infants have displayed decreased cognitive performance when subjected in utero to as little as three drinks per day ingested by their mother (Streissguth et al., 1983). Physicians, therefore, should counsel all women as to the potential danger to their fetuses of drinking this or even less alcohol during their pregnancy (USDHHS, 1991).

As noted earlier, certain psychiatric diagnoses, including antisocial personality, mania, drug abuse, panic disorder, depressive disorder, and schizophrenia, are found more frequently in conjunction with alcoholism than in patients without these disorders, and hence patients with these diagnoses should raise a psychiatrist's index of suspicion that alcoholism also may be present (Helzer et al., 1991).

It is important to emphasize that early phases of the disease may be marked by subtle or no physical, psychiatric, or laboratory signs and thus require a high index of suspicion by the physician coupled with a sensitive and thorough approach to history taking.

CASE HISTORY

J.W., a 35-year-old plant foreman, arrived at his physician's office with chief complaints of 3 weeks of intermittent epigastric pain, anorexia with a 5-lb (2.3-kg) weight loss, and nausea and vomiting. He related that these symptoms were worse in the morning and improved as the day progressed. He indicated that he was not too worried by the symptoms but had come at the urging of his supervisor, who was concerned because of his frequent absences from work.

He denied all other gastrointestinal symptoms, and review of systems was negative except for numerous "colds" in the past year, causing frequent work absence. Physical examination was within normal limits.

When questioned about his drinking practices, he said that he drank "no more than anyone else." When asked to elaborate, he stated that he went to a local tavern with fellow employees after work for "a few beers" and drank "a six pack or two on the weekends while watching football on TV." When asked about drinking at other times, he replied, "That's all. Why do you keep badgering me about my drinking?" He was then asked if others badgered him; he answered, "Yes, my wife—she thinks everybody drinks too much. Just because I was arrested for driving under the influence last year . . . but I'm here for my stomach, Doc. Can you help me?" He was scheduled for routine laboratory tests and endoscopy and was asked to return in 1 week.

J.W. may or may not be an alcoholic, but the pattern of his symptoms and his responses to questions about his drinking habits should raise his physician's index of suspicion.

LABORATORY FINDINGS

As is true of signs and symptoms, there are no pathognomonic laboratory measures that can be used to diagnose alcoholism. There are a number of laboratory findings, however, that, when present, should increase the physician's index of suspicion that alcohol may be a problem. These tests, in approximate order of their usefulness, include the following:

1. *Blood alcohol level.* The National Council on Alcoholism includes among its criteria for diagnosing alcoholism a blood alcohol level greater than 300 mg/dl at any time or a level greater than 100 mg/dl recorded during a routine clinical examination (NCA, 1972). It also has been noted that a blood alcohol level of more than 150 mg/dl in a patient not obviously intoxicated is strong evidence of significant tolerance to alcohol, and hence potentially of alcoholism. Blood alcohol levels may be obtained either by direct measurement of blood levels or by estimation from the amount of alcohol in expired air using a Breathalyzer. A recently developed saliva dipstick method to estimate serum ethanol concentration has been found to lack accuracy (Rodenberg et al., 1990).

2. *Mean corpuscular volume (MCV).* Macrocytosis, as indicated by an elevation of the MCV (commonly reported as part of a complete blood count), has been reported to occur in 35 to 95 percent of actively drinking alcoholics, with most studies reporting 35 to 40 percent. Although an elevated MCV can occur in folate and B_{12} deficiency, hypothyroidism, malignancies, and nonalcoholic liver disease, these causes are uncommon, especially in outpatient settings, giving the MCV a specificity of 90 to 95 percent, which is greater than most markers for alcoholism. The cause of the elevated MCV in alcoholics is unknown, and it is more marked in alcoholics who smoke. MCV returns to normal 2 to 4 months after alcohol ingestion ceases (Rosman and Lieber, 1990).

3. *Gamma glutamyl transpeptidase (GGTP).* GGTP has been reported to be elevated in 35 to 85 percent of alcoholics or heavy drinkers, and this finding is considered by some to be the earliest laboratory sign of heavy alcohol use (Holt et al., 1981; Chan, 1991). Its specificity is 50 percent (i.e., in 50 percent of those with elevated GGTP, the cause is not due to alcoholism or heavy alcohol intake). GGTP in alcoholics returns to normal after approximately 4 to 5 weeks of abstinence, and it takes about 2 weeks of heavy drinking to acquire abnormal GGTP levels (Harada et al., 1989).

4. *Aspartate aminotransferase (AST) and alanine aminotransferase (ALT).* AST and ALT are increased in liver damage from a variety of causes. AST and ALT have been reported elevated in 30 to 75 percent of inpatient alcoholics (Holt et al., 1981; Chan, 1991). AST exists in two forms, mitochondrial (m-AST) and soluble (s-AST) and the ratio of m-AST to s-AST has been found to be of value in distinguishing alcoholic hepatitis from other causes of elevated AST (Harada, 1989).

Various rules relating AST to ALT have been formulated to differentiate alcoholic from nonalcoholic liver disease. A ratio of AST to ALT of greater than 1 with AST plus ALT less than 300 IV/l to indicate alcohol liver disease was applied to patients with liver disease and correctly identified 90 percent of patients with alcoholic liver disease and 77 percent of patients with nonalcoholic liver disease (Ryback et al., 1982).

5. *Chest x-ray.* In one study, 28.9 percent of alcoholics had evidence of rib or vertebral fractures or both on routine chest x-rays, compared with 1.3 percent of an age-matched group of social drinkers (Israel et al., 1980).

6. *Uric acid.* Uric acid levels have been reported to be elevated in heavy drinkers and to return to normal several days after alcohol ingestion ceases (Holt et al., 1981).

7. The following routine laboratory tests have been reported to be abnormal in alcohol abusers, but because of poor sensitivity and/or specificity in detecting alcoholism, they are not considered of value as markers for alcoholism: HDL-cholesterol, glutamate dehydrogenase (GDH), lactic acid dehydrogenase (LDH), uric acid, blood urea nitrogen (BUN), ferritin, serum iron, plasma glucose, leukocytes, red blood cells, and thrombocytes (Chan, 1991; Harada, 1989).

Attempts have been made to distinguish alcoholics from nonalcoholics with a battery of common laboratory tests subjected to complex mathematical manipulations. Eckardt et al. (1981) carried out a quadratic multiple discriminant analysis on 24 common laboratory tests and compared 121 alcoholic males with 130 nonalcoholic males. The analysis correctly classified 100 percent of the nonalcoholics and 98 percent of the alcoholics. Ryback et al. (1982), using the same procedure, reported similar success in distinguishing among nonalcoholics without liver disease, alcoholics with presumed mild liver involvement, alcoholics with liver disease, and nonalcoholics with liver disease. Results with a younger less impaired group of alcoholics with fewer years of heavy drinking was less robust (Ryback and Rawlings, 1985). These results appear promising, but the validity and reliability of discriminant analysis for diagnosing and screening for alcoholism has yet to be established and must be tested in diverse normal and medically ill groups in diverse settings before its usefulness can be adequately assessed (Dolinsky and Schnitt, 1988).

In addition to the more traditional markers noted above, a variety of laboratory tests have been reported in the past several years as possible biochemical markers for alcoholism and/or alcohol abuse. None of these is available as a routine test, and although, generally, most were reported to have reasonable sensitivity and specificity on initial testing, such tests have usually been conducted in a limited population, using small numbers of subjects, and when replicated often lose a great deal of their initial specificity and sensitivity. These markers include urinary dolichol, serum carbohydrate-deficient transferrin, serum methanol, plasma carnitine, serum beta-hexosaminidase, plasma salsolinol, serum acetaldehyde-hemoglobin adducts, serum acetate, and serum 2,3-butanediol (Chan, 1991; Glass et al., 1989; Hultberg, et al., 1991; Farraj et al., 1989).

In addition to these markers, which hold promise for being helpful as sensitive and specific indicators of current or recent alcohol abuse and alcoholism, others markers are being explored as possible indicators of susceptibility to alcoholism. The hope is that biochemical markers will be found that are "trait" markers, able to identify individuals who may become alcoholic, before the onset of alcoholism or even drinking. Most of the research in this area is conducted by comparing children (usually sons) of alcoholics with individuals without a family history of alcoholism before either group has begun drinking heavily. Variations in serum acetaldehyde, prolactin, cortisol, monoamine oxidase, serotonin, and GABA have all been shown to be potential trait markers of alcoholism in a small number of studies, most unreplicated and conducted on a small number of patients (Chan, 1991; Rausch et al., 1991; Schuckit and Gold, 1988; Moss et al., 1990; Tabakoff et al., 1988). Several studies have indicated an association between alcoholism and/or severity of alcoholism and an allele of the D^2 dopamine receptor gene (Parsian et al., 1991). The pace of research in this area is developing rapidly, and other potential markers will undoubtedly be proposed. All such markers will require testing in alcoholic (or "prealcoholic"), normal, and nonalcoholic subjects in a variety of settings before their value as biologic markers can be asserted.

In summary, all laboratory tests may be normal early in the course of alcoholism. However, not infrequently, MCV, GGTP, AST, and ALT will be mildly elevated and blood alcohol levels markedly elevated in a clinically nonintoxicated patient. As alcoholism progresses, many laboratory tests are apt to be abnormal, reflecting the chronic effects of alcohol on a number of organ systems. There are promising approaches that may eventually allow the diagnosis of alcoholism at an early stage by the complex analysis of currently available laboratory tests. In addition, active research is under way to discover the elusive biochemical marker for alcoholism that may allow reliable early detection of alcoholism or, possibly, identification of those at risk for developing the disease.

CLINICAL COURSE

Understanding the clinical course of any disease requires longitudinal investigations of individuals with that illness. The clinical course of alcoholism is obscured by a dearth of such longitudinal studies and a lack of agreement on the definition of the illness. The studies that have been done have investigated a subset of patients with alcohol problems, e.g., felons (Goodwin et al., 1971), public hospital inpatients (Vaillant, 1983), private clinic outpatients (Hyman, 1976), patients attending various units of a large university hospital or its affiliates (Helzer et al., 1985), married or cohabiting residential treatment inpatients (Finney and Moos, 1991), college students (Vaillant, 1983) and untreated alcohol abusers (Ojesjo, 1981). Despite the limitations of these studies, there are enough of them to provide a reasonable idea of the various clinical courses alcoholism can take.

Historically, the first modern attempt to delineate the course of alcoholism was undertaken by Jellinek (1952). He analyzed questionnaires from 2000 Alcoholics Anonymous members, and from their responses he postulated that alcoholism is a progressive disease in which 43 distinct symptoms occur in more or less definite order. He grouped the symptoms into three phases: *prodromal*, the first symptom of which is blackouts; *crucial*, the first symptom of which is loss of control; and *chronic*, the first symptom of which is binge drinking. In a later work, Jellinek (1960) introduced the concept that there are five types of drinking patterns and complications, which he labeled alpha, beta, gamma, delta, and epsilon. He suggested that gamma (characterized by tolerance, craving, and loss of control) and delta (characterized by tolerance, craving, and inability to abstain) represented true diseases that followed most closely his 43 symptoms' progression. In Jellinek's view, once the disease of alcoholism was established, usually when an individual was in his or her early or middle 20s, its course was inexorable, with progression over 20 to 30 years, ending at any stage in death or abstinence. Many studies then followed, some supporting in part and some seriously questioning Jellinek's conclusions and methodology (Trice and Wahl, 1958; Park and Whitehead, 1973; Paredas et al., 1973; Clark, 1976; Pattison et al., 1977; Goodwin et al., 1969).

One of the first studies to challenge Jellinek's hypothesis of an inexorable progression of alcoholism was Lemere's 1953 study, in which he asked his patients about the drinking histories of their deceased relatives who had had alcohol problems. He thus collected information on 500 presumed alcohol abusers and found that 28 percent increased their alcohol use before death; 10 percent decreased alcohol use substantially, with 3 percent of the total sample returning to social drinking; 29 percent did not change their alcohol consumption; approximately 20 percent stopped drinking because they were too ill to drink; and approximately 10 percent achieved abstinence. Because of lack of treatment resources available, Lemere concluded that these results, with approximately 20 percent of those with alcohol problems becoming abstinent or reducing their drinking, represented the natural history of untreated alcoholism.

In 1968, Drew observed that first admissions for alcoholism increased steadily from ages 25 to 55 but that the predicted prevalence of alcoholism of those 40 and over, based on these admission figures, was consistently more than the actual prevalence figures for this age group. He did not believe that the literature supported the conclusion that this decreased prevalence was due to treatment effectiveness or to mortality and suggested that the decreased prevalence indicated that alcoholism is a self-limiting disease mainly of young and middle-aged individuals.

Vaillant (1983) reviewed 10 major follow-up studies of alcohol abusers, each of which followed patients for 7 years or longer. The studies had different methodologies and followed different subgroups of alcohol patients. These studies and others (Finney and Moos, 1991; Helzer et al., 1985), although methodologically disparate, are remarkably similar in indicating that approximately 2 to 6 percent of alcoholics remit (are abstinent or drinking in a controlled fashion) each year. These approximations hold for samples of both treated alcoholics (e.g., Vaillant, 1983; Voetglin and Broz, 1949; Sundby, 1967; Lundquist, 1973; Bratfos, 1974), "skid row" alcoholics (Myerson and Mayer, 1966), and untreated alcoholics (e.g., Goodwin et al., 1971; Ojesjo, 1981). Patients in successful remission are about two to three times more likely to be abstinent than drinking in a controlled fashion (Finney and Moos, 1991; Vaillant, 1983), although one study, which followed socially stable patients, found the reverse (Nordstrom and Berglund, 1987b). The majority of studies have concluded that remitted patients able to drink in a social manner at follow-up were mild cases to begin with (Taylor et al., 1986; Helzer et al, 1985), although not all studies concur with this conclusion (Nordstrom and Berglund, 1987b). These studies, therefore, partially support Davis's hypothesis that alcoholism is, for some, a self-limiting disorder. However, as is pointed out in studies by Vaillant (1983) and Pokorny et al. (1981), the more numerous and more severe the symptoms of alcoholism, the closer the clinical picture is to Jellinek's stages and the more alcoholism appears to be a progressive disease, ending in abstinence, serious morbidity, or death. Such conclusions, however, may be tautological; the more serious and intense the symptoms, the more serious and numerous the effects (many of which are also symptoms) unless halted by abstinence.

There have been further attempts to determine whether the 2 to 3 percent abstinence rate per year and the 1 percent annual rate of return to social drinking are due to spontaneous remission or to treatment. As Emrick (1974, 1975) points out in his reviews of the treatment outcome literature, most treatment studies have major methodological flaws, such as inadequate controls, failure to control for premorbid variables, and inadequate follow-up periods. However, he concludes that improvement rates at 6 months and longer are positively correlated with the amount of treatment. Conversely, several well-done studies since Emrick's reviews conclude that treatment does little to change the natural course of alcoholism (Orford and Edwards, 1977; Ojesjo, 1981; Vaillant, 1980, 1983; Finney and Moos, 1991; Taylor et al, 1986). The current evidence, therefore, appears to indicate that spontaneous remission, abstinence, and return to asymptomatic drinking rates are equivalent for treated and untreated alcoholics. Several investigators (Pattison, 1981; Sells, 1981) have suggested that therapy appears ineffective because all patients are expected to respond to the same treatment. They suggest that patients should be matched to the treatments best suited to them. Although this approach is logical, the method for matching patients to treatments has not been established, and the theory that such matching would be advantageous awaits verification.

It should be emphasized that the rate of improvement noted earlier applies to patients who are probably diagnosable as being alcohol-dependent. Many patients with alcohol problems, especially those in their teens and 20s, return to social drinking and abstinence at much higher rates. For example, Fillmore (1975), in her 20-year follow-up of college students, found that only 30 percent of 31 individuals who had been problem drinkers in college were still having problems with alcohol at follow-up.

All alcoholics, including those who become abstinent or return to social drinking, are at risk to experience significant medical and psychiatric morbidity from their illness. In addition to the medical and psychiatric complications alcoholics experience, which were noted earlier in this chapter and which frequently lead patients into outpatient or inpatient medical or psychiatric care, alcoholics also experience a great deal of psychosocial morbidity. Given that alcoholism is diagnosed in part by its psychosocial consequences, it is somewhat difficult and arbitrary to separate psychosocial complications from symptoms of alcoholism. It is worth emphasizing, however, that job difficulties and loss; marital tensions, separations, and divorces; and arrests for traffic offenses, disturbing the peace, and criminal behavior are all strongly associated with alcoholism (Taylor and Helzer, 1983).

Not only does a diagnosis of alcoholism carry a significant risk of various complications, but it is also strongly associated with increased mortality. Death rates in alcoholics (adjusted for age and sex) are 1.6 to 9.5 times higher than in controls (Finney and Moos, 1991). The lifetime risk of suicide in chronic alcoholism is estimated to be 3.4 percent, which is 60 to 120 times higher than in the nonpsychiatrically ill general population (Murphy and Wetzel, 1990). Alcohol use and probably abuse are strongly associated with violent deaths, accidents, and homicide. Alcoholism is strongly associated with death from cirrhosis and, in conjunction with cigarette smoking, with cancer of the oropharynx and esophagus (USDHHS, 1990). Moderately increased morbidity, 1.5 to 3.0 times that expected, in alcoholics from cardiovascular disease and infectious disease also has been reported (Vaillant, 1983; Taylor and Helzer, 1983). These various causes lead to an average age of death of 55 to 60 for alcoholics (Schuckit, 1989). Also of note is the finding of Vaillant (1983) that offering intense, readily available treatment to alcoholics does not lower their mortality rate and the finding of Pell and D'Alonzo (1973) that the mortality rate of recovered alcoholics is not significantly different from that of alcoholics who continue to drink. Although this latter finding has been supported recently (Finney and Moos, 1991), there are three studies that indicate that survival is greater in those alcoholics who are able to abstain or drink moderately than in those who continue as heavy and/or problem drinkers (Smith et al., 1983; Barr et al., 1984; Bullock et al., 1992).

An overall view of the natural history of alcoholism reveals that an alcoholic's first drink occurs at age 13, problem drinking begins between the ages of 18 and 25, first hospitalization for drinking problems occurs at about age 40, and death occurs between the ages of 55 and 60 (Glatt, 1959; Schuckit, 1989; Taylor and Helzer, 1983). This natural history differs somewhat for women, who begin problem drinking later than men and have a more rapid development of symptoms. Women also have been found to have the onset of physical complications at an earlier age, have more psychiatric disability, have a greater likelihood of co-occurring psychiatric disorders (especially depressive disorder), have a worse prognosis, (especially in relation to mortality), and have an equal response to treatment (Glatt, 1961; Gomberg, 1976; Winokur and Clayton, 1967; Liban and Smart, 1980; Ashley et al., 1977; Dahlgren, 1978; Wilsnack, 1982; Helzer et al., 1991; Schuckit, 1989; Blume, 1991).

There are many exceptions to this natural history for both men and women, as there are to the onset, order, and occurrence of specific signs and symptoms of alcoholism. The most severe alcoholic spends much of his or her time sober (Ludwig, 1972; Helzer et al., 1991), with concomitant decreases at such times in alcohol-related problems.

The disease appears to fit the pattern of a chronic relapsing illness, with periods of remission and exacerbation. Some alcoholics appear to have permanent remissions either spontaneously, through internal resolve, or with the help of various factors in their environment. Others continue a pattern of intermittent but not worsening problems, and still others inexorably deteriorate with increasingly severe, debilitating, and often fatal alcohol-related problems. A continuing challenge to those working in the field of alcoholism is to identify the patients with the more benign course and determine what factors lead to such a course and to identify those with a more malignant course and determine what interventions and treatments are effective for them.

DIFFERENTIAL DIAGNOSIS

Sometimes alcoholism is called *primary*, meaning that it is not associated with other psychiatric conditions. Twenty or thirty years ago, it seems, most hospitalized alcoholics were primary by this definition. More recently, however, it appears that most treated alcoholics do *not* have primary alcoholism. Their alcoholism is associated with other disorders, principally affective disorder, anxiety disorders, and nonalcoholic substance abuse. The so-called polydrug user has become a familiar figure in most treatment centers.

Studies indicate that between 30 and 50 percent of alcoholics fulfill criteria for affective disorder. About one-third of alcoholics fulfill criteria for one of the anxiety disorders, particularly social phobia in men and agoraphobia in women. Many alcoholics have antisocial personality disorder (sociopathy), although prevalence figures vary too widely to warrant citing (Goodwin, 1988).

The coexistence of alcoholism and drug addiction is increasing. A 1989 survey of Alcoholic Anonymous (AA) members (The Alcoholism Report, 1990) found that 38 percent of respondents reported addiction to drugs as well as alcohol—an increase over the 30 percent recorded in a 1986 survey, reflecting a trend first tracked in 1977, when the proportion of such respondents was 18 percent. Age and sex were major factors; about 75 percent of young people reported previous drug addiction, as did a greater percentage of women than men.

Chronic excessive use of alcohol produces a wide range of psychiatric symptoms that, in various combinations, can mimic other psychiatric disorders. *Therefore, while a person is drinking heavily and during the withdrawal period, it is difficult to determine whether he or she is suffering from a psychiatric condition other than alcoholism.*

Various personality disorders have been associated with alcoholism, particularly those in which "dependency" is a feature. The consensus at present is that alcoholism is not connected with a particular constellation of personality traits. Longitudinal studies help little in predicting what types of individuals are particularly susceptible to alcoholism (McCord and McCord, 1962; Vaillant, 1989).

ETIOLOGY

Most adults in Western countries drink alcohol. About 1 in 12 to 1 in 15 have serious problems from drinking. There is no scientifically acceptable explanation why some develop problems and most do not. Although the cause of alcoholism is unknown, a number of risk factors have been identified.

1. *Family history.* Alcoholism runs in families. Four times as many children of alcoholics become alcoholic as do children of nonalcoholics. There is evidence that they become alcoholic whether they are raised by their alcoholic parents or not. Whether "hereditary" or not, alcoholism in the family is probably the strongest predictor of alcoholism occurring in particular individuals.

2. *Sex.* More men are alcoholic than women. The difference is about five to one.

3. *Age.* Alcoholism in men usually develops in the twenties and thirties. In women it often develops later. People of either sex over 65 rarely become alcoholic.

4. Alcoholism is unevenly distributed geographically and among people of different occupations, racial backgrounds, nationality, income, and religion (see section on Epidemiology).

In recent years the familial nature of alcoholism has been intensively studied. Many family studies have been conducted in Western countries, and all show much higher rates of alcoholism among the relatives of alcoholics than in the general population. Children are usually raised by the same individuals who provide their genes, and nature–nurture studies have attempted to separate genetic from environmental influences. Among these are adoption and twin studies.

Adoption Studies

If there is alcoholism in the biological parents and the disorder has a partial genetic basis, children of alcoholics adopted in infancy by nonalcoholics should still have a relatively high rate of alcoholism. Four such studies have been conducted.

The first by Roe (1944) found no difference between children of alcoholics and children of nonalcoholics when both groups were raised by nonalcoholic adoptive parents. There were no alcoholics in either group. The sample size was small, and it was not clear that the biological parents would be classified as alcoholic today. Also, the adoptees were young, and some had not entered the age of risk for alcoholism.

The 1970s saw a renewed interest in biologic factors in alcoholism. Three adoption studies were conducted in three countries: Denmark (Goodwin et al., 1973), Sweden (Bohman, 1978), and the United States (Cadoret et al., 1979). Methodologically dissimilar, the three studies came to similar conclusions:

1. Grownup children of alcoholics raised by nonalcoholic adoptive parents continued to have a high rate of alcoholism—about as high as that found in children of alcoholics raised by alcoholic parents.
2. Having an alcoholic biological parent apparently did not increase the risk of adoptees having other psychiatric disorders.

In the Danish study, four groups of individuals were interviewed: sons and daughters of alcoholic parents who were adopted out and raised by nonalcoholic, unrelated adoptive parents and their brothers and sisters raised by the alcoholic parent. No differences in alcoholism rates in same-sex biological siblings were found. Nor did the adopted-out children of alcoholics have elevated rates of other psychiatric pathology compared with controls (adopted-out children of nonalcoholics). Alcoholism ran true to type. Having an alcoholic parent did not even increase the chance of the adopted-out offspring being classified as heavy drinkers.

The Swedish and U.S. studies initially reported similar findings. In the Swedish study, criminality in the biological parents did not predict criminality in the offspring, nor did alcoholism predict criminality. The data were later reanalyzed by Cloninger and colleagues (1981), who reported an increased prevalence of antisocial personality in a subset of alcoholics called *type II alcoholics*.

Originally, the U.S. study also found that alcoholism ran true to type; that is, a family history of alcoholism in the biological parents did not increase the likelihood of other psychiatric illnesses occurring in the adopted-out offspring. Further study found a tendency for the adopted-out children to misuse drugs and also found that alcoholism in the adoptive parents somewhat raised the chance of alcoholism occurring in their adopted children (Cadoret et al., 1987). Whether alcoholism in parents increases the chance of other psychiatric disorders in their adopted-out offspring remains uncertain.

Twin Studies

Single-egg monozygotic twins share the same DNA and presumably have identical susceptibility to genetic illnesses. Twin-egg dizygotic twins share a familial susceptibility to genetic illnesses to the extent to which they share the same genes.

Several twin studies have examined drinking patterns. A Swedish study (Kaij, 1960) found that identical twins were more concordant for alcoholism than fraternal twins. A Finnish study (Partanen et al., 1966) found similarities of drinking patterns but no difference between identical and fraternal twins regarding "loss of control" (believed by some to be the sine qua non of alcoholism). However, there was a discrepancy in concordance rates for younger twins, with young identical twins more likely to be concordant for alcoholism than young fraternal twins. A review of Veterans Administration (VA) records in the United States lent support to a genetic factor (Hrubec and Omenn, 1981), finding that identical twins were more often concordant for alcoholism than fraternal twins. Finally, an ongoing study in England has failed so far to find differences between identical and fraternal twins with respect to alcoholism (Murray and Gurlin, 1983; personal communication, 1991).

EDITORS' COMMENT

A treatment sample of 50 monozygotic (MZ) and 64 dyzygotic (DZ) men and 31 MZ and 24 DZ women found significantly higher concordance for DSM-III alcohol abuse and/or dependence in MZ twins compared with the dyzygotic twins. For female twins, MZ twins showed significantly higher concordance than DZ twins for alcohol dependence only (Pickens R et al., Arch Gen Psychiatry 48:19–28, 1991). A population-based interview study of 1033 pairs of female twins (Kendler KS et al., JAMA 268:1877–1882, 1992) reported different results. These authors found, using three definitions of alcohol abuse from broad to narrow, that in all three the proband-wise concordance for alcoholism was higher in monozygotic than dyzygotic twin pairs. Thus in both genders, genetic factors play a major role in the etiology of alcoholism. Although environment is important (one cannot become an alcoholic if one is not exposed to alcohol), high-risk children must be educated about risk, and women as well as men need to be included in studies related to abuse of alcohol.

Like adoption studies, most twin data are consistent with the presence of genetic factors in alcoholism, but they are not conclusive. The relative importance of environmental and genetic factors remains to be ascertained.

Two Alcoholisms

Reanalyzing Swedish adoption data, Cloninger and colleagues (1981) proposed the existence of two types of alcoholism: type I and type II. In a 1987 review, Cloninger expanded on the two types, adding personality traits. Space permits only a summary of the core features of this interesting dichotomy.

Type I is relatively mild, occurs in both sexes, and is influenced by environmental factors (e.g., low economic status). Type II, affecting mainly men, involves a more severe family history of alcoholism and is manifested by antisocial features but is not influenced by social or environmental factors.

The two-type hypothesis has attracted a good deal of attention. Nordstrom and Berglund (1987a)

found that type II alcoholics, like their biological parents, represent a more severe group with a lower frequency of abstinence and social drinking and a tendency to drinking bouts when compared with type I alcoholics.

There also have been nonreplicative studies. Penick et al. (1987), in a study of 360 VA alcoholics, found marked overlap in the symptom clusters associated with the two subtypes. Ninety-one percent satisfied criteria for both clusters. Schuckit and Irwin (1989), similarly failing to replicate Cloninger's symptom groups, suggested that type II alcoholics may be sociopaths who drink a lot.

Another typology involves dividing alcoholics into familial and nonfamilial alcoholics. Although alcoholism runs in families, it does not run in all families, and many alcoholics do not have a family history of alcoholism. By comparing alcoholics with a positive family history with those having a negative family history, interesting findings have been reported. These include an earlier age of onset and a more severe form of alcoholism in familial alcoholics (Penick et al, 1987).

Vaillant (1989) conducted one of the few studies failing to show a positive correlation between early age of onset and family history of alcoholism. This may be due to sample differences. The rate of parental alcoholism in Vaillant's study was low compared with most studies.

Similarities exist between Cloninger's type I and type II alcoholics and familial and nonfamilial alcoholics. Both the type II alcoholic and the familial alcoholic have an early onset and involve a more serious form of alcoholism than occurs in nonfamilial alcoholism. Cloninger's proposal that heavy-drinking parents and low occupational status have additive effects in increasing alcoholism in the offspring has been supported by a study by Parker and Harford (1988). Another environmental factor that might distinguish type I and type II alcoholism (or familial versus nonfamilial alcoholism) may involve maltreatment of children by the alcoholic parents. Alcoholics are overrepresented in the population of child abusers (Famularo et al., 1986), and child abuse may occur more often in familial alcoholics than in nonfamilial alcoholics.

The Serotonin Theory

Buydens-Branchey et al. (1989) reported findings supporting the concept that alcoholism has two subtypes: familial and nonfamilial. Once more, the observation was made that early onset and a positive family history were correlated. Moreover, the early-onset, positive-family-history group had reduced serotonin activity, as measured by a peripheral blood assay. Questions can be raised about a correlation between peripheral blood measures and central nervous system serotonergic activity, but the study supports a growing body of evidence that serotonin to some extent mediates consumption of alcohol. The evidence includes the following observations:

1. Persons with a genetic propensity for alcoholism may be deficient in certain forms of biochemical activity required for optimal well-being. These persons, given available alcohol, a suitable culture, and an absence of countervailing traits, may discover that alcohol temporarily corrects this hypothetical deficiency, producing an intensity of mood change foreign to those without the deficiency. The model thus requires that alcohol would have a biphasic effect, causing subsequent underactivity of the reward system.

There is some evidence that alcohol has a biphasic effect on serotonin metabolism that might correspond to the deficiency model (Kent et al., 1985). Alcohol appears to increase serotonergic activity during acute intoxication, followed by a reduction of serotonin activity to subnormal levels during the postintoxication period. The deficient person, then, would have two reasons for drinking: first to correct the deficiency and then to correct for an even greater deficiency resulting from the biphasic effect of alcohol on serotonin. Biochemically, this might explain the addictive cycle in which a person initially drinks to feel good and then later drinks to stop feeling bad from the substance that originally made him or her feel good.

2. Animals bred to have a high preference for alcohol have lower levels of serotonin in the limbic system and centers regulating emotion than do animals bred to have a low preference for alcohol (McBride et al., 1989).

3. Pharmacologic agents have been developed for the treatment of depression with a highly selective effect on serotonin activity. By blocking the reuptake of serotonin released into the synaptic cleft, more serotonin becomes available for postsynaptic receptors. Serotonin reuptake blockers cause reduced drinking in experimental animals (Zabik et al., 1985) and, in three double-blind, placebo-controlled studies (Naranjo et al., 1987), reduce drinking in nondepressed heavy drinkers.

Thus increasing evidence points to serotonin as having a critical role in consumption of alcohol and perhaps alcoholism.

Search for a Gene

Adoption and twin studies suggest a possible genetic role in the development of alcoholism. In the late 1980s, molecular biologists began searching for a specific gene or genes responsible for the putative genetic influence. The first studies focused on the dopamine D^2 receptor located on the long arm of chromosome 11. In 1990 and 1991, four studies reported an association between alcoholism and the A-1 allele of the D^2 receptor. Two studies failed to find this association. Failures to replicate the original findings of an association may be related to sample differences (Cloninger, 1991). In any event, funding by the federal government for exploration of a genetic basis for alcoholism, plus the increasing availability of genetic probes, has elevated genetic studies of alcoholism to the top rank of research in this area.

TREATMENT

The treatment of alcoholism and the management of alcohol withdrawal symptoms present separate problems.

In the absence of serious medical complications, the alcohol withdrawal syndrome is usually transient and self-limiting; the patient recovers within several days regardless of treatment (Victor and Adams, 1953). Insomnia and irritability may persist for longer periods (Gerard et al., 1962).

Treatment of withdrawal is symptomatic and prophylactic. Agitation and tremulousness can be relieved with a variety of drugs, including barbiturates, paraldehyde, chloral hydrate, the phenothiazines, and the benzodiazepines. The benzodiazepines currently are considered the drugs of choice for withdrawal. They have little, if any, synergistic action with alcohol and, compared with barbiturates and paraldehyde, relatively little abuse potential. They can be administered parenterally to intoxicated patients without apparent risk and continued orally during the withdrawal period. There is some evidence that mortality is increased when the phenothiazines are used, reportedly from hypotension or hepatic encephalopathy.

Administration of large doses of vitamins—particularly the B vitamins—is obligatory, given the role of these vitamins in preventing peripheral neuropathy and the Wernicke-Korsakoff syndrome. The B vitamins are water soluble, and there is no apparent danger in administering them in large doses.

Unless the patient is dehydrated because of vomiting or diarrhea, there is no reason to administer fluids parenterally. Contrary to common belief, alcoholics usually are not dehydrated; actually, they may be overhydrated from consumption of large volumes of fluid (Ogata et al., 1968). During the early stages of withdrawal, hyperventilation may cause respiratory alkalosis, and this, together with hypomagnesemia, has been reported to produce withdrawal seizures (Mendelson, 1970).

If the patient develops delirium, he or she should be considered dangerous to himself or herself and others, and protective measures should be taken. Ordinarily, tranquilizers calm the patient sufficiently to control agitation, and restraints are unnecessary. Administration of intravenous barbiturates or diazepam may be needed to control severe agitation. Most important, if delirium occurs, further exploration should be conducted to rule out serious medical illness missed in the original examination. When a patient is delirious, an attendant should always be present. It is sometimes helpful to have a friend or relative present.

The treatment of alcoholism should not begin until withdrawal symptoms subside. Treatment has two goals: (1) sobriety and (2) amelioration of psychiatric conditions associated with alcoholism. A small minority of alcoholics are eventually able to drink in moderation, but for several months after a heavy drinking bout, total abstinence is desirable for two reasons. First, the physician must follow the patient, sober, for a considerable period to diagnose a coexistent psychiatric problem. Second, it is important for the patient to learn that he or she can cope with ordinary life problems without alcohol. Most relapses occur within 6 months of discharge from the hospital; they become less and less frequent after that (Glatt, 1959).

Alcoholics Anonymous (AA) has been widely viewed as providing more help for alcoholics than any other approach. AA discourages research, and there has been little supporting data to confirm this assertion. However, AA has conducted a survey every 3 years since 1968, and some interesting observations have derived from it.

For example, there was a time in the 1970s and 1980s when more and more young people joined AA. This declined sharply in the 1989 survey. Those under age 21 made up 3 percent of the 1989 respondents (The Alcoholism Report, 1990).

A similar phenomenon involved women. There was a marked increase of women members (34 percent) in 1986, but women members increased by only 1 percent in the 1989 survey. Of members, 50 months was the average sobriety length. The survey underscored a continued problem—half of those who come to AA do not remain for more than 3 months. Former surveys have indicated that only about 15 percent continued attending meetings. The fate of alcoholics who reject AA is not clear, but treatment evaluation studies indicate that many of them reduce their drinking or stop altogether without the help of AA. Most of these improvements can be described as "spontaneous" inasmuch as professional help did not seem responsible.

The preceding almost completely encompasses the "hard data" about AA. However, subjective impressions should not be ignored. There is no question that AA provides help for many alcoholics that they cannot obtain elsewhere. No doubt it has saved many lives. Most clinicians who treat alcoholics commonly encourage their patients to attend AA meetings. It is not possible to predict in advance whether one patient will benefit from AA and another will not. AA—just about everyone agrees—should be given a fair opportunity.

For many patients, disulfiram (Antabuse) is helpful in maintaining abstinence. By inhibiting aldehyde dehydrogenase, the drug leads to an accumulation of acetaldehyde if alcohol is consumed. Acetaldehyde is highly toxic and causes nausea and hypotension. The latter condition leads to shock and may be fatal (Wright and Moore, 1989). In recent years, however, Antabuse has been prescribed in a lower dosage (250 mg) than was used previously, and no deaths from its use have been reported for a number of years. One study indicates that the dose is irrelevant; the deterrent effect is psychological and not dose-dependent (Fuller and Williford, 1980).

When Antabuse is discontinued after administration for several days or weeks, the deterrent effect still lasts for a 3- to 5-day period, since the drug takes that long to be excreted. Thus it may be useful to give patients Antabuse during office visits at 3- to 4-day intervals early in the treatment program.

It was once recommended that patients be given Antabuse for several days and then be challenged with alcohol to demonstrate the unpleasant effects that follow. This procedure was not always satisfactory because some patients showed no adverse effects after considerable amounts of alcohol were consumed and other patients became very ill after drinking small amounts of alcohol. The principal disadvantage of Antabuse is not that patients drink while taking the drug, but that they stop taking the drug after a brief period. This, again, is a good reason to give the drug on frequent office visits during the early crucial period of treatment.

A wide variety of procedures, both psychological and somatic, have been tried in the treatment of alcoholism. None has proved to be definitely superior to others (Blum and Blum, 1969). There is no evidence that intensive psychotherapy helps most alcoholics. Nor are tranquilizers or antidepressants usually effective in maintaining abstinence or controlled drinking (Goodwin, 1988). Aversive conditioning techniques have been tried with such agents as apomorphine and emetine to produce vomiting, succinylcholine to produce apnea, and electrical stimulation to produce pain. The controlled trials required to show that these procedures are effective have not been conducted, but a high rate of success has been reported for the apomorphine treatment in motivated patients (Smith et al., 1991). Although the number of alcoholics who benefit from participation in Alcoholics Anonymous is unknown, most clinicians agree that alcoholics should be encouraged to attend AA meetings on a trial basis.

In three double-blind studies, lithium carbonate was found to be superior to a placebo in reducing drinking in depressed alcoholics (Kline et al., 1974; Merry et al., 1976; Fawcett et al., 1987). The dropout rate was high in the three studies. A large multicenter VA study failed to confirm the efficacy of lithium for alcoholism (Dorus et al., 1989). Naltrexone, an opioid antagonist, has been reported to reduce drinking by alcoholics (Volpicelli et al., 1990).

Relapses are characteristic of alcoholism, and physicians treating alcoholics should avoid anger or excessive pessimism when such relapses occur. Alcoholics see nonpsychiatric physicians as often as they see psychiatrists (probably more often), and there is evidence that general practitioners and internists are sometimes more helpful (Gerard and Saenger, 1966). This may be particularly true when the therapeutic approach is warm but authoritarian, with little stress on "insight" or "understanding." Because the cause of alcoholism is unknown, "understanding," in fact, means acceptance of a particular theory. This may provide temporary comfort but probably seldom provides lasting benefit.

REFERENCES

The Alcoholism Report. June 1990, p 5.

American Psychiatric Association: Diagnostic and Statistical Manual of Mental Disorders, 3d ed. Washington, American Psychiatric Association, 1980.

American Psychiatric Association: DSM-IV Options Book: Work in Progress. Washington, American Psychiatric Association, 1991.

American Society of Addiction Medicine News. March–April 1990, p 2.

Ashley MJ, Olin JW, le Reiche WM, et al: Morbidity in alcoholics. Arch Intern Med 137:883–887, 1977.

Barr HL, Antes D, Ottenberg DJ, Rosen A: Mortality of treated alcoholics and drug addicts: The benefits of abstinence. J Stud Alcohol 45:440–452, 1984.

Benzer DG: Medical consequences of alcohol addiction. In Miller NS (ed): Comprehensive Handbook of Drug and Alcohol Addiction. New York, Marcel Dekker, 1991, pp 551–571.

Blum EM, Blum RH: Alcoholism. San Francisco, Jossey-Bass, 1969.

Blume S: Women, alcohol, and drugs. In Miller NS (ed): Comprehensive Handbook of Drug and Alcohol Addiction. New York, Marcel Dekker, 1991, pp 147–177.

Bohman M: Genetic aspects of alcoholism and criminality. Arch Gen Psychiatry 35:269–276, 1978.

Boyd JH, Weissman MM, Thompson WD, et al: Different definitions of alcoholism: I. Impact of seven definitions on prevalence rates in a community survey. Am J Psychiatry 140:1309–1313, 1983.

Bratfos O: The Course of Alcoholism: Drinking, Social Adjustment and Health. Oslo, Norway, Universitet Forlaget, 1974.

Brenner MH: Trends in alcohol consumption and associated illnesses: Some effects of economic changes. Am J Public Health 65:1279–1292, 1975.

Brenner MH: International trends in alcohol consumption, in Alcohol Consumption and Related Problems. NIAAA Alcohol and Health Mongraph No. 1 DHMS Pub. No. (ADM) 82-1190. Washington, D.C., Government Printing Office, 1982, pp. 157–176.

Bullock KD, Reed RJ, Grant I: Reduced mortality in alcoholics who achieve long-term abstinence. JAMA 267:668–672, 1992.

Buydens-Branchey L, Branchey MH, Noumair D, Lieber CS: Age of alcoholism onset: II. Relationship to susceptibility to serotonin precursor availability. Arch Gen Psychiatry 46:231–236, 1989.

Cadoret RJ, Cain CA, Grove WM: Development of alcoholism in adoptees raised apart from alcoholic biologic relatives. Arch Gen Psychiatry 37:561–563, 1979.

Cadoret RJ, Troughton E, O'Gorman TW: Genetic and environmental factors in alcohol abuse and antisocial personality. J Stud Alcohol 48:1–8, 1987.

Cahalan D: Problem Drinkers. San Francisco, Jossey-Bass, 1970.

Chan AWK: Biochemical markers for alcoholism. In Miller NS (ed): Comprehensive Handbook of Drug and Alcohol Addiction. New York, Marcel Dekker, 1991, pp 311–338.

Clark WB: Loss of control, heavy drinking and drinking problems in a longitudinal study. J Stud Alcohol 37:1256–1290, 1976.

Cloninger CR: Neurogenetic adaptive mechanisms in alcoholism. Science 236:410–416, 1987.

Cloninger CR: D² dopamine receptor gene is associated but not linked with alcoholism. JAMA 266:1833, 1991.

Cloninger CR, Bohman M, Sigvardsson S: Inheritance of alcohol abuse: Crossfostering analysis of adopted men. Arch Gen Psychiatry 36:861–868, 1981.

Dahlgren L: Female alcoholics: III. Development and pattern of problem drinking. Acta Psychiatr Scand 57:325–334, 1978.

Dolinsky ZS, Schnitt M: Discriminant function analysis of clinical laboratory data. In Galanter M (ed): Recent Development in Alcoholism, vol 6. New York, Plenum Press, 1988, pp 367–385.

Dorus W, Ostrow DG, Anton R, et al: Lithium treatment of depressed and nondepressed alcoholics. JAMA 262:1646–1652, 1989.

Drew LR: Alcoholism as a self limiting disease. Q J Stud Alcohol 29:956–967, 1968.

Eckardt MJ, Ryback RS, Rawlings RR, et al: Biochemical diagnosis of alcoholism: A test of the discriminating capabilities of gamma-glutamyl transpeptidase and mean corpuscular volume. JAMA 246:2707–2710, 1981.

Emrick CD: A review of psychologically oriented treatment of alcoholism: I. The use and interrelationship of outcome criteria and drinking behavior following treatment. Q J Stud Alcohol 35:523–549, 1974.

Emrick CD: A review of psychologically oriented treatment of alcoholism: II. The relative effectiveness of different treatment approaches and the effectiveness of treatment versus no treatment. J Stud Alcohol 36:88–109, 1975.

Famularo R, Stone K, Barnum R, Wharton R: Alcoholism and severe child maltreatment. Am J Orthopsychiatry 56:481–485, 1986.

Farraj BA, Camp VM, Davis DC, et al: Elevation of plasma salsolinol sulfate in chronic alcoholics as compared to nonalcoholics. Alcohol Clin Exp Res 13:155–163, 1989.

Fawcett J, Clark VC, Aagesen CA, et al: A double-blind placebo-controlled trial of lithium carbonate therapy for alcoholism. Arch Gen Psychiatry 44:248–256, 1987.

Fillmore KM: Relationship between specific drinking problems in early adulthood and middle age: An exploratory 20-year follow-up study. Q J Stud Alcohol 36:882–907, 1975.

Finney JW, Moos RH: The long-term course of treated alcoholism: I. Mortality, relapse, and remission rates and comparisons with community controls. J Stud Alcohol 52:44–54, 1991.

Fuller RK, Williford WO: Life-table analysis of abstinence in a study evaluating the efficacy of disulfiram. Alcoholism (NY) 4:298, 1980.

Geller A: Neurological effects of drug and alcohol addiction. In Miller NS (ed): Comprehensive Handbook of Drug and Alcohol Addiction. New York, Marcel Dekker, 1991, pp 599–621.

Gerard D, Saenger G, Wile R: The abstinent alcoholic. Arch Gen Psychiatry 6:83–95, 1962.

Gerard DL, Saenger G: Out-patient Treatment of Alcoholism. Toronto, University of Toronto Press, 1966.

Glass IB, Chalmers R, Bartlett S, Littleton J: Increased plasma carnitine in severe alcohol dependence. Br J Addiction 84:689–693, 1989.

Glatt MM: An alcoholic unit in a mental hospital. Lancet 2:397–398, 1959.

Glatt MM: Drinking habits of English (middle-class) alcoholics. Acta Psychiatr Scand 37:88–113, 1961.

Gomberg E: Alcoholism in women. In Kissin B, Begleiter H (eds): Biology of Alcoholism, vol 4. New York, Plenum Press, 1976, pp 117–166.

Goodwin DW, Schulsinger F, Hermansen L, et al: Alcohol problems in adoptees raised apart from alcoholic biological parents. Arch Gen Psychiatry 28:238–243, 1973.

Goodwin DW: Alcoholism and hereditary. Arch Gen Psychiatry 36:57–61, 1979.

Goodwin DW: Alcoholism. In Goodwin DW, Guze SB (eds): Psychiatric Diagnosis. New York, Oxford University Press, 1984, pp 147–178.

Goodwin DW: Is alcoholism hereditary? New York, Oxford University Press, 1988.

Goodwin DW, Hill SY: Chronic effects of alcohol and other psychoactive drugs on intellect, learning and memory. In

Rankin G (ed): Alcohol, Drugs, and Brain Damage. Toronto, Addiction Research Foundation, 1975, pp 55–69.

Goodwin DW, Crane JB, Guze SB: Alcoholic "black-outs": A review and clinical study of 100 alcoholics. Am J Psychiatry 126:191–198, 1969.

Goodwin DW, Crane JB, Guze SB: Felons who drink: An 8-year follow-up. Q J Stud Alcohol 32:136–147, 1971.

Grob GN: Origins of DSM-I: A study in appearance and reality. Am J Psychiatry 184:421–431, 1991.

Hagnell O, Tunving K: Prevalence and nature of alcoholism in a total population. Soc Psychiatry 7:190–201, 1972.

Harada S, Agarwal DP, Goedde HW: Biochemical and hematological markers of alcoholism. In Goedde HW, Agarwal DP (eds): Alcoholism Biomedical and Genetic Aspects. New York, Pergamon, 1989, pp 238–255.

Helzer JE, Burnam A, McEvoy LT: Alcohol abuse and dependence. In Robins LN, Regier DA (eds): Psychiatric Disorders in America. New York, Free Press, 1991, pp 81–115.

Helzer JE, Pryzbeck TM: The co-occurrence of alcoholism with other psychiatric disorders in the general population and its impact on treatment. J Stud Alcohol 49:219–224, 1988.

Helzer JE, Robins LN, Taylor JR, et al: The extent of long-term moderate drinking among alcoholics discharged from medical and psychiatric treatment facilities. N Engl J Med 312:1678–1682, 1985.

Hingson R, Howland J: Alcohol as a risk factor for injuries or death resulting from accidental falls: A review of the literature. J Stud Alcohol 48:212–219, 1987.

Holt S, Skinner HA, Israel Y: Early identification of alcohol abuse: II. Clinical and laboratory indicators. Can Med Assoc J 124:1279–1295, 1981.

Horgan MM, Sparrow MD, Brazeau RN: Alcoholic Beverage Taxation and Control Policies, 6th ed. Ottawa: Brewers Association of Canada, 1986.

Howland J, Hingson R: Alcohol as a risk factor for injuries or death due to fires and burns: Review of the literature. Public Health Rep 102:475–483, 1987.

Howland J, Hingson R: Issues in research on alcohol in nonvehicular unintentional injuries. Contemp Drug Probl (Spring): 95–106, 1988.

Hrubec Z, Omenn GS: Evidence of genetic predisposition to alcoholic cirrhosis and psychosis: Twin concordances for alcoholism and its biological end points by zygosity among male veterans. Alcohol Clin Exp Res 5:207–215, 1981.

Hultberg B, Isaksson A, Berglund M, Moberg AL: Serum betahexosaminidase isoenzyime: A sensitive marker for alcohol abuse. Alcohol Clin Exp Res 15:549–552, 1991.

Hyman MM. Alcoholics 15 years later. Ann NY Acad Sci 273:613–623, 1976.

Israel Y, Orrego H, Host S, et al: Identification of alcohol abuse: Thoracic fractures on routine chest x-ray as indicators of alcoholism. Alcohol Clin Exp Res 4:420–422, 1980.

Jellinek EM: Estimating the prevalence of alcoholism: Modified values in the Jellinek formula and an alternate approach. Q J Stud Alcohol 20:261–269, 1959.

Jellinek EM: Phases of alcohol addiction. Q J Stud Alcohol 13:673–684, 1952.

Jellinek EM: The Disease Concept of Alcoholism. New Haven, Hillhouse Press, 1960.

Jellinek EM, Keller M: Rates of alcoholism in the United States of America, 1940–1948. Q J Stud Alcohol 13:49–59, 1952.

Jones KL, Smith DW, Ulleland CN, et al: Patterns of malformation in offspring of chronic alcoholic mothers. Lancet 1: 1267–1271, 1973.

Kaij L: Studies on the etiology and sequels of abuse of alcohol. Thesis, University of Lund, Sweden, 1960.

Keller M: Problems of epidemiology in alcohol problems. Q J Stud Alcohol 36:1442–1451, 1975.

Keller M, Effron V: The prevalence of alcoholism. Q J Stud Alcohol 16:619–644, 1955.

Kent TA, Campbell JR, Goodwin DW: Blood platelet uptake of serotonin in men alcoholics. J Stud Alcohol 46:357–359, 1985.

Klatsky AL: The cardiovascular effects of alcohol. Alcohol Alcohol 22(suppl 1):117–124, 1987.

Kline NS, Wren JC, Cooper TB, et al: Evaluations of lithium therapy in chronic and periodic alcoholism. Am J Med Sci 268:15–22, 1974.

Lemere F: What happens to alcoholics? Am J Psychiatry 109:674–676, 1953.

Liban C, Smart RG: Generational and other differences between males and females in problem drinking and its treatment. Drug Alcohol Depend 5:207–221, 1980.

Ludwig AM: On and off the wagon: Reasons for drinking and abstaining by alcoholics. Q J Stud Alcohol 33:91–96, 1972.

Lundquist GAR: Alcohol dependence. Acta Psychiatr Scand 49:332–340, 1973.

McBride WJ, Murphy JM, Lumeng L, Li TK: Serotonin and ethanol preference. In Galanter M (ed): Recent developments in alcoholism, vol 7. New York, Plenum Press, 1989.

McCord W, McCord J: A longitudinal study of the personality of alcoholics. In Pittman D, Snyder C (eds): Society, Culture and Drinking Patterns. New York, Wiley, 1962.

Malin H. Coakley J, Klaeber C, et al: An epidemiologic perspective on alcohol use and abuse in the United States. In Alcohol Consumption and Related Problems (NIAAA Alcohol and Health Monograph No. 1, DHMS Pub. No. ADM 82-1190). Washington, US Government Printing Office, 1982, pp 99–153.

Mann RE, Smart RG: Alcohol problems, prevention, and epidemiology: Looking for the next questions. Br J Addict 85: 1385–1387, 1990.

Mardsden CD: Neurological disorders induced by alcohol. In Edwards G, Grant M (eds): Alcoholism: New Knowledge and New Responses. Baltimore, University Park Press, 1977, pp 189–197.

Mendelson JH: Biologic concomitants of alcoholism. N Engl J Med 283:24–32, 1970.

Merry J, Reynolds CM, Bailey J, Coppen A: Prophylactic treatment of alcoholism by lithium carbonate. Lancet 2:481–482, 1976.

Moss HB, Yao JK, Burns M, et al: Plasma GABA-like activity in response to ethanol challenge in men at high risk for alcoholism. Biol Psychiatry 27:617–625, 1990.

Murphy GL, Wetzel RD: The lifetime risk of suicide in alcoholism. Arch Gen Psychiatry 47:383–392, 1990.

Murray RM, Gurlin CC: Twin and alcoholism studies. In M. Galanter (ed), Recent Developments in Alcoholism, vol 1. New York, Gardner, 1983.

Myerson DJ, Mayer J: Origins, treatment and destiny of skid row alcoholic men. N Engl J Med 275:419–424, 1966.

Naranjo CA, Sellers EM, Sullivan JT, et al: The serotonin uptake inhibitor citalopram attenuates ethanol intake. Clin Pharmacol Ther 41:266–274, 1987.

National Council on Alcoholism, Criteria Committee: Criteria for the diagnosis of alcoholism. Am J Psychiatry 129:127–135, 1972.

National Institute on Alcohol Abuse and Alcoholism: Apparent Per Capita Alcohol Consumption: National, State, and Regional Trends, 1977–1987. Surveillance Report No. 13. Rockville, MD: NIAAA, 1989a.

National Institute on Alcohol Abuse and Alcoholism. Liver Cirrhosis: Mortality in the United States, 1972–1986, by Grant BF, Zobeck TS. Surveillance Report No. 11. Rockville, MD: NIAAA, 1989b.

National Institute on Drug Abuse. National Household Survey on Drug Abuse: Main Findings 1988 (DHHS Pub. No. ADM 90–1682). Washington, US Government Printing Office, 1990.

Ng SK, Hanser WA, Brust JC, Susser M: Alcohol consumption and withdrawal in new onset seizures. N Engl J Med 319: 666–673, 1988.

Nordstrom G, Berglund M: Type I and type II alcoholics (Cloninger and Bohman) have different patterns of successful long-term adjustment. Br J Addict 82:761–769, 1987a.

Nordstrom G. Berglund M: A prospective study of successful long-term adjustment in alcohol dependence: Social drinking versus abstinence. J Stud Alcohol 48:95–103, 1987b.

Ogata M, Mendelson J, Mello N: Electrolytes and osmolality in alcoholics during experimentally induced intoxication. Psychosom Med 30:463–488, 1968.

Ojesjo L: Long-term outcome in alcohol abuse and alcoholism among males in the Lundley general population, Sweden. Br J Addict 76:391–400, 1981.

Orford J, Edwards G: Alcoholism. New York, Oxford University Press, 1977.

Paredes A, Hood W, Seymour H, et al: Loss of control in alcoholism: An investigation of the hypothesis with experimental findings. Q J Stud Alcohol 34:1146–1161, 1973.

Park P, Whitehead PC: Developmental sequence and dimensions of alcoholism. Q J Stud Alcohol 34:887–904, 1973.

Parker DA, Harford TC: Alcohol-related problems, marital disruption and depressive symptoms among adult children of alcohol abusers in the United States. J Stud Alcohol 49:306–313, 1988.

Parsian A, Todd RD, Devor EJ, et al: Alcoholism and alleles of the human D² dopamine receptor locus. Arch Gen Psychiatry 48:655–663, 1991.

Partanen J, Bruun K, Markkanen T: Inheritance of Drinking Behavior: A Study of Intelligence, Personality, and Use of Alcohol of Adult Twins. Helinski, Finnish Foundation for Alcohol Studies, 1966, pp 14–159.

Pattison EM: Differential diagnosis of the alcoholism syndrome: Clinical implications of empirical research. In Gotheil E, McLellan AT, Druley KA (eds): Matching Patient Needs and Treatment Methods in Alcoholism and Drug Abuse. Springfield, IL, Charles C Thomas, 1981, pp 3–31.

Pattison EM, Sobell MB, Sobell LC: Emerging Concepts of Alcohol Dependence. New York, Springer, 1977.

Pell S, D'Alonzo CA: A five-year mortality study of alcoholics. J Occup Med 15:120–125, 1973.

Penick EC, Powell BJ, Bingham SF, et al: A comparative study of familial alcoholism. J Stud Alcohol 48:136–146, 1987.

Pokorny AD, Kanas T, Overall J: Order of appearance of alcoholic symptoms. Alcohol Clin Exp Res 5:216–220, 1981.

Rausch JL, Monteiro MG, Schuckit MA: Platelet serotonin uptake in men with family histories of alcoholism. Neuropsychopharmacology 4:83–86, 1991.

Rodenberg HD, Bennett JR, Watson WA: Clinical utility of a saliva alcohol dipstick estimate of serum ethanol concentrations in the emergency department. DICP Ann Pharmacother 24:350–361, 1990.

Roe A: The adult adjustment of children of alcoholic parents raised in foster homes. Q J Stud Alcohol 5:378–393, 1944.

Roizen J: Estimating alcohol involvement in serious events. In Alcohol Consumption and Related Problems (NIAAA Alcohol and Health Monograph No. 1, DHMS Pub. No. ADM 82-1190). Washington, US Government Printing Office, 1982, pp 179–219.

Rosman AS, Lieber CS: Biochemical markers of alcohol consumption. Alcohol Health Res World 14:210–218, 1990.

Ryback RS, Echardt MJ, Feisher, et al: Biochemical and hematologic correlates of alcoholism and liver disease. JAMA 248:2261–2265, 1982.

Ryback RS, Rawlings RR: Biochemical correlation of alcohol consumption. In Chang NC, Chao HM (eds): Early Identification of Alcohol Abuse (NIAAA Research Monograph No. 17). Washington, US Government Printing Office, 1985, pp 31–48.

Schmidt W, Popham R: Heavy alcohol consumption and physical health problems: A review of the epidemiological evidence. Drug Alcohol Depend 1:27–50, 1975/76.

Schuckit MA: Drug and Alcohol Abuse. New York, Plenum Press, 1989.

Schuckit MA, Gold EO: A simultaneous evaluation of multiple markers of ethanol/placebo challenges in sons of alcoholics and controls. Arch Gen Psychiatry 45:211–216, 1988.

Schuckit M, Irwin M: An analysis of the clinical relevance of type I and type II alcoholics. Br J Addict 84:869–876, 1989.

Sellers EM, Kalant H: Alcohol intoxication and withdrawal. N Engl J Med 294:757–762, 1976.

Sells SB: Matching clients to treatment: Problems, preliminary results, and remaining tasks. In Gotheil E, McLellan AT, Druley KA (eds): Matching Patient Needs and Treatment Methods in Alcoholism and Drug Abuse. Springfield, IL, Charles C Thomas, 1981, pp 33–50.

Smith EM, Cloninger CR, Bradford S: Predictors of mortality in alcoholic women: A prospective follow-up study. Alcohol Clin Exp Res 7:237–243, 1983.

Smith JW, Frawley PJ, Polissar L: Six- and twelve-month abstinence rates in inpatient alcoholics treated with aversion therapy compared with matched inpatients from a treatment registry. Alcohol Clin Exp Res 15:862–870, 1991.

Streissguth AP, Martin DC, Barr HM: Intrauterine alcohol exposure and attentional decrements in 4-year-old children. Alcohol Clin Exp Res 7:122, 1983.

Sundby P: Alcoholism and Mortality. Oslo, Norway, Universitets Forlaget, 1967.

Tabakoff B, Hoffman PL, Lee JM, et al: Differences in platelet enzyme activity between alcoholics and nonalcoholics. N Engl J Med 318:134–139, 1988.

Taylor JR, Helzer JE: The natural history of alcoholism. In Kissin B, Begleiter H (eds): The Biology of Alcoholism, vol 6. New York, Plenum Press, 1983, pp 17–65.

Taylor JR, Helzer JE, Robins LN: Moderate drinking in ex-alcoholics: Recent studies. J Stud Alcohol 47:115–121, 1986.

Trice HM, Wahl JR: A rank-order analysis of the symptoms of alcoholism. Q J Stud Alcohol 19:636–648, 1958.

U.S. Department of Health and Human Services: Seventh Special Report to the U.S. Congress on Alcohol and Health (DHHS Pub. No. ADM 90-1656). Washington, US Government Printing Office, 1990.

Vaillant G: Letter to editor. Arch Gen Psychiatry 46:1151, 1989.

Vaillant G: The Natural History of Alcoholism. Cambridge, MA, Harvard University Press, 1983.

Vaillant G: The doctor's dilemma. In Edwards GE, Grant M (eds): Alcoholism, Treatment and Transition. London, Croom Helm, 1980.

Victor M, Adams RD: The effects of alcohol on the nervous system. In Merritt H, Hare C (eds): Metabolic and Toxic Diseases of the Nervous System. Baltimore, Williams & Wilkins, 1953.

Voetglin WL, Broz WR: The conditioned reflex treatment of chronic alcoholism: X. An analysis of 3125 admissions over a period of ten and a half years. Ann Intern Med 30:580–597, 1949.

Volpicelli JR, O'Brien CP, Alterman AL: Naltrexone and the treatment of alcohol dependence: Initial observations. In Reid LB (ed): Opioids, Bulimia, Alcohol Abuse and Alcoholism. New York, Springer-Verlag, 1990, p 195.

Weissman MM, Myers JK, Harding PS: Prevalence and psychiatric heterogeneity of alcoholism in a United States urban community. Q J Stud Alcohol 41:672–681, 1980.

Wilsnack SC: Alcohol abuse and alcoholism in women. In Pattison EM, Kaufman E (eds): Encyclopedia Handbook of Alcoholism. New York, Gardner Press, 1982, pp 718–735.

Winokur G, Clayton P: Family history studies II. Sex differences and alcoholism in primary affective illness. Br J Psychiatry 113:973–979, 1967.

Winokur G, Tsuang M: Expectancy of alcoholism in a midwestern population. Q J Stud Alcohol 39:1964–1967, 1978.

Wright C, Moore RD: Disulfiram treatment of alcoholism. Ann Intern Med 111:943–944, 1989.

Zabik JE, Binkerd K, Roache JD: Serotonin and ethanol aversion in the rat. In Naranjo CA, Sellers EM (eds): Research Advances in New Psychopharmacological Treatments for Alcoholism. New York, Elsevier Science, 1985.

CHAPTER 15

Drug Abuse

JOSEPH WESTERMEYER

DEFINITION

Diagnostic criteria for drug abuse or (in DSM-IV terms) substance-related disorder are as follows:

A. A maladaptive pattern of substance use, leading to clinically significant impairment or distress, as manifested by the following:

1. Tolerance, as defined by any of the following:
   a. Need for markedly increased amounts of the substance to achieve intoxication or desired effect.
   b. Markedly diminished effect with continued use of the same amount of the substance.
   c. Has functioned adequately at doses or blood levels of the substance that would produce significant impairment in a casual user.
2. The characteristic withdrawal syndrome for the substance symptoms.
3. The same substance is often taken to relieve or avoid withdrawal symptoms.
4. The substance is often taken in larger amounts or over a longer period than intended.
5. Any unsuccessful effort or persistent desire to cut down or control substance use.
6. A great deal of time is spent in activities necessary to obtain the substance (e.g., visiting multiple doctors or driving long distances), take the substance (e.g., chain-smoking), or recover from its effects.
7. Recurrent substance use resulting in inability to fulfill major role obligations at work, school, or home (e.g., repeated absences or poor work performance related to substance use; substance-related absences, suspen-

sions, or expulsions from school; neglect of children or household).
8. Recurrent substance use in situations in which it is physically hazardous (e.g., driving an automobile or operating a machine when impaired by substance use).
9. Important social, occupational, or recreational activities given up or reduced because of substance use.
10. Recurrent substance-related legal or interpersonal problems (e.g., substance-related arrests and traffic accidents, physical fights related to substance use).
11. Continued substance use despite knowledge of a persistent or recurrent problem(s) caused or exacerbated by the use of the substance (e.g., keeps using heroin despite family arguments about it, cocaine use despite recognition of cocaine-induced depression, or continued drinking despite recognition that an ulcer was made worse by alcohol consumption).

Pharmacologic considerations also must be included in the diagnosis, but clinical judgment still must be applied regardless of dosage. For example, mixed drug abuse, mental retardation, organic brain syndrome, other psychiatric conditions, and extreme youth or older age may lead to drug-related problems at doses lower than usual. Even relatively mild psychoactive compounds, such as caffeine or nicotine, can lead to disabling symptoms in vulnerable patients or in large doses. Episodes of opioid or cocaine overdose, amphetamine delusional disorder, phencyclidine delirium, or cannabis delusional disorder exemplify other types of pathologic drug use.

Drug dependence is a special category of drug abuse. It involves the presence of either tolerance to the drug or withdrawal upon stopping use. With tolerance, the patient must consume markedly increased amounts of the drug to achieve the desired effect, or there is markedly diminished effect with regular use of the same amount. Sudden drug withdrawal results in abstinence symptoms if tolerance is present. Different drugs produce withdrawal symptoms as follows:

Opioids: Lacrimation, rhinorrhea, mydriasis, piloerection, sweating, abdominal cramps, diarrhea, yawning, anxiety, irritability, mild hypertension, tachycardia, fever, and insomnia

Sedatives: Nausea, vomiting, malaise, weakness, tachycardia, sweating, hypertension, anxiety, depressed mood or irritability, orthostatic hypotension, coarse tremor and possible disorientation, hallucinations, and convulsions in severe cases

Stimulants: Fatigue, disturbed sleep, increased dreaming

Tobacco: Craving, irritability, anxiety, difficulty concentrating

Onset of abstinence symptoms following the last dose varies with the drug's duration of action. Withdrawal can begin in 4 to 6 hours with short-acting drugs (e.g., sodium amytal, heroin, morphine), in 8 to 16 hours with intermediate-acting drugs (e.g., opium, methadone, phenobarbital), or in a few to several days with long-acting drugs (e.g., ethchlorvynol, diazepam).

Cannabis does not have a distinct withdrawal syndrome. However, chronic heavy users do experience a need for markedly increased doses to achieve the desired effect and/or markedly diminished effect from regular doses. Lack of abstinence symptoms may be due to storage of active cannabis fractions (such as tetrahydrocannabinal) in body fat stores, with gradual excretion over days or weeks.

DSM-IV includes the diagnosis of tobacco dependence, but not tobacco abuse. The latter diagnosis is made if the tobacco withdrawal syndrome occurs upon cessation, serious attempts to stop or reduce use have been unsuccessful, or use continues despite a serious tobacco-related physical disorder (e.g., emphysema, coronary artery disease, Berger's disease of leg arteries).

Other drug-related conditions include hallucinogen hallucinosis, hallucinogen or cannabis delusional disorder, and hallucinogen affective disorder. Substance-related amnestic disorder and organic affective syndrome are additional diagnostic categories which may be associated with drug use. Depending on duration and pattern of drug use, these diagnoses may or may not be accompanied by the diagnosis of drug abuse.

ETIOLOGY AND PATHOGENESIS

Other than excessive or problematic drug use as a final common pathway, there is no one cause of drug abuse. Rather it is multifactorial in its etiology. The public health model of agent (i.e., drug), host (i.e., the individual), and environment (i.e., society) has proven useful in conceptualizing the complex causes of drug abuse.

Host Factors

FAMILY–GENETIC INFLUENCES

Like many other psychiatric disorders, drug abuse tends to occur within the same family. This suggests that genetic factors may play a role in drug abuse. Offspring of heavy tobacco smokers are considerably more apt to become tobacco dependent than the general population (Sarvik et al., 1977, Krasnagor, 1979). Opium-dependent persons in Asia show a higher rate of opium dependence among their siblings and relatives than does the general population (Westermeyer, 1974). Similarly, drug-dependent persons in the United States often have alcoholic relatives, as well as depressed or manic relatives. Thus far, adoptive and twin studies have not established the extent to which family prevalence is due to genetics and/or environment.

NEUROTRANSMITTERS

Specific opiate receptors exist in several areas of the brain, including the limbic system. Endogenous morphine-like substances, called *endorphines*, have been shown to exist in several mammalian species. Opioid drugs probably interact with this system directly, thereby replacing endogenous or host rewards (e.g., from food, social approval, sex, exercise) with exogenous or drug rewards. This same mechanism also may operate for other drugs. For example, condensation products of alcohol metabolism with dopamine include tetra-hydroisoquinolines (TIQs), which are also intermediary products of morphine in opium poppy (Simon, 1980).

Benzodiazepine receptors in the brain also have been demonstrated. These probably play a role in sedative abuse. Like other biologic systems, these may be influenced by genetic as well as environmental factors.

Elucidation of these neurotransmitters and their loci of action in the brain has contributed much to current thinking regarding drug abuse. It has helped us to understand why drug-dependent persons often ignore other personal and social needs to seek drug-induced effects. As the drug-abusing person becomes increasingly reliant on drugs as a means of functioning and enjoying life, other means for enhancing life diminish. Consequently, the drug-dependent person pays increasingly less attention to food, exercise, work, recreation, friends, and family.

PSYCHOLOGICAL VARIABLES

Psychological and personality variations usually accompany drug abuse, although it is difficult to ascertain the extent to which these are primary and etiologic or secondary to drug abuse. Factors that initially lead a person to start drug use may change over time so that the original causes may be replaced by different or altered factors that drive continued or increased drug use (Gottheil et al., 1983). Most clinicians and researchers agree that no one personality type predates drug abuse, although those with chronic pain, anxiety, depression, impulsiveness, and/or antisocial attitudes appear to be at greater risk. Personality characteristics of drug abusers, perhaps as much acquired as primary, typically include hostile dependence, low frustration tolerance, limited flexibility and adaptiveness, and low self-esteem.

Several theories regarding host psychology, difficult to test in either laboratory or clinical settings, remain popular but still unproven. The "anxiety-reduction theory" states that some people take drugs initially to reduce tension, especially in social settings. The "field-dependent theory" holds that drug abusers rely more on external rather than internal cues in making decisions and adjusting to life and thus are vulnerable to exogenous drug administration as a means of modifying or controlling internal emotional or physiologic states. The "career-addict hypothesis" suggests that many drug-dependent persons cease their career of abusing drugs later in life as they "mature out" of a need to rely on drugs.

Agent or Drug Factors

PHARMACOLOGIC CONSIDERATIONS

Pharmacologic properties of drugs themselves affect their propensity to be abused. Opioids and sedatives produce rapid, albeit temporary relief of anxiety, fear, and insomnia. Stimulants similarly relieve boredom, somnolence, low energy, and fatigue. Drugs that alter perceptions may aid in blocking out undesirable thoughts or feelings. Physiologic symptoms relieved by drugs of potential abuse include pain, nausea, vomiting, cramps, diarrhea, and cough.

Drugs with more rapid onset of action (e.g., heroin, amytal) tend to be preferred for abusive purposes over more delayed drugs (e.g., methadone, phenobarbital). Modes of administration also govern rate of drug effect and thereby the liability for drug abuse. Intravenous injecting, smoking, and snuffing produce quicker drug effect than subcutaneous injection or ingestion.

Tolerance and withdrawal phenomena also contribute to drug abuse syndromes. Tolerance relates to the need for increasing doses to produce the same effect; it is particularly characteristic of opioids and sedatives but also has been observed with stimulants, cannabis, and tobacco. Cessation of drug use in the tolerant individual precipitates withdrawal, a morbid state that usually persists some days to weeks (depending on the drug) in its acute phase. Subclinical abstinence symptoms can continue for months in the second phase of withdrawal. These subacute abnormalities, best described for opioid drugs, consist of altered sleep patterns, vital signs, and endocrine functions which may persist for up to a year. Anxiety symptoms, panic attacks, irritability, suspiciousness, low pain tolerance, depressive symptoms, and sometimes manic symptoms may persist for several weeks to several months following a return to abstinence. Sedative and opioid withdrawal are accompanied by weakness, anorexia, tachycardia, agitation, insomnia, irritability, social withdrawal, and remorse. Stimulant withdrawal tends to be marked by fatigue, hyperphagia, bradycardia, and somnolence. In the chronic stages of drug dependence, drug usage is often continued more to avoid the withdrawal syndrome than to obtain the acute effects of the drug (Martin and Jasinsky, 1969; Wikler, 1971).

HOST–AGENT AND ENVIRONMENT–AGENT CONSIDERATIONS

Host factors may interact with drug factors in various ways. Insomniac, anxious, rageful, or chronic pain patients may seek relief of their symptoms in opioids and sedatives. Bored, fatigued, or depressed individuals may seek relief from stimulant drugs. Those seeking a pharmacologic "time out" from their ordinary cognitions may enjoy the effect of hallucinogens. Antisocial persons may find enjoyment in the deviant social role afforded by illicit drug use.

As availability of a drug increases in the environment, the prevalence of its use tends to increase (Hughes, 1972). Availability of licit drugs (such as tobacco) may be governed by such factors as distance between sales outlets, hours of sale, and restrictions on sale to minors. Prohibition of a substance by law usually leads to decreased availability, but this is not inevitably true. In the case of prescribed drugs, availability may be due largely to prescribing habits among physicians. The greatly increased use of benzodiazepines in the late 1960s and 1970s, and their waning use in the 1980s, has hinged largely on physician prescribing practices. This was formerly true of amphetamine prescribing, which was prevalent during the 1950s and 1960s in many countries, including the United States (Smart, 1980).

Cost for drugs of abuse influence their use also. As price increases, drug use tends to decrease, even if availability is held constant. This is one argument for drug prohibition laws, which often increase the cost of drugs considerably (since they are illicit) but may not greatly reduce availability. Both price and availability affect prevalence of drug abuse.

Environmental or Social Factors

SOCIAL TRADITIONS REGARDING DRUGS OF ABUSE

Cultures that effectively prohibit or preferentially ignore certain drugs have little or no problems with them. For example, alcohol abuse is rare in certain Moslem nations that forbid beverage alcohol for religious reasons. However, sanctions against one substance do not necessarily prohibit use of other drugs. For example, certain Middle Eastern countries have economic problems with widespread importation of khat, a stimulant somewhat stronger than caffeine but weaker than the amphetamines. Since khat must be consumed within 24 hours of being harvested from a bush, its distribution of use is limited to the rapidity of accessible commercial transportation. Currently raised only around the Red Sea, it has reached England and Atlanta, Georgia, via jet aircraft.

Patterns of use for a particular drug determine the likelihood that the drug will be associated with abuse. Problematic use is more apt to attend nonritual use away from family, in a surreptitious fashion, with intoxication as a goal. Use without abuse is more apt to occur when everyone in the society is introduced to the drug experience in a family-sponsored, multigenerational, socially approved setting, with ritual feasting and celebration.

A dilemma in today's world is that only one or a few drugs can be thus woven into the fabric of a society. Families cannot enculturate (and thereby "immunize") their offspring against all drugs to which they will probably be exposed. In general, cultures approve a few mild intoxicants (e.g., tobacco, caffeine drinks, betel-areca) and perhaps a few stronger intoxicants (e.g., alcohol, peyote, cannabis) but not the more addicting or potentially psychopathologic drugs (e.g., heroin, amphetamine, phencyclidine).

DRUG LAWS

Antidrug laws began to appear several hundred years ago. Prior even to the nineteenth century, the Aztecs, Chinese emperors, and several European kingdoms enacted legislation regarding alcohol, tobacco, and opium. Antidrug legislation accelerated in the eighteenth century during a time when many new drugs as well as new routes of drug administration were spreading around the world, following the newly established international trade routes of the time. We are still in the era of drug diffusion, as modified drugs (e.g., cocaine from coca, heroin from opium) and new manufactured drugs (e.g., synthetic opioids, sedatives, hallucinogens) spread rapidly from one part of the world to another.

Regulations governing or prohibiting drug use have been most successful in countries with strong centralized power, including both rightist and leftist police states. They have been weakest in the democratic and socialist countries that rely heavily on citizen support for law enforcement. Legislation alone, without other social interventions, can exacerbate drug problems by driving the drug user into a criminal subculture.

EPIDEMIOLOGY

Methods of Study

Epidemiologic assessment is a key step in measuring the extent of drug abuse in the population and in observing the results of treatment and prevention efforts over time. Self-report, blood and urine tests, withdrawal signs, and autopsy studies have been used as measures. Sampling methods have ranged from door-to-door surveys to studies of special populations (e.g., students, medical patients, arrested persons in jail).

One special technique used for drug-abuse epidemiology is the capture–recapture technique. For example, the number of diagnosed cases may be measured (e.g., those admitted to a treatment program, say, 100 over a period of time). Then the number of drug abuse cases surfacing to another facility is measured (e.g., deaths in a morgue or arrests by the police). If any 1 person out of 10 arrested addicts is previously known to the treatment facility and 100 addicts are arrested, then an estimate of 1000 drug-abuse persons in the community would be made. Other factors that must be considered in this extrapolation technique include duration of time and ingress into or egress from the addicted subgroup.

Another special method has been the registry, most often used for opioid abusers. One central agency collects data on opioid abusers admitted for treatment or rehabilitation, seeking help at social agencies, arrested, convicted for opioid possession, or dying from an opioid-related cause.

Complications of drug abuse also have been used. These include antibodies against serum hepatitis as epidemiologic indicators (from parenteral injection) and overdose deaths from opioids and sedatives. Since many nondrug factors can influence such data, they tend to have a low stability and thus a poor reliability over time (WHO, 1980).

Rates of Drug Abuse

Rates of drug abuse often fluctuate widely over time and from place to place in the United States. An epidemiologic study in the early 1980s indicated that 5 to 6 percent of adults had drug dependence at some point in their lives (Regier et al., 1984). There have been several opioid "epidemics" in the twentieth century, especially during and after war actions. An amphetamine "epidemic" occurred in the late 1950s and early 1960s. Tobacco dependence increased progressively over the last century, first among men and more recently among women. Cannabis abuse increased markedly during the late 1960s and did not begin to decline until the early 1980s. Cocaine abuse and dependence continued at stable levels during the 1970s, increased dramatically in the early 1980s, and then decreased in the early 1990s. Although sedatives are largely obtained from physicians by prescription, growing attention has been focused on excessive use. Pharmacists annually fill tens of millions of prescriptions for benzodiazepine alone.

Demographic Characteristics

Men generally engage in drug abuse more frequently than women, although there are exceptions. Betel-areca dependence in parts of Asia and sedative abuse in North America and Europe have occurred predominantly among women. In recent years, the rates of tobacco and alcohol dependence have been increasing more among American women than men.

Since World War II, drug abuse has begun to affect teenagers to a considerable extent, although it formerly began primarily in adulthood. Especially heroin, cannabis, tobacco, volatile hydrocarbons, cocaine, and hallucinogens have had a dramatic upsurge among youths. Amphetamines and sedative abuse still tend to begin later. Elderly people have shown increased rates of alcohol and sedative abuse, often in association with death of a marital partner, isolation from friends and family in residences for the elderly, major depression, chronic pain, or disabling medical conditions. (Cohen, 1981).

EDITORS' COMMENT:

Another emerging substance of abuse, anabolic steroids, is reviewed in Chapter 17, Other Psychiatric Syndromes.

Socioeconomic variables affect the availability and type of drugs. For example, successful drug smugglers, athletes, and entertainers have had both the money for and access to such drugs as cocaine and heroin. Because of the low rate of drug interdiction by law enforcement officers, even students have been able to afford cannabis, stimulants, and sedatives on their limited funds.

Medical workers are especially liable to abuse of prescription drugs. Of 10 substance-abusing physicians, 1 is usually abusing drugs only. The remaining 9 are abusing alcohol primarily, while often abusing other drugs to offset the effects of alcohol. Drug-dependent physicians have preferred the synthetic opioids in recent years, perhaps because these drugs have been incorrectly touted as less addicting than the opium-based drugs (e.g., morphine). Nurses, pharmacists, and dentists show similar patterns. Among younger health professionals, drug abuse with illicit or "street" drugs has appeared in recent years.

PATHOLOGY

Pathologic consequences from drug abuse vary widely with the drug, dosage, and duration of use. Route of administration is also an important consideration.

Opioids

Although opioid drugs differ considerably in dosage and duration of action, the maximal potencies of the stronger opioid drugs (e.g., morphine, heroin, fentanyl, methadone) are quite similar. Weaker opioids (e.g., codeine, propoxyphene) cannot equal them, even in large doses. Some opioids, such as pentazocine, have mixed agonist–antagonist effects. In order to ameliorate the antagonist effects, drug abusers may take such drugs with antihistamines. The recently popular "T's and blue's" among opioid dependents consist of Talwin along with an antihistamine in a blue capsule.

Opioids can relieve pain, anxiety, cough, and diarrhea. Especially in the naive user, they produce nausea and vomiting. While acute doses may relieve social and sexual inhibition, chronic use leads paradoxically to social withdrawal and decreased libido. Tolerance to analgesia begins with the first dose, so opioids are excellent for acute, severe pain but poor for chronic or recurrent pain.

Acute effects include meiosis or pinpoint pupils (which occurs with most but not all opioids), constipation, hypotension, and lethargy. Coma and possibly death by respiratory depression result from overdose. The withdrawal syndrome, beginning 4 to 12 hours after the last dose (depending on the drug), consists of agitation, piloerection, dilated pupils, muscle aches, and abdominal cramps. A subclinical withdrawal syndrome consisting of sleep disturbance, irritability, vital sign fluctuations, and autonomic system lability may persist for several months in tolerant individuals (Wikler, 1971; Jaffee, 1980).

Sedatives

These drugs include the benzodiazepines, barbiturates, glutethimide, methaqualone, chloral hydrate, paraldehyde, and ethchorvynol. Although showing cross-tolerance with alcohol, they are synthetic and chemically dissimilar to each other. Sedatives with rapid onset of action tend to be abused more readily. Longer-acting sedatives produce a more stable withdrawal regimen.

Sedative drugs are more apt to be abused by those presenting to physicians with symptoms of insomnia, palpitations, tachycardia, headache, epigastric burning, or similar psychophysiologic symptoms of anxiety. Much sedative abuse in the United States has an iatrogenic component. Careful psychiatric assessment and careful monitoring of sedative prescribing are key strategies in reducing sedative abuse.

Duration of action and margin of safety differ widely among the sedatives. Like the opioids and alcohol, they can produce tolerance if taken chronically in increasing doses. Acute effects include incoordination, dysarthria, lethargy, and somnolence; overdose leads to coma and death by respiratory depression. The withdrawal syndrome consists variably of tachycardia, fever, hypertension, headache, agitation, and tremor. Seizures, confusion, delusions, and hallucinations occur in severe cases. Onset of withdrawal can occur within several hours after the last dose in the case of short-acting barbiturates or within several days with the long-acting diazepines (Smith and Wesson, 1971; Maletzky and Klotter, 1976).

EDITORS' COMMENT

Early experience with the barbiturates revealed tolerance to both the sedative and the therapeutic effects of these drugs in the treatment of sleep disorders and anxiety symptoms. A recent assessment entitled, *Benzodiazepine Dependence, Toxicity, and Abuse* (Washington, American Psychiatric Association, 1990), suggests that the development of tolerance to the sedative and psychomotor effects of benzodiazepines has been found. The question, however, remains whether the data support tolerance of the effects of benzodiazepines on the symptoms of anxiety and panic attacks. Such a tolerance could lead to an increase in dosage and abuse. Here, the findings are conflicting. Some researchers have shown a dose reduction over time, and others have observed small increases. These increases are small enough that using benzodiazepines over the long-term does not lead to abuse. Thus, though there might be some tolerance to the anxiolytic effects of the drugs, these are not likely to cause any clinical difficulty.

Amphetamines and Similar Drugs

These drugs (including methylphenidate) are often abused by night workers, those doing prolonged repetitive work (e.g., truck driving), or chronically dysthymic individuals. Formerly obtained primarily from physicians, most amphetamines today come from illegal sources.

Amphetamines facilitate the release of nor-epinephrine, thereby increasing pulse, blood pressure, metabolic rate, and sometimes temperature. Stimulant effects on the central nervous system include mydriasis, tachycardia, elevated mood, heightened self-confidence, alertness, and wakefulness with a decrease in rapid-eye-movement (REM) sleep.

Tolerance and increased daily doses occur in chronic users. Confusion, panic, and paranoia may ensue, and a psychotic state similar to schizophrenia or mania can persist for days, weeks, or months. Hyperthermia, hypertension, arrythmias, convulsions, and cerebrovascular accidents accompany overdose. Withdrawal consists of lethargy and increased REM sleep. Depression often appears following withdrawal; this may be a withdrawal effect, emergence of a primary depression, or some combination of both (Ellinswood, 1967).

Cocaine

Like amphetamines, cocaine abuse is apt to ensue in the user who is bored, fatigued, or depressed. Since the intoxicant effect is extremely short compared with those of other drugs of abuse, the user may snort, smoke, or inject drugs several times an hour to obtain the drug effect. Under such circumstances, the cost of a cocaine habit mounts readily. The heavy user may become financially destitute or enter an illegal occupation (e.g., drug smuggling or selling, burglary, prostitution) to obtain the drug (Cohen, 1981).

One form of cocaine is the hydrochloride, taken by injection or snorting. The paste form, used for smoking, involves an extraction from coca leaves using kerosene and sulfuric acid. Cocaine potentiates catecholamine effect by interfering with reuptake. Its effects are similar to those of amphetamine, but with a half-life persisting over minutes rather than hours. Certain complications resemble those of amphetamine, such as paranoia, hallucinations, or hypertension.

Cannabis

Although numerous psychoactive compounds exist in cannabis, most of its effect appears due to delta-9-tetrahydrocannabinal. Potency of cannabis preparation varies with proximity to the equator, climate, plant species, part of the plant consumed, and procedures to increase potency (e.g., hashish). It may be consumed by eating or smoking. Effect persists for a few to several hours, depending on dose, tolerance, and pattern of use.

Many people appear able to consume small amounts of cannabis at infrequent intervals (i.e., weekly or monthly) without ill effect. Vulnerable individuals may experience hallucinations, delusions, or confusion at low doses. With chronic, heavy use, the percentage of impaired users probably increases.

Intoxication involves aspects of both stimulation and depression, sympathetic and parasympathetic manifestations. These include dry mouth, increased appetite, tachycardia, injected conjunctivae, and relaxation. Coordination for simple tasks is not impaired at lower doses, although balance and complex tasks become increasingly impeded with higher doses. Minutes may be perceived as hours. This may contribute to the enhanced sexual enjoyment reported by some. Short-term memory loss leads to disjointed thinking, with consequent silliness, social withdrawal, or panic.

Some tolerance occurs with chronic use, but a distinct withdrawal syndrome has not been described. Since tetrahydrocannabinal is stored in fat, chronic users may demonstrate cannabis effect and excrete the drug for days or even weeks following the last use (Jaffee, 1980).

Tobacco

Whether consumed by smoking, snuffing, or chewing, tobacco's psychoactive effect is largely due to nicotine. Like cocaine, the half-life of nicotine is brief (under an hour). Many carcinogens exist in tobacco. Nicotine, which mimics the effects of acetylcholine, acts as a mild stimulant. Although smoking produces almost instantaneous effect, absorption after oral ingestion is slow. Chewing produces intermediate onset. Effects include increased heart rate, gastric atony, and peripheral vasoconstriction. Large doses may produce nausea, emesis, and convulsions. One cigarette ingested by a small child can be lethal. Withdrawal effects include bradycardia, irritability, and increased appetite.

Heavy smokers maintain plasma nicotine levels by smoking tobacco about every half hour. Tobacco consumption in dependent persons may be linked to such biologic events as waking up, eating, and bowel movements. Smoking also reinforces activities (e.g., meeting with friends, sexual encounters). If the nicotine content in a cigarette is decreased, dependent smokers adjust by increasing their inhalations.

As a mild intoxicant with few or mild effects on cognition, mood, and coordination, tobacco rarely produces acute problems. However, it can produce numerous, sometimes catastrophic damage to health, including heart disease, emphysema, Berger's disease, and lung cancer. Health complications increase markedly after 20 pack-years of smoking (i.e., one pack per day, per year, over 20 years). Although tobacco dependence is notoriously difficult to reverse permanently, physician recommendations to cease tobacco use are effective (Russell, 1971).

Caffeine

In lower doses, caffeine reduces fatigue and enhances mental activity while causing some tachycardia, vasodilation, and diuresis. It produces these effects by stimulating catecholamine release (Bellet et al., 1969). Higher doses (i.e., over 600 mg/d) may produce excitement, agitation, headache, irritability, and insomnia. Withdrawal symptoms in high-dose users (i.e., over 1000–1200 mg/d) can include fatigue and somnolence (Dreisbach and Pfeiffer, 1943; Greden, 1981). Caffeine is present in many common beverages, including coffee (120–150 mg), tea (50–80 mg), cocoa, colas (50 mg), and other soft drinks. It is also present in many over-the-counter and prescription drugs taken for pain, appetite suppression, and the common cold.

Volatile Hydrocarbons

These substances have acute psychotoxic effects similar to alcohol, but with a shorter half-life, often under an hour. Effects include ataxia, dysparthesia, elation, and silliness. Special populations such as prisoners, industrial workers, or children sniff them, since they are available, inexpensive, and short acting. Aerosols, glue, cleaning and industrial solvents,

and paint thinners can produce hepatic, renal, hematologic, or neurologic damage depending on the chemical, pattern of use, and individual propensity. Early symptoms of chronic use, which may come to the attention of a pediatrician or psychiatrist, are irritability, declining academic or occupational performance, memory loss, and personality change. Health students and professionals have sometimes abused anesthetic agents, especially nitrous oxide. Amyl nitrate use for sexual enhancement has led to chronic abuse, especially in recent years. Endemic and epidemic use has prevailed among children over the last three decades. Originally reported in American Indian and Hispanic communities, it now occurs also in Afro-American and white communities (Easson, 1962; Lowry, 1979; Prockop, 1977).

Phencyclidine (PCP)

This versatile drug may be ingested, snuffed, smoked, or injected. Its effects are variable, so it may produce relaxation or panic, hypotension or hypertension, decreased reflexes or status epilepticus. In general, however, it potentiates adrenergic effects. Impurities from illicit production may cause anticholinergic effects. Body-image distortions, agitation, and hallucinations are common in PCP users coming to clinical attention. Vertical or horizontal nystagmus, muscular rigidity, and dystonic reactions are clues to the diagnosis. Half-life is relatively short, but after-effects can continue over hours or a few days due to enterohepatic recirculation. Acute and chronic users may present to emergency rooms with various psychiatric syndromes from panic attack, to mania, to schizophreniform psychosis, to delirium (Cohen, 1981).

Hallucinogens

These include natural substances (e.g., peyote, morning glory seeds) and synthetic compounds (e.g., D-lysergic acid, or LSD). Altered perceptual states are produced; panic, hallucinations, and delusions may occur. While the half-lives of these drugs are only a few hours, psychic effects may persist for 6 to 12 hours. Hallucinosis can continue for a few to several days in unusual cases. In vulnerable individuals, first episodes or recurrences of mania, schizophreniform psychosis, delusional disorder, or schizophrenia may ensue. Physical manifestations are few, except when anticholinergic properties are present (Cohen, 1981).

CLINICAL PICTURE

The Great Imitator

The clinical picture depends on the drug, duration of abuse, route of administration, the individual's nutrition, associated medical and psychiatric problems, and socioeconomic impairment. Impairment may be minimal, with early or mild signs or symptoms, or so severe that signs and symptoms irrefutably support the diagnosis. Patients may hide, alter, or accurately describe the drug use and its associated problems, depending on their openness, wish for help, and extent of discomfort. A key factor is the clinician's comfort and skill in aiding patients to relate their history. A nonjudgmental attitude toward patients is critical. Clinical skill as well as judgment in managing drug abuse cases requires supervised clinical training. Without training and experience, the clinician is not likely to perceive the clinical picture accurately nor to manage the case in a supportive and therapeutic fashion.

Substance abuse has been called the "great imitator" of our time for good reason. It may present with medical, psychiatric, or surgical pictures. Drug abusers are found in medical settings more frequently than expected from their number in the population. Drug-related problems are proportionately more common among inpatients than among outpatients. Patients may present quite early in their course or in severely advanced stages. The problem may be acute or chronic, life-threatening or minor, readily discerned or vague and difficult to define (Dupont et al., 1979).

Data Collection

Drug-abuse patients usually seek clinical help in response to some coercive force, either external (e.g., family, work supervisor) or internal (e.g., malaise, depression). An important step in management involves delineating this coercive force. Complicating this process is patient's frequent lack of awareness regarding the relationship between the current problem and the drug use. Another obstacle is the patient's tendency to blame others for the current problem rather than to take responsibility for the problem.

Since drug abuse may present with various surgical, medical, or psychiatric problems, the clinician will want to inquire routinely about each patient's use of drugs. In order to rule drug abuse in or out, the physician must know each patient's drug use type (if present), dose, duration, and pattern of use and route of administration.

Drug-abusing patients typically do not volunteer symptoms indicative of depression, anxiety, panic, or psychosis. Specific inquiry is necessary.

Formal mental status examination may reveal unsuspected deficits in orientation, memory, or cognition. Physical examination can demonstrate evidence of parenteral injection (e.g., venous tracks, skin-popping scars), chronic smoking (e.g., rales and rhonchi), malnutrition, infectious diseases, and traumatic sequelae. Neurologic findings (e.g., ataxia, dysarthria, pupillary changes), autonomic signs (e.g., flushing, perspiration, piloerection), and vital sign abnormalities (e.g., tachycardia, hypertension) provide valuable clues. Table 15-1 lists the signs associated with various drugs.

CASE REPORT

A 14-year-old girl had been sniffing gasoline for about 2 hours per day, two to four times per week, over the previous 3 years. She presented after having written a suicide note. Formerly an A-B student, her current school grades were D's and F's. Mental status examination revealed impaired orientation, memory impairment, concrete thinking, and extreme irritability.

Analysis of the Findings

Acute drug-related problems are generally related to pharmacologic actions of the drug itself or the route of administration. These include intoxication, overdose, withdrawal, and such medical emergencies as agitated delirium, malignant hyperthermia, or anaphylaxis. Unlike these acute problems, the initial problems associated with chronic use tend to be due to psychosocial complications. These are elicited by a careful history but may not be evident on physical examination. Socioeconomic deterioration, increasing family alienation and social withdrawal, progressive (rather than static) sociopathy, and legal problems should raise the index of suspicion for drug abuse. This is the opposite of many other disorders in which early manifestations are subjective and historical, while objective biomedical signs appear in later stages.

Special clinical pictures depend on the drug and the setting. Amotivational syndromes and decline in grades are seen among adolescents and young adults. Families report anger, oppositional behavior, and personality change. Monday morning absenteeism, reduced productivity, and injuries occur in the workplace. Family members and friends may observe social withdrawal or secretive behavior. Nurses or physicians may note drug-seeking behaviors, with symptomatic complaints out of proportion to physical or laboratory findings.

CLINICAL COURSE

The typical course of untreated, chronic drug abuse is deterioration over a period of years, often with periods of relative stabilization or brief improvement followed by further deterioration. Acute problems associated with recent drug abuse may cause the disorder to be self-limiting if the consequences motivate the user to moderate or cease drug usage. However, spontaneous abstinence from drugs occurs infrequently among those with recurrent episodes of drug abuse or with chronic drug dependence. Death or lifelong disability may complicate the picture even before drug dependence is established (Vaillant, 1970, 1973).

Duration of course, like the clinical picture, varies with the drug, route of administration, and various host and environmental factors. Other things being equal, routes with rapid drug onset (i.e., injection, smoking, snuffing) hasten the mor-

TABLE 15-1. *Drug Signs*

Vital signs	Intoxication						Overdose						Withdrawal			
	Alcohol	Stimulants	Sedatives	Opiates	Hallucinogens	Phencyclidine	Alcohol	Stimulants	Sedatives	Opiates	Hallucinogens	Phencyclidine	Alcohol	Stimulants	Sedatives	Opiates
Circulatory collapse							●		●	●	●		●		●	●
Hypertension		●				●	●		●	●			●		●	
Hyperthermia		●			●		●				●		●		●	
Orthostatic hypotension							●		●	●			●		●	●
Respiration, slow and shallow							●		●	●						
Tachycardia		●			●	●	●				●	●	●			●

APPEARANCE, BEHAVIOR, MENTAL STATUS

Vital signs	Alcohol	Stimulants	Sedatives	Opiates	Hallucinogens	Phencyclidine	Alcohol	Stimulants	Sedatives	Opiates	Hallucinogens	Phencyclidine	Alcohol	Stimulants	Sedatives	Opiates
Affect, labile	●	●	●	●	●	●	●	●	●	●	●	●	●	●	●	●
Comprehension, slow	●		●	●	●	●	●		●	●	●	●	●	●	●	
Delirium	●	●	●			●	●	●	●	●	●	●	●		●	
Delusions	●	●	●	●		●	●	●	●	●	●	●	●		●	
Depressed mood	●		●				●		●				●	●	●	●
Euphoria	●	●	●	●	●	●										
Hostile, assaultive	●	●	●			●		●			●	●			●	●
Irritability	●	●	●			●		●			●	●			●	●
Lethargy	●		●	●			●		●	●				●		
Memory, poor	●		●	●		●	●		●	●			●		●	●
Restlessness		●			●	●	●	●			●	●	●		●	●
Skin picking		●		●									●			
Suspiciousness		●			●	●	●				●	●	●	●	●	
Sweating							●						●		●	●
Talkativeness	●	●	●	●			●									
Vomiting	●				●		●			●	●	●	●		●	●
Yawning			●													●

EYES, EARS, NOSE, AND THROAT

Vital signs	Alcohol	Stimulants	Sedatives	Opiates	Hallucinogens	Phencyclidine	Alcohol	Stimulants	Sedatives	Opiates	Hallucinogens	Phencyclidine	Alcohol	Stimulants	Sedatives	Opiates
Coryza																●
Lacrimation																
Mouth, dry		●			●			●			●					
Nystagmus	●		●		●	●	●		●				●	●		
Pupils, dilated		●					●	●	●	●	●					●
Pupils, pinpoint				●						●						
Rhinorrhea														●		

NEUROLOGICAL EXAMINATION

Vital signs	Alcohol	Stimulants	Sedatives	Opiates	Hallucinogens	Phencyclidine	Alcohol	Stimulants	Sedatives	Opiates	Hallucinogens	Phencyclidine	Alcohol	Stimulants	Sedatives	Opiates
Analgesia to pinprick	●		●	●		●	●	●	●	●		●				
Coma							●		●	●		●				
Convulsions			●				●	●	●		●	●	●	●		●
Dysmetria	●		●	●		●	●		●	●		●				
Facial grimacing						●		●								
Hypotonia	●		●	●			●		●	●				●		
Muscle spasms (rigidity)						●		●					●	●	●	●
Reflexes, hyperactive		●				●		●			●	●	●		●	●
Speech, slurred	●		●	●		●	●		●	●		●				
Stare, blank	●		●	●	●	●	●		●	●	●	●				
Tremor	●	●	●						●		●		●		●	●

SKIN

Vital signs	Alcohol	Stimulants	Sedatives	Opiates	Hallucinogens	Phencyclidine	Alcohol	Stimulants	Sedatives	Opiates	Hallucinogens	Phencyclidine	Alcohol	Stimulants	Sedatives	Opiates
Flushing	●		●		●		●	●			●		●		●	
Piloerection (gooseflesh)																●

Adapted from Westermeyer J: Primer on Chemical Dependency: A Clinical Guide to Alcohol and Drug Problems. Baltimore, Williams & Wilkins, 1976.

bid course over slower routes of administration (e.g., ingestion, chewing). Drugs with shorter half-lives (e.g., heroin, amytal, cocaine) lead to a more rapid course than those with longer half-lives (e.g., opium, diazepam, amphetamine). More potent drugs (e.g., morphine, methadone) hasten and increase the morbid effects over weaker drugs in the same category (e.g., codeine, propoxyphene). Some drugs usually produce medical complications (e.g., tobacco) or neuropsychiatric complications (e.g., phencyclidine) as their first manifestation, while others are more apt initially to produce psychosocial consequences (e.g., sedatives, opioids). Despite these differences, most drug-dependent patients present for treatment within 3 years of initiating their drug abuse, although some individuals may go as long as 10 years or longer without treatment.

Age at onset influences the course, so opioid dependence beginning at age 15 affects the patient's life course differently from opioid dependence beginning at age 35. Younger individuals have not yet had the opportunity to complete their education, learn an occupation, become employed, marry, have children, or otherwise establish some social competency. Older drug abusers coming to treatment usually have more biomedical problems and social isolation; younger drug abusers gradually experience more legal, occupational, and marital problems. In many studies, women show a more rapid progression than men, but this is not always so (Wilsnack, 1982).

Individual differences also exist. In one large survey of opioid-dependent subjects, I encountered one subject who presented initially for treatment after 3 months of dependence and another who presented for his first treatment experience after 45 years of dependence. Despite these extremes, it was unusual for most opioid-dependent subjects to have their first treatment before 1 year or after 10 years of opioid dependence.

Tables 15-2 to 15-6 describe arbitrary phases in the course of drug abuse. Course progression is not always as consistent as shown in the tables, however. A patient may show early changes in some areas along with more advanced changes in other areas.

Treatment usually, but not always, alters the natural course of drug abuse. In general, treatment earlier in the course tends to be more effective and less costly. Later treatment, especially after occupational loss and alienation from family, is less apt to be effective. Even in advanced cases, however, treatment often reduces the patient's morbidity and may set the stage for eventual recovery.

Acute phases of recovery, from medical, psychiatric, or social crises, usually take place over several weeks. The intermediate phase of recovery from autonomic instability, remorse, and social isolation occurs over several months. Psychological well-being, social fulfillment, and occupational stability in the final phase of recovery may require a few to several years. Brief but increasingly less frequent return to drug abuse often persists during the early months of recovery. Although pharmacologic factors greatly influence the pretreatment course, the posttreatment relapse rates for heroin, alcohol, and tobacco (in the absence of ongoing outpatient treatment) are remarkably similar, as shown in Figure 15-1.

LABORATORY FINDINGS

Laboratory tests for drug abuse are of two kinds. One set of tests involves direct assessment of drugs or drug action in the body, such as drug levels in body fluids or administration of an antagonist to precipitate withdrawal (e.g., naloxone for opiate dependence). Another set of tests involves indirect biochemical, physiologic, and psychological tests to

TABLE 15-2. *Phases of Chemical Dependency: Behavioral Factors*

Characteristic	Early phase: problematic usage	Middle phase: chronic dependence, addiction	Late phase: deterioration
Drug usage	Increasing amounts and frequency of use	"Titer" or "binge" usage; attempts at abstinence	Continuous usage; uses "substitute" intoxicants
Control over usage	Begins attempts to decrease amounts or frequency of use	Begins to lose control (takes more than intended or for a longer period than intended)	Loses control most of the time
Drug-related behavior	Seeks occasions to use; chooses friends who use heavily; may begin to be secretive about usage	Increased need to use at specific times and places; develops ingenuity at obtaining, paying for, hiding, and using drug	Compulsive usage, despite many problems associated with usage and decreased enjoyment from drug or alcohol; plans daily activities around usage
Drug effects on behavior	Episodic intoxication, dysarthria, emotional lability; attempts to hide drug or alcohol effects from others	Impairment between intoxication episodes: trite expressions and "non sequiturs" prevail in conversation; fatigue; decreased productivity	Poor grooming, disheveled dress; lack of interest in appearance; unconcern with opinions of others

TABLE 15-3. *Phases of Chemical Dependency: Psychologic Factors*

Characteristic	Early phase: problematic usage	Middle phase: chronic dependence, addiction	Late phase: deterioration
Motivation	Uses to enjoy, build up confidence, relieve insomnia, anxiety, etc.; use becomes increasingly important	Uses to feel normal; use is as important as family, friends, work	Enjoys usage less, but cannot stop; use becomes the central element of person's life
Emotional concomitants	Mood swings related to usage: anger, remorse, anxiety; shamed or anxious regarding usage; feels weak, remorseful	Personality change, increasing emotional lability; ambivalent about usage; feels guilty, resentful, inadequate, inferior	Erratic, suspicious, often apathetic; defensive regarding usage; feels alone, deserted
Cognitive processes	Obsesses regarding next usage; reduced interests and ambition; focuses thoughts and conversation on chemical usage	Increasing self-pity, deteriorating self-image; self-deception regarding usage and its effects; loses sense of time	Confused, projects own problems onto others; unable to conceptualize current status objectively
Judgment, insight	Begins to exercise poor judgment; still able to extricate self from most problems; episodic insight and concern with drug or alcohol usage	Large proportion of decisions lead to problems; problem solving increasingly ineffective; avoids being insightful, although capable of insight	Extremely poor judgment in most matters; unable to solve own problems; is not insightful even during abstinent intervals

TABLE 15-4. *Phases of Chemical Dependency: Social Factors*

Characteristic	Early phase: problematic usage	Middle phase: chronic dependence, addiction	Late phase: deterioration
Interpersonal relationships	Changes associates, from abstainers and moderate users to heavy users	Alienates others by arguing, embarrassing, taking advantage; breaks promises, lies	Manipulates others to obtain drug or alcohol; compensatory bragging
Family	Argues with family over usage; spends less time at home; neglects family emotionally	Abuses family by lying, stealing, or fighting; spends most of time away from home	Alienated from family; lives away from family
Employment	"Monday morning" absenteeism; conflict with boss	Decreased job efficiency; changes jobs often or is fired; decreasing job prestige; holds jobs for shorter periods	Day labor; unemployed, on relief or social welfare
Residence	Stable residence; lives with others	Begins moving from place to place; loses roommates, family members	Lower socioeconomic neighborhood; lives alone
School*	Decreasing grades; complaints from teachers	Suspension from school; school dropout	Requires special educational and rehabilitation facilities
Legal effects	May have legal problems; driving while intoxicated, disorderly, assault	Usually has legal problems and large attorney fees; may be litigious	Defaults on contractual obligations; may be imprisoned for property offenses, manslaughter
Finances	Spends family funds on drug or alcohol; may take extra job to support habit; may become extravagant	Spends 1/4 to 1/2 of annual income on drug or alcohol; heavily in debt, bankruptcy	Spends most of income on drugs or alcohol; destitute
Social affiliations	Discontinues social activities not involving usage (e.g., church, hobby, theater, sports)	Drops formal group affiliations (e.g., union, guild, club); begins short-lived companionship with chemically dependent persons	Becomes an involuntary client of social institutions

*For chemically dependent persons of school age.

assess the extent of impairment produced by drugs. These tests augment but cannot substitute for a thorough history, psychiatric interview, mental status assessment, and physical examination. Another important assessment technique is the "test of time," in which the individual is observed and reassessed over time in order to assess the severity of the condition and the potential for recovery.

Many drugs of abuse can be found in urine for 12 to 48 hours after the last dose and sometimes longer in the case of chronic use (e.g., cannabis). Qualitative urine tests are useful for screening in

TABLE 15-5. *Phases of Chemical Dependency: Biomedical Factors*

Characteristic	Early phase: problematic usage	Middle phase: chronic dependence, addiction	Late phase: deterioration
Pharmacology	Tolerance increases; larger doses used to relax, relieve insomnia or other symptoms	Withdrawal effects; blackout (for alcohol); morning or daytime usage to alleviate withdrawal	Decreased tolerance (early onset of intoxication or blackout); delirium tremens or withdrawal seizure (with alcohol or sedatives)
Common health problems	Injuries: vehicular or industrial, accidents, falls, burns	Infections: respiratory, urogenital, skin; injuries; accidental overdosage; suicide attempts	Parenteral users: septicemia, pulmonary edema, endocarditis; alcoholics: cirrhosis, pancreatitis, myocarditis; violence: injuries, homicide, suicide; nutritional problems: vitamin, protein, mineral deficiency
Sexual effects	May initially enhance sexual function	Sexual problems: impotence, frigidity, promiscuity or extramarital liaisons, venereal disease	Difficulty obtaining sexual partner; purchase of sexual services; loss of interest in sex; prostitution to obtain funds for drug
Common symptoms	Insomnia, boredom, chronic anxiety, headache, palpitation, tachycardia, flatulence, belching, cramps, epigastric distress, irritability, puffy face or extremities	Sweating, apprehension, decreased libido, visual disturbances, myalgia, malaise, obesity, diarrhea, weight change (loss or gain), memory lapses, weak, fatigues easily, "dry heaves," depression, panic, fears	Bad taste, impotence, halitosis, cachexia, persistent abdominal pain, seizures

TABLE 15-6. *Phases of Chemical Dependency: Treatment Approaches*

Characteristic	Early phase: problematic usage	Middle phase: chronic dependence, addiction	Late phase: deterioration
Prognosis without treatment	Some spontaneously improve, some progress to later stages (percentages unknown)	Small percentage (<10%) spontaneously improve; most progress to later stage	Virtually no spontaneous improvement; a few "plateau"; most deteriorate rapidly
Most effective treatment modalities	Self-help groups; marital, family therapy; selective use of pharmacotherapy for 1–2 years (e.g., antidepressants, Antabuse); partial hospitalization (e.g., day only, evening only, weekend only)	Initial residential treatment: hospital unit, therapeutic community, halfway house, followed by some outpatient treatment methods as in "early phase"	Long-term residential treatment: special long-term units, nursing home, quarterway house, followed by "middle" and "early" treatment methods in selected cases
Prognosis with treatment	Optimal: 60%–80% "significantly improved" at 1 year posttreatment	Fairly good: 40%–60% "significantly improved" at 1 year posttreatment	Poor: 10%–20% improved at 1 year; high mortality and morbidity rate in remainder
Cooperation with treatment	Willing to undertake a prolonged period of abstinence, see physician regularly, follow treatment recommendations	Does not enter treatment unless pressured by family, employer, court, friends, physician	Will not undertake abstinence voluntarily; must be coerced by society (e.g., incarceration, legal commitment into treatment)

high-risk situations, such as emergency rooms, orthopedic and psychiatric hospital admissions, and certain target groups (e.g., trauma victims, brittle diabetics, treatment failures). Quantitative blood measures are usually required only for special instances, such as management of overdose or forensic evaluation. Naloxone challenge, specific for the diagnosis of opioid dependence, consists of administering parenteral naloxone and observing for the opioid withdrawal syndrome.

Other laboratory tests not specifically measuring drugs can aid in assessing the severity of the drug-abuse problem. Acute intoxication or recent withdrawal may produce abnormalities on the electroencephalogram, which can suggest specific drug effects to the experienced electroencephalographer.

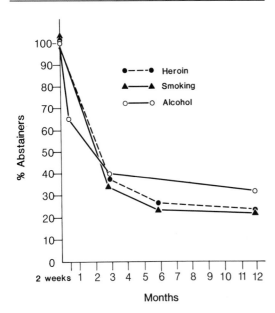

FIGURE 15-1. *Relapse Rate Over Time for Heroin, Smoking, and Alcohol. From: Hunt, W.A., Barnett, L.W., Branch, L.G.: Relapse rates in addiction programs. J. Clin. Psychol. 27:455–456, 1971.*

Biochemical tests for renal and hepatic function reflect drug-related tissue damage to these organs. Vitamin (e.g., carotene or folic acid), serum iron, and serum protein levels can reveal nutritional neglect. With chronic drug abuse, many patients experience mild to moderate endocrine dysfunctions reflected in thyroid tests, electrolyte disturbances, hyperglycemia, or hypoglycemia and/or an abnormal dexamethasone suppression test. Chronic smoking produces physiologic changes in respiratory dead space, vital capacity, rate of timed expiration, and blood gases. Parenteral injection of drugs can give rise to positive blood cultures, an elevated sedimentation rate, high white blood cell count, or an increased gamma globulin fraction in the serum protein. Depending on the psychiatric picture, abnormalities may occur on personality tests (e.g., the Minnesota Multiphasic Personality Inventory), intelligence tests (e.g., Wechsler Intelligence Scales), and organicity tests (e.g., Bender-Gestalt). Traumatic injuries (from fights or falls) may show up on x-rays as healing fractures of the ribs or extremities.

Response to treatment can be assessed by following both the first category of tests (e.g., direct drug measures) and the second category (e.g., tests of impairment or secondary complications), especially when these have been abnormal previously.

DIFFERENTIAL DIAGNOSIS

Differentiating drug abuse from other psychiatric disorders is often difficult. Substance abuse and psychiatric disorder coexist in one-quarter to one-third of psychiatric inpatients and in about the same proportion of substance-abuse patients. Drug abuse may develop as an attempt at self-treatment for a preexisting disorder (e.g., stimulant abuse for depression, sedative abuse for anxiety or mania). Or secondary psychiatric disturbances (e.g., depression, panic attacks) may appear during the course of drug abuse. Secondary sociopathy may attend the disinhibiting effects of certain drugs. Hostile-dependent behavior is a common secondary behavioral manifestation that usually clears with successful recovery.

Drug effects may mimic psychiatric disorder. For example, caffeine, cocaine, or amphetamine intoxication can produce symptoms like those of anxiety or mania (Greden, 1974). Withdrawal from these drugs may resemble depression or, less often, paranoia. Acute cannabis, phencyclidine, or hallucinogen intoxication may present clinically as acute schizophreniform psychosis, manic psychosis, or organic delirium.

Drugs also may precipitate psychiatric syndromes, which persist well beyond the drug effect in the body. Acute or chronic use of cocaine, amphetamine, cannabis, phencyclidine, and the hallucinogens may bring about a lengthy illness indistinguishable from schizophrenia or bipolar illness. In some cases, the disorder (once successfully treated) does not recur. In other cases, the disorder may recur even without subsequent drug abuse, as in this case:

A 19-year-old college student became acutely and floridly psychotic following her first use of hashish. She failed to respond to high doses of neuroleptics prescribed over several weeks but did recover with a course of ECT and subsequent neuroleptic treatment. A discharge diagnosis of schizoaffective schizophrenia was made. Over the subsequent year, her medication was reduced without incident. She later completed graduate school, worked for a few years, and married. Within weeks following the birth of her third child, at age 31, she developed insomnia, racing thoughts, euphoric mood, grandiose plans, and poor judgment (but without hallucinations or delusions). Neuroleptics (in low doses) along with lithium, prescribed on an outpatient basis, led to resolution of her symptoms over several weeks.

In this case it appears that drug abuse may have precipitated as well as exacerbated the first episode. The second episode, without drug abuse, was milder and responded more readily to treatment. The patient's course suggests that hashish alone did not produce the first illness but rather precipitated the illness in a person with a premorbid potential for affective disorder.

Drug effect from opioids, sedatives, stimulants, cannabis, phencyclidine, and the hallucinogens, as well as the volatile hydrocarbons, may produce an organic brain syndrome, with confusion and delirium. Chronic organic brain syndrome is less common but can occur. Certain volatile hydrocarbons can, with chronic use, produce dementia pictures similar to alcohol. Sedative and opioid abusers also may demonstrate it, probably from recurrent hypoxia secondary to respiratory depression. The milder, although dependency-producing drugs—such as caffeine and tobacco—do not directly produce chronic brain syndromes, although they may indirectly do so as a result of secondary medical complications (e.g., hypertension, emphysema).

TREATMENT

Drug-Related Emergencies

Intoxication is managed simply by observing and protecting the individual until the drug is metabolized or excreted. It is important to ensure that the patient does not injure self or others while the drug is being metabolized and/or excreted. Involuntary hospitalization may be necessary for 2 or 3 days during this phase.

Overdose is managed on medical or psychiatric units, depending on the nature of the problem and the type of drug. Specific antidotes are available for two drug types liable to abuse: opioids and anticholinergics. Naloxone for opioid overdose and physostigmine for anticholinergic overdose share two common features. First, dosage must be individualized for each patient, and second, repeated doses at 2- to 3-hour intervals are necessary because their duration of action is considerably shorter than those of many drugs of abuse (particularly when taken in large doses). Gastric lavage and charcoal remain cornerstones for most drug overdoses. Rarely, dialysis may be necessary for sedative overdose; very high blood levels, rapidly progressing stupor, and depression of vital signs comprise indications for dialysis. Acidifying the urine hastens the excretion of phencyclidine and amphetamines, while alkalinization aids excretion of some barbiturates (Bourne, 1976).

Withdrawal treatment hastens recovery, reduces mortality, and can aid in establishing the doctor–patient relationship. It also may induce the suffering patient, still ambivalent about giving up drug dependence, to enter treatment. Opioid and sedative withdrawal are managed by using one or another drug that is cross-tolerant with the drug being abused. Some clinicians use tricyclic drugs for stimulant withdrawal. The first step consists of administering enough drug to make the patient comfortable, even to the point of mild intoxication. For patients in severe withdrawal, most clinicians prefer to administer the first dose intravenously, since oral ingestion or subcutaneous injection of the drug may not be well absorbed. The half-life of the drug used should be at least as long as that of the drug being abused, and preferably longer (e.g., phenobarbital for seconal dependence, methadone for heroin dependence). Otherwise, the patient will be in and out of withdrawal, frequent doses will be necessary, and the withdrawal will be stormy. For barbiturate withdrawal, some clinicians prefer to administer a shorter-acting drug initially in case the patient requires respiratory assistance with the stabilizing dose. It is important to remember that 30 mg phenobarbital is equivalent to 100 mg seconal and pentobarbital. Duration of the withdrawal is shorter for short-acting drugs and longer for longer-acting drugs. For short-acting drugs, such as amytal or heroin, 5- to 10-day withdrawal regimens are adequate for resolution of acute symptoms. Intermediate-acting drugs, such as seconal or opium, require 10 to 20 days depending on the degree of dependence and the patient's medical condition. Longer withdrawal regimens, lasting up to several weeks or a few months, may be needed for the long-acting drugs, such as diazepam and ethchorvynol. Doses should be administered on a routine basis rather than as requested by the patient. For example, a 20 percent daily reduction would cover a 5-day withdrawal or 10 percent daily for a 10-day withdrawal. Some mild insomnia or discomfort may still occur during withdrawal treatment. Patients should be dissuaded from seeking sedatives, analgesics, antiemetics, and other symptom-relieving drugs, since these may mask underlying medical or psychiatric disorders which should be identified and managed appropriately.

Common medical complications associated with drug abuse should be considered early during patient assessment. These include nutritional abnormalities, acute and chronic infections, and occult trauma (e.g., subdural hematoma).

Referral to special drug treatment programs may be necessary if those providing early medical care do not have resources for further treatment. Patients commonly view such a referral as a rejection by the physician. This can be avoided by making an appointment for the patient in a few weeks or months after the referral. Should the patient be dissatisfied with or no longer working with the referral resource, the follow-up appointment provides an opportunity to assess this and consider other alternatives with the patient.

Treatment Modalities

Modalities for treatment of drug abuse are numerous and include the following:

Residential: General hospital units, special residential facilities, halfway houses, and therapeutic communities

Psychotherapies and sociotherapies: Individual, couples, family, and group; verbal aversion; contingency contracting; social skills learning; and day, evening, or weekend programs

Self-help: Narcotics Anonymous (primarily for illicit drug abusers), Alcoholics Anonymous (primarily for abusers of prescribed or licit drugs, as well as alcohol), Alanon (for relatives of drug abusers)

Pharmacotherapies: methadone (for opioid-dependent patients who have failed other modalities), tricyclic antidepressant medication (especially for amphetamine- or cocaine-dependent patients and those with persistent depressive symptoms)

Somatotherapies: Electrical or chemical aversion, electroacupuncture (Lowinson and Ruiz, 1981; Patterson, 1974)

If major psychiatric problems persist beyond a few to several days, they will probably not resolve spontaneously. Continuation of major depression, schizophreniform psychosis, mania, and other major disorders beyond 2 weeks almost always calls for specific treatment rather than expectant observation. If the patient responds rapidly and completely to low doses of medication, a lengthy course of medication may not be needed.

Minor or less disabling psychiatric syndromes are common in the early weeks of recovery. These include adjustment reactions, generalized anxiety, and panic disorder. If these are decreasing in severity and becoming less frequent, specific treatment may not be necessary. On the other hand, increasing, severe, or disabling symptoms generally require psychiatric treatment.

Treatment Goals, Outcome, and Efficacy

Treatment for drug abuse may be aimed at total abstention, reduction of drug use, or removal of problematic aspects of continued drug use. Generally, abstention, temporary or permanent, is the explicit goal. Simple reduction in dose, with continued use, is rarely effective over the long term but may result in a temporary reduction in symptoms or problems. Licit substitution of illicit opioid consumption in methadone maintenance programs can be helpful in selected patients.

Treatment success is related to many factors besides treatment modalities themselves. Patients who are doing better at the end of 1- and 2-year follow-up studies show the following characteristics:

Occupied as employees or students at the time of entering treatment.

Living with their families at the time of entering treatment.

Come earlier rather than later in their course to treatment.

Collaborate with treatment recommendations (i.e., manifest compliance).

Their families are involved in treatment.

Ongoing outpatient treatment or self-help activities continue on a regular basis over 1 or more years.

Receive indicated pharmacotherapies, especially when other modalities have been ineffective (Hunt and Azrin, 1973; Senay, 1983; Westermeyer, 1976).

Acute management alone tends to have limited efficacy. This is also true of residential treatment alone without outpatient after-care. Under such circumstances, the rate of abstinence 1 year following discharge is low, usually around 0 to 15 percent. With after-care, the rate of abstinence can range up to 80 percent under optimal conditions, although rates half that are more common. Since those abstinent and doing well at the end of 1 year have good outcomes in most cases, the first year of outpatient care is most critical (McLellan et al., 1982).

Cost/benefit from treatment also must be considered. Effective treatment over an adequate period of time is expensive. For unemployed or destitute patients, society must provide the care, and society must be assured that its funds are well spent. Ethical considerations also intrude. For example, methadone maintenance is the most cost-effective modality in many cases of opioid dependence (Dole and Nyswander, 1965; Newman and Whitehill, 1979), but most clinicians believe that these patients should have other treatment alternatives available.

REFERENCES

Bellet S, Roman L, DeCastro O, et al: Effect of coffee ingestion on catecholamine release. Metabolism 18:288, 1969.

Bourne P (ed): Acute Drug Abuse Emergencies: A Treatment Manual. New York, Academic Press, 1976.

Cohen S: The Substance Abuse Problems. New York, Haworth Press, 1981.

Dole VP, Nyswander ME: A medical treatment of diacetylmorphine (heroin) addiction. JAMA 193:646–650, 1965.

Dreisbach RH, Pfeiffer C: Caffeine-withdrawal headache. J Lab Clin Med 28:1212, 1943.

Dupont R, Goldstein A, O'Donnell J (eds): Handbook on Drug Abuse. Washington, National Institute on Drug Abuse, 1979.

Easson W: Gasoline addiction in children. Pediatrics 29:250, 1962.

Ellinwood E: Amphetamine psychosis: I. Description of the individuals and process. J Nerv Ment Dis 144:273–283, 1967.

Gottheil E (ed.): Etiological Aspects of Alcohol and Drug Abuse. Springfield, IL, Charles C Thomas, 1983.

Greden JF: Anxiety or caffeinism: A diagnostic dilemma. Am J Psychiatry 131:1089, 1974.

Greden JF: Caffeinism and caffeine withdrawal. In Lowinson JH, Ruiz P (eds): Substance Abuse: Clinical Problems and Perspectives. Baltimore, Williams & Wilkins, 1981, pp 274–286.

Hughes PH, Barker NW, Crawford GA, Jaffee H: The natural history of a heroin epidemic. Am J Public Health 62: 995–1001, 1972.

Hunt GM, Azrin NH: A community-reinforcement approach to alcoholism. Behav Res Ther 11:91–104, 1973.

Hunt WA, Barnett LW, Branch LG: Relapse rates in addiction programs. J Clin Psychol 27:455–456, 1971.

Jaffee JH: Drug addiction and drug abuse. In Gilman AG, Goodman LS, Gilman A (eds): The Pharmacological Basis of Therapeutics, 6th ed. New York, Macmillan, 1980.

Krasnagor NA (ed): The Behavioral Aspects of Smoking (NIDA Research Monograph No 26). Washington, US Government Printing Office, 1979.

Lowinson JH, Ruiz P (eds): Substance Abuse: Clinical Problems and Perspectives. Baltimore, Williams & Wilkins, 1981.

Lowry TP: The volatile nitrites as sexual drugs: A user survey, J Sex Ed Ther 1:8, 1979.

Maletzky BM, Klotter J: Addiction to diazepam. Int J Addict 11:95–115, 1976.

Martin WR, Jasinski DR: Physiological parameters of morphine dependence in man: Tolerance, early abstinence, protracted abstinence. J Psychiatr Res 7:9–17, 1969.

McClellan AT, Lubovsky L, O'Brien CP, et al: Is treatment for substance abuse effective? JAMA 247:1423–1428, 1982.

Newman RG, Whitehill WB: Double-blind comparison of methadone and placebo maintenance treatments of narcotic addicts in Hong Kong. Lancet 11:485–488, 1979.

Patterson MA: Electro-acupuncture in alcohol and drug addictions. Clin Med 81:9–13, 1974.

Prockop L: Multifocal nervous system damage from volatile hydrocarbon inhalation. J Occup Med 19:139, 1977.

Regier D, Meyers JK, Kramer M, et al: The NIMH Epidemiologic Catchment Area program. Arch Gen Psychiatry 41:934–958, 1984.

Russell MAH: Cigarette smoking: Natural history of a dependence disorder. Br J Med Psychol 44:1, 1971.

Sarvik ME, Cullen JW, Gritz E, et al (eds): Research on Smoking Behavior (NIDA Research Monograph No 17). Washington, US Government Printing Office, 1977.

Senay EC: Substance Abuse Disorders in Clinical Practice. Littleton, MA, John Wright PSG, 1983.

Simon EJ: Opiate receptors and their implications for drug abuse. In Lettieri J, Sayers M, Pearson HW (eds): Theories on Drug Abuse, Selected Contemporary Perspectives (NIDA Research Monograph No 30). Washington, US Government Printing Office, 1980, pp 303–308.

Smart RG: An availability-proneness theory of illicit drug abuse. In Lettieri J, Sayers M, Pearson HW (eds): Theories on Drug Abuse, Selected Contemporary Perspectives (NIDA Research Monograph No 30). Washington, US Government Printing Office, 1980, pp 46–49.

Smith DE, Wesson DR: Phenobarbital technique for treatment of barbiturate dependence. Arch Gen Psychiatry 24:56–60, 1971.

Vaillant GE: The natural history of narcotic drug addiction. Semin Psychiatry 2(4):486–498, 1970.

Vaillant GE: A 20-year follow-up of New York narcotic addicts. Gen Arch Psychiatry 19:237–241, 1973.

Westermeyer J: Opium smoking in Laos: A survey of 40 addicts. Am J Psychiatry 13:165–170, 1974.

Westermeyer J: A Clinical Guide to Alcohol and Drug Problems. New York, Praeger, 1986.

Wikler A: On the nature of addiction and habituation. Br J Addict 57:73–79, 1961.

Wikler A: Some implications of conditioning therapy for problems of drug abuse. Behav Sci 16:92–97, 1971.

Wilsnack SC: Alcohol abuse and alcoholism in women. In Pattison E, Kaufman E (eds): Encyclopedic Handbook of Alcoholism. New York, Gardner Press, 1982, chap 57.

World Health Organization: Review of general population surveys of drug abuse (WHO Offset Publication No. 52). Geneva, WHO, 1980.

CHAPTER 16

Sexual Disorders

GENE G. ABEL
JOANNE L. ROULEAU
CANDICE A. OSBORN

INTRODUCTION

Sexual disorders include three major categories: (1) sexual dysfunctions, problems that interfere with an individual's attempts to perform various sexual behaviors, (2) gender identity disorders, problems with the individual's self-concept as male or female, and (3) paraphilic disorders, interest in sexual behaviors that are outside the range of what our culture considers appropriate.

SEXUAL DYSFUNCTIONS

Definition

Accurate definitions are essential to any science to allow communication regarding our understanding, assessment, treatment, and prognosis of specific conditions. The current standard of classification of sexual dysfunctions is the *Diagnostic and Statistical Manual of Mental Disorders*, third edition revised (DSM-IIIR), of the American Psychiatric Association (American Psychiatric Association, 1987). *Sexual dysfunctions* are defined as inhibition in the appetitive or psychophysiologic changes that characterize the complete sexual response cycle. Table 16-1 lists the nine DSM-IIIR categories of sexual dysfunction subdivided into sexual desire disorders, sexual arousal disorders, orgasm disorders, sexual pain disorders, and sexual dysfunction not otherwise specified.

Incidence and Prevalence

According to Spector and Carey (1990), *incidence* refers to the number of new cases of dysfunction occurring in a specific population during a discrete period of time. *Prevalence* refers to how often the disease occurs (i.e., its incidence) as well as how long it lasts (i.e., its duration). Prevalence rates can be determined for any period of time. Tracking of incidence facilitates the investigation of causal factors of sexual dysfunction and can provide outcome data to assess the efficacy of prevention strategies, while prevalence data can be used to determine the need of clinical resources to alleviate a given problem (Schuman, 1986).

In order to evaluate the incidence and prevalence of the sexual dysfunctions, Spector and Carey (1990) reviewed 23 studies conducted over the past 50 years. With community samples, the completed prevalence studies indicated that 5 to 10 percent of females experience orgasmic difficulties, whereas 4 to 9 percent of males experience erectile disorders, 4 to 10 percent experience inhibited orgasm, and 36 to 38 percent experience premature ejaculation. These authors report that the current prevalence rates of female sexual arousal disorders, vaginismus and dyspareunia, are not available. Recent clinical studies suggest a slight decrease for arousal disorders and a slight increase for orgasmic dysfunction in females; for males there has been a decrease in premature ejaculation and an increase in erectile dysfunction. Furthermore, during the last decade, males outnumber females seeking help for desire disorders.

At the end of their review, Spector and Carey propose four suggestions to the fields of epidemiology and sexuality for the collection of data on sexual dysfunction: (1) obtain stratified samples representative of the general population, (2) devise psychometrically sound assessment techniques to facilitate

TABLE 16-1.   *Categorization of Sexual Dysfunctions*

Sexual desire disorders*

Diagnostic criteria for *hypoactive sexual desire disorder* (302.71)
  This disorder is characterized by a persistent or recurrent deficiency or absence of sexual fantasies and desire for sexual activity.
  The clinician should take into account other factors that affect sexual functioning, such as age, gender, and the context of the
  patient's life.
Diagnostic criteria for *sexual aversion disorder* (302.79)
  This disorder is characterized by persistent or recurrent extreme aversion to, and/or avoidance of, all or almost all, genital sexual
  contact with a sexual partner.

Sexual arousal disorders

Diagnostic criteria for *female sexual arousal disorder* (302.72)
  This disorder is characterized by either a persistent or recurrent partial or complete failure to attain or maintain the lubrication-
  swelling response of sexual excitement until completion of the sexual activity or a persistent or recurrent lack of a subjective
  feeling of sexual excitement and pleasure during sexual activity.
Diagnostic criteria for *male erectile disorder* (302.72)
  This disorder is characterized by either a persistent or recurrent partial or complete failure to attain or maintain erection until
  completion of the sexual activity or persistent or recurrent lack of a subjective feeling of sexual excitement and pleasure during
  sexual activity.

Orgasm disorders

Diagnostic criteria for *inhibited female orgasm* (302.73)
  This disorder is characterized by a persistent or recurrent delay in, or absence of, orgasm in a female following a normal sexual
  excitement phase during sexual activity which the clinician has judged to be of adequate focus, intensity, and duration. Some
  females are unable to experience orgasm during coitus but are able to experience orgasm during noncoital clitoral stimulation.
  This should be considered a normal variation of female sexual response and should not be classified as a disorder. However, in
  some cases, failure to achieve orgasm during intercourse does represent a psychological inhibition that justifies this diagnosis.
  This difficult judgment requires thorough evaluation and may require a trial of treatment.
Diagnostic criteria for *inhibited male orgasm* (302.74)
  This disorder is characterized by a persistent or recurrent delay in, or absence of, orgasm in a male following a normal sexual
  excitement phase during sexual activity which the clinician determines to be of adequate focus, duration, and intensity,
  allowing for the person's age. This diagnosis is usually applied when such failure occurs only during vaginal insertion but not
  during other types of stimulation, such as masturbation.
Diagnostic criteria for *premature ejaculation* (302.75)
  This disorder is characterized by persistent or recurrent ejaculation following minimal sexual stimulation or before, upon, or
  shortly after penetration and before the person, or partner, wishes it. The clinician should consider the person's age, novelty of
  the sexual partner or situation, and frequency of sexual activity.

Sexual pain disorders

Diagnostic criteria for *dyspareunia* (302.76)
  This disorder is characterized by persistent or recurrent genital pain in either males or females before, during, or after sexual
  intercourse, and this pain is not caused exclusively by lack of lubrication or by vaginismus.
Diagnostic criteria for *vaginismus* (306.51)
  This disorder is characterized by a persistent or recurrent involuntary spasm of the musculature of the outer third of the vagina
  that interferes with coitus and is not exclusively caused by a physical disorder.

Sexual dysfunction not otherwise specified

Diagnostic criteria for *sexual dysfunction not otherwise specified* (302.70)
  Sexual dysfunctions that do not meet the criteria for any of the specific sexual dysfunctions listed above.

*This and all other diagnostic categories of sexual dysfunction include the criteria of "occurrence not exclusively during the course of
another Axis 1 disorder (other than a sexual dysfunction)."
From American Psychiatric Association: Diagnostic and Statistical Manual of Mental Disorders, 3d ed revised. Washington, American
Psychiatric Association, 1987.

interpretation and replication of findings, (3) create a common classification system to aid comparison across studies, and finally, (4) develop a collection of incidence data.

Etiology

In order to determine the etiology of sexual dysfunctions, valid and reliable assessment procedures are needed. In the past, etiologic studies have failed to assess the source of various dysfunctions, often assuming that they were caused by a current disease process present in their patients.

Jensen and colleagues (1990) systematically studied a population of 86 epileptic outpatients, 38 men and 48 women. Their sexual functioning was compared with results from an earlier study on a group of patients with diabetes mellitus and a nonpatient control group.

Following sexologic, biologic, psychological,

and social assessments, Jensen and colleagues observed that only 8 percent of the epileptic men reported a sexual dysfunction compared with 13 percent of the controls and 44 percent of the diabetic; no significant differences in sexual dysfunction were observed between epileptic, control, and diabetic women: 29, 25, and 28 percent, respectively. The hormonal status was within normal limits in both women and men, and only a few minor differences were observed, which were not correlated with sexual dysfunction. Jensen and colleagues concluded that "epilepsy does not necessarily increase the risk of sexual dysfunction in male or female patients." Their results differ from previous studies of epileptic men (Taylor, 1969), in which the frequency of hyposexuality in male patients varied from 30 to 70 percent. Jensen and colleagues attributed their different results to a more rigorous methodology, the selection of epileptic patients without accompanying disorders, and the inclusion of female subjects and control groups.

The incidence and correlates of erectile problems in patients with Alzheimer's disease were studied by Zeiss and associates (1990). They reported that 53 percent of 55 male Alzheimer's disease patients, with an average age of 70 years, reported a loss of erectile ability. Patients with erectile problems did not have a greater incidence of concurrent physical problems and did not take more medications than those without sexual problems. The onset of erectile problems was concurrent with the onset of Alzheimer's symptoms, and Zeiss and associates concluded that "there may be an elevated incidence of erectile failure in patients with Alzheimer's disease as a primary problem not attributable to other age-related factors."

Clinical Course

Because sexual behavior results from an interaction of our cultural training, biologic function, and psychological state, it is not surprising that the clinical course of sexual dysfunctions is highly varied. When sexual dysfunctions develop, they are likely to disappear spontaneously or become resistant to common home remedies. Collins and associates (1981), for example, studied 200 males with erectile impotence and found that 13 percent had the dysfunction less than 6 months, 24 percent 6 to 12 months, 29 percent 1 to 2 years, 22 percent 3 to 5 years, and 12 percent longer than 5 years. Clinically, acute sexual symptoms either resolve themselves or the dysfunctions persist chronically.

It is also apparent that an isolated sexual dysfunction is rather unusual. Table 16-2 lists the various sexual symptoms in a group of nonorganically impaired males seeking sexual dysfunction treatment (Rouleau et al., 1984). These data reflect the percentage of occurrence of various sexual dysfunctions. Earlier clinical reports about sexual dys-

TABLE 16-2. *Prevalence of Sexual Symptoms in Males*

Sexual symptoms	Percent ($n = 92$)
1. Continuous (not intermittent) impotence	42.9
2. No morning erection	44.0
3. Retarded ejaculation	23.9
4. Impotence during nonintercourse sex	48.9
5. Decreased ejaculation	26.1
6. No premature ejaculation	53.8
7. Failure to achieve erection	77.2
8. Slow (longer than 1 month) onset of problem	70.3
9. Loss of sex drive	27.5
10. No emotional stress at onset	57.1
11. Sex problem not partner-specific	74.5
12. Decreased sensitivity to pain in T10 area	8.8
13. No climax during intercourse	10.3
14. Loss of erection	73.9
15. Retrograde ejaculation	7.6
16. Partial erection	79.1
17. No climax with any type stimulation	8.8
18. Loss of desire	27.2

functions categorized patients in broad diagnostic categories, such as impotence, frigidity, or erection problems. However, broad classification and the lack of a detailed history conceal the variety of sexual symptoms present in most patients.

Not only do patients present with multiple sexual symptoms, but their symptoms also do not fall into discrete etiologic categories. There appears to be a sequence in which these symptoms develop. In non-organically impaired males, the sequence is premature ejaculation, followed by an episodic inability to achieve a full erection, increased incidence of partial or incomplete erections, loss of erection, loss of sexual desire, retarded ejaculation, and decreased ejaculate. In a group of male diabetics with erectile difficulties, the sequence also begins with premature ejaculation but is followed by partial erections, loss of erections, inability to achieve a full erection, loss of sexual desire, and decreased ejaculate (Rouleau et al., 1984).

The interaction between the various sexual dysfunctions is beginning to be identified. Inhibited sexual desire in males or females appears in two clinical forms. In a small percentage of individuals, the loss of sexual desire is the patient's first symptom and is often followed by the development of either erectile dysfunction in males or excitement and orgasmic dysfunction in females. More commonly, however, erectile dysfunction is the first symptom observed in males (excitement or orgasmic dysfunction in females), which then leads to an increased avoidance of sexual relationships based on the belief that the person is no longer able to function sexually. Removed from sexual interactions, such people begin to change their cognitions that support active participation in sexual activities, and they develop a loss of desire. As a result, their low sexual desire matches their functional capacity. Although their partners may be displeased with decreased frequency of sex, the patients themselves suffer less depression and lowered self-esteem because their desire equals their performance.

The clinical course of inhibited sexual excitement appears to run differently in females and males. In females, increased sexual experience is likely to reduce the incidence of sexual symptoms. In males, increased sexual experience also may reduce the incidence of sexual symptoms as the individual learns to adapt to new partners. In many cases, however, males will attempt home remedies or will seek new partners with the expectation of resolving their erection difficulty. These attempts tend to aggravate, rather than resolve, the erectile difficulties, resulting in more inhibited sexual excitement.

Inhibited female orgasm either persists throughout a woman's lifetime, or more commonly, there is steady improvement in her sexual functioning and reduction of her inhibited orgasms as she becomes more experienced at self-stimulation and teaches her partner how to stimulate her. Inhibited orgasm in the male is a more difficult problem than in the female. The symptom does not result from a lack of experience but from a more deeply rooted, chronic fear of sexual functioning. Its subsequent course is more resistant to increased knowledge about sexual stimulation.

Premature ejaculation in the male is a relatively common problem, occurring early in patients' sexual lives. It also may follow chronic erectile impotence. In some cases, the symptom spontaneously resolves itself as the patient increases the frequency of his sexual encounters. In a large percentage of males, however, it persists throughout their sexual lives if untreated. The remaining sexual dysfunctions have a varied course.

Assessment

Recently, tremendous efforts have been made to develop and refine diagnostic procedures for sexual dysfunctions, especially for male erectile dysfunction. Twenty years ago, the work of Masters and Johnson (1970) concluded that 95 percent of erectile problems were psychogenic; however, recent studies have reported that 50 percent of all patients with erectile failure have neurologic, vascular, and/or hormonal causes (Melman et al., 1988).

In their excellent review of diagnostic and treatment procedures for erectile dysfunction, Mohr and Beutler (1990) classified the assessment procedures as either physical or psychological measures. Since there have not been significant new developments in psychological measures for sexual dysfunction, we will focus on the new physical diagnostic measures, beginning with the role of nocturnal penile tumescence (NPT) monitoring as a diagnostic tool to differentiate psychogenic from organic causes of erectile dysfunction.

Nocturnal penile tumescence (NPT) monitoring is based on the assumption that males without erectile difficulties or with exclusively psychogenic erectile difficulties obtain full erections four to six times per night during rapid eye movement (REM) sleep. Males with organic disease, by contrast, fail to achieve full erections during the night. Mohr and Beutler reported two significant problems with NPT evaluation: a 15 to 20 percent rate of false-positive responses (men with NPT deficits without organic disease) and a 17 percent rate of false-negative responses (men with no NPT deficits but without enough rigidity for penetration).

In the search for reliable, economical, and cost-effective methods to differentiate between psychogenic and organic erectile problems, two other methodologies have been developed that the patient can carry out at home to determine changes in circumference and rigidity: the snap gauge and the poten test. The snap gauge is an inexpensive loop fastened together with Velcro. The two halves of the loop are connected with cellophane strips of known tensile strength. If the patient achieves a significant erection, the various cellophane strips break. In the poten test, the patient places a loop of stamps around his penis. Again, if the patient achieves a significant erection the loop is broken. According to Condra and associates (1986), the snap gauge is more reliable than the poten test because the latter was found unreliable when correlated with NPT findings and corporal calibration testing (CCT).

The Rigi-Scan portable device to assess erectile rigidity provides information, including rigidity at the base and the shaft of the penis, as well as duration of erection. However Beutler and Gleason (1981) suggested that Rigi-Scan, like the other portable devices, has "a high likelihood of interpretive error when the findings are positive (i.e., diminished erections) because of the unassessed effects of REM sleep disturbance, equipment failure, and/or malingering."

In the last 10 years, several vascular assessment strategies have been developed to study erectile dysfunction. The penile blood pressure examination is a widely used method to screen vascular involvement. However, Mellinger and colleagues (1987) reported that such assessment failed to identify 54 percent of men with vascular causes of erectile problems. Venous leakage can be evaluated by a radiologic procedure: cavernography. An artificial erection also can be produced by the injection of papaverine or prostaglandin into the corpus cavernosum of the penis. In a man with venous leakage, it will result in a prolonged erection (Wespes et al., 1984). Wespes and colleagues (1987) suggested that papaverine injection performed while the patient is standing can be the most effective method to identify vascular involvement.

The new methods of assessment of erectile dysfunction have not been matched by the same level of development in assessing inorgasmia in women.

McCabe and Delaney (1992) indicate that little attention has been paid to the use or development of pre- and posttherapy measures of orgasmic experience and other associated factors in females. This limitation in assessment procedures prevents objective evaluation of therapeutic success with female sexual dysfunction.

Differential Diagnosis

The differential diagnosis of sexual dysfunction is a complex process. Although NPT testing has become a standardized method of evaluation to differentiate organically and psychogenically impotent males, several factors can interfere with its sensitivity and specificity. For example, psychological disturbances such as depression can result in erectile difficulties comparable with those experienced by individuals with organic dysfunction. Mohr and Beutler (1990) point out the problem of confounds of extraneous factors in NPT evaluation. These authors suggest, for example, that NPT norms for smokers should be different from those for nonsmokers. In addition to nicotine, several other drugs are also associated with erectile problems: antihypertensive agents, some antidepressants, antipsychotics, alcohol, and marijuana. Wincze and colleagues (1988) observed that males with erectile deficits during NPT evaluation were able to achieve erections during the day in response to erotic stimuli. These observations suggest that the relationship between nocturnal and erotic erections has to be further investigated.

It is clear that recent work on erectile failure has focused primarily on the differential diagnosis of psychological and physiologic factors in erectile difficulties. According to Lo Piccolo (1985), not one simple differential diagnosis procedure has been identified; unfortunately, a complex and expensive multidimensional evaluation is required for accurate diagnosis.

The clinician is frequently faced with the reality that the newer, expensive diagnostic studies to differentiate organic from psychogenic erectile difficulties are not available to him or her. However, specific elements of a clinical history can strongly suggest an organic or psychogenic etiology of erectile disorders. The clinician can ask the following questions to assist in the differential diagnosis:

1. Did you used to get full, 100 percent erections in the early morning or during the night, and do you still get them now that you are having erectile dysfunction? Organically impaired males will report the lack of sensation of full erections, while psychogenically impaired males report continuing to have erections on awakening during the night or in the morning. Such information may preclude the necessity for NPT monitoring.

2. When you are with another partner, in the shower touching your penis to see if it works, or during oral sex, are you able to get full, 100 percent erections? When a patient reports that different partners, different sexual activities, or different environments allow for the development of full erections while other settings or environments preclude same, this is strongly suggestive of a psychogenic etiology of the erectile disorder.

3. Are your daytime erections greater than, equal to, or less than the erections that you have on awakening, during the night, or early morning? In exclusively organic erectile disordered patients, daytime erections match or exceed their erections on awakening, apparently because an organically impaired individual can augment his erection responses by sexual fantasies or thoughts during the day. Individuals with exclusive psychogenic erection difficulties frequently get less of an erection during the day when compared with erections on awakening, presumably because emotional factors contributing to erectile disorder are active when awake but not active during sleep.

4. Was the onset of your erectile dysfunction specifically temporally related to use of medication, medical illness, specific psychological stress, or specific concerns about performing sexually? This question is less accurate than others at discriminating organic from psychogenic erection difficulties. A number of medications and organic illnesses (Segraves and Schoenberg, 1985) can lead to erectile disorders. Likewise, specific emotional stress closely associated with the onset of erectile dysfunctions can identify psychological factors as contributors to erectile dysfunction. Unfortunately, erectile dysfunctions that began as a result of organic factors can then be furthered by psychological causes as the patient attempts to cope with the organic dysfunction. If the possible etiologic agent can be removed (discontinuation of a medication temporarily), it is important not only to clinically determine if erectile dysfunction continues but also to get snap gauge measurements or NPT monitoring while the patient is off the medication.

5. Do you have delayed, retrograde or absent ejaculation, or decreased genital sensation? Individuals with organic erectile dysfunction sometimes report significant ejaculatory or sensation disturbances. These ejaculatory disturbances point to an organic etiology for the erectile disorder.

As Mohr and Beutler (1990) have suggested, attempts to draw a clear dichotomy between organic and psychogenic erectile failure may not accurately reflect the realities of this erectile problem. A diagnosis of psychological involvement does not rule out organic involvement, and vice versa; furthermore, many patients present with a mixed etiology in which organic problems may mask or confound psychological factors, and vice versa. Mohr and Beutler concluded that an assessment procedure measuring multiple causes will aid in identifying the focus of treatment and the development of several intervention strategies for each case of erectile dysfunction.

Treatment

According to Lo Piccolo and Stock (1986), orgasm and arousal problems are the most common presenting sexual complaints from women. Primary orgasmic dysfunction responds well to a directed masturbation training program; however, lack of coital orgasm, which is not clearly a true dysfunction, is more resistant to change. In vaginismus, a progressive dilation program has proven to be very effective.

Male premature ejaculation is easily treated by the "pause" and "squeeze" procedures developed by Semans (1956) and Masters and Johnson (1970), although little is known about the causes of premature ejaculation or the mechanisms that account for treatment effectiveness.

It appears that the recent work in differential diagnosis of physical and psychological causes of erectile failure has led to more somatic treatment of impotence. No new psychological treatments for psychogenic erectile disorders have been developed beyond the standard Masters and Johnson treatment techniques.

One of the most invasive of physiologic treatments is the implantation of a rigid or semirigid rod or an inflatable penile implant device. Beutler and colleagues (1986) reported that patients receiving the inflatable device were significantly more satisfied and had a higher level of sexual functioning, a greater improvement in mood, and shorter recovery times than those receiving the noninflatable penile implants.

According to Goldstein (1987), revascularization for patients with vasculogenic erectile dysfunctions can lead to restored sexual functioning in 80 percent of cases, but other authors report much poorer success rates.

Intracavernosal papaverine or prostaglandin injections have been used to produce an erection lasting from 1 to 4 hours; however, some evidence has shown that a prolonged use of intracavernosal injection can be related to development of nodules and fibrosis in the penis, priapism, bruising, and a decrease in the quality of erections over time (Girdley et al., 1988). Nonetheless, chronic corporal injections have been recommended increasingly by urologists and appear to be replacing penile implants as the treatment of choice in some organically impaired patients.

According to Nadig and associates (1986), a promising noninvasive, somatic treatment of erectile dysfunction is the vacuum construction device (VCD). The VCD is a cylinder placed over the penis and pressed against the body to create an airtight seal. A vacuum is then created in the cylinder, leading to penile engorgement. Rubber bands are slipped from the end of the cylinder onto the base of the penis, obstructing venous return and maintaining the erection for up to 30 minutes for intercourse. For this procedure, the more responsive patients have been those with vasculogenic erectile dysfunction due to diabetes, vascular surgery, medication, or alcohol abuse.

Unfortunately too little attention has been paid to psychological and interpersonal variables associated with physiologic intervention, encouraging a simplistic and antipsychological view of erectile failure.

It is still recommended, in cases of suspected psychogenic involvement, that the patient undergo sex therapy treatment before considering a surgical procedure. Furthermore, to have a "working penis" after surgery does not necessarily provide the skills to approach a partner and to be comfortable in sexual intimacy. In other words, sex therapy treatment also should be available to assist the patient following surgery.

GENDER IDENTITY DISORDERS

Definition

Since 1960, individuals with gender identity disorders have been requesting sex-reassignment surgery (SRS). Therefore, the primary role of clinicians is to formulate diagnostic criteria that lead to safe decisions regarding whether patients should or should not have surgery. To address this problem, the classification system of DSM-IIIR divides gender identity disorders into transsexualism and gender identity disorder of childhood and adolescence, or adulthood, nontranssexual type. Table 16-3 presents the DSM-IIIR diagnostic criteria for gender identity disorders.

In DSM-IIIR, transsexualism and gender identity disorder of childhood are classified under a large category entitled "disorders usually first evident in infancy, childhood, or adolescence." The members of the Subcommittee on Gender Identity Disorders, a subcommittee of the Child Psychiatry Work Group for DSM-IV, have recognized some advantages to the DSM-IIIR classification, since clinicians can differentiate gender identity disorders from childhood and adolescence. However, they found that the same classification criteria were inappropriate for transsexualism, since behavioral precursors in some cases of transsexualism are not identifiable in childhood (Bradley et al., 1990).

As a result of their discussions, the subcommittee has decided to develop a set of criteria for gender identity disorder that include a dichotomy between children and adults to take into account developmental differences (Table 16-4).

Prevalence

The prevalence of gender identity disorder of childhood (GIDC) has not been measured in the general population. Estimates of prevalence are made from individuals attending clinics in order to be admitted

TABLE 16-3. *Categorization of Gender Identity Disorders*

Diagnostic criteria for *gender identity disorder of childhood* (302.60)

For *females:* This disorder is characterized by a long-standing intense distress about being a girl and a stated desire to be a boy (not merely wanting the perceived cultural advantages of being a boy) or an insistence that the girl is actually a boy. In addition to the above, the girl has a significant aversion to wearing feminine clothing and insists on wearing masculine clothing and/or the girl repudiates her female anatomy by at least one of the following: (1) an assertion that she has, or will grow, a penis, (2) rejection of urinating in a sitting position, or (3) assertion that she does not want to menstruate or grow breasts. This disorder occurs before the child has reached puberty.

For *males:* This disorder is characterized by long-standing distress about being a boy and a stated desire to be a girl or, more rarely, insistence that he is a girl. In addition to the above, the boy has a preoccupation with stereotypical female activities (e.g., cross-dressing, playing with female toys or games) or persistent repudiation of male anatomy as indicated by asserting at least one of the following: (1) that he will grow up to be a woman, (2) that his penis and testicles are repugnant or will disappear, or (3) that it would be preferable not to have a penis or testicles. This disorder occurs prior to the individual reaching puberty.

Diagnostic criteria for *transsexualism* (302.50)

This disorder is characterized by long-standing discomfort and a sense of inappropriateness about one's assigned gender. Additionally, there is a persistent preoccupation (at least 2 years' duration) with eliminating one's primary and secondary sex characteristics and acquiring the sex characteristics of the opposite gender. This disorder occurs once the individual has reached puberty.

Diagnostic criteria for *gender identity disorder of adolescence or adulthood, nontranssexual type* (302.85)

This disorder is characterized by persistent or recurrent discomfort regarding one's assigned gender; persistent or recurrent cross-dressing, either in fantasy or reality, but not for the purpose of sexual excitement as in transvestic fetishism; and/or a lack of preoccupation (of at least 2 years' duration) with eliminating one's primary and secondary sex characteristics and acquiring those of the opposite gender. This disorder occurs in individuals who have reached puberty. The clinician should specify the individual's sexual orientation.

Diagnostic criteria for *gender identity disorder not otherwise specified* (302.85)

This diagnosis includes disorders of gender identity that are not classifiable as a specific gender identity disorder, as specified above.

From American Psychiatric Association: Diagnostic and Statistical Manual of Mental Disorders, 3d ed revised. Washington, American Psychiatric Association, 1987.

TABLE 16-4. *Proposed DSM-IV Diagnostic Criteria for Gender Identity Disorder*
by the Subcommittee of the Child Psychiatric Work Group for DSM-IV

A. A profound and persistent cross-gender identification.

In *children*, as manifested by at least four of the following:

1. Repeatedly stated desire to be, or insistence that he or she is, the opposite sex.
2. In girls, insistence on wearing stereotypical masculine clothing; in boys, preference for cross-dressing or simulating female attire.
3. Strong and persistent preferences for cross-sex roles in fantasy play or persistent fantasies of being the opposite sex.
4. Intense desire to participate in the games and pastimes of the opposite sex.
5. Strong preference for playmates of the opposite sex.

In *adolescents and adults*, as manifested by symptoms such as a stated desire to be the opposite sex, frequent passing as the opposite sex, desire to live as or be treated as the opposite sex, or the conviction that one has the typical feelings and reactions of the opposite sex.

B. Persistent discomfort with one's assigned sex or sense of inappropriateness in that gender role.

In *children*, manifested by any of the following:

In *boys*, assertion that his penis or testes are disgusting or will disappear, or assertion that it would be better not to have a penis, or aversion toward rough and tumble play and rejection of male stereotypical toys, games, and activities

In *girls*, rejection of urinating in a sitting position or assertion that she does not want to grow breasts or menstruate, assertion that she has or will grow a penis, or persistent marked aversion toward normative feminine clothing

In *adolescents and adults*, manifested by symptoms such as preoccupation with getting rid of one's primary and secondary sex characteristics (e.g., request for hormones, surgery, or other procedures to physically alter sexual characteristics to simulate the opposite sex) or belief that one was born the wrong sex

For *sexually mature individuals*, specify history of sexual attraction: toward males, females, both, neither, unspecified.

for surgical and/or hormonal sex reassignment. This method tends to underestimate the prevalence of gender identity disorder. Nevertheless, Meyer-Bahlburg (1985) reported that the number of transsexuals is exceedingly small: 1 in 24,000 to 37,000 men and 1 in 103,000 to 150,000 women.

According to Bradley and Zucker (1990), it has been consistently observed that boys are referred more often than girls for concerns about gender identity. Their clinic has the most systematic data on this subject, with a referral ratio of 5.6:1. They also considered that social factors appear to influence a

higher rate of referral for boys, since cross-gender behavior is more likely to be tolerated in girls than in boys.

According to the same authors, DSM-IIIR does not properly address the range of psychosexual concerns during the adolescent years. Based on their clinical experience, Bradley and Zucker developed a more practical classification system with four categories: (1) about 25 percent of their sample were transsexuals with a request for sex reassignment, (2) about 30 percent were transvestites engaged in various degrees of fetishistic cross-dressing, (3) about 25 percent of their adolescents experienced homosexual attraction, and (4) the remaining 20 percent clinically showed behavioral characteristics resembling the transsexual and homosexual groups.

Etiology

Both psychological and biologic factors have been considered relevant in the etiology of GIDC. The most interesting studies have been of girls and women with congenital adrenal hyperplasia (CAH). In this condition, the adrenal gland does not produce normal amounts of corticosteroids, which causes an increase in testosterone production and the subsequent masculinization of the external genitalia. Although the girls with CAH are more masculine in gender role behavior, the evidence of frank identity disorder is not clear (Zucker et al., 1987). A recent long-term follow-up study of girls with CAH shows a higher than expected rate of homosexual and bisexual fantasy and behavior and a lower rate of marriage and sexual experience (Mulaikal et al., 1987).

From experiments with animals, Dorner (1988) has suggested that both homosexuality and transsexualism (homosexual type) are the result of "a hormonal abnormality in utero which produces a differentiation of the hypothalmic center contrary to the individual's genetic sex." Despite the relevance of this work, Bradley and Zucker (1990) point out that it is rare for a specific hormonal anomaly to be found in children with gender identity disorder of childhood.

The role of biologic factors in psychosexual development is widely accepted by sex researchers. The work of Money and colleagues (1987) with intersex children suggests that certain aspects of psychological process may have the upper hand during psychosexual development. Psychosocial factors also have been investigated in the development of GIDC. Stoller (1968) has suggested that some of these boys had "an overly close, blissfully symbiotic" relationship with a mother who herself had gender identity problems. To our knowledge, there have not been any empirical studies evaluating parent–child relationships in girls; however, in his clinical work, Stoller (1972) suggests that the mother–daughter relationship is often impaired, leading to a "disidentification" from the mother.

Clinical Course

The onset of cross-gender behaviors is generally noted by parents, before the child reaches age 2. In boys, the most commonly observed behaviors are wearing the mother's clothing, shoes, and jewels and preference for stereotypical feminine toys. Over time, such boys prefer girls as playmates and avoid playing with boys. By middle childhood, their high-pitched voice and exaggerated dorsiflexion of the

wrist (Rekers and Morey, 1989) often produce peer ostracism, which then results in depression and social withdrawal. At the threshold of adolescence, many boys with GIDC continue to show effeminate mannerisms and, in more severe cases, continue to fantasize about being a girl. Social isolation becomes more and more severe.

In girls, the most commonly observed behaviors are repetitive requests for a penis, or insistence that they have one, and aversion to wearing culturally feminine clothing. Over time, girls with GIDC prefer boys as playmates and typically masculine activities. They will often have temper tantrums if obliged to wear feminine clothing. At the threshold of adolescence, the course of GIDC in girls has been evaluated less extensively. Because of the greater flexibility in the gender role behavior of girls, it is easily possible for girls with GIDC to experiment with opposite-sex friendships. However, in severe cases, girls with GIDC will socialize exclusively with boys, where their masculine appearance is accepted. Conflicts with parents will intensify as the girls demonstrate acute uncertainty about their sexual orientation and gender status.

Differential Diagnosis

In children, a major diagnostic dilemma related to GIDC currently exists. In boys, cross-dressing in GIDC helps enhance the fantasy of being like the opposite sex. Boys who avoid athletics and other conventional masculine activities may feel uncomfortable about being males but do not wish to be girls. Friedman (1988) used the term *juvenile unmasculinity* to describe such boys and suggests that it is not clear whether this behavior pattern actually constitutes a distinct syndrome or a mild form of GIDC.

In girls, according to Green and colleagues (1982), the primary differential diagnostic issue concerns the distinction between tomboyism and GIDC. In their study of a community sample of tomboys, they observed that many cross-gender traits were present that are also observed in clinic-referred gender-disturbed girls. The modification of the DSM-IIIR criteria (see Table 16-4) for GIDC should help to make a clearer differentiation between these two groups of girls.

Assessment

FEMININE BOYS AND MASCULINE GIRLS

Green (1974) compared a population of feminine boys, masculine boys, and typical girls. The groups were comparable for age, IQ, ethnic background, and extent of their fathers' formal education. The standard tests given to the subjects were the It-Scale for Children, the Draw-a-Person Test, the Family-Doll Preference Test (Green, 1971a), and the Parent and Activity Preference Test (Green, 1971b). When both biological parents were available, they were tested with their child with the Family Communication Test. According to Green, the overall psychological results supported the subjective impressions obtained from clinical interviews. For example, one of the most striking observations was the degree of similarity between feminine boys and girls. With this more objective method for collecting data, feminine boys did not emerge as a "third sex."

ADULT TRANSSEXUALS

As reported by Lothstein (1984), over the past 30 years, 41 studies have been published on the psychological testing of transsexuals, in which 699 self-labeled transsexuals have been evaluated. A summary of these studies shows that 80 percent focused on male-to-female transsexuals.

The most commonly used tests are the Minnesota Multiphasic Personality Inventory, the Draw-a-Person Test, and several cognition tests or intellectual functioning tests. Contrary to the assessment of feminine boys and masculine girls, the methodologies for assessment of adult transsexuals are not designed to evaluate the psychological treatment needs of the transsexuals. Rather, they are mainly designed to be used as predictors of success of surgical reassignment.

As also pointed out by Lothstein (1984), a considerable amount of psychological information has been obtained about transsexuals without providing a real understanding of the phenomenon itself. More psychological forms of testing should be used with transsexuals in order to provide a profile of psychological characteristics of transsexualism, a description of their treatment needs, and a means of evaluating their treatment needs and treatment outcome.

A newer method of assessing transsexuals involves direct measurement of sexual responses while presenting various stimuli depicting the subject as heterosexual, homosexual, lesbian, or a transvestite. Using the penile transducer, Abel and associates (1975) described the assessment of a male seeking sex-reassignment surgery. Contrary to the subject's self-report, the psychophysiologic erection responses demonstrated his major arousal pattern to be that of masochism, including themes of being changed into a female against his will. Cunningham-Rathner and Abel (1984) described a similar psychophysiologic assessment of a female-to-male transsexual using the vaginal photoplethysmograph (a device that measures female sexual arousal by quantifying vaginal engorgement in biologic females) while concomitantly presenting various sexual stimuli. Standards for such psychophysiologic measurement have not been established, but these preliminary studies suggest that objective psychophysiologic assessment can be an important adjunct to traditional clinical interviews and paper-and-pencil testing for potential transsexuals.

Treatment

At the Gender Identity Treatment Program at UCLA, many approaches to treatment of feminine boys and masculine girls have been developed (Green, 1974). Three specific strategies for intervention have been used: (1) individual sessions with the patient and separate sessions with his or her parent(s), (2) group sessions with several patients and individual sessions for each parent, and (3) identifying to parents specific aspects of behavior in their child to be systematically reinforced or extinguished at home. The aims of these clinical interventions are to (1) develop a relationship of trust and affection between a patient and a therapist of the sex opposite to that of the patient, (2) inform the child of the impossibility of changing his or her sex, (3) demonstrate to the child the positive aspects of participating in some of the activities engaged in by same-sex peers and promote comfort in such activities, (4) teach the parents how they may be fostering sexual identity conflicts in their child, (5) make the parents aware of the importance of consistent disapproval of opposite-sex behaviors performed by the child and consistent approval of appropriate behaviors, and (6) increase the same-sex parent's involvement in the child's life.

Regarding the treatment of adult transsexuals, as psychiatrists and psychologists, what meaningful alternative help (other than surgical sex reassignment) have we been able to offer to the transsexual patient? Clinical interviews and psychological testing of transsexuals seem to exclusively target the narrow issue of predicted success of sex-reassignment surgery. However, recent developments raise some questions about this approach, since recent reports describe patients so dissatisfied with sex-reassignment surgery that they discard their biologic gender role despite the physical irreversibility of the surgery (Van Putten and Fawzy, 1976).

A few reports now suggest that behavioral procedures can be effective in changing gender identity in some patients. Barlow and colleagues (1973) have reported the first successful change of gender identity in a diagnosed transsexual using a behavioral approach. Six years later, Barlow and colleagues (1979) reported a follow-up study on this case in which the 17-year-old male transsexual's gender-specific motor behavior, appropriate sex-role social behavior, cognitive sexual activity, and sexual arousal patterns were defined, measured, and sequentially modified. In the 6 years after treatment, the patient remained completely sexually reoriented, denied desire for sex-reassignment surgery, and reported masturbation approximately four times a week to heterosexual fantasies. His memories of treatment were fuzzy, but he recalled this period as an unhappy time in his life. Two additional cases are also reported in this study.

THE SURGICAL PROCESS

According to Brown (1990), sex-reassignment surgery in male-to-female transsexuals largely consists of surgical interventions to transform the male physique to the closest approximation of the female, both in form and function. The basic procedure costs between $7500 and $20,000. Following good surgical results and good patient compliance, the neovagina can function during sexual intercourse, including retained capacity for orgasm. Several months after the operation, the neovagina can be indistinguishable from the external genitalia of an adult female. The sex reassignment of female-to-male transsexuals is more difficult, since there are major deficits in aesthetic appearance and sexual functioning. (Readers who are interested in an illustrated review of this technical topic are referred to the article by Gilbert and colleagues, 1988.)

As reported by Brown (1990), recent studies suggest that 10 to 15 percent of patients who receive sex-reassignment surgery failed and 7 percent suffered a tragic outcome (e.g., requests for reversal, psychotic episode, hospitalization, or suicide). Approximately 20 gender identity clinics have been established in the Western Hemisphere, but only an estimated 12 currently remain open. (Again, we refer the reader to a well-delineated standard of care published by an international group of experts: Walker and colleagues, 1985). Referral to an established gender identity clinic should only be considered for patients with a severe disorder that warrants potential somatic interventions.

PARAPHILIAS[1]

Definition

All of us are sexually interested in specific targets, objects, and/or acts. Some categories of sexual target choice (e.g., 4-year-old children), sexual objects (e.g., stolen lingerie), and sexual activities (e.g., sadism) are either inappropriate within our culture, deny the rights of others, or ignore their inability to give informed consent. These varieties of sexual behavior have been categorized as psychiatric disorders, specifically *paraphilias*. The categories of paraphilias and their criteria for diagnosis are listed in Table 16-5. The current DSM-IIIR criteria indicate that in order to be classified as a paraphiliac, the individual must have persistent, recurrent fantasies or urges regarding the paraphilic behavior for a period of at least 6 months and/or have engaged in the behavior. In the majority of cases, the paraphiliac can function successfully in appropriate sexual activities. However, a few paraphiliacs can only attain orgasm through paraphilic fantasies or acts.

[1] Although this section focuses on male paraphiliacs, most of the information also applies to females (with the exception of penile plethysmography and specific studies focusing on males).

Over 50 percent of paraphiliacs report the onset of their paraphilic interest prior to age 18. Transvestism has the earliest average age of onset of all the paraphilias (13.6 years), followed by fetishism, bestiality, voyeurism, and the other common paraphilias. Pedophilia involving incest has the latest average age of onset (23.5 years for female targets; 27.1 years for male targets) (Abel et al., in press).

Prevalence

Accurate information regarding the prevalence of paraphilias is unavailable because deviant sexual behavior is generally not revealed to others. Discussion of one's paraphilic interests or acts may lead to ostracism at the very least and frequently leads to arrest, conviction, and/or incarceration, thus intensifying the difficulty of collecting accurate information. One way to measure the frequency of various paraphilias is through information regarding victims. Data gathered from a large number of outpatient paraphiliacs suggest that, in terms of victimizations, the acts of the highest incidence are those of frottage (sexual touching without the victim's permission), exhibitionism, and child molestation (Abel, 1991a).

Criminal justice records are poor reflections of the incidence of various paraphilias because (1) some paraphilic acts considered by the police to be of minor consequence are unreported, (2) paraphilic acts that offend the general decency of our culture are more likely to be reported and pursued, and (3) during the course of criminal disposition of sex offense crimes, plea bargaining conceals the true frequencies of various paraphilias.

PARAPHILIAS IN THE GENERAL POPULATION

Individuals with paraphilic interests are, by definition, generally ostracized by society because their behaviors are seen as inappropriate and morally wrong. Because of social ostracism and potential legal consequences of reporting paraphilic interests or behaviors, determining the occurrence of paraphilias in the general population has always been problematic. Briere and Runtz (1989) investigated college students' interests in children by means of an anonymous questionnaire. Twenty-one percent of the sample reported some sexual attraction to children, 9 percent reported sexual fantasizing about children, 5 percent reported masturbating to sexual fantasies of children, and 7 percent indicated that if assured that they would not be found out for having had sex with a child, they would want to have sex with a child. Templeman and Stinnett (1991) also reported on the paraphilic experiences of male college students. Three percent of their sample reported having been arrested for a sexual offense, 3 percent having been in trouble because of their sexual behavior, 3 percent having been sexual with a girl under 12 years of age, 42 percent voy-

TABLE 16-5. *Categorization of Paraphilias*

Paraphilia	Diagnostic criteria
Zoophilia (302.10)	The act or fantasy of engaging in sexual activity with animals is a repeatedly preferred method of achieving sexual excitement.
Pedophilia (302.20)	The act or fantasy of engaging in sexual activity with prepubertal children is a repeatedly preferred method of achieving sexual excitement.
Transvestism (302.30)	Recurrent and persistent cross-dressing by a heterosexual. Use of cross-dressing for the purpose of sexual excitement, at least initially in the course of the disorder. Intense frustration when the cross-dressing is interfered with.
Exhibitionism (302.40)	Repetitive acts of exposing the genitals to an unsuspecting stranger for the purpose of achieving sexual excitement, with no attempt to further sexual activity with the stranger.
Fetishism (302.81)	The use of nonliving objects is a repeatedly preferred method of achieving sexual excitement. The fetishes are not limited to articles of female clothing used in cross-dressing or to objects designed to be used for the purpose of sexual stimulation.
Voyeurism (302.82)	The individual repeatedly observes unsuspecting people who are naked, in the act of disrobing, or engaging in sexual activity, and no sexual activity with the observed people is sought. The observing is the repeatedly preferred method of achieving sexual excitement.
Sexual masochism (302.83)	Either a preferred or exclusive mode of producing sexual excitement is to be humiliated, bound, beaten, or otherwise made to suffer, or the individual has intentionally participated in an activity in which he or she was physically harmed or his or her life was threatened in order to produce sexual excitement.
Sexual sadism (302.84)	One of the following: (1) on a nonconsenting partner, the individual has repeatedly intentionally inflicted psychological or physical suffering in order to produce sexual excitement, (2) with a consenting partner, the repeatedly preferred mode of achieving sexual excitement combines humiliation with simulated or mildly injurious bodily suffering; (3) on a consenting partner, bodily injury that is extensive, permanent, or possibly mortal is inflicted in order to achieve sexual excitement.
Frotteurism (302.89)	The act of fantasy or touching and rubbing against a nonconsenting person.
Atypical paraphilia (302.90)	Paraphilias not otherwise categorized.

From American Psychiatric Association: Diagnostic and Statistical Manual of Mental Disorders, 3d ed revised. Washington, American Psychiatric Association, 1987.

euristic behavior, 8 percent making obscene phone calls, 35 percent frottage, 5 percent coercive sexual behavior, 2 percent exhibitionism, and a full 65 percent of the sample having been involved in some type of sexual misconduct. These two studies point out that "normal" college males are frequently involved in paraphilic behavior.

In a study of the prevalence of paraphilic interests (either current or previous interest) in health care professionals, Abel (1991b) found that 31.3 percent reported a current or past history of paraphilic behaviors, 1.3 percent pedophilia with boys, 2.5 percent pedophilia with girls, 8.8 percent exhibitionism, 8.8 percent fetishism, 11.3 percent frottage, and 15 percent voyeuristic activity.

In summary, random samples of the general population have not been conducted to determine the prevalence of paraphilic behaviors. However, studies examining nonrepresentative subgroups suggest that past or present occurrences of paraphilic behaviors are relatively common in the general population. A fruitful avenue of research would be to examine why and how individuals previously involved in paraphilic behaviors stopped these activities.

Etiology

A number of theories have been postulated to explain the etiology of deviant sexual arousal. One theory proposed by Malmquist (1972) suggests that sexual deviancy results from the persistence beyond childhood of earlier forms of sexuality. Deviant sexual behavior is viewed as an alternative to neurotic development, with the difference being attributed to ego acceptance of particular unrepressed infantile sexual fantasies. According to this theory, paraphiliacs are viewed as developmentally impaired.

A second theoretical model of sexually deviant behavior is the cognitive model. This model purports that individuals engage in inappropriate sexual behaviors due to cognitive distortions. These distortions, or thinking errors, provide a rationale for the justification of such behaviors, allowing the perpetrator to continue to engage in his inappropriate sexual behavior. In addition to these cognitive distortions, a number of characteristics have been found to be common among male sexual offenders. These include a low self-esteem, objectification of females, hostility or rage, feelings of powerlessness and/or emptiness, poor impulse control, gender identity confusion, a fear of intimacy, and poor coping and problem-solving skills (Davis and Leitenberg, 1987; Groth, 1977; Hains et al., 1986). Together, the cognitive distortions and these offender characteristics enable perpetrators to continue their paraphilic behavior with minimal regard for their victim(s).

A third theoretical model of deviant sexual behavior is the conditioning and social learning model

(Laws and Marshall, 1990). This model suggests that individuals learn deviant sexual arousal/behaviors in the same way they learn other behaviors, i.e., through observational learning or modeling and through the pairing and association of deviant thoughts or behaviors with a positive reinforcer (sexual arousal and/or orgasm).

According to this model, the early developmental years encompass a variety of exploratory sexual behaviors for most individuals. Some of these early sexual behaviors are instigated by watching others (modeling) either in vivo or through the mass media. Other deviant sexual behaviors are expressions of actual experiences that the perpetrator has had in the past (e.g., incestuous activities). Finally, some deviant sexual behavior is normal exploratory sexual behavior practiced by adolescents, but due to their lack of knowledge or misinformation, these behaviors sometimes continue into adulthood (Bandura, 1973).

Laws and Marshall (1990) propose 10 fundamental learning principles underlying the acquisition of deviant sexual behavior based on classical and operant conditioning principles and social learning influences. Basically, they contend that as deviant sexual thoughts and behaviors are paired with positive reinforcers (sexual arousal and/or orgasm), they tend to be repeated. Laws and Marshall also propose three fundamental learning principles to explain the maintenance of deviant sexual behavior: intermittent reinforcement, differential reinforcement, and differential punishment. Maintenance of the paraphilic behavior depends on its consequences to the offender. For example, if the paraphiliac leaves the scene and avoids arrest, he not only fails to suffer negative consequences for the actions but also fails to see the consequences of the behavior on the victim.

A major contributor to the maintenance of paraphilic behavior is the paraphiliac's use of his memories or fantasies of the deviant experience during masturbation (Abel and Blanchard, 1974). If the paraphiliac recalls and relives the deviant experience(s) during masturbation, the fantasies or images recalled become associated with the positive experience of orgasm. As repeated pairings occur over time, these fantasies become more and more erotic, and paraphilic interests become more entrenched, possibly developing into a chronic condition.

Marshall and Barbaree (1990a) contend that the learning model alone is not sufficient to explain the etiology of deviant sexual behavior and propose an integration of the role of learning experiences, sociocultural factors, and biologic processes to account for sexual offending. According to this viewpoint, "biologic inheritance confers upon males a ready capacity to sexually aggress which must be overcome by appropriate training to instill social inhibitions toward such behavior. Variations in hormonal functioning may make this task more or less difficult" (pp. 270–271). Social influences such as poor parenting and sociocultural attitudes may increase the likelihood of sexual offending. In combination with the learning paradigms described above and identification of situational factors, this integrated theory provides the most comprehensive explanation of the etiology of paraphilias to date.

Developmentally delayed individuals are especially at risk to carry out paraphilic behaviors if they fail to receive appropriate sex education. Not knowing exactly how to provide sex education to the developmentally delayed, society frequently attempts to conceal sexual knowledge and information from this group, and they, in turn, fail to develop social inhibitions to engaging in inappropriate sexual behaviors. As a result, the individual is more likely to initiate sexual behavior which is unacceptable within our culture.

Some paraphiliacs reflect poor impulse control resulting from other DSM-IIIR, Axis I conditions, such as schizophrenia. Treatment of the underlying Axis I disorder frequently leads to effective control of the paraphilic behavior, although there are some individuals who develop an organic brain syndrome or schizophrenia and who also have a concomitant diagnosis of paraphilia.

A final category of individuals commits a variety of antisocial acts, including some paraphilic acts. Individuals with antisocial personalities may commit paraphilic acts simply to gratify their immediate need for a sexual outlet. Most of these individuals do not have a true paraphilia, i.e., a recurrent, intense urge for sexual involvement with culturally prohibited objects, targets, or behaviors. As with other conditions, there will be some antisocials who have a true paraphilia.

Clinical Course

The behavior of most paraphiliacs follows a recurrent cycle. Urges to participate in paraphilic behavior usually develop during adolescence. As the paraphiliac asks others about his fantasies or acts on these urges, he or she learns that such acts may be inappropriate or harmful to others. The paraphiliac attempts to develop internal controls to inhibit the interest. Lacking the knowledge that the use of paraphilic fantasies during masturbation will intensify his interest and lead to a stronger desire to commit the acts, the paraphiliac inadvertently pairs and associates the paraphilic fantasies with masturbation and orgasm in an attempt to satisfy these urges through masturbation alone. The paraphilic arousal becomes strengthened during the course of these learning trials, and as time passes, the paraphiliac's control breaks down, and he or she acts (once or a number of times) until orgasm is attained or until the negative consequences of commission of the acts outweigh the expected benefits.

Immediately after arrest or discovery, there is frequently a total cessation of interest in the deviant act or behavior that unfortunately gives the para-philiac a false impression that the arrest/discovery experience has eradicated the problem. In actuality, this can be an exceedingly dangerous time for the offender, since marked reduction of the fantasies is misinterpreted as a cure, and the paraphiliac is more likely to place himself in situations where recommission of the act is probable.

As negative consequences follow expression of the paraphilic interests or the patient's internal analysis of the impropriety of the behavior becomes more powerful, the paraphiliac temporarily curtails his urges. As time passes, however, and the memory of these negative consequences weakens, control breaks down, and the cycle repeats itself.

Cognitive distortions serve an especially important role in the maintenance of paraphilic behavior. Paraphiliacs are raised in a culture that prohibits the commission of deviant sexual behavior. However, as the paraphiliac repeatedly carries out an inappropriate behavior, he must balance the commission of the behavior with his cognitions or attitudes about its appropriateness.

When a marked disparity exists between the paraphiliac's behavior and his perception of that behavior as inappropriate, anxiety and depression are likely to follow. To protect against these negative emotional responses, the paraphiliac alters the cognitions. Exhibitionists, for example, conclude that exposing their genitals is actually an enjoyable sexual experience for the victim. The victim's laughter or confusion upon seeing the exhibitionist's genitals is reinterpreted as sexual interest. Individuals who molest children will interpret their behavior as non-harmful to the child unless physical violence occurs. When the child does not violently object to participation in the act or fails to report the crime, the paraphiliac interprets this as an expression of the child's desire to continue to participate in the behavior. Incest offenders likewise falsely believe that if their marriage partner is cold and distant from them, it is better to be sexual with their own children than become involved with extramarital sex. Indeed, it appears that all paraphiliacs develop cog-

nitive distortions that support or justify their continued involvement in the paraphilic behavior.

Table 16-6 reflects the typical lifetime course of various paraphilias. As can be seen, the majority of paraphilic arousal patterns begin during adolescence and start to decrease in frequency in the late 30s and early 40s. Paraphilic arousal patterns that can be enjoyed without a sexual partner tend to be more persistent, such as transvestism, and fetishism.

Assessment

Assessment of paraphiliacs requires (1) evaluation to quantify the presence or absence of arousal to paraphilic stimuli, (2) clarification of behavioral excesses or deficits that are closely correlated with deviant sexual behavior (cognitive distortion, deficits of sexual knowledge, insufficient social and assertive skills, and inadequate arousal to nondeviant stimuli), and (3) factors less closely associated with paraphilic arousal and yet reported as contributors to the expression of paraphilic behavior (anxiety, deficit coping skills, and boredom). Assessment includes a clinical interview or history, paper and pencil tests, and more recently, psychophysiologic laboratory measurements.

CLINICAL INTERVIEW

Paraphiliacs are frequently under coercion to participate in assessment and treatment as a result of a recent arrest. Frequently, the paraphiliac fears that accurate reporting of the extent of the sexual crime may put him at greater risk for incarceration. Consequently, the paraphiliac is reluctant to reveal the scope, intensity, and frequency of his paraphilic interest. Without this information, the clinician is severely limited in defining the treatment needs of the paraphiliac. This major difficulty with valid reporting explains the marked discrepancies between the reports of deviant sexual behavior by the paraphiliac when confidentiality is protected and when confidentiality is not protected (Kaplan et al., 1990).

TABLE 16-6. *Lifetime Course of Paraphilias*

Paraphilia	Clinical course
Zoophilia	Onset at early age, usually ceases during late teens.
Pedophilia	Onset at early age, suppressed for 5 to 10 years, or onset at early age and continues throughout adolescence. In both situations, pedophilic acts peak in the late 20s and early 30s and decrease in frequency by age 40, although behavior may continue into the 90s.
Transvestism	Onset at early age with continuation throughout adulthood.
Exhibitionism	Onset at early age with gradual reduction during the 40s, but behavior may continue through the 80s.
Fetishism	Onset at early age with continuation throughout adulthood.
Voyeurism	Onset at early age with reduction of symptoms by late 20s.
Sexual masochism	Onset at early age, fluctuating course throughout adulthood if compliant sexual partner permits.
Sexual sadism	Onset in early life, fluctuating course throughout adulthood.
Atypical paraphilia	The majority have an early onset, with reduction in frequency of paraphilic acts by age 40.

Abel describes various steps the clinician can take to obtain a more accurate clinical history (Abel, 1985; Abel and Osborn, 1992). The therapist should be extremely active in the interview in order to stop or divert patients if they begin to deny that they have committed the current offense, because once patients have committed themselves in detail to denial, it is extremely difficult for them to retreat from that position. A common error by the clinician is failure to assess the multiplicity of categories of paraphilic behavior in which offenders may be involved. Unless questioned about each paraphilia specifically, paraphiliacs are unlikely to reveal their complete arousal patterns. A structured interview should explore each paraphilic category and include the patient's age at the time of onset of each paraphilia, the frequency of paraphilic acts, the number of victims, the amount of force used during the commission of the act(s), the extent of present control over paraphilic arousal, the amount of masturbatory fantasies that involve paraphilic behaviors, and a comparison of the relative arousal to each of the various paraphilic interests. Interviews should incorporate developmental milestones that help offenders identify the chronology of their paraphilic histories.

Particular attention should be paid to the behavioral antecedents and consequences of the paraphiliac's use of deviant fantasies or commission of deviant acts because these factors strongly affect maintenance of the arousal. Appropriate therapy can then be devised to reduce the frequency of these antecedents and negative consequences can be arranged to follow use of deviant fantasies or acts.

PAPER AND PENCIL TESTS

A number of paper and pencil tests have been developed specifically for use with paraphiliacs to outline the extent of deviant interests by various paraphilic categories (Sexual Interest Cardsort, Salter, 1988; Clarke Sexual History Questionnaire, Langevin, 1983), measures of cognitive distortions associated with child molesters and incest offenders (Abel-Becker Cognition Scale, Salter, 1988), and measures of appropriate social skills (Barlow et al., 1977), assertiveness, and anxiety and sexual knowledge. Each of these tests helps to quantify various aspects contributing to paraphilic behavior.

LABORATORY MEASURES

The greatest advance in the assessment of paraphilias has been in the area of psychophysiologic assessment. Kurt Freund's pioneering work (1981) in the measurement of sexual arousal using the penile transducer has contributed immensely to the quantification of deviant interests. This measurement procedure involves the paraphiliac wearing a penile transducer (that quantifies penile circumference) while listening to or looking at depictions of paraphilic and nonparaphilic stimuli. Using this technology, it has been possible to quantify an individual's interest in virtually every category of paraphilic arousal. Quantification of interests in child molestation, sadism, rape, masochism, and exhibitionism have been substantiated (Abel et al., 1981). This scientific advancement has provided the clinician, for the first time, with a means of quantifying treatment needs before, during, and after therapy by repeated objective measures of deviant interest.

Annon (1988) reviewed the reliability and validity of penile plethysmography in measuring sexual arousal patterns of sexual offenders. He concluded that there is sufficient research indicating that penile plethysmography is the most reliable measure of sexual arousal in males and that this measure provides valid determination of sexual preferences. He admits that the weakest data results from minimal responses across all stimulus categories presented to the offender. However, the use of differential response measures (standard or z scores) rather than the amplitude of individual responses has solved this particular problem in most cases.

Psychophysiologic assessment is also extremely useful in cutting through the patient's denial. Many paraphiliacs reveal or admit their paraphilic interest(s) when they are shown their positive physiologic responses to paraphilic stimuli. A controlled study has shown that 62 percent of paraphiliacs so confronted with their physiologic measures admitted to paraphilic behaviors or interests that they had previously denied or failed to reveal. This increased reporting of paraphilic interests makes treatment outcome far more effective because treatment can encompass all the patient's deviant sexual interests rather than overlooking those the patient has failed to reveal (Abel et al., 1983a).

Differential Diagnosis

Differentiation of paraphilic behavior resulting from schizophrenia or organic disease is relatively straightforward because of the clinical presentation of the organic brain syndrome or schizophrenia and because the expression of paraphilic behavior resulting from these two conditions is usually different from the expression of deviant behavior by paraphiliacs. The individual with an organic brain syndrome does not have a history of early interest in paraphilic behaviors, and the first expression of paraphilic behavior follows the development of the organic brain syndrome. Paraphilia resulting from poor control associated with schizophrenia is likewise unusual in its presentation. The schizophrenic develops idiosyncratic interpretations of the meaning of his behavior and frequently openly admits involvement for reasons idiosyncratic to him. The true paraphiliac, on the other hand, attempts to conceal his deviant behavior.

Developmentally delayed individuals whose paraphilic behavior is more a reflection of their limited intellectual functioning and limited sex education also can be identified by the existence of their primary intellectual deficit.

One of the most difficult differential diagnostic problems is evaluating whether deviant sexual behavior committed by adolescents is caused by a true paraphilic interest or is an exploratory behavior devoid of an underlying paraphilic interest. Abel and associates (1983b) reported preliminary data on the penile tumescence monitoring of adolescent sex offenders to assist in this differential diagnosis. Results indicate that the same psychophysiologic assessment used with adults can be used effectively with adolescents to assist in the differential diagnosis.

Treatment

COGNITIVE-BEHAVIORAL TREATMENT

Treatment of the paraphilias resulted in minimal success until the advent of more direct, behavioral interventions in the early 1970s. Instead of exploring the possible early developmental factors and interpersonal conflicts that may lead to the patient's earliest interest in paraphilic behavior, the behavioral approach addresses the directly observable behavioral excesses and deficits of the paraphiliac. The development of psychophysiologic assessment allows direct observation of the patient's interest in deviant stimuli and possible deficits of nondeviant arousal.

Early behavioral interventions focused exclusively on decreasing paraphilic arousal (Quinsey and Marshall, 1983). Marshall (1971) was the first behavior therapist to recognize the need to add social skills training to the treatment package. Other treatment components have been added gradually as additional deficits in paraphiliacs have been identified. Procedures aimed at modifying the cognitive distortions that paraphiliacs employ to justify their deviant behavior (Abel et al., 1985) have been identified as a critical component in comprehensive treatment packages. The cognitive-behavioral treatment approach is now the model for the majority of specialized sex offender treatment programs.

The components of comprehensive cognitive-behavioral treatment programs can be divided into two primary categories: those which target the reduction of deviant sexual arousal and the development or enhancement of appropriate sexual arousal and those which target the development of prosocial and effective coping skills.

There are several behavioral treatment strategies designed to decrease deviant sexual arousal and/or increase appropriate sexual arousal. Olfactory aversion pairs previously pleasant deviant sexual thoughts and behaviors with an unpleasant event, inhalation of a noxious odor. Covert sensitization scripts pair these antecedents to deviant sexual behavior with imagined negative social consequences (e.g., being arrested or incarcerated, being abandoned by family members or friends, losing a job, etc.). Masturbatory satiation requires the offender to masturbate to orgasm while verbalizing an appropriate sexual fantasy and then, while in the refractory phase and thus unable to orgasm again, to continue to masturbate for a concentrated period of time to deviant sexual fantasies. Repeated experiences of deviant sexual fantasies without the reinforcing experience of orgasm results in a pairing of deviant sexual fantasies with boredom rather than pleasure (Abel et al., 1984). Orgasmic reconditioning requires the offender to substitute an appropriate sexual fantasy, just prior to orgasm, during his usual deviant sexual fantasy. This technique is especially helpful for those offenders who have minimal or absent arousal to appropriate sexual behaviors.

Components targeting prosocial and effective coping skills include the following: (1) social skills training to increase or expand paraphiliacs' social and/or dating skills so that they are able to communicate more effectively with potential peer partners, (2) assertive skills training to expand paraphiliacs' ability to express their wants and needs, request behavior changes from others, and express positive or negative feelings toward others, (3) cognitive restructuring to identify and challenge the faulty cognitions that paraphiliacs have used to justify their deviant sexual behavior, (4) sex education to debunk myths, clarify appropriate sexual behaviors, identify the components of healthy sexual relationships, etc., (5) victim sensitization to assist offenders in comprehending the consequences of their deviant behavior on the victim(s), the victim's family and friends, the offender's family and friends, and society, (6) reduction of stress and anxiety, which are frequently antecedents to deviant sexual behavior, (7) improvement in daily living skills and reduction of unstructured leisure time that is likely to lead to paraphilic behavior, (8) treatment of substance-abuse problems, (9) impulse control, (10) anger management, (11) treatment of sexual dysfunctions, and (12) establishment of a surveillance system so that others in the paraphiliacs' environment can assist them and the therapist in identification of early signs of renewed or continued paraphilic interest. Not all specialized sex offender treatment programs include all the components listed above, but most comprehensive programs address at least some elements of each of these.

One of the most significant recent trends in the comprehensive treatment of paraphiliacs is the recognition of the need for long-term maintenance or follow-up treatment strategies for the prevention of reoffending. Relapse prevention, a treatment strategy originally developed as a method for enhancing maintenance of change in substance abusers (Marlatt, 1982; Marlatt and Gordon, 1980; 1985), has been incorporated very effectively into the treatment of paraphiliacs (Nelson et al., 1988; Pithers, 1990). This treatment strategy focuses on strengthening self-control by providing paraphiliacs with methods for identifying situations that place them at risk for reoffending, analyzing decisions that set up situations enabling resumption of inappropriate sexual behaviors, and developing strategies to avoid or cope more effectively with these situations. Relapse prevention is a method of enhancing self-management skills.

Treatment of paraphilias is an ongoing process throughout the paraphiliac's life span. To have an effective impact on this problem, treatment programs must address a wide variety of patient deficits, retrain sexual arousal patterns, and address the long-term treatment needs of the patient.

DRUG TREATMENT

Some paraphiliacs pose more extensive dangers than others because they are at high risk to relapse and/or their paraphilic behavior is potentially highly injurious to the victim. Although cognitive-behavioral treatment is the most commonly used type of treatment of paraphiliacs, these treatments require time to have an impact on the patient, and thus more rapid, vigorous treatment may be needed for high-risk patients. Two categories of drugs have been used under these circumstances, fluoxetine and hormonal treatment.

Recently, case reports have described the effective use of fluoxetine, but the mode of action of the drug is unclear (Emmanuel et al., 1991; Kafka, 1991; Perilstein et al., 1991). As an antidepressant, its effect could result from the paraphiliac being depressed and responding to its antidepressant effect. Since fluoxetine also has been effective with obsessive-compulsive behaviors, this is another potential mechanism of action. Still a third is that, in some cases, fluoxetine reduces sex drive as a side effect of the medication. This reduction of the patient's overall sex drive would include reduction of the paraphilic sex drive and thereby provide the patient increased control over paraphilic urges. Further research is needed to more clearly delineate the method by which this drug is helpful with paraphilias.

Hormonal treatment has a much more extensive history. Two drugs are currently available in North America, cyproterone acetate (not available in the United States) and medroxyprogesterone acetate (MPA). Since first reported as effective at reducing male sex drive in 1958, MPA has been used in a number of studies of paraphiliacs. The method of action of MPA appears to be in accelerating the metabolic breakdown of testosterone and thereby reducing the level of plasma testosterone. As testosterone decreases, there is a concomitant decrease in the frequency of paraphilic fantasy, followed by decreased erection and decreased ejaculation. As their sex drives decrease, patients develop a

sense of better control over their paraphilic interests. Studies by Money (1970), Blumer and Migeon (1975), Money et al. (1976), and Gagne (1981) all indicate significant reduction of paraphilic behavior following treatment, but with the return of paraphilic interest following discontinuation of the medication.

Despite its limitations, MPA can serve a critical role in the treatment of those paraphiliacs with a high likelihood for relapse and at greater risk to harm their victims. Given in the depo form, the drug ensures a continued administration of MPA for 7 to 10 days. The side effects of weight gain, lethargy, nightmares, dyspnea, hypoglycemia, hypogonadism, and leg cramps are relatively minor when compared with the relatively rapid effectiveness of reduction of paraphilic interest while taking the medication (Bradford, 1983). In this respect, hormonal treatment provides a very useful component to the treatment of some patients.

Treatment Outcome

Evaluating treatment outcome of paraphiliacs is problematic. The validity of such studies is first of all hampered by the difficulty of having nontreated control groups of paraphiliacs. This poses a significant ethical dilemma. Second, since many paraphilic behaviors are felonies, accurate reporting is problematic in that acknowledgment of a relapse could lead to the offender's incarceration or revocation of probation. A third factor is that there is tremendous variance in baseline rates of the various categories of paraphilia. Comparison of a treatment group with a high incidence of baseline paraphilic behavior (e.g., exhibitionism) cannot be equivocally compared with a group of paraphiliacs with a low frequency of paraphiliac behaviors (e.g., pedophilia). Studies on the hormonal treatment of paraphiliacs (Bradford, 1983) also suffer from a lack of outcome studies with untreated control groups or with a variety of categories of paraphiliacs in the treated versus untreated control group.

Cognitive-behavioral treatment of groups of pedophiles stand out as the most valid measure of treatment outcome to date. Table 16-7 reflects the outcome of cognitive-behavioral treatment of pedophiles. Of note are the studies by Davidson (1979), Marques (1990), Marshall and Barbaree (1990b), and Rice et al. (in Marshall, 1991), in which the recidivism of treated molesters can be compared with the recidivism of untreated molesters. The studies of Marshall and Barbaree are especially important because the recidivism of the treated molesters was determined using arrest and nonarrest records gathered from a number of official and unofficial sources. In general, recidivism in treated molesters is approximately 20 percent lower than that in untreated molesters. The exception is the study by Rice et al. reporting recidivism rates from a particularly severe group of paraphiliacs

TABLE 16-7.   *Treatment Outcome with Child Molesters*

Victim category	Recidivism of treated molesters (%)	Recidivism of untreated molesters (%)	Author, year
Girls and boys	11	35	Davidson, 1979
Girls and boys	8	20	Marques, 1990
Girls/nonincest	17.9	42.9	Marshall et al., 1991
Boys/nonincest	13.3	42.9	Marshall et al., 1991
Girls and boys/incest	8	21.7	Marshall et al., 1991
Girls and boys	37 (NGBRI)	31	Rice et al., 1991
Girls and boys	12.2		Abel et al., 1988
Girls and boys	10		Gordon, 1989
Girls and boys	20		Leger, 1989
Girls	12.7		Maletzky, 1987
Boys	13.6		Maletzky, 1987
Girls and boys	3		Pithers et al., 1989

From Marshall WL: Effectiveness of treatment with sex offenders. Paper presented at Second International conference on the Treatment of Sex Offenders, Minneapolis, MN, September 1991.

also considered not guilty by reason of insanity (NGBRI). These molesters appear to have had not only severe paraphilic diagnoses but other major psychiatric disorders. Currently, recidivism rates of treated molesters range from 10 to 12 percent, with the exception of the results from Pithers and Cumming (1989), who report a 3 percent recidivism rate.

Success of cognitive-behavioral treatment is even more impressive when one examines the cost savings and the reduction in subsequent victims of child molestation. The current cost in the United States for bringing one child molester and his victim through the criminal justice system, plus 1 year of incarceration for the offender, is $185,000. Since treatment reduces recidivism rates by 20 percent below untreated recidivism rates, for every 100 child molesters treated, the cost savings would be 20 times $185,000, or $3.7 million. This cost savings would provide resources to treat at least 925 child molesters (Prentky and Burgess, 1990).

At a more human cost level, by the time a pedophile has been apprehended, on average, he has molested two children. As a result, cognitive-behavioral treatment, by reducing recidivism by 20 percent, would reduce the number of children molested by 40 victims for every 100 pedophiles treated (Marshall, 1990). These results strongly suggest the economic and humane advantages of treatment for child molesters in the prevention of child molestation.

In conclusion, programs involving the assessment and treatment of paraphiliacs have made tremendous gains in the last 10 years. Cost-effective treatment is already available. The major remaining obstacle is society's attitude regarding the sex offender. We, as a society, are so angry with the sex offender that we ignore what our goal should be—to stop sex offenses before they occur, before anyone is victimized. This approach demands treating the initiator of paraphilic acts, the paraphiliac himself. Unfortunately, this humane approach, to date, has been overpowered by society's desire for vengeance on the paraphiliac, and as a consequence, more victims needlessly suffer.

REFERENCES

Abel GG: A clinical evaluation of possible sex offenders. In The Incest Offender, the Victim, the Family: New Treatment Approaches. White Plains, NY, Mental Health Association of Westchester County, 1985.

Abel GG: The assessment and treatment of child molesters (CME Workshop). Presented at the 144th Annual Meeting of the American Psychiatric Association, New Orleans, LA, May 1991a.

Abel GG: Assessment of paraphilic in non-patient populations. Paper presented at the 10th Annual Research and Treatment Conference of the Association for the Treatment of Sexual Abusers, Fort Worth, TX, November 1991b.

Abel GG, Blanchard EB: The role of fantasy in the treatment of sexual deviation. Arch Gen Psychiatry 30:467–475, 1974.

Abel GG, Osborn CA: Stopping sexual violence. Psychiatr Ann 22:301–306, 1992.

Abel GG, Blanchard EB, Barlow DH: Measurement of sexual arousal in several paraphilias: The effects of stimulus modality, instructional set and stimulus control on the objective. Behav Res Ther 19:25–33, 1981.

Abel GG, Mittelman MS, Becker JV: Sex offenders: Results of assessment and recommendations for treatment. In Ben-Aron MH, Hucker SJ, Webster CD (eds): Clinical Criminology: The Assessment and Treatment of Criminal Behavior. Toronto, M&M Graphics, 1985, pp 191–205.

Abel GG, Osborn CA, Twigg DA: Sexual assault through the lifespan: Adult offenders with juvenile histories. In Barbaree HE, Marshall WL, Laws DR (eds): The Juvenile Sexual Offender. New York, Guilford Publications, in press.

Abel GG, Rouleau JL, Cunningham-Rathner J: Sexually aggressive behavior. In Curran W, McGarry AL, Shah SA (eds): Modern Legal Psychiatry and Psychology. Philadelphia, FA Davis, 1985.

Abel GG, Blanchard EB, Barlow DH, Mavissakalian M: Identifying specific erotic cues in sexual deviation by audiotaped description. J Appl Behav Anal 8:247–260, 1975.

Abel GG, Cunningham-Rathner J, Becker JV, McHugh J: Motivating sex offenders for treatment with feedback of the psychophysiologic assessment. Paper presented at the World Congress of Behavior Therapy, Washington, DC, December 1983a.

Abel GG, Becker JV, Cunningham-Rathner J, et al: Treatment of Child Molesters. Atlanta, GA, Behavioral Medicine Institute of Atlanta, 1984.

Abel GG, Mittelman MS, Becker JV, et al: The characteristics of men who molest young children. Paper presented at the World Congress of Behavior Therapy, Washington, DC, December 1983b.

American Psychiatric Association: Diagnostic and Statistical Manual of Mental Disorders, 3d ed revised. Washington, American Psychiatric Association, 1987.

Annon JS: Reliability and validity of penile plethysmography in rape and child molestation cases. Am J Forensic Psychol 6:11–26, 1988.

Bandura A: Aggression: A Social Learning Analysis. Englewood Cliffs, NJ, Prentice-Hall, 1973.

Barlow DH, Abel GG, Blanchard EB: Gender identity change in transsexuals: Follow-up and replications. Arch Gen Psychiatry 36:1001–1007, 1979.

Barlow DH, Reynolds EH, Agras WS: Gender identity change in a transsexual. Arch Gen Psychiatry 28:569–579, 1973.

Barlow DH, Abel GG, Blanchard EB, et al: Heterosocial skills checklist for males. Behav Ther 8:229–239, 1977.

Beutler LE, Gleason DM: Integrating the advances in the diagnosis and treatment of male potency disturbance. J Urol 126:338–342, 1981.

Beutler LE, Scott FB, Rogers RR, et al: Inflatable and non-inflatable penile prostheses: Comparative follow-up evaluation. Urology 28:136–143, 1986.

Blumer D, Migeon C: Hormone and hormonal agents in the treatment of aggression. J Nerv Ment Dis 160:127–137, 1975.

Bradford JMW: Research on sex offenders: Recent trends. Psychiatr Clin North Am 6:715–731, 1983.

Bradley J, Blanchard R, Coates S, et al: Interim Report of the DSM-IV Subcommittee on Gender Identity Disorders. Arch Sex Behav 20:333–344, 1990.

Bradley SJ, Zucker KJ: Gender identity disorder and psychosexual problems in children and adolescents. Can J Psychiatry 35:477–486, 1990.

Briere J, Runtz M: University males' sexual interest in children: Predicting potential indices of "pedophilia" in a nonforensic sample. Child Abuse Neglect 13:65–75, 1989.

Brown GR: A review of clinical approaches to gender dysphoria. J Clin Psychiatry 51:57–64, 1990.

Collins WE, McKendry SBR, Silverman M, et al: Multidisciplinary survey of erectile impotence. Can Med Assoc J 28:1393–1399, 1981.

Condra M, Morales A, Owen JA, et al: Prevalence and significance of tobacco smoking in impotence. Urology 6:495–498, 1986.

Cunningham-Rathner J, Abel GG: Psychophysiologic measurements of sexual arousal in females. In Fisher M, Fishkin R, Jacobs J (eds): Sexual Arousal. Springfield, IL, Charles C Thomas, 1984, pp 70–87.

Davis GE, Leitenberg H: Adolescent sex offenders. Psychol Bull 101:417–427, 1987.

Davidson P: Outcome data for a penitentiary-based treatment program for sex offenders. Paper presented at the Conference on the Assessment and Treatment of the Sex Offender, Kingston, Ontario, March 1979.

Dorner G: Neuroendocrine response to estrogen and brain differentiation in heterosexuals, homosexuals, and transsexuals. Arch Sex Behav 17:57–75, 1988.

Emmanuel NP, Lydiard RB, Ballenger JC: Fluoxetine treatment of voyeurism. Am J Psychiatry 148:950, 1991.

Freund K: Assessment of pedophilia. In Cook M, Howell SK (eds): Sexual Interest in Children. London, Academic Press, 1981, pp 139–179.

Friedman RC: Male homosexuality: A contemporary psychoanalytic perspective. New Haven, Yale University Press, 1988.

Gagne P: Treatment of sex offenders with medroxyprogesterone acetate. Am J Psychiatry 138:644–646, 1981.

Gilbert DA, Winslow B, Gilbert DM: Transsexual surgery in the genetic female. Clin Plast Surg 15:471–487, 1988.

Girdley FM, Bruskewitz RC, Feyzi J, et al: Intracavernous self-injection for impotence: A long-term option? Experience in 78 patients. J Urol 140:972–974, 1988.

Goldstein I: Penile revascularization. Urol Clin North Am 14:805–813, 1987.

Green R: Family-Doll Preference Test. Copyright 1971, Richard Green, M.D., 1971a.

Green R: Parent and Activity Preference Test. Copyright 1971, Richard Green, M.D., 1971b.

Green R: Sexual Identity Conflicts in Children and Adults. New York, Basic Books, 1974.

Green R, Williams K, Goodman M: Ninety-nine "tomboys" and "non-tomboys": Behavioral contrasts and demographic similarities. Arch Sex Behav 11:247–266, 1982.

Groth, AN: The adolescent sexual offender and his prey. Int J Off Ther Comp Crim 21:249–254, 1977.

Hains AA, Herrman LP, Baker KL, Graber S: The development of a psycho-educational group program for adolescent offenders. J Off Couns Ser Rehab 11:63–75, 1986.

Jensen P, Jensen SB, Sorensen PS, et al: Sexual dysfunction in male and female patients with epilepsy: A study of 86 outpatients. Arch Sex Behav 19:1–14, 1990.

Kafka MP: Successful treatment of paraphilic coercive disorder (a rapist) with fluoxetine hydrochloride. Br J Psychiatry 158:844–847, 1991.

Kaplan MS, Abel GG, Cunningham-Rathner J, Mittelman MS: The impact of parolee's perception of confidentiality of their self-reported sex crimes. Ann Sex Res 3:293–304, 1990.

Langevin R: Sexual Strands: Understanding and Treating Sexual Anomalies in Men. Hillsdale, NJ, Erlbaum Associates, 1983.

Laws DR, Marshall WL: A conditioning theory of the etiology and maintenance of deviant sexual preference and behavior. In Marshall WL, Laws DR, Barbaree HE (eds): Handbook of Sexual Assault: Issues, Theories, and Treatment. New York, Plenum Press, 1990, pp 209–229.

Lo Piccolo J: Diagnosis and treatment of male sexual dysfunction. J Sex Marital Ther 11:215–232, 1985.

Lo Piccolo J, Stock WE: Treatment of sexual dysfunction. J Consult Clin Psychol 54:158–167, 1986.

Lothstein LM: Psychological testing with transsexuals: A 30-year review. J Pers Assess 48:5, 1984.

Malmquist CP: Juvenile sex offenders. In Resnick HL, Wolfgang ME (eds): Sexual Behaviors: Social, Clinical, and Legal Aspects. Boston, Little, Brown, 1972, pp 76–77.

Marlatt GA: Relapse prevention: A self-control program for the treatment of addictive behaviors. In Stuart RB (ed): Adherence, Compliance, and Generalization in Behavioral Medicine. New York, Bruner/Mazel, 1982, pp 329–378.

Marlatt GA, Gordon JR: Determinants of relapse: Implications for the maintenance of change. In Davidson PO, Davidson SM (eds): Behavioral Medicine: Changing Health Lifestyles. New York, Bruner/Mazel, 1980, pp 410–452.

Marlatt GA, Gordon JR (eds): Relapse Prevention. New York, Guilford Press, 1985.

Marques, J: The relapse prevention model: Is it working with sexual offenders? Paper presented at the 9th Annual Clinical and Research Conference on the Assessment and Treatment of Sexual Abusers, Their Families and Victims, Toronto, Ontario, October 1990.

Marshall WL: A combined treatment method for certain sexual deviations. Behav Res Ther 9:293–294, 1971.

Marshall WL: A review of treatment outcome studies for the sexual offender. Paper presented at the 9th Annual Clinical and Research Conference on the Assessment and Treatment of Sexual Abusers, Their Families and Victims, Toronto, Ontario, October 1990.

Marshall WL: Effectiveness of treatment with sex offenders. Paper presented at Second International conference on the Treatment of Sex Offenders, Minneapolis, MN, September 1991.

Marshall WL, Barbaree HE: An integrated theory of the etiology of sexual offending. In Marshall WL, Laws DR, Barbaree HE (eds): Handbook of Sexual Assault: Issues, Theories, and Treatment of the Offender. New York, Plenum Press, 1990a, pp 257–275.

Marshall WL, Barbaree HE: Outcome of comprehensive cognitive-behavioral treatment programs. In Marshall WL, Laws DR, Barbaree HE (eds): Handbook of Sexual Assault: Issues,

Theories, and Treatment of the Offender. New York, Plenum Press, 1990b, pp 363–385.

Masters WH, Johnson V: Human Sexual Inadequacy. Boston: Little, Brown, 1970.

McCabe MP, Delaney SM: An evaluation of therapeutic programs for the treatment of secondary inorgasmia in women. Arch Sex Behav 21:69--90, 1992.

Mellinger BC, Vaughan ED, Thompson SL, Goldstein M: Correlation between intracavernous papaverine injection and Doppler analysis in impotent men. Urology 30:416–419, 1987.

Melman A, Tiefer L, Pedersen R: Evaluation of first 406 patients in urology department–based center for male sexual dysfunction. Urology 32:6–10, 1988.

Meyer-Bahlburg HFL: Gender identity disorder of childhood: Introduction. J Am Acad Child Psychiatry 24:681–683, 1985.

Mohr DC, Beutler LE: Erectile dysfunction: A review of diagnostic and treatment procedures. Clin Psychol Rev 10:123–150, 1990.

Money J: Use of androgen-depleting hormone in the treatment of male sex offenders. J Sex Res 6:165–172, 1970.

Money J, Hampson JG, Hampson JL: Imprinting and the establishment of gender role. Arch Neurol Psychiatry 77:333–336, 1987.

Money JM, Wiedeking C, Walker PS, et al: Combined antiandrogen and counseling program for treatment of 46 XY and 47 XYY sex offenders. In Sachar EJ (ed): Hormones, Behavior, and Psychopathology. New York, Raven Press, 1976.

Mulaikal RM, Migeon CJ, Rock JA: Fertility rates in female patients with congenital adrenal hyperplasia due to 21-hydroxylase deficiency. N Engl J Med 316:178–182, 1987.

Nadig PW, Ware JC, Blumoff R: Noninvasive device to produce and maintain an erection-like state. Urology 27:126–131, 1986.

Nelson C, Miner M, Marques J, et al: Relapse prevention: A cognitive-behavioral model for treatment of the rapist and child molester. J Soc Work Human Sex 7:125–143, 1988.

Perilstein RD, Lipper S, Friedman LJ: Three cases of paraphilias responsive to fluoxetene treatment. J Clin Psychiatry 52:169–170, 1991.

Pithers WD: Relapse prevention with sexual aggressors: A method for maintaining therapeutic gain and enhancing external supervision. In Marshall WL, Laws DR, Barbaree HE (eds): Handbook of Sexual Assault: Issues, Theories, and Treatment of the Offender. New York, Plenum Press, 1990, pp 343–361.

Pithers WD, Cumming GF: Can relapses be prevented? Initial outcome data from the Vermont Treatment Program for Sexual Aggressors. In Laws DR (ed): Relapse Prevention with Sex Offenders. New York, Guilford Press, 1989.

Prentky R, Burgess AW: Rehabilitation of child molesters: A cost benefit analysis. Am J Orthopsychiatry 60:108–117, 1990.

Quinsey VL, Marshall WL: Procedures for reducing inappropriate sexual arousal: An evaluation review. In Greer JG, Stuart IR (eds): The Sexual Aggressor: Current Perspectives on Treatment. New York, Van Nostrand Reinhold, 1983, pp 267–289.

Rekers GA, Morey SM: Sex-typed body movements as a function of severity of gender disturbance in boys. J Psychol Human Sex 2:183–196, 1989.

Rouleau JL, Abel GG, Mittelman MS, et al: Sexual symptoms specific to diabetes. Paper presented at the World Meeting on Impotence, Paris, June 1984.

Salter, AC: Treating Child Sex Offenders and Victims: A Practical Guide, Appendix F. Newbury Park, CA, Sage Publications, 1988, pp 278–280.

Schuman SH: Practice-Based Epidemiology: An Introduction. New York, Gordon and Breach Science, 1986.

Segraves RT, Schoenberg HW: Diagnosis and treatment of erectile problems: Current status. In Segraves RT, Schoenberg HW (eds): Diagnosis and Treatment of Erectile Disturbances: A Guide for Clinicians. New York, Plenum Medical Book Company, 1985, pp 1–22.

Semans JH: Premature ejaculation: A new approach. South Med J 49:353, 1956.

Spector IP, Carey MP: Incidence and prevalence of the sexual dysfunctions: A critical review of the empirical literature. Arch Sex Behav 19:374–389, 1990.

Stoller RJ: Sex and Gender, vol 1: The Development of Masculinity and Femininity. New York, Science House, 1968.

Stoller RJ: Etiological factors in female transsexualism: A first approximation. Arch Sex Behav 2:47–64, 1972.

Taylor DC: Sexual behavior and temporal lobe epilepsy. Arch Neurol Psychiatry 21:510–516, 1969.

Templeman TL, Stinnett RD: Patterns of sexual arousal and history in a "normal" sample of young men. Arch Sex Behav 20:137–150, 1991.

Van Putten T, Fawzy FI: Sex conversion surgery in a man with severe gender dysphoria: A tragic outcome. Arch Gen Psychiatry 33:751–754, 1976.

Walker P, Berger J, Green R: Standards of care: The hormonal and surgical sex reassignment of GD persons. Arch Sex Behav 70:79–90, 1985.

Wespes E, Delcour C, Rondeux C, et al: The erectile angle: Objective criterion to evaluate the papaverine test in impotence. J Urol 138:1171–1173, 1987.

Wespes E, Delcour C, Struyven J, Schulman CC: Cavernometry-cavernography: Its role in organic impotence. Eur Urol 10:229–232, 1984.

Wincze JP, Bansal S, Malhotra C, et al: A comparison of nocturnal penile tumescence and penile response to erotic stimulation during waking states in comprehensively diagnosed groups of males experiencing erectile difficulties. Arch Sex Behav 17:333–348, 1988.

Zeiss AE, Davies HD, Wood M, Tinklenberg JR: The incidence and correlates of erectile problems in patients with Alzheimer's disease. Arch Sex Behav 19:325–333, 1990.

Zucker KJ, Bradley SJ, Hughes HE: Gender dysphoria in a child with true hermaphroditism. Can J Psychiatry 32:602–609, 1987.

CHAPTER 17

Other Psychiatric Syndromes: Adjustment Disorder, Factitious Disorder, Illicit Steroid Abuse

WILLIAM R. YATES

Several additional topics merit consideration as psychiatric syndromes. This chapter covers four additional topics: adjustment disorder, factitious disorder, psychiatric effects of illicit anabolic steroid abuse, and special psychiatric syndromes identified by eponyms or cultural ties.

Adjustment disorder and factitious disorder are psychiatric syndromes important in the medical setting. Adjustment disorder occurs commonly in the medically ill patient presenting for psychiatric consultation. Patients with factitious disorder, although rare, present a challenge for medical personnel in assessment and management. The psychiatric aspect of anabolic steroid use is an emerging area of study and clinical relevance. Most understanding of the psychiatric effects of illicit steroid use has occurred recently. Finally, psychiatric eponyms and cultural syndromes describe unique clinical profiles and provide a method to classify certain clinical presentations. A glossary of these eponyms increases awareness of the history of psychiatric classification. Culture-bound syndromes highlight the role of environment and society in the presentation of psychiatric disorders.

ADJUSTMENT DISORDER

Definition

Adjustment disorder constitutes a group of disorders defined by a maladaptive response to a stressor. Adjustment disorders are subclassified according to the dominant clinical symptoms. Table 17-1 defines the categories of adjustment disorder according to DSM-IIIR (American Psychiatric Association, 1987).

By definition, the predominant symptoms must evolve within 3 months of the stressor. Symptom duration may not exceed 6 months. The disorder is transient, with resolution over time or with development into a more severe syndrome such as major depressive disorder.

The maladaptive reaction to a stressor is confirmed by either impairment in occupational or social functioning or symptoms that exceed a normal response. Additionally, the symptom complex must not meet criteria for any other specific psychiatric disorder. For example, a patient displaying a full major depressive disorder following a divorce is diagnosed with major depressive disorder and not with adjustment disorder with depressed mood. The role of the stressor in the major depressive disorder is noted with a reference to the psychosocial stressor severity rating on Axis IV.

Epidemiology

The prevalence of adjustment disorder in various populations has been the subject of limited attention. This limited attention results from several factors. Standardized interviews and operationalized criteria are recent developments. Nevertheless, several studies in various populations exist. These studies suggest that adjustment disorder is a frequent clinical condition worthy of further study. Several prevalence studies of adjustment disorder are noted in Table 17-2.

Clinical Picture

The clinical profile of symptoms in adjustment disorder is quite variable and appears dependent on

TABLE 17-1. *Classification of Adjustment Disorders*

Adjustment disorder with anxious mood
Adjustment disorder with depressed mood
Adjustment disorder with disturbance of conduct
Adjustment disorder with disturbance of emotions and conduct
Adjustment disorder with mixed emotional features
Adjustment disorder with physical complaints
Adjustment disorder with withdrawal
Adjustment disorder with work or academic inhibition
Adjustment disorder not otherwise specified

the age of the individual. Adolescents appear to be more likely to develop behavioral problems with acting-out symptoms. Adults appear more likely to respond in a maladaptive fashion with depressive and anxiety symptoms.

Generally, the clinical picture reflects mild to moderate distress in the context of significant psychosocial difficulties. Symptom severity is less than most other Axis I disorders. Nevertheless, the symptom severity in adjustment disorder is significant enough to distinguish this population from community samples free from psychiatric illness (Fabrega et al., 1987).

ILLUSTRATIVE CASE

Mrs. K was a 64-year-old married white woman who was admitted to the coronary care unit for congestive heart failure and atrial fibrillation. The attending physician requested a psychiatric consultation for episodes of nervousness and anxiety.

Mrs. K reported persistent anxiety since being admitted to the hospital. She felt her symptoms stemmed from confinement to her hospital room. Her usual daily activities included plenty of activity and movement. Being restricted to her room made her feel trapped and out of control. She had difficulty sleeping and felt keyed up with rumination about her physical condition.

The patient denied depressed mood. There was no history of past or current panic attacks. She denied obsessions, compulsions, or phobias. She did not drink alcohol. She had no major significant psychiatric history. She did undergo a brief trial of hypnosis after a divorce. There was no history of psychotropic medication use, psychiatric hospitalization, or suicide attempts. There was no family history of psychiatric disorder.

Her medications at the time of her psychiatric evaluation included sucralfate qid, warfarin 5 mg daily, sublingual nitroglycerin, furosemide 40 mg daily, captopril 37.5 mg tid, digoxin 0.125 mg daily, metoclopramide 10 mg qid, and diazepam 5 mg every 6 hours prn. Mrs. K reported that the diazepam relieved her anxiety symptoms, but she had received only one dose over the last 72 hours. Onset of her anxiety symptoms did not coincide with the initiation of any new medication during her hospital stay.

Laboratory and medical testing revealed normal thyroid function studies. Complete blood count, arterial blood gases, and general chemistry screen were within normal limits. Her electrocardiogram revealed atrial fibrillation.

On mental status examination, Mrs. K appeared well groomed and was dressed in a hospital gown. A handshake demonstrated the presence of perspiring palms. She appeared anxious in facial expression and bodily movements. She did not appear depressed. Her thoughts were logical and goal directed without a formal thought disorder. There were no hallucinations, delusions, or suicidal or homicidal thoughts. Her insight and judgment were unimpaired. Cognitive testing revealed no abnormalities of orientation, memory, concentration, or comprehension.

The psychiatric consultant considered the following diagnoses in the differential diagnosis: generalized anxiety disorder, obsessive-compulsive personality disorder, organic anxiety syndrome secondary to medication, delirium, and adjustment disorder with anxious mood. Adjustment disorder with anxious mood was diagnosed after ruling out the other diagnostic considerations. Recommendations included a trial of diazepam 5 mg bid and an additional 5 mg prn during hospitalization. Continued diazepam treatment after discharge was felt unlikely to be necessary. A psychiatric nurse visited Mrs. K regularly during her hospitalization and provided relaxation exercises. The cardiology team was encouraged to allow ambulation and physical therapy as soon as medically possible to allow the patient to return to her active lifestyle.

The patient's anxiety responded well to the combination of diazepam and relaxation training. At discharge, the diazepam was tapered and discontinued. In a follow-up visit 3 weeks after discharge, the patient's anxiety symptoms had essentially resolved.

Clinical Course

The duration limitation of less than 6 months reflects a generally good prognosis for adjustment disorder. Outcome studies of adults with adjustment disorder have found over 70 percent without

TABLE 17-2. *Prevalence Estimates of Adjustment Disorder in Various Populations*

Category	n	Site	Contact	Prevalence (%)	Author, year
Children	386	Community	Survey	4.2–7.6	Bird et al., 1988
Adolescent suicides	56	Urban	Postmortem	14	Runeson, 1989
Suicide attempters	127	Inpatient	Consult	24.4	Hale et al., 1990
Gunshot wounds	260	Inpatient	Consult	10	Frierson and Lippman, 1990
Consultation series	1048	Inpatient/outpatient	Consult	11.5	Popkin et al., 1990
Geriatric	197	Nursing home	Consult	16	Loebel et al., 1991
Psychiatric clinic	5573	Outpatient	Diagnostics	12.3	Fabrega et al., 1987
Psychiatric hospital	2699	Inpatient	Admissions	5	Andreasen and Wasek, 1980

significant impairment or psychiatric illness 5 years after the index diagnosis (Andreasen and Hoenck, 1982.) This follow-up study found that those with a psychiatric disorder were likely to have antisocial personality, alcoholism, or a major depressive disorder. However, the generally favorable prognosis is tempered by a 4 percent suicide rate in this study population.

The prognosis of adjustment disorder appears less optimistic in the adolescent population. Andreasen and Hoenck's study (1982) found that only 44 percent of adolescents were well 5 years after an index diagnosis of adjustment disorder. The most frequent follow-up psychiatric diagnoses in the adolescent populations included major depressive disorder, antisocial personality disorder, alcoholism, drug abuse, schizophrenia, and bipolar disorder. The 5-year follow-up of adolescent adjustment disorder also found a 2 percent suicide rate. Masterson (1967) also documented the poor prognosis in adolescents with adjustment disorder. Sixty-two percent of adolescents displayed moderate to severe impairment 5 years after an index diagnosis. The prognosis for adjustment disorder in adolescents appears to be especially poor when there is a disturbance of conduct (Chess and Thomas, 1984).

Etiology

The cause of adjustment disorder stems from the interaction between a stressor and the adaptive mechanisms of the individual. The type of stressor responsible for the initiation of an adjustment disorder can be quite variable and mimics the types of stressors commonly seen in everyday life. In a series of adult patients receiving psychiatric care with a diagnosis of adjustment disorder, the most common types of precipitants included marital problems, divorce or separation, a move to a new location, financial problems, and school or work problems (Andreasen and Hoenck, 1982). The type of stressor precipitating symptoms reflects the clinical setting of contact. For psychiatric consultations in the general hospital, a frequent precipitant is acute and chronic medical illness.

The severity of the stressor appears also to play a role in the etiology of adjustment disorder. The risk of developing psychiatric symptoms appears to increase with increased stressor severity. However, the response does need to meet the maladaptive and excessive responses criteria noted in the adjustment disorder.

The individual's pattern of response to stress has some stability over time. Therefore, individuals with previous maladaptive responses are more likely to display repeated maladaptive responses. The reason some individuals are more vulnerable to stressors is not completely known. Genetic and environmental factors probably influence individual risks for maladaptive response to stressors.

Differential Diagnosis

The differential diagnosis for adjustment disorder focuses on the primary complaint. For example, differential diagnoses in a patient with marked anxiety prior to a surgical procedure would include adjustment disorder with anxious mood, generalized anxiety, panic disorder, simple phobia, organic anxiety syndrome, or a mood, substance abuse, or personality disorder. Generally, it is best to begin the differential diagnosis with attention to the predominant symptom and include disorders likely to produce the target symptom in the differential diagnosis.

Adjustment disorder is not diagnosed when the target symptoms are only one instance of a pattern of overreaction. Personality disorders encompass behaviors or traits that are personal characteristics stable for long time periods. Under stress these traits may increase target symptoms or behaviors similar to those of an adjustment disorder. The differentiation of adjustment disorder and personality disorder is difficult during time-limited assessments of new patients.

Another stress-related diagnostic category in DSM-IIIR is the category of psychological factors affecting physical condition. In this disorder, the focus of attention is worsening of a physical condition due to a psychosocial stressor. Adjustment disorder with physical complaints is diagnosed when no physical cause of the complaints is identified. In contrast, a patient with rheumatoid arthritis experiencing increased pain following the death of a relative exemplifies psychological factors affecting physical condition.

A final stress-related category in DSM-IIIR is the category posttraumatic stress disorder (PTSD). This category differs from adjustment disorder in several ways. In PTSD, the stressor must be of sufficient severity to be considered an "event that is outside the range of usual human experience and that would be markedly distressing to almost anyone" (American Psychiatric Association, 1987). Note that this category places a greater emphasis on the extreme nature of the stressor compared with the adjustment disorder. Additionally, in PTSD, the traumatic event must be persistently reexperienced with avoidance and arousal symptoms. With PTSD there is no limit on symptom duration. The onset of symptoms can be delayed for more than 6 months.

Mood or anxiety disorders are frequent differential diagnosis concerns in patients displaying symptoms related to an identifiable stressor. It is important to question for major depression, dysthymia, panic disorder, and generalized anxiety disorder in patients seen for conditions in which adjustment disorder is being considered. Clinical factors appear to distinguish adjustment disorder with depressed mood from major depression (Bronisch and Hecht, 1989). In a general hospital psychiatry series, major depression was linked to older age, widowed marital status, and living alone (Snyder et al., 1990). Psychosocial stressors can exacerbate nearly any chronic psychiatric disorder, and the resultant increase in symptoms may appear to be due to an adjustment disorder. The key to differential diagnosis between adjustment disorders and an anxiety or a mood disorder is to elicit sufficient information to confirm whether a full anxiety or mood disorder is present.

Treatment

Treatment recommendations for adjustment disorder are based primarily on clinical experience. Few treatment studies focus on adjustment disorder. Although the often transient nature of the condition suggests that treatment has limited importance, treatment can significantly reduce distress. Additionally, identification and treatment may prevent development of a more chronic condition.

Identification of the individual causes of adjustment reactions is the beginning of treatment planning. For patients demonstrating acute anxiety or depressive symptoms, it is beneficial to question the patient about the most distressing source of stress. This precipitating stressor may be a misunderstanding or an overestimation of danger or risk. Simple acknowledgment of the stressor sources, along with education and support, provides the basis for beginning intervention.

It is helpful to consider the individual's usual coping strategies for dealing with stressors. Facilitating the use of past successful strategies can prevent the need for new strategies. For example, allowing hospitalized patients to contact trusted friends, family, or clergy and discuss their condition and receive support may be quite beneficial.

Psychotherapy principles for adjustment disorder focus more on crisis-intervention principles than on a particular psychotherapy model. A BICEPS (brevity, immediacy, centrality, expectancy, proximity, and simplicity) model successfully limits the functional impairment following exposure to significant military stressors (Salmon and Fenton, 1929). This model uses a brief intervention approach beginning as soon as possible following stressor exposure. Patients receive notice that they are expected to return quickly to their previous level of function. The intervention occurs without transfer to another location. Attention focuses on symptom reduction without attention to underlying personality or neurotic issues.

This strategy has implications for general hospital patients experiencing adjustment disorders in the hospital setting. Symptom identification begins as soon as possible—brief intervention strategies follow immediately after symptom identification. Treatment occurs on the medical ward rather than on transfer to the psychiatric unit. Physicians can encourage and expect quick symptom resolution.

Psychotherapy strategies remain basic, using approaches such as relaxation training.

Medication approaches for adjustment disorder target the primary presenting complaint (Schatzberg, 1990). The majority of adjustment disorder diagnoses are subclassified with anxious, depressed, or mixed emotional features. Many adjustment disorders respond to support and the passage of time—some more severe and persistent syndromes merit consideration for medication trials. Treatment studies have suggested adjustment disorder with depressed mood responds as well as major depressive disorder to a trial of antidepressant medication (Schwartz et al., 1989).

In the case study, short-term benzodiazepine administration alleviated a significant adjustment disorder with anxious mood. Benzodiazepines have the advantage of rapid onset of anxiolytic effect. Concern about long-term dependence and withdrawal symptoms minimizes when the course of treatment is 6 weeks or less. Rational strategies for benzodiazepine use in adjustment disorder include alprazolam, 0.75 to 3 mg, in three divided doses, lorazepam, 1.5 to 6 mg, in three divided doses, or diazepam, 10 to 30 mg, in a single or divided dose. Doses can be titrated to the symptom level. In hospitalized patients it is better to use regularly scheduled administration rather than rely on an as-needed or prn administration schedule. Physicians should notify patients that the medication is for short-term use and that the development of tolerance and dependence will be medically monitored.

Prevention

Adjustment disorders in the medical setting often arise out of fear or anxiety about medical illnesses, hospitalization, and medical procedures. Miscommunication between medical personnel and the hospitalized patient can contribute to the development of adjustment disorders. Clear communication about the diagnosis, prognosis, and treatment plan can prevent significant adjustment disorder problems. Physicians, nurses, and ancillary medical staff efforts at education and support for the acutely and chronically hospitalized patient are important. Anticipatory education decreases adjustment symptomatology and increases patient satisfaction with medical care.

FACTITIOUS DISORDER

The voluntary production of physical or psychological symptoms or signs of illness represents the core for disorders classified as *factitious disorders*. This disorder is another problem encountered in the hospital setting. Although much less common than adjustment disorder, factitious disorder presents a significant challenge for medical physicians and psychiatric consultants. Along with the challenge of documenting the voluntary production of symptoms, factitious disorder patients often evoke strong negative emotional responses in members of the health care team. The management of factitious disorder also adds to the challenging character of these disorders.

Definition

DSM-IIIR defines three categories of factitious disorder. The first category is factitious disorder with physical symptoms. This is the category covering the earliest described factitious disorder—Munchausen syndrome (Asher, 1951). The essential features of Munchausen's syndrome include pseudologica fantastica (pathologic lying), peregrination (traveling or wandering), and recurrent feigned or simulated illness. By definition, the physical symptoms or signs in factitious disorder are intentionally produced or feigned. The motive for this symptom production is a "psychological need to assume the sick role." Motivation by an obvious external incentive is absent. By definition, the symptoms cannot occur exclusively as part of another major mental disorder. Another category in DSM-IIIR is factitious disorder with psychological symptoms. The definition of this disorder is identical to that for factitious disorder with physical symptoms except for the psychological character of the intentional symptom. A residual category of factitious disorder not otherwise specified defines patients with both physical and psychological symptoms or atypical presentations. Factitious disorder with psychological symptoms has less clinical history and less acceptance in psychiatry. Some have suggested that this disorder is not a valid diagnostic entity because of unresolved issues in motivation, inclusion and exclusion criteria, and outcome (Rogers et al., 1989).

A form of factitious disorder in childhood exists. Referred to as *Munchausen syndrome by proxy*, this clinical disorder involves a parent–child interaction. For this disorder, parents fabricate symptoms or signs of illness in their children to maintain their child in a sick role. Various presentations in the pediatric setting exist (Meadow, 1982).

Epidemiology

No community information exists for the general population prevalence of this disorder. Most estimates of the prevalence of this disorder originate from hospital and psychiatry consultation series. Table 17-3 notes the prevalence findings for factitious disorder in the medical setting.

Clinical Picture

The presenting clinical sign or symptom for factitious disorder can be quite variable. Despite this variability, certain symptoms encourage aggressive pursuit of factitious disorder in the medical differential diagnosis. These high-risk situations include recurrent skin infection, especially with fecal flora contamination; recurrent unexplained hypoglycemia in diabetics and others with access to insulin; unexplained bruises or dermatologic conditions; fever of unknown origin; and surreptitious use of prescribed and over-the-counter medication. Particular medical diagnoses such as cancer have been the focus of feigned illness. Predictably as new conditions arise and become more prevalent, factitious variants arise. For example, recent reports of factitious AIDS have developed (Sno et al., 1991). Feigned psychosis and feigned posttraumatic stress disorders exemplify factitious disorder with psychological symptoms (Pope et al., 1982; Sparr and Pankratz, 1983).

In Munchausen syndrome by proxy, several similarities exist compared with adult factitious disorder (Meadow, 1982). Common fabricated signs included bleeding, neurologic problems, rashes, glycosuria, and fever. Medical occupations are frequently noted in the mothers of these children, similar to the adult factitious disorder series.

ILLUSTRATIVE CASE

Ms L was a 20-year-old single unemployed woman seen by her primary-care physician for recurrent right leg swelling. The recurrent swelling had occurred over a period of 18 months, resulting in several hospitalizations for "thrombophlebitis." The patient was taking anticoagulants. Despite anticoagulant therapy, the right leg continued to be intermittently swollen. The swelling resolved with elevation, rest, and compression stockings.

At one point during the patient's illness, while she was taking anticoagulants, an acute gastrointestinal bleed occurred. Bleeding resulted in anemia (hemoglobin level 5 mg/dl). The patient's prothrombin time was in the therapeutic range prior to the acute bleed. However, at the time of the acute bleed, the prothrombin time was elevated to greater than 30 seconds. Although the patient denied taking an excessive dose of warfarin, a pill count by the physician documented excessive daily dosing. The patient required transfusion to correct the anemia.

TABLE 17-3. *Prevalence of Factitious Disorder in Treatment Populations*

Category	n	Site	Contact	Prevalence (%)	Author, year
Teaching hospital	1361	Inpatient	Consult	1	Sutherland and Rodin, 1990
Fever of unknown origin	343	Inpatient	Referral	9.3	Aduan et al., 1979
Psychotic disorder	219	Inpatient	Series	4.2	Pope et al., 1982

Ms L denied any significant psychological distress. She did not appear depressed or anxious or have any psychotic symptoms. She did not respond to the intermittent swelling with anxiety or increased concern about her condition. There was no previous psychiatric history. Ms L was an only child who lived at home with her parents. Her mother had been somewhat overbearing and dominant, to the point of completing all the patient's high school homework and paper assignments. Following graduation from high school, Ms L briefly attended a secretarial training course at a school 65 miles from home. She was unable to complete the course because of her recurrent leg difficulties. When her leg became intermittently worse, Ms L received care by her mother. Her mother constantly checked her condition and provided assistance with daily cares.

During one acute swelling episode, the patient presented to the primary-care physician's office. A physical examination was done in the usual fashion with the patient gowned. However, further examination of the proximal right leg revealed a half-inch-deep circumferential tourniquet mark.

Ms L was confronted. Her physician noted the voluntary production of leg swelling and offered to arrange a psychiatric evaluation. She was not punished or humiliated for her behavior. She refused psychiatric referral and left the physician's office without returning for any scheduled follow-up appointments.

Ms L's primary-care physician called her mother to determine the reason for noncompliance with recommendations for follow-up. She reported that Ms L had transferred her care to another physician in a town 25 miles away. Additionally, she later began work at the new physician's office as a medical transcriptionist.

Clinical Course

Separating factitious disorder into those with a Munchausen syndrome and those without defines two different prognostic groups. Munchausen syndrome has a very poor prognosis, with only one case report of successful treatment (Yassa, 1978). Factitious disorder without a Munchausen's syndrome appears to have a better prognosis. Good prognosis correlates with patients who also have a major depressive disorder. Combined medical and psychiatric management also decreases the morbidity of the disorder.

Ten patients with factitious disorder with hypoglycemia have been the subject of an outcome study (Gruenberger et al., 1988). Following identification of surreptitious insulin use, confrontation, and psychiatric treatment, only three patients showed complete resolution of their condition. Remarkably, two patients died during follow-up, presumably due to self-induced hypoglycemia.

The outcome of factitious disorder with psychological symptoms has received limited attention. In the study by Pope et al. (1982) of factitious disorder with psychological symptoms, the outcome was poor. Nine patients were followed for 4 to 7 years. One had committed suicide. Seven of the remaining eight had significant histories of frequent hospitalizations. Factitious disorder with psychosis predicted a poorer outcome than true psychoses such as schizophrenia or mania.

Nineteen children with Munchausen syndrome by proxy received longitudinal study (Meadow, 1982). Two died presumably from the effects of the factitious disorder. Eight children were removed from their parents with resolution of the feigned signs. Nine children remained with their parents after confrontation and with close supervision by social workers. Of these nine children, seven were completely well without symptoms on follow-up. Two children continued with frequent physician visits for minor complaints not considered harmful factitious problems.

Etiology

The etiology of factitious disorder is unknown. The risk factor and personality studies in this disorder present some basis for theoretical attempts to define the etiology of the disorder. Because factitious disorder patients often have severe personality disorders, the role of personality development and deficits appears to be important. Case studies of factitious disorder have described significant drives for dependency. The production of serious medical signs and symptoms mobilizes a medical care structure that often places patients in a dependent relationship. Significant angry affect is documented in case studies of factitious disorder. Borderline personality disorder is common. Patients may receive satisfaction at deceiving their health care team and getting revenge for previous interpersonal conflicts.

The common finding of a medical background in factitious disorder suggests that medical knowledge facilitates the disorder in patients who have vulnerable personality structures.

Differential Diagnosis

The primary difficulty in the differential diagnosis of factitious disorder is confirming the voluntary production of signs and symptoms. Many patients never demonstrate their factitious behavior to others. This lack of proof is often frustrating and leaves an element of diagnostic doubt.

Malingering constitutes a disorder similar to factitious disorder. Both disorders involve the voluntary production of symptoms. The primary distinction in malingering is evidence that the intent of the feigned symptoms or illness is to obtain an external incentive. This external incentive, or "secondary gain," is often financial reimbursement through disability or through liability damages. Nonmonetary secondary gain also can be the motive for malingering. Nonmonetary incentives include evasion of military duty, evasion of criminal charges or jail sentences, or becoming eligible for better living circumstances.

Personality disorders in the medical setting mimic some of the characteristics of factitious disorder. Borderline personality disorder patients often evoke some of the same anger and frustration in health care professionals as the factitious disorder patient. The self-mutilation behaviors found with borderline personality tend to be stereotypical—an example being repeated superficial lacerations over the forearm. Although such behavior is voluntary, the patient acknowledges the behavior as being self-inflicted.

True medical illnesses deserve careful consideration in presumed factitious disorder. Follow-up series of patient's diagnosed with factitious disorder have included some who went on to have the "factitious" symptoms explained by medical disease (Sutherland and Rodin, 1990).

Other somatoform disorders also involve unexplained somatic complaints. Somatization disorder differs from factitious disorder in the number of presenting complaints. Although multiple symptoms occur in factitious disorder, single symptoms or signs are more often the focus of attention. Somatization disorder symptoms are more likely to involve subjective pain complaints, while factitious disorder target symptoms and signs often involve objective signs, i.e., hypoglycemia, skin infection, or fever.

Psychiatric comorbidity presents an additional challenge in the assessment of factitious disorder. It is possible for the patient to have more than one psychiatric disorder including factitious disorder. Treatable psychiatric comorbid conditions should receive attention. Diagnoses in this category include mood disorders, anxiety disorders, psychotic disorders, organic mental disorders, and substance abuse.

Careful consideration of the psychiatric and medical differential diagnoses of factitious disorder can lead to accurate diagnosis of the syndrome. Management of the syndrome can be as complicated as the diagnostic process.

Laboratory Tests

Laboratory tests can occasionally provide supporting evidence for the diagnosis of factitious disorder. This is particularly true with the surreptitious use of insulin. For patients without diabetes and without a medical cause for insulin treatment, the identification of insulin antibodies provides evidence of exogenous insulin use (Gruenberger et al., 1988). Additionally, monitoring C-peptide levels during episodes of hypoglycemia also may confirm suspicions of surreptitious insulin use to produce factitious hypoglycemia.

Self-induced infections may produce cultures revealing multiple organisms commonly found in feces. For example, recurrent wound or skin infections growing such organisms as *Escherichia coli*, group D enterococcus, and *Klebsiella* is highly suggestive of the use of feces to feign recurrent infections. However, fecal sources of bacteria are not the only source of possible infectious agents. Factitious infections from pure cultured bacteria also have been reported (Aduan et al., 1979). Other pyogenic substances such as tetanus toxoid and milk proteins can produce a clinical picture of fever of unknown origin.

Bleeding and clotting factor studies provide assistance in evaluating the patient with unexplained bleeding problems. As in the case example, pill counting for factitious use of anticoagulants also can be helpful in confirmation of factitious disorder.

Treatment

The treatment of factitious disorder involves a coordinated medical and psychiatric assessment and treatment plan. Treatment of concurrent psychiatric disorders can assist in management. Factitious disorder is not a contraindication for somatic treatment of comorbid mood or anxiety disorders.

Early studies of the treatment and natural history of factitious disorder promoted confrontation of the patient as the key to beginning treatment. There is less consensus that confrontation, especially in a punitive fashion, is an effective treatment approach. There is no evidence that the patient must admit the self-injurious behavior has occurred in order for the clinical picture to improve.

After collecting sufficient evidence to confirm a factitious disorder diagnosis, a coordinated plan to notify the patient and provide follow-up care is needed. An example of a method of notifying the patient in a nonpunitive fashion follows. This example is taken as a hypothetical approach to the illustrative case prior to the primary care physician scheduling psychiatric consultation.

Ms L, I would like to give you some information about my assessment and treatment recommendations. I know your leg swelling has caused you a significant amount of discomfort. I have tried my best to provide quality care for your condition. The observation of a tourniquet mark on your leg leads me to believe your behaviors have contributed to the problem. I understand behaviors like this have complex meanings but generally can be seen as a cry for help, for understanding, and for a needed more comprehensive evaluation of emotional factors involved in your life.

I will continue to care for your medical problems. I know that these behaviors have served some purpose for you, but as your physician I must tell you they must now stop. I expect that with help and support you will be able to discontinue these behaviors. To provide assistance for you I will arrange for you to see a psychiatrist who will provide an expert evaluation and behavioral management plan for us. Together I believe we can provide you with a strategy to improve your physical and emotional health.

The role of psychotherapy in factitious disorder has received only minimal attention. The treatment is tailored to the individual patient and his or her individual psychiatric presentation. For patients with concurrent borderline personality disorder, cognitive therapy strategies for personality disorders exist (Beck and Freeman, 1990). For the factitious disorder behaviors, behavioral management plans provide a method of intervention. Behavioral strategies should eliminate positive reinforcement in the home and hospital for the factitious behaviors. Behavioral strategies can allow the patient to minimize embarrassment and shame. Positive reinforcement for reducing factitious behaviors is also helpful.

In Munchausen syndrome by proxy, the safety and health of the child are a priority for management. This syndrome is a form of child abuse. Notification of social services and the initiation of child abuse evaluations must begin when the syndrome becomes apparent.

ILLICIT ANABOLIC STEROID USE

Anabolic steroids (ASs) are a group of natural and synthetic hormones with masculinizing as well as anabolic (tissue-building) properties. Illicit use of ASs began with their discovery and synthesis in the 1940s. The illicit use of ASs occurs primarily in the context of athletic competition—the goal of their use is to increase size, speed, and performance, thereby gaining a competitive edge. Illicit use is defined as use without a physicians' prescription. Illicit procurement of supplies occurs through black-market sources. Although the illicit use of AS compounds has a 50-year history, their use appears to be increasing and their effect on mental status is receiving increased attention. In 1990, ASs were added to schedule III of prescription drugs covered by the Controlled Substances Act. This assignment has stimulated discussion of the addiction potential of the compounds. In this section, the scope, mental status effects, and addiction hypothesis for illicit AS use will be examined.

Epidemiology

Various population groups surveyed for the prevalence of illicit AS use include high school and college students and participants in specific sports. The surveys have been predominantly self-report with limited reliability and validity testing. Despite this, the surveys suggest that AS use is common, begins frequently during the adolescent years, and is primarily a problem in men. Reviews of the epidemiology of AS use allow some general conclusions about the epidemiology of AS use (Yesalis, 1992). Table 17-4 summarizes several of the surveys with the best methodologies.

Yesalis (1992) argues that survey methods probably underestimate the prevalence rates of anabolic steroid use. Nonresponse bias is likely to play a role in underestimation due to the legal and sports sanctions attached to illicit use. The prevalence estimates of AS use double or triple when athletes estimate the use of AS in their peer group (Yesalis et al., 1990). This suggests that self-reported use of ASs is a lower bound of the prevalence rates. Despite using this lower bound, estimates suggest that 250,000 adolescents in the United States are using or have used ASs.

Several risk factors appear related to anabolic steroid use. Male gender predominates in this problem. Specific sports and specific positions within sports have higher rates of AS use. Table 17-5 displays the rank order of AS use among Division I National Collegiate Athletic Association male athletes.

AS use typically occurs in 8- to 16-week cycles. AS use cycles are interspersed with periods of AS abstinence. The specific steroids ingested and durations of use are variable. The methods and patterns of use develop through user experience and are disseminated through word-of-mouth and underground publications (Duchaine, 1989). Typically, the AS use pattern involves the use of multiple compounds. Compounds can include oral as well as injectable drugs. Although ASs were used for therapeutic indications for many years, illicit users typically employ doses much higher than the therapeutic replacement dose. This high-dose pattern has limited the generalization of current knowledge. Medical and psychiatric effects of ASs in therapeutic doses do not necessarily predict effects at supratherapeutic doses.

Psychiatric Effects

The apparent increased prevalence of AS use has brought the psychiatric effects of these compounds under attention. Early studies with testosterone and related steroids proposed an antidepressant effect for these compounds (Kopera, 1978). These studies tended to be small and uncontrolled. AS treatment studies for depression decreased following the ad-

TABLE 17-4. *Prevalence Rates of AS Use in Various Populations*

Category	n	Period	Males (%)	Females (%)	Author, year
High school students (12th grade)	2350	Lifetime	5.0	0.5	Johnston et al., 1990–1991
High school students (12th grade)	3403	Lifetime	6.6	N/A	Buckley et al., 1988
College athletes	12	months	6.2	0.6	Anderson et al., 1991
Elite power lifters	45	Lifetime	55	N/A	Yesalis et al., 1988
Elite multiple-sport athletes	271	Lifetime	N/A	2	Newman, 1987

TABLE 17-5.   *Rank Order (Highest to Lowest)*
Use of AS in Last Year by Collegiate Sport

Football	9.6%
Baseball	2.6%
Track/field	2.3%
Basketball	1.6%
Tennis	0.05%

From Anderson WA, Albrecht MA, McKeng DB, et al: A national survey of alcohol and drug abuse by college athletes. Phys Sportsmed 19:91, 1991.

vent of tricyclic compounds. With the increased use of high-dose AS compounds in athletes, the adverse psychiatric effects of these compounds became more the focus of attention and research.

The types of psychiatric effects reported with high-dose AS use fall into three categories: mood syndromes, psychotic syndromes, and behavioral syndromes, especially the development of violent and aggressive behavior. Reviews of the psychological and behavioral aspects of use of the AS compounds describe complex psychiatric effects (Bahrke et al., 1991; Pope and Katz, 1992). Some individuals using high doses experience minimal psychiatric effects, while others may develop full-blown mood or psychotic disorders. Individual vulnerability to the psychiatric effects may be influenced by past psychiatric history, family history of psychiatric disorder, type of steroid used, pattern of cycling, other psychoactive drug use, and other factors.

Mood syndromes of depression and mania have been reported in case series and controlled studies of AS use. During the cycling phase when ASs are being used, a feeling of enhanced self-esteem and euphoria with increased energy and other mania-like features has been described. Depressive symptoms have been reported during on- and off-cycle periods of use. Case reports of suicide in AS users also have been published (Brower et al., 1989; Elofson and Elofson, 1990). The frequency that these mood syndromes meet criteria for a psychiatric diagnosis is unclear. Pope and Katz (1988) argue for full affective syndromes in up to 12 percent of users, while other studies suggest that although psychiatric symptoms are common, the production of a syndrome characteristic of a full psychiatric disorder is rare (Perry et al., 1990).

Psychotic symptoms reported with AS use have included ideas of reference, paranoid delusions, grandiose delusions, and visual and auditory hallucinations. These psychotic symptoms have been noted during cycles of AS use as well as during periods of withdrawal. AS compounds with a 17-alkylated structure appear to be most likely to induce psychotic symptoms. Compounds in this class include oxandrolone, methandrostenolone, and oxymethalone. In all cases reported, psychotic symptoms have responded to antipsychotic medica-

tion and remitted with prolonged abstinence from AS compounds.

The psychiatric effect of AS use best documented is aggressive behavior. The link of aggressiveness to AS use has the advantage of correlates in the nonhuman primates and other animal species. Numerous studies in mammalian species have documented the role of testosterone in the increase in aggressive behavior (Svare, 1983). Animal studies report that the aggressive effects of testosterone appear to be male-specific—this suggests that the presence or absence of testosterone during specific developmental periods controls later response to testosterone. Other social factors appear important in determining the pattern and severity of response in males exposed to exogenous ASs. Rejeski et al. (1988) studied a group of cynomolgus monkeys given equal amounts of exogenous testosterone. Increase in aggressive behaviors was seen primarily in monkeys that displayed significant aggression at baseline. This link may have significant human implications since there is some indication that AS users are more likely to have premorbid antisocial personality disorder (Yates et al., 1990).

The study of the aggressive effects of ASs in humans is limited primarily to observational studies and small experimental design studies. An AS-induced link to aggression has been used in court cases of AS-related assault and homicide. This legal approach has been labeled the "dumbbell defense." Case studies suggest that the violent behavior associated with AS use is primarily in response to some provocation, but the behavioral response is excessive and extremely deviant from what would be expected.

In addition to case reports, the psychometric effects of AS use have been the subject of investigation. Yates et al. (1992) examined the role of AS use in a group of AS users and controls using the Buss-Durkee Hostility Inventory (BDHI) (Buss and Durkee, 1957). This inventory measures several aspects of aggression and hostility. AS users reported elevated responses to scales measuring verbal aggression and direct and indirect aggression. Typical questions from elevated BDHI subscales illustrate differences between AS users and nonuser controls. (True responses scored positively.) For the assault scale, a typical question is: "Once in a while I cannot control my urge to harm others." For the indirect aggression subscale, a typical question is: "I can remember being so angry that I picked up the nearest thing and broke it." For the verbal aggression scale, a typical question is: "When I get mad, I say nasty things." These behavioral characteristics of AS users are likely to increase the risk for significant legal and interpersonal difficulties. Mean scores for AS users on the BDHI are higher than reported means for a group of psychiatric patients and a group prison inmates (Buss et al., 1962; Hall, 1989). The responses from AS users in this study showed some psychometric specificity. AS users had elevated scores on the aggression factor of the BDHI but not on a separate hostility factor.

Most studies of aggression in AS use have focused on retrospective designs, relying on the self-report of AS use to identify cases and controls. Two small prospective studies have monitored the effects of ASs (Choi et al., 1990; Su et al., 1991). In one study, volunteers received an AS compound from the research team. Both studies confirm the aggressive effect of AS compounds. The Choi et al. study confirmed the relationship of AS use with the aggression subscale of the BDHI found in the Yates et al. study (1992). Interestingly, a subject in the Su et al. study (1991) asked to be placed in seclusion to prevent aggressive behaviors from getting out of control and resulting in harm to others.

Significant questions about the exact role of AS in mental status and behavioral changes remain to be answered. Significant uncontrolled factors could affect the interaction of ASs within individual users. Some of these factors include previous and family history of psychiatric disorder, individual personality traits and disorders, the concurrent effects of alcohol and other psychoactive agents, the effect of expectancy in response to use, and the environment in which mental status and behavioral changes occur.

Despite the limitations of the knowledge of the effects of AS use, several clinical implications appear warranted at this time. High-risk groups presenting with new-onset psychiatric disorders should have an AS use history obtained. Urinary AS assays can be used to confirm the patient's history. Although AS use appears common, the majority of users appear to have subclinical mental status effects. Despite this, documented significant clinical mental status and behavioral effects of AS use do appear to be present in a minority of users. Clinical suspicion regarding the mental status and behavioral effects of AS use in high-risk subjects is likely to lead to better understanding of the psychopharmacology of AS compounds.

In addition to the psychiatric effects of AS compounds, the phenomenology of AS use compares in many ways with the phenomenology of DSM-IIIR psychoactive substance abuse and dependence. Similarities and differences in AS use compared with other drugs of abuse have implications about our understanding and treatment of AS use.

A New Drug of Abuse?

The underground pathway for the distribution of illicit steroids presents a law enforcement challenge. This distribution system has many similarities to illicit systems developed for drugs such as cocaine and heroin. AS compounds are often obtained from sources outside the United States and brought across the border with supplies assigned to dealers who distribute to individual users for monetary

gain. Recognizing this pathway, in November of 1990 the U.S. Congress placed ASs in schedule III of the Controlled Substances Act. This addition classifies ASs in the same category as compounds such as acetaminophen with codeine. Illegal possession and distribution of these agents are now subject to felony arrest and prosecution.

Although AS compounds now are classified with other prescription psychoactive substances of abuse and dependence, the implication of this classification is unclear. The potential for AS use to develop into an uncontrolled habit with withdrawal and psychological and physical dependence is unknown and speculative. Kashkin and Kleber (1989) have hypothesized that some individuals may be susceptible to an "unrecognized sex steroid hormone–dependence disorder" and that such a disorder may be modulated through the relationship of ASs to the opioid and aminergic neurotransmission network. The possible classification of ASs as psychoactive substances of abuse and dependence has implications for the clinical assessment and treatment of AS users. The lines of evidence supporting this hypothesis as well as those not supporting it will be reviewed.

Support for the addiction hypothesis of ASs will be dependent on linking the phenomenology and biologic mechanisms of AS use with those of the use of existing psychoactive substances such as alcohol and cocaine. Table 17-6 presents some comparisons of these issues in addressing the AS hypothesis.

TABLE 17-6. *Comparison of Use of AS Compounds with Alcoholism and Cocaine Abuse*

	Phenomenology		
Comparison categories	Alcoholism	Cocaine abuse	AS use
Male gender predominant	Yes	Yes	Yes
Early age of onset	Yes	Yes	Yes
Linked to antisocial personality	Yes	Yes	Yes
DSM-IIIR abuse/dependence criteria	Yes	Yes	Yes
Polysubstance abuse common	Yes	Yes	?
Controlled Substance Act	No	Yes	Yes
Family history of abuse/dependence	Yes	Yes	?
Used primarily for psychoactive effect	Yes	Yes	No
Seek treatment for discontinuation	Yes	Yes	?/No
	Biologic mechanism		
Intoxicating mood effect	Yes	Yes	?
Withdrawal symptoms/craving	Yes	Yes	?
Animal model for self-administration	Yes	Yes	No

had elevated scores on the aggression factor of the BDHI but not on a separate hostility factor.

Most studies of aggression in AS use have focused on retrospective designs, relying on the self-report of AS use to identify cases and controls. Two small prospective studies have monitored the effects of ASs (Choi et al., 1990; Su et al., 1991). In one study, volunteers received an AS compound from the research team. Both studies confirm the aggressive effect of AS compounds. The Choi et al. study confirmed the relationship of AS use with the aggression subscale of the BDHI found in the Yates et al. study (1992). Interestingly, a subject in the Su et al. study (1991) asked to be placed in seclusion to prevent aggressive behaviors from getting out of control and resulting in harm to others.

Significant questions about the exact role of AS in mental status and behavioral changes remain to be answered. Significant uncontrolled factors could affect the interaction of ASs within individual users. Some of these factors include previous and family history of psychiatric disorder, individual personality traits and disorders, the concurrent effects of alcohol and other psychoactive agents, the effect of expectancy in response to use, and the environment in which mental status and behavioral changes occur.

Despite the limitations of the knowledge of the effects of AS use, several clinical implications appear warranted at this time. High-risk groups presenting with new-onset psychiatric disorders should have an AS use history obtained. Urinary AS assays can be used to confirm the patient's history. Although AS use appears common, the majority of users appear to have subclinical mental status effects. Despite this, documented significant clinical mental status and behavioral effects of AS use do appear to be present in a minority of users. Clinical suspicion regarding the mental status and behavioral effects of AS use in high-risk subjects is likely to lead to better understanding of the psychopharmacology of AS compounds.

In addition to the psychiatric effects of AS compounds, the phenomenology of AS use compares in many ways with the phenomenology of DSM-IIIR psychoactive substance abuse and dependence. Similarities and differences in AS use compared with other drugs of abuse have implications about our understanding and treatment of AS use.

A New Drug of Abuse?

The underground pathway for the distribution of illicit steroids presents a law enforcement challenge. This distribution system has many similarities to illicit systems developed for drugs such as cocaine and heroin. AS compounds are often obtained from sources outside the United States and brought across the border with supplies assigned to dealers who distribute to individual users for monetary gain. Recognizing this pathway, in November of 1990 the U.S. Congress placed ASs in schedule III of the Controlled Substances Act. This addition classifies ASs in the same category as compounds such as acetaminophen with codeine. Illegal possession and distribution of these agents are now subject to felony arrest and prosecution.

Although AS compounds now are classified with other prescription psychoactive substances of abuse and dependence, the implication of this classification is unclear. The potential for AS use to develop into an uncontrolled habit with withdrawal and psychological and physical dependence is unknown and speculative. Kashkin and Kleber (1989) have hypothesized that some individuals may be susceptible to an "unrecognized sex steroid hormone–dependence disorder" and that such a disorder may be modulated through the relationship of ASs to the opioid and aminergic neurotransmission network. The possible classification of ASs as psychoactive substances of abuse and dependence has implications for the clinical assessment and treatment of AS users. The lines of evidence supporting this hypothesis as well as those not supporting it will be reviewed.

Support for the addiction hypothesis of ASs will be dependent on linking the phenomenology and biologic mechanisms of AS use with those of the use of existing psychoactive substances such as alcohol and cocaine. Table 17-6 presents some comparisons of these issues in addressing the AS hypothesis.

TABLE 17-6. *Comparison of Use of AS Compounds with Alcoholism and Cocaine Abuse*

Comparison categories	Phenomenology		
	Alcoholism	Cocaine abuse	AS use
Male gender predominant	Yes	Yes	Yes
Early age of onset	Yes	Yes	Yes
Linked to antisocial personality	Yes	Yes	Yes
DSM-IIIR abuse/dependence criteria	Yes	Yes	Yes
Polysubstance abuse common	Yes	Yes	?
Controlled Substance Act	No	Yes	Yes
Family history of abuse/ dependence	Yes	Yes	?
Used primarily for psychoactive effect	Yes	Yes	No
Seek treatment for discontinuation	Yes	Yes	?/No

	Biologic mechanism		
Intoxicating mood effect	Yes	Yes	?
Withdrawal symptoms/ craving	Yes	Yes	?
Animal model for self-administration	Yes	Yes	No

TABLE 17-5. *Rank Order (Highest to Lowest) Use of AS in Last Year by Collegiate Sport*

Football	9.6%
Baseball	2.6%
Track/field	2.3%
Basketball	1.6%
Tennis	0.05%

From Anderson WA, Albrecht MA, McKeng DB, et al: A national survey of alcohol and drug abuse by college athletes. Phys Sportsmed 19:91, 1991.

vent of tricyclic compounds. With the increased use of high-dose AS compounds in athletes, the adverse psychiatric effects of these compounds became more the focus of attention and research.

The types of psychiatric effects reported with high-dose AS use fall into three categories: mood syndromes, psychotic syndromes, and behavioral syndromes, especially the development of violent and aggressive behavior. Reviews of the psychological and behavioral aspects of use of the AS compounds describe complex psychiatric effects (Bahrke et al., 1991; Pope and Katz, 1992). Some individuals using high doses experience minimal psychiatric effects, while others may develop full-blown mood or psychotic disorders. Individual vulnerability to the psychiatric effects may be influenced by past psychiatric history, family history of psychiatric disorder, type of steroid used, pattern of cycling, other psychoactive drug use, and other factors.

Mood syndromes of depression and mania have been reported in case series and controlled studies of AS use. During the cycling phase when ASs are being used, a feeling of enhanced self-esteem and euphoria with increased energy and other mania-like features has been described. Depressive symptoms have been reported during on- and off-cycle periods of use. Case reports of suicide in AS users also have been published (Brower et al., 1989; Elofson and Elofson, 1990). The frequency that these mood syndromes meet criteria for a psychiatric diagnosis is unclear. Pope and Katz (1988) argue for full affective syndromes in up to 12 percent of users, while other studies suggest that although psychiatric symptoms are common, the production of a syndrome characteristic of a full psychiatric disorder is rare (Perry et al., 1990).

Psychotic symptoms reported with AS use have included ideas of reference, paranoid delusions, grandiose delusions, and visual and auditory hallucinations. These psychotic symptoms have been noted during cycles of AS use as well as during periods of withdrawal. AS compounds with a 17-alkylated structure appear to be most likely to induce psychotic symptoms. Compounds in this class include oxandrolone, methandrostenolone, and oxymethalone. In all cases reported, psychotic symptoms have responded to antipsychotic medica-tion and remitted with prolonged abstinence from AS compounds.

The psychiatric effect of AS use best documented is aggressive behavior. The link of aggressiveness to AS use has the advantage of correlates in the nonhuman primates and other animal species. Numerous studies in mammalian species have documented the role of testosterone in the increase in aggressive behavior (Svare, 1983). Animal studies report that the aggressive effects of testosterone appear to be male-specific—this suggests that the presence or absence of testosterone during specific developmental periods controls later response to testosterone. Other social factors appear important in determining the pattern and severity of response in males exposed to exogenous ASs. Rejeski et al. (1988) studied a group of cynomolgus monkeys given equal amounts of exogenous testosterone. Increase in aggressive behaviors was seen primarily in monkeys that displayed significant aggression at baseline. This link may have significant human implications since there is some indication that AS users are more likely to have premorbid antisocial personality disorder (Yates et al., 1990).

The study of the aggressive effects of ASs in humans is limited primarily to observational studies and small experimental design studies. An AS-induced link to aggression has been used in court cases of AS-related assault and homicide. This legal approach has been labeled the "dumbbell defense." Case studies suggest that the violent behavior associated with AS use is primarily in response to some provocation, but the behavioral response is excessive and extremely deviant from what would be expected.

In addition to case reports, the psychometric effects of AS use have been the subject of investigation. Yates et al. (1992) examined the role of AS use in a group of AS users and controls using the Buss-Durkee Hostility Inventory (BDHI) (Buss and Durkee, 1957). This inventory measures several aspects of aggression and hostility. AS users reported elevated responses to scales measuring verbal aggression and direct and indirect aggression. Typical questions from elevated BDHI subscales illustrate differences between AS users and nonuser controls. (True responses scored positively.) For the assault scale, a typical question is: "Once in a while I cannot control my urge to harm others." For the indirect aggression subscale, a typical question is: "I can remember being so angry that I picked up the nearest thing and broke it." For the verbal aggression scale, a typical question is: "When I get mad, I say nasty things." These behavioral characteristics of AS users are likely to increase the risk for significant legal and interpersonal difficulties. Mean scores for AS users on the BDHI are higher than reported means for a group of psychiatric patients and a group prison inmates (Buss et al., 1962; Hall, 1989). The responses from AS users in this study showed some psychometric specificity. AS users

Several of the phenomenologic features of AS use mimic alcoholism and drug abuse. Use of AS compounds is primarily a male gender phenomenon. Although found in women, the male/female ratio for AS use appears to be about 10:1. The ratio for AS users who could be considered dependent is unknown. Results from the National Institute of Mental Health's Epidemiologic Catchment Area (ECA) study suggest that the male/female ratio for alcohol abuse and dependence is 6:1 and for non-alcohol abuse and dependence is 1.6:1 (Robins et al., 1984). The age of onset for AS use is adolescence and early adulthood; this also corresponds with the age of onset for alcohol and drug use. Also similar to alcoholism and cocaine abuse, antisocial personality disorder has been found at higher rates in AS users (Yates et al., 1990).

Several case reports highlight the possibility of a dependence syndrome associated with AS use. Individual users have reported feeling that their AS use became out of control. Despite a desire to quit AS use, some users have described continued use as a result of withdrawal dysphoria or fear of losing weight, strength, or muscle mass. According to DSM-IIIR criteria for psychoactive substance dependence, at least three of nine criteria are necessary for diagnosis of a dependence syndrome.

Brower et al. (1991) completed a survey of 49 AS users to determine the prevalence of DSM-IIIR dependence criteria for ASs. Ninety-four percent of the users reported at least one dependence syndrome, with 57 percent reporting three or more dependence symptoms with AS use. The most prevalent dependence symptoms reported by the AS users were withdrawal symptoms, more substance taken than intended, large quantities of time spent in AS-related activities, and continued AS use despite AS problems. Users who reported dependence symptoms were more likely to have had more cycles of ASs, used higher doses, felt they were still not big enough, and had aggressive symptoms.

There is limited evidence to support a family history of alcoholism or drug dependence in AS users and also not enough data to determine the prevalence of polysubstance abuse in AS users. Investigation of both these factors is necessary.

Despite the phenomenologic similarities, some important differences remain between alcohol, cocaine, and AS use. The primary reason for AS use is not for a psychoactive effect. Motivation varies for initiation and maintenance of AS use but primarily reflects the user's drive for development of strength, muscle mass, and improved physical appearance. Although users report increased self-esteem and energy, the compounds are not used primarily for a

TABLE 17-7. *Psychiatric Syndromes Identified with Eponyms*

Eponym	Description	Found in	Reference
Capgras delusion	One of the delusions of doubles. A belief that a person, usually a close family member, has been replaced by an imposter	Schizophrenia, affective psychosis, and dementia	Capgras et al., 1923
Clerambault's delusion	A delusion usually held by a woman that a famous or wealthy person is in love with her; also known by the term *pure erotomania*	Paranoid schizophrenia, paranoid disorder, and organic psychoses	Clerambault, 1942
Cotard's delusion	A delusion that all has been lost including money, possessions, and parts of the body such as the heart or other organs; the delusion may include the belief that the person is dead	Schizophrenia, affective psychoses, and organic psychoses	Cotard, 1888
Couvade syndrome	The experience of signs and symptoms of pregnancy or labor by the husband of a wife who is pregnant or in labor	No psychiatric disorder and possibly anxiety disorders	Trethowan, 1965
DaCosta's syndrome	The syndrome, also known as *neurocirculatory asthenia*, characterized by easy fatiguability, chest pain, dyspnea, and palpitations	Many cases probably panic disorder	Da Costa, 1871
Fregoli's delusion	The reverse of Capgras delusion; strangers are identified as familiar friends or family members	Schizophrenia, affective psychosis, and dementia	Courbon and Fail, 1927
Ganser's syndrome	A syndrome where responses to questions are approximate but not correct; also described as *hysterical pseudodementia*	Schizophrenia, bipolar disorder, organic psychoses, malingering	Ganser, 1898
Kleine-Levin syndrome	Periodic episodes of hypersomnia accompanied by bulimia	Thalamic lesions	Carpenter et al., 1982
Kluver-Bucy syndrome	The loss of facial recognition, rage reactions, hypersexuality, and memory deficits	Surgical removal of both temporal lobes	Cummings and Duchen, 1981
Othello's delusion	The delusion of infidelity by the spouse	Paranoid disorder, schizophrenia or affective psychoses, organic psychoses, alcoholism	Enoch and Trethowan, 1979

TABLE 17-8. *Cultural Psychiatric Syndromes*

Cultural syndrome	Description	Culture	Reference
Amok	Unexpected rapid development of agitation; accompanied by obtaining a weapon and attacking everything in sight until apprehended	Malaysia	Westermeyer, 1972
Dhat	Delusion that sperm is leaking from the body through urination, resulting in weakness	India	Carstairs, 1956
Koro	An acute anxiety state characterized by fear that the penis will retract into the abdomen, resulting in death	China and Malaysia	Arieti and Meth, 1959
Latah	A syndrome of echopraxia, echolalia, and coprolalia; behaviors may involve putting one's self in dangerous situations	Malaysia, similar syndromes described in Africa, Japan, and Russia	Yap, 1952
Piblokto	Attacks of bizzare behavior, including screaming, running about, and tearing off clothing	Eskimo	Ackerknecht, 1948
Voodoo	A delusion of possession by devils or evil spirits.	Haiti and Africa	Sargant, 1973
Windingo	A delusion of being possessed by a cannabalistic monster (windingo)	Canadian Indians	Teicher, 1961

euphoric effect. This difference remains a significant challenge to the AS addiction hypothesis.

Although case reports have documented substance-dependence treatment seeking in AS users, the extent of this treatment-seeking behavior appears small. Clancy and Yates (1992) reported results from a national survey of substance-abuse treatment directors. Eighty-one percent of surveyed directors reported no patients with AS use presenting for treatment at their facilities over a 1-year period. Those reporting AS-using patients did note DSM-IIIR psychoactive substance dependence for ASs. However, the limited treatment-seeking behavior in AS users also challenges the validity of the AS addiction hypothesis.

Biologic mechanisms for addiction with AS compounds have received limited research attention. There is no current animal model for addiction to ASs. Further study of the physiologic and psychoactive effects of AS use will need to address the effects of high-dose use, withdrawal, and evidence for development of craving.

Presently, the AS addiction hypothesis is unproven. Further epidemiologic, clinical, and basic science study will be necessary to more completely understand the psychopharmacology and psychiatric effects of these compounds.

EPONYMS AND CULTURAL SYNDROMES

Eponyms and cultural syndromes important in psychiatry are summarized in Tables 17-7 and 17-8. These categories have been the subject of review (Nasrallah, 1986). Knowledge of these descriptive syndromes underscores the role of the history of psychiatric nosology. Knowledge of cultural syndromes underscores the effect of environmental and cultural influences on the phenomenology of psychiatric syndromes.

REFERENCES

Ackerknecht BH: Medicine and disease among Eskimos. Ciba Symp 10:916, 1948.

Aduan RP, Fauci AS, Pale DC: Factitious fever and self-induced infection. Ann Intern Med 90:230–242, 1979.

American Psychiatric Association: Diagnostic and Statistical Manual of Mental Disorders, 3d ed revised. Washington, American Psychiatric Association, 1987.

Anderson WA, Albrecht MA, McKeag DB, et al: A national survey of alcohol and drug use by college athletes. Phys Sportsmed 19:91–106, 1991.

Andreasen NC, Hoenck PR: The predictive value of adjustment disorder in adolescents and adults. Am J Psychiatry 139:584–590, 1982.

Andreasen NC, Wasek P: Adjustment disorders in adolescents and adults. Arch Gen Psychiatry 37:1166–1170, 1980.

Arieti S, Meth JM: Rare, unclassifiable, collective and exotic psychotic syndromes. In Arieti S (ed): American Handbook of Psychiatry. New York, Basic Books, 1959.

Asher R: Munchausen's syndrome. Lancet 1:339–341, 1951.

Bahrke MS, Yesalis CE, Wright JE: Psychological and behavioural effects of endogenous testosterone levels and anabolic-androgenic steroids among males: A review. Sports Med 10:303–337, 1990.

Beck AT, Freeman A: Cognitive Therapy of Personality Disorders. New York, Gilford Press, 1990, pp 176–205.

Bird HR, Canino G, Rubio-Stipec M, et al: Estimates of the prevalence of childhood maladjustment in a community survey in Puerto Rico. Arch Gen Psychiatry 45:1120–1126, 1988.

Bronisch T, Hecht H: Validity of adjustment disorder, comparison with major depression. J Affective Disord 17:229–236, 1989.

Brower KJ, Blow FC, Eliopulos GA, Beresford TP: Anabolic androgenic steroids and suicide. Am J Psychiatry 146:1075, 1989.

Brower KJ, Blow FC, Young JP, Hill EM: Symptoms and correlates of anabolic-androgenic steroid dependence. Br J Addict 86:759–768, 1991.

Buckley W, Yesalis C, Friedl K, et al: Estimated prevalence of anabolic steroid use among male high school seniors. JAMA 260:3441–3445, 1988.

Buss AH, Durkee A: An inventory for assessing different kinds of hostility. J Consult Psychol 21:343–349, 1957.

Buss AH, Fischer H, Simmons AJ: Aggression and hostility in psychiatric patients. J Consult Psychol 26:84–89, 1962.

Capgras J, Reboul-lachaud J: L'illusion des sosies dans un delire systematique chronique. Bull Soc Clin Med Ment 2:6, 1923.

Carpenter S, Yassa R, Ochs R: A pathologic basis for Kleine-Levin syndrome. Arch Neurol 39:25–28, 1982.

Carstairs GM: Hinjra and Jiryan. Br J Med Psychol 29:128–132, 1956.

Chess S, Thomas A: Origins and Evolution of Behavior Disorders. New York, Brunner Mazel, 1984.

Choi PYL, Parrott AC, Cowan D: High-dose anabolic steroids in strength athletes: Effects upon hostility and aggression. Human Psychopharmacol 5:349–356, 1990.

Clancy GP, Yates WR: Anabolic steroid use among substance abusers in treatment. J Clin Psychiatry 53:97–100, 1992.

Clerambault GG: Ouvre Psychiatrique. Paris, Presses Universitaires, 1942.

Cotard M: Du delire de negations. Arch Neurol Paris 4:152–170, 282, 1882.

Courbon P, Fail G: Syndrome "d'illusion de Fregoli" et schizophrenie. Bull Soc Clin Med Ment 15:121, 1927.

Cummings JL, Duchen LW: Kluver-Bucy syndrome in Pick's disease. Neurology 31:1415–1422, 1981.

Da Costa JM: An irritable heart: Clinical study of functional cardiac disorder and its consequences. Am J Med Sci 61:17, 1871.

Duchaine D: Underground Steroid Handbook, vol 2. Venice, CA, HLR Technical Books, 1989.

Elofson G, Elofson S: Steroids claimed our son's life. Phys Sportsmed 18:15–16, 1990.

Enoch MD, Trethowan WH: Uncommon Psychiatric Syndromes. Bristol, England, John Wright's Sons, 1979.

Fabrega H, Mezzich JE, Mezzich AC: Adjustment disorder as a marginal of transitional illness category in DSM-III. Arch Gen Psychiatry 44:567–572, 1987.

Frierson RL, Lippman SB: Psychiatric consultation for patients with self-inflicted gunshot wounds. Psychosomatics 31:67–74, 1990.

Ganser SJM: Uber einen eigenartigen hysterischen Dammerzustand. Arch Psychiatr Nervenkr 38:633, 1898.

Grunberger G, Weiner JL, Silverman R, et al: Factitious hypoglycemia due to surreptitious administration of insulin: Diagnosis, treatment, and long-term follow-up. Ann Intern Med 108:252–257, 1988.

Hale M, Jacobsen J, Carson R: A database review in C-L psychiatry: Characteristics of hospitalized suicide attempters. Psychosomatics 31:282–286, 1990.

Hall GCN: Self-reported hostility as a function of offense characteristics and response style in a sexual offender population. J Consult Clin Psychol 57:306–308, 1989.

Johnston L, Bachman J, O'Malley P: Monitoring the Future: Continuing Study of the Lifestyles and Values of Youth. Ann Arbor, University of Michigan Institute for Social Research, 1990–1991.

Kaskin KD, Kleber HD: Hooked on hormones? An anabolic steroid addiction hypothesis. JAMA 262:3166–3170, 1989.

Kopera H: Miscellaneous uses of anabolic steroids. In Kochakian CD (ed): Anabolic-Androgenic Steroids. New York, Springer-Verlag, 1976.

Loebel JP, Borson S, Hyde T, et al: Relationships between requests for psychiatric consultations and psychiatric diagnoses in long-term care facilities. Am J Psychiatry 148:898–903, 1991.

Masterson JF: The symptomatic adolescent five years later: He didn't grow out of it. Am J Psychiatry 123:1338–1345, 1967.

Meadow R: Munchausen syndrome proxy. Arch Dis Child 57:92–98, 1982.

Nasrallah HA: Special and unusual psychiatric syndromes. In Winokur G, Clayton P (eds): The Medical Basis of Psychiatry. Philadelphia, W.B. Saunders Co., 1986.

Newman M: Elite Women Athletes Survey Results. Center City, MN, Hazelden Research Services, 1987.

Perry PJ, Yates WR, Andersen KH: Psychiatric effects of AS: A controlled retrospective study. Ann Clin Psychiatry 2:11–17, 1990.

Pope HG, Katz DL: Psychiatric effects of anabolic steroids. Psychiatr Ann 22:24–29, 1992.

Pope HG, Katz DL: Affective and psychotic symptoms associated with anabolic steroid use. Am J Psychiatry 145:482–490, 1988.

Pope HG, Jonas JM, Jones B: Factitious psychosis: Phenomenology, family history, and long-term outcome of nine patients. Am J Psychiatry 139:1480–1483, 1982.

Popkin MK, Callies AL, Colon EA, et al: Adjustment disorders in medically ill inpatients referred for consultation in a university hospital. Psychosomatics 31:410–414, 1990.

Rejeski WJ, Brubaker PH, Herb RA, et al: Anabolic steroids and aggressive behavior in cynomolgus monkeys. J Behav Med 11:95–105, 1988.

Robins LN, Helzer JE, Weissman MM, et al: Lifetime prevalence of specific psychiatric disorders in three sites. Arch Gen Psychiatry 41:949–958, 1984.

Rogers R, Bagby RM, Rector N: Diagnostic legitimacy of factitious disorder with psychological symptoms. Am J Psychiatry 146:1312–1314, 1989.

Runeson B: Mental disorders in youth suicide: DSM-IIIR Axes I and II. Acta Psychiatr Scand 79:490–497, 1989.

Salmon TW, Fenton N: Neuropsychiatry, vol 10: The American Expeditionary Forces. Washington, U.S. Government Printing Office, 1929.

Sargant W: The Mind Possessed. London, Heineman, 1973.

Schatzberg AF: Anxiety and adjustment disorder: A treatment approach. J Clin Psychiatry 51(suppl):20–24, 1990.

Schwartz JA, Speed N, Beresford TP: Antidepressants in the medically ill: Prediction of benefits. Int J Psychiatry Med 19:363–369, 1989.

Sno HN, Storosum JG, Wortel CH: Psychogenic "HIV infection." Int J Psychiatry Med 21:93–98, 1991.

Snyder S, Strain JJ, Wolf D: Differentiating major depression from adjustment disorder with depressed mood in the medical setting. Gen Hosp Psychiatry 12:159–165, 1990.

Sparr L, Pankratz LD: Factitious posttraumatic stress disorder. Am J Psychiatry 140:1016–1019, 1983.

Su TP, Rubinow DR, Pagliaro RN, et al: Neuropsychiatric effects of anabolic steroids. New Research Abstract NR148, 1991. New Research Program and Abstracts, American Psychiatric Association, 1991, p 83.

Sutherland AJ, Rodin GM: Factitious disorders in a general hospital setting: Clinical features and a review of the literature. Psychosomatics 31:392–399, 1990.

Svare B (ed): Hormones and Aggressive Behavior. New York, Plenum Press, 1983.

Teicher M: Windingo psychosis: A study of a relationship between belief and behavior among the Indians of Northeastern Canada. Proc Am Ethnol Soc 11:1, 1961.

Trethowan WH: The Couvade syndrome. Br J Psychiatry 111:57–66, 1965.

Westermeyer JA: Comparison of amok and other homicides in Laos. Am J Psychiatry 129:703–708, 1972.

Yap PM: The latah reaction: Its pathodynamics and nosological position. J Ment Sci 98:515, 1952.

Yassa R: Munchausen's syndrome: A successfully treated case. Psychosomatics 19:242–243, 1978.

Yates WR, Perry PJ, Andersen KH: Illicit anabolic steroid use: A controlled personality study. Acta Psychiatr Scand 81:548–550, 1990.

Yates WR, Perry PJ, Murray S: Aggression and hostility in anabolic steroid users. Biol Psychiatry 31:1232–1234, 1992.

Yesalis C, Herrick R, Bucklye W, et al: Self-reported use of anabolic-androgenic steroids by elite power lifters. Phys Sportsmed 16:90–100, 1988.

Yesalis CE, Buckley WA, Wang MO, et al: Athletes' projections of anabolic steroid use. Clin Sports Med 2:155–171, 1990.

Yesalis CE: Epidemiology and patterns of anabolic-androgenic steroid use. Psychiatr Ann 22:7–18, 1992.

UNIT 2

Child Psychiatry

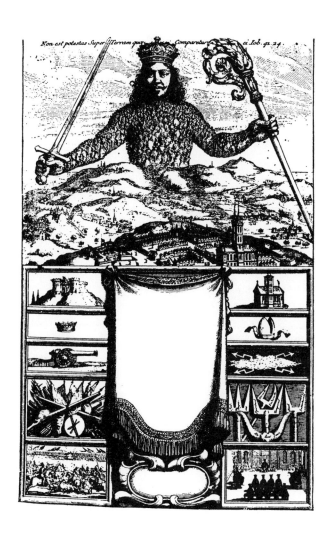

CHAPTER 18

The Disruptive Behavior Disorders: Attention Deficit Disorders, Oppositional Disorder, and Conduct Disorder

DENNIS P. CANTWELL

INTRODUCTION

The disruptive behavior disorders are a group of childhood and adolescent psychiatric disorders that are characterized by socially disruptive behaviors producing more distress to the patient's environment than to the patient. The group of disruptive behavior disorders consists of three specific psychiatric diagnoses: attention deficit (hyperactivity) disorder (ADD), oppositional (defiant) disorder (ODD), and conduct disorder (CD).

These disorders constitute an extremely important set of clinical problems in childhood and adolescence for a number of reasons. First, they are among the most prevalent of childhood and adolescent psychiatric disorders. Second, they produce a good deal of morbidity in childhood and adolescence. And third, they tend to be very persistent over time. There is evidence that these disorders may predispose a youngster to the later development of adult antisocial spectrum disorders (e.g., antisocial personality disorder and substance abuse).

Issues of definition and classification are particularly problematic with the disruptive behavior disorders because the different disorders share a number of features in common and tend to be comorbid. Among the features that the disruptive behavior disorders share are outcome characteristics, responses to various types of therapeutic interventions, etiologic (biologic and psychosocial) factors, and other medical, developmental neurologic, or psychiatric disorders that are associated. For example, the DSM-IIIR grouping together of ODD with ADD and CD into a single category was motivated by recognition of a substantial amount of overlap between these disorders in clinical symptomatology, outcome, comorbidity, and shared risk factors.

In terms of comorbidity, not only do children often present with ADD, ODD, and CD in various combinations, but they also may present with any or all three conditions along with other psychiatric disorders as well.

The exact amount and nature of the overlap between the various disruptive behavior disorders is still a matter of controversy. The degree of overlap found in different studies is influenced by various methodologic aspects of the studies, such as the diagnostic criteria used, the sample studied, and the methods of assessment employed. Nonetheless, both clinical studies (Biederman et al., 1987) and epidemiologic studies (Anderson et al., 1987) have demonstrated some overlap between ODD, CD, and ADD.

In this chapter it will be assumed that there are pure cases of ODD, CD, and ADD. It is also recognized that there is a significant overlap between the three disorders. Consequently, the following discussions of associated conditions, epidemiology, etiologic factors, outcome, and management will summarize findings general to all three of the disruptive behavior disorders. In addition, discussion will be provided to highlight known (empirically demonstrated) differences between the three separate conditions. Since the core symptomatology is quite different for each of the three disorders, the clinical pictures of the three disorders is discussed separately below.

CLINICAL PICTURE/
PHENOMENOLOGY

Attention Deficit Hyperactivity Disorder (ADHD)

Attention deficit disorder (ADD) is one of the best studied of all child psychiatric disorders. A variety of names have been attached to it over the years. The early terms (such as *brain damage behavior syndrome*, the *minimal brain damage syndrome, minimal brain dysfunction,* and *minimal cerebral dysfunction*) all emphasized some type of underlying organic etiology generally of a nonspecific nature. Later terms (such as the *hyperkinetic reaction of childhood* and the *hyperactive child syndrome*) focused on what was then considered the major clinical symptom, namely, hyperactivity. The most recent terms for the disorder (ADD, ADHD) have focused on an attentional deficit as the key symptom.

Current definitions of ADD still recognize both motor overactivity and attentional difficulties as key symptoms of the disorder. Generally, the ADD syndrome is now viewed as consisting of various combinations of symptoms having to do with inattention (e.g., being easily distracted, having difficulty sustaining attention in tasks), impulsivity (e.g., often blurting out answers to questions before they have been completed, often interrupting or intruding on others), and hyperactivity (e.g., often fidgeting with hands or feet or squirming in seat, having difficulty remaining seated when required to do so).

However, there is no consensus on a definition of the disorder. For example, there is no consensus as to how many symptoms must be present or whether certain types or combinations of types of symptoms must be present.

Like DSM-III, DSM-IV will probably recognize three major forms of ADD: attention deficit hyperactivity disorder, attention deficit disorder without hyperactivity, and a residual category attention deficit disorder not otherwise specified. At this writing, it is not clear how DSM-IV will define these different subtypes of ADD. There are two possible approaches being considered: one recognizing two parameters of symptomatology (inattention and hyperactivity/impulsivity) and the other recognizing three parameters (inattention, hyperactivity, and impulsivity), very similar to DSM-III. Most, but not all, of the empirical data suggest that the inattention and hyperactivity/impulsivity (two groupings) approach is better. However, field trials of the criteria will be used to help decide between two or three groupings and to determine the best number of symptoms to be required for the diagnosis. Currently, it has been suggested that there be 8 inattention symptoms and 10 impulsivity/hyperactivity symptoms.

One diagnostic problem with ADD is that some of its symptoms may only be manifested in certain settings. The issue of these "setting specific" symptoms could be handled in two different ways. One approach is to specify that the symptoms must be present in a structured environment, such as school or work. Another approach would not require the presence of symptoms in any specific setting.

Another major problem with defining ADD has to do with the clinical description of ADD without hyperactivity. It is not clear from presently available data whether the inattention symptoms of ADD *with* hyperactivity are sufficient to characterize ADD *without* hyperactivity. One suggestion for DSM-IV is to include additional inattention items for ADD without hyperactivity. Such symptoms include "often stares into space and reports daydreaming," "is often forgetful in daily activities," "often appears to be low in energy level, sluggish, or drowsy," and "often appears to be apathetic or unmotivated to engage in goal-directed activities (school work, chores, or job-related activities), although motivation to engage in favored or passive activities (e.g., hobbies, watching television, or listening to music) is unimpaired."

Conduct Disorder (CD)

Conduct disorder is characterized by a persistent pattern of behavior that violates the basic rights of others or that violates major age-appropriate norms and rules of society. Children with conduct disorder have symptoms that are usually present not only in the home but also in school and the community at large. Their symptoms are generally of a serious nature. Children with CD show both reactive and proactive aggression, fight frequently, bully others, and are often described as cruel to other people and animals. They may destroy the property of others intentionally by fire setting or other means. They generally steal, initially in a covert fashion, then in a more overt fashion. Truancy, running away from home, lying, and cheating are also common symptoms. Later in life, physical violence may be present, including mugging, robbery, rape, assault, and rarely homicide.

The diagnosis and subclassification of conduct disorder has always been somewhat controversial. In DSM-III, conduct disorders were conceptualized as a set of problems characterized by repetitive and persistent patterns of conduct in which either the basic rights of others, major age-appropriate societal norms, or rules were violated regularly. The essential features of the disorder remained the same in DSM-IIIR. However, there are different views as to the subtypes of CD.

At issue are how symptoms of aggression and socialization/peer relationships cluster. For example, conduct-disordered children could be "socialized" (having social attachment to others) or "undersocialized" (lacking a normal degree of affection, empathy, or bonding to others). Similarly, they could be aggressive (confronting others in assaults, muggings, or physical violence) or nonaggressive.

DSM-III listed four subtypes of CD: under-socialized aggressive, undersocialized nonaggressive, socialized aggressive, and socialized nonaggressive conduct disorder. In DSM-IIIR, three subtypes of CD were specified: group CD (in which conduct symptom problem occurred mainly in group activities with peers), solitary/aggressive CD (involving aggressive physical behavior initiated individually toward adults and peers), and undifferentiated CD (a mixed or grab bag category).

It is not clear how conduct disorder will be defined and subtyped in DSM-IV. However, based on the literature, two new symptoms have been suggested for inclusion in the diagnostic criteria: "onset of alcohol or other substance use before age 13 and recurrent use during the past six months" and "engaging in sexual activities in order to obtain money, goods, or drugs."

Oppositional Defiant Disorder (ODD)

Oppositional defiant disorder is characterized by a pattern of negativistic, defiant, and hostile behaviors. However, the more serious violations present in conduct disorder are not present. Rather, children with ODD resist direction by authority figures. They are stubborn and unwilling to compromise, to give in, or to negotiate with adult figures or peers. Chronic arguing and blaming others for mistakes also may be present. Quick temper toward adults and peers and the deliberate annoyance of peers also may be present. Symptoms are always present in the home, even if not present in school or in other settings. Some cases begin with symptoms in the home and spread to other settings.

Oppositional disorder was first defined in DSM-III as a mild condition characterized by opposition to authority figures. DSM-IIIR changed the name to *oppositional defiant disorder* and modified the diagnostic criteria such that ODD more closely resembled CD. As a result, it is becoming increasingly controversial whether ODD and CD are manifestations of the same disorder or are distinct clinical syndromes (Rey et al., 1988). The possibility that ODD is an earlier or milder form of CD is supported by the fact that, in many cases, ODD precedes CD. Also, CD and ODD also have very similar patterns of association with known risk factors.

An interesting but radical proposal for DSM-IV is to combine ODD and CD into a single generic category involving different severity levels. This approach has the advantage of being able to account for possible developmental relationships that may exist between ODD and CD. For example, one possible developmental relationship is that the symptoms of both disorders may emerge on a continuum with the less severe symptoms occurring first and the more serious symptoms occurring later. A second possible developmental relationship is that ODD symptoms occur early and to some degree predict later CD symptoms. A third possible relationship is that the same risk factors and the same forms of impairment are related to both ODD and CD, with various factors being stronger for CD than they are for ODD.

However, there are also disadvantages to subsuming ODD and CD into a single category. The most serious problem is that many children who manifest the symptoms of ODD do not progress into more serious symptomatology. The concern has been raised that if ODD and CD are grouped together, what might be a mild condition with no progression could become a stigmatizing diagnosis if lumped with a more serious disorder.

COMORBIDITY AND ASSOCIATED CONDITIONS

As described above, the disruptive behavior disorders (DBDs) tend to be associated with each other. Other conditions or symptoms that are frequently associated with the disruptive behavior disorders include peer relationship problems, academic achievement problems, speech/language disorders, substance abuse, and depressive disorders. These associated conditions are relevant to the differential diagnosis and to the treatment of disruptive behavior disorders.

Poor peer relationships and/or social skills deficits are common problems for DBD children. They may be the result of any or all of the following: immature interactional skills, egocentric/selfish behavior, poor awareness of and regard for the consequences of one's own behavior, low frustration tolerance coupled with increased sensitivity to environmental stimuli, and exaggerated emotional reactions. In addition, some DBD children may be avoidant in their interpersonal relationships, showing schizoid or schizotypal characteristics. Whatever factors may contribute to peer problems, it is generally true that DBD children will have difficulty in making and keeping friends.

Academic achievement problems (i.e., not performing at the academic level appropriate for one's chronologic age and IQ levels) are also common in children with DBD. It is important to recognize that there may be different etiologies for the academic achievement problems. In some cases they may be a direct result of the core symptoms of DBD, while in other cases there may be other reasons for the academic problems.

Speech and language disorders are very common in children with DBD. The association is best documented for ADD; the literature suggests that as many as 50 percent of ADD patients may have associated speech/language disorders (Baker and Cantwell, 1992). However, there is also a substantial literature indicating an association between speech/language disorders and "juvenile delinquency" (or conduct disorder).

The nature of the relationship between speech/language disorders and DBD is not understood but is of considerable theoretical interest (Cantwell and Baker, 1991). From a clinical standpoint, the association is of interest because of the need for early remediation. The long-term outcome of children with speech and language disorders is fairly good with respect to the speech and language disorder itself. However, there is a high likelihood of learning disorders developing as a residual effect of an early speech and language difficulty.

Older children with DBD are at risk for substance abuse. This includes the abuse of alcohol and other drugs. Available data suggest that it is those DBD children whose DBD symptoms persist into adolescence and adult life who are most at risk for substance abuse. Apparently, the choice of drug may be at least partially environmentally determined in that some studies have found high rates of alcohol abuse and others have found high rates of other forms of substance abuse. Genetic factors also may play a role in the predisposition to the development of both forms of substance abuse.

Carlson and Cantwell (1989) have found high rates of both major depressive disorder and dysthymic disorder in children who carry a diagnosis of DBD. Biederman and associates (1987) have found the same thing and also have reported on an increased rate of mood disturbance in the family members of those children with ADD who also had comorbid mood disturbance. Some authors (Wender et al., 1981) have suggested that there may be a rather unique form of mood disturbance that develops as a result of ADD. This mood disturbance begins in childhood with a brief period of ups and downs that are generally related to environmental circumstances. As the child moves into adolescence and adult life, the up periods become less frequent, and the down periods become more frequent and more prolonged.

DIFFERENTIAL DIAGNOSIS

The task of differential diagnosis in child psychiatry requires distinguishing between various disorders having similar symptom complexes as well as considering various possible etiologic factors that will lead to the same symptoms. Differential diagnosis is particularly difficult with the disruptive behavior disorders because there are many psychiatric and other conditions that can produce inattention, overactivity, and antisocial behaviors. Some of these difficulties are illustrated in our comprehensive discussion of the differential diagnosis of hyperactivity (Cantwell and Baker, 1987).

One method for organizing differential diagnosis is to use the multiaxial system of DSM-IIIR, considering in turn Axis I clinical psychiatric conditions, Axis II developmental and personality disorders, Axis III physical and neurologic disorders, and Axis IV psychosocial factors. With regard to Axis I, the clinical psychiatric conditions that involve symptoms of the disruptive behavior disorders include anxiety and affective disorders, pica, Tourette's syndrome, and childhood-onset schizophrenia. Borderline personality disorder is coded in Axis II with or without an Axis I diagnosis. All these disorders share some of the core symptoms of "inattention," "impulse control," and "motor activity" disturbance characteristic of the ADD syndrome. For example, children and adolescents with bipolar disorder often manifest agitation and hyperactivity; adolescents with borderline personality disorder may manifest excitability, mood lability, and impulsivity; and children with separation anxiety disorder may manifest episodic symptoms of inattention, motor activity, and impulsivity in association with their anxiety. Likewise, children with schizophrenia with onset below the age of 12 also may present with symptoms of attention impairment, but they may not be overactive and are not necessarily impulsive.

Bipolar disorder in a younger child or adolescent may present with irritability and antisocial behavior which can be misdiagnosed as CD, ODD, ADD, or all three. Given the stigmatizing effect of the CD diagnosis, it is particularly important that isolated instances or adolescent onset of antisocial behavior not be confused with the persistent pattern of antisocial behaviors necessary for the CD diagnosis.

Pica may result in lead being ingested, and the lead poisoning may, in turn, cause ADD-like symptoms. Many Tourette's syndrome patients present initially with ADD symptomology and develop tics and obsessive-compulsive symptoms later in life. It is unclear whether the ADD that occurs with Tourette's syndrome is etiologically distinct from the ADD that occurs without Tourette's.

The key to the differential diagnosis of these disorders is the core clinical picture of the disorders themselves and the distinction between episodic versus persistent symptomatology. In most of the non-DBD conditions, the relevant DBD symptoms are episodic in nature and have not been present from early childhood.

The ADD symptoms of poor attention, poor impulse control, and motor overactivity are associated with a number of Axis II conditions, including mental retardation, infantile autism, pervasive developmental disorders, developmental speech or language disorders, and academic skills disorders. The association with ADD symptoms is particularly strong for mentally retarded children whose IQs are in the moderately to profoundly retarded ranges. These Axis II disorders are also characterized by developmental immaturity and frustration associated with poor communicative skills, both of which may lead to acting-out or antisocial behaviors. In such cases, care must be taken to determine whether children meet the diagnostic criteria for both the DBD and the Axis II disorder.

There is a voluminous list of Axis III physical and neurologic disorders that may present with motor activity and attentional symptoms. Neurologic disorders associated with ADD symptoms include brain injury due to head trauma; seizure disorders; central nervous system infections and encephalitis; prematurity with significantly low birth weight; various forms of pre- , peri- , and postnatal difficulties (e.g., asphyxia, maternal infection during pregnancy); movement disorders (e.g., Sydenham's chorea); hyperthyroidism; and sleep apnea syndrome. With these disorders, the symptoms of hyperactivity, inattentiveness, and poor impulse control only mimic the syndrome of ADD. The comorbid diagnosis of ADD can usually be ruled out on grounds of the episodic nature of the core symptoms of ADD and the absence of an early history of the ADD core symptoms.

Axis IV psychosocial or environmental factors (including a wide variety of stressors, chaotic and disorganized homes, physical or sexual abuse, and/or neglect) may lead to symptoms of the ADD syndrome. The symptoms seen with these problems do not generally have the driven and disorganized quality that is characteristic of children with the ADD syndrome. However, true ADD may occur in chaotic environments. Understimulation, inadequate parental control, and other environmental factors also may trigger hyperactive behavior that can be misdiagnosed as ADD.

The same situation is true with ODD and CD. That is, a transient occurrence of some of the symptoms of ODD or CD may be seen in the face of the disorder's various psychosocial stressors. As mentioned above, it is particularly important that isolated instances of antisocial behavior not be confused with the persistent pattern of antisocial behaviors required for the CD diagnosis.

EPIDEMIOLOGY

The prevalence of DBDs has not been studied systematically. Prevalence estimates vary widely across studies because of different definitions and methodologies being employed.

A number of studies have examined the presence of hyperactivity in school children. Prevalence estimates range from 3 to 20 percent, with the estimates tending to be higher in younger children and in boys. In various clinical studies, ADD has been found to be the most common childhood psychiatric disorder. Barkley (1990) suggests that its prevalence rate is between 3 and 5 percent of the general population of children.

Certain conduct symptoms (e.g., arguing, disobedience, fighting, lying) are rather common in children, especially among clinically referred children. However, most children with these symptoms would not receive a CD diagnosis. Kazdin (1987a) has reviewed the literature and suggests that the rate of CD is between 4 and 10 percent of the general population.

ODD is a relatively common accompaniment of disorders in children who are referred to psychiatric clinics for evaluation. However, since it is a relatively new psychiatric diagnosis, its prevalence has not been documented. The childhood ECA study now in progress should go a long way toward answering some of the questions we now have regarding the exact prevalence rate of specific psychiatric disorders in the general population.

ETIOLOGY AND RISK FACTORS

To truly be considered a risk factor, a particular variable must be associated with an increased prevalence of a disorder, must have been present before the onset of the disorder, and must show strong evidence of playing a causal role in the disorder. The fact that a variable is associated with an increased prevalence of a disorder may mean that the variable is causal, but it also may be simply a correlate or a consequence of the disorder. Thus, to show that the variable is truly causal, it must be demonstrated that a change in the severity of the variable being studied is followed by a change in the prevalence of the disorder. Alternatively, if it can be demonstrated that there is a specific mechanism of causation between the variable and the disorder, then a causal relationship can be proven.

Many factors have been studied as possible risk and etiologic factors for the DBDs. Familial factors are particularly important and seem to suggest both genetic and environmental components to the disorders. For CD and ODD, environmental factors seem to play major roles, whereas for ADD, biologic factors seem more important. Findings specific to the different DBDs are summarized below.

Conduct Disorder

There is an extensive literature on the factors associated with juvenile delinquency and a less extensive literature specifically examining factors associated with CD. Among the factors that have been proposed as etiologic in the development of CD are gender, chronic physical illness, brain damage, personality or temperamental characteristics, race, body build, physiologic characteristics (e.g., autonomic reactivity), family characteristics, and community and socioeconomic factors (e.g., geographic area of residence, social class, nature of peer groups, types of schools, exposure to television). For many of these factors, the data are limited, and a causal relationship has not been established.

It has been clearly demonstrated that CD is more common in males and that it is strongly associated with chronic physical illness and with brain damage. It is also clear that CD is familial in nature, in that it is significantly more common in children whose parents have a diagnosis of antisocial personality disorder, attention deficit hyperactivity disorder, or alcoholism.

There are also data to suggest that nonhereditary environmental risk factors are equally as important if not more important than hereditary risk factors. For example, causal relationships have been reported between CD and the following family factors: parental deviance, parental psychopathology, poor parenting skills, the presence of marital discord, parental rejection, neglect, inconsistent parental management with harsh discipline, a lack of parental supervision, early institutionalization, frequent changes in the parenting figures, absence of a father, paternal alcoholism, large family size, and family history of disruptive behavior disorders (Loeber, 1990).

Oppositional Defiant Disorder

There are no comprehensive longitudinal studies examining the etiologic factors associated with ODD. It is thought that the risk factors for ODD are essentially similar to those for CD.

For example, like CD, ODD shows some degree of familiality. It appears to be more prevalent in families whose parents had a childhood diagnosis of ODD or ADD, and it may be more common in families where the mother has a diagnosis of depression. A ''difficult temperament'' and motor hyperactivity in the preschool years also seem to be predisposing factors for ODD. Some parent–child factors, such as disruptive childrearing practices with a succession of different caretakers or childrearing practices which are either harsh or neglectful also may predispose a child to ODD.

Attention Deficit Disorder

For ADD, environmental factors seem less significant etiologically than they are for ODD or CD, although they may play a role in determining how the specific symptoms are manifested in an individual child. In general, there is a growing general consensus that biologic factors are the major etiologic determinants of ADD.

Originally, ADD was viewed as the result of a form of brain damage. We now know that only a small number of children with a well-defined ADD have documented evidence of brain damage. Furthermore, the great majority of children who *do* have well-documented structural abnormalities of the brain do not exhibit ADD symptomatology. The currently more popular view is that some type of central nervous system dysfunction may be present in a local area.

Although early CT scans failed to demonstrate significant differences between ADD patients and controls (Shaywitz et al., 1983), subsequent work has identified some differences. For example, a series of studies by Lou and colleagues (1989, 1990) using single-photon and xenon-133 emission tomographic scans found hypoperfusion in frontal lobes and caudate nuclei and hypoperfusion of the right striatal region in children with pure ADD. There is some suggestion of reversal of this hypoperfusion with methylphenidate (Lou et al., 1989).

Another study using a positron-emission tomographic (PET) technique (Zametkin et al., 1990) found lowered cerebral glucose metabolism in adults with ADD who had never been treated with medication, all of whom had children with ADD. The greatest reductions were in the premotor cortex and in the superior prefrontal area.

A large number of psychophysiologic and neurochemical studies also have produced evidence of organic differences between ADD children and other children. The psychophysiologic studies suggest a pattern of underreactivity in certain areas, particularly those involving the frontal-limbic regions and the mesial-frontal regions (Barkley, 1990). The neurochemical studies tentatively indicate the involvement of dopamine and/or norepinephrine systems (Zametkin and Rapoport, 1986). These tentative neurochemical findings are consistent with the psychophysiologic findings and the hypoperfusion studies. Neuropsychological tasks sensitive to brain dysfunction suggest differences in ADD children in performance of tasks which are sensitive to frontal lobe dysfunction.

The family and adoption studies suggest a familial and possibly a genetic factor in some, but not all, children with ADD. The mechanism of genetic transmission is unknown.

There is also evidence that the etiology of ADD is multifactorial. A number of different biologic factors (e.g., genetic predisposition, exposure to toxins) may singly or in combination lead to a final common pathway of the clinical picture of ADD.

While certain patterns in family interaction appear characteristic in families with ADD children, these are not thought to be etiologic in the disorder. Rather, they are considered to be reactions of the parents to the difficult type of behavior that is presented by their ADD child. However, it may be that certain aspects of family interaction and other family factors may be involved in the maintenance or in the worsening of ADD symptomatology over time and/or in the development of an associated ODD or CD.

CLINICAL COURSE AND OUTCOME

There are several study designs that can be used to trace the clinical course of a disorder. The first is a true or ''real time'' prospective study in which the investigator selects patients with a defined clinical picture and follows them up at a later time. In this way, the pathways of the clinical disorder can be delineated. This design is very effective, especially for assessing treatment effectiveness, since patients can be randomly assigned to different treatment conditions. However, this design has the disadvantages of being time-consuming, costly, and vulnerable to problems of subject attrition. Nonetheless, there are a number of studies of ADD children that used this format.

The second major study design is the follow-back study or true retrospective design in which an adult or adolescent is selected and his or her previously existing records or retrospective diagnoses are used for earlier data. This design has more reliability problems than the true prospective study design, but it has the major advantage that there is no need to wait for the sample to "age." The major disadvantage is that the prior reports may be inadequate. Follow-back studies of juvenile delinquents and convicted criminals are common.

The third study design is the catch-up prospective design. It combines elements of both of the preceding types of designs; the sample is identified in childhood, selected from existing records that have already been collected. This eliminates the aging factor. Robins' (1966) classic follow-up study of delinquent children is an example of this type of research.

Data from all of these types of studies suggest that the DBDs have high rates of persistence and morbidity. Although patients with mild cases may show improvement over time, most patients remain ill for years. Over time, there is a strong likelihood of developing associated psychiatric disorders (including other DBDs, substance abuse, and affective disorders) and learning disorders. Levels of adaptive functioning tend to be impaired in all areas of functioning (family, social relationships, educational achievement, and career/employment).

Conduct Disorder

Angry, aggressive, and defiant behaviors in children tend to be very stable, particularly across the early childhood years.

EDITORS' COMMENT

In a longitudinal Finnish study, peer nominations and teacher ratings of 8-year-olds for aggressiveness predicted criminal behavior at age 20 (Pulkkinen Lea: J Youth Adolescence 12:253–283, 1983).

However, the diagnostic criteria for the full syndrome of CD are generally not met before the prepubertal age range. Nonetheless, onset is typically before age 16. Postpubertal onset is rare but relatively more common in females.

The outcome of CD is somewhat variable, but it tends to be chronic. Milder forms of the disorder are less chronic. The disorder is also less chronic in girls than in boys.

Robins (1978) has done some comprehensive longitudinal studies involving both children and adults with antisocial behavior problems. She found that while adult antisocial behavior virtually requires childhood antisocial behavior, most antisocial children do not become antisocial adults. An-

other important finding was that the variety of antisocial behavior in childhood is a better predictor of adult antisocial behavior than are any particular childhood symptoms.

More recently, Kazdin (1987a) reviewed the literature on children who were clinically referred for antisocial behavior. Several factors that were associated with persistence of antisocial behavior were found: earlier onset, greater number of different types of antisocial behaviors, greater number of situations (e.g., home, school, community) in which the conduct symptomatology is shown, and greater number of persons and/or organizations against which antisocial behavior is demonstrated. Such family factors as marital discord, large family size, parental psychopathology, paternal arrest history, unemployment, alcoholism, and poor parental discipline also were associated with continuation of antisocial behavior over time. Several studies also have identified childhood attention deficits, impulsivity, and overactivity as predictors of persistent antisocial problems.

Psychiatric, social, and educational complications are frequent serious sequelae of CD. Substance abuse and antisocial personality disorder are among the major psychiatric sequelae. Psychiatric hospitalizations, criminal behaviors, arrests and convictions, and employment problems are also common in adulthood. In the adolescent years, there are high rates of school drop out and poor educational achievement. Relationship problems are also a common consequence of CD, including high rates of marital conflicts, divorce, remarriage, and separation. Social isolation (e.g., limited participation in community organizations and churches and limited contact with relatives, friends, and neighbors) is another outcome of CD.

The extreme seriousness of CD is shown by elevated rates of mortality and of hospitalizations (both physical and psychiatric). The elevated mortality rate is associated with higher rates of physical injury from accidents and fights and with higher rates of suicidal behavior.

Attention Deficit Disorder

ADD symptoms in the form of increased motor activity and possibly temperamental difficulties such as feeding, sleeping, and adaptability problems generally are noticeable by the toddler age. Although symptoms begin earlier in life, diagnosis is often not made until the child is in a structured school setting.

The clinical course of ADD is also variable. However, the idea that children outgrow ADD in adolescence or at puberty is clearly not accurate. The ADD symptoms generally remain present across settings, although the child may appear to be less symptomatic during the school vacation times because of the unstructured nature of the setting and less demand for cognitively effortful activity. It is now believed that 60 to 70 percent of children with ADD will continue to demonstrate significant symptomatology in late adolescence and early adult life. Although motor activity problems sometimes diminish with age, attentional problems tend to persist over time.

CD and ODD alone or together may develop as complications as well as academic difficulty. It is unclear whether anxiety and affective disorders are also complications of ADD, but it seems that adults who identify themselves as having had ADD in childhood have elevated rates of these disorders. However, prospective studies by Mannuzza and associates (1989) suggest that ADD in childhood leads to antisocial personality disorder, drug abuse disorders, and impairment in educational and occupational achievement but not to other disorders. There is some suggestion that the combination of ADD, ODD, and CD speeds up the progression of the severity of antisocial behavior, but this has not been definitely established.

Oppositional Defiant Disorder

There are few studies of the clinical course and outcome of ODD. One, by the present author (Cantwell and Baker, 1989), followed 15 children with oppositional disorder 4 years after initial diagnosis. The data revealed a generally poor prognosis, with only 1 child becoming psychiatrically well, 6 retaining the ODD diagnosis, and the remaining 8 having developed a variety of other behavioral, emotional, and psychiatric illnesses.

In another study, Loeber and colleagues (1989) reported that a third of boys with DSM-IIIR ODD developed CD over a 3-year period. If criteria other than DSM-IIIR were used with the same subjects, approximately 50 percent would have developed a CD diagnosis. Thus there is clear evidence that in some cases ODD is a developmental precursor to later CD.

TREATMENT AND MANAGEMENT

Children with DBDs have been a major focus of clinical psychiatric service for many years. Thus there is a relatively large literature about various types of interventions that have been attempted with these children. With ADD in particular, there is a large literature on psychopharmacologic and psychosocial interventions. There is also a relatively large clinical literature on the treatment of CD and antisocial disorder, but little is known about the treatment of ODD. In the absence of empirical data, it is currently presumed that the techniques that are beneficial in the management of CD also will prove useful in the management of ODD.

The best research has been done on psychopharmacologic interventions with ADD children. Aside from these studies, much of the literature is uncontrolled and anecdotal in nature. Many of the studies do not provide enough detail about what was done for what group of subjects for what length of time. Also, important details, such as who provided the various types of interventions and the quality, nature, and duration of the interventions, often were not specified. There are very few studies that have used random allocation of patients and careful matching, especially matching on key data that are known to predict outcome. Often only gross measures of outcome (e.g., arrest rate, reconviction rate, parole violations) have been used in a number of studies.

Conduct Disorder

Kazdin (1987b) reviewed the literature on treatment of antisocial behavior in children and adolescents and found that no clear conclusions could be drawn about the effects of various types of individual and group psychotherapy. Insight-oriented or relationship therapy did not appear to be the treatment of choice for children with CD.

Since family factors are related to the development of antisocial behavior in children, it would seem likely that some type of family therapy would be an effective treatment. However, there is a shortage of outcome studies to substantiate that any particular form of family therapy should be considered the treatment of choice. Behavioral family therapy, however, seems more promising.

Behavioral therapy (i.e., reinforcement and punishment, multifaceted operant-conditioning programs, social skills training, and behavioral family therapy) focuses directly on CD behaviors and their removal. The literature supports the view that behavioral interventions are effective in removing some specific conduct symptomatology in children and adolescents in a variety of settings, including homes, schools, and institutional settings. Unfortunately, many studies have reported only on the treatment of isolated symptoms. Demonstrations that change has occurred in isolated symptoms are not the same as showing that CD itself has changed. Most of the behavioral literature also has failed to demonstrate generalization of changes from one setting to another (e.g., from home to school or from school to the general environment).

Parent management techniques within the home setting are effective in helping children with various degrees of CD. Short-term changes have been demonstrated in the home and in school, and follow-up studies suggest that the improvement may persist for a year or more. Unfortunately, many conduct-disordered children come from severely dysfunctional families with significant socioeconomic disadvantages. These families are not as likely to benefit from parent management training, since the parents tend to have difficulties in attending appointments and in complying with treatment activities (such as reading detailed manuals of therapeutic information, collecting observational data on the child's behavior, and carrying out specific behavioral procedures).

More recently, cognitive psychotherapy, or cognitive-behavioral psychotherapy, has been aimed at thought processes, self statements, problem-solving skills, and other cognitive strategies that are postulated to underlie CD symptoms in some children. Clinical studies show that such training can alter specific cognitive deficits and can lead to positive changes in the psychosocial adjustment. Impulsive hyperactive children have been trained to approach tasks in a more reflective fashion and also how to monitor and evaluate their performance. Studies have shown that changes over time toward normality on impulsivity measures, in problem-solving skills, in role-taking ability, and on other cognitive processes. However, the research is not as clear on significant changes in behavior at home, at school, or in the community, especially with seriously disturbed antisocial conduct–disordered children.

There are no solid data on pharmacologic management of children with CD. However, a variety of different types of psychotropic medications have been used with children whose symptomatology includes aggressive behavior. Neuroleptics, stimulants, lithium, propanolol, and carbamazepine may all be effective for aggressive behavior in certain types of children. The effect of these medications on other aspects of CD symptomatology is not known.

Attention Deficit Disorder

There is a relatively large literature on the treatment of ADD. Because ADD is frequently accompanied by a myriad of social, behavioral, emotional, and developmental difficulties, treatment programs need to be tailored to the individual child. Depending on the needs of the child, such programs can include educational tutoring, behavioral training, cognitive training, parent training, or other approaches. Stimulants are the medications of choice, with the antidepressants (particularly the tricyclics) being second-choice drugs for those children who cannot take stimulants because of side effects or for whom the stimulants are ineffective. Newer medications such as bupropion and clonidine also have been used for some ADD children. They may have some unique effects on children with ADD who also have ODD or CD symptomatology.

From the clinical standpoint, the following can be stated about the effect of stimulants in ADHD. They have behavioral effects, including decreased activity, more focused and more coordinated activity, more selective and better sustained attention, less impulsive, oppositional, and intense social behavior, better integration of the self, and increased self-esteem. Cognitive effects include improvement on rate, accuracy, and consistency of processing, as measured by laboratory procedures and also by classroom performance. Social effects include improved peer acceptance and in some cases less aggressive and less provocative social behavior. There is an improvement in communication with others (giving and receiving instructions); medicated children receive less criticism and corrections from parents and teachers.

The guidelines for the use of the stimulants include the recognition that when used in equivalent dosages, all the stimulants are approximately equally effective. For a single dose of methylphenidate, dosages range from 0.15 to 1.0 mg/kg per dose, for dextroamphetamine 0.15 to 0.5 mg/kg per dose, and for pemoline 0.5 to 2.0 mg/kg per dose. An average low dose of methylphenidate is 0.3 mg/kg per dose, a medium dose is 0.6 mg/kg, and high dose is 1.0 mg/kg. Pelham (1989) recently completed a series of studies comparing the efficacy of standard methylphenidate given twice a day, methylphenidate in a sustained-release preparation, a sustained-released form of dextroamphetamine, and magnesium pemoline. He found that all the medications at equivalent dosages were generally equally effective on all parameters, including social behaviors during a group recreational activity, performance in the classroom, and scores on a continuous-performance task.

Standard methylphenidate and standard amphetamines have about a 4-hour duration of action. Magnesium pemoline and longer-acting dexedrine and ritalin probably last from 6 to 9 hours in different children. Common side effects of stimulants include insomnia, anorexia, abdominal distress, and headaches. Monitoring should include parent and teacher ratings at baseline and periodically during treatment; measures of height, weight, resting pulse, and blood pressure several times during the year; and a complete blood count and blood chemistries once a year or more often if clinical symptoms indicate. Systematic studies suggest that in the absence of clinical symptoms, routine blood studies are unlikely to turn up any problems. Pemoline does have a side effect that other stimulants do not in that it may cause liver function tests to be abnormal in a small number of patients.

If stimulants are not completely effective, or if negative side effects occur that lead to discontinuation, the antidepressants are the next drugs of choice. The tricyclics have been studied the most. With dosages of up to 3 mg/kg per day of drugs such as desipramine, the percentage of children who respond is not quite as good as the response to stimulants. With dosages of up to 5 mg/kg per day of desipramine, the percentage of children who respond approximates the percentage of children who respond to stimulants. The available literature suggests that greatest effects of the tricyclics are on behavior, and the effect on cognitive function is less direct. Behavioral effects include more organized behavior and decreased aggression and oppositionality. Recommended desipramine dosage is 50 mg bid at least twice daily and possibly three times daily with blood levels of 150 mg ± 30 ng/ml. No true relationship between clinical effect and plasma effect has been demonstrated in ADD patients, although this has been reported in some studies of depressed patients. One of the more significant problems is that the initial effectiveness of tricyclic antidepressants may disappear over time. One of the advantages compared with the stimulants is less rebound and a more even effect across the day.

Considerably less evidence exists for the effect of other antidepressants such as bupropion, fluoxetine, and monoamine oxidase inhibitors. Buproprion at a dosage of 150 to 300 mg/day (or 3–6 mg/kg) has been reported to positively affect behavior and most likely have some effect on cognitive function, although the data are not as clear. The cognitive effects of the newer antidepressants seem to be greater organization and improved attention; the behavior effects include calmer behavior and improvement on parent and teacher ratings with less aggressive behavior. Fluoxetine has been used in dosages as low as 5 mg/day up to 80 mg/day. Both tranylcypromine and corgyline have been reported to improve behavior rapidly and to improve performance on laboratory tests of cognitive functions. They are very similar to the stimulants in their effects. However, the potential for side effects is greater, and this limits their utility.

Clonidine may have a special role for children with ADD who also have tic disorders. It also should be considered a third-line drug after the stimulants and antidepressants in those without tics. Effects of clonidine include improved frustration tolerance, less excessive arousal or hyperactivity, less oppositionality and aggressive behavior, an increase in social skills and social adjustment, and less explosive behavior, with children being described as having a longer fuse and less extreme rage reactions. If the child is cognitively intact, clonidine allows for a greater focus of attention and improved task orientation, and the child seems less overwhelmed by demands; the drug also may improve problem solving of complex tasks. It may be combined with stimulant medication, and some authors suggest that a lower dose of stimulants may be used and that there are fewer side effects. ADD children with Tourette's, with low frustration tolerance, with significant aggression, and with oppositional behavior and hyperarousal are those considered most likely to benefit from clonidine. With oral clonidine there should be a slow increase and decrease with one-half tablet per day up to 0.05 mg qid. The equivalent dose is 3 to 10 mg/kg given qid. The uneven response and a very short half-life of the oral drug necessitate frequent dosing during the day. Clonidine also comes in patch form with the transthermal system (TTS) patches of 0.1, 0.2 and 0.3 mg/day. These skin patches last for about 5 days, but there may be variable absorption.

A variety of other medications, including carbamazepine, lithium, propanol and other beta blockers, caffeine, fenfluramine, L-deprenyel, and amantadine, have some clinical suggestion of effectiveness for individual children. However, there is no really substantial evidence from controlled studies that they have any role in straight-forward ADD. As noted earlier, some have been suggested as drugs that might affect aggressive behavior that may accompany ADD and very often accompanies CD.

In summary, the literature on management of the DBDs is relatively lacking compared with the literature on phenomenology, possible etiologic factors, and clinical course. This is true to some degree of the literature on all forms of childhood psychopathology. More carefully controlled studies with well-defined populations of children are needed, since children with DBDs do make up a large proportion of those children referred for clinical intervention to child psychiatric services throughout the United States.

REFERENCES

Anderson JC, Williams S, McGee R, Silva PA: DSM-III disorders in preadolescent children. Arch Gen Psychiatry 44:69–76, 1987.

Baker L, Cantwell DP: Attention deficit disorder and speech/language disorders. Compr Mental Health Care 2(1):3–16, 1992.

Barkley RA: Attention Deficit–Hyperactivity Disorder: A Handbook for Diagnosis and Treatment. New York, Gilford Press, 1990.

Biederman J, Munir K, Knee D: Conduct and oppositional disorder in clinically referred children with attention deficit disorder: A controlled family study. J Am Acad Child Adolesc Psychiatry, 26(5):724–727, 1987.

Cantwell DP, Baker L: Differential diagnosis of hyperactivity. J Dev Behav Pediatr 8(3):159–165, 1987.

Cantwell DP, Baker L: Stability and natural history of DSM-III childhood diagnoses. J Am Acad Child Adolesc Psychiatry 28:691–700, 1989.

Cantwell DP, Baker L: Psychiatric Developmental Disorders in Children with Communication Disorder. Washington, American Psychiatric Press, 1991.

Carlson GA, Cantwell DP: Unmasking masked depression in children and adolescents. Am J Psychiatry 137:445–449, 1980.

Kazdin AE: Conduct Disorders in Childhood and Adolescence. Beverly Hills, CA, Sage Publications, 1987a.

Kazdin AE: Treatment of antisocial behavior in children: Current status and future directions. Psychol Bull 102(2):187–203, 1987b.

Loeber R: Development and risk factors of juvenile antisocial behavior and delinquency. Clin Psychol Rev 10(1):1–42, 1990.

Loeber R, Tremblay RE, Gagnon C, Charebois P: Continuity and desistance in disruptive boys' early fighting at school. Dev Psychopathol 1:39–50, 1989.

Lou HC, Henriksen L, Bruhn P, et al: Striatal dysfunction in attention deficit and hyperkinetic disorder. Arch Neurol 46:48–52, 1989.

Lou HC, Henriksen L, Bruhn P: Focal cerebral dysfunction in developmental learning disabilities. Lancet 335(8680):8–11, 1990.

Mannuzza S, Klein RG, Konig PH, Giampino TL: Hyperactive boys almost grown up: IV. Criminality and its relationship to psychiatric status. Arch Gen Psychiatry 46(12):1073–1079, 1989.

Pelham WE: Behavior therapy, behavioral assessment and psycho-stimulant medication in the treatment of attention deficit disorders: An interactive approach. In Bloomingdale LM, Swanson JM (eds): Attention Deficit Disorder IV: Emerging Trends in Attentional and Behavioral Disorders of Childhood. New York, Pergamon Press, 1989, pp 169–202.

Rey JM, Bashir MR, Schwarz M, et al: Oppositional disorder: Fact or fiction? J Am Acad Child Adolesc Psychiatry 27:157–162, 1988.

Robins LN: Deviant Children Grown Up. Baltimore, Williams & Wilkins, 1966.

Robins LN: Sturdy childhood predictors of adult antisocial behavior: Replications from longitudinal studies. Psychol Med 8:611–622, 1978.

Shaywitz BA, Shaywitz SE, Byrne T, et al: Attention deficit disorder: Quantitative analysis of CT. Neurology 33:1500–1503, 1983.

Wender PH, Reimherr FW, Wood DR: Attention deficit disorder (minimal brain dysfunction) in adults. Arch Gen Psychiatry 38:449–456, 1981.

Zametkin AJ, Rapoport JL: The pathophysiology of attention deficit disorder with hyperactivity: A review. In Lahey BB, Kazedin AE (eds): Advances in Clinical Child Psychology, vol. 9. New York, Plenum Press, 1986, pp 177–216.

Zametkin AJ, Nordahl TE, Gross M, et al: Cerebral glucose metabolism in adults with hyperactivity of childhood onset. N Engl J Med 323(20):1361–1366, 1990.

Major Affective Disorders in Children and Adolescents

BARRY D. GARFINKEL

INTRODUCTION

The investigation and understanding of child and adolescent affective disorders have historically been hampered by a series of theoretical misconceptions. Psychoanalytic theory originally stressed that children could not experience depression because they had not completely progressed through and resolved the oedipal conflict (Mendelson, 1972). It was postulated that only after childhood and the complete resolution of the oedipal conflict, a superego or conscience results, allowing for the capacity to experience guilt and remorse (Rie, 1966). Because guilt, self-blame, and remorse were among the central feelings said to characterize adult depression, it was assumed that children could not have depression without a fully formed superego (Rochlin, 1959; Sandler and Joffe, 1965). Many empirical reports, as well as substantial clinical experience derived from interviews with depressed children, indicated that self-blame, remorse, guilt, and low self-esteem all indeed occur at younger ages. Despite the incongruity between psychoanalytic theory and actual clinical observation, theory continued to dominate psychodynamic psychiatric perspectives on childhood affective disorders.

The second major hurdle in understanding child and adolescent affective disorders was the concept that developmental stages altered the presentation of clinical symptoms so that totally different symptoms were expressed at different ages (Bemporad and Wilson, 1978). It was postulated that particular symptoms were only observed in children with major affective disorder. Such concepts as "depressive equivalents" (Malmquist, 1971) and "masked depression" (Glaser, 1967;

Cytryn and McKnew, 1972) became terms that described vastly divergent behaviors that were assumed to be expressions of an underlying depression. These terms made depression incomprehensible from direct patient interview and observation. Depression became a diagnosis that was discernible only by clinicians who were astute enough to identify underlying affective states. From encopresis and enuresis to promiscuity and drug abuse, vastly discrepant behaviors were viewed as behavioral manifestations of affective disorders in children and adolescents (Frommer, 1968).

Infancy, a specific developmental stage, was thought to influence the expression of depression. Spitz (1946) coined the term *anaclitic depression*, and Bowlby (1973, 1980) described concepts concerning attachment and loss. Although these terms describe marked behavioral and, at times, physiologic responses to grieving, mourning, or loss, it is impossible to discern a unique relationship to affective disorders. These concepts and the conditions they describe are not representative of affective disorders, and thus, on the basis of their presumed presence, it cannot be assumed that an underlying affective disorder exists other than grief and mourning (Carlson and Cantwell, 1980b).

Adolescence has been characterized by specific stages of development associated with concerns about identity, relationships, and communication (Erikson, 1950), all of which have been theorized to influence the expression of depression at this age. Early adolescents have been described as normally reflecting low self-esteem, guilt, remorse, and a poor self-concept (Anthony and Scott, 1960). Identity concerns, fearfulness, multiple somatic complaints, dysphoria, and irritability have been identified (Blos, 1962). Worries of a pervasive nature have been described, reflecting thoughts of pessimism and incompetence. It has been concluded, however, that these observations have not been systematically derived and do not represent normal characteristics of this stage of development but, in fact, may represent clinically derived symptoms. Similarly, these symptoms alone do *not* satisfy the criteria for the presence of an affective disorder (McConville et al., 1973).

Concepts concerning separation (Harlow and Harlow, 1965; Bowlby, 1973; Spitz, 1946) and developmental models do not describe affective disorders in children but demonstrate the developing individual's response to attachment, grief, and mourning in response to breaks in the attachment to a significant figure in the child's life (Bowlby, 1980). The proper conclusion derived from these studies is that stages of development may be associated with some of the features resembling the criteria of affective disorders. There is, however, no stage of development that has either as its primary characteristics or in the routine reaction to stresses associated with that stage the manifestation of sufficient criteria to fulfill the diagnosis of an affective disorder.

Research has suggested that the identification of symptoms during a clinical interview with a child may depend on specialized interview techniques and that the interview process may be more difficult to conduct. At each stage of development, consideration should be given to the fact that without exception the adult criteria for major affective disorder can be identified in children and adolescents. Numerous studies (Poznanski and Zrull, 1970; Puig-Antich et al., 1978; Chambers and Puig-Antich, 1982; Carlson and Cantwell, 1981) have identified the presence of symptoms, in children and in adolescents, that are equivalent to those found in adults, and it has been shown that the adult criteria can be applied satisfactorily for child and adolescent affective disorders.

DEFINITION

In the past 20 years, it has been demonstrated that symptoms constituting the adult criteria for affective disorders have been observed in children and adolescents (Annell, 1971). Because children and adolescents do not easily or accurately verbalize their affective states, these symptoms are harder to recognize. A number of classification systems showing little overlap with the diagnostic criteria for affective disorder in children and adolescents have been unsuccessfully proposed. In general, the earlier diagnostic systems incorporated two conceptual errors: First, the criteria were far too broad, and second, the diagnosis was determined by developmental stage rather than by clinical presentation.

The Weinberg et al. (1973) criteria are an example of a major effort at a systematic classification

system that was far too inclusive. The original classification system was based on the Feighner et al. (1972) criteria adapted for children. A study by Carlson and Cantwell (1981) comparing the Weinberg criteria with that of the *Diagnostic and Statistical Manual of Mental Disorders*, third edition (DSM-III), showed that most children who met DSM-III criteria for depression also met Weinberg criteria. Many more children were diagnosed by Weinberg criteria as being depressed; however, approximately 40 percent of them did not meet the DSM-III criteria for depression. Most of these children had oppositional, conduct, and attention deficit disorders.

Another example of an exceptionally broad concept of depression was held by Frommer (1968). The approach postulated three types of depressed children: enuretic, pure, and phobic. Enuretic depressed children were characterized by immaturity, developmental delays, and learning disabilities, as well as conduct-disorder forms of behavioral problems. The pure depressives were characterized by profound periods of sadness, irritability, crying, anger, hostility, suicidal ideation, and sleep disturbances. Antisocial and anxiety symptoms were not commonly observed in such children. The phobic depressives were seen as being severely depressed, with multiple somatic symptoms, lack of energy, and overwhelming feelings of anxiety. The latter group was predominantly female, with a young age of onset and without a family history of significant psychiatric disorders. The other two groups had an approximately equal representation of boys and girls and a significant family history for psychiatric disorders. The three subtypes of depression were thought to respond to different pharmacologic and behavioral forms of treatment.

Two other descriptive classifications of depression are worth noting—those by Malmquist (1971) and McConville et al. (1973). Malmquist (1971) suggested five types of depression. The first group consists of those depressions resulting from an organic etiology, the second group resulting from severe deprivation, and the three remaining types related to three stages of development: toddler, primary school age, and adolescence. These forms of depression confounded three independent features: etiology, developmental stage, and analytic theory. For example, a child of a certain age, because of the intrafamilial relationships and real and symbolic past experiences, appears depressed in a unique way. This classification reinforced the notion that development altered the causation as well as the presentation of depressive symptomatology. It was thought impossible to separate the stage of development from the acute disorder, since maturation not only altered symptom presentation but also influenced the psychosocial etiology of an affective disorder.

McConville et al. (1973) established a classification system based on cognitive development, repeated loss, and interpersonal relationships. They linked development to three types of depression. Early childhood depression (ages 6 to 8 years) was said to be characterized by dysphoria, guilt, and low self-esteem. The second type of depression was thought to occur in children between ages 8 and 11 and was primarily characterized by significant low self-esteem and cognitive changes, such as guilt, self-reproach, pessimism, preoccupation with failure, and helplessness. In this stage, feelings of worthlessness were thought to be derived from repeated loss. The third type of childhood depression was theorized to occur in children older than 11 and was typified by significant feelings of guilt and self-blame.

Cytryn and coworkers (1972, 1980) postulated a classification system based on developmental stage, the time course of the disorder, and the patient's family history. The three types that were observed were acute, chronic, and "masked" (Glaser, 1967). Acute depression was said to be associated with a good premorbid adjustment, minimal family history of psychiatric disorders, and a brief duration of the affective disorder. The chronic type was said to be associated with significant preexisting psychopathology and a family history for psychiatric disorders. The "masked" depression group, on reexamination, was predominantly a group of conduct-disordered children (Cytryn et al., 1980).

The classification that most professionals have adopted for children is the same as that for adults. Poznanski et al. (1976), Puig-Antich et al. (1978), and Carlson and Cantwell (1980a) have all demonstrated that affective disorders in prepubertal children are best conceptualized and defined according to a schema that includes all the diagnostic criteria observed in adults. To date, not every adult form of affective disorder has been systematically observed in children. The greatest number of children have been placed in one of four categories: major depression, bipolar disorder, dysthymia, or adjustment disorder with depressed mood. It is not known whether schizoaffective disorder or cyclothymic disorder will be systematically documented in children. These disorders may be viewed as occurring as one acute episode, as recurrent episodic disorders, or as chronic unremitting states (see Table 19-1). It is important to determine the time course, as well as the primary or secondary nature, of the affective disorder. Any physical or psychiatric condition that predates the affective disorder determines that it would be a secondary affective disorder. The distinction between primary and secondary affective disorders is not well established for children and adolescents and has not led to different approaches to treatment and management for the two types.

ETIOLOGY AND PATHOGENESIS

There are four major explanations that contribute to our understanding of the etiology of affective disor-

TABLE 19-1. *Affective Disorders in Children and Adolescents*

A. Primary affective disorders in children and adolescents
 1. Chronic unremitting
  a. Dysthymia (habitual pattern resembling a chronic depression)
 2. Multiple recurrent episodes
  a. Unipolar depression
  b. Bipolar disorder (manic and depressive episodes)
  c. Manic episodes
 3. Acute single episode
  a. Major depressive disorder
  b. Adjustment disorder with depressed mood (an environmental precipitant present or duration too short to be a major depressive disorder, i.e., reactive type of depression)

B. Secondary affective disorders
 1. Physical etiology: medication usage (e.g., steroids, reserpine) and endocrine disorder (e.g., hypothyroidism)
 2. Other primary psychiatric disorder present: e.g., attention deficit disorder, conduct disorder, eating disorder (anorexia nervosa)

ders in children and adolescents. These models do not represent mutually exclusive formulations but in effect describe interactive factors that predispose an individual to a specific affective disorder. The disorder itself represents a final common pathway through which all or many of these factors exert their influence (Akiskal and McKinney, 1975). Because major affective disorders have been studied much more extensively in children, this condition will be used as a model for understanding these etiologic factors. The four main models are (1) reinforcement, (2) cognition, (3) life stresses, and (4) genetic/biochemical factors (Lewinsohn and Hoberman, 1982).

The first model, behavioral reinforcement (Lewinsohn, 1979), assumes that depression results from and is augmented by limited social reinforcement. This may include a poor living situation with an actual insufficiency of positive reinforcers, fewer social skills that elicit less positive reinforcement from the child's environment, or a punishing and aversive environment that creates a deficiency in reinforcements in life situations. These three circumstances would decrease the frequency and impact of the positive reinforcers with which the child has contact. Included in this model are family factors, such as cohesion (Reinherz et al., 1989) and conflict (Burke et al., 1990). Living with a depressed mother has been associated with higher rates of affective symptoms in the children (Gelfand and Teti, 1990); however, genetic, economic, and other social factors were not controlled. This model does not explain why the child originally is lacking in the social skills that create opportunities for positive reinforcement. Also, all children exposed to these circumstances do not develop an affective disorder. Similarly, this is a purely psychosocial model, which would imply that with the correction of the reinforcement situation, depression would invariably go away. Increasing positive reinforcement is one component of an intervention program of therapy, but in itself, it is not always sufficient in the treatment of major affective disorder. Pleasant interactions, positive responses from others, and the avoidance of punishing and unpleasant experiences generally enhance the medical treatment of depression. Positive experiences for children include enjoyable games, competition in sports, and the pursuit of skill development.

The second model assumes that depression is a result of negative cognition that the child has concerning himself or herself, the world, or his or her personal future (Beck, 1970). Cognitive patterns occur that lead to a selective and negative view of current and past events. At times, it appears that the child "rewrites history" to support a negative self-perception. Self-control is deficient in depressed individuals, with inadequate self-monitoring, self-evaluation, and self-reinforcement. These tasks are always used to further depreciate the individual and support a pessimistic view of oneself and the world. "Learned helplessness," a concept developed in laboratory animals, is an aspect of this overall model in which features of depression occur when an organism experiences that it has no control over reinforcers from its environment (Seligman and Maier, 1967). A balance between the locus of control of internal and external events is also a function of this model, with individuals feeling controlled both by others and by external events, creating a greater sense of inadequacy and failure. For depressed individuals, internal control and responsibility are assumed when something negative occurs, whereas external factors are thought to create positive events. Longitudinal studies have not indicated that these cognitive styles predate the onset of depression but rather that they are probably a consequence of depression and may perpetuate depression once it occurs. After the remission of depression, these cognitive symptoms disappear, and the individual returns to a more optimistic and positive cognitive style (Lewinsohn and Hoberman, 1982).

The life stress, or third model, has two major theoretical orientations. The first is psychoanalytic, with the original Freudian model (1917) emphasizing the symbolic or metaphorical loss of a significant, highly valued person or thing that results in depression. The lost object was ambivalently regarded, and the negative feelings that were formerly directed to the lost object are subsequently internalized and self-directed. According to this theory, all losses, irrespective of how trivial they may appear to objective scrutiny, can be a cause of a major depression because of the personalized significance with which the lost object was regarded.

The other life stress model, proposed by Graham (1974) and Lefkowitz and Burton (1978), indicates that childhood depression is a consequence of actual environmental stress and loss, primarily based within the family. Family stress, in the form of critical expressed emotion by mothers, was associated with higher rates of children's depressive symptomatology, especially when there was a higher rate of parental psychiatric disorder (Schwartz et al., 1990). This model does not take into account individual variability and the fact that depression is not associated with significant stress or loss in all families. Clearer distinction between major affective disorder and mourning or grief must be established. These three theoretical models do not adequately explain individual vulnerability, onset, morbidity, or the recurrent and episodic course of a specific affective disorder.

The fourth model proposes a genetic predisposition that alters the neurochemical regulation of mood. For affective disorders, the concordance rates for monozygotic twins is approximately 76 percent and for dizygotic twins 19 percent. Monozygotic twins reared apart had a concordance rate of 67 percent (Tsuang, 1978). Welner et al. (1977), Tsuang (1978), Kuyler et al. (1980), and Cantwell and Baker (1983) established a strong genetic predisposition for psychiatric disorders in children of parents with affective disorder. The Welner et al. study showed that children of depressed mothers had more symptoms of an affective disorder than did children of normal mothers. The family history of affective disorder in parents is associated with a much greater likelihood of affective disorder in the children (Puig-Antich et al., 1978; McKnew and Cytryn, 1979). Although no definitive neurochemical pathway has been established, there is some evidence to suggest that monoamine metabolism and neuroendocrine regulation in children may be altered (Kashani et al., 1981; Steingard et al., 1990; Jensen and Garfinkel, 1990).

In general, a final common pathway exists for childhood depression, with multiple determinants that include social, genetic, environmental, life events, and neurochemical factors all interacting to create the clinical condition of major affective disorder (Akiskal and McKinney, 1975). Subsequent study of children with affective disorder must determine what psychological, biologic, and social abnormalities are a consequence of the depression and which factors predate the clinical disorder, as well as how these factors interact with one another. Similarly, it will be important to establish the permanence of these features after the remission of the acute illness. Depression alters family life, school performance, skill attainment, and the internal subjective view the child has about himself or herself. Because affective disorders have such a profound impact on the individual, it is not surprising that multiple psychosocial factors that reflect these effects have been identified.

EPIDEMIOLOGY

The studies of specific clinical samples of children for affective disorders have been influenced by the unique qualities defining the subjects and the criteria by which affective disorder was diagnosed. In general, the criteria for affective disorder have been varied and there are few studies using DSM-IIIR criteria. The studies can be divided into two broad categories: those investigating the prevalence of this disorder in a normal population and those identifying its specific representation in a clinical sample of children. Rutter et al. (1970), in the Isle of Wight study, found 1.4 cases per 1000 children. Nissen (1971), in Germany, observed severe depression in 1.8 percent of the 6000 children he studied. Kashani and Simonds (1979), in the United States, found that 1.9 percent of 103 children had major affective disorder. Preschool children were found to have major affective disorder at a rate of approximately one-sixth that of school aged children (0.3 versus 1.9 percent) (Garrison et al., 1990). Kashani et al. (1983), in New Zealand, demonstrated a rate of 1.8 percent for major affective disorder in 641 9-year-old children. Another 2.5 percent met criteria for minor affective disorder.

In various clinical samples of both inpatient and outpatient psychiatrically treated children, studies have demonstrated that between 13.7 and 58 percent of the patients had a major affective disorder (Bauersfeld, 1972; McConville et al., 1973; Weinberg et al., 1973; Pearce, 1977; Carlson and Cantwell, 1981).

The risk for major depression increases with age, and there is a threefold greater likelihood of depression being identified at age 14 than at age 10 (Rutter et al., 1970). The rate of major depression and dysthymia in high school students (ages 14 to 17 years) was found to be 4.0 and 4.9 percent, respectively. Girls had rates twice that of boys in this age group (Whitaker et al., 1990). It is also significant that children showed a higher rate of minor depressive disorder, whereas adults consistently are found to have a greater proportion of major affective disorder (Kashani et al., 1983). In general, children with affective disorders are recognized as being in need of help more often by parents than by teachers. This is in contrast to recognizing disruptive disorders in children, which are readily identified by teachers.

Kuperman and Stewart (1979) demonstrated a major affective disorder rate of 13 percent for girls seen in their clinic and 5 percent for boys. Weinberg et al. (1973), Poznanski and Zrull (1970), and Kashani et al. (1981) found more boys than girls to be affected. In a comprehensive report by Kashani et al. (1983), similarly, there was a higher rate for boys in the nonreferred sample. This finding is in contrast to the female predominance in adults and adolescents. The switch to the adult gender ratio, with the higher female rate, occurs sometime after the onset of puberty.

CLINICAL PICTURE

In describing major affective disorders of children and adolescents, four main disorders are commonly observed. They include major depression with or without psychotic features, bipolar affective disorder, dysthymia, and adjustment disorder with depressed mood. Kovacs et al. (1984) studied 65 children who met criteria for major depression, dysthymic disorder, and adjustment disorder with depressed mood. It was shown that these three disorders had a similar age of onset and that the adjustment disorder had episodes of shortest duration (25 ± 18 weeks), with a peak recovery occurring at 6 to 9 months after diagnosis; the dysthymic disorder lasted for approximately 3 years (±68 weeks), and maximal recovery rate was 89 percent at 6 years. The major depression lasted for 32 weeks (±28 weeks), which was not significantly different from the adjustment disorder, with the maximal recovery rate approximately 1 1/2 years from onset. The dysthymic disorder also was the purest illness, being least likely to be associated with other common childhood psychiatric disorders. Anxiety disorder and other psychiatric diagnoses were most frequently associated with the other two diagnoses. In general, dysthymic disorder is a more chronic, severer disorder, with the potential for other affective disorders developing subsequently. Both dysthymic disorder and major depressive disorder showed a high rate of recurrence, with dysthymic children showing a high rate of major depressive disorder occurring within the first 5 years after the onset of the dysthymia. However, children originally diagnosed with major depressive disorder do not show the later development of dysthymic disorder.

Major depression is characterized by the symptoms listed in Table 19-2. This disorder has been

TABLE 19-2. *Symptom Clusters of Major Depression in Children and Adolescents*

Dysphoria or anhedonia (loss of interest or pleasure in usual activities)
   Tearfulness
   Sadness*
   Irritability*
   Sulkiness

Cognitive change—conscience
   Low self-esteem
   Guilt/remorse*
   Helplessness/hopelessness
   Self-reproach*
   Suicidal ideation*

Cognitive change—psychomotor
   Psychomotor retardation/agitation*
   Loss of energy/fatigue*
   Restlessness
   Decreased concentration*
   Apathy
   Aggressivity*

Vegetative
   Sleep disturbance*
   Somatic complaints*
   Appetite change*
   Weight loss/gain*

Note: Either dysphoria or anhedonia and at least four of the remaining symptoms must be present nearly every day for at least a 2-week duration while interfering with everyday functioning.
*Found in DSM-IIIR.

well established in both children and adolescents. It may be associated with psychotic features, as documented by Puig-Antich et al. (1978) and Carlson and Cantwell (1979, 1980a). Other disorders, such as learning disabilities, attention deficit disorder, conduct disorder, anxiety, and anorexia, also may be recognized. The somatic complaints of affective disorder children have long been recognized, with pediatricians and surgeons acknowledging that somatic complaints without organic etiology result most often from an affective disorder (Weinberg, 1970). Compared with adults, children and adolescents with major affective disorder have higher rates of anxiety and somatic, aggressive, and irritability symptoms, as well as mood-congruent hallucinations (Carlson and Kashani, 1988).

Bipolar affective disorder has been recognized and well documented in both children and adolescents (Strober and Carlson, 1982; Strober et al., 1981; Feinstein and Wolpert, 1973; Thompson and Schindler, 1976; Weinberg and Brumback, 1976). The cyclic nature of mood swings is much more difficult to document in children than in adults. The younger the child, the less prominent are typically manic features such as elation and grandiosity (Strober and Carlson, 1982). The depression in bipolar adolescents, when compared with nonbipolar depression, is characterized by a more rapid, acute onset, more severe dysphoria, trouble concentrating, psychomotor retardation, and psychotic features. In addition, the family history is positive for affective disorder (Strober, 1991). Marked increase in psychomotor activity is the most readily observable and consistently noted symptom in the premorbid child. Manic or hypomanic children are most often confused with ADHD and conduct-disordered children (Carlson, 1990).

The cyclothymic or extroverted personality is not commonly observed in children and adolescents with this disorder. Strober and Carlson (1982) showed that 20 percent of the hospitalized early adolescents with major depressive disorder later developed bipolar affective disorder. Those children who developed bipolar affective disorder, when compared with the other children with major depressive disorder, more frequently responded with manic or hypomanic symptoms to antidepressant medication. In general, the bipolar patients appeared more severely affected than the unipolar depressed adolescents. Carlson et al. (1977), however, were unable to demonstrate that adolescent-onset bipolar disorder had a worse prognosis than adult-onset bipolar disorder.

CLINICAL COURSE

Two prospective studies have examined the clinical outcome of a clinic sample of children with major affective disorder. On follow-up, Poznanski et al. (1976) demonstrated that during adolescence, approximately 6½ years later, the children had almost a 50 percent chance of being depressed and that the depression was indistinguishable from other adult forms of affective disorder. Herjanic et al. (1976) followed 20 children with a clinical diagnosis of depression. Those children who met specific systematic criteria for depression had some form of an affective disorder at follow-up, whereas those who were simply given various clinical diagnoses at the time of discharge were less likely to have a psychiatric diagnosis on follow-up and, if diagnosed, had diagnoses other than depression.

Two European studies also should be noted because of their opposite findings. Nissen (1971) followed 105 severely depressed children and adolescents and found that they had a poor prognosis, unrelated to the type of depression they had. Dahl (1971) showed that on follow-up of a large Danish sample of child psychiatric patients, few developed major affective disorder.

In the Chess et al. (1983) longitudinal study of 133 children, 6 were diagnosed as having an affective disorder, 2 with primary affective disorder, with an early severe onset and a recurrent course. Four had secondary affective disorder, also with early onset, but for these children, the primary diagnoses were varied, and precipitating events also were noted. There was a tendency for recurrence and a chronic history in this group of young people as well.

In one study, approximately 80 children who were diagnosed with depression in either childhood or adolescence were followed for approximately 18 years and were found to have adult rates of any depressive disorder and major depressive disorder of 58 and 31 percent, respectively. The prepubertal depressed children had a better adult outcome than those who were diagnosed with depression in adolescence (Harrington et al., 1990). It can be concluded that affective disorders whose onset is in either the childhood and adolescent years may be more chronic, with a worse prognosis.

Retrospective studies of adults with major affective disorder have revealed that in childhood, there was marked family disruption, discord, and parental neglect. Parents were viewed as having high rates of psychiatric disorders (Perris, 1968; Jacobson et al., 1975; Raskin, 1977; Orvaschel et al., 1979). In general, these adults did not have a specific psychiatric disorder during their childhood. Furthermore, only a small proportion of adult affective disorders have their onset during the prepubertal years.

LABORATORY FINDINGS

A child can be evaluated for depression using standardized and reliable techniques (Kazdin, 1981). The diagnosis is based on five methods of clinical investigation (Table 19-3). They include (1) struc-

TABLE 19-3. *Laboratory Investigation of Major Affective Disorders in Children and Adolescents*

I. Structured interviews with children
   a. Diagnostic Interview for Children and Adolescents (DICA) (Herjanic, 1975)
   b. Diagnostic Interview Schedule for Children (DISC) (Costello, 1984)
   c. Kiddie-SADS (E and L) (Puig-Antich, 1978)
   d. Interview Schedule for Children (SCI) (Kovacs, 1978)
II. Structured interviews with parents
   a. Diagnostic Interview for Children and Adolescents— Parent (DICA-P)
   b. Diagnostic Interview Schedule for Children—Parent (DISC-P)
   c. Kiddie-SADS (Puig-Antich, 1978)
III. Rating scales
   a. Children's Depression Rating Scale (CDRS) (Poznanski et al., 1979)
   b. Children's Depression Scale (CDS) (Lang and Tisher, 1978)
   c. Children's Depression Inventory (CDI) (Kovacs and Beck, 1978)
   d. SCDI (Carlson and Cantwell, 1979)
   e. Montgomery-Asberg (1979)
   f. Child Behavioral Checklist (Achenbach, 1979)
   g. Birleson (1981)
   h. Teacher Affect Rating Scale (TARS) (Petti, 1981)
   i. Bellevue Index of Depression (Petti, 1981)
   j. Peer Nomination Inventory (PNID) (Lefkowitz and Terri, 1981)
IV. Neuroendocrine
   a. Cortisol—dexamethasone suppression test (Carroll, 1982)
   b. Growth hormone—clonidine or ITT challenge (Puig-Antich et al., 1984)
V. Psychometric tests
   a. Minnesota Multiphasic Personality Inventory
   b. Personality Inventory for Children (Wirt et al., 1977)

tured interviews, (2) rating scales (self-report, parent, and clinician), (3) personality inventories, (4) neuroendocrinologic investigation, and (5) clinical pharmacologic trials (i.e., a trial of medication with a positive response being weak support for the clinical diagnosis). Chambers et al. (1978) have demonstrated the utility of the Kiddie-SADS (schizophrenia affective diagnosis schedule). This structured interview has successfully identified children with major depression, according to Research Diagnostic Criteria (Endicott and Spitzer, 1978). The Diagnostic Interview for Children and Adolescents (DICA) (Herjanic et al., 1975; Reich et al., 1982) was developed as a structured interview for parent and child. It systematically reviews specific DSM-III criteria. The Interview Schedule for Children (ISC) was developed by Kovacs (1978) and includes both a parent and a child interview for depression. The DISC and DISC-P were developed at the National Institute for Mental Health and are a children's version of the adult DIS (diagnostic interview schedule) interview (Brent et al., 1984).

The Children's Depression Inventory (CDI) (Kovacs and Beck, 1977) is a simple self-report method of identifying depression in children between ages 7 and 17 and is somewhat effective. The

Short Children's Depression Inventory (SCDI) (Carlson and Cantwell, 1979) is a modification of the CDI. Birleson (1981) developed an 18-item self-rating scale, which is a reliable instrument and is strongly associated with the clinical diagnosis. The Children's Depression Scale (CDS) (Lang and Tisher, 1978), a 48-item card-sorting task, addresses symptoms that are most-to-least like the patient. The Inventory to Diagnose Depression (IDD) has been shown to be effective in establishing the diagnosis of depression without gender bias (Ackerson et al., 1990). All these techniques have both a high false-positive and false-negative error rate but are found to compliment structured and clinical interviews.

The Children's Depression Rating Scale (CDRS) was developed by Poznanski et al. (1979) to be used during an interview by clinicians to assess the child according to items similar to those in the Hamilton Rating Scale for Adults (Hamilton, 1960). The Montgomery-Asberg Depression Rating Scale (1979) also has been used by clinicians after an interview with children and adolescents. Parent rating of children by the Personality Inventory for Children (Wirt et al., 1977) also may be useful in detecting depression.

During the past 15 years, scientists using the dexamethasone suppression test (DST) have studied the presence of cortisol hypersecretion in adult depression (Brown et al., 1979; Carroll, 1982; Carroll et al., 1981; Meltzer et al., 1982). Carroll et al. (1976) found that depressed individuals responded to dexamethasone in one of two ways; they showed either a normal 24-hour cortisol suppression or a morning cortisol suppression followed by elevated cortisol levels in the afternoon and evening. Few studies have examined cortisol hypersecretion in childhood affective disorders. Puig-Antich et al. (1979a) found evidence for adrenocortical hyperactivity in depression, but this study was limited to four subjects. On follow-up of 20 depressed children, 20 percent were found to be hypersecretors (Puig-Antich, 1980). Poznanski et al. (1982) examined 18 outpatient children, 6 to 12 years of age, and reported DST sensitivity and specificity that were similar to those in adult studies. Weller et al. (1983) found that 70 percent of 20 hospitalized depressed children were nonsuppressors. In contrast, Geller et al. (1983) found a low sensitivity of 17 percent in their sample of depressed 6- to 12-year-old children. Extein et al. (1982) compared postdexamethasone cortisol levels for 15 depressed and 12 nondepressed postpubertal patients. This study reported a sensitivity of 53 percent and a specificity of 92 percent. Similarly, Robbins et al. (1982), in a study of 9 children and adolescents, reported a DST sensitivity of 50 percent and a specificity of 100 percent. Klee and Garfinkel (1984) demonstrated a 40 percent sensitivity and a 92 percent specificity for 33 inpatient children and adolescents. Depressed outpatients do not show the same nonsuppression rate as hospitalized children and adolescents with depression (Birmeyer et al., 1992). These preliminary studies involving both prepubertal and postpubertal hospitalized children and adolescents have demonstrated a range for sensitivity and specificity comparable with that of adult patients. Puig-Antich et al. (1984) also studied growth hormone in response to insulin-induced hypoglycemia. Major depression in children was associated with a hyposecretion of growth hormone. In contrast, sleep studies, as reviewed by Puig-Antich (1980), have not revealed comparable findings to those in adults for children with affective disorder.

DIFFERENTIAL DIAGNOSIS

There are six major diagnoses that are often confused with major affective disorders in children and adolescents. They are attention deficit disorder, conduct disorder, anxiety disorders—especially school phobia or school refusal—eating disorders, substance abuse, and early stages of schizophrenia. Other organic syndromes that have affective disorder symptoms as part of their clinical presentation are endocrinopathies (e.g., hyperthyroidism, hypothyroidism, hypercalcemia), viral infections (e.g., infectious mononucleosis, infectious hepatitis, cytomegalovirus, and respiratory syncitial virus), and severe chronic illness (e.g., cystic fibrosis, inflammatory bowel disease, rheumatoid arthritis, and diabetes mellitus).

Attention deficit disorder may resemble depression or hypomania in children because these youngsters exhibit increased psychomotor activity, difficulty concentrating, mood lability and may have some of the vegetative symptoms, especially sleep disturbance. Attention deficit disorder children also have a high rate of depressive spectrum disease in their families, presenting with family psychopathology similar to that of depressed children (Cantwell, 1972; Biederman et al., 1987). The low self-esteem in attention deficit disorder children is secondary to school failure and is not a primary feature of the cognitive state and self-perceptions of the attention deficit disorder syndrome. Attention deficit disorder children most resemble children with dysthymic disorder because both disorders are chronic. In contrast, the main differentiating feature of major affective disorder is its episodic nature, with completely euthymic and symptom-free periods between episodes. Attention deficit disorder is a chronic, unremitting, and continuous disorder of childhood, with onset in the preschool years. Further research will be necessary to provide more differentiating features.

Conduct disorders in children and adolescents have for many years been confused with major affective disorders. Antisocial and delinquent behavior has often been interpreted as a "depressive equivalent" and as covering over, or "masking," an underlying depression (Cytryn et al., 1980). Antisocial behaviors have often obscured hypomanic and manic behaviors in bipolar disorder adolescents. Lying, running away, promiscuity, hypersexuality, drug overdoses, school truancy, gambling, and other aggressive or antisocial behaviors have been frequent methods by which young people have expressed themselves when significantly depressed or elated. Poor impulse control and immature judgment have resulted in a high rate of these behaviors occurring in depressed youngsters. Puig-Antich (1982) and Carlson and Cantwell (1980a) demonstrated that one-third of all major affective disorder children met the criteria for conduct disorder. If the criteria for affective disorder are not satisfied, these behaviors would likely represent an unsocialized, nonaggressive conduct disorder. Conduct-disordered children without an affective disorder exhibit an uninterrupted, continuous progression of more serious misbehavior, a disregard for others and their property. In affective-disordered children with disturbing behavior the behavior is directed more toward themselves than to others.

The studies by Hershberg et al. (1982) and Bernstein and Garfinkel (1986) indicate that many children and adolescents who refuse to attend school are actually depressed. These depressed individuals also have symptoms of anxiety disorders but meet the criteria for major affective disorder as well. In the school-refusing population, affective disorder and anxiety disorders overlap to a large extent, especially in the older, more chronic school refuser. Children with severe anxiety disorders and school refusal have many of the symptoms of depression as well as family histories positive for anxiety and affective disorders. In general, anxiety disorders are frequently confused with affective disorders, and only with precise, systematic interviews is one able to differentiate these two disorders.

Recent research indicates that a number of patients with anorexia nervosa may have a major affective disorder and that anorexia symptoms may be simply vegetative symptoms of the depression (Cantwell et al., 1977). Related to this are the clinical observations that treatment with tricyclic antidepressants, fluoxetine, and monoamine oxidase inhibitors has been efficacious in some patients with eating disorders, especially bulimia. To differentiate between a primary eating disorder and undereating or overeating associated with an affective disorder, one looks for chronic symptoms rather than episodic symptoms; the absence of a family history for affective disorder and the preoccupation with food and body size predominate over affective symptoms.

Dysphoria and other primary symptoms of depression have long been recognized as early features of the onset of schizophrenia in adolescents. A disorder of thought process, severe social isolation, first-rank characteristics of schizophrenia and bizarre thoughts or behaviors distinguish the early schizophrenic adolescent from the depressed adolescent.

Alcoholism and substance abuse also have been associated with affective disorders. Depressed children and adolescents may use street drugs or alcohol in an effort to self-medicate themselves and treat their depression. The affective symptoms predominating at the time of the *onset* of alcohol or drug use are the best way to differentiate between these two disorders. Unfortunately, when the depressed individual chronically uses alcohol in this manner, dependency may develop. Frequently, adolescent depression coexists with either conduct disorder or substance abuse, complicating the diagnosis and treatment of the depression.

SUICIDE IN CHILDREN AND ADOLESCENTS

Self-destructive behavior in children and adolescents is under greater scientific scrutiny than ever before. HIV infection aside, no other fatal medical condition has increased to the same extent as suicide in children and adolescents. Each year in the United States approximately 5000 young persons 24 years old and younger commit suicide (Frederick, 1978; Holinger, 1982). It has become the second leading cause of death for this age group, exceeded only by motor vehicle accidents (Holinger, 1978). Since 1960, completed suicide has increased more than 200 percent for young people between ages 10 and 24 (Holinger, 1978). Furthermore, research has shown that for every one completed suicide, there are at least 30 to 40 attempts (Weissman, 1974; Wexler et al., 1978). In adolescents, there may be as many as 50 to 100 suicide attempts for every young person who commits suicide (Otto, 1966).

Epidemiologic findings reflect an underestimate of the true occurrence of the problem, with current government statistics underreporting the extent of suicide by 10 to 15 percent and incompletely documenting the problem below age 10 (Garfinkel and Golombek, 1983). Most, if not all, suicides in children 10 years of age or younger are recorded as accidental deaths because suicide is not recorded in government statistics below this age. In other words, our understanding, knowledge, and description of suicidal children and adolescents may in fact be based on a smaller and more incomplete data set than actually exists.

The unique features of completed suicide in children and adolescents not only distinguish it from suicide in adults but also provide specific characteristics that allow clinicians to identify the young individual at risk for self-destructive behavior. Suicide below age 10 does occur but is uncommon. Suicide increases rapidly to peak by ages 18, 19, and 20, the late teenage years, followed by a plateau that

occurs for the remainder of the early young adult years, 20 through 24 (Holinger, 1978; Garfinkel and Golombek, 1983). The age at greatest risk is the time during which adolescents are leaving high school, going off to college, or seeking employment for the first time, a time when there is a natural ending of the family and community-based support systems that provide guidance, direction, and problem resolution when serious psychiatric disorders arise. Two-thirds of all suicides occur in the 20 to 24 age group, appearing during the late teenage years and early young adult years; 30 percent occur in the middle teen years (16 to 19 years); approximately 8 percent of all youthful suicide occurs in children younger than 15 years.

Suicide appears to depend on maturation (Weininger, 1979). Various factors reflecting cognitive development must be present, such as judgment, abstract reasoning, formulation of a suicide plan, self-blame, and the age at risk for the onset of significant depression. Young people who commit suicide are not only reacting to a seriously depressed mood and the impulse to end their suffering. They also must have sufficient cognitive abilities to determine which of their actions will likely be fatal (Schneidman, 1976; Garfinkel et al., 1982). To this extent, various investigators have studied the role of intelligence and academic achievement as they influence the suicide rate and have demonstrated that the number of suicides is greater in students doing well at school and for students attending more prestigious schools and universities (Rook, 1959; Hawton et al., 1978). The question persists whether there are more environmental stressors and expectations placed on students at the schools with the highest standards or whether brighter students are more prone to feelings of failure, depression, and self-criticism. Similarly, individuals who are intelligent are more able to plan on not being rescued. There is no evidence to date that suggests that the better universities studied provide fewer support systems, are more stressful, and are more alienating than less prestigious institutions. More intelligent youngsters can conceptualize what is lethal and what is not and will likely succeed on the first attempt. The identification of a successful plan is a critical factor that is both intelligence- and age-dependent and explains the steep increase in the suicide rate according to age.

For every girl who completes suicide, four boys succeed (Garfinkel and Golombek, 1983). This gender difference has only been observed for completed suicide, whereas suicide attempts receiving medical attention may occur more often in girls than in boys. If cultural and societal factors create these gender differences, it would appear that with the changing role of women in North America from the mid-1970s onward, one would expect a trend toward an equalization of the completed and attempt rates for both genders. This has not occurred. What was observed from 1975 onward was a significant trend for girls and young women to use methods of self-destruction that were more similar to those that males were using (firearms, carbon monoxide, and jumping from buildings) (Garfinkel and Golombek, 1983). When males experience depression, there is a much greater internal perception of the irreversibility and irrevocable nature of their sense of failure and pessimism. Boys do not seek help or medical attention as often as girls, limiting the opportunity for intervention. The observed higher rate of suicide attempts for females indicates that the self-destructive action is probably undertaken ambivalently, with only a limited amount of resolve.

Suicide is much more common in Caucasian young people than in African-American youth (Murphy and Robins, 1967). Similarly, the number of Protestant children and adolescents committing suicide is disproportionate to the number of Catholics and Jews committing suicide (Lukianowicz, 1968) and attempting suicide (Garfinkel and Golombek, 1983). Some authors suggest that religious taboos and strongly supportive families may be factors that result in a lower suicide rate.

Completed suicide is unevenly distributed throughout the country and is much more common in urban centers than in rural settings (Mintz, 1970). Some regions and states have a suicide rate that is two to three times higher than in other areas (e.g., Nevada, Alaska) (Liberakis and Hoenig, 1978; Frederick, 1978). Areas with a high Native American population have high suicide rates, with studies indicating that the suicide rate among Native Americans is 10 times higher than that in the Caucasian American population (Dizmang et al., 1974). African-American youth have a suicide rate one-third that of Caucasian youth.

Young people who commit suicide have a much lower unemployment rate than the youthful population in general (Garfinkel and Golombek, 1983). Completed suicide is much more common in college students, high school students, and young people pursuing gainful employment. Socioeconomic factors also play a role in suicide for children and adolescents, with middle- to upper-middle-class youth having a higher rate of suicide than do children of lower socioeconomic groups.

Completed suicide in young people appears to be related to a family history of alcoholism, substance abuse, antisocial personality disorder, and major affective disorder (Murphy, 1983). A definite family pattern emerges, with suicide occurring in specific families. Both suicide and suicide attempts occurred more frequently in the families of young people who attempted suicide than in a comparison group. These families also had more substance abuse and affective disorder. Family breakdown was much more common, with most suicidal young people coming from single-parent families or having experienced placement in foster care, group homes, and institutions. Whether the effect of the family is a result of modeling, a genetic predisposi-

tion, or a breakdown of the support provided by adults is not clear at this time; however, it is likely that all three interact. There is a strong association between suicide and psychiatric disorders that have a known genetic predisposition (such as depression, anxiety, antisocial personality disorder, and alcoholism). For example, it is not uncommon to find completed suicide in two or three first-degree family members from two generations in a family of a child who committed or attempted suicide.

Child and adolescent suicide does not occur randomly throughout the year (Sanborn et al., 1973; Eastwood and Peacocke, 1976). Just as recent research has indicated that serious psychiatric disorders occur at peak times, so the same may be said of suicide in children and adolescents. For this age group, suicide occurs much more often in the late fall, winter, and early spring. These findings are in contrast to adults, who commit suicide most often in the late spring. Self-destructive behavior in youth most often occurs in the afternoon and evening hours, unlike adult suicides, which occur primarily in the early morning hours, before dawn (Garfinkel et al., 1982).

In North America, completed suicide is primarily a function of firearm use. Forty-five to 55 percent of all completed suicides in young people are attributed to firearms (Boyd, 1983). The second most common method is hanging, followed by drug overdoses. Carbon monoxide poisoning, jumping from high places, jumping in front of moving vehicles, and drowning are the next most common methods. The choice of specific methods is determined by many factors, including gender, age, demographic factors (e.g., urban versus rural, geographic location, race, socioeconomic status), and psychopathology (Garfinkel and Golombek, 1983). It is apparent from these findings that a major means of prevention may be to curtail the availability of the various methods of self-destruction for specific risk groups. Figure 19-1 is a schematic depiction of the vulnerable individual undergoing stress, not using help from others, and having a method of injury readily available. This figure represents the key temperamental and psychosocial elements determining suicidal behavior.

Suicide Attempts

A *failed suicide* or *suicide attempt* occurs when the individual is fully intent on dying as a result of the self-inflicted injury but for some unforeseen circumstance was prevented from doing so; a *suicide gesture* is self-inflicted injury with no intention of dying as a result of the injury; the action is primarily "a cry for help." Because there are many more attempts and suicide gestures than there are completed suicides, it is important to distinguish those failed suicides from less lethal behavior. In general, all attempts must be taken seriously, and a complete psychiatric workup is often necessary. It has been

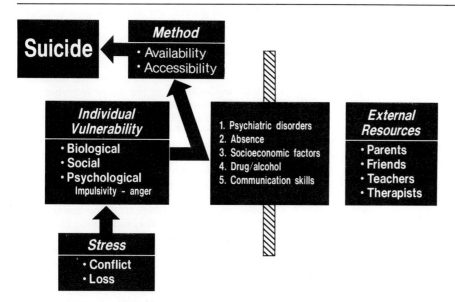

FIGURE 19-1.   *Major factors determining suicidal behavior.*

demonstrated that 1 of 10 individuals who attempt suicide will ultimately succeed (Otto, 1971; Dahlgren, 1977). Our follow-up research indicated that when suicide attempters were compared with medically and surgically ill children and adolescents, they had a higher mortality rate despite the fact that the nonsuicidal group was significantly physically ill (Garfinkel et al., 1982). A severe suicide attempt is commonly preceded by symptoms of depression, hostility, nihilism, and self-depreciation. Those who attempt suicide often have a history of substance abuse and antisocial conduct disorder behavior (Kandel, 1991). Homosexual and bisexual youth report suicide attempts at a much higher rate than do a matched control group (Remafedi et al., 1991). Young people who make serious attempts are often those with a clinical depression in combination with a large amount of rage, hostility, and impulsivity.

It is often possible to identify specific crises, precipitants, and environmental stressors that led to the suicide attempt (Garfinkel et al., 1982). Most often conflict with parents, nonspecific conflict within the family, or conflict between boyfriend and girlfriend precedes the attempt. Surprisingly, 1 in 10 suicide attempts have been related to problems at school. It is often difficult to determine just how stressful a particular event is, since adolescents may view such occurrences idiosyncratically. An apparently nontraumatic event may become overwhelming to a young person because she or he is already overburdened with a preexisting depression. The stress may be related to the depression, result from it, or be coincidental in time. Nevertheless, at that

particular time, the individual is exquisitely sensitive to that event and cannot cope with the feelings and thoughts generated by it. Often the environmental stressor or precipitant has been identified as a "loss" (Stanley and Barter, 1978). The loss may be based in reality, such as losing one's girlfriend, or peer status, or the loss may be internal and not readily recognized, such as loss of self-esteem, reputation, or sense of worth. It is during the adolescent years of development that private, closely guarded personal perceptions of oneself can be painfully destroyed by life's events, and this can intensify an already existing mood disorder. For example, a varsity basketball star who was forced to miss a season because of a knee injury committed suicide. It is possible that he was experiencing a major depression previously, with the injury further affecting his mood and representing the "straw that broke the camel's back." The athlete perceived loss of self-esteem when he could not play on the team.

Unlike completed suicides, suicide attempts most often result from overdoses, with approximately 90 percent of all attempts receiving medical attention in the child and adolescent age group attributed to this method. As shown in Table 19-4, household analgesics, benzodiazepines, and barbiturates are the most common medications used in such attempts (Garfinkel et al., 1982).

Suicidal individuals often talk about a desire to die or say that they would be better off dead. The psychiatrist working with depressed and suicidal children must be able to determine the mental status of the individual and the severity of the attempt. Some warning before the self-destructive behavior

TABLE 19-4. *Drugs Used by Children and Adolescents in Suicide Attempt*

Attempts by ingestion n = 532*	Percent
Analgesics	36.8
Benzodiazepines	23.7
Barbiturates	18.6
Phenothiazines	5.6
Solvents/Inhalants	5.5
Street drugs (LSD, speed, opiates)	5.1
Antibiotics	4.5
Patent medicines	3.9
Antihistamines	3.6
Bizarre ingestion (perfume, soap, etc.)	3.4
Hypnotics	3.4
Anticonvulsants	2.4
Alcohol	2.3
Antidepressants	2.1
Other	3.2
Unknown	3.0

*144 patients used two drugs.

occurs is often recognized only after the event. In young people, it may take the form of giving away a prized possession or giving inappropriate advice (Connell, 1972).

A severe attempt has the following characteristics: (1) the amount of planning associated with the attempt, (2) the timing and the isolation of the actions, with no one nearby, (3) the method chosen (hanging, jumping, etc. are severer than wrist slashing or drug overdoses), (4) leaving of a suicide note, (5) a family history of suicide, and (6) symptoms of depression (Garfinkel et al., 1982). Of all the features that identify severe suicidal behavior in children and adolescents, one of the strongest predictors of a serious attempt is the family history of suicide (Dabbagh, 1977). In our 1982 study, completed suicide occurred only in the families of those young people who attempted suicide, and not in a matched control group, and suicide attempts were six times more common in the attempters' families compared with the families of the control group of children.

TREATMENT

The literature on the pharmacologic management of affective disorders in children has only recently reflected systematic scientifically controlled studies. This literature is reviewed in Tables 19-5 and 19-6 as to methodology, design and controls of the research, the instruments of evaluating improvement, the degree of improvement, duration of treatment, and side effects. There have been 44 published reports describing tricyclic antidepressants, fluoxetine, monoamine oxidase inhibitors, and lithium carbonate treatment of childhood major affective

disorders. In general, the methodology is limited to 18 case reports in which no experimental control was implemented. Characteristically, these studies did not have a placebo phase, patient or clinician blindness, or objective review of therapeutic response. In most of these 18 studies, the diagnostic criteria for inclusion in the study were not presented. The duration of treatment recorded in the studies is also a significant factor, with 6 studies not recording length of treatment, 5 studies for 1 to 3 weeks, and only 16 studies using tricyclic antidepressants for longer than 4 weeks.

There were only 10 double-blind studies. After excluding Frommer's (1967) study, because of diagnostic imprecision, the remaining 9 double-blind studies included children receiving imipramine, amitriptyline, nortriptyline, and lithium carbonate. Puig-Antich et al. (1979b) conducted a crossed double-blind study with a placebo phase. Kashani et al. (1980) and Petti and Unis (1981) each had one patient who was in a double-blind, placebo-controlled crossover study.

Clinical improvement was measured in 12 studies by nonspecific clinician judgment alone, in 7 by an unspecified method, and in 16 by a combination of rating scales, clinical judgment, and serial psychometric tests. With these limitations in mind, the reported efficacy for tricyclic antidepressants, fluoxetine, and monoamine oxidase inhibitors was between 57 and 100 percent, with a mean of 65 percent. There are a number of reasons why medication has not proved efficacious in children and adolescents. There are diagnostic factors, including comorbidity with conduct disorder, bipolar and delusional disorders, concurrent medical illness, and severe psychosocial stress. Pharmacologic factors primarily include too small dosage, inadequate duration of treatment, and changing neuroendocrine and neurochemical mediation of drug response in the developing central nervous system. Tricyclic antidepressants have been augmented with lithium, resulting in a good therapeutic response (Ryan, 1988). Puig-Antich et al. (1979b) and Weller et al. (1982) have correlated serum levels of desipramine and imipramine with therapeutic efficacy and have unequivocally demonstrated that only with levels within the 150 to 250 ng/ml range will a positive therapeutic response be observed. Nortriptyline serum levels within the range of 50 to 150 ng/ml correlate with clinical therapeutic response.

Side effects observed were hypomania and aggression (Berg et al., 1974; Pallmeyer and Petti, 1979; Kashani et al., 1980) and rapid eye movement suppression (Kupfer et al., 1979). Puig-Antich et al. (1978) have documented cardiac arrhythmias as a function of tricyclic antidepressant dosage. Because there have been deaths of ADHD children being treated with desipramine, cardiac arrhythmias have been suggested as the primary explanation of the cause of death (Biederman, 1991). Monitoring for electrocardiographic abnormalities when

Text continued on page 317

TABLE 19-5. *Tricyclic Antidepressant Use in Children and Adolescents*

Author (year)	No. in study	Drug	Daily dosage	Duration of drug trial	Use of placebo	Double blind	Diagnosis	Assessment procedures	Improvement	Side effects
Lucas (1965)	14	Amitriptyline	30–50 mg	42 days	Yes	Yes	Mixed	Clinical rating	60%	Sedation
Frommer (1967)	32	Phenelzine, chlordiazepoxide, phenobarbitane	30 mg 20 mg 60 mg	14+ days	Yes	Yes	Affective/depression	Clinical impression	88%—combination of phenelzine and chlordiazepoxide	NR
Annell (1969)	8	Amitriptyline and/or lithium carbonate	30 mg 300 mg 600 mg	Varied	No	No	Affective/manic depression	Parent, teacher, and clinician's impression	100%	NR
Ling (1970)	10	Amitriptyline or imipramine	Varied	Varied	No	No	Depression	Clinical impression	70%–90%	NR
Frommer (1971)	200	Amitriptyline	NR	NR	No	No	Affective/depression	Clinical impression	67%	NR
Kuhn and Kuhn (1971)	100	Imipramine, desmethylimipramine, clomipramine, opipramol	NR	NR	No	No	Affective/phasic, chronic depression	NR	76%	Nausea, vomiting, dizziness, headaches, gastric upset
Stack (1971)	116	Opipramol, amitriptyline, imipramine	50 mg 2–5 mg 10 mg	28–730 days	No	No	Affective/depression (preschool)	NR	Imipramine especially effective	Drowsiness; fatigue with opipramol and amitriptyline
Stack (1971)	75	Nortriptyline, amitriptyline, opipramol, phenelzine	30 mg 2–25 mg 50–150 mg NR	NR	No	No	Affective/depression (school-age)	NR	80%	Drowsiness; fatigue with opipramol and amitriptyline
Stack (1971)	64	Phenelzine	NR	NR	No	No	Affective/phobic obsession with depressive states	NR	94%	NR
Stack (1971)	150	Nortriptyline, imipramine	75 mg	NR	No	No	Affective/mixed depression	NR	67%	NR
Stack (1971)	85	Opipramol, amitriptyline	100–150 mg 75 mg	NR	No	No	Affective/depression-related psychosis	NR	57%	Drowsiness; fatigue with opipramol and amitriptyline
Polvan and Cebiroglu (1971)	29	Pyrithioxin and amitriptyline, or nortriptyline and levomepromazine	According to age and weight	56 days	No	No	Affective/depression	NR	90%	NR
Petti and Campbell (1975)	1	Imipramine	75 mg	20 days	No	No	Affective/manic depression	Clinical impression, EEG	Seizures occurred; IMI discontinued	Extensive seizures
Brumback et al. (1977)	19	Imipramine or amitriptyline	25–125 mg	28 days	No	No	Affective/depression	Clinical impression	95%	NR

Table continued on following page

TABLE 19-5. *Tricyclic Antidepressant Use in Children and Adolescents (Continued)*

Author (year)	No. in study	Drug	Daily dosage	Duration of drug trial	Use of placebo	Double blind	Diagnosis	Assessment procedures	Improvement	Side effects
Puig-Antich et al. (1978)	8	Imipramine	3–5 mg/kg	42–56 days	No	No	Affective/depression	RDC CPRS	75%	(Elicited interview) nausea, constipation, somnolence, tachycardia, anorexia
Puig-Antich et al. (1979b)	6 7	Imipramine	4 mg/kg	35 days	Yes Yes	No Yes Cross-over	Affective/manic depression	Kiddie-SADS, RDC	Plasma levels indicated good response	NR
Kupfer et al. (1979)	12	Imipramine	4.3 mg/kg	21 days	No	No	Affective/depression	EEG, sleep observation, clinical assessment	REM suppression	Sleep disturbance
Pallmeyer and Petti (1979)	2	Imipramine	3.5–5 mg/kg	51 days	No	No	Affective/depression	CBI	Anger and hostility increased with IMI	Hostility, anger
Kashani et al. (1980)	1	Amitriptyline	1.5 mg/kg	28 days	Yes	Yes	Affective/depression	Clinical impression	Hypomanic reaction (dose reduced)	Hypomanic
Petti et al. (1980)	1	Imipramine	5 mg/kg	40 days	No	No	Affective/depression	CBI, SoSAD	Behavioral symptoms improved	NR
Petti and Unis (1981)	1	Imipramine	5 mg/kg	7 days	Yes	No	Affective/depression, borderline psychosis	Clinical, and parent assessment, PALS-C	Marked improvement	NR
Staton et al. (1981)	11	Amitriptyline, desipramine	1.1–3.5 mg/kg 3.4 mg/kg	90–100 days	No	No	Affective/depression	CDRS, CDI, WISC-R	100%	NR

Study	N	Medication	Dose	Duration			Affective/major depression	Plasma IMI levels, CGI rating scales	100%	Minimal—tachycardia, syncope, diaphoresis
Weller et al. (1982)	11	Imipramine	5 mg/kg	20 days	No	No	Affective/major depression	Plasma IMI levels, CGI rating scales	100%	Minimal—tachycardia, syncope, diaphoresis
Conners and Petti (1983)	21	Imipramine	5 mg/kg	53–202 days	No	No	Affective/depression	BID, CBI	66%	NR
Geller et al. (1983)	12	Nortriptyline		172 days	No	No	Affective/depression	RDC, CDI	75%	Minimal
Ryan et al. (1988)	23	Phenelzine Tranylcypromine	45 mg 30mg	14 days	No	No	Major depression	Clinician	57%	Lethargy, dizziness, headache, insomnia
Hughes et al (1988)	64	Imipramine	NR	42 days	Yes	Yes	Major depression	CGI CDRS-R GDI	Based on: CGI severity, age, school behavior, CDI Score	NR
Walling and Pfefferbaum (1990)	1	Methylphenidate	35 mg	NR	No	No	AIDS dementia/ depression Major depression	NR CDRS	Marked	None Tired Headache
Geller et al (1990)	31	Nortriptyline	91.1 ng/ml	56 days	Yes	Yes	Major depressive disorder	GAS CDRS	8%	Headache Sleep
Strober (1990)	34	Imipramine	222 mg Or 180 ng/ml	42 days	Yes	Yes	Major depression with and without delusions Major Depression	HAM-D CGI	10% (delusional) 30% (nondelusional)	NR
Simeon et al (1990)	6	Fluoxetine Clomipramine	20 mg 50 mg	17.5 weeks	Yes	Yes	OCD/depression	CGI-IS		Hand tremors, night awakenings, weight loss
Boulos et al (1991)	30	Desipramine	200 mg	42 days	Yes	Yes	Major depression	BDI HAM-D	50%	Cardiovascular, rash

Note: NR, not reported; RDC, Research Diagnostic Criteria; CPRS, Children's Psychiatric Rating Scale; Kiddie-SADS, Schedule for Affective Disorders and Schizophrenia for School Aged Children; CBI, Children's Behavior Inventory; SoSAD, Scale of School Age Depression; CDRS, Children's Depression Rating Scale; CDI, Children's Depression Inventory.

315

TABLE 19-6. *Lithium Use in Children and Adolescents*

Author (year)	No. in study	Drug	Daily dosage	Duration of drug trial	Use of placebo	Double blind	Diagnosis	Assessment procedures	Improvement	Side effects
Berg et al. (1974)	1	(Amitriptyline) lithium carbonate	2400 mg/1 mEq/l	365 days	No	No	Affective/bipolar, manic-depressive psychosis	Clinical impressions	Caused switch from depression to hypomania	NR
Sovner (1975)	1	(Haloperidol, mesoridazine) lithium carbonate	2400 mg/1 mEq/l	18+ days	No	No	Affective/manic depression	WAIS, Bender-Gestalt Test	Dramatic improvement	NR
Warneke (1975)	1	(Haloperidol, doxepin) lithium carbonate	1800 mg/1.2 mEq/l	21 days	No	No	Affective/manic depression	Clinical impression	Marked improvement	NR
Horowitz (1977)	8	Lithium carbonate	1500–2400 mg/0.5–1.2 mEq/l	14–90 days	No	No	Affective/manic depression	Clinical impression	Marked improvement	NR
White and O'Shanick (1977)	1	(Haloperidol) lithium carbonate	1200 mg/1 mEq/l	42 days	No	No	Affective/manic depression	Clinical impression	Marked improvement	NR
Brumback and Weinberg (1977)	6	Lithium carbonate	30–40 mg/kg/0.6–1.2 mEq/l	5–110 days	No	No	Affective manic/depression	Clinical impression	33%	Nausea, anxiety, increased depression, EEG abnormalities
DeLong (1978)	4	Lithium carbonate	450–1200 mg	80–1000 days	Yes	Yes	Affective/manic depression	Conner's PSQ	Behaviorally effective	Minimal hand tremors, increased urination, blunted motivation
Engstrom et al. (1978)	1	Lithium carbonate	2100–2400 mg/1.0–1.5 mEq/l	14+ days	No	No	Affective/manic depression	Clinical impression	Marked improvement	NR
Davis (1979)	4	Lithium carbonate	0.8–1.0 mEq/l serum level	180 days	No	No	Affective/manic depression	Parental symptom assessment	Marked improvement	NR
Mayo et al. (1979)		Lithium carbonate	NR	730 days	No	No	Affective/bipolar manic depression	RDC, CGI, CPRS	Substantial decrease in stress events during treatment	NA
Ryan et al. (1988)	14	Lithium carbonate plus tricyclic.	0.5–1.2 mEq/l	42 days	No	No	Major affective disorder—depressed	CGI, CAD	43%	Secondary to tricyclic

Note: NR, not reported; WAIS, Wechsler Adult Intelligence Scale; Conner's PSQ, Conner's Parent Symptom Questionnaire; RDC, Research Diagnostic Criteria; CGI, Clinical Global Impression Scale; CPRS, Children's Psychiatric Rating Scale; NA, not applicable.

one exceeds 3.0 mg/kg is mandatory, since first-degree heart block is common beyond this dosage.

Psychotherapy of Major Affective Disorders in Children and Adolescents

The major principles for managing and treating affective disorders in children and adolescents are similar to those for adults (Lewinsohn, 1979). The literature supports combination treatment as the most efficacious management (i.e., psychotherapy in combination with medication). Individual therapy or drugs alone are less effective in adults. Consideration must be given to the age of the child, cognitive development, and verbal skill attainment before psychotherapy is provided. Psychotherapy need not be entirely verbal but may rely on activity or play as well. Concurrent family therapy is often provided to families of depressed children. Such therapy should include child management techniques. The overall goal is to teach children how to increase pleasant experiences and decrease negative reinforcement (Ross, 1981).

Behavioral, interpersonal, and cognitive-behavioral therapies for affective disorders in children and adolescents reflect the underlying behavioral principles assumed to affect the cognitive and perceptual state of the individual. These include graduated task assignment with cognitive rehearsal, assertiveness training, and role playing (Leon et al., 1980). Children also benefit from a psychoeducational approach (Lewinsohn, 1979). Therapy for children is time limited, with sufficient direction, control, and encouragement to undertake new activities, enabling skill attainment and positive reinforcement. However, little empirical work has been conducted as to the nature and efficacy of cognitive-behavioral therapy for depression in children and adolescents.

REFERENCES

Achenbach TM, Edelbrock CS: The child behavior profile: II. Boys aged 12–16 and girls aged 6–11 and 12–16. J Consult Clin Psychol 47:223–233, 1979.

Ackerson LM, Dick RW, Namson SM, et al: Properties of the inventory to diagnose depression in American Indian adolescents. J Am Acad Child Adolesc Psychiatry 29:601–607, 1990.

Akiskal HS, McKinney WT Jr: Overview of recent research in depression. Arch Gen Psychiatry 32:285–305, 1975.

Annell AL: Manic-depressive illness in children and effect of treatment with lithium carbonate. Acta Paedopsychiatrica (Basel) 36:292–301, 1969.

Annell AL (ed): Depressive States in Childhood and Adolescence. New York, Halsted Press, 1971.

Anthony J, Scott P: Manic depressive psychosis in childhood. J Child Psychol Psychiatry 1:52–72, 1960.

Bauersfeld KH: Diagnosis and treatment of depressive conditions at a school psychiatric center, in Annell AL (ed): Depressive States in Childhood and Adolescence. Stockholm, Almquist & Wiksell, 1972.

Beck AT: Cognitive therapy: Nature and relation to behavior therapy. Behav Ther 7:184–200, 1970.

Bemporad JR, Wilson A: A developmental approach to depression in childhood and adolescence. J Am Acad Psychoanal 6:325–352, 1978.

Berg I, Hullin R, et al: Bipolar manic depressive psychoses in early adolescence: A case report. Br J Psychiatry 125:416–417, 1974.

Bernstein GA, Garfinkel BD: School phobia: The overlap of affective and anxiety disorders. J Am Acad Child Psychiatry 25:235–241, 1986.

Biederman J, Munirk, Knee D, et al: High rate of affective disorders in probands with attention deficit disorder and in their relatives: a controlled family study. Am J Psychiatry 144: 330–333, 1987.

Birleson P: The validity of depressive disorder in childhood and the development of a self-rating scale: A research report. J Child Psychol Psychiatry 22:73–88, 1981.

Birmaher B, Dahl R, Ryan N, et al: The dexamethasone suppression test in adolescent outpatients with major depressive disorder. Am J Psychiatry 149:1040–1045, 1992.

Blos P: The Psychology of Adolescence—A Psychoanalytic Interpretation. Glencoe, NY, Free Press of Glencoe, 1962.

Boulos C, Kutcher S, Marton P, et al: Response to desipramine treatment in adolescent major depression. Psychopharmacol Bull 27:59–65, 1991.

Bowlby J: Separation: Attachment and Loss, vol 2. New York, Basic Books, 1973.

Bowlby J: Attachment and Loss, vol 3: Loss: Sadness and Depression. London, Hogarth Press and the Institute of Psychoanalysis, 1980.

Boyd JH: The increasing rate of suicide by firearms. N Engl J Med 308:872–874, 1983.

Brent DA, Kalas R, Edelbrock C, et al: Nosologic correlates of the severity of suicidal ideation in children and adolescents. Paper presented at the Annual Meeting of the American Academy of Child Psychiatry, Toronto, 1984.

Brown GL, Goodwin FK, Ballenger JC, et al: Aggression in humans: Correlates with cerebrospinal fluid amine metabolites. Psychiatry Res 1:131–139, 1979.

Brumback RA, Dietz-Schmidt SG, Weinberg WA: Depression in children referred to an educational diagnostic center: Diagnosis and treatment and analysis of criteria and literature review. Dis Nerv Syst 38:529–535, 1977.

Brumback RA, Staton RD: Depression-induced neurologic dysfunction (letter). N Engl J Med 10:305:642.

Brumback RA, Weinberg WA: Mania in childhood: II. Therapeutic trial of lithium carbonate and further description of manic-depressive illness in children. Am J Dis Child 131:112–126, 1977.

Burke P, Kocoshis SA, Shandra R, et al: Determinants of depression in recent onset pediatric inflammatory bowel disease. J Am Acad Child Adolesc Psychiatry 29:608–610, 1990.

Cantwell DP, Baker L: Parental psychiatric illness and psychiatric disorder in at-risk children. Paper presented at the 30th Annual Meeting of the American Academy of Child Psychiatry, San Francisco, October 26–30, 1983.

Cantwell DP: Psychiatric illness in the families of hyperactive children. Arch Gen Psychiatry 27:414–417, 1972.

Cantwell DP, Carlson G: Problems and prospects in the study of childhood depression. J Nerv Ment Dis 167:522–529, 1979.

Cantwell D, Sturzenberger S, Burroughs J, Salkin B, Green J: Anorexia nervosa: An affective disorder. Arch Gen Psychiatry 34:1087–1091, 1977.

Carlson GA: Annotation: Child and adolescent mania-diagnostic considerations. J Child Psychol Psychiatry 31:331–341, 1990.

Carlson GA, Davenport YB, Jamison K: A comparison of outcome in adolescent and late onset bipolar manic depressive illness. Am J Psychiatry 134:919–922, 1977.

Carlson GA, Cantwell DP: A survey of depressive symptoms in a child and adolescent psychiatric population: Interview data. J Am Acad Child Psychiatry 18:587–599, 1979.

Carlson GA, Cantwell DP: A survey of depressive symptoms, syndrome and disorder in a child psychiatric population. J Child Psychol Psychiatry 21:19–25, 1980a.

Carlson GA, Cantwell DP: Unmasking masked depression in children and adolescents. Am J Psychiatry 137:445–449, 1980b.

Carlson GA, Cantwell DP: Diagnosis of childhood depression—A comparison of Weinberg and DSM-III criteria. J Am Acad Child Psychiatry 21:247–250, 1981.

Carlson GA, Kashani JH: Phenomenology of major depression from childhood through adulthood: Analysis of three studies. Am J Psychiatry 145:1222–1225, 1988.

Carroll BJ: Use of the dexamethasone suppression test in depression. J Clin Psychiatry 43:44–48, 1982.

Carroll BJ, Curtis GC, Mendels J: Neuroendocrine regulation in depression: II. Discrimination of depressed from nondepressed patients. Arch Gen Psychiatry 33:1051–1058, 1976.

Carroll BJ, Feinberg M, Greden JF, et al: A specific laboratory test for the diagnosis of melancholia. Arch Gen Psychiatry 38:15–22, 1981.

Chambers WJ, Puig-Antich J: Psychiatric symptoms in prepubertal major depressive disorder. Arch Gen Psychiatry 39:921–927, 1982.

Chambers W, Puig-Antich J, Tabrizi MA: The ongoing development of the Kiddie-SADS. Paper presented at the 25th Annual meeting of the American Academy of Child Psychiatry, San Diego, 1978.

Chess S, Thomas A, Hassibi M: Depression in childhood and adolescence: A prospective study of six cases. J Nerv Ment Dis 171:411–420, 1983.

Connell HM: Depression in childhood. Child Psychiatry Hum Dev 4:70–85, 1972.

Cytryn L, McKnew DH Jr: Proposed classification of childhood depression. Am J Psychiatry 129:149–155, 1972.

Cytryn L, McKnew DH Jr, Bunney WE Jr: Diagnosis of depression in children: A reassessment. Am J Psychiatry 137:22–25, 1980.

Dabbagh F: Family suicide. Br J Psychiatry 130:159–161, 1977.

Dahl V: A follow-up study of a child psychiatric clientele with special regard to manic depressive psychosis. In Annell AL (ed): Depressive States in Childhood and Adolescence. Stockholm, Almquist & Wiksell, 1971, pp 534–541.

Dahlgren KG: Attempted suicides—35 years afterward. Suicide Life Threat Behav 7:75–79, 1977.

Davis RE: Manic-depressive variant syndrome of childhood: A preliminary report. Am J Psychiatry 136:702–705, 1979.

DeLong GR: Lithium carbonate treatment of select behavior disorders in suggesting manic-depressive illness. J Pediatrics 93:689–694, 1978.

Dizmang LH, Watson J, May PA, et al: Adolescent suicide at an Indian reservation. Am J Orthopsychiatry 44:43–49, 1974.

Eastwood MR, Peacocke J: Seasonal patterns of suicide, depression and electroconvulsive therapy. Br J Psychiatry 129:472–475, 1976.

Endicott J, Spitzer RL: A diagnostic interview: The schedule for affective disorders and schizophrenia. Arch Gen Psychiatry 35:837–844, 1978.

Engstrom FW, Robbins DR, May JG: Manic-depressive illness in adolescence. J Am Acad Child Psychiatry 17:514–520, 1978.

Erikson EH: Childhood and Society. New York, WW Norton, 1950.

Extein I, Rosenberg G, Pottash ALC, Gold MS: Preliminary data on the dexamethasone suppression test in depressed adolescents. Am J Psychiatry 139:1617–1618, 1982.

Feighner JP, Robins E, Guze SB, et al: Diagnostic criteria for use in psychiatric research. Arch Gen Psychiatry 26:57–63, 1972.

Feinstein SC, Wolpert EA: Juvenile manic-depressive illness clinical and therapeutic considerations. J Am Acad Child Psychiatry 12:123–136, 1973.

Frederick C: Current trends in suicidal behavior in the United States. Am J Psychother 32:169–200, 1978.

Freud S: Mourning and melancholia. In Gaylin W (ed): The Meaning of Despair: Psychoanalytic Contributions to the Understanding of Depression. New York, Science House, 1968.

Frommer EA: Treatment of childhood with antidepressant drugs. Br Med J 1:729–732, 1967.

Frommer EA: Depressive illness in childhood. In Coppens A, Walk A (eds): Recent Developments in Affective Disorders. Ashford, Kent, Headley Bros, 1968, pp 117–136.

Frommer EA: Indications for antidepressant treatment with special reference to depressed preschool children. In Annell AL (ed): Depressive States in Childhood and Adolescence. Stockholm, Almquist & Wiskell, 1971.

Garfinkel BD, Froese AM, Hood J: Suicide attempts in children and adolescents. Am J Psychiatry 139:1257–1261, 1982.

Garfinkel BD, Golombek H: Suicidal behavior in adolescence. In Golombek H, Garfinkel BD (eds): The Adolescent and Mood Disturbance. New York, International University Press, 1983.

Garrison ZZ, Jackson KL, Marteller F, et al: A longitudinal study of depressive symptomatology in young adolescents. J Am Acad Child Adolesc Psychiatry 29:581–585, 1990.

Gelfand DM, Teti DM: The effects of maternal depression on children. Clin Psychol Rev 10:329–353, 1990.

Geller B, Rogol AA, Knitter EF: Preliminary data on the dexamethasone suppression test in children with major depressive disorder. Am J Psychiatry 140:620–622, 1983.

Geller B, Cooper TB, Graham DI, et al: Double-blind, placebo-controlled study of nortriptyline in depressed adolescents using a "fixed plasma level" design. Psychopharmacol Bull 26:85–90, 1990.

Glaser K: Masked depression in children and adolescents. Am J Psychother 21:565–574, 1967.

Graham P: Depression in prepubertal children. Dev Med Child Neurol 136:1203–1205, 1974.

Hamilton M: A rating scale for depression. J Neurol Neurosurg Psychiatry 23:56–62, 1960.

Harlow HF, Harlow MIC: The affectional systems. In Schrier AM, Harlow HF, Stollnitz F (eds): Behavior of Nonhuman Primates. New York, Academic Press, 1965.

Harrington R, Fudge H, Rutter M, et al: Adult outcomes of childhood and adolescent depression: I. Psychiatric status. Arch Gen Psychiatry 47:465–473, 1990.

Hawton K, Crowle J, Simkin S, Bancroft J: Attempted suicide and suicide among Oxford University students. Br J Psychiatry 132:506–509, 1978.

Herjanic B, Herjanic M, Brown F, Wheatt T: Are children reliable reporters? J Assoc Child Psychol 3:41–48, 1975.

Herjanic B, Hudson R, Kotloff K: Does interviewing harm children? Res Commun Psychol Psychiatr Behav 1:523–531, 1976.

Herjanic B, Reich W: Development of a structured psychiatric interview for children: Agreement between child and parent on individual symptoms. J Abnorm Child Psychol 10:307–324, 1982.

Hershberg SG, Carlson GA, Cantwell DP, Strober M: Anxiety and depressive disorders in psychiatrically disturbed children. J Clin Psychiatry 43:358–361, 1982.

Holinger PC: Adolescent suicide: An epidemiologic study of recent trends. Am J Psychiatry 135:754–756, 1978.

Holinger PC, Offer D: Prediction of adolescent suicide: A population model. Am J Psychiatry 139:302–307, 1982.

Horowitz HA: Lithium and the treatment of adolescent manic-depressive illness. Dis Nerv Syst 38:480–483, 1977.

Hughes C, Preskorn S, Weller, E, et al: Imipramine versus placebo studies of childhood depression: Baseline predictors of response to treatment and factor analysis of presenting symptoms. Psychopharmacol Bull 24:275–279, 1988.

Hughes CW, Preskorn SH, Wrona M, et al: Follow-up of adolescents initially treated for prepubertal onset major depressive disorder with imipramine. Psychopharmacol Bull 26:245–248, 1990.

Jacobson S, Fasman J, DiMascio A: Deprivation in the childhood of depressed women. J Nerv Ment Dis 166:5–14, 1975.

Jensen JB, Garfinkel BD: Growth hormone dysregulation in children with major depressive disorder. J Am Acad Child Adolesc Psychiatry 29:295–301, 1990.

Johnson GFS, Leeman MM: Ancestral secondary cases on paternal and maternal sides of bipolar affective illness. Br J Psychiatry 133:68–72, 1978.

Kandel D, Raveis V, Davies M: Suicidal ideation in adolescence: Depression, substance use, and other risk factors. J Youth Adolesc 20:289–309, 1991.

Kandel DB, Kessler RC, Margulies RZ: Antecedents of adolescent initiation to stages of drug use: A developmental analysis. In Kandel DB (ed): Longitudinal Research on Drug Use: Empirical Findings and Methodological Issues. Washington, Hemisphere, 1978, pp 73–99.

Kashani JH, Hodges KK, Shekim WO: Hypomanic reaction to amitriptyline in a depressed child. Psychosomatics 21:867–872, 1980.

Kashani JH, Carlson GA, Beck NC, et. al: Depression, depressive symptoms, and depressed mood among a community sample of adolescents. Am J Psychiatry 144:931–939, 1987.

Kashani JH, Husain A, Shekim WO, et al: Current perspectives on childhood depression: An overview. Am J Psychiatry 135:143–153, 1981.

Kashani JH, McGee RO, Clarkson SE, et al: Depression in a sample of 9-year-old children. Arch Gen Psychiatry 40:1217–1223, 1983.

Kashani JH, Simonds JF: The incidence of depression in children. Am J Psychiatry 136:1203–1205, 1979.

Kazdin AE: Assessment techniques for childhood depression: A critical appraisal. J Am Acad Child Psychiatry 20:358–375, 1981.

Klee SH, Garfinkel BD: Identification of depression in children and adolescents: The role of the DST. J Am Acad Child Psychiatry 4:410–415, 1984.

Kovacs M, Beck AT: Maladaptive cognitive structures in depression. Am J Psychiatry 135:525–533, 1978.

Kovacs M: Interview Schedule for Children (ISC). Unpublished document. Pittsburgh, University of Pittsburgh, 1978.

Kovacs M: Rating scales to assess depression in school age children. Acta Paedopsychiatr 46:305–315, 1981.

Kovacs M, Beck AT: An empirical clinical approach toward a definition of childhood depression. In Schulterbrandt JG (ed): Depression in Childhood: Diagnosis, Treatment and Conceptual Models. New York, Raven Press, 1977, pp 1–25.

Kovacs M, Feinberg TL, Crouse-Novak MA, Paulavskas SL, Finkelstein R: Depressive disorders in childhood. Arch Gen Psychiatry 41:229–237, 1984.

Kuhn V, Kuhn R: Drug therapy for depression in children: Indications and methods. In Depressive States in Childhood and Adolescence, Proc. 4th U.E.P. Congress. Stockholm, Almquist & Wiskell, 1971, pp 455–459.

Kuhn V, Kuhn R: Drug therapy for depression in children. Indications and methods. In Annell AL (ed): Depressive States in Childhood and Adolescence. Stockholm, Almquist & Wiskell, 1972, pp 455–459.

Kuperman S, Stewart MA: The diagnosis of depression in children. J Affect Disord 1:117–123, 1979.

Kupfer DJ, Cable P, Kane J, Petti T, Conners CK: Imipramine and EEG sleep in children with depressive symptoms. Psychopharmacology 60:117–123, 1979.

Kuyler PL, Rosenthal L, Igel G, et al: Psychopathology among children of manic-depressive illness. Biol Psychiatry 15:589–597, 1980.

Lang M, Tisher M: Children's Depression Scale. Victoria, Australia, Australian Council for Educational Research, 1978.

Lefkowitz MM, Burton N: Childhood depression: A critique of the concept. Psychol Bull 85:716–726, 1978.

Lefkowitz M, Monroe M, Tesiny EP: Assessment of childhood depression. J Consult Clin Psychol 48:43–50, 1980.

Lefkowitz MM, Tesiny EP: Assessment of childhood depression. J Consult Clin Psychol 48:43–50, 1980.

Leon GR, Kendall PC, Garber J: Depression in children: Parent, teacher and child perspectives. J Abnorm Child Psychol. 8:221–235, 1980.

Lewinsohn PM: Depression: A social learning perspective. Paper presented at Western Psychiatric Institute and Clinic, Pittsburgh, 1979.

Lewinsohn PM, Hoberman H: Depression. In Bellack AS, Hersen M, Kazdin AE (eds): International Handbook of Behavior Modification and Therapy. New York, Plenum Press, 1982, pp 397–431.

Liberakis EA, Hoenig J: Recording of suicide in Newfoundland. Psychiatr J Univ Ottawa 3:254–259, 1978.

Ling W, Oftdahl G, Weinberg W: Depressive illness in childhood presenting as severe headache. Am J Dis Child 120:122–124, 1970.

Lucas AR, Lockett HJ, Grimm F: Amitriptyline in childhood depressions. Dis Nerv Syst 26:105–110, 1965.

Lukianowicz N: Attempted suicide in children. Acta Psychiatr Scand 44:415–435, 1968.

Malmquist C: Depression in childhood and adolescence. Pts I and II. N Engl J Med 284:887–955, 1971.

Mayo JA: Marital therapy with manic-depressive patients treated with lithium. Comp Psychiatry 20:419–426, 1979.

McConville BJ, Boag LC, Purohit AP: Three types of childhood depression. Can J Psychiatry 18:133–138, 1973.

McKnew DH, Cytryn L: Urinary metabolites in chronically depressed children. J Am Acad Child Psychiatry 18:608–615, 1979.

Meltzer HY, Fang VS, Tricou BJ, et al: Effect of dexamethasone on plasma prolactin and cortisol levels in psychiatric patients. Am J Psychiatry 139:763–768, 1982.

Mendelson M: Psychoanalytic Concepts of Depression, 2d ed. New York, Spectrum Publications, 1972.

Mintz RS: Prevalence of persons in the city of Los Angeles who have attempted suicide: A pilot study. Bull Suicidal 7:9–16, 1970.

Montgomery SA, Asberg M: A new depression scale disagreed to be sensitive to change. Br J Psychiatry 134:382–389, 1979.

Murphy GE: Problems in studying suicide. Psychiatr Dev 4:339–350, 1983.

Murphy GE, Robins E: Social factors in suicide. JAMA 199:303–308, 1967.

Nissen G: Symptomatik und prognose depressive vertimmungszwstande in Kindes und Jungendelter. In Arnell A (ed): Depressive States in Childhood and Adolescence. Stockholm, Almquist & Wiskell, 1971, pp 517–524.

Orvaschel H, Mednick S, Schulsinger F, Rock D: The children of psychiatrically disturbed parents: Differences as a function of the sex of the sick parent. Arch Gen Psychiatry 36:691–695, 1979.

Otto U: Suicide attempts made by children. Acta Psychiatr Scand 55:64–72, 1966.

Otto U: Suicidal attempts in childhood and adolescence—today and after 10 years. A follow-up study. In Annell AL (ed): Depressive States in Childhood and Adolescence. Stockholm, Almquist & Wiskell, 1971, pp 357–366.

Pallmeyer T, Petti TA: Effects of imipramine on aggression and dejection in depressed children. Am J Psychiatry 136:1472–1473, 1979.

Pearce J: Depressive disorder in childhood. J Child Psychol Psychiatry 18:79–82, 1977.

Perris C: The course of depressive psychoses. Acta Psychiatr Scand 44:238–248, 1968.

Perris C: Abnormality on paternal and maternal sides: Observations in bipolar (manic-depressive) and unipolar depressive psychoses. Br J Psychiatry 118:207–210, 1971.

Petti TA, Campbell M: Imipramine and seizures. Am J Psychiatry 132:538–540, 1975.

Petti TA, Bornstein M, Delameter A, Conners CK: Evaluation and multimodality treatment of a depressed prepubertal girl. J Am Acad Child Psychiatry 19:690–702, 1980.

Petti, TA, Conners CK: Changes in behavioral ratings of depressed children treated with imipramine. J Am Acad Child Psychiatry 22:355–360, 1983.

Petti TA, Unis A: Imipramine treatment of borderline children's case reports with a controlled study. Am J Psychiatry 134:516–518, 1981.

Polvan O, Cebiroglu R: Treatment with psychopharmacologic agents in childhood depressions. In Annell AL (ed): Depressive States in Childhood and Adolescence. Stockholm, Almquist & Wiskell, 1971.

Poznanski E, Krahenbuhl V, Zrull J: Childhood depression. J Am Acad Child Psychiatry 15:491–501, 1976.

Poznanski E, Zrull J: Childhood depression: Clinical characteristics of overtly depressed children. Arch Gen Psychiatry 23:8–15, 1970.

Poznanski EO, Carroll BJ, Banegar MC, et al: The dexamethasone suppression test in prepubertal depressed children. Am J Psychiatry 139:321–324, 1982.

Poznanski EO, Cook SC, Carroll BJ: A depression rating scale for children. Pediatrics 64:442–450, 1979.

Puig-Antich J, Blau S, Marx N: A pilot open trial of imipramine in prepubertal depressive illness (proceedings). Psychopharmacol Bull 14:40–42, 1978.

Puig-Antich J: Affective disorders in childhood: A review and perspective. Psychiatr Clin North Am 3:403–424, 1980.

Puig-Antich J: Major depression and conduct disorder in prepuberty. J Am Acad Child Psychiatry 21:118–123, 1982.

Puig-Antich J, Blau S, Marx N, et al: Prepubertal major depressive disorder: Pilot study. J Am Acad Child Psychiatry 17: 695–707, 1978.

Puig-Antich J, Chambers W, Halpern F, et al: Cortisol hypersecretion in prepubertal depressive illness: A preliminary report. Psychoneuroendocrinology 4:191–197, 1979a.

Puig-Antich J, Gittleman R: Depression in childhood and adolescence. In Paykel ES (ed): Handbook of Affective Disorders. London, Churchill Livingstone, 1980.

Puig-Antich J, Novecenko H, Davies M, et al: Growth hormone secretion in prepubertal children with major depression: I. Final report on response to insulin-induced hypoglycemia during a depressive episode. Arch Gen Psychiatry 41: 455–460, 1984.

Puig-Antich J, Perel JM, Lupatkin W, et al: Plasma levels of imipramine (IMI) and desmethylimipramine (DMI) and clinical response in prepubertal major depressive disorders. J Am Acad Child Psychiatry 18:616–627, 1979b.

Raskin A: Depression in children: Fact or fallacy. In Schulterbrandt JG, Raskin A (eds): Depression in Childhood: Diagnosis, Treatment, and Conceptual Models. New York, Raven Press, 1977, pp 141–146.

Reich W, Herjanic B, Welner Z, et al: Development of a structured interview for children: Agreement on diagnosis comparing child and parent interviews. J Abnorm Child Psychol 10:325–336, 1982.

Reinherz HZ, Stewart-Berghauer G, Pakiz B, et al: The relationship of early risk and current mediators to depressive symptomatology in adolescents. J Am Acad Child Adolesc Psychiatry 28:942–947, 1989.

Remafedi G, Farrow JA, Deisher RW: Risk factors for attempted suicide in gay and bisexual youth. Pediatrics 87:869–875, 1991.

Rie HE: Depression in childhood: A survey of some pertinent contributors. J Am Acad Child Psychiatry 5:653–685, 1966.

Robbins DR, Alessi NE, Yanchyshyn GW, Colfer MV: Preliminary report on the dexamethasone suppression test in adolescents. Am J Psychiatry 139:942–943, 1982.

Rochlin G: The loss complex. J Am Psychoanal Assoc 7:299–316, 1959.

Rook A: Student suicides. Br Med J 1:599–603, 1959.

Ross AO: Child behavior therapy: Principles, procedures, and empirical basis. New York, Wiley, 1981.

Rutter M, Tizard J, Whitmore K: Education, Health and Behavior. London, Longman, 1970.

Ryan N, Meyer V, Dachille S, et al: Lithium antidepressant augmentation in TCA-refractory depression in adolescents. J Am Acad Child Adolesc Psychiatry 3:371–376, 1988.

Ryan N, Puig-Antich J, Rabinovich H, et al: MAOIs in adolescent major depression unresponsive to tricyclic antidepressants. J Am Acad Child Adolesc Psychiatry 6:755–758, 1988.

Sallee FR, Pollock BG, Perel JM, et al: Intravenous pulse loading of clomipramine in adolescents with depression. Psychopharmacol Bull 25(1):114–118, 1989.

Sanborn DE, Sanborn CJ, Cimbolie P: Two years of suicide: A study of adolescent suicide. In NH Child Psychiatry and Human Development, 1973, pp 234–242.

Sandler J, Joffe WG: Notes on childhood depression. Int J Psychoanal 46:88–96, 1965.

Schaffer D: Suicide in childhood and early adolescence. J Child Psychol Psychiatry 15:275–291, 1974.

Schneidman ES: Suicide among the gifted. In Schneidman ES (ed): Suicidology: Contemporary Developments. New York, Grune & Stratton, 1976.

Schwartz CE, Dorer DJ, Beardslee WR, et al: Maternal expressed emotion and parental affective disorder: Risk for childhood depressive disorder, substance abuse, or conduct disorder. J Psychiatr Res 24:231–250, 1990.

Seligman M, Maier S: Failure to escape traumatic shock. J Exp Psychol 74:1–9, 1967.

Simeon JG, Dinicolav F, Ferguson HB, Copping W: Adolescent depression: A placebo-controlled fluoxetine treatment study and follow-up. Prog Neuropsychopharmacol Biol Psychiatry 14:791–795, 1990.

Sovner R: The diagnosis and treatment of manic-depressive illness in childhood and adolescence. Psych Opinion 12:37–42, 1975.

Spitz RA: Anaclitic depression. Psychoanal Study Child 11: 313–342, 1946.

Stack JJ: Chemotherapy in childhood depression. In Depressive States in Childhood and Adolescence. Proc. 4th U.E.P. Congress. Stockholm, Almquist & Wiskell, 1971, pp 460–466.

Stanley EJ, Barter JT: Adolescent suicidal behavior. Am J Orthopsychiatry 132:180–185, 1978.

Strain PS, Hill AD: Social interaction. In Wehrman P (ed): Recreation Programming for Developmentally Disabled Persons. Baltimore, University Park Press, 1979.

Steingard R, Biederman J, Keenan K, Moore C: Co-morbidity in the interpretation of dexamethasone suppression test results in children: A review and report. Biol Psychiatry 28: 193–202, 1990.

Strober M, Carlson GA: Bipolar illness in adolescents with major depression. Arch Gen Psychiatry 39:349–355, 1982.

Strober M, Freeman R, Rigali J: The pharmacotherapy of depressive illness of adolescents: I. An open-labeled trial of Imipramine. Psychopharmacol Bull 26:80–84, 1990.

Strober M, Green J, Carlson GA: Reliability of psychiatric diagnosis in adolescents: Interrater agreement using DSM-III. Arch Gen Psychiatry 38:141–145, 1981.

Strober M, Salkin B, Burroughs J, Morrell W: Validity of the bulimia-restricter distinction in anorexia nervosa: Parental personality characteristics and family psychiatric morbidity. J Nerv Ment Dis 170:345–351, 1982.

Thompson RJ, Schindler FH: Embryonic mania. Child Psychiatry Hum Dev 6:149–154, 1976.

Tsuang MT: Genetic counseling for psychiatric patients and their families. Am J Psychiatry 135:1465–1475, 1978.

Walling VR, Pfefferbaum, B: The use of methylphenidate in a depressed adolescent with AIDS. Dev Behav Pediatr 11: 195–197, 1990.

Warneke L: A case of manic-depressive illness in childhood. Can Psychiatry Assoc J 20:195–200, 1975.

Weinberg S: Suicidal intent in adolescence: A hypothesis about the role of physical illness. J Pediatr 77:579–586, 1970.

Weinberg WA, Brumback RA: Mania in childhood. Am J Dis Child 130:380–385, 1976.

Weinberg WA, Rutman J, Sullivan L, et al: Depression in children referred to an educational diagnostic center: Diagnosis and treatment. J Pediatr 83:1065–1072, 1973.

Weininger O: Young children's concept of dying and dead. Psychol Rep 44:395–407, 1979.

Weissman MM: The epidemiology of suicide attempts, 1960–1971. Arch Gen Psychiatry 30:737–746, 1974.

Weller EB, Weller RA, Carr S: Imipramine treatment of trichotillomania and coexisting depression in a seven-year-old. J Am Acad Child Adolesc Psychiatry 6:952–953, 1989.

Weller EB, Weller RA, Fristad M: Dexamethasone suppression test in prepubertal depressed children. Paper presented at the American Psychiatric Association Meeting, New York, May 1983.

Weller EB, Weller RA, Fristad MA, et al: Dexamethasone suppression test in prepubertal depressed children. Am J Psychiatry 141:290–291, 1984.

Weller EB, Welner A, McCrary H, et al: Psychopathology in children of inpatients with depression: A controlled study. J Nerv Ment Dis 164:408–413, 1977.

Weller EB, Weller RA, Preskorn SH, Glotzbach R: Steady state plasma imipramine levels in prepubertal depressed children. Am J Psychiatry 139:506–508, 1982.

Welner A, Welner A, McCray MD, et al: Psychopathology in children of inpatients with depression: A controlled study. J Nerv Ment Dis 164:408–413, 1977.

Wexler L, Weissman MM, Kasl SV: Suicide attempts 1970–1975: Updating a United States study and comparisons with international trends. Br J Psychiatry 132:180–185, 1978.

Whitaker A, Johnson J, Shaffer D, et al: Uncommon troubles in young people. Arch Gen Psychiatry 47:487–496, 1990.

White JH, O'Shanick G: Juvenile manic-depressive illness. Am J Psychiatry 134:1035–1036, 1977.

Wirt RD, Lachar D, Klinedinst JK, Seat PD: Multidimensional Description of Child Personality Manual for the Personality Inventory for Children. Los Angeles, Western Psychological Services, 1977.

CHAPTER 20

Autistic Disorder and Schizophrenia in Childhood

LUKE Y. TSAI

AUTISTIC DISORDER

Definition

Ever since Kanner (1943) published his first description of autism, views of the etiology and nature of autism have evolved and changed. During the past four decades, despite the significant advances in the understanding of autism, disagreements over the validity and definition of autism have never ceased. Kanner (1943) used the term *early infantile autism* to describe a group of 11 children with a previously unrecognized disorder. He noted a number of characteristic features in these children, such as an inability to develop relationships with people, extreme aloofness, a delay in speech development, noncommunicative use of speech after it developed, a lack of imagination, insistence on preserving sameness, repeated simple patterns of play activities, and islets of ability. He noted that these children had extreme autistic aloneness and that they had an innate inability to form the usual biologically provided affective contact with people. Despite the variety of individual differences that appeared in the case descriptions, Kanner believed that only two features were of diagnostic significance. These were *autistic aloneness* and *obsessive insistence on sameness*. He adopted the term *early infantile autism* to describe the disorder and called attention to the fact that its symptoms were already evident in infancy.

During the next decade, clinicians in the United States and Europe reported cases with similar features (Despert, 1951; Van Krevelen, 1952; Bakwin, 1954). However, there was considerable controversy over the definition of the disorder because the name *autism* was ill-chosen. It led to confusion with Bleuler's (1911) use of the same term to describe schizophrenia in adults. This confusion led many clinicians to use childhood schizophrenia (Bender, 1956; American Psychiatric Association, 1968), borderline psychosis (Ekstein and Wallerstein, 1954), symbiotic psychosis (Mahler, 1952), infantile psychosis (Rutter and Lockyer, 1967) as interchangeable diagnoses. Each label had its roots in a particular view of the nature and causation of autism.

In 1968, Rutter critically analyzed the existing empirical evidence and proposed four essential characteristics of infantile autism: (1) a lack of social interest and responsiveness, (2) impaired language, ranging from absence of speech to peculiar speech patterns, (3) bizarre motor behavior, ranging from rigid and limited play patterns to more complex ritualistic and compulsive behavior, and (4) early onset, before 30 months of age. These features were present in nearly all autistic children. There also were many other specific features, but they were unevenly distributed. In 1978, the Professional Advisory Board of the National Society for Children and Adults with Autism (NSAC) further formulated a "Definition of the Syndrome of Autism." The NSAC defines autism as a behavioral syndrome which manifested itself before 30 months of age and has the following essential features: (1) disturbances of developmental rates and sequences, (2) disturbances of responses to sensory stimuli, (3) disturbances of speech, language, cognition, and nonverbal communication, and (4) disturbances of the capacity to relate appropriately to people, events, and objects (Ritvo and Freeman, 1978). This definition and the definitions of Kanner (1943) and Rutter (1968) paved the way for two sets of criteria that are widely used by clinicians all over the world: the *International Classification of Disease*, 9th revision: *Clinical Modification* (ICD-9-CM) (USDHHS, 1980) and the *Diagnostic and Statistical*

Manual of Mental Disorders, third edition revised (DSM-IIIR) (American Psychiatric Association, 1987).

Although the ICD-9 and the DSM-IIIR have similar definitions for infantile autism, there are apparent differences in the concept of autism. In ICD-9, infantile autism is classified as a subtype of "psychoses with origin specific to childhood," whereas in DSM-IIIR, infantile autism is viewed as a type of pervasive developmental disorder (PDD). The PDDs are defined as a group of severe, early developmental disorders characterized by delays and distortions in the development of social skills, cognition, and communication. There are only two subcategories under PDDs, namely, autistic disorder (roughly corresponding to infantile autism) and pervasive developmental disorder not otherwise specified (PDDNOS) (referring to individuals who have some of the characteristics of PDD but not enough to qualify for a diagnosis of autistic disorder). The menu-like scheme of DSM-IIIR diagnostic criteria requires the presence of a minimum number of criteria in each of the three cardinal features described above. The revised criteria are concrete, observable, and operational. They do not require raters to subjectively determine whether there is a "pervasive impairment" or a "gross deficit." Hence the clinicians' hesitation to use the diagnosis of autistic disorder in older and higher-functioning autistic individuals has been removed. DSM-IIIR has broadened the diagnostic concept of autistic disorder/autism from DSM-III (American Psychiatric Association, 1980), allowing for the gradation of behavior seen in autistic individuals. Thus it is not surprising that studies using DSM-IIIR criteria have yielded higher prevalence rates of autistic disorder than those using the DSM-III criteria for infantile autism (Volkmar et al., 1988; Factor et al., 1989; Hertzig et al., 1990). On the other hand, the "lumpers" approach of defining PDDNOS results in netting a very heterogeneous group of individuals with autistic-like symptoms, hence a problem for the study of external validity. In other words, it is likely to lead to all the different groups (e.g., atypical autism, residual autism, Asperger syndrome, Rett syndrome, etc.) being bundled together in a way that will lose crucial diagnostic distinctions. It also will cause poor replication of research findings. What is needed is a system that can break down symptom clusters into smaller, homogeneous, and meaningful subgroups (i.e., "splitters" approach). Such a system would enhance and ensure both reliability and validity of mental disorders under study. The ICD-10 diagnostic classification (World Health Organization, 1988) takes exactly such an approach.

The ICD-10 definition of autistic disorder/autism shows that it also has adopted the diagnostic term of *pervasive developmental disorders*. In the ICD-10 system, PDDs include (1) childhood autism, (2) atypical autism, (3) Asperger syndrome, (4) Rett syndrome, (5) childhood disintegrative disorders, (6) overactive disorders associated with mental retardation and stereotyped movements, (7) other pervasive disorders, and (8) unspecified pervasive disorder. The ICD-10 definition of PDDs is based on the belief that there is taxonomic validity of each subtype of PDDs.

The ICD-10 system defines childhood autism as "a type of pervasive developmental disorder that is defined by the presence of abnormal and/or impaired development that is manifested before the age of three years, and by the characteristic type of abnormal functioning in all three areas of social interaction, communication, and restricted, repetitive behavior." The ICD-10 system further defines the following *research diagnostic criteria* for childhood autism:

A. Presence of abnormal/impaired development from before the age of 3 years. Usually there is no period of unequivocally normal development but, when present, the period of normality does not extend *beyond age 3 years*. Delay and/or abnormal patterns of functioning before 3 years (whether or not recognized as such at the time) in at least one of the following areas is required:
   1. Receptive and/or expressive language as used in social communication.
   2. The development of selective social attachments and/or of reciprocal social interaction.
   3. Functional and/or symbolic play.
B. Qualitative impairments in reciprocal social interaction. Diagnosis requires demonstrable abnormalities in at least three of the following five areas:
   1. Failure to adequately use eye-to-eye gaze, facial expression, body posture, and gesture to regulate social interaction.
   2. Failure to develop (in a manner appropriate to mental age, and despite ample opportunities) peer relationships that involve a mutual sharing of interests, activities, and emotions.
   3. Rarely seeking and using other people for comfort and affection at times of stress or distress and/or offering comfort and affection to others when they are showing distress or unhappiness.
   4. Lack of shared enjoyment in terms of vicarious pleasure in other people's happiness and/or a spontaneous seeking to share their own enjoyment through joint involvement with others.
   5. A lack of socioemotional reciprocity, as shown by an impaired or deviant response to other people's emotions, and/or lack of modulation of behavior according to social context and communicative behaviors.
C. Qualitative impairments in communication. Diagnosis requires demonstrable abnormalities in at least two of the following five areas:

1. A delay in or total lack of development of spoken language that is not accompanied by an attempt to compensate through the use of gesture or mime as alternative modes of communication (often preceded by a lack of communicative babbling).
2. Relative failure to initiate or sustain conversational interchange (at whatever level language skills are present) in which there is reciprocal to and from responsiveness to the communications of the other person.
3. Stereotyped and repetitive use of language and/or idiosyncratic use of words or phrases.
4. Abnormalities in pitch, stress, rate, rhythm, and intonation of speech.
5. A lack of varied spontaneous make-believe play or (when young) in social imitative play.

D. Restricted, repetitive, and stereotyped patterns of behavior, interests, and activities. Diagnosis requires demonstrable abnormalities in at least two of the following six areas:

1. An encompassing preoccupation with stereotyped and restricted patterns of interest.
2. Specific attachments to unusual objects.
3. Apparently compulsive adherence to specific nonfunctional routines or rituals.
4. Stereotyped and repetitive motor mannerisms that involve either hand/finger flapping or twisting or complex whole-body movements.
5. Preoccupations with part objects or nonfunctional elements of play materials (such as their odor, the feel of their surface, or the noise/vibration that they generate).
6. Distress over changes in small nonfunctional details of the environment.

E. The clinical picture is not attributable to the other varieties of pervasive developmental disorder, specific developmental disorder of receptive language with secondary socioemotional problems, reactive attachment disorder or disinhibited attachment disorder, mental retardation with some associated emotional/behavioral disorder, schizophrenia of unusually early onset, or Rett syndrome.

It should be pointed out here that the proposed ICD-10 diagnostic criteria of PDDs are not based on any systematically collected data. Therefore, it is expected that the new criteria of ICD-10 will not satisfy everyone and will no doubt be revised when improved understanding and further knowledge of autism is gained. Nonetheless, further research of refinement of the criteria would ensure more reliable diagnoses of autism and would provide further support of the taxonomic validity of autism.

The United States is under a treaty obligation with the World Health Organization (WHO) to maintain a coding and terminologic consistency with the ICD. The American Psychiatric Association (APA) has already appointed several committees to develop DSM-IV and to publish it in 1993. It is quite certain that the DSM-IV will continue to adopt the concept that autistic disorder is a subtype of PDDs, as well as to continue the use of menu-like scheme of diagnostic criteria. It also will adopt the ICD-10 "splitters" approach to include several other subtypes in the PDDs. However, it is uncertain at the present time how many subtypes will be contained in the PDDs and what will be the diagnostic criteria for these subtypes of PDDs. The present author agrees that every attempt should be made to achieve compatibility with ICD-10 so that a common language will be used throughout the world. However, the present author feels that the diagnostic term *autistic disorder* should be used in DSM-IV instead of the proposed ICD-10 category of "childhood autism" because this disorder does not occur only in children.

This chapter will focus mainly on autistic disorder and schizophrenia in childhood. However, information on the other subtypes of PDDs also will be described briefly in the section on differential diagnosis. For the purpose of convenience, the term of *autism* will be used for autistic disorder in the remaining sections of this chapter.

Etiology

PSYCHOGENIC FACTORS

Kanner's (1943) original descriptions of autism, as well as a number of subsequent reports by other workers, suggested that parents of autistic children were highly intelligent, were preoccupied with abstractions, had limited interest in people, and were emotionally cold. Some studies reported findings of disturbances in family dynamics (Reiser, 1963a, 1963b), unconscious parental hostility and rejection (Bettelheim, 1967), parental perplexity (Meyers and Goldfarb, 1961), and lack of parent–child communicative clarity (Goldfarb et al., 1972). These investigators had suggested that autism might be a response to these parental personality characteristics, deviant parent–child interactions, or a variety of severe early stress. However, findings that support these psychogenic hypotheses have come from samples that did not make any distinction between autism and schizophrenia in childhood and that were based on projective tests and selected family observations. Similar techniques and other well-controlled studies have produced largely negative findings (Ornitz and Ritvo, 1976). There is no evidence to suggest that the parents of autistic children are unkind or uncaring or that poor parenting results in autism. If this were so, many children who suffer from poor parenting would have developed autism.

Thus there are good grounds for concluding that no psychological factors can cause infantile autism. Although some people may still believe in the psychogenic hypothesis of autism, most authorities now agree that biologic and not psychological factors are of crucial importance.

ORGANIC FACTORS

Genetic Factors

Genetic factors seem to play a major role in the etiology of autism. Several studies have shown that siblings of autistic persons have increased rates of the disorder (Rutter, 1967; Tsai et al., 1981; Minton et al., 1982). It has been estimated that the pooled frequency of autism in the sibs is about 3 percent (Smalley et al., 1988; Rutter, 1990), which is about 50 times higher than that of the general population (based on 4 to 5 per 10,000 rate of autism).

Twin studies also provide support to the etiologic role of genetic factors in autism. However, in view of the fact that twin births are rather uncommon in the general population, few major studies have been done. A carefully designed study was undertaken by Folstein and Rutter in 1977. They studied 21 same-sex autistic twin pairs and found that 4 of the 11 (36 percent) monozygotic (MZ) twin pairs were concordant for autism, as compared with none of the dizygotic (DZ) pairs. In addition, they found an 82 percent concordance for serious cognitive abnormalities in MZ pairs and 10 percent in DZ pairs. On the basis of this finding, they suggested that what was inherited in autism was a pattern of cognitive deficits that included, but was not restricted to, autism (Folstein and Rutter, 1977). Autism was hypothesized as lying on an extreme pole of a spectrum of cognitive language disorders, with some learning, and/or language disorders being milder variants of the same continuum (Folstein, 1985). A follow-up of Folstein and Rutter's sample has revealed that the nonautistic MZ co-twins in discordant pairs tend to show marked social deficits in adult life, suggesting that the inherited deficit is social as well as cognitive (Le Couteur et al., 1989).

Ritvo and associates (1985a) studied 23 pairs of MZ and 17 pairs of DZ twins drawn from the UCLA Registry for Genetic Studies in Autism. Of the 23 MZ pairs, 22 were found to be concordant for autism compared with 4 of the 17 DZ pairs. This yields a 96 percent concordance rate for MZ pairs and 24 percent for DZ pairs. The higher concordance for DZ pairs (24 percent) probably reflects the fact that the sample studied was not representative of twinships in the population of autistic patients. Also, only 12 pairs of MZ twins and 5 of the 12 pairs of same-sex DZ twins had blood grouping done (Smalley et al., 1988; Folstein and Rutter, 1987). Other twin studies also have found higher concordance rates for MZ pairs and no concordance for DZ pairs, supporting the role of genetic factors in autism (Steffenburg et al., 1989).

Apart from the increased prevalence of autism in siblings and the MZ–DZ differences in concordance, additional support for the importance of ge-

netic factors comes from the finding of increased rate of cognitive disabilities in siblings of autistic persons. August et al. (1981) found a 15 percent rate of cognitive abnormalities in the siblings of autistic probands as compared with 3 percent among the siblings of Down syndrome controls. Of the 11 siblings of autistic probands, 4 showed problems in the comprehension or production of language, 9 had IQs below 80, and 2 had reading disabilities. Similar observations have been made by other investigators (Ritvo et al., 1985b). In another study, Minton et al. (1982) found that nonautistic siblings of autistic children had significantly lower verbal scores than performance scores on Wechsler Intelligence Scales, and 10 percent were mentally retarded. It has been suggested that the familial loading for cognitive disabilities is most evident in the families of mentally retarded autistic children (Baird and August, 1985). However, other studies have shown that most of the familial loading for cognitive disabilities is not accounted for by mental retardation (Piven et al., 1990b) and that a family history of reading or language disabilities is present in a quarter of families with an autistic child whose IQ is 70 or more (Bartak et al., 1975). A recent study has confirmed that most of the cognitive disabilities in siblings consist of specific disorders of speech and language rather than global mental retardation (Macdonald et al., 1989).

Association of autism with certain genetic syndromes also provides support to the importance of genetic factors in this disorder. Thus a proportion of autistic individuals has been found to exhibit a fragile site on the X chromosome (Brown et al., 1986; Levitas et al., 1983). Some investigators have suggested that the rate of chromosomal anomalies in autistic individuals is at least 47 percent, with about 20 to 25 percent showing the fragile X chromosome (Gillberg and Wahlstöm, 1985). While the issue is not yet decided, most recent studies have produced figures of below 5 percent (Payton et al., 1989; Piven et al., 1991). In addition to fragile X syndrome, occasional reports have described the association of autism with single-gene disorders such as phenylketonuria (Knoblock and Pasamanick, 1975) and tuberous sclerosis (Lawlor and Maurer, 1987). These reports, though not based on systematic series of cases of these single-gene disorders, do provide further support to the importance of genetic factors in autism.

Based on the preceding studies, possible modes of inheritance have been proposed. Ritvo et al. (1985b), on the basis of a segregation analysis of 46 families with multiple cases of autism, produced results that were consistent with autosomal recessive inheritance. However, this is inconsistent with the observed marked excess of autistic males. Tsai and colleagues (August et al., 1981; Tsai et al., 1981; Tsai and Beisler, 1983) proposed a multifactorial model with different thresholds for males and females. Vertical transmission has been implied by some authors (Ritvo et al., 1988); however, most studies have found no evidence of personality abnormalities in parents (Cantwell et al., 1978).

Thus, while familial aggregation noted in case series and the data from the twin studies indicate that genetic factors are likely to be important in autism, these studies tell us little about the nature of the genetic defect, whether one or more genetic mechanisms are operating, or whether the genetic mechanism(s) operate(s) in the whole group of autism or just in some subgroups. A delineation of just what is inherited will provide a better understanding of genetic implications in autism. Now that "gene maps" are being made of the positions of genes on human chromosomes, new possibilities are arising for studies called *linkage studies*, which can determine whether genes for a given disorder lie on a chromosome in close proximity to known genetic markers, such as the gene for color blindness or certain blood types. If two genes lie together, the two traits they cause are likely to be inherited together. Finding clear evidence of linkage between a given psychiatric disorder and a trait caused by a known genetic marker would provide hard evidence that the psychiatric disorder is genetically caused and would lay to rest any doubts left by loopholes in twin and adoption studies. Furthermore, through the identification of genetic markers, a clearer pattern of genetic transmission may be elucidated, etiologic subgroups may be identified, and the pathophysiology of a disorder may be determined (Smalley et al., 1988). For example, utilizing this approach in medical genetics, different enzymatic defects have been identified to elucidate the existence of many subtypes of mucopolysaccharidoses.

To date there is one linkage study of autism using blood polymorphisms in a subset of multiple-incidence families (Spence et al., 1985). Spence and colleagues (1985) found no evidence for linkage for autism with 30 blood polymorphisms and could rule out linkage with 19 of these markers. They also found no evidence for an association of HLA and autism. However, they did suggest that potential markers might be found on chromosome 9 in the region of the ABO blood group.

The finding of fragile X chromosome among autistic patients led Tsai and colleagues (1988) to use six DNA probes in the Xq26–q28 region to search for DNA markers for autism. Although clinically useful markers have not been found, such a research approach may provide a potentially fruitful means of increasing our understanding of the relationship between genetic factors and autism.

In *summary*, the last decade of genetic research in autism has found strong evidence suggesting that there may be different genetic mechanisms that result in the syndrome of autism, hence suggesting genetic heterogeneity in autism. Several different kinds of studies are needed to sort out the various mechanisms. It should begin with a detailed family study based on a systematically ascertained sample. Each autistic proband and all first-degree relatives should have a detailed clinical examination and laboratory tests, including social, cognitive, and language assessment. The goal is to identify genetic markers so that the autism phenotype can be redefined using such markers. Then comparative studies of autistic and nonautistic individuals who have the same subclinical marker (e.g., unaffected relatives) should be conducted. In this way, genotype–genotype interaction or genotype–environment interactions may be elucidated in the etiology of autism (Smalley et al., 1988). The ultimate goal is to be able to apply gene therapy to those who are affected with autism, as well as to be able to practice prevention of autism.

Obstetric and Postnatal Factors

There is strong evidence that complications of pregnancy and delivery are associated with autism. A wide variety of neurologic disorders have been reported: cerebral palsy, congenital rubella, toxoplasmosis, tuberous sclerosis, cytomegalovirus infection, lead encephalopathy, meningitis, encephalitis, severe brain hemorrhage, many types of epilepsy, and others. Many of these neurologic or congenital disorders derive from unfavorable prenatal, perinatal, and neonatal complications (reviewed by Fish and Ritvo, 1979). On the other hand, twin pairs discordant for autism also provide strong evidence for an association between obstetric/postnatal factors and autism. For example, in the Folstein and Rutter study quoted above (1977) the authors found that the nonautistic but cognitively disabled MZ cotwins had normal or near-normal birth histories compared with their autistic cotwins, several of whom had a history of significant perinatal problems. Steffenburg et al. (1989) confirmed this finding in a more recent study. They described 11 twin pairs in which only one twin was autistic. In eight of these discordant pairs, the autistic twin had suffered more perinatal and neonatal complications than the nonautistic cotwin.

In addition to twin studies, other data also suggest that autistic singletons experience significantly more obstetric and neonatal complications than matched controls, with complications of pregnancy being more common than complications of delivery (Deykin and MacMahon, 1980; Gillberg and Gillberg, 1983). A number of pre-, peri-, and neonatal factors appear to be more frequent in autistic subjects than in their siblings or matched controls (see review by Tsai, 1987). These include increased maternal age, birth order (first and fourth or later born), bleeding after the first trimester, use of medication, and meconium in amniotic fluid. However, due to the lack of uniformity in applying diagnostic criteria for autism, as well as in the selection of obstetric complications, these findings should be received with caution. Nonetheless, it has been suggested that pre- or perinatal insults to the brain are the biologic causation of autism in persons whose autistic symptoms are present from birth and that postnatal cerebral infections or injuries cause the disorder when symptoms appear after a period of apparent normal development. However, research done so far does not indicate a causal relationship between obstetric and neonatal factors and autism. Nor does it suggest that the association is specific, in the sense that a number of factors of a variable severity have been implicated. This implies that either obstetric and neonatal factors can sometimes convert an entirely normal fetus into an autistic person (Steffenburg et al., 1989) or can sometimes unmask or potentiate a preexisting genetic liability (Folstein and Rutter, 1977). Clearly, more research is needed before a causal link can be proposed between autism and obstetric/postnatal complications.

Neurologic Factors
Neurologic abnormalities have been reported in 30 to 75 percent of several series of autistic patients (Gittelman and Birch, 1967; DeMyer et al., 1973; Tsai et al., 1981). These include abnormalities of hypotonia or hypertonia, disturbance of body schema, clumsiness, choreiform movements, pathologic reflexes, myoclonic jerking, drooling, abnormal posture and gait, dystonic posturing of hands and fingers, tremor, ankle clonus, emotional facial paralysis, and strabismus. These are all signs of dysfunction in the basal ganglia, particularly the neostriatum, and closely related structures of the mesial aspects of the frontal lobe or limbic system. Based on the analogy to signs and conditions seen in adults with certain forms of brain damage, Damasio and Maurer (1978) proposed that autism results from dysfunction in a system of bilateral central nervous system structures that includes the ring of mesolimbic cortex located in the mesial frontal and temporal lobes, the neostriatum, and the anterior and medial nuclear groups of the thalamus. They suggested that such dysfunction might involve macroscopic or microscopic cerebral changes consequent to a variety of causes, such as perinatal viral infection, insult to the periventricular watershed area, or genetically determined neurochemical abnormalities. This hypothesis, though plausible, needs to be verified.

Neuroanatomic Factors
In view of the high prevalence of neurologic signs in persons with autism, attempts have been made to relate these signs to underlying brain pathology. However, because of various ethical and practical reasons, very few neuropathologic studies in autism have been done. Initial postmortem brain studies of seven cases were largely negative (Darby, 1976; Williams et al., 1980). Bauman and Kemper (1985) reported the autopsy findings of a 29-year-old man with clear autism who had died by drowning. The findings included major cellular and structural

changes in hippocampus, amygdala, and cerebellum (including Purkinje cell loss). In the following year, Ritvo and colleagues (1986) reported autopsy findings in four autistic patients. They too found Purkinje cell loss in the cerebellum of all the patients. Kemper and Bauman and associates (Arin et al., 1991; Bauman, 1991; Kemper, 1990) reported further autopsy results in six autistic individuals. The forebrain in all six showed a reduction in neuronal size and increased cell packing density in the hippocampal formation, entorhinal cortex, amygdala, and medial septal nuclei. In the hindbrain, there was a decreased number of Purkinje and granule cells in the cerebellum. However, in view of the small numbers involved, it is not clear what weight should be attached to the findings of these studies. Nevertheless, these findings provide some direction (i.e., posterior cerebral fossa) for in vivo neuroanatomical imaging studies of autism.

Computed tomographic (CT) studies have identified gross abnormalities (e.g., porencephalic cyst) in a minority of autistic patients (Damasio et al., 1980; Gillberg and Svendsen, 1983). However, CT studies remain contradictory and inconsistent. Some studies showing abnormalities such as reversed hemispheric asymmetry (Hier et al., 1979) and ventricular enlargement (Rosenbloom et al., 1984) have been challenged by others which fail to observe such findings (Prior et al., 1984; Creasey et al., 1986; Rumsey et al., 1988).

Magnetic resonance imaging (MRI) is rapidly replacing CT as the method of choice of obtaining detailed anatomic information about the brain. Because many autistic subjects require sedation to remain still for scanning, only a few head MRI studies have been carried out. Minshew et al. (1986) found that the cerebellum and fourth ventricle were normal in all 10 autistics with IQs of 70 or greater. However, 3 of the 6 patients with IQs of 70 to 85 had other abnormalities.

Gaffney et al. (1987a, 1987b) studied the head MRIs of 14 autistic patients aged 4 to 22 years with IQs of 60 or greater. Six of the 14 patients had brain lesions seen on the MRI scans, but there was no single, circumscribed lesion common to all the autistic patients. Midsagittal MRI scans showed the fourth ventricle to be significantly larger and the entire brainstem to be significantly smaller in the autistic group compared with the control group. In the coronal scans, the cerebella of the autistic patients were proportionally smaller and the fourth ventricles proportionally larger. Piven et al. (1990a) found the presence of cerebral cortical malformations in 7 of 13 high-functioning autistic males. Courchesne et al. (1988) reported cerebellar hypoplasia in a group of 18 autistic patients compared with normal controls. However, Garber et al. (1989, 1992) found no difference on measures of the posterior fossa structures between the autistic subjects and the normal controls. The finding of abnormalities of the cerebellum is consistent with microscopic postmortem findings described earlier. Although the link between the cerebellar abnormalities and autism is yet to be determined, MRI technology has provided an exciting new avenue for future in vivo studies of the brain.

Only a few positron emission tomographic (PET) studies have been done in autism because of the risk of radiation exposure in children. In one study, Rumsey and associates found elevated utilization of glucose throughout many parts of the brains of 10 autistic men as compared with normal controls (Rumsey et al., 1985). Similar findings were reported in a group of 18 autistic children by DeVolder et al. (1988), although the mean brain glucose metabolism did not differ significantly between autistic patients and controls. Heh et al. (1989) used PET to examine the cerebellum in a group of seven adult autistic patients and eight age-matched controls. The results showed no significant differences in mean cerebellar glucose metabolism between the two groups, although all mean glucose rates of autistic patients were either equal to or greater than those of the controls. Although the meaning of these findings remains to be determined, it appears that PET should become increasingly important for researchers studying autism.

Neurophysiologic Factors
There are two rather disparate neurophysiologic hypotheses of autism. The first, which considers a *primary cortical dysfunction* in autism, emphasizes the autistic symptoms of language and communication and assumes an underlying specific cognitive disorder that is presumably of cortical origin. More specifically, this hypothesis considers that autism results from a disorder of hemispheric lateralization, that is, that the neural substrates in the left hemisphere necessary for sequential forms of information processing fail to develop (Prior, 1979).

The second hypothesis suggests a rostrally directed sequence of pathophysiologic influences originating in the brainstem and diencephalic structures, particularly the reticular formation of pontine and midbrain, substantia nigra, and the nonspecific nuclei of thalamus (Ornitz, 1985). This hypothesis has been developed through observation of the impaired ability of autistic children in modulating their own responses to sensory input and consequently their own motor output (Ornitz, 1974, 1983).

Support for cortical dysfunction in autism comes from studies of event-related potentials (ERPs) in which a reduced P3b wave has been found (Courchesne et al., 1984, 1985). This component represents purely cognitive functions and occurs 300 to 900 ms after stimulus. In addition, another long-latency evoked potential component, Nc, also appears to be smaller in autism (Courchesne, 1987).

Further support for the cortical dysfunction hypothesis comes from electroencephalographic (EEG) studies in autism. In general, these studies have found bilateral hemispheric abnormalities (Tsai and Tsai, 1984) and are characterized by focal or diffuse spike, slow wave, or slow dysrhythmic patterns. However, no abnormalities have been found to be specific. Unusually low voltage patterns suggesting a state of chronic hyperarousal also have been found in some studies (Kolvin, 1971; Hutt et al., 1965), a finding not confirmed by others (Hermelin and O'Connor, 1968; Creak and Pampiglione, 1969). Sleep EEG studies in autistic children have found that the eye movements of these children resemble those of normal infants more than those of age-matched controls, suggesting immaturity (Ornitz, 1965; Tanguay et al., 1976). Computerized EEG studies in autism also indicate abnormal patterns of cerebral lateralization (Small, 1975; Tanguay et al., 1976; Ogawa et al., 1982; Cantor et al., 1986). Studies on measurement of ongoing EEG activity during the administration of various cognitive tasks, such as those involving language or other left hemisphere mediated functions, also suggest abnormal patterns of functional brain lateralization (Dawson et al., 1982, 1983).

Auditory evoked response (AER) studies also have been done in autism. By and large, these studies have shown maturational deviation in a subgroup of autistic children (Student and Sohmer, 1978; Skoff et al., 1980; Fein et al., 1981; Tanguay et al., 1982; Gillberg et al., 1983a). Studies also have suggested that AERs are irregular and variable in autistic subjects with smaller amplitudes (Lelord et al., 1973). These findings suggest defective integration between visual and auditory pathways in autism.

Studies exploring the role of brainstem dysfunction in autism have focused on autonomic response studies. A variety of disturbances in autonomic function have been found to occur in autistic children. These include cardiac arrhythmias (Hutt et al., 1975), inadequate galvanic skin responses to auditory and visual stimuli (Bernal and Miller, 1970), etc. Dysfunctions of the vestibular system, which is said to be involved with self-monitoring, also have been reported. For example, Ritvo et al. (1969) found a decrease in duration of nystagmus after vesticular stimulation by rotation or by caloric irrigation in a group of autistic children. Prolongation of brainstem transmission time also has been reported in autism (Rosenblum et al., 1980; Taylor et al., 1982), although some investigators have failed to replicate this finding (e.g., Rumsey et al., 1984).

Biochemical Factors
Studies focusing on the neurochemical and neurotransmitter substances secreted in the brains of autistic persons also have been done. Three main reasons are responsible for the recent increase in interest in this area of autism research: (1) lack of gross brain pathology suggesting that microscopic

or functional factors may be responsible, (2) relative success in the pharmacologic treatments for certain limited aspects of autism, and (3) recent advances in basic neurosciences as applied to psychiatric disorders. Accordingly, all the major neurotransmitters have been studied in autism. Although the studies are usually preliminary, often compounded by problems inherent in neurochemical research (such as assay methods, measurements of body fluids, confounding variables of age, sex, etc.), overall evidence strongly suggests that neurochemical factors play a major role in the presentation of autism. This section will focus on each of the major neurotransmitters separately, although there is a considerable overlap between their functions.

SEROTONIN. Serotonin (5-hydroxytryptamine, or 5-HT) is an important neurotransmitter whose activity has been implicated in a variety of important processes such as temperature regulation, pain, sensory perception, sleep, sexual behavior, appetite, learning and memory (Young et al., 1982). Many studies have consistently reported that about one-third of autistic individuals have hyperserotonemia (reviewed by Anderson et al., 1987). There are three possible explanations of the hyperserotonemia: (1) enhanced platelet uptake, storage, or volume, (2) increased synthesis, and (3) decreased catabolism.

Studies of intestinal synthesis of 5-HT have focused on the measurement of the urinary excretion rates of the endpoint metabolite, 5-hydroxyindoleacetic acid (5-HIAA), with or without tryptophan loading. The results have been conflicting. Most studies have not found any difference between autistic and normal subjects (Minderaa et al., 1987). Thus it appears that increased intestinal synthesis of 5-HT is not the mechanism underlying the increased levels of serotonin seen in some autistic individuals.

Degradation of 5-HT occurs as a result of the activity of the enzyme monoamine oxidase (MAO). Several studies have reported that the functioning of this enzyme is normal in autism, as reflected by the lack of differences in the urinary excretion rates between autistic and normal subjects (Minderaa et al., 1987; Boullin et al., 1982). Thus the occurrence of increased serotonin blood levels in autistic persons does not appear to be the result of decreased catabolism of serotonin.

Previous studies found that the handling of 5-HT by platelets is normal in autism (Anderson et al., 1985; Boullin et al., 1982). However, recent work has suggested that this may not be so (Rotman et al., 1980; Katsui et al., 1986).

No consistent correlations have yet been found between blood serotonin level and any autistic behaviors or symptoms. Moreover, hyperserotonemia also has been found in some children who are severely retarded. Clearly, the mechanism and importance of hyperserotonemia in autism remains unclear.

DOPAMINE. The brain dopaminergic system is considered to affect several functions and behaviors, including cognition, motor function, eating and drinking behaviors, sexual behavior, neuroendocrine regulation, and selective attention. Young et al., (1982) and Campbell (1977) reported that neuroleptics, which are dopamine receptor–blocking agents, modulated several symptoms involving the motor system (e.g., hyperactivity, stereotypies, aggression, and self-injury) and made autistic children more compliant and receptive to special education procedures. On the other hand, dopamine agonists, such as stimulants, cause a worsening of preexisting stereotypies, aggression, and hyperactivity in autistic children (Young et al., 1982). These findings strongly suggest a role of dopamine in autism.

Studies of dopamine in autism have focused on the measurement of the homovanillic acid (HVA), the main metabolite of dopamine. Cohen et al. (1977) found that autistic children did not differ from other diagnostic groups in cerebrospinal fluid (CSF) level of HVA. However, the CSF level of HVA was found to be higher in the more severely impaired children, especially those with greater locomotor activity and more severe stereotypies. Leckman et al. (1980) also failed to find a difference in CSF HVA between "child psychosis (largely autism)" and "perceptual cognitive disorder" diagnostic groups. Gillberg and Svennerholm (1987) found elevated CSF HVA in autistic subjects. Two studies find no difference for plasma HVA between the autistic children and controls (Launay et al., 1987; Minderaa et al., 1989). However, HVA concentrations have not been shown to correlate with any autistic behaviors or symptoms.

EPINEPHRINE AND NOREPINEPHRINE. These two neurotransmitters are often discussed together because of their overlapping actions. Both these neurotransmitters are associated with the regulation of cardiovascular function, attention, memory, anxiety, sleep and learning (Young et al., 1982). Some studies have reported increased plasma norepinephrine levels in autistic patients (Lake et al., 1977), while others have found lower levels (Launay et al., 1987).

MHPG (3-methoxy-4-hydroxyphenylethylene glycol) levels in the urine have been found to be decreased in autistic subjects (Young et al., 1982), which is not consistent with the hypothesis that levels of norepinephrine might be increased in autism. So far as CSF MHPG is concerned, three recent studies have found no difference between autistic subjects and controls (e.g., Gillberg et al., 1983b).

Levels of the enzyme DBH (dopamine-beta-hydroxylase), which controls the conversion of dopamine to norepinephrine, also have been studied, but the results have been, again, conflicting. Thus Goldstein et al. (1976) and Lake et al. (1977) found decreased DBH levels in autistic subjects, while Young et al. (1980) found no difference between autistic and control groups.

Since the level of norepinephrine activity is also affected by two metabolic enzymes, catechol-*O*-methyl transferase (COMT) and MAO, Giller et al. (1980) studied COMT activity in cultured fibroblasts and in red blood cells of autistic children and found no difference compared with controls. MAO activity also appears normal in autism (Young et al., 1982; Lake et al., 1977).

PEPTIDES. Certain peptides have been shown to act as neurotransmitters and to affect pain perception, emotion, appetite, and sexual behavior. Certain peptides such as enkephalins and endorphins appear to act as endogenous opioids. It has been observed that some opiate-induced psychosocial distortions in animals resemble autistic behaviors, which has led to the clinical use of opiate antagonists, such as naltrexone, for the control of severe self-injurious behaviors (Deutsch, 1986). Weizman et al. (1984) reported low *H*-endorphin levels in the blood of a group of autistic children as compared with schizophrenic children or normal controls. However, Gillberg et al. (1985) reported that the mean CSF endorphin fraction II levels were higher in autistic children compared with normal children. Thus the limited evidence for the role of peptides in autism is, again, conflicting. Nevertheless, there is a need for further research in this field because of the clinical efficacy of opioid antagonists in the control of some autistic symptoms.

Trygstad et al. (1980) described a number of different urinary peptides profile patterns each said to be characteristic of a different behavioral abnormality. The characteristic profile for autism was initially shown in 20 patients with a variation of ± 30 percent for each peak. However, in an attempt to replicate such a finding from 69 urine samples obtained from three groups of young-adult males (autistic, mentally handicapped, and normal), no consistent patterns of urinary chromatographic profile were identified (Couteur et al., 1988). Nevertheless, the findings are intriguing, and further study may develop patterns with high specificity that may be used as diagnostic markers. Isolation and identification of any factors present in the chromatographic fractions also may contribute to the understanding of the pathogenesis of autism.

Other Biomedical Factors

A number of other abnormal biomedical measures in autistics have been reported. In one study, Sankar (1971) reported significantly lower blood adenosine triphosphatase activity in assays of red blood cells from autistic children. In another study, Katz and Liebman (1970) found an elevated CSF creatine phosphokinase (CPK) activity in some autistic children, as well as in children with meningitis, a finding suggesting that autistic children with an increased CSF CPK activity may represent a subgroup of children whose autism is due to brain insult from infection. On the whole, the significance of these findings is far from clear, but these studies merit further exploration.

Immunologic Factors

Immune system dysfunction also has been implicated in autism. Chess (1977) reported an increased frequency of autism in individuals with congenital rubella. Deykin and MacMahon (1979) found that autism was associated with prenatal rubella or influenza infection in about 5 percent of cases. Other studies also have confirmed this low rate of maternal infections during pregnancy in autistic individuals (Finegan and Quarrington, 1979; Gillberg and Gillberg, 1983; Mason-Brothers et al., 1987).

Young et al. (1977) studied the CSF immunoglobulin levels in 15 autistic children and found no abnormalities of glucose, protein cells, or folate, concluding that the hypothesis of slow virus playing a role in autism could not be supported. Stubbs (1976) gave rubella vaccine challenge to 15 autistic children and 8 age-matched controls in order to retrospectively diagnose prenatal rubella and found that the challenge did not differentiate autistic children from controls. However, 5 of the 13 autistic children had undetectable hemagglutination inhibition antibody titers despite previous vaccination. The author speculated that these autistic children might have an altered immune response. Warren et al. (1986, 1990) found several immune system abnormalities, including a decreased number of T-lymphocytes, an altered ratio of helper to suppressant T cells, etc. They further reported (1987) impaired activity of natural killer (NK) cells, which are large granular lymphocytes active against virus-infected cells and malignancy. Weizman et al. (1982) suggested that a cell-mediated immune response to brain antigen occurred in some autistic individuals. However, Todd et al. (1988), in an attempt to test for the presence of a generalized antibrain antibody response in autistic patients, failed to find such a response, while others (Westall and Root-Bernstein, 1983; Todd and Ciaranello, 1985) emphasized the role increased serotonin levels may play in the immune response of some autistic individuals.

Thus a variety of immune system abnormalities occur in autism. More studies are needed to link these abnormalities to the etiology and presentation of the syndrome.

SUMMARY OF ETIOLOGY

Previous studies have shown convincingly that neurobiologic factors are of critical importance in the causation of autism. However, despite several important discoveries, it must be admitted that no abnormalities have been found to be specific for the disorder. Besides, the etiologic implications of quite a few of the findings are not clear, nor is it clear if some of the abnormalities reflect chance associations without any significance. While some of the inconsistencies are due to methodologic shortcomings, they also reflect that autism is a heterogeneous behavioral disorder with several different but distinct subtypes. Future research in autism should continue to emphasize the further subclassification of autism. Such an approach will enable investigators to select more homogeneous groups of subjects for future neurobiologic research. From this approach, more consistent results could be derived from various independent research groups to further clarify the role of the various factors that contribute to autism.

Epidemiology

PREVALENCE

Epidemiologic studies in North America, Asia, and Europe have estimated the prevalence of autism to be between 2 and 15 per 10,000 children (Bryson et al., 1988; Cialdella and Mamelle, 1989; Gillberg, 1984; Hoshino et al., 1982; Lotter, 1966; Ishii and Takahashi, 1983; Matsuishi et al., 1987; McCarthy et al., 1984; Ritvo et al., 1989; Steffenburg and Gillberg, 1986; Steinhausen et al., 1986; Sugiyama and Abe, 1989; Treffert, 1970; Wing and Gould, 1979) (Table 20-1). There was a tendency for Japanese investigators to report higher prevalence rates than those reported by other researchers. It is not clear why such a difference exists. At the moment, DSM-IIIR suggests the prevalence of autistic disorder to be 2 to 4 cases per 10,000 children and 10 to 15 children in every 10,000 for PDDNOS.

It is also not clear whether prevalence rates of autism in cities differ from those in rural districts. Treffert (1970) reported that there was no statistically significant difference between the rural and urban prevalence rates. However, some studies have found higher rates in urban areas (Hoshino et al., 1982; Steffenburg and Gillberg, 1986).

SEX RATIO

All studies of autism have shown a predominance of boys over girls. Ratios from 3 to 4 boys to 1 girl have been reported consistently (reviewed by Tsai, 1986). In addition, several recent studies have found that autistic girls tend to suffer a greater degree of morbidity; that is, a greater proportion of the autistic females are more often severely impaired than are autistic males (Tsai, 1986). The findings indicate that there are significant sex differences in the occurrence and severity of autism.

SOCIAL CLASS

Kanner (1943) originally indicated that the families of his patients were predominantly of an upper socioeconomic status. A number of studies also had suggested that autistic children tended to come from upper socioeconomic families (reviewed by Tsai et al., 1982). The finding has not been confirmed by other investigators (see Table 20-2). Furthermore, several recent studies have shown that selection bias accounts largely for the previous notion of social class bias in autism (Schopler et al., 1979; Wing, 1980; Tsai et al., 1982). As pointed out by the present author (Tsai et al., 1982), most of the studies showing high social class bias were con-

TABLE 20-2. *Social Class Distribution in Studies of Autistic Children*

Author	No. of subjects	Social class (%)		
		I & II	III	IV & V
Kanner (1943)	11	91	9	0
Creak and Ini (1960)	102	59	31	9
Lotter (1967)	32	44	41	13
Rutter and Lockyer (1967)	63	56	41	3
Ritvo et al. (1971)	74	36	15	49
Campbell et al. (1978a)	99	31	13	56
Schopler et al. (1979)	264	22	17	61
Tsai et al. (1982b)	102	21	18	61

Note: I & II, upper class; III, middle class; IV & V, lower class

TABLE 20-1. *The Prevalence of Autistic Disorder*

Authors	Reported year	Country	Ages	Criteria	Survey population	Prevalence (per 10,000)
Lotter	1966	Great Britain	8–10	Creak	78,000	4.5
Treffert	1970	USA	3–12	Kanner	899,750	0.7
Wing and Gould	1979	Great Britain	5–14	Kanner	35,000	4.9
Hoshino et al.	1982	Japan	0–18	Kanner	609,848	2.3
Ishii and Takahashi	1983	Japan	6–12	DSM-III	34,987	16
McCarthy et al.	1984	Ireland	8–10	Rutter	65,000	4.3
Gillberg	1984	Sweden	4–18	Rutter	128,584	3.9
Steinhausen et al.	1986	Germany	0–15	Rutter	279,616	1.9
Steffenburg and Gillberg	1986	Sweden	0–10	DSM-III	78,413	6.6
Matsuishi et al.	1987	Japan	4–12	DSM-III	32,834	15.5
Bryson et al.	1988	Canada	6–14	DSM-IIIR	20,800	10.1
Cialdella and Mamelle	1989	France	3–9	DSM-III	135,180	4.5
Sugiyama and Abe	1989	Japan	1.5–3	DSM-III	12,263	13
Ritvo et al.	1989	USA	8–12	DSM-III	—	4

ducted before 1970, and those showing no bias were carried out after that date. When the possible effects of parental educational and occupational achievements and patterns of referral were controlled, autistic persons were found in all social classes.

Clinical Features

AGE AT ONSET

Kanner (1943) described the syndrome as beginning shortly after birth. Subsequent observations by other workers, however, have found that in perhaps one-third of the autistic children parents reported a clinical picture indistinguishable from Kanner's original autism, which arose after a period of apparently normal development (up to 2 years of age). Whether early development in these children had been truly normal in all aspects is hard to decide. Subtle signs occurring during the first 2 years of life may be forgotten, overlooked, or denied by parents because of difficulty in recall, anxiety, or lack of knowledge of normal child development.

A few investigators have reported the onset of autistic behavior beginning in the third to fifth year of life. In Rutter and Lockyer's (1967) series of 63 autistic children, 4 had an onset between the ages of 3 and 5^1/$_2$ years. Lotter (1966) found similar histories among the autistic children identified in his survey: 3 of 32 children with a "setback in development" occurring between 3 and 4^1/$_2$ years. Little is known about these cases in terms of etiology and outcome. In the ICD-10 classification, such cases will be described as having "atypical autism." According to ICD-10, all cases of childhood autism should have an onset before age 3 years.

IMPAIRMENTS IN RECIPROCAL SOCIAL INTERACTION

Social deficits were regarded by Kanner to be central to the pathogenesis of autism. In infancy, autistic babies tend to avoid eye contact and demonstrate little conventional interest in the human voice. They do not assume an anticipatory posture or put up their arms to be picked up in the way that normal children do. They are indifferent to affection and seldom show facial responsiveness. As a result, parents often suspect that the child is deaf. In the more intelligent autistic individuals, lack of social responsiveness may not be obvious until well into the second year of life.

In early childhood, autistic children continue to show deviation in eye contact, but they may enjoy a tickle or may passively accept physical contact, such as lap sitting. They do not develop attachment behavior, and there is a relative failure to bond. They generally do not follow their parents around the house. The majority of them do not show normal separation or stranger anxiety. Adults usually are treated as interchangeable, so such children

may approach a stranger almost as readily as they do their parents. There is a lack of interest in being with or playing with other children, or they may even actively avoid other children.

In middle childhood, greater awareness of the attachment to parents and other familiar adults may develop. However, serious social difficulties continue. Such children show a disinterest in playing group games, and there is an inability to form peer relationships. Some of the least handicapped may become passively involved in other children's games or physical play. However, this apparent sociability is usually superficial.

As autistic children grow older, they may become affectionate and friendly with their parents and siblings. However, they seldom initiate social contact and show an apparent lack of positive interest in people. Some of the less severely impaired autistic individuals may have a desire for friendships. But a lack of response to other people's interests and emotions, as well as a lack of appreciation of humor, often results in the autistic youngster saying or doing socially inappropriate things that usually prevents the development of friendships.

IMPAIRMENTS IN COMMUNICATION

IMPAIRMENT IN NONVERBAL COMMUNICATION. Autistic infants show their needs through crying and screaming. In early childhood, they may develop the concrete gesture of pulling adults by the hand to the object that is wanted. This is often done without a socially appropriate facial expression. Nodding and shaking of the head are seldom seen either as a substitute for or as an accompaniment of speech. Autistic children generally do not participate in imitative games. They are less likely than other normal children to copy or follow their parents' activity.

In middle and late childhood, autistic children use gestures infrequently, even when they understand other people's gestures fairly well. A small number of autistic children do develop the stage of imitative play, but this tends to be stereotyped and repetitive actions of their own experience.

Generally speaking, autistic children are able to show their emotions of joy, fear, or anger, but they tend to show only the extreme of emotions. Facial expressions that ordinarily reinforce meaning are usually absent. Some autistic people appear wooden and expressionless much of the time.

IMPAIRMENT IN UNDERSTANDING OF SPEECH. Comprehension of speech is impaired to a varying degree. Severely retarded autistic persons may never develop any awareness of the meaning of speech. Children who are less severely impaired may follow simple instructions if given in an immediate present context or with the aid of gestures. When impairment is mild, only the comprehension of subtle or abstract meanings may be affected. Humor and idiomatic expressions can be confusing for even the brightest autistic person.

IMPAIRMENT IN SPEECH DEVELOPMENT. Many autistic persons have an impaired amount or pattern of babble in their first year. Nearly half of Kanner's subjects (Eisenberg and Kanner, 1956) were still mute by age 5. About half of autistic patients remain mute all their lives (Ricks and Wing, 1976). When speech has developed, it usually exhibits many abnormalities. Meaningless, immediate, and delayed echolalia may be the only kind of speech that is acquired in some autistic individuals. However, while the echolalic speech may be produced quite accurately, the child often has little or no comprehension of the meaning. When echolalia is extreme, distorted syntax and fragmented speech patterns result. Other autistic people may develop appropriate use of phrases copied from others. This is often accompanied by pronoun reversal in the early stages of language development.

Often the mechanical production of speech is impaired. The speech may be like that of a robot, characterized by a monotonous, flat delivery with little lability, change of emphasis, or emotional expression. Some children may use speech primarily for self-stimulatory purpose. Such speech tends to be repetitive in nature, with words, phrases, or sounds being produced over and over without any apparent relation to the environment or ongoing activity (Lovaas et al., 1977). Problems of pronunciation are common in young autistic children, but these tend to diminish with increasing age. There may be a marked contrast between clearly enunciated echolalic speech and poorly pronounced spontaneous speech. There may be chanting or singsong speech, with odd prolongation of sounds, syllables, and words. A question-like intonation may be used for propositional statements. Odd respiratory rhythms may produce staccato speech in some autistic individuals.

Immature and abnormal grammatical constructions are often present in autistic persons' spontaneous speech. Words and phrases may be used idiosyncratically, or phrases may be telegraphic and distorted. Words of similar sound or related meaning may be muddled. They may label objects by their use or else coin words of their own. Prepositions, conjunctions, and pronouns are often dropped from phrases or used incorrectly.

When functional speech develops, it tends not to be used in the usual way for social communication. Usually autistic people rely on stereotyped phrases and repetition when they talk. Their speech almost always fails to convey imagination, abstraction, or subtle emotion. They are generally poor in talking about anything outside the immediate context. They tend to talk excessively about their special interests, and the same pieces of information tend to recur whenever the same subject is raised. The most advanced autistic persons may be able to exchange concrete pieces of information that interest them, but once the conversation departs from this level, they become lost and may withdraw from social contact. In general, the ordinary to-and-fro chatter of a reciprocal interaction is lacking. Thus they give the impression of talking "to" someone rather than "with" someone.

UNUSUAL PATTERNS OF BEHAVIOR

Autistic children's unusual responses to their environment may take several forms. All the items of behavior mentioned in this section are common in autistic children, but a single child seldom shows all the features at one time.

RESISTANCE TO CHANGE. Autistic children are disturbed by changes in the familiar environment, and tantrums may follow even a minor change of everyday routine. Many autistic children line up toys or objects and become very distressed if these are disturbed. The behavior is twice as common in retarded autistic children as in autistic youngsters with normal intelligence (Bartak and Rutter, 1976). Almost all autistic children show a resistance to learning or practicing a new activity.

RITUALISTIC OR COMPULSIVE BEHAVIORS. Ritualistic or compulsive behaviors usually involve rigid routines (e.g., insistence on eating particular foods) or stereotyped, repetitive motor acts, such as hand clapping or finger mannerisms (e.g., twisting, flicking movements carried out near the face). Some children develop preoccupations, such as spending a great deal of time memorizing weather information, state capitals, or birth dates of family members. In adolescence, some of these behaviors may develop into obsessional symptoms (e.g., repeatedly asking the same question, which must be answered in a specific manner) and compulsive behaviors (e.g., compulsive touching of certain objects). Ritualistic or compulsive behaviors are more often displayed by normally intelligent autistics than by retarded autistics (Bartak and Rutter, 1976).

ABNORMAL ATTACHMENTS. Many autistic children develop intense attachments to odd objects, such as pipe cleaners, small plastic toys, etc. The child may carry the object at all times and protest or throw tantrums if it is being removed, but if the object is not eventually returned to the child, a new object is frequently chosen.

UNUSUAL RESPONSES TO SENSORY EXPERIENCES. There may be a fascination with lights, patterns, sounds, spinning objects, and tactile sensations. Objects often are manipulated without regard for their usual functions. Thus young autistic children may perseveratively line up, stack, or twirl objects. They may repetitively flush toilets or turn on and off light switches. There may be a perseverative preoccupation with certain features of objects, such as their texture, taste, smell, color, or shape. There often is either an underresponsiveness or an overresponsiveness to sensory stimuli. Thus they may be suspected of being deaf, short-sighted, or blind. Autistic children may actively avoid gentle physical contact but react with intense pleasure to rough games. Some autistic children may follow extreme food fads.

DISTURBANCE OF MOTILITY

The typical motor milestones may be delayed but are often within normal range. Young autistic children usually have difficulties with motor imitation, especially when they have to learn by watching and the movements have to be reversed in direction. Many young autistic children are markedly overactive but tend to become underactive in adolescence. The autistic child often displays grimacing, hand flapping or twisting, toe walking, lunging, jumping, darting or pacing, body rocking and swaying, and head rolling or banging. These movements do not appear to be involuntary. In some cases they may appear intermittently, whereas in other cases they are continuously present. They are usually interrupted by episodes of immobility and odd posturing with head bowed and arms flexed at the elbow. Many children exhibit body-tensing movements when they are excited about or absorbed in some sensory experience, such as watching a spinning toy.

INTELLIGENCE AND COGNITIVE DEFICITS

Most autistic children are mentally retarded (Rutter, 1978). About 40 to 60 percent of autistic children have an IQ below 50; only 20 to 30 percent have an IQ of 70 or more. Because a significant number of autistic children are either without functional speech or untestable, the validity of testing intelligence in autistic children is questionable. Several observations argue against the notion that autism masks the intellectual potential of autistic children. First, Hingtgen and Churchill (1971) showed that low IQ scores are not a function of poor motivation because even when motivation was greatly increased through operant techniques, intellectual performance still remained well below normal. Second, both short-term (Alpern and Kimberlin, 1970) and long-term studies (Lockyer and Rutter, 1969) have shown that autistic children who failed to score on IQ tests do so because they are severely retarded, not because of an unwillingness to attempt the tasks. Third, a number of autistic children had major improvements in autism during the follow-up period, but there was no change in IQ (Lockyer and Rutter, 1969). Fourth, follow-up studies have shown that retardation present at the time of initial diagnosis tends to persist (Freeman et al., 1985).

Although both low-IQ and high-IQ autistic children are similar in terms of the main symptoms associated with autism, those with a low IQ show a more severely impaired social development and are more likely to display deviant social responses, such as touching or smelling people, stereotypies, and self-injury (Bartak and Rutter, 1976). A third of mentally retarded autistic youngsters develop a sei-

zure disorder; this condition is less prevalent in those of normal intelligence (Rutter, 1978). The prognosis is both worse and different for low-IQ autistics (Rutter, 1970). As the difference in outcome according to IQ is so marked, it is essential to obtain an accurate assessment of intelligence during the initial evaluation of every autistic child.

Earlier studies (Creak et al., 1961) suggested that the retardation accompanying autism is differentiated from general retardation by islets of normal or near-normal intellectual function, revealed particularly on performance tests or in special abilities of the idiot savant kind. Kanner (1943) noted the excellent rote memories of autistic children. The most common areas of special skill tend to be musical, mechanical, and mathematical abilities. Rutter and Lockyer (1967) noted that in contrast to a clinic control group matched for IQ, autistic children were generally superior on the subtests requiring manipulative or visuospatial skills or immediate memory, while they did poorly on tasks demanding symbolic or abstract thought and sequential logic. Other studies have shown that cognition in autistic children is impaired, most particularly in capacity for imitation, comprehension of spoken words and gestures, flexibility, inventiveness, rule information and application, and information utilization. The impairment is both more severe and more extensive than in nonautistic children of comparable IQ (reviewed by Werry, 1979). On the other hand, mentally retarded autistic children tend to have a wider cognitive deficit that involves general difficulties in sequencing and feature extraction, whereas in normally intelligent autistic children the deficits mainly affect verbal and coding skills (Rutter, 1977).

ASSOCIATED FEATURES

The affective expression of autistic persons may be flattened, excessive, or inappropriate to the situation. Their mood often is labile; sobbing, crying, or screaming may be unexplained or inconsolable; hysterical laughing and giggling may occur for no obvious reason. Real dangers, such as moving vehicles or heights, may not be appreciated by a young autistic child, but the same child may be terrified of harmless objects or situations, such as a stuffed animal or visiting a relative's house. Peculiar habits, such as hair pulling or biting parts of the body, are sometimes present, particularly in mentally retarded autistic children. Lack of dizziness after spinning has often been observed, and some autistic children love to spin themselves for long periods. Epilepsy has been noted in between one-quarter and one-third of autistic persons. Several reports have suggested that many autistic individuals develop first seizures in adolescence (Deykin and MacMahon, 1979; Rutter, 1984). Recently, Volkmar and Nelson (1990) reported that risk for developing seizures in the autistic subjects is highest during early childhood. The seizure types are varied. However, the most common type is the generalized, major motor (tonic-clonic) seizure.

Clinical Course and Prognosis

The general picture is of a disorder with a chronic course. Although social, conceptual, linguistic, and obsessive difficulties frequently persist, they do so in forms that are rather different from those shown in early years. A small number of autistic children (7 of 64 cases) in Rutter and Lockyer's (1967) study showed a progressive deterioration in adolescence, characterized by a general intellectual decline. Between 7 and 28 percent of autistic children who had shown no clinical evidence of neurologic disorder in early childhood developed seizures for the first time in adolescence or early adult life. The seizures are usually major in type but tend to occur infrequently (Rutter, 1977).

During adolescence, hyperactivity is often replaced by marked underactivity and lack of initiative and drive. Some autistics may have increased anxiety and tension. There may be inappropriate sexual curiosity that may lead to socially embarrassing behavior, such as masturbation in public or self-exposure.

In an extensive review of follow-up studies of psychotic children, Lotter (1978) found that between 5 and 17 percent of the autistic children had a good outcome as assessed from a judgment of overall social adjustment; that is, they had a normal or near-normal social life and demonstrated satisfactory functioning at school or work. But even those with a good adjustment generally continued to have difficulties in relationships and some oddities of behavior. Between 1 in 6 and a quarter of the autistics had an intermediate outcome; that is, they had some degree of independence and only minor problems in behavior. But they still needed supervision and could not hold a job. Between 61 and 74 percent had a generally poor outcome, remaining severely handicapped and unable to lead any kind of independent life. Between 39 and 74 percent of the autistic persons were placed in institutions. These studies, however, followed the autistics up to the age of about 30 years only. Obviously, placement depends on age and on local patterns of available services. The effect of age on institutional placement is evident in the study of Rutter and Lockyer (1967); at the first follow-up, 44 percent were so placed; the proportion had risen to 54 percent 6 years later. Nonetheless, the program for the Treatment and Education of Autistic and Related Communication Handicapped Children (Division TEACCH) of the University of North Carolina has demonstrated that when community service is available and provides adequate educational and vocational trainings, only a minority (i.e., 8 percent) of the autistic individuals would be placed in institutions (Schopler et al., 1982).

Three factors were consistently found to be related to outcome: IQ, the presence or absence of speech, and the severity of the disorder (Lotter, 1978). IQ alone predicts best to those with poor outcome. A high nonverbal score with no subsequent language is of no predictive value, whereas if language subsequently does develop, the nonverbal score is a useful guide to later general IQ scores (Rutter, 1970). One additional factor, work–school status, was found to be the best predictor of academic or work performance at follow-up (DeMyer et al., 1973). Four other variables have been reported to be significantly associated with outcome, but the correlations are less strong than the variables already described. These are (1) amount of time spent in school, (2) rating of social maturity, (3) rating of social behavior, and (4) developmental milestones.

Conflicting findings have been reported on a number of variables in relation to outcome. These are sex, brain dysfunction or damage, and the category "untestable" child. Factors that were unrelated to outcome included birth weight, perinatal complications, age of onset, history of a period of normal development before onset, late development of seizures, social class, broken home, family mental illness, and type of treatment.

Differential Diagnosis

In the ICD-10 classification, *atypical autism* is defined as a subtype of PDDs that differs from childhood autism in terms of either age of onset (i.e., at or after age 3 years) or of failing to fulfill all three sets of diagnostic criteria for childhood autism. Many children with atypical autism appeared to be highly anxious and tense, often expressing their confusions and preoccupations in repetitive and stereotypical verbalizations. Although they also had severe impairments in social relatedness, deviant and/or delayed language development, and bizarre and stereotypic behavior, they had some age-appropriate cognitive skills, more social relatedness, and a greater ability to communicate than the children with infantile autism (Rescorla, 1988).

The validity of this diagnostic entity and its relationship to childhood autism and other PDDs remain unclear. It is highly possible that there is great heterogeneity, and it may be further divided into smaller groups in the future.

Asperger syndrome was first described in 1944 by Hans Asperger, a Viennese child psychiatrist. Asperger regarded the syndrome he described as a personality disorder, and he used the term *autistic psychopathy* to describe the syndrome. According to Asperger's observations, individuals with Asperger syndrome usually began to speak at the expected age, as in normal children. A full command of grammar was acquired sooner or later. There might be difficulty in using pronouns correctly. The content of speech was usually abnormal and pedantic and consisted of lengthy disquisitions on favorite subjects. Often a word or phrase was repeated over and over again in a stereotyped fashion. Other features he described were the impairment of a two-way social interaction, totally ignoring demands of the environment, repetitive and stereotyped play, and isolated areas of interests. Asperger believed that the condition was never recognized in infancy and that those with the syndrome had excellent logical abstract thinking and were capable of originality and creativity in chosen fields.

Wing (1981) indicated that half her sample of 34 cases had been slow to talk, that careful questioning often elicited a history of a lack of communication behaviors in infancy, and that the apparent originality and special abilities were best explained by reliance on rote memory skills. Wing suggested that Asperger syndrome be considered as a part of the "autistic continuum." She believes that Asperger syndrome is possibly a mild variant of autism in relatively bright children. This view of Asperger syndrome has received support from several prominent researchers in the field of autism research (Gillberg, 1989; Rutter and Schopler, 1987; Szatmari et al., 1989).

Asperger (1979) disagrees that Asperger syndrome is a variant of autism. He maintains that the two conditions are differentiated by age of onset, speech delay, clinical features, and prognosis. This view has gained some support from Rutter, who recently reassessed this issue and wrote to the DSM-IV Advisors on Pervasive Developmental Disorders, stating, "My own clinical research has been concerned with Asperger's syndrome, and I do think that there might be enough valid data at this point to support this as a valid subtype." He continued, "Our data suggests that children with autism and Asperger's syndrome differ on both early history and outcome. It is this difference on outcome, it seems to me, that would justify the specification of an Asperger's syndrome subgroup in ICD-10" (Rutter, 1989, personal communication).

Neither Asperger nor Wing has offered detailed specific diagnostic criteria for Asperger syndrome, and they both refer to partial or spectrum cases. Both DSM-III and DSM-IIIR schemes consider Asperger syndrome a mild variant of autism and hence offer no specific definition and diagnostic criteria for it. The ICD-10 system considers Asperger syndrome as a distinct subtype of PDDs and defines it as a disorder characterized by the same type of qualitative impairment of reciprocal social interaction and restricted, stereotyped, repetitive repertoire of interests and activities that typifies autism. There is no general delay or retardation in language or in cognitive development.

Specifically, the ICD-10 classification emphasizes "a lack of any clinically significant general delay in language development," whereas other investigators allowed for delay in language development as one of the inclusion criteria for Asperger syndrome. Nonetheless, there is general agreement on the clinical features of the syndrome.

Rett syndrome was originally described by Rett (1966), who reported (in German) his findings in 22 patients. However, it did not gain wide recognition until 1983, when a series of 35 cases from a pooled study of French-Portuguese-Swedish patients was reported in English (Haas, 1988). Rett syndrome is a progressive neurologic disorder, and there is variability of clinical presentation which depends on patient's age and stage of the disease. Hagberg and Witt-Engerstrom (1986) proposed a four-stage model: (1) the early-onset stagnation stage is present between 6 months and 1½ years of age, (2) the rapid developmental regression stage usually appears at 1 to 2 years of age, (3) the pseudostationary stage usually occurs at 3 to 4 years of age but can be delayed and may persist many years or even decades, and (4) the late motor deterioration stage often occurs during school age or early adolescence.

Many investigators reported that "autistic features" developed during rapid developmental regression stage. The features include no sustained interest in persons or objects, stereotypic responses to environmental stimuli, absent or very limited interpersonal contact, manifestation of great anxiety and apparent fear when confronted with an unfamiliar situation or even without evident stimulation, loss of already acquired elements of language, stereotypic hand movements (including especially "hand-washing" movements in front of the mouth or chest and rubbing motions of the hands), and repetitive blows on the teeth, grabbing of the tongue, and other movements. In addition, most patients develop seizures. Some patients have self-abusive behavior such as chewing fingers and slapping face (Trevathan and Moser, 1988). However, the clinical course is quite different, with Rett syndrome progressing from relatively normal development until about 6 months of age to various forms of progressive neurologic impairment that is not seen in autism.

Disintegrative disorders are a group of childhood disorders that roughly fit Heller's account of dementia infantilis (Heller, 1954): a progressive intellectual deterioration with, ultimately, the appearance of neurologic signs. Individuals with disintegrative disorder demonstrate quite remarkable consistency in their clinical features. Characteristically, their general development usually is normal or near normal up to the age of 3 or 4 years. In most instances, without any obvious antecedent illness, these children became anxious, irritable, negativistic, and disobedient, having frequent outbursts of temper without provocation and throwing their toys. In some cases, the disorder develops after measles, encephalitis, or some other clear-cut brain disease that damages the central nervous system (Rutter, 1985). Over the course of a few months, these children had a complete loss of speech and language. There was impoverishment of comprehension of language as well as cognitive function. They lost their social skills, and their interpersonal relationships were impaired. These children became disinterested in the environment. They also developed motor restlessness and stereotyped repetitive movements and mannerism with grimacing and tics. During this regressive period, the children became incontinent and needed to be fed. Functionally, all these children were severely mentally retarded, but in some cases there is retention of "islands" of relatively good abilities in some areas. General physical and neurologic examination usually reveals no abnormal physical signs. After the regression phase, the children are stable for many years. However, they are overactive with poor attention span, isolation, and obsessive behavior. Their comprehension of language is rather limited, as is their expressive language. However, they generally have relatively good motor abilities. The prognosis is usually very poor. In the cases with neurolipoidoses and leukodystrophies, there is progressive deterioration leading to death. In the other instances, the children remain without speech and are severely mentally retarded. They will remain wholly dependent individuals. Thus the patterns of symptomatology and clinical course differ in crucial aspects from autism.

Children with a *developmental language disorder, receptive type,* may show some autistic behavior, especially before age 5 (Wing, 1969). They may develop disturbances in relating and social responses, but they do not manifest the perceptual disturbances (e.g., sensory hyperreactivity or hyporeactivity) that are characteristic of autistic children (Ornitz and Ritvo, 1976). They are much more likely to be able to relate to others by nonverbal gestures and expressions. When they do acquire speech, they also demonstrate communicative intent and emotion, characteristics that are not present in verbal autistic children. Furthermore, children with a receptive language disorder have some imaginative play, which is markedly deficient in autistic children (Bartak et al., 1975). Recently, Cantwell et al. (1989) reported an interim follow-up study of a group of "higher functioning" boys with autism and a control group of boys with severe receptive developmental language disorder. They noted that in middle childhood very few of the autistic boys had good language skills at follow-up, whereas nearly half the language-disorder group were communicating well, a striking difference in view of the initial general similarity.

Courchesne et al. (1989), studied event-related brain potential (ERP) in nonretarded autistic children, children with a receptive developmental language disorder, and normal children. Their findings suggest that higher-functioning autism may be differentiated from receptive developmental language disorder using quantitative neurophysiologic measures.

In recent years a group of children has been identified as having *developmental learning disabilities of the right hemisphere* (Weintraub and Mesulam,

1983) or *social-emotional learning disability* (Baron, 1987). The problems of these children encompass both academic and social spheres, and often present through channels of pediatric neurology or educational psychology. These children usually have at least average intelligence but generally with some academic failure, particularly in arithmetic. Examination usually reveals neurologic and neuropsychologic signs consistent with right hemisphere dysfunction. Most of these children avoid eye contact and lack the gesture and prosody that normally accompany and accentuate speech. They exhibit monotonic and/or exaggerated speech patterns. They also show serious difficulties with interpersonal relationships; an idiosyncratic, concrete, and perseverative style of responding; and deficient processing of nonverbal, visual–spatial stimuli. Some of them cannot express their feelings but appear to be sensitive and aware of the emotions of others.

Unfortunately, neither the DSM-III nor the DSM-IIIR classifications were applied to the children included in the studies (Weintraub and Mesulam, 1983; Baron, 1987). It is unclear whether these children would meet the diagnostic criteria of autism or atypical autism. Baron (1987), however, felt that these children with social-emotional learning disability might in fact be the continuum of Asperger syndrome.

In *general mental retardation*, there are often behavioral abnormalities similar to those seen in autism. Wing (1975) found that about one-quarter of the severely retarded children in one area of London demonstrated a lack of affect, resistance to change, stereotypies, and bizarre responses to sensory input, but few could be called classically autistic. Furthermore, in general mental retardation, generalized delays in development occur across many areas. Some children, especially those with Down syndrome, are quite sociable and can communicate in gesture and mime. Moreover, there are studies in which autistic children were found to be different from matched groups of children with mental retardation. The autistic children made less use of meaning in their memory processes, were impaired in their use of concepts, and were limited in their abilities of coding and categorizing (Schopler, 1966; Hermelin and O'Connor, 1970).

Children with a *congenital peripheral blindness* or *partial sightedness* may show self-stimulation and stereotyped movements like those seen in autism. Blind children, however, usually develop an interest in their environment and do not have disturbances in relating with other people.

Many verbal and higher-functioning autistic people speak more in a familiar than in new or strange environment. Others become mute when they do not know how to respond or answer certain questions. It is not clear whether there is an underlying anxiety disorder, or this is just a part of the autistic disorder (i.e., difficulty in adjusting to new situations). This behavior, however, may cause a diagnostic difficulty with elective mutism. In *elective mutism*, the child refuses to speak in almost all social situations, despite the ability to comprehend spoken language and to speak. The child may communicate by gestures, nodding or shaking the head, or in some cases by monosyllabic or short monotone utterances. The same child talks normally at home with family members. Autistic people retain their characteristic language and speech abnormalities in all situations. Thus the whole pattern of behavior is markedly different in the two conditions.

Bartak and Rutter (1976) noted that about 68 percent of the normally intelligent autistic children had shown rituals. About 80 percent of these children also had "quasi-obsessive behaviors." Difficult adaptation to new situations were found in about 74 percent of these children. Although Mesibov and Shea (1980) describe ritualistic and compulsive behaviors as most intense during middle childhood and tending to decrease during adolescence and adulthood, Rumsey et al., (1985a) reported that stereotyped, repetitive movements were highly prevalent (78 percent) and were directly observable among the higher functioning autistic men they studied. The movement most frequently observed involved the hands or arms with individual finger movement, rotating movements of whole-body rocking and pacing.

Some of these obsessive and/or compulsive symptoms have obvious similarities to those seen in obsessive-compulsive disorder (OCD). It is conceivable that in some higher-functioning autistic people, "quasi-obsessive behaviors" reflect true symptoms of a coexisting OCD. Because of the difficulties in communicating with other people, as well as in showing appropriate affect, autistic individuals do not seem to resist their compulsions or to complain about the compulsive acts or to manifest distress. This raises the possibility that clinicians may hesitate to diagnose superimposed OCD in persons with autism.

On the other hand, in the classic OCD, the developmental history is usually within normal limits. People with an OCD struggle against their compulsions, often develop a dysphoric mood, and become irritable, tense, and depressed. Although their symptoms may interfere with their usual social activities or relationships with others, individuals with an OCD almost always develop and maintain an interest in their environment and do not have deviant social skills in terms of relating with other people.

Compulsive and ritualistic behaviors (e.g., keeping objects neatly arranged and routines unchanged, compulsive touching of people and things nearby, compulsive shouting and swearing, echoing of words, sounds, and actions) that can occur in the syndrome of *Gilles de la Tourette* (or the syndrome of chronic multiple tics) resemble some phenomena occurring in autism. Sometimes separating

symptoms of Tourette syndrome from the symptoms of autism can be difficult. However, the examination of the total behavior pattern and developmental history should make the diagnosis clear. The individuals with Tourette syndrome are aware of their disorder. They are frightened and are distressed because they do not feel that they can control it. They usually do not have significantly delayed and deviant language and speech development, and their tics often have a waxing and waning pattern.

However, some recent studies have described the development of Tourette's syndrome in autistic individuals (Barabas and Matthews, 1983; Burd et al., 1987; Realmuto and Main, 1982). The author also has seen a few such cases. It is unclear how frequently the two disorders might occur coincidentally. It is also uncertain how this finding might be linked to the etiology of the two disorders. This remains one of many areas requiring further investigation.

The relationship between autistic disorder and *schizophrenia* has long been the subject of controversy. There were isolated reports of children originally diagnosed as having autism who later exhibited "schizophrenic symptomatology" (Howells and Guirguis, 1984; Petty et al., 1984). However, a recent study (Howells and Guirguis, 1984) has demonstrated that whether an autistic child develops schizophrenia in adulthood may depend on which set of diagnostic criteria is used. Rutter and Schopler (1987) also question what weight to attach to these reports, since the systematic studies of autistic individuals have not found this transition. They suspect that the "supposed autism to schizophrenia change reflects a broader concept of autism or of schizophrenia or a difference in the interpretation of the odd thinking that is quite common in older autistic individuals" (p. 176).

Most autistic individuals do manifest prodromal or residual symptoms of schizophrenia such as social isolation, impairment in role functioning or grooming, inappropriate affect, and so on. Many higher-functioning autistic people exhibit illogical thinking, incoherence, and poverty in content of speech. Their lack of nonverbal communication may be seen as exhibiting blunt affect. Autistic people's inappropriate laughing or weeping due to inability to comprehend the meaning of events may be interpreted as labile or abnormal affect. Some higher-functioning verbal autistic persons have strange beliefs (e.g., some may believe there is no air in other states), idiosyncratic interests (e.g., spending enormous amount of time studying dinosaurs), or sensory experiences (e.g., seeing other people's faces in the air when alone in the room) bordering on delusions or hallucinations. These symptoms, however, are qualitatively different from those shown in schizophrenic patients. These "schizophrenic symptoms" may be caused by underdevelopment of cognitive and language/speech functions in autistic individuals, whereas the schizophrenic symptoms in schizophrenic patients are a deviance of previously relative normal cognitive and language/speech development. Autistic persons tend to answer "yes" to questions they do not quite understand or tend to literally interpret meanings of words. Often an autistic person may talk or laugh to himself or herself while looking at something the observer cannot identify or having some funny thoughts he or she does not know how to share with the observer. This tends to be interpreted as "listening to voices or seeing visions." Some autistic adolescents or adults continue to have childish fantasies of being an inanimate object, an animal, or a character of a fairy tale, which may be mistaken for "delusions," while the tendency of others to make irrelevant remarks or to talk excessively on their favorite topics may lead to a mistaken diagnosis of "thought disorder."

Nevertheless, individuals with schizophrenia can be differentiated from higher-functioning autistic people on the basis of such factors as age of onset, developmental history, clinical features, and family history. Almost all autistic people have an onset before 5 years, whereas the onset of schizophrenia in childhood is most often during the preadolescent or adolescent period. Eggers (1978) reported that the early development in slightly half the schizophrenic children was unremarkable. While there is no evidence that schizophrenic children diagnosed by DSM-IIIR criteria manifest severe developmental deficits, all autistic people, including those with a higher-functioning disorder, have a history of "pervasive developmental disorder."

Furthermore, there is an increased incidence of schizophrenia in the families of children with schizophrenia but not of autistic disorder (Kolvin et al., 1971). Moreover, a recent study of patterns involving intellectual functioning (WISC-R factor scores) by Asarnow and colleagues (1987) found that schizophrenic and autistic children did not differ significantly on the verbal and perceptual organization factors but that the schizophrenic children had significantly lower scores on the freedom from distraction factor (including attention, short-term memory, visual–motor coordination, speed of responding, and mental arithmetic) than the non-retarded (higher-functioning) autistic children. The only subtest on which the autistic children scored significantly lower than the schizophrenic children was the comprehension subtest.

Although *psychosocial deprivation* is not infrequently mentioned as a possible cause of autistic disorder, no data from systematic studies have yet been presented to support such a view. On the other hand, there are reports of children who had been deprived over several years, resulting in severe retardation of all aspects of development, who then made rapid strides when they were rescued and put in a caring and stimulating environment. They showed no evidence of autistic disorder (Wing,

1976). Thus a careful history and observation of a rapid response to environmental stimulation should differentiate this condition from autistic disorder.

Treatment

The primary aim of medical and psychiatric care of autistic persons is to ensure physical and psychological health. To accomplish this goal, preventive medical care is crucial. Generally speaking, a good preventive health care system should include regular physical checkup to monitor somatic growth, vision, hearing, and blood pressure; administering immunization according to schedule; arranging regular visits to the dentist; and paying attention to diet and hygiene.

The secondary aim is early detection and treatment of the unappealing and irritating behaviors (e.g., hyperactivity, stereotypies, self-injury, aggressiveness) which interfere with or are incompatible with the child's functioning and learning, disturb sleep, result in eating problems, and cause discomfortable medical/dental conditions associated with autistic disorder—hence to improve the quality of life of individuals with autism.

As mentioned earlier, specific biologic markers have not been identified in autistic disorder. Hence, in the absence of an understanding of the causes of autistic disorder, it is not surprising that attempts at treatment have inevitably been haphazard and poorly organized. So far, no single treatment modality has been shown to be effective in *curing* autistic disorder. However, the comprehensive treatment program (comprising parental counseling, behavior modification, and special education in a highly structured environment) has demonstrated significant treatment effect on behavioral symptoms of many individuals with autistic disorder.

Extensive research in behavior therapy since the 1960s has shown that many autistic children can be taught special skills in the areas of social adaptation and cognitive and motor skills. Their maladaptive behavior also can be ameliorated significantly. Lovaas et al. (1976) have reviewed the principles involved in behavior therapy with autistic children. A few points are emphasized here. First, behavior therapy programs should be designed for individual children because autistic children vary greatly in their handicaps and family circumstances. Some treatment approaches that work in certain patients may not work in others. Second, autistic children are handicapped in generalizing from one situation to another, so the skills they have learned in a hospital or school tend not to transfer to the home or other settings. It is crucial in treatment to plan the approach specifically to ensure that the changes in the child's clinical state are being carefully monitored, that the problems in each setting are dealt with, and that steps are taken to encourage generalization of behavior changes. Third, because one of the treatment goals is to promote the child's social development, long-term residential treatment is a definite drawback. A home community–based approach, which trains parents and local special education teachers to carry out behavior therapies, has been instrumental in achieving maximum results (Hemsley et al., 1978).

Parents of autistic children and other caregivers who work with autistic people rarely have any grave concern in terms of accepting the preceding comprehensive treatment approach. However, they often feel uneasy about medical treatment, particularly drug treatment/pharmacotherapy for their autistic children/clients. Such feelings, no doubt, come from past abuses of psychotropic drugs in persons with developmental disabilities. Today, in the eyes of many parents and other caregivers, drug therapy is often seen as a treatment of last resort to be used only when other types of treatment have been unsuccessful. However, there is enough evidence to suggest that certain drugs may be effective as a first-line treatment in other mental disorders, as well as some maladaptive behaviors caused by organic brain disease in the autistic people. In addition, an effective drug will increase the response of these patients to other forms of treatment.

The following clinical conditions in autism and associated psychiatric disorders are potentially drug responsive. In some of the conditions, the administration of certain drugs has been based on well-documented research. However, the efficacy of drug therapy in other conditions requires further research. Here suggestions are made based on the limited clinical and empirical experiences of the present author and a few other investigators, since little research has been done in this area.

In unusual behaviors such as resistance to change, stereotypies or ritualistic/compulsive behaviors, and abnormal attachments, *haloperidol (Haldol)* (at doses ranging from 0.25 to 4.0 mg/day), *clomipramine (Anafranil)* (3 mg/kg per day), or *fluoxetine (Prozac)* (40 to 60 mg/day) should be considered (Anderson et al., 1984; Gordon et al., 1990; Mehlinger et al., 1990; Bregman et al., 1991).

In the cases with severe hyperactivity, attention deficit, and impulsiveness, *Haldol* should be considered in the low- or middle-functioning individuals with or without other neurologic disorders such as seizure disorders, Tourette disorder, etc. *Clonidine (Catapres)* (0.025 to 0.25 mg/day) (Jaselskis et al., 1990; Ghaziuddin et al., 1991) or *imipramine (Tofranil)* should be considered in the patients who do not respond to Haldol or become a Haldol nonresponder. In *high-functioning* individuals without other neurologic disorders, *stimulants* such as *methylphenidate (Ritalin)* should be tried first. *Haldol, Catapres*, and *Tofranil* should be considered in the patients who do not respond to stimulants or in those who have other neurologic disorders. Recently, naltrexone (0.5 to 2.0 mg/kg per day) also has shown selective decreases in hyperactivity in autistic subjects (Herman et al., 1991).

In the autistic patients with ticlike symptoms, *Haldol* or *diphenylbutylpiperidine (Pimozide* or *Orap)* should be tried first because they are more potent than *Catapres*. For treatment of social withdrawal in autistic people, *naltrexone* may be considered (Campbell et al., 1988).

In autistic individuals with a strong family history of unipolar affective illness, tricyclic antidepressants such as *desipramine (Norpramine)* or other antidepressants such as *Prozac* should be considered. *Lithium* may be the drug of choice in patients with a family history of bipolar affective illness.

Some autistic individuals may become aggressive and physically attack other people. Some of the aggressive behaviors may relate to the frustrations of these individuals. Most of the aggressive behaviors, however, do not seem to have any clear cause. They are of great concern because of their more devastating effect. In individuals who exhibit frequent aggressive behaviors and who do not respond to behavioral interventions, *Haldol* may be the drug of choice. *Lithium* and *propranolol* may be considered in patients who fail to respond to Haldol treatment.

Self-injurious behavior, such as head banging; finger, hand, or wrist biting; or face or extremities scratching, may occur in lower-functioning autistic individuals. *Naltrexone* (at doses of 0.5 to 2.0 mg/kg per day) should be the drug of first choice (Campbell et al., 1988; Herman, 1987). *Haldol* (at doses ranging from 0.25 to 4.0 mg/day) may be considered in individuals who do not respond to naltrexone treatment.

Unusual sleeping patterns are common in autistic children. Many autistic children seem to need much less sleep than most normal children. These children tend to keep the whole family awake every night because of their sleep disturbances. Some children develop a completely reversed sleep pattern; that is, they sleep during the day and stay up during the night. *Chloral hydrate* may be the drug of first choice. Some autistic children may respond to antihistamines such as *diphenhydramine* and *hydroxyzine*. In other, more severe cases, tricyclic antidepressants such as *imipramine* may be considered.

In the autistic individuals who develop clear delusions, hallucinations, and bizarre behaviors including catatonia, *Haldol* (in doses ranging from 2 to 16 mg/day) would be the drug of first choice (Pool et al., 1976). Other antipsychotic medications such as *thiothixene (Navan)* and *loxapine (Loxitane)* are the second-line drugs of choice.

In *summary*, the preceding information was developed mainly from autistic children treated with neuroleptics. A great deal of work remains to be done with other drugs, as well as with adolescents and adults with autism. Future research also should put more emphasis on studying the efficacy of combined treatments such as pharmacotherapy with behavioral therapy or group therapy with drug therapy. It is highly unlikely that certain medication(s) can be developed that would be curative for autism.

SCHIZOPHRENIA IN CHILDHOOD

Definition

The term *schizophrenic syndrome of childhood* or its synonym, *childhood schizophrenia,* has a different meaning than the term *schizophrenia in childhood.* The former is a term proposed by the British Working Party (Creak et al., 1961) to apply to a wide spectrum of patients, including autistics, schizophrenics, disintegrative psychotics, and other childhood psychotics. The latter is a term to be applied to children only if clear schizophrenic symptoms, as found in adult schizophrenia, are present. Thus it is clear that data derived from the studies that use childhood schizophrenia diagnostic criteria (most of these studies were conducted before 1970) are not very meaningful because they fail to make any distinction between autism and schizophrenia in childhood.

For the purpose of this chapter, the definition and diagnostic criteria for schizophrenia in childhood are the same as those described in the DSM-IIIR for adult schizophrenia. There are at least three good reasons to do so. First, there is now convincing evidence supporting the view that infantile autism and schizophrenia in childhood are two distinct disorders (Rutter, 1978). Second, it is clear that schizophrenia, as described in adult literature, can begin in childhood (Kolvin, 1971; Vrono, 1974). Third, according to DSM-IIIR, children and adolescents display the same symptoms as do adults diagnosed as schizophrenic (American Psychiatric Association, 1987). Hence the definition and diagnostic criteria of schizophrenia in childhood and adolescence include hallucinations, delusions, incoherence or loosening of associations, catatonic behavior, and affective disturbance during the active phase. Drafts of ICD-10 and DSM-IV diagnostic criteria for schizophrenia have been published.

Etiology

Because schizophrenia in childhood is so similar symptomatically, genetically, and epidemiologically to the adult form, readers are referred to current theories of this disorder. Suffice it to say that most of the theories are now centering on biochemical or neuropathophysiologic abnormalities of genetic origin, triggered in some instances by psychological stress.

Epidemiology

The true incidence of schizophrenia in childhood is unknown. It was suggested that the prevalence of schizophrenia with onset in childhood is 50 times less frequent than that of schizophrenia with onset in adulthood (Karno and Norquist, 1989). Population studies have suggested that the prevalence may be less than 1 per 1000 (reviewed by Werry, 1979). Kydd and Werry (1982) reviewed schizophrenic children admitted as inpatients to a child psychiatric unit in Auckland, New Zealand. They found only 15 cases over a period of 10 years (the at-risk population served by the unit was approximately 130,000). On the other hand, Makita (1966) found that only 3 of the 32 schizophrenics in his study had an onset before age 13 (2 at age 10 and 1 at age 11). Similar findings have been reported by Loranger's (1984) study of the age at first treatment of 100 males and 100 females with a DSM-III diagnosis of schizophrenia. Loranger found that 18 percent of male and 11 percent of female schizophrenics were first treated under 15 years of age.

Kydd and Werry (1982) noted a nearly equal sex ratio (i.e., 8 boys and 7 girls), and Eggers (1978) found a slight female preponderance (i.e., 25 boys and 32 girls) in their respective samples. However, as far as schizophrenic children under 10 years of age are concerned, Kydd and Werry's study, like that of Kolvin (i.e., ratio of 2.7:1) (1971), showed a preponderance of boys. It appears that the age of the child may determine the sex ratio in schizophrenia occurring in childhood.

Although Kydd and Werry (1982) found that the social class distribution of the schizophrenic children's families resembles that of the base population, schizophrenic children probably tend to come from lower social class families, just as adult schizophrenics do (Kolvin et al., 1971; Rutter, 1972). The exception is a study by Russell and associates (1984), in which 54 percent of the subjects came from families of socioeconomic status I and II.

Parents of schizophrenic children often do have psychopathology (e.g., isolation, introversion, neurosis, aggressiveness, suicide, affective disorder) and an increased family prevalence of schizophrenia (Kolvin et al., 1971; Eggers, 1978; Kydd and Werry, 1982).

Clinical Features

The age at onset is most often during the preadolescent or adolescent period, and the condition seldom becomes manifest in children before 9 years of age (Makita 1966; Russell et al., 1989). On the other hand, the onset may be as early as 7 years and, rarely, even before that (Rutter, 1977). There is some evidence suggesting that schizophrenia in males starts at an earlier age than in females (Loranger, 1984). In Loranger's study, by the age of 19 years, 49 percent of males and only 28 percent of females had developed schizophrenia.

Eggers (1978) noted that in the schizophrenic children who had manifested the disorder in or before the tenth year of life, the acute course was less frequent than the chronic. Conversely, in patients with age of onset in the prepubertal phase, the acute type was seen more frequently than the chronic type. On the whole, more than two-thirds of the schizophrenic children had experienced a gradual development of symptoms (Asarnow and Ben-Meir 1988; Green et al., 1984; Kolvin et al., 1971; Kydd and Werry, 1982; Russell et al., 1989). Eggers (1978) noted that in slightly more than half the cases (55 percent), the manifestation of the schizophrenia was preceded by prodromal features, characterized by depressive mood and delusions. The risk of suicide increases during the prodromal phase. Kolvin et al., (1971) observed that almost 90 percent of schizophrenic children had been shy, different, withdrawn, sensitive, or timid before their psychosis developed. Russell et al. (1989) reported that 26 percent of the children displayed autistic-like developmental delays and behavioral abnormalities prior to the onset of schizophrenia. However, the findings were drawn from retrospective review of charts. On the other hand, Eggers (1978) reported that the early development in slightly half the schizophrenic children was unremarkable and that slightly more than half the schizophrenic children had a fair to good adaptive functioning before the first presentation of the disorder.

Nevertheless, obvious psychological precipitating factors (e.g., change to a new school, brief hospitalization, death of a close relative, a disturbed parental relationship) were present in about half the cases (Kolvin et al., 1971; Kydd and Werry, 1982).

Schizophrenic children, although less studied, would appear to be mostly of dull-normal intelligence (Werry, 1979), with IQs ranging from 50 to 125 (Green and Padron-Gayol 1986; Green et al., 1984). They probably tend to exhibit a substantial excess of perinatal, developmental, soft neurologic, and EEG abnormalities as compared with normal children (Werry, 1979). The work of Goldfarb and associates (1972) and that of Kolvin (reviewed by Werry, 1979), suggest that while speech and language difficulties also can be associated with schizophrenia in children, they are more variable, more bizarre, and less related to fundamental defects of the comprehension of language so characteristic of autism.

The symptomatology may be determined by the stage of development. Generally speaking, the clinical picture in younger schizophrenic children is similar to that of hebephrenic schizophrenia in adults. It is characterized by an increasing loss of contact with reality, diminishing of interests, disturbed motility (e.g., stereotypies, peculiar mannerisms, grimacings, bizarre posture), echolalia, neologism, disintegration of speech, moodiness, excessive anxiety, and blunting of affect. Some children become compulsively disinhibited and destructive, defecate or masturbate openly, or injure

themselves. Delusions and hallucinations are uncommon in younger children. The delusional symptoms in younger children often appear in the form of irrational and diffuse fears or even cosmic threats (e.g., "the sun won't come out again"). Delusion of loss of identity or of being poisoned also may be observed, although rarely.

Schizophrenia in later childhood and the prepubertal phase is characterized by more persistent, abstract, and systematized delusions and hallucinations. Hallucinations are the most frequently reported symptoms, and the most frequent type of hallucinations are auditory. Auditory hallucinations were reported in about 80 percent of cases (Russell et al., 1989) and in up to about 94 percent of children aged 13 years or younger (Green and Padron-Gayol, 1986). Nearly half the patients with auditory hallucinations also had bodily or visual hallucinations (Kolvin et al., 1971). Visual hallucinations were reported in about 50 percent of cases (Green and Padron-Gayol, 1986), and they were usually accompanied by auditory hallucinations. Tactile hallucinations were reported in a small percentage of children (Green and Padron-Gayol, 1986; Russell et al., 1989).

In children aged 4 to 13 years, delusions are less frequent than hallucinations. The frequency of delusions ranges from about 44 percent (Green and Padron-Gayol, 1986) to 63 percent (Russell et al., 1989). In general, ideas of reference (Eggers, 1978) and persecutory and somatic delusions (Russell et al., 1989) are the most frequent among the delusions. Thought control and religious delusions were rare, about 3 percent (Russell et al., 1989).

Assessing thought disorder in children is problematic. Nevertheless, disorders of thought association and thought blocking were present in three-fifths of schizophrenic patients with an age of onset in later childhood (Kolvin et al., 1971). More recent studies showed that thought disorder was present in 40 percent (Russell et al., 1989) to 100 percent (Watkins et al., 1988) of schizophrenic children aged 13 years or younger.

Affective disturbance was common in this age group of schizophrenic children, ranging from about 71 percent (Volkmar et al., 1988) to about 84 percent (Green et al., 1984). Eggers (1978) noted that 65 percent of the patients were preoccupied by problems connected with death. During their illness, 25 percent of the patients expressed death thoughts, 15 percent had suicidal intentions without autoaggressive actions, 20 percent attempted suicide, and 5 percent committed suicide. The average time between onset of the disorder and attempted suicide was 8.5 years.

Course and Prognosis

As already mentioned, studies conducted before 1970 are not very meaningful in terms of data on course and prognosis because they made no distinction between groups. Most of the recent work, however, has centered on autistic children. There are few well-documented, long-term outcome studies of schizophrenia in childhood that are based on criteria similar to that of the DSM-III. Eggers (1978) reported a follow-up study of 57 clearly diagnosed schizophrenic children, aged 7 to 13 years at initial evaluation, and admitted between 1925 and 1961 to a West German university psychiatric service. At an average of 15 years after onset of the disorder, 20 percent were rated to be in complete remission, 30 percent had made a very good or good to satisfying social adaptation, and 50 percent had moderate or poor outcome. Kydd and Werry (1982) reported a follow-up study of 10 schizophrenic children, aged 6 to 15 years at first presentation, diagnosed according to the DSM-III criteria. The follow-up interval ranged from 1 to 9 years, with a mean of 4.6 years and a median of 5 years. Forty percent of the patients were found to be in remission at follow-up, and deterioration after the active phase of the illness occurred in only 4 patients. The authors felt that the outcome in schizophrenic children may be more favorable than generally assumed. They also cautioned that better results possibly reflect the brief follow-up interval, as well as the small sample sizes.

On the whole, the best predictors of favorable outcome are later age at onset, a good premorbid adaptive functioning, an above-average intelligence, and the presence of precipitating factors. Factors that are unrelated to outcome include family history of psychiatric disorders, socioeconomic status and intactness of the family, frequency of psychotic episodes, occurrence of cyclothymic phase and prodromal episodes, and patterns of psychopathologic symptoms.

Differential Diagnosis

The differential diagnosis between *autistic disorder* and *schizophrenia* has already been described in detail in an earlier section. Patients with *major depressive disorder* or *bipolar affective disorder* may exhibit hallucinations or delusions (Carlson and Strober, 1978; Chambers et al., 1982). Comprehensive evaluation using a variety of measures is necessary to clarify whether schizophrenic symptoms are present.

Other relatively rare conditions may present problems in differential diagnosis, e.g., acute psychotic-like episodes induced by drugs such as amphetamine, phencyclidine, artane, etc. (e.g., organic delusional syndrome). However, the persistent disorientation or memory impairment strongly suggests an organic delusional disorder.

Treatment

Treatment of children and adolescents with schizophrenia has not been as thoroughly studied as it has with adults. Although there are indications that

pharmacotherapies may prove effective, in daily clinical practice, treatment of these children and adolescents involves a multifaceted approach (i.e., parental counseling, family therapy, behavioral management, cognitive therapy, individual psychotherapy, group psychotherapy, special education, and the use of psychotropic medications). It is up to the physician to employ the various combined treatments as deemed appropriate.

Regarding the use of psychotropic drugs, there is a suggestion that different forms of schizophrenia in children may respond differently to drugs, and when the age at onset is before 15 years, prognosis with drug treatment tends to be poor (Werry, 1982). Winsberg and Yepes (1978) hold that when antipsychotics are used in children, they are useful for behavioral management through sedating effects but are not really controlling the disorder. Kydd and Werry (1982) noted that acute positive symptoms (delusions, hallucinations, thought disorder) seem to respond better to the neuroleptics, but negative symptoms (withdrawal, blunting of affect) less so. They suggest that it may be that the effect of the antipsychotics in well-defined schizophrenic children is the same as in adults. In terms of the average daily dose of psychoactive drugs administered to the schizophrenic children and adolescents, Pool and associates reported the use of 87.5 mg for loxapine and 9.8 mg for Haldol (Pool et al., 1976); Realmuto and associates reported the optimal dosage to be 0.3 mg/kg for thiothixene and 3.3 mg/kg for thioridazine (Realmuto et al., 1984); and Spencer and colleagues suggested low doses (1.5 to 2.5 mg) for Haldol (Spencer et al., 1990).

REFERENCES

Alpern GD, Kimberlin CC: Short intelligence test ranging from infancy levels through childhood levels for use with the retarded. Am J Ment Deficiency 75:65–71, 1970.

American Psychiatric Association: Diagnostic and Statistical Manual of Mental Disorders (DSM-II), 2d ed. Washington, American Psychiatric Association, 1968.

American Psychiatric Association: Diagnostic and Statistical Manual of Mental Disorders (DSM-III), 3d ed. Washington, American Psychiatric Association, 1980.

American Psychiatric Association: Diagnostic and Statistical Manual of Mental Disorders (DSM-IIIR), 3d ed. revised. Washington, American Psychiatric Association, 1987.

Anderson GM, Schlicht KR, Cohen DJ: Two-dimensional high-performance liquid chromatographic determination of 5-hydroxyindoleacetic acid and homovanillic acid in urine. Anal Biochem 144:27–31, 1985.

Anderson GM, Freedman DX, Cohen DJ, et al: Whole blood serotonin in autistic and normal subjects. J Child Psychol Psychiatry 28:85–900, 1987.

Anderson LT, Campbell M, Grega DM, et al: Haloperidol in the treatment of infantile autism: Effects on learning and behavior symptoms. Am J Psychiatry 141:1195–1202, 1984.

Arin DM, Bauman ML, Kemper TL: The distribution of Purkinje cell loss in the cerebellum in autism. Neurology 41(Suppl 1):307, 1991.

Asarnow JR, Ben-Meir S: Children with schizophrenia spectrum and depressive disorders: A comparative study of premorbid adjustment, onset pattern and severity of impairment. J Child Psychol Psychiatry 29:477–488, 1988.

Asarnow RF, Tanguay PE, Bott L, et al: Patterns of intellectual functioning in non-retarded autistic and schizophrenic children. J Child Psychol Psychiatry 28:273–280, 1987.

Asperger H: Die autistischen psychopathen im kindesalter. Arch Psychiatr Nervenkr 117:76–136, 1944.

Asperger H: Problems of infantile autism. Communication 13:45–52, 1979.

August GJ, Stewart MA, Tsai L: The incidence of cognitive disabilities in the siblings of autistic children. Br J Psychiatry 138:416–422, 1981.

Baird TD, August GJ: Familial heterogeneity in infantile autism. J Autism Dev Disord 15:315–321, 1985.

Bakwin H: Early infantile autism. Pediatrics 45:492–497, 1954.

Barabas G, Matthews WS: Coincident infantile autism and Tourette syndrome: A case report. J Dev Pediatr 4:280–281, 1983.

Baron IS: The childhood presentation of social-emotional learning disabilities: On the continuum of Asperger's syndrome. Paper presented at the 15th Annual International Neuropsychological Society Meeting, February, Washington, 1987.

Bartak L, Rutter M: Differences between mentally retarded and normally intelligent autistic children. J Autism Child Schizophr 6:109–120, 1976.

Bartak L, Rutter M, Cox A: A comparative study of infantile autism and specific developmental receptive language disorder: I. The children. Br J Psychiatry 126:127–145, 1975.

Bauman M: Microscopic neuroanatomic abnormalities in autism. Pediatrics 87:791–796, 1991.

Bauman M, Kemper TL: Histoanatomic observations of the brain in early infantile autism. Neurology 35:866–874, 1985.

Bender L: Schizophrenia in childhood—its recognition, description, and treatment. Am J Orthopsychiatry 26:499–506, 1956.

Bernal ME, Miller WH: Electrodermal and cardiac responses of schizophrenic children in sensory stimuli. Psychophysiology 7:155–168, 1970.

Bettelheim B: The Empty Fortress—Infantile Autism and the Birth of the Self. New York, Free Press, 1967.

Bleuler E: Dementia Praecox Oder Gruppe der Schizophrenien. Deutiche, 1911; trans J. Zinkin. New York, International University Press, 1950.

Boullin DJ, Freeman BJ, Geller E, et al: Toward the resolution of conflicting findings. J Autism Dev Disord 12:97–98, 1982.

Bregman J, Volkmar F, Cohen D: Fluoxetine in the treatment of autistic disorder. In Scientific Proceedings of the Annual Meeting of American Academy of Child and Adolescent Psychiatry, 1991, p 52.

Brown WT, Jenkins EC, Cohen IL, et al: Fragile-X and autism: A multicenter survey. Am J Med Genet 23:341–352, 1986.

Bryson SE, Clark BS, Smith IM: First report of Canadian epidemiological study of autistic syndromes. J Child Psychol Psychiatry 29:433–445, 1988.

Burd L, Fisher WW, Kerbeshian J, et al: Is development of Tourette disorder a marker for improvement in patients with autism and other pervasive developmental disorders? J Am Acad Child Adolesc Psychiatry 26:162–165, 1987.

Campbell M: Treatment of childhood and adolescent schizophrenia. In Weiner JM (ed): Psychopharmacology in Childhood and Adolescence. New York, Basic Books, 1977.

Campbell M, Adams P, Perry R, et al: Naltrexone in infantile autism. Psychopharmacol Bull 24:135–139, 1988.

Cantor DS, Thatcher RW, Hrybyk M, Kaye H: Computerized EEG analyses of autistic children. J Autism Dev Disord 16:169–187, 1986.

Cantwell D, Baker L, Rutter M: Family factors. In Rutter M, Shopler E (eds): Autism: A Reappraisal of Concepts and Treatment. New York, Plenum Press, 1978.

Cantwell DP, Baker L, Rutter M, et al: Infantile autism and developmental dysphasia: A comparative follow-up into middle childhood. J Autism Dev Disord 19:19–31, 1989.

Carlson GA, Strober M: Manic-depressive illness in early adolescence. J Am Acad Child Adolesc Psychiatry 17:138–153, 1978.

Chambers WJ, Puig-Antich J, Tabrizi MA, et al: Psychotic symptoms in prepubertal major depressive disorder. Arch Gen Psychiatry 39:921–927, 1982.

Chess S: Follow-up report on autism in congenital rubella. J Autism Dev Disord 7:69–81, 1977.

Cialdella P, Mamelle N: An epidemiological study of infantile autism in a French Department (Rhone): A research note. J Child Psychol Psychiatry 30:165–175, 1989.

Cohen DJ, Caparulo BK, Shaywitz BA, Bowers M: Dopamine and serotonin metabolism in neuropsychiatrically disturbed children: CSF homovanillic acid and 5-hydroxyindoleacetic acid. Arch Gen Psychiatry 34:545–550, 1977.

Courchesne E: A neurophysiological view of autism. In Schopler E, Mesibov GB (eds): Neurobiological Issues in Autism. New York, Plenum Press, 1987.

Courchesne E, Kilman BA, Galambos R, Lincoln AJ: Autism: Processing of novel auditory information assessed by event-related brain potentials. Electroencephalogr Clin Neurophysiol 59:238–248, 1984.

Courchesne E, Lincoln AJ, Kilman BA, Galambos R: Event-related brain potential correlates of the processing of novel visual and auditory information in autism. J Autism Dev Disord 15:55–75, 1985.

Courchesne E, Lincoln AJ, Yeung-Courchesne R, et al: Pathophysiologic findings in nonretarded autism and receptive developmental language disorder. J Autism Dev Disord 19:1–17, 1989.

Courchesne E, Yeung-Courchesne BA, Press GA, et al: Hypoplasia of cerebellar vermal lobules VI and VII in autism. N Engl J Med 318:1349–1354, 1988.

Couteur AL, Trygstad O, Evered C, et al: Infantile autism and urinary excretion of peptides and protein-associated peptide complexes. J Autism Dev Disord 18:181–190, 1988.

Creak M, Pampiglione G: Clinical and EEG studies in a group of 35 psychotic children. Dev Med Child Neurol 11:218–227, 1969.

Creak M, Cameron K, Cowie V, et al: Schizophrenic syndrome in childhood. Br Med J 2:889–890, 1961.

Creasey H, Rumsey J, Schwartz M, et al: Brain morphometry in autistic men as measured by volumetric computed tomography. Arch Neurol 43:669–672, 1986.

Damasio AR, Maurer RG: A neurological model for childhood autism. Arch Neurol 35:777–786, 1978.

Damasio H, Maurer RG, Damasio AR, et al: Computerized tomographic scan findings in patients with autistic behavior. Arch Neurol 37:504–510, 1980.

Darby JC: Neuropathologic aspects of psychosis in children. J Autism Child Schizophr 6:339–352, 1976.

Dawson G, Warrenburg S, Fuller P: Cerebral lateralization in individuals diagnosed as autistic in early childhood. Brain Language 15:353–368, 1982.

Dawson G, Warrenburg S, Fuller P: Hemisphere functioning and motor imitation in autistic persons. Brain Cognition 2:346–354, 1983.

DeMyer M, Barton S, DeMyer W, et al: Prognosis in autism: a follow-up study. J Autism Child Schizophr 3:199–246, 1973.

Despert JL: Some considerations relating to the genesis of autistic behavior in children. Am J Orthopsychiatry 21:335–350, 1951.

Deutsch SI: Rationale for the administration of opioid antagonists in treating infantile autism. Am J Ment Deficiency 90:631–635, 1986.

DeVolder AG, Bol A, Michel C, et al: Cerebral glucose metabolism in autistic children. Acta Neurol Belg 88:75–90, 1988.

Deykin E, MacMahon B: The incidence of seizures among children with autistic symptoms. Am J Psychiatry 126:1310–1312, 1979.

Deykin EY, MacMahon B: Pregnancy, delivery, and neonatal complications among autistic children. Am J Dis Child 134:860–864, 1980.

Eggers C: Course and prognosis of childhood schizophrenia. J Autism Child Schizophr 8:21–36, 1978.

Eisenberg L, Kanner L: Early infantile autism 1943–55. Am J Orthopsychiatry 26:556–566, 1956.

Ekstein R, Wallerstein J: Observations on the psychology of borderline and psychotic children. In Psychoanalytic Study of the Child, vol 9. New York: International University Press, 1954.

Factor DC, Freeman NL, Kardash A: A comparison of DSM-III and DSM-IIIR criteria for autism. J Autism Dev Disord 19: 637–640, 1989.

Fein D, Skoff B, Mirsky AF: Clinical correlates of brainstem dysfunction in autistic children. J Autism Dev Disord 11: 303–315, 1981.

Finegan JA, Quarrington B: Pre-, peri-, and neonatal factors and infantile autism. J Child Psychol Psychiatry 20:119–128, 1979.

Fish B, Ritvo ER: Psychoses of childhood. In Noshpitz JD (ed): Basic Handbook of Child Psychiatry. New York, Basic Books, 1979.

Folstein SE: Genetic aspects of infantile autism. Annu Rev Med 36:415–419, 1985.

Folstein SE, Rutter M: Infantile autism: a genetic study of 21 twin pairs. J Child Psychol Psychiatry 18:297–321, 1977.

Folstein SE, Rutter M: Autism: Familial aggregation and genetic implications. J Autism Dev Disord 18:3–30, 1987.

Freeman BJ, Ritvo ER, Needleman R, et al: The stability of cognitive and linguistic parameters in autism: A five-year prospective study. J Am Acad Child Psychiatry 24:459–464, 1985.

Gaffney G, Tsai L, Kuperman S, et al: Cerebellar structure in autism. Am J Dis Child 141:1330–1332, 1987a.

Gaffney G, Kuperman S, Tsai L, et al: Midsagittal magnetic resonance imaging of autism. Br J Psychiatry 151:831–833, 1987b.

Garber HJ, Ritvo ER: Magnetic resonance imaging of the posterior fossa in autistic adults. Am J Psychiatry 149:245–247, 1992.

Garber HJ, Ritvo ER, Chiu LC, et al: A magnetic resonance imaging study of autism: Normal fourth ventricle size and absence of pathology. Am J Psychiatry 146:532–534, 1989.

Ghaziuddin M, Tsai, LY, Ghaziuddin N: An open trial of clonidine in autism. In Proceedings of the Annual Meeting of American Academy of Child and Adolescent Psychiatry, 1991, p 54.

Gillberg C: Infantile autism and other childhood psychoses in a Swedish urban region: Epidemiological aspects. J Child Psychol Psychiatry 25:35–43, 1984.

Gillberg C: Asperger syndrome in 23 Swedish children. Dev Med Child Neurol 31:520–531, 1989.

Gillberg C, Gillberg IC: Infantile autism: A total population study of reduced optimality in the pre-, peri- and neonatal periods. J Autism Dev Disord 13:153–166, 1983.

Gillberg C, Svendsen P: Childhood psychosis and computed tomographic brain scan findings. J Autism Dev Discord 13: 19–32, 1983.

Gillberg C, Svennerholm L: CSF monoamines in autistic syndromes and other pervasive developmental disorders of early childhood. Br J Psychiatry 151:89–94, 1987.

Gillberg C, Wahlström J: Chromosome abnormalities in infantile autism and other childhood psychoses: A population study of 66 cases. Dev Med Child Neurol 27:293–304, 1985.

Gillberg C, Rosenthall U, Johansson E: Auditory brainstem responses in childhood psychosis. J Autism Dev Disord 13: 181–195, 1983a.

Gillberg C, Svennerholm L, Hamilton-Hellberg C: Childhood psychosis and monoamine metabolite in spinal fluid. J Autism Dev Disord 13:383–396, 1983b.

Gillberg C, Terenius L, Lönnerholm G: Endorphin activity in childhood psychosis. Arch Gen Psychiatry 42:780–783, 1985.

Giller EL Jr, Young JG, Breakfield XO, et al: Monoamine oxidase and catechol-O-methyltransferase activities in cultured fibroblasts and blood cells from children with autism and the Gilles la Tourette syndrome. Psychol Res 2:187–197, 1980.

Gittelman M, Birch G: Childhood schizophrenia: Intellect, neurologic status, perinatal risk, prognosis and family pathology. Arch Gen Psychiatry 17:16–25, 1967.

Goldfarb W, Levy DM, Meyers DI: The mother speaks to her schizophrenic child: Language in childhood schizophrenia. Psychiatry 35:217–226, 1972.

Goldstein M, Mahanand P, Lee J, Coleman M: Dopamine-beta-hydronylase and endogenous total 5-hydroxyindate levels in autistics and controls. In Coleman M. (ed): The Autistic Syndrome. Amsterdam, Elsevier, 1976.

Gordon C, Rapoport J, Hamburger MS, Mannheim G: Differential response of autistic disorder to clomipramine. In Scientific Proceedings of the Annual Meeting of American Academy of Child And Adolescent Psychiatry, 1990, p 48.

Green WH, Padron-Gayol M: Schizophrenic disorder in childhood: Its relationship to DSM-III criteria. In Shagass C, Josiassen RC, Bridger WH, et al (eds): Biological Psychiatry 1985. New York, Elsevier, 1986, pp 1484–1486.

Green WH, Campbell M, Hardesty AS, et al: A comparison of schizophrenic and autistic children. J Am Acad Child Adolesc Psychiatry 23:399–409, 1984.

Haas RH: The history and challenge of Rett syndrome. J Child Neurol 3(suppl):S3–S5, 1988.

Hagberg BA, Witt-Engerstrom I: Rett syndrome: A suggested staging system for describing impairment profile with increasing age toward adolescence. Am J Med Genet 24:47–59, 1986.

Heh CWC, Smith R, Wu J, et al: Position emission tomography of the cerebellum in autism. Am J Psychiatry 146:242–245, 1989.

Heller T: Uber Dementia infantalis. Z Kinderforsch 37:661–667, 1930. Reprinted in Howells JG (ed): Modern Perspectives in International Child Psychiatry. Edinburgh, Oliver & Boyd, 1969.

Hemsley R, Howlin P, Berger M, et al: Treating autistic children in a family context. In Rutter M, Schopler E (eds): Autism: A Reappraisal of Concepts and Treatment. New York, Plenum Press, 1978.

Herman BH, Asleson GS, Borghese IF, et al: Acute naltrexone in autism: Selective decreases in hyperactivity. In Proceedings of the Annual Meeting of American Academy of Child and Adolescent Psychiatry, 1991, p 52.

Herman BH, Hammock MK, Arthur-Smith A, et al: Naltrexone decrease self-injurious behavior. Ann Neurol 22:550–552, 1987.

Hermelin B, O'Connor N: Measures of the occipital alpha rhythm in normal, subnormal and autistic children. Br J Psychiatry 114:603–610, 1968.

Hermelin B, O'Connor N: Psychological Experiments with Autistic Children. Oxford, Pergamon Press, 1970.

Hertzig ME, Snow ME, New E, et al: DSM-III and DSM-IIIR diagnosis of autism and pervasive developmental disorder in nursery school children. J Am Acad Child Adolesc Psychiatry 29:123–126, 1990.

Hier DE, LeMay M, Rosenberger PB: Autism and unfavorable left-right asymmetrics of the brain. J Autism Dev Disord 9:153–159, 1979.

Hingtgen JN, Churchill DW: Differential effects of behavior modification in four mute autistic boys. In Churchill DW, Alpern CD, DeMyer M (eds): Infantile Autism. Springfield, IL, Charles C Thomas, 1971.

Hoshino Y, Kumashiro H, Yshima Y, et al: The epidemiological study of autism in Fukushima-Ken. Folia Psychiatr Neurol Jpn 36:115–124, 1982.

Howells JG, Guirguis WR: Childhood schizophrenia 20 years later. Arch Gen Psychiatry 41:123–128, 1984.

Hutt C, Forrest SJ, Richer J: Cardiac arrhythmia and behavior in autistic children. Acta Psychiat Scand 51:361–372, 1975.

Hutt S, Hutt C, Lee D, Ounsted C: A behavioral and electroencephalographic study of autistic children. J Psychiat Res 3:181–197, 1965.

Ishii T, Takahashi O: The epidemiology of autistic children in Toyota, Japan: Prevalence. Jpn J Child Adolesc Psychiatry 24:311–321, 1983.

Jaselskis CA., Cook EH, Leventhal BL: Clonidine treatment of hyperactive and impulsive children with autistic disorder. In Scientific Proceedings of the Annual Meeting of American Academy of Child And Adolescent Psychiatry, 1990, pp 46–47.

Kanner L: Autistic disturbances of affective contact. Nerv Child 2:217–250, 1943.

Karno M, Norquist GS: Schizophrenia: Epidemiology. In Kaplan HI, Sadock BJ (eds): Comprehensive Textbook of Psychiatry V, vol 1. Baltimore, Williams & Wilkins, 1989, pp 699–705.

Katsui T, Okuda M, Usuda S, Koizumi T: Kinetics of H-serotonin uptake by platelets in infantile autism and developmental language disorder (including five pairs of twins). J Austism Dev Disord 16:69–76, 1986.

Katz RM, Liebman W: Creatine phosphokinase activity in central nervous system disorders and infections. Am J Dis Child 120:543–546, 1970.

Kemper TL: Neuropathology of infantile autism. In Program and Abstract of Conference on Neurobiology of Infantile Autism, a satellite meeting of the 5th International Child Neurology Congress, Tokyo, Japan, November 1990.

Knoblock H, Pasamanick B: Some etiologic and prognostic factors in early infantile autism and psychosis. Pediatrics 55: 182–191, 1975.

Kolvin I: Psychoses in childhood—A comparative study. In Rutter M (ed): Infantile Autism: Concepts, Characteristics and Treatment. London, Churchill Livingston, 1971.

Kolvin I, Ounsted C, Humphrey M, et al: Six studies in the childhood psychoses. Br J Psychiatry 118:381–419, 1971.

Kydd RR, Werry JS: Schizophrenia in children under 16 years. J Autism Dev Disord 12:343–357, 1982.

Lake R, Ziegler MG, Murphy DL: Increased norepinephrine levels and decreased DBH activity in primary autism. Arch Gen Psychiatry 35:553–556, 1977.

Launay JM, Bursztejn C, Ferrari P, et al: Catecholamine metabolism in infantile autism: A controlled study of 22 autistic children. J Autism Dev Disord 17:333–347, 1987.

Lawlor, BA, Maurer RG: Tuberous sclerosis and the autistic syndrome. Br J Psychiatry 150:396–397, 1987.

Leckman JF, Cohen DJ, Shaywitz BA, et al: CSF monoamine metabolites in child and adult psychiatric patients. Arch Gen Psychiatry 37:677–681, 1980.

Le Couteur A, Bailey AJ, Rutter M, Gottesman I: An epidemiologically based twin study of autism. Paper given at the First World Congress on Psychiatric Genetics, Churchill College, Cambridge, August 3–5, 1989.

Lelord G, Laffont F, Jusseaume P, Stephant JL: Comparative study of conditioning of averaged evoked responses by coupling sound and light in normal and autistic children. Psychophysiology 10:415–425, 1973.

Levitas A, McBogg P, Hagerman R: Behavioral dysfunctions in the fragile X syndrome. In Hagerman R, McBogg P (eds): The Fragile X Syndrome: Diagnosis, Biochemistry and Intervention. Dillon, CO, Spectra Publications, 1983.

Lockyer L, Rutter M: A five to fifteen year follow-up study of infantile psychosis: III. Psychological aspects. Br J Psychiatry 115:865–882, 1969.

Loranger AW: Sex difference in age at onset of schizophrenia. Arch Gen Psychiatry 41:157–161, 1984.

Lotter V: Epidemiology of autistic conditions in young children: I. Prevalence. Soc Psychiatry 1:124–137, 1966.

Lotter V: Follow-up studies. In Rutter M, Schopler E (eds): Autism: A Reappraisal of Concepts and Treatment. New York, Plenum Press, 1978.

Lovaas OL, Schreibment L, Koegel RL: A behavior modification approach to the treatment of autistic children. In Schopler E, Reichler RJ (eds): Psychopathology and Child Development. New York, Plenum Press, 1976.

Lovaas OL, Varni J, Koegel RL, et al: Some observations on the nonextinguishability of children's speech. Child Dev 48: 1121–1127, 1977.

Macdonald H, Rutter M, Rios P, Bolton P: Cognitive and social abnormalities in the siblings of autistic and Down's syndrome probands. Paper given at the First Word Congress on Psychiatric Genetics; Churchill College, Cambridge, August 3–5, 1989.

Mahler M: On child psychosis and schizophrenia. In Autistic and Symbiotic Psychoses: Psychoanalytic Study of the Child, vol 7. New York, International University Press, 1952.

Makita K: The age of onset of childhood schizophrenia. Folia Psychiatr Neurol Jpn 20:111–121, 1966.

Mason-Brothers A, Ritvo E, Guze B, et al: Pre-, peri-, and postnatal factors in 1981 autistic patients from single and multiple incidence families. J Am Acad Child Adolesc Psychiatry 26:39–42, 1987.

Matsuishi T, Shiotsuki Y, Yoshimura K, et al: High prevalence of infantile autism in Kurume City, Japan. J Child Neurol 2:268–271, 1987.

McCarthy P, Fitzgerald M, Smith MA: Prevalence of childhood autism in Ireland. Irish Med J 77:129–130, 1984.

Mehlinger R, Scheftner WA, Poznanski E: Fluoxetine and autism. J Am Acad Child Adolesc Psychiatry 29:985, 1990.

Mesibov GB, Shea V: Social and interpersonal problems of autistic adolescents and adults. Paper presented at the meeting of the Southeastern Psychological Association, Washington, March 1980.

Meyers D, Goldfarb W: Studies of perplexity in mothers of schizophrenic children. Am J Orthopsychiatry 3:551–564, 1961.

Minderaa RB, Anderson GM, Volkmar FR, et al: Neurochemical study of dopamine functioning in autistic and normal subjects. J Am Acad Child Adolesc Psychiatry 28:190–194, 1989.

Minderaa RB, Anderson GM, Volkmar FR, et al: Urine 5-hydroxyindoleacetic acid, whole blood serotonin and tryptophan in autistic and normal subjects. Biol Psychiatry 22:933–940, 1987.

Minshew NJ, Payton JB, Wolf GL, et al: H NMR imaging of autistics: Implication for neurobiology. Ann Neurol 20:417, 1986.

Minton J, Campbell M, Green WH, et al: Cognitive assessment of siblings of autistic children. J Am Acad Child Adolesc Psychiatry 21:256–261, 1982.

Ogawa T, Sugiyama A, Ishiwa S, et al: Ontogenic development of EEG asymmetry in early infantile autism. Brain Dev 4:439–449, 1982.

Ornitz EM: Dreaming sleep in autistic twins. Arch Gen Psychiatry 12:77–79, 1965.

Ornitz EM: The modulation of sensory input and motor output in autistic children. J Autism Dev Disord 4:197–215, 1974.

Ornitz EM: The functional neuroanatomy of infantile autism. Int J Neurosci 19:85–124, 1983.

Ornitz EM: Neurophysiology of infantile autism. J Am Acad Child Adolesc Psychiatry 24:251–262, 1985.

Ornitz EM, Ritvo ER: The syndrome of autism: A critical review. Am J Psychiatry 133:609–621, 1976.

Payton JB, Steele MW, Wenger SL, Minshaw NJ: The fragile X marker in perspective. J Am Acad Child Adolesc Psychiatry 28:417–421, 1989.

Petty LK, Ornitz EM, Michelman JD, et al: Autistic children who become schizophrenic. Arch Gen Psychiatry 41:129–135, 1984.

Piven J, Berthier ML, Starkstein SE, et al: Magnetic resonance imaging evidence for a defect of cerebral cortical development in autism. Am J Psychiatry 147:734–739, 1990a.

Piven J, Gayle J, Chase G, et al: A family history of neuropsychiatric disorders in adult siblings of autistic individuals. J Am Acad Child Adolesc Psychiatry 29:177–183, 1990b.

Piven J, Gayle J, Landa R, et al: The prevalence of fragile X in a sample of autistic individuals diagnosed using a standardized interview. 30:825–830, 1991.

Pool D, Bloom W, Mielke DH, et al: A controlled evaluation of loxitane in seventy-five adolescent schizophrenic patients. Curr Ther Res 19:99–104, 1976.

Prior MR: Cognitive abilities and disabilities in infantile autism: A review. J Abnorm Child Psychol 7:357–380, 1979.

Prior MR, Tress B, Hoffman WL, et al: Computed tomographic study of children with classic autism. Arch Neurol 41: 482–484, 1984.

Realmuto GM, Main B: Coincidence of Tourette's disorder and infantile autism. J Autism Dev Disord 12, 367–372, 1982.

Realmuto GM, Erickson WD, Yellin AM, et al: Clinical comparison of thiothixene and thioridazine in schizophrenic adolescent patients. Am J Psychiatry 141:440–442, 1984.

Reiser DE: Psychosis of infancy and early childhood, as manifested by children with atypical development, part I. N Engl J Med 269:790–798, 1963a.

Reiser DE: Psychosis of infancy and early childhood, as manifested by children with atypical development, part II. N Engl J Med 269:844–850, 1963b.

Rescorla L: Cluster analytic identification of autistic preschoolers. J Autism Dev Disord 18:475–492, 1988.

Rett A: Ueber ein cerebral-atrophisches syndrome bei hyperammonamie. Vienna, Bruder Hollinek, 1966.

Ricks DM, Wing L: Language communication and the use of symbols. In Wing L (ed): Early Childhood Autism. Oxford, Pergamon Press, 1976, pp 93–134.

Ritvo ER, Freeman BJ: Current research in the syndrome of autism: Introduction—The National Society of Autistic Children's definition of the syndrome of autism. J Am Acad Child Adolesc Psychiatry 17:565–575, 1978.

Ritvo ER, Mason-Brothers A, Freeman BJ: Eleven possibly autistic parents. J Autism Dev Disord 18:139–143, 1988.

Ritvo ER, Freeman BJ, Mason-Brothers A, et al: Concordance for the syndrome of autism in 40 pairs of afflicted twins. Am J Psychiatry 142:74–77, 1985a.

Ritvo ER, Freeman BJ, Pingree C, et al: The UCLA–University of Utah epidemiologic survey of autism: Prevalence. Am J Psychiatry 146:194–196, 1989.

Ritvo ER, Freeman BJ, Scheibel AB, et al: Lower Purkinje cell counts in the cerebella of four autistic subjects: Initial findings of the UCLA–NSAC autopsy research report. Am J Psychiatry 143:862–866, 1986.

Ritvo ER, Ornitz EM, Evitar A, et al: Decreased postrotatory nystagmus in early infantile autism. Neurology 19:653–658, 1969.

Ritvo ER, Spence A, Freeman BJ, et al: Evidence of autosomal recessive inheritance in 46 families with multiple incidences of autism. Am J Psychiatry 142:187–192, 1985b.

Rosenbloom S, Campbell M, George AE, et al: High-resolution CT scanning in infantile autism: a quantitative approach. J Am Acad Child Adolesc Psychiatry 1:72–77, 1984.

Rosenblum SM, Arick JR, Krug DA, et al: Auditory brainstem evoked responses in autistic children. J Autism Dev Disord 10:215–225, 1980.

Rotman A, Caplan R, Szekeley GA: Platelet uptake of serotonin in psychotic children. Psychopharmacology 67:245–248, 1980.

Rumsey JM, Rapoport JL, Sceery WR: Autistic children as adults: Psychiatric, social and behavioral outcomes. J Am Acad Child Adolesc Psychiatry 24:465–473, 1985a.

Rumsey JM, Creasy H, Stepanek JS, et al: Hemispheric asymmetries, fourth ventricular size, and cerebellar morphology in autism. J Autism Dev Disord 18:127–137, 1988.

Rumsey JM, Duara R, Grady C, et al: Brain metabolism in autism: Resting cerebral glucose utilization rates measured with positron emission tomography. Arch Gen Psychiatry 42:448–455, 1985b.

Rumsey TM, Grimes AM, Pikus AM, et al. Auditory brainstem responses in pervasive developmental disorders. Biol Psychiatry 19:1403–1418, 1984.

Russell AT, Bott L, Sammons C: The phenomenology of schizophrenia occurring in childhood. J Am Acad Child Adolesc Psychiatry 28:399–407, 1989.

Rutter M: Psychotic disorders in early childhood. Br J Psychiatry 1:133–158, 1967.

Rutter M: Concepts of autism: a review of research. J Child Psychol Psychiatry 9:1–25, 1968.

Rutter M: Autistic children: Infancy to adulthood. Semin Psychiatry 2:435–450, 1970.

Rutter M: Childhood schizophrenia reconsidered. J Autism Child Schizophr 2:315–337, 1972.

Rutter M: Infantile autism and other child psychoses. In Rutter M, Henson L (eds): Child Psychiatry: Modern Approach. Oxford, Blackwell, 1977.

Rutter M: Diagnosis and definition. In Rutter M, Schopler E (eds): Autism—A Reappraisal of Concepts and Treatment. New York, Plenum Press, 1978.

Rutter M: Autistic children growing up. Dev Med Child Neurol 26:122–129, 1984.

Rutter M: Infantile autism and other pervasive developmental disorder. In Rutter M, Hersov L (eds): Child and Adolescent Psychiatry. London, Blackwell, 1985.

Rutter M: Autism as a genetic disorder. In McGuffin P (ed): The New Genetics of Mental Illness. London, Heinemann Medical, 1990.

Rutter M, Lockyer L: A five to fifteen year follow-up study of infantile psychosis: Description of sample. Br J Psychiatry 113:1169–1182, 1967.

Rutter M, Schopler E: Autism and pervasive developmental disorders: concept and diagnostic issues. J Autism Dev Disord 17:159–186, 1987.

Sankar DV: Studies on blood platelets, blood enzymes, and leukocyte chromosome breakage in childhood schizophrenia. Behav Neuropsychiatry 2:2–10, 1971.

Schopler E: Visual versus tactual receptor preference in normal and schizophrenic children. J Abnormal Psychol 71:108–114, 1966.

Schopler E, Andrews CE, Strupp K: Do autistic children come from upper-middle class parents? J Autism Dev Disord 9:139–152, 1979.

Schopler E, Mesibov GB, Baker A: Evaluation of treatment for autistic children and their parents. J Am Acad Child Adolesc Psychiatry 21:262–267, 1982.

Skoff BF, Mirsky A, Turner D: Prolonged brainstem transmission time in autism. Psychiatry Res 2:157–166, 1980.

Small JG: EEG and neurophysiological studies of early infantile autism. Biol Psychiatry 10:385–397, 1975.

Smalley SL, Asarnow RF, Spence MA: Autism and genetics: A decade of research. Arch Gen Psychiatry 45:953–961, 1988.

Spence MA, Ritvo ER, Marazita ML, et al: Gene mapping studies with the syndrome of autism. Behav Genet 15:1–13, 1985.

Spencer E, Padron-Gayol M, Kafantaris V, et al: Haloperidol in schizophrenic children. In Scientific Proceedings of the Annual Meeting of the American Academy of Child and Adolescent Psychiatry, 1990, pp 64–65.

Steffenburg S, Gillberg C: Autism and autistic-like conditions in Swedish rural and urban area: a population study. Br J Psychiatry 149:81–87, 1986.

Steffenburg S, Gillberg C, Hellgren L, et al: A twin study of autism in Denmark, Finland, Iceland, Norway and Sweden. J Child Psychol Psychiatry 30:405–416, 1989.

Steinhausen HC, Göbel D, Breinlinger M, Wohlleben B: A community survey of infantile autism. J Am Acad Child Adolesc Psychiatry 25:186–189, 1986.

Stubbs EG: Autistic children exhibit understandable hemagglutination-inhibition titers despite previous rubella vaccination. J Autism Child Schizophr 6:269–274, 1976.

Student M, Sohmer H: Evidence from auditory nerve and brainstem evoked responses for an organic brain lesion in children with autistic traits. J Autism Dev Disord 8:13–20, 1978.

Sugiyama T, Abe T: The prevalence of autism in Nagoya, Japan: A total population study. J Autism Dev Disord 19:87–96, 1989.

Szatmari P, Bremner R, Nagy J: Asperger's syndrome: a review of clinical features. Can J Psychiatry 34:554–560, 1989.

Tanguay PE, Edwards RM, Buchwald J, et al: Auditory brainstem evoked responses in autistic children. Arch Gen Psychiatry 39:174–180, 1982.

Tanguay PE, Ornitz EM, Forsythe AB, et al: Rapid eye movement (REM) activity in normal and autistic children during REM sleep. J Autism Child Schizophr 6:275–288, 1976.

Taylor MJ, Rosenblatt B, Linschoten L: Auditory brainstem response abnormalities in autistic children. Can J Neurol Sci 9:429–433, 1982.

Todd RD, Ciaranello RD: Demonstration of inter- and intraspecies differences in serotonin binding sites by antibodies from an autistic child. Proc Natl Acad Sci USA 82:612–616, 1985.

Todd RD, Hickok JM, Anderson GM, et al: Antibrain antibodies in infantile autism. Biol Psychiatry 23:644–647, 1988.

Treffert DA: Epidemiology of infantile autism. Arch Gen Psychiatry 22:431–438, 1970.

Trevathan E, Moser HW: Diagnostic criteria for Rett syndrome. Ann Neurol 23:425–428, 1988.

Trygstad OE, Reichelt KL, Foss I, et al: Patterns of peptides and protein-associated peptide complexes in psychiatric disorders. Br J Psychiatry 136:59–72, 1980.

Tsai LY: Infantile autism and schizophrenia in childhood. In Winokur G, Clayton P (eds): The Medical Basis of Psychiatry. Philadelphia, WB Saunders Co, 1986.

Tsai LY: Pre-, peri, and neonatal factors in autism. In Schopler E, Mesibov GB (eds): Neurobiological Issues in Autism. New York, Plenum Press, 1987.

Tsai LY, Beisler JM: The development of sex differences in infantile autism. Br J Psychiatry 142:273–378, 1983.

Tsai LY, Stewart MA, August G: Implication of sex differences in the familial transmission of infantile autism. J Autism Dev Disord 11:165–173, 1981.

Tsai LY, Crowe RR, Patil SR, et al: Search for DNA markers in two autistic males with the fragile X syndrome. J Autism Dev Disord 18:681–685, 1988.

Tsai LY, Tsai MC: Using EEG diagnosis to subtype autistic syndrome. Proceedings, 1984 International Conference of the Naional Society for Children and Adults with Autism. San Antonio, Texas, July.

Tsai LY, Stewart MA, Faust M, et al: Social class distribution of fathers and children enrolled in the Iowa autism program. J Autism Dev Disord 12:211–222, 1982.

US Department of Health and Human Services: International Classification of Disease, 9th revision: Clinical Modification. Washington, US Department of Health and Human Services, 1980.

Van Krevelen DA: Early infantile autism. Acta Paedopsychiatry 91:81–97, 1952.

Volkmar FR, Bregman J, Cohen DJ, et al: DSM-III and DSM-IIIR diagnosis of autism. Am J Psychiatry 145:1404–1408, 1988.

Volkmar FR, Cohen DJ, Hoshino Y, et al: Phenomenology and classification of the childhood psychoses. Psychol Med 18:191–201, 1988.

Volkmar FR, Nelson DS: Seizure disorders in autism. J Am Acad Child Adolesc Psychiatry 29(1):127–129, 1990.

Vrono M: Schizophrenia in childhood and adolescence. Int J Ment Health 2:7–116, 1974.

Warren RP, Foster A, Margaratten NC: Reduced national killer cell activity in autism. J Am Acad Child Adolesc Psychiatry 26:333–335, 1987.

Warren RP, Margaratten NC, Pace NC, Foster A: Immune abnormalities in patients with autism. J Autism Dev Disord 16:189–197, 1986.

Warren RP, Yonk LJ, Burger RA, et al: Deficiency of suppressor-inducer (CD4 + CD45RA +) T cells in autism. Immunol Invest 19:245–251, 1990.

Watkins JM, Asarnow RF, Tanguay PE: Symptom development in childhood onset schizophrenia. J Child Psychol Psychiatry 29:865–878, 1988.

Weintraub S, Mesulam MM: Developmental learning disabilities of the right hemisphere: Emotional, interpersonal, and cognitive components. Arch Neurol 40:463–468, 1983.

Weizman A, Weizman R, Szekely GA, et al: Abnormal immune response to brain tissue antigen in the syndrome of autism. Am J Psychiatry 139:1462–1465, 1982.

Weizman R, Weizman A, Tyano S, et al: Humoral endorphine blood levels in autistic, schizophrenic and healthy subjects. Psychopharmacology 82:368–370, 1984.

Werry JS: The childhood psychoses. In Quay HC, Werry JS (eds): Psychopathological Disorders of Childhood, 2d ed. New York, Wiley, 1979.

Westall FC, Root-Bernstein RS: Suggested connection between serotonin, and myelin basic protein. Am J Psychiatry 140:1260–1261, 1983.

Williams RS, Hauser SL, Purpura DP, et al: Autism and mental retardation. Arch Neurol 37:749–753, 1980.

Wing L: The handicaps of autistic children—A comparative study. J Child Psychol Psychiatry 10:1–40, 1969.

Wing L: A study of language impairments in severely retarded children. In O'Conner N (ed): Language, Cognitive Deficits and Retardation. London, Butterworths, 1975.

Wing L: Diagnosis, clinical description and prognosis. In Wing L (ed): Early Childhood Autism. Oxford, Pergamon Press, 1976.

Wing L: Childhood autism and social class: A question of selection. Br J Psychiatry 137:410–417, 1980.

Wing L: Asperger's syndrome: A clinical account. Psychol Med 11:115–129, 1981.

Wing L, Gould J: Severe impairments of social interaction and associated abnormalities in children: Epidemiology and classification. J Autism Dev Disord 9:11–29, 1979.

Wolff S, Barlow A: Schizoid personality in childhood: A comparative study of schizoid, autistic and normal children. J Child Psychol Psychiatry 20:19–46, 1979.

Wolff S, Chick J: Schizoid personality in child hood: A controlled follow-up study. Psychol Med 10:85–100, 1980.

World Health Organization: ICD-10 1988, draft of chapter V: Categories F00–F99, mental behavioral and developmental disorders. Clinical descriptions and diagnostic guidelines. Geneva: World Health Organization, 1988.

Young JG, Caparulo BK, Shaywitz BA, et al: Childhood autism: Cerebrospinal fluid examination and immunoglobulin levels. J Child Psychiatry 16:174–179, 1977.

Young JG, Kavanagh ME, Anderson GM, et al: Clinical neurochemistry of autism and associated disorders. J Autism Dev Disord 12:147–165, 1982.

Young JG, Kyprie RM, Ross NT, et al: Serum dopamine-beta-hydroxylase activity: Clinical applications in child psychiatry. J Autism Dev Disord 10:1–14, 1980.

CHAPTER 21

Anxiety, Phobia, and Obsessive Disorders in Children

GAIL A. BERNSTEIN

Recent epidemiologic studies document that anxiety disorders are one of the most prevalent categories of childhood and adolescent psychopathology. The research investigations into childhood anxiety disorders have lagged behind the research into adult anxiety disorders. However, the number and quality of studies providing data about these disorders are rapidly increasing. Currently, this is a topic of high interest.

The anxiety disorders are separated into two different sections of the DSM-IIIR manual. The anxiety disorders section contains criteria for panic disorder, agoraphobia, social phobia, simple phobia, obsessive-compulsive disorder, post-traumatic stress disorder, generalized anxiety disorder, and anxiety disorder not otherwise specified. All these diagnoses can be applied to children, adolescents, and adults. In addition, there is a section for the anxiety disorders of childhood and adolescence, including separation anxiety disorder, overanxious disorder, and avoidant disorder. This chapter begins with the latter group of disorders but in addition reviews fears and simple phobias and obsessive-compulsive disorder in children.

DEFINITION

The primary feature of separation anxiety disorder is excessive anxiety about separation from attachment figures and anxiety about leaving home and familiar surroundings. The separation reactions are marked, beyond that expected for the child's stage of development. In some cases, the children's distress at separation approaches panic level (Gittelman-Klein, 1988). Three of the following nine criteria are

needed to make the DSM-IIIR diagnosis. These criteria include unrealistic worry about harm to self during periods of separation, unrealistic worry about harm to attachment figures during separations, school refusal, reluctance to sleep without an attachment figure nearby or to sleep away from home, avoidance of being alone, recurrent nightmares with themes of separation, somatic complaints, signs of distress in anticipation of separation, and distress at the time of separation (American Psychiatric Association, 1987).

The essential feature of overanxious disorder is excessive, generalized anxiety that is not focused on a specific situation or object and is not due to a recent stressor. These children are worriers. Four of the following seven criteria are necessary to make a diagnosis: excessive worry about future events, worry about past behavior, concern about competence, physical complaints, marked self-consciousness, continual need for reassurance, and feelings of tension with the inability to relax (American Psychiatric Association, 1987).

In avoidant disorder of childhood or adolescence, the main criterion is avoidance of contact with unfamiliar persons which is severe enough to interfere with social functioning. However, in addition, there is a desire for social contact with family members and other familiar persons (American Psychiatric Association, 1987). Prior to age 2½ years, this diagnosis is not made because stranger anxiety is a normal developmental phenomenon up to this age. There is overlap in symptoms between

Dr. Bernstein's effort on this chapter was supported in part by Grant R29 MH46534 from the National Institute of Mental Health.

children who meet criteria for social phobia and those who meet criteria for avoidant disorder.

ETIOLOGY

Precipitants and environmental stressors appear to be associated with the manifestation of anxiety symptoms. Children (Kashani et al., 1990) and adolescents (Bernstein et al., 1989) with high levels of anxiety compared with those reporting low levels identify a significantly greater number of psychosocial stressors, as measured on the Life Events Checklist (Johnson and McCutcheon, 1980). In fact, it has been suggested that conditioning by environmental stress is prominent in the development of simple phobias (Sheehan et al., 1981; Thyer et al., 1985).

There is an increasing number of studies demonstrating the familial patterns in anxiety disorders. Several studies indicate that children of adults with anxiety disorders have an increased likelihood of having an anxiety disorder. Weissman and colleagues (1984) demonstrated an elevated rate of separation anxiety disorder in children of mothers with major depression plus panic disorder or agoraphobia compared with children of mothers with major depression only or children of normal mothers. In this study, diagnoses in children were made by family history data rather than by direct interviews of the children, which is a shortcoming of the investigation.

Structured interviews of offspring of adults with anxiety disorder (agoraphobia or obsessive-compulsive disorder), of adults with dysthymia, and of adults with no psychiatric diagnoses were compared with structured interviews of normal children (Turner et al., 1987). There was a sevenfold increased likelihood of having a DSM-IIIR anxiety diagnosis in the children of parents with anxiety disorders when compared with children in the two control groups and a twofold increased likelihood of meeting criteria for an anxiety disorder in the children of parents with dysthymia.

A prospective, longitudinal study of children of adults with panic disorder or agoraphobia and children of normal adults reveals intriguing results (Rosenbaum et al., 1988). This study is important because it identifies an early familial risk factor for childhood anxiety disorders. The offspring of parents with an anxiety disorder are more likely to manifest behavioral inhibition to the unfamiliar (Kagan et al., 1984) than offspring of parents without anxiety disorders (Rosenbaum et al., 1988). *Behavioral inhibition*, a temperamental category, is the tendency to exhibit excessive withdrawal and shyness in unfamiliar situations.

Stable behavioral inhibition appears to be a marker for the later development of childhood anxiety disorders (Hirschfeld et al., 1992). Comparisons were made among offspring of parents with panic disorder and agoraphobia, previously categorized as behaviorally inhibited versus not behaviorally inhibited, an epidemiologic sample of children initially described at 21 months as inhibited or not inhibited, and a group of normal children. Rates of having any anxiety disorder and of having multiple anxiety disorders were higher in those children previously identified as having behavioral inhibition (Biederman et al., 1990; Hirshfeld et al., 1992).

Mothers of children with anxiety disorders are more likely to have anxiety disorders than mothers of control children. There were significantly higher rates of current and lifetime anxiety disorders in mothers of anxiety disorder children ($n = 58$) compared with the mothers of children with other psychiatric disorders ($n = 15$) (Last et al., 1987b). A specific relationship was found between overanxious disorder in children and their mothers but not between separation anxiety disorder in children and their mothers (Last et al., 1987c). A higher prevalence rate of overanxious disorder in childhood (42 percent) was reported retrospectively by mothers of children with overanxious disorder compared with mothers of children with separation anxiety disorder and mothers of psychiatric control patients. Mothers of children with separation anxiety disorder did not show a higher rate of separation anxiety disorder than the other two groups.

Structured interviews of parents and siblings of a small group of children and adolescents with school refusal with both major depression and anxiety disorder showed high prevalence rates of anxiety and depressive disorders compared with rates in parents and siblings of children in the psychiatric control group (Bernstein and Garfinkel, 1988). However, probands in the control group had disruptive behavior disorders rather than pure anxiety or depressive disorders. Therefore, the type of comparison in the Weissman et al. (1984) study was not possible.

While these studies document the familial pattern in anxiety disorders, they do not evaluate biologic versus environmental factors and their contribution to anxiety disorders in children. Family studies demonstrate that "if a higher frequency of a disorder is not observed among biological relatives, then genetic factors can not be involved" (Klein and Last, 1989, p. 97). Twin studies, adoption studies, segregation analyses, and genetic linkage studies are needed to clarify the hereditary component of childhood anxiety disorders.

Inheritance studies of Tourette's disorder suggest a biologic relationship between Tourette's disorder and some cases of obsessive-compulsive disorder (Pauls and Leckman, 1986). There is an increased rate of obsessive-compulsive disorder in children with Tourette's disorder (Grad et al., 1987) and in their first-degree relatives (Pauls et al., 1986) compared with controls and first-degree relatives of the controls. Segregation analyses of data collected by direct family interviews of first-degree relatives of probands with Tourette's syndrome (Pauls and

Leckman, 1986) suggest that Tourette's syndrome is transmitted as a sex-influenced, autosomal dominant trait and obsessive-compulsive disorder is part of the genetically mediated spectrum of Tourette's syndrome.

EPIDEMIOLOGY

A number of large, well-designed epidemiologic studies employing structured psychiatric interviews indicate that anxiety disorders are one of the most prevalent categories of childhood and adolescent psychopathology (Anderson et al., 1987; Bird et al., 1988; Costello, 1989; Kashani and Orvaschel, 1990; McGee et al., 1990).

In evaluating the results of these epidemiologic studies, the age range of the subjects needs to be kept in mind. Studies of referred patients indicate that certain anxiety disorders are more common in young children and other anxiety disorders are more common in adolescents (e.g., separation anxiety disorder is more prevalent in children than adolescents) (Geller et al., 1985; Ryan et al., 1987). In addition, epidemiologic studies suggest different prevalence rates of disorders in different age groups of children and adolescents (McGee et al., 1992).

Two large studies investigate rates of anxiety disorders in children (Anderson et al., 1987; Costello, 1989). Costello (1989) reported that 8.9 percent of a sample of general pediatric patients met criteria for a least one anxiety disorder. The rates for specific disorders were as follows: 4.1 percent with separation anxiety disorder, 4.6 percent with overanxious disorder, 1.6 percent with avoidant disorder, 9.2 percent having simple phobia, 1.0 percent with social phobia, and 1.2 percent with agoraphobia. Anderson and colleagues (1987) evaluated children in New Zealand and found rates as follows: 3.5 percent having separation anxiety disorder, 2.9 percent with overanxious disorder, 2.4 percent with simple phobia, and 0.9 percent with social phobia.

The prevalence rates appear somewhat different in adolescents when compared with the distribution in children. Kashani and Orvaschel's study (1988) of a representative sample of 150 adolescents found an overall rate of 17.3 percent for subjects meeting criteria for at least one anxiety disorder. This rate decreased to 8.7 percent when the criterion of clinical dysfunction requiring treatment was added, including 7.3 percent with overanxious disorder, 4.7 percent with simple phobia, and 0.7 percent with separation anxiety disorder. Whitaker et al. (1990) completed a two-stage study, first screening over 5000 adolescents and subsequently interviewing 356 subjects. Weighted prevalence estimates included lifetime rates of 3.7 percent for generalized anxiety disorder and 0.6 percent for panic disorder. In the same sample, there was a weighted prevalence rate of 1.0 percent for current episode of obsessive-compulsive disorder and 1.9

percent for lifetime obsessive-compulsive disorder (Flament et al., 1988). In a follow-up study of the children in the Anderson et al. (1987) study, 1000 adolescents in New Zealand were evaluated. Overanxious disorder was the most prevalent disorder (5.9 percent), the second was nonaggressive conduct disorder (5.7 percent), and the third was simple phobia (3.6 percent) (McGee et al., 1990).

Finally, several epidemiologic studies include both children and adolescents (Bird et al., 1988; Bowen et al., 1990). Bird et al. (1988) reported that 6.8 percent met criteria for separation anxiety disorder; however, the rate decreased to 4.7 percent if the criterion of functional impairment was added. In addition, 3.9 percent had simple phobias, and the number decreased to 2.6 percent if a maladjustment criterion was used (Bird et al., 1988). Bowen et al. (1990) reported rates of 3.6 percent for overanxious disorder and 2.4 percent for separation anxiety disorder.

SEPARATION ANXIETY DISORDER

Clinical Picture

Attachment theory suggests that separation anxiety is an innate, instinctual system that has evolved to promote close social bonds and to precipitate anxiety during maternal–child separation, thus ensuring survival (Husain and Kashani, 1992). It should be emphasized that separation anxiety is a normal developmental phenomenon beginning around age 6 to 7 months and continuing throughout the early preschool years. At 6 to 7 months, infants begin to show distress upon their mothers' leaving them; this indicates the infant's ability to form strong specific attachments. Normal separation anxiety peaks at approximately 18 months of age. At around age 3, children develop the cognitive capacity to perceive that separation is temporary. Thus normally between ages 3 and 5 years the frequency and intensity of separation anxiety decrease.

Separation anxiety is considered a disorder if the symptoms are more severe than expected for the child's age and if the symptoms interfere with the child's functioning (e.g., the child is not attending school). Many children with separation anxiety manifest school refusal. In a study by Last and associates (1987d), approximately 75 percent of those who met criteria for separation anxiety disorder also were refusing to go to school.

Separation anxiety disorder is probably the most common of the childhood anxiety disorders in nonreferred children (Anderson et al., 1987). The prevalence rate of separation anxiety disorder is higher in children than in adolescents (Kashani and Orvaschel, 1988, 1990).

Demographic data about children with separation anxiety disorder are as follows: The average age at presentation of children with separation anxiety disorder is significantly younger (9.1 years) than the average age of presentation of children with over-anxious disorder (13.4 years) (Last et al., 1987a). This study identified a predominance of female children and primarily Caucasian children from lower socioeconomic families (Last et al., 1987a). In an epidemiologic study (Velez et al., 1989), lower socioeconomic status was a significant risk factor for having separation anxiety disorder.

Developmental differences in the expression of separation anxiety disorder were identified in a study of 45 children and adolescents with this disorder (Francis et al., 1987). Young children with separation anxiety disorder endorsed a greater number of symptoms than adolescents, who generally reported the minimum of three symptoms (Francis et al., 1987). There were no significant differences between the responses of boys and girls to each of the DSM-IIIR criteria. However, different age groups were more likely to endorse different criteria. Young children (ages 5 to 8) most commonly reported concern about unrealistic harm to attachment figures and school refusal. Children aged 9 to 12 most often endorsed excessive distress at times of separation, and adolescents (ages 13 to 16) most frequently described school refusal and physical complaints.

In a recent study designed to evaluate anxiety symptoms in normal children, 62 subjects in the general population were administered the Schedule for Affective Disorders and Schizophrenia for School-Age Children (K-SADS) Present Episode Version (Chambers et al., 1985), a semistructured interview. Isolated subclinical separation anxiety fears of harm to self or to attachment figures were reported by 16 percent of the nonreferred children (Bell-Dolan et al., 1990). Subclinical fears were identified with K-SADS severity ratings of 2. Two percent of the nonreferred children endorsed isolated separation anxiety fears at a clinical level determined by a severity rating of 3 or above on K-SADS interviews. More studies are necessary to determine the prevalence of separation anxiety symptoms in children in the general population.

Outcome

In their prospective, longitudinal study of 151 children presenting to a speech and language clinic, Cantwell and Baker (1989) initially diagnosed 9 children with separation anxiety disorder. At follow-up, an average of 4 years later, 4 of these 9 children had no psychiatric diagnosis, indicating a remission rate of 44 percent. Only 1 child (11 percent) still met criteria for separation anxiety disorder. The remaining 4 subjects met criteria for overanxious disorder and/or disruptive behavior disorders. Since the number of children initially diagnosed with separation anxiety disorder was small, conclusions about outcome from this study must be considered tentative. Furthermore, the children with separation anxiety disorder had the

youngest average age at baseline (3.6 years); thus a possible explanation for the high recovery rate is that some of these children had normal separation anxiety.

A continuum between separation anxiety disorder in childhood and agoraphobia or panic disorder in adulthood has been suggested (Ayuso et al., 1989; Gittelman and Klein, 1984; Klein, 1964; Zitrin and Ross, 1988). In retrospective studies, 50 percent of adult inpatients with agoraphobia (Klein, 1964) and 22 percent of adult outpatients with agoraphobia reported a history of separation anxiety in childhood (Berg et al., 1974). Furthermore, children who manifest severe distress at times of separation from their parents may look panicky (Gittelman-Klein, 1988). Prospective, longitudinal studies of children with separation anxiety disorder are needed to determine if this disorder is a precursor of agoraphobia or panic disorder in adulthood.

OVERANXIOUS DISORDER

Clinical Picture

Demographic information indicates that referred children with overanxious disorder have an older age at presentation than children with separation anxiety disorder (Last et al., 1987a). In this sample of overanxious children, Caucasians were overrepresented. In addition, children from middle- and upper-class families were overrepresented. The gender ratio was equal, with approximately the same number of girls and boys in this study meeting criteria for overanxious disorder. In reviewing the literature on overanxious disorder, Werry (1991) concludes that the gender ratio is approximately equal in clinic and community samples until adolescence. After adolescence, more females have the disorder.

Strauss and colleagues (1988b) evaluated developmental differences in the expression of this disorder by comparing the number and type of symptoms endorsed by younger children (ages 5 to 11) and older children and adolescents (ages 12 to 19). The older group reported a greater number of symptoms than subjects in the younger group. Subjects in the older group compared with subjects in the younger group were significantly more likely to endorse the criterion of worry about past behavior (Strauss et al., 1988b). In both age groups, the criterion of unrealistic worries about future events was most commonly reported. Fifty-three of the 55 children and adolescents with overanxious disorder endorsed this criterion (Strauss et al., 1988b).

The criterion of somatic symptoms may be the least frequent and least specific (Werry, 1991). Isolated subclinical overanxious disorder symptoms are common in nonreferred children (Achenbach et al., 1989; Bell-Dolan et al., 1990).

To investigate the validity of the overanxious diagnosis, Mattison and Bagnato (1987) administered the Revised Children's Manifest Anxiety Scale (RCMAS) (Reynolds and Richman, 1978) to boys aged 8 to 12 with overanxious disorder ($n = 16$), to those with dysthymia ($n = 15$), and to children with attention deficit hyperactivity disorder (ADHD) ($n = 26$). Parents of subjects completed the Child Behavior Checklist (CBCL) (Achenbach and Edelbrock, 1983). The boys with overanxious disorder showed greater elevations than boys with dysthymia or those with ADHD on the worry/over-sensitivity and physiological anxiety factors of the RCMAS. In addition, on the CBCL, boys with overanxious disorder most often manifested a profile type of schizoid or anxious, with none of the overanxious boys showing the hyperactive or delinquent profile types. The boys with ADHD showed the greatest percentage of hyperactive profiles, and some manifested the delinquent profile. This study provides some evidence for the convergent and discriminant validity of the overanxious diagnosis.

A recent study compared children with overanxious disorder ($n = 11$), children with social phobia ($n = 18$), and normal, matched controls ($n = 11$) on self-report instruments and daily diary data (Beidel, 1991). In addition, children performed two behavioral tasks (taking a vocabulary test and reading aloud before an audience). At baseline and at intervals during the preceding two tasks, pulse rates were recorded. After the tasks, cognitions of the child were reported and later categorized. The results indicated that the children with social phobia were differentiated from the other two groups on most measures, with few variables distinguishing the overanxious children. The author concluded that the study supports the validity of the diagnosis of social phobia in children but provides less support for overanxious disorder as currently defined. Since the number of children with overanxious disorder in this study is small, conclusions about overanxious disorder need to be viewed cautiously. However, the author raises the idea that overanxious disorder is not a clear clinical syndrome but rather a constellation of symptoms of somatic and cognitive anxiety that represents a prodromal state preceding the onset of other anxiety disorders.

Outcome

The follow-up study of 151 young children referred to a speech and language clinic (Cantwell and Baker, 1989) included 8 children with overanxious disorder. This anxiety disorder had the lowest recovery rate; only 2 of the overanxious children (25 percent) were completely well at 4-year follow-up. At follow-up, 2 were diagnosed with overanxious disorder (25 percent stability). The mean age of presentation of overanxious disorder in this study was 7.3 years, while in Last and colleagues' study (1987a) the mean age was 13.4 years. Therefore,

the young sample studied by Cantwell and Baker (1989) probably is not representative of all referred overanxious children. Furthermore, the initial sample of children with overanxious disorder is small, therefore limiting the conclusions about the outcome of children with overanxious disorder.

Overanxious disorder usually does not prevent a child from meeting basic academic and social demands (Husain and Kashani, 1992). In the study of Beidel (1991) comparing children with overanxious disorder and children with social phobia, the children meeting criteria for overanxious disorder had higher trait anxiety than social phobics and normals, yet the anxiety did not seem to interfere with their daily functioning. The children with overanxious disorder were not significantly different from normal controls in their perceptions of their competence, the number of daily events they found distressing, or the severity of the distress they experienced when the events occurred.

The data indicate that in some cases the symptoms remit (Beitchman et al., 1987; Cantwell and Baker, 1989; Verhulst et al., 1985; Verhulst and Althaus, 1988). However, it has been suggested that some children with overanxious disorder may have a chronic course (Husain and Kashani, 1992; Werry, 1991).

While DSM-IIIR suggests that overanxious disorder may continue into adulthood as generalized anxiety disorder, prospective longitudinal studies are not yet available. One retrospective study indicated that only 20 percent of adults with generalized anxiety disorder reported onset of this disorder in childhood or adolescence (Thyer et al., 1985).

AVOIDANT DISORDER

Clinical Picture

A study including 19 children with avoidant disorder referred to an anxiety disorders clinic provides preliminary data about the demographics of this disorder (Francis et al., 1992). The mean age at intake was 11.3 years with an age range from 6 to 17 years. Close to three-fourths were female, and 94 per cent were Caucasian. Sixty per cent of the sample were from upper or middle socioeconomic status families and forty per cent were from lower socioeconomic status families (Francis et al., 1992).

This disorder is reported to be comorbid with other anxiety disorders. In a clinic sample, 4.5 percent of the children and adolescents with separation anxiety disorder also had avoidant disorder, and 27.3 percent of those with overanxious disorder also met criteria for avoidant disorder (Last et al., 1989). It appears that children with avoidant disorder commonly have an additional comorbid anxiety disorder, especially overanxious disorder (Klein and Last, 1989).

Outcome

Fourteen children (mean age of 5.0 years) of the 151 in the Cantwell and Baker study (1989) were initially diagnosed with avoidant disorder. Five (36 percent) had no diagnosis at 4-year follow-up, and 4 (29 percent) met criteria for avoidant disorder. It has been suggested that the high percentage (9 percent) of children in the Cantwell and Baker study (1989) with avoidant disorder was due to the fact that children with speech and language disorders were studied (Husain and Kashani, 1992).

FEARS AND SIMPLE PHOBIAS

Clinical Picture

A *fear* is a subjective, unpleasant feeling that is the response to an imagined or real danger (Husain and Kashani, 1992). A *simple phobia* is the specific, isolated, persistent fear of a circumscribed stimulus. The associated avoidant behavior interferes with the child's normal functioning (American Psychiatric Association, 1987). Because of their cognitive level of development, children, unlike adults, may not realize the irrational aspects of their phobias (Silverman and Nelles, 1990).

Fears, common in children of all ages, are often transient and part of the normal process of development (Silverman and Nelles, 1990). Younger children report more fears than older children (Ollendick et al., 1989). Girls report more fears than boys (Ollendick et al., 1985; Silverman and Nelles, 1988). Further research is needed to determine whether gender-role expectations influence reporting of fears (Silverman and Nelles, 1988).

The Revised Fear Survey Schedule for Children (FSSC-R) (Ollendick, 1983), a widely used self-report instrument, identifies five fear factors: fear of failure and criticism, fear of the unknown, fear of minor injury and small animals, fear of danger and death, and medical fears. Use of this instrument has demonstrated that certain common fears (e.g., being hit by a car, falling from a high place, a burglar breaking into the house) are consistent across different age, gender, and cultural groups (Ollendick et al., 1989), suggesting that not all fears are transitory (Ollendick et al., 1985).

Evaluation of 325 children and adolescents using data from multiple sources revealed the following prevalence rates: phobias—7.7 percent, of which 0.2 percent were reported to be "severe" phobias (Agras et al., 1969). Epidemiologic studies report prevalence rates of simple phobias of 2.4 percent in children (Anderson et al., 1987), 3.6 percent in adolescents (McGee et al., 1990), and 2.6 percent in a study of children and adolescents (Bird et al., 1988). The children of adults with panic disorder and agoraphobia who have stable behavioral inhibition (marked withdrawal and excessive shyness in new situations) appear to be at risk for phobic disorders (Hirschfeld et al., 1992).

A retrospective study indicated that 31 percent of adults had the onset of their simple phobias before age 9, with 26 percent reporting an onset between 10 and 19 years (Sheehan et al., 1981). Different types of phobias appear to have different ages of onset. A retrospective study indicated that phobias of animals began before the age of 5, with social phobias such as fear of eating in public starting after puberty (Marks and Gelder, 1966). Other phobias, including fear of heights, darkness, and storms, had variable ages of onset (Marks and Gelder, 1966).

Outcome

A subset of children with simple phobias continues to have symptoms as adults. In following 30 untreated children and adults with simple phobias, Agras et al. (1972) reported that only 43 percent of the adults improved, whereas 100 percent of those under age 20 improved. Ollendick (1979) reinterpreted the data and found that only 40 percent of those younger than 20 were truly symptom free. Thus some simple phobias appear to persist from childhood into adulthood.

OBSESSIVE-COMPULSIVE DISORDER

Clinical Picture

Obsessions are recurrent, persistent ideas that are experienced as intrusive and senseless, and *compulsions* are repetitive, intentional behaviors or rituals. In DSM-IIIR, either obsessions or compulsions with the associated characteristics are needed to qualify for a diagnosis of obsessive-compulsive disorder (American Psychiatric Association, 1987). The clinical picture of obsessive-compulsive disorder is virtually identical in children and adults (Berg et al., 1989). One-fourth to over half of adults with obsessive-compulsive disorder report the onset in childhood or adolescence (Lo, 1967; Pollitt, 1957).

Minor obsessions and compulsions frequently occur in young children and are not considered pathologic (Husain and Kashani, 1992). Normal developmental rituals such as bedtime routines are not associated with distress or dysfunction (Husain and Kashani, 1992).

The reported prevalence rates for obsessive-compulsive disorder may be underestimates. Children with obsessive-compulsive disorder often appear to minimize or hide their symptoms. The intrusive, unacceptable nature of the obsessional thoughts and embarrassment associated with the rituals cause children to be secretive about their symptoms. Children attempting to minimize their symptoms or those with mild symptoms are often difficult to identify. Symptoms suggestive of obsessive-compulsive disorder include long periods of time spent on homework assignments, including frequent erasures and doing parts of the assignments over and over again, insistence on wearing clothes or using a towel only one time, requesting that family members repeat phrases, preoccupation with having an illness, and hoarding of useless objects (Leonard and Rapoport, 1991b). Parents may become aware of the problem when children become dysfunctional due to the frequency and complexity of the rituals (e.g., a child who is late to school due to repeated handwashing and checking behavior before leaving the house).

Several studies report a male predominance in this disorder in clinical samples of children and adolescents (Hollingsworth et al., 1980; Last and Strauss, 1989; Rapoport, 1986; Swedo et al., 1989). Rapoport reported males manifesting the disorder an average of 2.5 years earlier than females (Rapoport, 1986). Similarly, boys in another sample reported onset of their disorder an average of 3.1 years earlier than girls (age 9.5 versus age 12.6) (Last and Strauss, 1989). However, approximately equal numbers of males and females with obsessive-compulsive disorder were reported in an epidemiologic study of adolescent obsessive-compulsive disorder (Flament et al., 1988) and in a study of referred children and adolescents with this disorder (Riddle et al., 1990).

As part of an epidemiologic study, 20 high school students with obsessive-compulsive disorder were identified (Flament et al., 1988). The mean age of the adolescents was 16.2 years, with average age of onset of obsessive-compulsive disorder at 12.8 years. In most cases, onset was gradual, although in some cases it was sudden. It had previously been described that the disorder occurs in some children with no premorbid obsessive-compulsive traits (Rapoport, 1986). Of the 20 teenagers in the epidemiologic sample, only 4 had received any psychiatric intervention. This included 3 for associated anxiety and/or depressive symptoms, and they did not reveal any of their obsessive-compulsive symptoms (Flament et al., 1988). This illustrates the secretive approach the teenagers were taking to their obsessive-compulsive symptoms.

In the Flament et al. study (1988), having multiple obsessions and compulsions was the most common presentation. Obsessions alone were rare, occurring in only 1 of the 20 adolescents. The most commonly reported obsessions were fear of contamination and thoughts of harm to self and familiar persons. The most frequent compulsions included washing and cleaning rituals, checking behavior, and straightening.

Twenty-one children with obsessive-compulsive disorder were studied by Riddle and colleagues (1990). Four of these children had a parent with obsessive-compulsive disorder, and an additional 11 children had a parent with obsessive-compulsive symptoms. The majority of the sample ($n = 19$) reported both obsessions and compulsions. The remaining 2 subjects reported only compulsions. The most prevalent obsessions were thoughts of contamination, aggressive or violent thoughts, and somatic preoccupations. The most common rituals included repeating, washing, ordering, and checking.

Twenty referred children with obsessive-compulsive disorder were assessed by Last and Strauss (1989). The mean age at evaluation was 12.7 years, and the mean age of onset was 10.7 years. Sixteen of 20 reported rituals, most commonly washing, arranging objects, checking, and counting. Of those with rituals, half reported multiple rituals. Four children reported obsessions only.

In the National Institute of Mental Health sample of 70 children and adolescents with primary severe obsessive-compulsive disorder, the average age of onset was 10 years (Leonard and Rapoport, 1991b). Boys reported onset approximately 2 years earlier than girls. While Tourette's disorder was an exclusionary criterion for the study, 20 percent of the patients had a history of simple motor or vocal tics. The most common rituals included cleaning (i.e., handwashing, toothbrushing, showering) in 85 percent, repeating behaviors in 51 percent, and checking in 46 percent. There were 3 subjects (4 percent) with obsessions only. A small subgroup had compulsions only; these subjects were unable to identify any obsessional thoughts associated with their rituals. Most of the subjects reported that their symptoms had periods of remissions and exacerbations and that the main symptom changed over time.

Outcome

A follow-up study of a community-based sample of adolescents initially diagnosed with obsessive-compulsive disorder and a control group demonstrated that an initial diagnosis of obsessive-compulsive disorder or another psychiatric disorder with obsessive-compulsive features predicted obsessive-compulsive disorder 2 years later (Berg et al., 1989).

Obsessive-compulsive disorder in childhood frequently continues into adulthood. Elkins and associates (1980) reviewed outcome studies and concluded that 50 percent of children with obsessive-compulsive disorder do not show improvement. However, this report preceded the availability of the treatment option of the serotonin reuptake inhibitors, fluoxetine, and clomipramine.

Several authors have commented on positive prognostic indicators, including good premorbid functioning, mild symptoms, and short duration of symptoms. Poor prognostic indicators in adults are noncompliance with treatment protocols (Baer and Minichiello, 1986), the presence of a personality disorder (Baer and Minichiello, 1986), and the belief that the symptoms are necessary and must be performed to avoid bad consequences (Foa, 1979).

DIFFERENTIAL DIAGNOSIS

The three childhood anxiety disorders need to be differentiated from each other. In separation anxiety disorder and avoidant disorder, the anxiety is situation-specific: anxiety about separation from attachment figures and anxiety about unfamiliar people, respectively. In overanxious disorder, the anxiety is generalized and present in a variety of situations. While it is important to differentiate among the childhood anxiety disorders, it is not uncommon to meet criteria for more than one anxiety disorder. Approximately a third of children with anxiety disorders meet criteria for two or more anxiety disorders (Kashani and Orvaschel, 1988; Last et al., 1987d).

Separation Anxiety Disorder

Since separation anxiety is a normal developmental stage up to preschool age, developmentally normal separation anxiety needs to be differentiated from separation anxiety disorder. When the separation reactions are extreme, beyond those which are considered normal for the particular age, and when the symptoms interfere with functioning, then separation anxiety disorder is diagnosed.

School refusal secondary to separation anxiety disorder is to be differentiated from school refusal associated with conduct disorder. These two groups of school refusers have different patterns of behavior. Children with separation anxiety disorder generally are eager to please, quiet, compliant, and follow rules at school, while those with conduct disorder are disruptive and defiant. Children with conduct disorder manifest behaviors such as lying, stealing, running away from home overnight, and fighting. The patterns of nonattendance are different. When not in school, children with separation anxiety are usually at home with a parent or with parental knowledge. On the other hand, conduct-disordered children and adolescents may be roaming the community engaging in antisocial activities without parental knowledge.

There is often an overlap between anxiety and depressive symptoms in children. For example, somatic complaints and insomnia may be present in both types of disorders. Major depression is a common comorbid disorder with separation anxiety disorder (Bernstein, 1991; Strauss et al., 1988a). If full criteria for both disorders are met, then both are diagnosed. Children with pervasive developmental disorder may have symptoms of separation anxiety disorder. While the anxiety may be overwhelming, it is secondary to the underlying condition, so the diagnosis of separation anxiety disorder is not made.

Overanxious Disorder

Children with attention deficit hyperactivity disorder are often on the go, busy, and overly active. They may appear jittery or tense. However, unlike children with overanxious disorder, they do not present with multiple worries about future and past events and concern about competence. Generalized anxiety disorder in adults has some similarities to overanxious disorder. Both disorders are characterized by feelings of tension. If the patient is age 18 or older and criteria for both are met, generalized anxiety disorder is diagnosed. In adjustment disorder with anxious mood, onset of anxiety symptoms follows within 3 months of an identifiable stressor, and the duration of symptoms is less than 6 months.

Avoidant Disorder

Avoidant disorder is different from schizoid disorder of children and adolescents (DSM-III) (American Psychiatric Association, 1980), which describes children who withdraw from all people. Unlike children with avoidant disorder, schizoidal children do not desire warm relationships with family and familiar people. In adjustment disorder with withdrawal, social inhibition is linked to a recent precipitant, and the children do not have a chronic history of avoiding contact with unfamiliar people.

Fears and Simple Phobias

Fears are transitory, developmental phenomena. Phobias are associated with more marked anxiety and are accompanied by avoidant behavior. Exposure to the phobic object invokes an immediate anxiety response. In patients with obsessive-compulsive disorder, there may be avoidance of certain objects, but avoidance is associated with obsessive thoughts or compulsive rituals. In post-traumatic stress disorder, a child or adolescent may avoid situations that invoke or are associated with recollection of a previous traumatic event.

Obsessive-Compulsive Disorder

Young children engaging in minor rituals such as bedtime rituals are differentiated from those with obsessive-compulsive disorder by the lack of associated obsessive thoughts and absence of associated distress and dysfunction. Simple phobias are circumscribed, isolated fears with avoidant behavior. With simple phobias, it is uncommon for germs to be the primary stimuli avoided (Leonard and Rapoport, 1991a). In addition, the fears of the child with a simple phobia decrease when not confronted with the object, which is not characteristic of a child with obsessive-compulsive disorder (Leonard and Rapoport, 1991a). Children with chronic motor tics or Tourette's disorder manifest repetitive, involuntary actions that do not serve the purpose of allaying the individual's anxiety. Children with separation anxiety disorder report unrealistic worry about harm to self and to attachment figures but do not engage in rituals to allay their fears.

LABORATORY FINDINGS

There is no laboratory test for diagnosing anxiety disorders in children. However, several tests and physiologic parameters have been explored in an attempt to identify a biologic marker for childhood anxiety. Children with separation anxiety disorder had higher pulse rates compared with children without an anxiety disorder in a study of hospitalized children with different psychiatric diagnoses (Rogeness et al., 1990). In addition, there was a positive correlation between systolic blood pressure and anxiety symptoms. The researchers found their data to be consistent with the hypothesis that anxiety disorders are associated with increased noradrenergic function.

A study of the dexamethasone suppression test in 15 prepubertal inpatients indicated that this test may be positive in children with separation anxiety disorder as well as in children with depression (Livingston et al., 1984). All subjects received a careful diagnostic assessment by several independent clinicians prior to the dexamethasone suppression test. Seven positive dexamethasone suppression tests included three children with separation anxiety disorder, one with simple phobia, and three with depression. Two borderline positive tests were obtained from one child with separation anxiety disorder and one with depression. The dexamethasone suppression test was 60 percent sensitive to separation anxiety disorder and 75 percent sensitive to depression.

There is preliminary evidence for neurologic differences in some children and adolescents with obsessive-compulsive disorder. Behar et al. (1984) reported a significantly higher ventricular/brain ratio on CT scan in 16 children and adolescents with severe obsessive-compulsive disorder in comparison with a matched control group. The obsessive-compulsive disorder sample also displayed spatial-perceptual deficits on neuropsychological assessment compared with the control group. In another study, subtle abnormalities of right hemispheric functions on neuropsychological testing were found in children and adolescents with obsessive-compulsive disorder (Cox et al., 1989). Neurologic findings, including left hemisyndrome, choreiform syndrome, and neurodevelopmental differences have been described in children and adolescents with obsessive-compulsive disorder (Denckla, 1989). Rapoport et al. (1981) reported that the sleep electroencephalograms of nine children with obsessive-compulsive disorder, all of whom had a history of major depression, were similar to those of young adults with primary depression.

While serotonin, epinephrine, and dopamine dysfunction have all been implicated in the etiology of obsessive-compulsive disorder, serotonin has been viewed as most important. Clomipramine, a serotonin reuptake blocker, is effective in the treatment of children and adolescents with obsessive-compulsive disorder (Flament et al., 1985a, 1985b; Leonard et al., 1988). A recent study evaluated the level of cerebrospinal fluid somatostatin in 10 children with disruptive behavior disorders and 10 children with obsessive-compulsive disorder (Kruesi et al., 1990). Somatostatin is a peptide that stimulates serotonin release and inhibits the release of growth hormone. A lower level of somatostatin was found in the cerebrospinal fluid of children with disruptive behavior disorders in comparison with the level in children with obsessive-compulsive disorder, even after controlling for Tanner stage.

TREATMENT

The treatment of child and adolescent anxiety disorders generally involves a multimodal approach (McDermott et al., 1989). Possible treatment modalities include education of the parent and child about the disorder, behavioral treatment, family therapy, individual therapy, and pharmacotherapy.

Behavioral Treatment

Behavioral therapy focuses on the behavior of the child or adolescent and views treatment in the context of family and school instead of emphasizing intrapsychic conflict (Leonard and Rapoport, 1991a). Cognitive-behavioral therapy includes techniques to change maladaptive cognitions associated with the individual's anxiety state as well as behavioral interventions (Kendall et al., 1991).

In school refusal secondary to separation anxiety disorder, the overall goal is to implement a plan for separation of parent and child and a return to school as quickly as possible. Several case studies report the successful treatment of school refusers with systematic desensitization and exposure (classical conditioning based interventions) (Croghan, 1981; McNamara, 1988; Miller, 1972). Other case reports describe success treating school refusers with operant behavioral techniques (Ayllon et al., 1970; Brown et al., 1974; Doleys and Williams, 1977; Hersen, 1970; Kolko, 1987; McNamara, 1988; Patterson, 1965). Operant techniques include positive reinforcement for desired behaviors and negative consequences for undesirable behavior.

Cognitive-behavioral therapy was reported to be efficacious in the treatment of two children with separation anxiety (Mansdorf and Lukens, 1987). It was emphasized in this report that the evaluation and treatment phases should involve the family and the school. Kearney and Silverman (1990) reported that six of seven school refusers were attending school regularly 6 months after receiving cognitive-behavioral treatment. In a study of cognitive-behavioral treatment in four children with over-anxious disorder, all showed improvement on self-report and parent and clinician ratings of anxiety (Kane and Kendall, 1989). In general, gains were maintained at 3- and 6-month follow-ups.

There are two comparative studies of treatment approaches for school refusal. Blagg and Yule (1984) compared behavioral treatment, hospitalization, and a combination of home tutoring and psychotherapy. The average length of treatment was shortest for the behavioral therapy group. At follow-up 1 year later, 83, 31, and 0 percent, respectively, of the three treatment groups were attending school more than 80 percent of the time. However, a major criticism of this study is that subjects were not randomly assigned to the three treatments. This may have introduced a bias into the results. Miller and colleagues (1972) compared systematic desensitization, psychotherapy, and waiting list control in the treatment of childhood phobias (69 percent with school phobia). Parental ratings suggested that both active treatments were superior to waiting list in reducing fears in the children. However, the clinician ratings demonstrated no differences among the three groups after treatment. In the Miller et al. study (1972), subjects were randomized to the three treatment groups.

The case reports and two comparative studies indicate that behavioral interventions play a role in the treatment of anxiety disorders of children and adolescents.

Family Therapy

Family dynamic issues are often prominent in homes with a child diagnosed as having an anxiety disorder. For example, in separation anxiety disorder, the mother and child may have an enmeshed relationship (Johnson et al., 1941; Waldfogel et al., 1957) and the father may be distant and not involved with the family. Sometimes there is role reversal between a parent and child. Family therapy is often recommended to address these types of issues.

While there are some data that family therapy is effective in the treatment of conduct disorder, substance use disorders, and schizophrenia (Gurman et al., 1986), there are no controlled studies evaluating the efficacy of family therapy for anxiety disorders.

Psychodynamic Psychotherapy

Psychodynamic therapy that emphasizes exploration of underlying fears and anxieties is often an important component in the treatment of a child with an anxiety disorder (Leonard and Rapoport, 1991a). Involvement of parents in the therapy process is beneficial so that parents learn to understand a child's symptoms and need for reassurance and begin to model and encourage independence. Since mothers of children with anxiety disorders have an increased rate of anxiety disorders (Last et al., 1987b), they may need individual therapy, as well.

Pharmacologic Treatment

Medication may be used in conjunction with behavioral, family, or individual therapy. Psychopharmacology is considered if the level of symptomatology is severe. Two classes of medications have been used most commonly: tricyclic antidepressants and benzodiazepines. Scientific studies supporting the efficacy of either of these classes of medications are limited. However, clinical experience suggests that some individuals benefit from such agents in treating their anxiety symptoms. Further controlled studies are clearly needed.

TRICYCLIC ANTIDEPRESSANTS

Since tricyclic antidepressants such as imipramine have been demonstrated to be effective in treating anticipatory anxiety and panic attacks in adults (Zitrin et al., 1983), it has been suggested that this class of drug might be effective for treatment of separation anxiety disorder in children which is often associated with panic-like reactions.

Placebo-controlled studies of tricyclic antidepressants in treating school refusal associated with separation anxiety indicate contrasting results. The original study by Gittelman-Klein and Klein (1971, 1973) included 35 children with separation anxiety. Children on imipramine were significantly more successful in returning to school in comparison with those on placebo (81 and 47 percent returned to school in the imipramine and placebo groups, respectively). Furthermore, those on imipramine had a significant improvement in symptoms when rated by self-report, by mothers, and by psychiatrists.

A study by Berney et al. (1981) showed no significant difference between clomipramine and placebo in facilitating a return to school or in decreasing symptomatology. The 51 subjects in the study with anxiety symptoms included 44 percent with comorbid depressive symptoms. The dosage of 40 to 75 mg clomipramine was probably subtherapeutic.

Imipramine, alprazolam, and placebo were compared in the treatment of 24 children and adolescents with school refusal and no significant differences between active medications and placebo were found (Bernstein et al., 1990). While there were trends for both alprazolam and imipramine to produce greater improvement in anxiety and depression symptomatology, it was unclear whether the improvement was secondary to medication effects or baseline differences in symptom severity among groups. A recent attempt to replicate the results of the Gittelman-Klein and Klein study (1971, 1973) indicated no superiority for imipramine over placebo in treating separation anxiety disorder, with half of the subjects in each treatment group improving (Klein et al., 1992).

Thus the four controlled studies do not provide conclusive evidence to support the use of tricyclic antidepressants in the treatment of anxiety disorders associated with school refusal. However, clinical experience suggests that some children with anxiety-based school refusal benefit from the addition of tricyclic antidepressants.

There are case reports describing effective treatment of panic attacks in children and adolescents with tricyclic antidepressants (Ballenger et al., 1989; Black and Robbins, 1990; Garland and Smith, 1990).

BENZODIAZEPINES

An open trial in 12 children and adolescents with avoidant and/or overanxious disorders showed that just over half had at least moderate improvement in symptoms on alprazolam, a benzodiazepine (Simeon and Ferguson, 1987). A subsequent double-blind, placebo-controlled trial of 30 children and adolescents with avoidant or overanxious disorder showed trends toward greater improvement on alprazolam based on global improvement ratings at the end of the study. However, these findings did not demonstrate statistically significant differences between alprazolam and placebo (Simeon et al., 1992).

Several case reports support the use of benzodiazepines in children with anxiety symptoms. Clonazepam was reported to be effective in treating anxiety symptoms in one child with overanxious disorder, one with separation anxiety disorder, and one with avoidant disorder and separation anxiety disorder (Biederman, 1987). All three children also had panic attacks, and the clonazepam alleviated the panic symptoms as well as anticipatory anxiety (Biederman, 1987). Single, small doses of alprazolam have been reported to be useful in treating anticipatory and acute situational anxiety in pediatric cancer patients undergoing painful procedures in an open trial (Pfefferbaum et al., 1987).

In general, benzodiazepines are tolerated by children with minimal side effects (Bernstein et al., 1990; Biederman, 1987, 1990; Simeon and Ferguson, 1987; Simeon et al., 1992). Common side effects include sedation, drowsiness, and decreased mental acuity (Biederman, 1991). Behavioral disinhibition has been reported with clonazepam in children (Graae et al., 1991). Because of the possible addiction potential, it is suggested that duration of treatment be short term. However, tolerance to and dependence on ben-

zodiazepines are yet to be systematically evaluated in children (Biederman, 1991).

An example of short-term use of a benzodiazepine would be using the medication to allay anxiety symptoms in a child with school refusal secondary to separation anxiety disorder as he or she attempts to return to school. After the child has successfully reentered the classroom and demonstrates several weeks of regular attendance, the medication can be tapered. Gradual tapering is recommended to avoid withdrawal effects which may be associated with rapid cessation (Biederman, 1991; Coffey, 1990).

REFERENCES

Achenbach TM, Conners CK, Quay HC, et al: Replication of empirically derived syndromes as a basis for taxonomy of child/adolescent psychopathology. J Abnorm Child Psychol 17:299–323, 1989.

Achenbach TM, Edelbrock C: Manual for the Child Behavior Checklist and the Revised Child Behavior Profile. Burlington: Department of Psychiatry, University of Vermont, 1983.

Agras S, Chapin HN, Oliveau DC: The natural history of phobia: Course and prognosis. Arch Gen Psychiatry 26:315–317, 1972.

Agras S, Sylvester D, Oliveau D: The epidemiology of common fears and phobia. Compr Psychiatry 10:151–156, 1969.

American Psychiatric Association: Diagnostic and Statistical Manual of Mental Disorders, 3rd ed. Washington, American Psychiatric Association, 1980.

American Psychiatric Association: Diagnostic and Statistical Manual of Mental Disorders, 3d ed revised. Washington, American Psychiatric Association, 1987.

Anderson JC, Williams S, McGee R, Silva PA: DSM-III disorders in preadolescent children: Prevalence in a large sample from the general population. Arch Gen Psychiatry 44:69–76, 1987.

Ayllon T, Smith D, Rogers M: Behavioral management of school phobia. J Behav Ther Exp Psychiatry 1:125–138, 1970.

Ayuso JL, Alfonso S, Rivera A: Childhood separation anxiety and panic disorder: A comparative study. Prog Neuropsychopharmacol Biol Psychiatry 13:665–671, 1989.

Baer L, Minichiello WE: Behavior therapy for obsessive-compulsive disorder. In Jenike M, Baer L, Minichiello WE (eds): Obsessive-Compulsive Disorder. Littleton, MA, PSG Publications, 1986, pp 45–75.

Ballenger JC, Carek DJ, Steele JJ, Cornish-McTighe D: Three cases of panic disorder with agoraphobia in children. Am J Psychiatry 146:922–924, 1989.

Behar D, Rapoport JL, Berg CJ, et al: Computerized tomography and neuropsychological test measures in adolescents with obsessive-compulsive disorder. Am J Psychiatry 141:363–369, 1984.

Beidel D: Social phobia and overanxious disorder in school-age children. J Am Acad Child Adolesc Psychiatry 30:545–552, 1991.

Beitchman JH, Wekerle C, Hood J: Diagnostic continuity from preschool to middle childhood. J Am Acad Child Adolesc Psychiatry 26:694–699, 1987.

Bell-Dolan DJ, Last CG, Strauss CC: Symptoms of anxiety disorders in normal children. J Am Acad Child Adolesc Psychiatry 29:759–765, 1990.

Berg CZ, Rapoport JL, Whitaker A, et al: Childhood obsessive-compulsive disorder. A two-year prospective follow-up of a community sample. J Am Acad Child Adolesc Psychiatry 28:528–533, 1989.

Berg I, Marks I, McGuire R, Lipsedge M: School phobia and agoraphobia. Psychol Med 4:428–434, 1974.

Berney T, Kolvin I, Bhate SR, et al: School phobia: A therapeutic trial with clomipramine and short-term outcome. Br J Psychiatry 138:110–118, 1981.

Bernstein GA: Comorbidity and severity of anxiety and depressive disorders in a clinic sample. J Am Acad Child Adolesc Psychiatry 30:43–50, 1991.

Bernstein GA, Garfinkel BD: Pedigrees, functioning and psychopathology in families of school phobic children. Am J Psychiatry 145:70–74, 1988.

Bernstein GA, Garfinkel BD, Borchardt CM: Comparative studies of pharmacotherapy for school refusal. J Am Acad Child Adolesc Psychiatry 29:773–781, 1990.

Bernstein GA, Garfinkel BD, Hoberman HM: Self-reported anxiety in adolescents. Am J Psychiatry 146:384–386, 1989.

Biederman J: Clonazepam in the treatment of prepubertal children with panic-like symptoms. J Clin Psychiatry 48(suppl): 38–41, 1987.

Biederman J: Psychopharmacology. In Wiener JM (ed): Textbook of Child and Adolescent Psychiatry. Washington, American Psychiatric Press, 1991, pp 545–570.

Biederman J, Rosenbaum JF, Hirshfeld DR, et al: Psychiatric correlates of behavioral inhibition in young children of parents with and without psychiatric disorders. Arch Gen Psychiatry 47:21–26, 1990.

Bird HR, Canino G, Rubio-Stipec M, et al: Estimates of the prevalence of childhood maladjustment in a community survey in Puerto Rico. Arch Gen Psychiatry 45:1120–1126, 1988.

Black B, Robbins DR: Panic disorder in children and adolescents. J Am Acad Child Adolesc Psychiatry 29:36–44, 1990.

Blagg NR, Yule W: The behavioural treatment of school refusal: A comparative study. Behav Res Ther 22:119–127, 1984.

Bowen RC, Offord DR, Boyle MH: The prevalence of overanxious disorder and separation anxiety disorder: Results from the Ontario child health study. J Am Acad Child Adolesc Psychiatry 29:753–758, 1990.

Brown R, Copeland RE, Hall RV: School phobia: Effects of behavior modification treatment applied by an elementary school principal. Child Study J 4:125–133, 1974.

Cantwell DP, Baker L: Stability and natural history of DSM-III childhood diagnoses. J Am Acad Child Adolesc Psychiatry 28:691–700, 1989.

Chambers WJ, Puig-Antich J, Hirsch M, et al: The assessment of affective disorders in children and adolescents by semistructured interview: Test-retest reliability of the Schedule for Affective Disorders and Schizophrenia for School-Age Children, Present Episode Version. Arch Gen Psychiatry 42:696–702, 1985.

Coffey BJ: Anxiolytics for children and adolescents: Traditional and new drugs. J Child Adolesc Psychopharmacol 1:57–83, 1990.

Costello EJ: Child psychiatric disorders and their correlates: A primary care pediatric sample. J Am Acad Child Adolesc Psychiatry 28:851–855, 1989.

Cox CS, Fedio P, Rapoport JL: Neuropsychological testing of obsessive-compulsive adolescents. In Rapoport JL (ed): Obsessive-Compulsive Disorder in Children and Adolescents. Washington, American Psychiatric Press, 1989, pp 73–85.

Croghan LM: Conceptualizing the critical elements in a rapid desensitization to school anxiety: A case study. J Pediatr Psychol 6:165–170, 1981.

Denckla MB: Neurological examination. In Rapoport JL (ed): Obsessive-Compulsive Disorder in Children and Adolescents. Washington, American Psychiatric Press, 1989, pp 107–115.

Doleys DM, Williams SC: The use of natural consequences and a make-up period to eliminate school phobic behavior: A case study. J School Psychol 15:44–50, 1977.

Elkins R, Rapoport JL, Lipsky A: Obsessive-compulsive disorder of childhood and adolescence. J Am Acad Child Psychiatry 19:511–524, 1980.

Flament MF, Rapoport JL, Berg CJ, Kilts C: A controlled trial of clomipramine in childhood obsessive-compulsive disorder. Psychopharmacol Bull 21:150–152, 1985a.

Flament FM, Rapoport JL, Berg CJ, et al: Clomipramine treatment of childhood obsessive-compulsive disorder. Arch Gen Psychiatry 42:977–983, 1985b.

Flament MF, Whitaker A, Rapoport JL, et al: Obsessive-compulsive disorder in adolescence: An epidemiological study. J Am Acad Child Adolesc Psychiatry 27:764–771, 1988.

Foa EB: Failures in treating obsessive-compulsives. Behav Res Ther 17:169–176, 1979.

Francis G, Last CG, Strauss CC: Expression of separation anxiety disorder: The roles of age and gender. Child Psychiatry Hum Dev 18:82–89, 1987.

Francis G, Last CG, Strauss CC: Avoidant disorder and social phobia in children and adolescents. J Am Acad Child Adolesc Psychiatry 31:1086–1089, 1992.

Garland EJ, Smith DH: Case study: Panic disorder on a child psychiatric consultation service. J Am Acad Child Adolesc Psychiatry 29:785–788, 1990.

Geller B, Chestnut EC, Miller MD, et al: Preliminary data on DSM-III associated features of major depressive disorder in children and adolescents. Am J Psychiatry 142:643–644, 1985.

Gittelman R, Klein DF: Relationship between separation anxiety and panic and agoraphobic disorders. Psychopathology 17(suppl 1):56–65, 1984.

Gittelman-Klein R: Childhood anxiety disorders. In Kestenbaum CJ, Williams DT (eds): Handbook of Clinical Assessment of Children and Adolescents, vol 2. New York, New York University Press, 1988, pp 722–742.

Gittelman-Klein R, Klein DF: Controlled imipramine treatment of school phobia. Arch Gen Psychiatry 25:204–207, 1971.

Gittelman-Klein R, Klein DF: School phobia: Diagnostic considerations in the light of imipramine effects. J Nerv Ment Dis 156:199–215, 1973.

Graae F, Milner J, Rizzotto L, Klein R: Clonazepam and childhood anxiety disorders: A pilot study. In Scientific Proceedings of the Annual Meeting of the American Academy of Child and Adolescent Psychiatry, vol 7, 1991.

Grad LR, Pelcovitz D, Olson M, et al: Obsessive-compulsive symptomatology in children with Tourette's syndrome. J Am Acad Child Adolesc Psychiatry 26:69–73, 1987.

Gurman AS, Kniskern DP, Pinsof WM: Research on the process and outcome of marital and family therapy. In Garfield SL, Bergin AE (eds): Handbook of Psychotherapy and Behavior Change, 3d ed. New York, Wiley, 1986, pp 565–624.

Hersen M: Behavior modification approach to a school phobia case. J Clin Psychol 26:128–132, 1970.

Hirshfeld DR, Rosenbaum JR, Biederman J, et al: Stable behavioral inhibition and its association with anxiety disorder. J Am Acad Child Adolesc Psychiatry 31:103–111, 1992.

Hollingsworth CE, Tanguay PE, Grossman L, Pabst P: Long-term outcome of obsessive-compulsive disorder in childhood. J Am Acad Child Psychiatry 19:134–144, 1980.

Husain SA, Kashani JH: Anxiety Disorders in Children and Adolescents. Washington, American Psychiatric Press, 1992.

Johnson AM, Falstein EI, Szurek SA, Svendsen M: School phobia. Am J Orthopsychiatry 11:702–711, 1941.

Johnson JH, McCutcheon SM: Assessing life stress in older children and adolescents: Preliminary findings with the Life Events Checklist. In Sarason IG, Spielberger CD (eds): Stress and Anxiety, vol 7. Washington, Hemisphere, 1980.

Kagan J, Reznick JS, Clarke C, et al: Behavioral inhibition to the unfamiliar. Child Dev 55:2212–2225, 1984.

Kane MT, Kendall PC: Anxiety disorders in children: A multiple-baseline evaluation of a cognitive-behavioral treatment. Behav Ther 20:499–508, 1989.

Kashani JH, Orvaschel H: Anxiety disorders in midadolescence: A community sample. Am J Psychiatry 145:960–964, 1988.

Kashani JH, Orvaschel H: A community study of anxiety in children and adolescents. Am J Psychiatry 147:313–318, 1990.

Kashani JH, Vaidya AF, Soltys SM, et al: Correlates of anxiety in psychiatrically hospitalized children and their parents. Am J Psychiatry 147:319–323, 1990.

Kearney CA, Silverman WK: A preliminary analysis of a functional model of assessment and treatment for school refusal behavior. Behav Modif 14:340–366, 1990.

Kendall PC, Chansky TE, Freidman M, et al: Treating anxiety disorders in children and adolescents. In Kendall PC (ed): Child and Adolescent Therapy: Behavioral Procedures. New York, Guilford Press, 1991, pp 131–164.

Klein DF: Delineation of two drug-responsive anxiety syndromes. Psychopharmacologia 5:397–408, 1964.

Klein RG, Last CG: Anxiety Disorders in Children. Newbury Park, CA, Sage Publications, 1989.

Klein RG, Koplewicz HS, Kanner A: Imipramine treatment of children with separation anxiety disorder. J Am Acad Child Adolesc Psychiatry 31:21–28, 1992.

Kolko DJ: Positive practice routines in overcoming resistance to the treatment of school phobias: A case study with follow-up. J Behav Ther Exp Psychiatry 18:249–257, 1987.

Kruesi MJP, Swedo S, Leonard H, et al: CSF somatostatin in childhood psychiatric disorders: A preliminary investigation. Psychiatry Res 33:277–284, 1990.

Last CG, Strauss CC: Obsessive-compulsive disorder in childhood. J Anxiety Disord 3:295–302, 1989.

Last CG, Francis G, Strauss CC: Assessing fears in anxiety-disordered children with the revised fear survey schedule for children (FSSC-R). J Clin Child Psychol 18:137–141, 1989.

Last CG, Phillips JE, Statfeld A: Childhood anxiety disorders in mothers and their children. Child Psychiatry Hum Dev 18:103–112, 1987c.

Last CG, Strauss CC, Francis G: Comorbidity among childhood anxiety disorders. J Nerv Ment Dis 175:726–730, 1987d.

Last CG, Hersen M, Kazdin AE, et al: Comparison of DSM-III separation anxiety and overanxious disorders: Demographic characteristics and patterns of comorbidity. J Am Acad Child Adolesc Psychiatry 26:527–531, 1987a.

Last CG, Hersen M, Kazdin AE, et al: Psychiatric illness in the mothers of anxious children. Am J Psychiatry 144:1580–1583, 1987b.

Leonard HL, Rapoport JL: Separation anxiety, overanxious and avoidant disorders. In Wiener JM (ed): Textbook of Child and Adolescent Psychiatry. Washington, American Psychiatric Press, 1991a, pp 311–322.

Leonard HL, Rapoport JL: Obsessive-compulsive disorder. In Wiener JM (eds): Textbook of Child and Adolescent Psychiatry. Washington, American Psychiatric Press, 1991b, pp 323–329.

Leonard H, Swedo S, Rapoport JL, et al: Treatment of childhood obsessive-compulsive disorder with clomipramine and desmethylimipramine: A double-blind crossover comparison. Psychopharmacol Bull 24:93–95, 1988.

Livingston R, Reis CJ, Ringdahl IC: Abnormal dexamethasone suppression test results in depressed and nondepressed children. Am J Psychiatry 141:106–108, 1984.

Lo WH: A follow-up study of obsessional neurotics in Hong Kong Chinese. Br J Psychiatry 113:823–832, 1967.

Mansdorf IJ, Lukens E: Cognitive-behavioral psychotherapy for separation anxious children exhibiting school phobia. J Am Acad Child Adolesc Psychiatry 26:222–225, 1987.

Marks IM, Gelder MG: Different ages of onset in varieties of phobia. Am J Psychiatry 123:218–221, 1966.

Mattison RE, Bagnato SJ: Empirical measurement of overanxious disorder in boys 8 to 12 years old. J Am Acad Child Adolesc Psychiatry 26:536–540, 1987.

McDermott JF, Werry J, Petti T, et al: Anxiety disorders of childhood or adolescence. In Karasu TB (ed): Treatments of Psychiatric Disorders, vol 1. Washington, American Psychiatric Association, 1989, pp 401–446.

McGee R, Feehan M, Williams S, Anderson J: DSM-III disorders from age 11 to age 15 years. J Am Acad Child Adolesc Psychiatry 31:50–59, 1992.

McGee R, Feehan M, Williams S, et al: DSM-III disorders in a large sample of adolescents. J Am Acad Child Adolesc Psychiatry 29:611–619, 1990.

McNamara E: The self-management of school phobia: A case study. Behav Psychother 16:217–229, 1988.

Miller LC, Barrett CL, Hampe E, Noble H: Comparison of reciprocal inhibition, psychotherapy and waiting list control for phobic children. J Abnorm Psychol 79:269–279, 1972.

Miller PM: The use of visual imagery and muscle relaxation in the counterconditioning of a phobic child: A case study. J Nerv Ment Dis 154:457–460, 1972.

Ollendick TH: Fear reduction techniques with children. In Miller P, Eisler R (eds): Progress in Behavior Modification, vol 8. New York, Academic Press, 1979.

Ollendick TH: Reliability and validity of the revised fear survey schedule for children (FSSC-R). Behav Res Ther 21:685–692, 1983.

Ollendick TH, King NJ, Frary RB: Fears in children and adolescents: Reliability and generalizability across gender, age and nationality. Behav Res Ther 27:19–26, 1989.

Ollendick TH, Matson JL, Helsel WJ: Fears in children and adolescents: Normative data. Behav Res Ther 23:465–467, 1985.

Patterson GR: A learning theory approach to the problem of the school phobia child. In Ullmann LP, Krasner L (eds): Case Studies in Behavior Modification. New York, Holt, Rinehart & Winston, 1965.

Pauls DL, Leckman JF: The inheritance of Gilles de la Tourette's syndrome and associated behaviors: Evidence for autosomal dominant transmission. N Engl J Med 315:993–997, 1986.

Pauls DL, Towbin KE, Leckman JF, et al: Gilles de la Tourette's syndrome and obsessive-compulsive disorder: Evidence supporting a genetic relationship. Arch Gen Psychiatry 43:1180–1182, 1986.

Pfefferbaum B, Overall JE, Boren HA, et al: Alprazolam in the treatment of anticipatory and acute situational anxiety in children with cancer. J Am Acad Child Adolesc Psychiatry 26:532–535, 1987.

Pollitt J: Natural history of obsessional states: A study of 150 cases. Br Med J 5012:194–198, 1957.

Rapoport JL: Annotation childhood obsessive-compulsive disorder. J Child Psychol Psychiatry 27:289–295, 1986.

Rapoport JL, Elkins R, Langer DH, et al: Childhood obsessive-compulsive disorder. Am J Psychiatry 138:1545–1554, 1981.

Reynolds CR, Richman BO: What I think and feel: A revised measure of children's manifest anxiety. J Abnorm Child Psychol 6:271–280, 1978.

Riddle MA, Scahill L, King R, et al: Obsessive-compulsive disorder in children and adolescents: Phenomenology and family history. J Am Acad Child Adolesc Psychiatry 29:766–772, 1990.

Rogeness GA, Cepeda C, Macedo CA, et al: Differences in heart rate and blood pressure in children with conduct disorder, major depression and separation anxiety. Psychiatry Res 33:199–206, 1990.

Rosenbaum JF, Biederman J, Gersten M, et al: Behavioral inhibition in children of parents with panic disorder and agoraphobia: A controlled study. Arch Gen Psychiatry 45:463–470, 1988.

Ryan ND, Puig-Antich J, Ambrosini P, et al: The clinical picture of major depression in children and adolescents. Arch Gen Psychiatry 44:854–861, 1987.

Sheehan DV, Sheehan KE, Minichiello, WE: Age of onset of phobic disorders: A reevaluation. Compr Psychiatry 22:544–553, 1981.

Silverman WK, Nelles WB: The influence of gender on children's ratings of fear in self and same-aged peers. J Gen Psychol 148:17–21, 1988.

Silverman WK, Nelles WB: Simple phobia in childhood. In Hersen M, Last CG (eds): Handbook of Child and Adult Psychopathology: A Longitudinal Perspective. New York, Pergamon Press, 1990, pp 183–196.

Simeon JG, Ferguson HB: Alprazolam effects in children with anxiety disorders. Can J Psychiatry 32:570–574, 1987.

Simeon JG, Ferguson HB, Knott V, et al: Clinical, cognitive and neurophysiological effects of alprazolam in children and adolescents with overanxious and avoidant disorders. J Am Acad Child Adolesc Psychiatry 31:29–33, 1992.

Strauss CC, Last CG, Hersen M, Kazdin AE: Association between anxiety and depression in children and adolescents with anxiety disorders. J Abnorm Child Psychol 16:57–68, 1988a.

Strauss CC, Lease CA, Last CG, Francis G: Overanxious disorder: An examination of developmental differences. J Abnorm Child Psychol 16:433–443, 1988b.

Swedo SE, Rapoport JL, Leonard H, et al: Obsessive-compulsive disorder in children and adolescents. Arch Gen Psychiatry 46:335–341, 1989.

Thyer BA, Parrish RT, Curtis GC, et al: Ages of onset of DSM-III anxiety disorders. Compr Psychiatry 26:113–122, 1985.

Turner SM, Beidel DC, Costello A: Psychopathology in the offspring of anxiety disorders patients. J Consult Clin Psychol 55:229–235, 1987.

Velez CN, Johnson J, Cohen P: A longitudinal analysis of selected risk factors for childhood psychopathology. J Am Acad Child Adolesc Psychiatry 28:861–864, 1989.

Verhulst FC, Althaus M: Persistence and change in behavioral/emotional problems reported by parents of children aged 4–14: An epidemiological study. Acta Psychiatr Scand 339:1–28, 1988.

Verhulst FC, Berden GFMG, Sanders-Woudstra JAR: Mental health in Dutch children: II. The prevalence of psychiatric disorder and relationship between measures. Acta Psychiatr Scand 324:1–45, 1985.

Waldfogel S, Coolidge JC, Hahn PB: The development, meaning and management of school phobia. Am J Orthopsychiatry 27:754–780, 1957.

Weissman MM, Leckman JF, Merikangas KR, et al: Depression and anxiety disorders in parents and children. Arch Gen Psychiatry 41:845–852, 1984.

Werry JS: Overanxious disorder: A review of its taxonomic properties. J Am Acad Child Adolesc Psychiatry 30:533–544, 1991.

Whitaker A, Johnson J, Shaffer D, et al: Uncommon troubles in young people: Prevalence estimates of selected psychiatric disorders in a nonreferred adolescent population. Arch Gen Psychiatry 47:487–496, 1990.

Zitrin CM, Klein DF, Woerner MG, Ross DC: Treatment of phobias: I. Comparison of imipramine hydrochloride and placebo. Arch Gen. Psychiatry 40:125–138, 1983.

Zitrin CM, Ross DC: Early separation anxiety and adult agoraphobia. J Nerv Ment Dis 176:621–625, 1988.

UNIT 3

Symptom Clusters

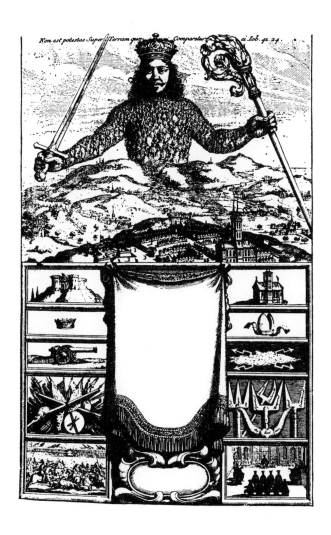

CHAPTER 22

Mood Disturbances

HAGOP S. AKISKAL

AFFECTS AND MOODS

Disturbances in the sphere of affect and mood—especially depressive manifestations—are among the most common signs and symptoms prompting medical consultation, both in psychiatry and in general medical practice. This is not surprising given the fact that, from an evolutionary perspective, affective arousal serves essential communication functions. Affect is something that moves us to appraise, for instance, whether another person is content, dissatisfied, or in danger. *Affect* refers to that aspect of emotion that is expressed through facial expression, vocal inflection, words, gestures, posture, and so on, whereas *mood* denotes more enduring emotional expressions. Joy, sadness, fear, and anger are basic affects, and their expression tells us how an individual feels at any given moment. Mood, on the other hand, relates to how one has been feeling over a period of time.

An individual's affective "tone" is thus the barometer of his or her inward emotional well-being. Each individual has a characteristic pattern of basal affective oscillations that defines his or her temperament. For instance, some people are minimally touched by adversity or reward and tend to remain placid. In contrast, others are easily moved to tears by sad or happy circumstances, and still others are more prone to fear, worry, or anger. Normally, oscillations in affective tone are relatively minor, tend to resonate with day-to-day events, and do not interfere with functioning.

We speak of affective disturbances when the amplitude and duration of affective change are beyond adaptive demands and lead to impaired function. Such impairment entails disturbances that go beyond subjective mood change and involves pathologic alterations in activity and thought as well. Mood disturbances leading to clinically diagnosable disorders arise in two patterns. The first pattern manifests in episodes which are sustained conglomerations of affective signs and symptoms typically lasting for months at a time and which tend to recur after variable intervals (typically measured in years). Episodes can be either depressive in nature (where depressive and associated signs and symptoms dominate the clinical picture), manic (where euphoric and associated signs and symptoms dominate the clinical picture), or mixed (where depressive and manic manifestations coexist simultaneously). In DSM-IV, patients with single or recurrent depressive episodes are said to have *major depressive disorder;* another name for this is *unipolar,* which happens to be the most prevalent of mood disorders and which can occur at any age. Almost all patients with manic and mixed episodes have depressive episodes as well, and for this reason, the illness is known as *bipolar disorder;* like its unipolar counterpart, this mood disorder also can occur at any age, but on average, it begins a decade earlier. Although both unipolar and bipolar forms of mood disorders can be precipitated by social or biologic stressors—and this is particularly true for episodes in the early course of these disorders—what characterizes them is that episodes persist autonomously even after these stressors are no longer operative. In brief, major depressive and bipolar disorders are characterized by pathologically sustained moods and related signs and symptoms that cannot be justified by external circumstances.

The second pattern of affective disturbances consists of "up" and "down" periods which do not cluster into discrete episodes but instead fluctuate in a low-grade intermittent pattern, typically beginning in late childhood or adolescence and continuing throughout much of adulthood. *Dysthymia* is characterized by low-grade depressive manifestations, *hyperthymia* with milder periods of frequent highs known as *hypomania*, and *cyclothymia* by a variability of moods which alternates between up and down periods. These three conditions are also known as *subaffective disorders* in the sense that they represent clinically attenuated expressions of affective disorders. They can exist throughout life as isolated temperamental extremes without significant pathology, but they often do produce at least some impairment in functioning in view of their tendency to be intermittently chronic. Others represent the precursors of major depressive or bipolar disorder or constitute the interepisodic manifestations to which patients return after recovering from depressive, manic, or mixed episodes (Akiskal and Akiskal, 1992).

Although current research tends to support the distinction between depressive and manic-depressive disorders (Winokur, 1991), a large territory exists between the two. Thus between the extremes of strict unipolar depressives (who have no high periods whatsoever) and bipolar I disorder (depression alternating with full-blown mania or mixed states) there are conditions termed as *unipolar II* (in which patients develop hypomanic or mild excitements upon antidepressant treatment) and *bipolar II* (in which patients have spontaneous hypomania, typically at the tail end of episodes). In some bipolar II patients, the high periods are so frequent that the patients are best described as being of cyclothymic temperament. Finally, to complicate matters, there are some unipolar patients who should actually be considered "pseudo-unipolar" because they descend into major depressive episodes from the higher than normal plane of a hyperthymic temperament (Akiskal and Akiskal, 1988; Cassano et al., 1989). Much more research needs to be conducted on these intermediate affective conditions for better nosologic assignment. At the moment, the unipolar–bipolar dichotomy remains a useful clinical and a heuristic research strategy.

In its pathologic expression, angry affect is not elaborated into a distinct psychopathologic disorder and is generic to a wide variety of psychiatric disorders. Fear, on the other hand, in its pathologic expression known as anxiety, is seen not only secondary to many psychiatric conditions but also elaborated into a spectrum of anxiety disorders. Because DSM-IV limits the rubric of mood disorder to conditions characterized by pathologic depression and elation, the discussion of anxiety and anger in this chapter is only to the extent that they represent manifestations of mood disorders.

The primary aim of this chapter, then, is to describe the signs and symptoms of disturbed affect and mood in such detail as to permit their differentiation from normal affective states and the manifestations of other psychiatric disorders.

Whatever their primary specialty, all physicians must be competent in the proper diagnosis and treatment of the more common depressive conditions not only because of their high prevalence but also in view of emerging data on the disabling nature of unrecognized protracted depressions. Indeed, Wells and colleagues (1989) have demonstrated that the functional disability induced by such depressions exceeds that of most medical conditions and equals that of cardiac disease. Social consequences appear equally disabling (Coryell et al., 1993).

THE DEPRESSIVE SYNDROME

As in other medical conditions, signs and symptoms of depression tend to cluster together in the form of a syndrome. Depression as a medical syndrome has been known since Hippocratic times, for nearly 2500 years. Excellent recent reviews are provided by Lewis (1934) and Jackson (1986). Multiple etiologic factors—some genetic, others environmental—can give rise to the final common pathway of depression (Akiskal and McKinney, 1973). One group of causative factors that should always be considered in the etiology of depression, especially in patients over the age of 40, is somatic disease or drugs used in their treatment (see Table 22-1). It is not always clear, however, that such diseases are sufficient causes of depression. Typically, not more than 15 percent of those with one of the conditions listed in the table will suffer from clinical depression. Further, eliminating the offending physical condition (e.g., reserpine) does not necessarily cure

TABLE 22-1. *Medical Conditions and Pharmacologic Agents Commonly Associated with Onset of Depression*

Medical conditions
  Hypothyroidism
  Cushing's disease
  Systemic lupus erythematosus
  Avitaminosis
  Cancer (especially abdominal)
  Tuberculosis
  Influenza; viral pneumonia
  Infectious mononucleosis
  General paresis (tertiary syphilis)
  Acquired immunodeficiency syndrome (AIDS)
  Cerebral tumor
  Head trauma
  Complex partial seizures (temporal lobe epilepsy)
  Stroke
  Parkinson's disease
  Multiple sclerosis
  Alzheimer's disease
  Sleep apnea
Pharmacologic agents
  Reserpine, alphamethyldopa, other antihypertensives
  Anticancer chemotherapy
  Corticosteroids, oral contraceptives
  Cimetidine, indomethacin
  Phenothiazines, other classes of neuroleptics
  Anticholinesterase insecticides
  Alcohol, barbiturates
  Stimulant withdrawal
  Psychedelics (?)

the depression. Indeed, those who succumb to depression secondary to reserpine and other medical factors seem to have past personal or familial history for depression. Thus some form of underlying predisposition, often of genetic nature, seems to be required, especially for recurrent mood disorders. However, the prognosis of the depressive syndrome may vary, depending on whether or not it is superimposed on a medical or a nonaffective psychiatric disorder, such as panic disorder, sociopathy, or schizophrenia (Robins and Guze, 1972). These secondary depressions tend to have somewhat atypical clinical features owing to the underlying disorder and often linger for many months (and sometimes years) beyond the usual duration of the depressive syndrome. It is in the syndrome occurring as a primary mood disorder that one observes the most typical manifestations of depressive illness, and whereas the course of secondary depressions is generally dictated by the underlying disorder, many primary depressions tend to recur on the basis of an inherent biologic rhythmicity.

The depressive syndrome is conveniently discussed by considering disturbances in four areas that characterize it: mood, vegetative, psychomotor, and cognitive.

Mood Change

The mood disturbance is usually considered the sine qua non of the syndrome and may manifest either in painful arousal or loss of the capacity for pleasurable experiences (anhedonia).

The painful arousal can take the form of depression, irritability, or anxiety and, in the extreme, is indescribably agonizing. The irritability and anxiety are often qualitatively different from their "neurotic" counterparts and take the form of severe inner turmoil and groundless apprehensions. In the full-blown form of the malady, the sustained nature of the painful mood does not permit distraction even for a moment. The psychic pain of depression is so agonizing that patients often describe it as being beyond ordinary physical pain. William James (1902), a sufferer of the malady, referred to his depression as "psychical neuralgia." Suicide often represents an attempt to find deliverance from such tormenting psychic pain. A more recent literary portrayal of the depressive's anguish is William Styron's memoir of his severe bout with the illness (1990). Other patients, suffering from a milder form of the malady and typically seen in primary-care settings, deny experiencing such mental pain and instead complain of physical agony in the form of, for example, headache, epigastric pain, and precordial distress, in the absence of any evidence of organically diagnosable pathology. Such conditions have been described as *depressio sine depressione*, or *masked depression* (Kielholz et al., 1982). In these situations, the physician can corroborate the presence of mood change by the depressed affect in the facial expression, the voice, and the patient's overall appearance.

Paradoxically, this heightened perception of pain so characteristic of clinical depression is often accompanied by an inability to experience normal sadness and grief, as well as joy and pleasure. Thus anhedonia, the loss of the ability to experience pleasure, is a special instance of a more generalized inability to experience normal emotions. Patients exhibiting this disturbance often lose the capacity to cry—an ability that may return as the depression is lifting.

During the clinical interview, it is not enough to inquire whether the patient has lost the sense of pleasure; the clinician must document that the patient has given up previously enjoyed pastimes. In the extreme, patients may complain that they have lost all feeling for their children, who once were a source of great joy. The impact of the loss of emotional experience can be so pervasive that patients may give up values and beliefs that had previously given meaning to their lives. This is well described by Tolstoy in his autobiographical *My Confessions* (1887), in which he describes how his bouts of depression later in life led to "spiritual crises." The depressive's inability to experience normal emotions is different from the blunting seen in schizophrenia in that the loss of emotions is itself experienced as painful; that is, the depressive suffers immensely from his or her inability to experience emotions.

Vegetative Disturbances

The ancients believed that depression was a somatic illness and ascribed it to black bile, hence the term *melancholia*, from the Greek word for this substance. Indeed, the mood change in depressive illness is accompanied by several physiologic disturbances that implicate limbic-diencephalic dysfunction (Akiskal and McKinney, 1973). These include changes in libido and menstruation, appetite and sleep, as well as other circadian rhythms. DSM-IV now uses the term *melancholia* for a special cluster of depressive symptomatology that includes marked vegetative and psychomotor disturbances, anhedonia, and self-reproach; these manifestations persist autonomously, showing no reactivity to psychosocial contingencies. It replaces the term *endogenous depression*, which carried the connotation of lack of precipitation, a notion not supported by current evidence. The melancholic cluster is generally believed to predict response to tricyclic antidepressants and electroconvulsive therapy.

Although decreased sexual desire occurs in both men and women, women are more likely to complain of infrequent menses or cessation of menses. Their unwillingness to participate in sex often leads to marital conflict. Therapists may mistakenly ascribe the depression to the marital conflict, leading to unnecessarily zealous psychotherapeutic attention to the marital situation and a prolongation of the depressive agony. Decrease or loss of libido in men often results in erectile failure, which may prompt endocrinologic or urologic consultation. Again, depression may be ascribed to the sexual dysfunction rather than the reverse, and definitive treatment is often delayed because of the physician's focus on the sexual complaint.

Disturbed appetite and sleep have been described since Hippocrates' classic case (Jackson, 1986):

In Thesus a woman, of a melancholic turn of mind . . . became affected with loss of sleep, aversion to food . . . frights . . . despondency . . . pains frequent, great and continued.

Most characteristically, there is a diminution in sleep and appetite, but not uncommonly, one may see an increase or, in rare cases, an alternation between them. Weight gain may be due to overeating, decreased activity, or both. Weight changes secondary to depression can have serious consequences. Inanition, especially in the elderly, can lead to malnutrition and electrolyte disturbances that represent medical emergencies, often requiring electroconvulsive therapy. Weight gain in middle-aged patients, on the other hand, may aggravate preexisting diabetes, hypertension, or coronary artery disease. In younger patients, especially women, weight problems may conform to a bulimic pattern. This is sometimes the expression of the depressive phase of a bipolar disorder with infrequent hypomanic periods (bipolar II disorder) and may benefit from specific therapies available for this disorder.

Like appetite, sleep may be increased or decreased. Insomnia is one of the major manifestations of depressive illness and is characterized more by multiple awakenings, especially in the early hours of the morning, than by difficulty falling asleep. This was described in "Waking up in the Blue," a verse by the American poet Robert Lowell, who had a documented history of bipolar swings (Hamilton, 1982). The "light" sleep of the depressive is a reflection of the painful arousal and prolongs the agony of the patient. Deep stages of sleep (3 and 4) are either decreased or deficient. The understandable attempt to drown the sorrow in alcohol, as the poet Lowell did, may initially have some success but ultimately leads to an aggravation of the insomnia. The same applies to sedative-hypnotic drugs, which are often prescribed by the busy medical practitioner who has not spent adequate time to diagnose the depressive condition. (Sedatives, including alcohol, although effective in reducing the number of awakenings in the short term, are not effective in the long run because of a further diminution of stage 3 and 4 sleep.)

Young depressives, especially those with bipolar tendencies, typically complain of hypersomnia, sleeping as long as 15 hours a day. Obviously, such patients will have difficulty getting up in the morning; this may lead to their being labeled "lazy." Whether suffering from insomnia or hypersomnia, nearly two-thirds of melancholic patients exhibit a shortening of rapid eye movement (REM) latency, the period from the onset of sleep to the first REM period (Kupfer and Thase, 1983). This abnormality is seen throughout the depressive episode and, in recurrent depressives, may be seen in relatively euthymic periods as well (Akiskal, 1983a). Other REM abnormalities include longer REM periods and increased density of eye movements in the first half of the night. These abnormalities in REM sleep are rather specific to primary depressive disorders in that they do not occur in most schizophrenic, anxious, and personality-disordered subjects. Figure 22-1 contrasts the sleep electroencephalogram (EEG) of a major depressive with insomnia with that of a normal control.

Other circadian abnormalities in depression include feeling worse in the morning, periodicity of episodes, and seasonal precipitation (Wehr and Rosenthal, 1989). The last two abnormalities are most commonly associated with bipolar II disorder. As with other vegetative abnormalities, these, too, point to the limbic-diencephalic dysfunction as the pathophysiologic substrate of the illness. Abnormal response to the dexamethasone suppression test (DST) (i.e., early escape from suppression of elevated plasma cortisol on overnight dexamethasone), seen in 50 percent of melancholic patients (Carroll et al., 1981), can be considered another indirect indicator of disturbed midbrain function.

In summary, vegetative dysfunction in depressive illness has lent itself to laboratory evaluation that has opened windows into the midbrain origins of the disorder. The sleep EEG and neuroendocrine

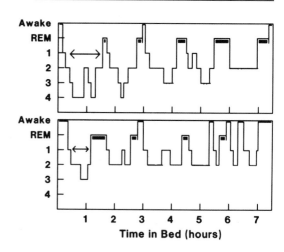

FIGURE 22-1. *Comparison of sleep in normal (top) and clinically depressed (bottom) subjects.*

abnormalities in depression, irrespective of their etiologic significance, are among the most replicated biologic findings in all of psychiatry and herald psychiatry's new momentum as a medical specialty.

Psychomotor Disturbances

Depressed patients exhibit characteristic abnormalities in the execution of motor functions in relation to psychological tasks. Although agitation (pressured speech, restlessness, wringing of hands, and, in the extreme, pulling of one's hair) is the more commonly described abnormality, it is less specific to the illness than retardation (slowing of psychomotor activity). Indeed, such slowing often coexists with agitation. Psychomotor retardation underlies many of the psychiatric deficits seen in depression and is considered the best predictor of response to tricyclic antidepressants (Nelson and Charney, 1981). According to Widlöcher (1983), psychomotor slowing is manifested by the following disturbances:

- Paucity of spontaneous movements
- Slumped posture with downcast gaze
- Overwhelming fatigue—patients complain that "everything is an effort"
- Reduced flow and amplitude of speech and increased latency of responses—often giving rise to monosyllabic speech
- Subjective feeling that time is passing slowly or has actually stopped
- Poor concentration and forgetfulness
- Painful rumination—or thinking that dwells on few (usually unpleasant) topics
- Indecisiveness—inability to make simple decisions

DSM-IV places greater emphasis on the more easily measurable objective or physical aspects of retardation. For the patient, however, the subjective sense of slowing is often the more pervasive and disabling aspect of retardation. This more "psychological" dimension of retardation is not always easy to elicit from patients, and only those with unusually good premorbid verbal skills can provide reliable descriptions, as documented in the following vignette.

A 47-year-old moderately depressed physics professor gave the following self-report: I am weary with a "leaden" feeling. Manual dexterity is diminished—writing legibly seems like an impossible task. What is most disabling, however, is a kind of staring or stoppage of mental functions. . . . I have great difficulty with the retention of facts and especially words. Recall is sluggish, frustrating. The brain feels "muddled"—thought processes slowed and confused. My mind simply "cuts off" at times—often in midsentence or midthought. Yet it seems to dwell on painful subjects. I think about how inadequate I am—and I cannot get rid of that idea, it keeps on coming back. In the morning I feel literally paralyzed with inadequacy and indecision—I cannot even decide which necktie to wear—or whether to wear one at all. I seem to lack any sense of direction or purpose. I have such an inertia—I cannot assert myself, I cannot fight. I do not seem to have any will at all.

It is because of such psychomotor deficits that depressed patients are often unable to continue to work or do so with much diminished efficiency; the household is typically disorganized; and students fail their classes or drop courses. In the elderly, the slowing of mental functions can be so pronounced that the patient may appear "demented" because of memory difficulties, disorientation, and confusion. This clinical picture is known as *depressive pseudodementia* (Roth, 1976) and may respond dramatically to a course of electroconvulsive therapy. Although appropriate neurologic evaluation may sometimes be necessary before instituting such therapy, the differentiation of pseudodementia from dementia can often be accomplished on primarily clinical grounds (Table 22-2). In some instances, a therapeutic trial with an antidepressant that possesses minimal or no anticholinergic side effects may be the only way to arrive at a differential diagnosis.

In young depressives, especially bipolars, psychomotor slowing may in the extreme manifest stupor—the patient is unable to participate even in basic biologic functions like feeding himself or herself. History is the most reliable way to distinguish depressive stupor from its hysterical and schizophrenic counterparts. Again, electroconvulsive therapy is often lifesaving in such cases, but somatic causes of stupor (e.g., metabolic, neurologic) must first be ruled out by appropriate clinical and laboratory evaluation.

Cognitive Disturbances

The term *cognitive* refers to such things as memory, thinking processes, and thought content. In depression, abnormalities in these areas are often secondary to psychomotor disturbances and, for this reason, were described under that heading. In addition

TABLE 22-2. *Clinical Features Useful in Differential Diagnosis of Depressive Pseudodementia from Primary Dementia*

	Pseudodemented depression	Primary dementia
Onset	Acute	Insidious
Past affective episodes	Common	Uncharacteristic
Self-reproach	Yes	Uncharacteristic
Diurnality	Worse in A.M.	Worse at night
Memory deficit	Recent = remote	Recent > remote
Responses	"Don't know"	Near miss
Reaction to failure	Tend to give up	Catastrophic reaction
Practice effects	Can be coached	Consistently poor

to difficulties in concentration and memory, the depressive exhibits a characteristic thought abnormality consisting of negative evaluations of the self, the world, and the future (Beck, 1967). Clinically, these are manifested as

- Ideas of deprivation and loss
- Low self-esteem and self-confidence
- Self-reproach and pathologic guilt
- Helplessness, hopelessness, and pessimism
- Recurrent thoughts of death and suicide

The main characteristic of the depressive's thinking is that he or she views everything in an extremely negative, gloomy light. The self-accusations are typically unjustified or grotesquely blown out of proportion, as in the case of a woman who was tormented by guilt because on one occasion 20 years previously she permitted someone other than her fiancé to kiss her on the lips. Some of these symptoms verge on the delusional. For instance, a world-famous artist presented to his physician with the complaint that he was "nothing." In what is termed *psychotic depression*, negative thinking acquires grossly delusional proportions, being maintained with such conviction that patients are not amenable to change by evidence to the contrary. Thus severely depressed patients may manifest delusions of worthlessness and sinfulness, reference, and persecution. They believe that they are being singled out for their past "transgressions" and that everyone is aware of these grievous errors. Persecutory ideation in depression is often prosecutory and derives from belief in the necessity of punishment for such transgressions. Other depressives believe that they have lost all their means and that their children will starve (delusions of poverty), or that they harbor an occult and "shameful" illness, such as cancer or AIDS (delusions of ill health), or that parts of their bodies are missing (nihilistic delusions). A minority of depressives may have fleeting auditory or visual hallucinations with extremely sions). A minority of depressives may have fleeting (e.g., accusatory voices or seeing themselves in coffins or graveyards). All these psychotic experiences are considered mood-congruent in the sense that they are understandable in light of the prevailing pathologic mood.

Given the fact that the depressives typically find themselves locked in the private hell of their negative thoughts, it is not surprising that 15 percent of untreated patients give up hope that they will ever be free of such torments and kill themselves. However, they do not do this at the depth of their melancholia.

The author once asked a severely depressed woman if suicide had crossed her mind, to which she replied, "Doctor, I am already dead. I have no existence." Such a patient is unlikely to undertake suicidal action.

It is when psychomotor activity is improving either spontaneously or with antidepressants—yet mood and thinking are still dark—that the patient is most likely to have the requisite energy to undertake the suicidal act.

THE DISTINCTION BETWEEN GRIEF AND MELANCHOLIA

Depression in its full-blown form is sharply demarcated from the "blues" (Akiskal, 1983a). The patient and his or her family will tell the doctor that the depressed state represents a break from his or her usual self. The sustained nature of the mood disturbance, the often disabling characteristic signs and symptoms in vegetative, psychomotor, and cognitive areas, the tendency for recurrence (especially in a periodic and seasonal fashion), and, in many cases, the presence of "loaded" (three consecutive generations) family histories for the same type of illness serve to distinguish this clinical disorder from the ordinary disappointments that are part of the fabric of human existence.

It is in deciding whether a given patient is suffering from ordinary grief or has progressed to clinical depression that the doctor will encounter the greatest difficulty. Since bereaved individuals manifest many depressive symptoms within the first year (Clayton et al., 1974), how does one decide whether grief has progressed to melancholia, as it does in 2 to 5 percent of such individuals? Clayton and associates have suggested the following criteria as a guideline:

- Preoccupation with suicidal ideation does not occur in normal grief except in some men during the first month or so of bereavement.
- Marked psychomotor retardation is not observed in normal grief.
- Although bereaved individuals sometimes experience guilt about having *omitted* to offer certain services that may have saved the life of the deceased loved one, they typically do not experience the more pathologic form of guilt known as *guilt of commission* (i.e., guilt about having done something bad to their loved one).
- *Mummification*, which refers to maintaining the belongings of the deceased person exactly as they were before his or her death, is abnormal and indicative of psychopathology.
- Severe anniversary reaction should, likewise, alert the clinician to the possibility of psychopathology.

Although dexamethasone suppression test and REM latency findings have not been systematically studied in this context, they also might assist, especially when extremely deviant values are obtained, in the differential diagnostic process. The following vignette (taken from Akiskal and Lemmi, 1983) on the joint use of clinical and biologic indices in the differential diagnosis of affective syndromes illustrates the features of pathologic grief.

A 75-year-old widow was brought by her daughter because of severe insomnia and loss of interest in daily routines after her husband's death 1 year earlier. She had been agitated for the first 2 or 3 months and thereafter "sank into total inactivity—not wanting to get out of bed, not wanting to do anything, not wanting to go out." According to her daughter, she had been married at 21, had four children, and had been a housewife until her husband's death from a heart attack. Past psychiatric history was negative; premorbid adjustment had been characterized by compulsive traits.

During the interview, she was dressed in black, appeared moderately slowed, and sobbed intermittently, saying, "I search everywhere for him—I don't find him." When asked about life, she said, "Everything I see is black." Although she expressed no interest in food, she did not seem to have lost an appreciable amount of weight. Her DST was 18 µg/dl. The patient declined psychiatric care, stating that she "preferred to join her husband rather than get well." She was too religious to commit suicide, but by refusing treatment, she felt that she would "pine away—find relief in death and reunion."

THE DISTINCTION BETWEEN ANXIETY AND DEPRESSIVE STATES

Anxiety is a common symptom of depressive illness, and depression is a common complication of anxiety states. Separating these two alternatives on strictly clinical grounds is not always easy. Systematic studies by Roth and Mountjoy (1982) have shown that early-morning awakening, psychomotor retardation, self-reproach, hopelessness, and suicidal ideation represent the most solid clinical markers of depression in this differential diagnosis. On follow-up of depressed patients, these manifestations tend to remit, whereas patients with anxiety states continue to exhibit a spectrum of signs and symptoms consisting of marked tension, phobias, panic attacks, vasomotor instability, feelings of unreality, perceptual distortions, as well as paranoid and hypochondriacal ideas. A predominance of such anxiety features antedating the present bout of illness suggests the diagnosis of an anxiety disorder. It must be kept in mind, however, that anxiety disorders seldom make their first appearance after age 40. Therefore, it is best to consider patients who present with marked anxiety features for the first time after age 40 as suffering from major depression and treat them accordingly (Watts, 1966).

A 52-year-old married teacher with unremarkable previous psychiatric history was referred by his internist to "rule out sleep apnea." Over the previous 3 weeks, he had begun to awaken several times at night, gasping for air and sweating, with palpitations and intense fear. There was no special dream recall. History revealed that a colleague, to whom the patient was not particularly close, had recently

suffered a severe coronary attack and underwent bypass surgery. Additional complaints of the patient included early-morning awakening, feeling tired in the morning, and tension, irritability, and apprehension throughout the day, rendering classroom teaching difficult. Appetite and libido were unchanged. The patient denied subjective depression. During psychiatric interview, his face expressed worry and gloom, and he was visibly agitated; he was tormented by the fear that he might die suddenly, although he could not say from what. Family history was unremarkable. The patient had not responded to a 3-week trial of diazepam, 20 mg/day. After drug washout, polysomnographic evaluation ruled out sleep apnea while demonstrating a REM latency of 38 minutes, middle and terminal insomnia with a sleep efficiency of 64 percent. Within 15 days, the patient showed a dramatic response to trazodone, 300 mg/day.

Such agitated patients represent variants of unipolar depression and, in former classifications, were termed *involutional melancholics.*

Currently, the differential diagnosis of anxiety and depressive states is not fully resolved. Although recurrent (especially retarded) major depressive illness is most certainly a distinct disorder from anxiety states, at least some forms of depression may share a common diathesis with panic disorder (Leckman et al., 1983). Biologic markers may contribute to the resolution of this nosologic problem:

- Sleep EEG studies indicate that short REM latency is uncharacteristic of anxiety states, even when complicated by depression (Akiskal et al., 1984). Furthermore, arecoline challenge shortens the REM latency in depression but not in anxiety states (Dube et al., 1985).
- DST findings are generally negative in anxiety states (Curtis et al., 1982). However, corticotropin-releasing factor (CRF) activity appears elevated in both depressive and anxiety states (Butler and Nemeroff, 1990).
- Basal forearm blood flow is elevated in anxiety but not depressive states (Kelly and Walter, 1969). By contrast, baseline skin conductance, another psychophysiologic measure, is lowered in depressive states (Ward and Doerr, 1986).

These promising biologic considerations cannot substitute for clinical judgment. Table 22-3 summarizes clinical considerations which the weight of the literature suggests to be most discriminatory between anxiety and depressive states.

EDITORS' COMMENT

Another possible distinction is family history (Clayton PJ, et al: Follow-up and family study of anxious depression. Am J Psychiatry 148:1512–1517, 1991; Diagnosis and Treatment of Anxiety Disorders: A Physician's Handbook. Washington, American Psychiatric Press, 1991, pp 8–11). Patients exhibiting anxiety symptoms during a depression have family members with depression and not anxiety

TABLE 22-3. *Cross-Sectional Differentiating Clinical Features of Anxiety and Depressive States*

Anxiety	Depression
Hypervigilance	Psychomotor retardation
Severe tension and panic	Severe sadness
Perceived danger	Perceived loss
Phobic avoidance	Loss of interest—anhedonia
Doubt and uncertainty	Hopelessness—suicidal
Insecurity	Self-depreciation
Performance anxiety	Loss of libido
	Early morning awakening
	Weight loss

Reproduced, with permission, from Akiskal HS: Toward a clinical understanding of the relationships between anxiety and depressive disorders. In Maser J, Cloninger R (eds): Comorbidity in Anxiety and Mood Disorders. Washington, American Psychiatric Press, 1990, pp. 597–607.

disorders. The opposite is true for patients whose primary diagnosis is an anxiety disorder.

A final issue in discussing the relationship between anxiety and depressive states is what have been termed *atypical depressions* (Davidson et al., 1982). As originally described in the British literature, these were mild, fluctuating outpatient depressions (which sometimes reached full syndromal depth) seen mostly in young women referred from the cardiology service, where they had been seen because of manifestations of autonomic nervous system overactivity. Against this background of somatic anxiety symptoms, which often led to phobias, these patients suffered from initial insomnia (yet slept deeply and too long once they fell asleep), daytime fatigue and lethargy, overeating, and feeling worse in the evening. Current experience supports the British suggestions that monoamine oxidase inhibitors (MAOIs) are more likely to be effective in such patients. Furthermore, Liebowitz et al. (1984) have shown that response to MAOIs is most likely in those atypical patients who give a history of panic attacks. It would therefore appear that atypical depression, as defined earlier, is in effect atypical panic disorder, presenting with or complicated by depressive symptoms. To compound matters, atypical depressions without the anxiety component seem to represent a heterogeneous group of disorders that range from mild hypothyroidism to mild bipolar disorder, both of which manifest with extreme lethargy, hypersomnia, and overeating.

THE HETEROGENEITY OF DYSTHYMIC DISORDERS

As defined in DSM-IV, *dysthymia* refers to chronic, low-grade, fluctuating depressions of at least 2 years' duration. Except for the requirement of chronicity, this group of patients is similar to what,

in former classifications, was termed *neurotic depression*. This is a heterogeneous grouping that subsumes several nosologically unrelated categories (Akiskal, 1983b). Most patients manifesting low-grade depressive mood swings are not suffering from primary mood disorder; their gloom is secondary to other psychiatric conditions, such as anxiety disorders, anorexia nervosa, or ego-dystonic homosexuality, hysteria, sociopathy, and their variants. In a special subgroup, however, low-grade depression represents the residual phase of incompletely remitted primary major depressions; such residuals are most commonly seen in late-onset unipolar illness (>40 years).

There is also an early-onset primary dysthymic pattern. It begins insidiously in teenage years—or even in late childhood—in the absence of other psychiatric disorders and pursues an intermittent course. If major depressions are superimposed, the patient returns to the low-grade, intermittent baseline on recovery. Such patients tend to be introverted, self-sacrificing, and self-denigrating. They are habitually brooding, anhedonic, and hypersomnolent; suffer from psychomotor inertia; and tend to feel worse in the morning. REM latency is reduced to less than 70 minutes, and family history can be positive for bipolar disorder. For this reason, such patients may respond to various antidepressants with hypomanic episodes. In brief, this form of dysthymia appears to be a true subaffective disorder (i.e., an attenuated clinical expression of primary mood disorder) or, alternatively, cyclothymia minus spontaneous hypomania. The vignette that follows is a self-description given by a 34-year-old nurse of her "depressive self"; it exemplifies the concept of dysthymia as a true subaffective disorder:

Suffering is so much part of me that it defines my personality. This is manifested by a profound sense of inadequacy which is almost physical. I feel as though a stone is suspended from a long chain inside me dangling over a dark bottomless well. I sense the futility of effort—though not where work is concerned, which, over the years, has been the major principle of my life. My suffering is endured in personal isolation. It has never been possible for me to describe to anyone the overwhelming sadness that almost paralyzes me in the mornings. I have never timed the periods of depression, as they seem to come and go irregularly. My appetite is usually unchanged, but I sleep more, sometimes 15 hours per day.

These black periods have been my share in life for as long as I can remember. I have never taken medication for them. Onset is insidious, but return to normal mood can come on suddenly, like the snapping of a light switch, and I will be well for a week or so, and if I am lucky, for several weeks.

My mother suffered a mood disorder. I remember days when she would cry for no reason—when I would come home from school to find her still huddled in bed. My aunt said she was "lazy." And then I remember her becoming hyperactive, grandiose, expansive. Her father also suffered periods of depression. So it would seem almost by destiny that I have been sentenced to a life of suffering. My major question is why I have been denied the highs that my mother enjoyed so much—even though at such times she gave hell to my father.

This is one of the unresolved questions in the riddle of the mood disorders—why some of the relatives of bipolar individuals suffer from depressive episodes alone and from depressive "personality" developments, as in the case of this patient. As described in a subsequent section of this chapter, in reality such patients are pseudo-unipolar in the sense that they are at risk for pharmacologically induced hypomanic periods.

THE MANIC SYNDROME

As with the depressive syndrome, mania manifests in disturbances in mood, vegetative, psychomotor, and cognitive functions. It has been known for two millennia, with a compelling description provided by Aretaeus of Capadocia in the first century A.D. (reviewed in Jackson, 1986). The monographs by Winokur et al., (1969) and by Goodwin and Jamison (1990) provide encyclopedic coverage of the explosion of research along clinical and biologic fronts since Kraepelin's classic treatise (1921). Destigmatization of manic–depressive illness has been recently achieved by self confessions of celebrities (e.g. Patty Duke, 1992). Clinical manifestations in mania are often, although not always, opposite in direction from those seen in depression. Mild degrees of mania (hypomania) can be useful in business, leadership roles, and the arts (Akiskal and Akiskal, 1988; Goodwin and Jamison, 1990). A powerful literary portrayal of hypomania is provided by Bellow's *Herzog* (1964). Many creative people have had such elevated periods, without necessarily reaching clinical proportions (Andreasen, 1987). Others appear to have suffered from psychotic mood swings; for instance, Van Gogh, who painted almost 200 masterpieces in his Arles period before committing suicide in 1890, wrote the following description in his letters to his brother Theo (1927): "Ideas for my work are coming to me in swarms . . . continued fever to work . . . an extraordinary feverish energy . . . terrible lucidity." In the case of Van Gogh, who suffered from extreme lows and highs, the unstable moods could have had epileptic basis (Monroe, 1992).

Although mania can be symptomatic of several medical conditions or precipitated by catecholaminergic drugs (Krauthammer and Klerman, 1978), the syndrome most typically develops in those with the familial manic-depressive diathesis. (Symptomatic manias are listed in Table 22-4.) One of many reasons that mania is considered an illness is that it often leads to personal disaster and tragedy, as it did in the case of Van Gogh. Fortunately, current treatments can often attenuate bipolar swings with no appreciable effect on creativity, which may even be enhanced, thanks to freedom from inca-

TABLE 22-4. *Medical and Pharmacologic Factors Commonly Associated with Onset of Mania*

Medical conditions
  Thyrotoxicosis
  Systemic lupus erythematosus
  Rheumatic chorea
  Influenza
  St. Louis encephalitis
  General paresis (tertiary syphilis)
  Huntington's chorea
  Multiple sclerosis
  Diencephalic and third ventricular tumors
  Complex partial seizures (temporal lobe epilepsy)
  Stroke
  Head trauma
Pharmacologic agents
  Corticosteroids
  Levodopa
  Bromocriptine
  Amphetamines
  Methylphenidate
  Cocaine
  Monoamine oxidase inhibitors
  Antidepressants

pacitating mood swings (Schou, 1979). This is not universal, however, and each patient who derives benefits from hypomanic bursts should be considered individually. Such consideration is important because creativity and achievement appear related to temperamental characteristics most affected by lithium salts (Akiskal and Akiskal, 1992).

Mood Change

The mood in mania is classically one of elation, euphoria, and jubilation, often associated with laughing, punning, and gesturing. The mood is not stable, and momentary tearfulness is not uncommon. Also, for many patients, the high is so excessive that it is dysphoric. When crossed, the patient can become extremely irritable and hostile. Thus lability is as much a feature of the manic's mood as the mood elevation.

Vegetative Disturbances

The cardinal sign here is decreased amount of sleep, the patient needing only a few hours of sleep and feeling energetic on awakening. Some patients may go without sleep for 48 hours at a time and feel even more energetic.

There does not seem to be a primary disturbance of appetite as such, but weight loss may occur because of increased activity and inattention to nutritional needs. The sexual appetite is increased and may lead to much sexual indiscretion. Married women with previously unblemished sexual histories may associate with men below their social station. Men may overindulge in alcohol and sex—frequenting bars and prostitutes on whom they squander their savings. The sexual adventures of manic patients characteristically result in marital disasters and multiple separations or divorces. The poor judgment and the impulsivity leading to such behavior are particularly problematic in the era of AIDS and dictate early diagnosis and treatment.

Psychomotor Disturbances

Increased psychomotor activity, the hallmark of mania, is characterized by increased energy and activity level and by rapid and pressured speech. These are coupled with a subjective sense of physical well-being known as *eutonia* and by flight of ideas; thinking and perception are unusually sharp or brilliant. Sometimes the patient speaks with such pressure that it is difficult to follow his or her associations; termed *clang associations*, these are often based on rhyming or chance perceptions and flow with great rapidity.

Manic patients are typically impulsive, disinhibited, and meddlesome. They are intrusive in their increased involvement with people, leading to much friction with colleagues, friends, and family. They are distractible and quickly move not only from one thought to another but also from one person to another, showing heightened interest in every new activity that strikes their fancy. They are indefatigable and engage in various and sundry activities, in which they usually display poor social judgment. Examples include preaching or dancing in the streets; abuse of long-distance calling; buying new cars, hundreds of records, expensive jewelry, or other unnecessary items; engaging in risky business ventures; gambling; and sudden trips. Obviously, these pursuits can lead to personal and financial ruin. In severe mania, known as *delirious mania*, frenzied physical activity continues unabated, leading to a medical emergency requiring daily electroconvulsive therapy.

Cognitive Disturbances

The manic has an inflated self-esteem and a grandiose sense of confidence and achievements. Underneath this facade, however, the patient sometimes has a painful recognition that these positive self-concepts do not represent reality. Such insight, if present at all, is, unfortunately, transient. Indeed, manic patients are notoriously refractory to self-examination and insight. As a result, manic delusions are often maintained with extraordinary fervor. These include delusions of exceptional mental and physical fitness; exceptional talent; wealth, aristocratic ancestry, or other grandiose identity; assistance (i.e., well-placed people or supernatural powers are assisting in their endeavors); or reference and persecution (i.e., enemies are observing them or following them out of malignant jealousy).

THE DISTINCTION BETWEEN BIPOLAR AND SCHIZOPHRENIC PSYCHOSES

As in depressive psychoses, fleeting auditory or visual hallucinations involving the mood-congruent themes mentioned earlier can be seen in a sizable minority of manic patients. Furthermore, severely ill manic patients can exhibit such a degree of psychotic disorganization that mood-incongruent symptoms pervade the clinical picture, and cross-sectionally, it may prove difficult to distinguish them from schizophrenic patients. They may even exhibit isolated schneiderian symptoms, although this is typically fleeting and occurs at the height or depth of affective psychosis (Carlson and Goodwin, 1973). Thinking may be so rapid that it may appear "loosened," but unlike schizophrenia, this will be in the setting of expansive and elated affect. By contrast, the severely retarded bipolar depressive, whose affect may superficially seem flat, will almost never exhibit major fragmentation of thought. The clinician should therefore consider the clustering of symptoms—rather than individual symptoms—in the differential diagnosis of affective and schizophrenic psychoses. Because the two psychotic conditions entail radically different pharmacologic treatments on a long-term basis, this differential diagnosis (Table 22-5) is of major clinical import.

In the past, many bipolar patients, especially those with prominent manic features at onset, were considered "acute schizophrenics" or "schizoaffective schizophrenics" (Cooper et al., 1972). This often resulted from exclusive reliance on the cross-sectional clinical picture. Although modern treatments tend to keep many schizophrenics out of the hospital, the illness still pursues a downhill course; by contrast, the intermorbid periods in bipolar illness are characterized by temperamental oscillations that can be dysthymic, hyperthymic, or cyclothymic; in a selected few, the interepisodic periods are marked by supernormal functioning, although in other patients some social impairment may come, over time, from the accumulation of divorces, financial catastrophes, and ruined careers. Genetic studies tend to separate the two disorders; e.g., discordance in identical twins for schizophrenia and bipolar illness is never due to the presence of

TABLE 22-5. *Clinical Features Distinguishing Bipolar from Schizophrenic Psychoses*

	Bipolar disorder	Schizophrenia
Cross sectional		
Affect	"Contagious"	"Praecox feeling"
Thought	Accelerated or retarded	Poverty of content and bizarre
Autism	Uncharacteristic	Characteristic
Hallucinations	Fleeting	Intermittent or continuous
Schneiderian symptoms	Few (≤ 2)	Numerous
Longitudinal		
Premorbid	Cyclothymic	Schizotypal
Intermorbid	Tempestuous, "supernormal"	Withdrawn or low functioning
Course	Biphasic	Fluctuating, downhill

the other disorder. Laboratory markers have not yet been systematically applied in the two disorders in the clinical setting; it is of clinical interest, however, that thyroid-stimulating hormone (TSH) blunting in response to thyrotropin-releasing hormone (TRH) challenge is almost never positive in schizophrenia, at least not in chronic schizophrenia (Loosen and Prange, 1982). This means that a blunted TSH response would essentially rule out schizophrenia.

Schizoaffective (or *cycloid*) *psychosis* refers to an uncommon form of recurrent psychosis with full affective and schizophrenic symptoms during each episode (Perris, 1974). Such a diagnosis should not be considered in an affective psychosis where mood-incongruent psychotic features (e.g., schneiderian and bleulerian symptoms) can be explained on the basis of one of the following: (1) affective psychosis superimposed on mental retardation, giving rise to extremely hyperactive and bizarre manic behavior, (2) affective psychosis complicated by concurrent medical or neurologic diseases, substance abuse, or withdrawal, giving rise to numerous schneiderian symptoms, or (3) mixed episodes of bipolar illness, which are notorious for signs and symptoms of psychotic disorganization.

Although mixed *features* (i.e., crying while manic) commonly occur in the course of bipolar disorder, mixed *states* with the full complement of depressive and manic syndromes occur in 40 percent of bipolar patients (Goodwin and Jamison, 1990), who exhibit the following signs and symptoms: crying, euphoria, racing thoughts, grandiosity, hypersexuality, suicidal ideation, irritability-anger, psychomotor agitation, severe insomnia, persecutory delusions, auditory hallucinations, and confusion. Such an episode, if it is the patient's first psychotic break, can be extremely difficult to characterize diagnostically unless it is immediately followed by more typical retarded depressive or manic episodes or family history is positive for bipolar illness. The following vignette (reprinted from Akiskal and Puzantian, 1979) exemplifies these points.

A 19-year-old boy was admitted to a state psychiatric facility because of social withdrawal, insomnia, severe headaches, and the obsession of sticking a knife into his heart in order to punish himself for rape fantasies. While in the hospital, he heard the devil's voice telling him that he should hang himself before a misfortune killed his entire family. His mood was extremely labile; his mental status shifted to an irritable-cantankerous mood; he expressed thoughts of cutting someone's cheeks with a knife (which he eventually did); he entered women's lavatories and said he could "seduce all of them at once"; he started communicating with God (but he wouldn't say how) and expressed the idea that his biologic father was Jesus Christ. At this juncture, he was physically accelerated, spoke constantly, did not experience any need for sleep, flirted with the nurses, joked with everybody, and danced naked in front of other patients "to aid in a campaign to help the poor." On full remission on lithium carbonate, he expressed great guilt over his aggressive behavior during the

intermediate mixed state of transition from depression into mania; as a matter of fact, he donated all of his savings to aid his victim in recovering from cosmetic surgery.

A subacute mixed state (i.e., one without psychotic features) can be confused with a severe anxiety state. Accurate diagnosis is essential, since mixed states tend to be notoriously refractory to antidepressants as well as neuroleptics, and lithium may work too slowly; electroconvulsive therapy is usually the more definitive treatment.

HYPOMANIA AND ITS DIAGNOSTIC SIGNIFICANCE

Setting the threshold for clinically significant hypomania is not only important for differentiating normal merriment and creative moods from illness but also for diagnosing bipolar II disorder. The following criteria, developed at the University of Tennessee Mood Clinic (Akiskal, 1983a), may assist in setting the clinical threshold for hypomania:

- It is often dysphoric in its drivenness.
- It is labile; i.e., the elation is unstable and easily alternates with irritability and anger.
- It may lead to substance abuse as a means to control the experienced high.
- It may impair social judgment.
- It is preceded or followed by retarded depression, typically with abrupt transition.
- It often springs from familial background of bipolar disorder.

Hypomania is a recurrent condition forming part of several overlapping "soft" bipolar subtypes (Fig. 22-2) of which bipolar II disorder is the most

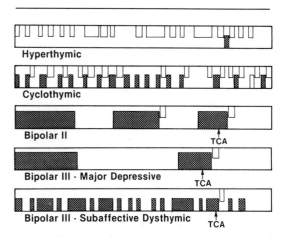

FIGURE 22-2. *Patterns of hypomania within the spectrum of "soft" bipolar disorders.*

common. Bipolar II patients who seek psychiatric help are usually women in their twenties and thirties who have suffered recurrent bouts of retarded depression. Because their highs are short-lived and typically not perceived as disruptive—indeed, the patient often finds them enjoyable—these individuals seldom present for help during such periods. The illness usually begins in the mid or late teens and leads to much interpersonal chaos. This facet of the illness can so impress the clinician that he or she may embark on a long-term psychotherapeutic endeavor, when in reality the tempestuous biography represents a complication of the recurrent mood disorder. It is therefore critical to document hypomanic swings in such patients in order to bring them the benefit of lithium carbonate. Another reason why accurate early diagnosis is important here lies in the fact that the continued high antidepressant doses in such patients may not only precipitate hypomanic periods but also tend to lead to increased cycling in the long term (Kukopulos et al., 1983). *Cycles* refer to the period from the onset of one episode to that of a subsequent one. In so-called rapid-cycling patients, who often come from the rank of bipolar II disorder, cycle frequency increases to at least four per year (Dunner, 1979).

The vignette that follows describes the subtle nature of the hypomanic periods in bipolar II patients and the ease of its induction by antidepressant pharmacotherapy.

A 26-year-old medical secretary who was separated from her third husband presented for outpatient psychiatric care with the chief complaint of "lack of hope, joy, meaning, and focus in life." She said she lacked the energy and motivation to take care of daily routines and slept 12 to 14 hours nightly. She said she would rather die than go through another divorce. She could not concentrate at work, and her typing speed had deteriorated. Since her teens she had had numerous similar periods that lasted from 2 to 12 weeks. These episodes often terminated abruptly, at which time she felt such an "intense relief and joy that I would sleep with the first man who happened to be around." It is this behavior that has led to repeated marital conflict and intermittent psychotherapy with little tangible benefit. On further questioning, she revealed that during the sudden recovery period, which lasted for four to five days, she sometimes felt no need for sleep, felt such "ecstasy from being alive again that I would cry," and had to drink whiskey to be able to "calm down my mind and body galloping with new life." Her husbands and numerous lovers were often irritated by her increased zeal, which led to new sexual misadventures. Family history revealed that a maternal uncle who had never received psychiatric help but who was known to be an alcoholic had hanged himself in his early 40s. An older sister had been treated for "mild depressions." Their mother had been periodically treated for excited psychotic states that had been labeled "paranoid schizophrenia," but little evidence could be found to substantiate that diagnosis; she had been married five times, indulged in much gambling, and associated with people in art circles. Given that the mother's illness suggested mania, and given the abundance of historical evidence for hypomanic episodes in the

patient, lithium carbonate was recommended. The patient refused to consider this treatment. Ten days later she was seen in the emergency department in an accelerated state and complained that she had not slept for two nights; she also revealed that she had been taking her sister's "tranquilizer," which turned out to be imipramine tablets.

Cyclothymic disorder often presents clinically in a similar fashion, except that the depressive periods are shorter, lasting for 3 to 10 days rather than for weeks, and are not of full syndromal depth. These rapid and tempestuous mood swings render the differential diagnosis from personality disorder even more problematic. Table 22-6 summarizes the main features of cyclothymia that need to be taken into account in such differential diagnosis.

In still another variant of the bipolar spectrum known as *bipolar III*, the patient suffers from early-onset repeated bouts of retarded depression—which can be either major episodes or intermittent minor depressions with the pattern of subaffective dysthymia as described earlier—but without evidence for spontaneous hypomanic periods; the bipolar tendency in these patients becomes manifest on pharmacologic challenge with antidepressants. Family history is often positive for frank bipolar illness. These pseudounipolar patients, who are sometimes referred to as *unipolar II*, represent either a less penetrant genetic form of bipolar disorder or simply the earliest depressive beginnings of bipolar disorder. The question then becomes, Can one predict which depressives will eventually switch into bipolar disorder? The following clinical features have been found useful in this regard in prospective followup studies (Strober and Carlson, 1982; Akiskal et al., 1983):

TABLE 22-6. *Clinical Features of Cyclothymic Disorder*

General characteristics
  Onset before 21 years
  Short cycles (days), which are recurrent in an irregular fashion, with infrequent euthymia
  May not attain full syndrome for depression and hypomania during any one cycle, but entire range of affective symptoms occur at various times
  Abrupt and unpredictable mood change
Subjective symptoms
  Lethargy alternating with eutonia
  Pessimism and brooding alternating with optimism and carefree attitudes
  Mental confusion and apathy alternating with sharpened and creative thinking
  Shaky self-esteem alternating between low self-confidence and grandiose overconfidence
Behavioral signs
  Hypersomnia alternating with decreased need for sleep
  Introverted self-absorption alternating with uninhibited people-seeking
  Taciturn versus talkative behavior
  Unexplained tearfulness alternating with excessive punning and jocularity

Modified from Akiskal HS, Khani MK, Scott-Strauss A: Cyclothymic temperamental disorders. Psychiatr Clin North Am 2:527–554, 1979, with permission.

- Onset before age 25
- Psychotic depression in a teenager
- Abrupt onset
- Postpartum onset
- Hypersomnic-retarded depression
- Pharmacologic mobilization of hypomania
- Bipolar family history
- Loaded (especially three consecutive generations) family history for mood disorder

This section on the milder end of the bipolar spectrum would be incomplete without mentioning chronically or intermittently hypomanic individuals termed *hypomanic personality* or *hyperthymic disorder* (Akiskal and Akiskal, 1992). This condition is characterized by intermittent subsyndromal hypomanic features with infrequent intervening euthymia (see Fig. 22-2). They are typically short sleepers (4 to 6 hours per night) and are high achievers. Although irritability is often seen in these individuals, depression as such is extremely uncommon; in other words, hyperthymia is cyclothymia with the minimum amount of depression, characterized by excessive use of denial, and given their successes in leadership positions or business, such individuals, unless suffering from a superimposed major depression, rarely present for psychiatric treatment. They are more often seen in sleep disorders centers, where they seek help because of sleep difficulty.

MOOD DISORDER IN DIFFERENT CLINICAL SETTINGS

This chapter has presented the manifold clinical picture of mood disorders that embrace a broad range of somatic, psychomotor, emotional, and cognitive manifestations, as well as certain personality disturbances representing complications of the illness. For this reason, the differential diagnosis of affective signs and symptoms interfaces with the "blues," bereavement reactions, anxiety states, primary character disorders, substance use disorders, schizophrenia, and dementia. Furthermore, depending on clinical setting, one set of manifestations may dominate the clinical presentation. Common examples include the following:

- Primary-care–somatic complaints and substance abuse
- Sleep disorders center–insomnia and hypersomnia
- Urology–impotence
- Neurology–memory disturbances
- Emergency department–psychosis and suicide attempts
- Educational counseling–scholastic failure
- Psychology and social work–marital problems
- Psychoanalysis–character pathology
- Courts–violence and murder
- City morgue–suicide

Since primary mood disorders are eminently treatable disorders—and because the complications of untreated depression or mania can be extremely serious—all physicians, as well as mental health professionals, should be competent in determining whether a given set of affectively tinged signs or symptoms are due to a primary mood disorder. The clinician should always inquire:

- Are unexplained somatic complaints and substance abuse alternative expressions of a primary mood disorder?
- Are insomnia and hypersomnia part of an affective syndrome, acute or chronic?
- Did depression precede the impotence?
- Are memory disturbances secondary to a reversible melancholia?
- Despite "schizophrenic" coloring, is the psychosis one phase of a recurrent bipolar disorder?
- Is school failure in a teenager or a young adult caused by a retarded depression heralding the onset of a bipolar disorder?
- Are marital problems secondary to depression, cyclothymia, or frank bipolar disorder in one or both spouses?
- What appears to be borderline character pathology—is it due to a cyclothymic or related temperament?
- Was the violent act committed during a psychotic depression or manic excitement?

It is necessary to inquire along these lines because it is obviously too late to do so in the city morgue.

These are serious clinical issues and necessitate a systematic approach to determine the affective basis of a patient's presenting complaints in different settings:

- To elicit other clinical features of the affective syndrome under consideration
- To document history of more typical major affective episodes in the past
- To assess if the presenting complaints recur in a periodic or cyclic fashion
- To substantiate relatively good social functioning between periods of illness
- To obtain positive family history for mood disorder and construct a family pedigree
- To document an unequivocal therapeutic response to thymoleptic agents or electroconvulsive therapy

In summary, the physician or mental health worker who engages in a systematic differential diagnosis of affective disturbances will soon find that many clinical enigmas will be solved in favor of a primary affective diagnosis. Because mood disorders are the most common and treatable of the serious psychiatric disorders, the practitioner is statistically admonished to err on the side of such diagnosis.

REFERENCES

Akiskal HS: Diagnosis and classification of affective disorders: New insights from clinical and laboratory approaches. Psychiatr Dev 1:123–160, 1983a.

Akiskal HS: Dysthymic disorder: Psychopathology of proposed chronic depressive subtypes. Am J Psychiatry 140:11–20, 1983b.

Akiskal HS: The bipolar spectrum: New concepts in classification and diagnosis. In Grinspoon L (ed): Psychiatry Update: The American Psychiatric Association Annual Review, vol 2. Washington, American Psychiatric Press, 1983c, pp 271–292.

Akiskal HS: Toward a clinical understanding of the relationship between anxiety and depressive disorders. In Maser J, Cloninger R (eds): Comorbidity in Anxiety and Mood Disorders. Washington, American Psychiatric Press, 1990, pp 597–607.

Akiskal HS, Akiskal K: Re-assessing the prevalence of bipolar disorders: Clinical significance and artistic creativity. Psychiatrie Psychobiol 3:29s–36s, 1988.

Akiskal HS, Akiskal K: Cyclothymic, hyperthymic and depressive temperaments as subaffective variants of mood disorders. In Tasman A, and Riba M, (eds): American Psychiatric Association Review. Washington, American Psychiatric Press, 1992, pp 43–62.

Akiskal HS, McKinney WT Jr: Depressive disorders: Towards a unified hypothesis. Science 182:20–28, 1973.

Akiskal HS, Puzantian VR: Psychotic forms of depression and mania. Psychiatr Clin North Am 2:419–439, 1979.

Akiskal HS, Khani MK, Scott-Strauss A: Cyclothymic temperamental disorders. Psychiatr Clin North Am 2:527–554, 1979.

Akiskal HS, Lemmi H, Dickson H, et al: Chronic depressions: 2. Sleep EEG differentiation of primary dysthymic disorders from anxious depressions. J Affect Disord 6:287–297, 1984.

Akiskal HS, Walker PW, Puzantian VR, et al: Bipolar outcome in the course of depressive illness: Phenomenologic, familial and pharmacologic predictors. J Affect Disord 5:115–128, 1983.

Andreasen NC: Creativity and mental illness: Prevalence rates in writers and their first-degree relatives. Am J Psychiatry 144:1288–1292, 1987.

Beck AT: Depression: Causes and Treatment. Philadelphia, University of Pennsylvania Press, 1967.

Bellow S: Herzog. New York, Viking Press, 1964.

Butler PD, Nemeroff CB: Corticotropin-releasing factor as a possible cause of comorbidity in anxiety and depressive disorders. In Maser J, Cloninger R (eds): Comorbidity in Anxiety and Mood Disorders. Washington, American Psychiatric Press, 1990, pp 413–435.

Carlson G, Goodwin F: The stages of mania. Arch Gen Psychiatry 28:221–288, 1973.

Carroll BJ, Feinberg M, Greden JF, Tarika J, et al: A specific laboratory test for the diagnosis of melancholia. Arch Gen Psychiatry 38:15–22, 1981.

Cassano GB, Akiskal HS, Musetti L, et al: Psychopathology, temperament, and past course in primary major depressions. 2. Toward a redefinition of bipolarity with a new semistructured interview for depression. Psychopathology 22:278–288, 1989.

Clayton PJ, Herjanic M, Murphy GE, Woodruff R: Mourning and depression: Their similarities and differences. J Can Psychiatr Assoc 19:309–312, 1974.

Cooper JE, Kendell RE, Gurland BJ, et al: Psychiatric Diagnosis in New York and London. London, Oxford University Press, 1972.

Coryell W, Scheftner W, Keller M, et al: The enduring psychosocial consequences of mania and depression. Am J Psychiatry 150:720–727, 1993.

Curtis GC, Cameron OG, Nesse RM: The dexamethasone suppression test in panic disorder and agoraphobia. Am J Psychiatry 139:1043–1046, 1982.

Davidson JRT, Miller RD, Turnbull CD, Sullivan JL: Atypical depression. Arch Gen Psychiatry 39:527–534, 1982.

DSM-IV: Diagnostic and statistical manual of mental disorders, 4th ed. Washington, American Psychiatric Press, 1994.

Dubé S, Kumar N, Ettedgui E, et al: Cholinergic REM-induction response: Separation of anxiety and depression. Biol Psychiatry, 20:408–418, 1985.

Duke P and Hochman G: A Brilliant Madness: Living with Manic-Depressive Illness. New York, Bantam Books, 1992.

Dunner D: Rapid cycling bipolar manic depressive illness. Psychiatr Clin North Am 2:461–467, 1979.

Goodwin F, Jamison K: Manic-Depressive Illness. New York, Oxford University Press, 1990.

Hamilton I: Robert Lowell—A biography. New York, Random House, 1982.

Himmelhoch JM, Mulla D, Neil JF, et al: Incidence and significance of mixed affective states in a bipolar population. Arch Gen Psychiatry 33:1062–1066, 1976.

Jackson SW: Melancholia and Depression: From Hippocratic Times to Modern Times. New Haven, Yale University Press, 1986.

James W: The Varieties of Religious Experience (lectures). Edinburgh, Scotland, 1902.

Kelly D, Walter CJS: A clinical and physiological relationship between anxiety and depression. Br J Psychiatry 115:401–406, 1969.

Kielholz, Poldinger, Adams C (eds): Masked Depression. Köln-Lövenich, Deutscher Arzte-Verlag Gmb, 1982.

Kraepelin E: Manic-Depressive Insanity and Paranoia. Edinburgh, E & S Livingstone, 1921.

Krauthammer C, Klerman GL: Secondary mania: Manic syndromes associated with antecedent physical illness or drugs. Arch Gen Psychiatry 35:1333–1339, 1978.

Kukopulos A, Caliari B, Tundo A, et al: Rapid cyclers, temperament, and antidepressants. Compr Psychiatry 24:249–258, 1983.

Kupfer DJ, Thase ME: The use of the sleep laboratory in the diagnosis of affective disorders. Psychiatr Clin North Am 6:3–21, 1983.

Leckman JF, Weissman MM, Merikangas KR, et al: Panic disorder and major depression. Arch Gen Psychiatry 40:1055–1060, 1983.

Lewis A: Melancholia: A clinical survey of depressive states. J Ment Sci 80:277–378, 1934.

Liebowitz MR, Quitkin FM, Stewart JW, et al: Phenelzine vs imipramine in atypical depression. Arch Gen Psychiatry 41:669–680, 1984.

Loosen PT, Prange AJ: Serum thyrotropin response to thryotropin-releasing hormone in psychiatric patients: A review. Am J Psychiatry 139:405–416, 1982.

Monroe RR: Creative Brainstorms: The relationship between madness and genius. New York, Irvington Publishers, Inc, 1992.

Nelson JC, Charney DS: The symptoms of major depressive illness. Am J Psychiatry 138:1–13, 1981.

Perris C: A study of cycloid psychoses. Acta Psychiatr Scand Suppl 253, 1974.

Pitts FN, McClure JN: Lactate metabolism in anxiety neurosis. N Engl J Med 277:1329–1336, 1967.

Robins E, Guze SB: Classification of affective disorders: The primary-secondary, the endogenous-reactive, and the neurotic-psychotic concepts. In Williams TA, Katz DM, Shield JA (eds): Recent Advances in the Psychobiology of the Depressive Illnesses. Washington, Government Printing Office, 1972, pp 283–292.

Roth M: The psychiatric disorders of later life. Psychiatr Ann 6:417–444, 1976.

Roth M, Mountjoy Q: The distinction between anxiety states and depressive disorders. In Paykel ES (ed): Handbook of Affective Disorders. New York, Guilford Press, 1982, pp 70–92.

Schou M: Artistic productivity and lithium prophylaxis in manic-depressive illness. Br J Psychiatry 135:97–103. 1979.

Strober M, Carlson G: Clinical, genetic and psychopharmacologic predictors of bipolar illness in adolescents with major depression. Arch Gen Psychiatry 39:549–555, 1982.

Styron W: Darkness Visible: A Memoir of Madness. New York, Random House, 1990.

Tolstoy L: My Confessions. New York, Crowell, 1887.

Van Gogh V: The Letters of Van Gogh to His Brother 1872–1886: With a Memoir by His Sister-in-Law—J. vanGogh-Bonger. London, Constable & Co, Ltd; Boston and New York, Houghton-Mifflin, 1927.

Ward NG, Doerr HO: Skin conductance: A potentially sensitive and specific marker for depression. J Nerv Ment Dis 174: 553–559, 1986.

Watts CAH: Depressive Disorders in the Community. Bristol, John Wright & Sons, 1966.

Wehr TA, Rosenthal NE: Seasonality and affective illness. Am J Psychiatry 146:829–839, 1989.

Wells KB, Stewart A, Hays RD, et al: The functioning and well-being of depressed patients: Results from the medical outcomes study. JAMA 262:914–919, 1989.

Widlöcher DJ: Psychomotor retardation: Clinical, theoretical, and psychometric aspects. Psychiatr Clin North Am 6:27–40, 1983.

Winokur G: Mania and Depression: A Classification of Disease and Syndrome. Baltimore, Johns Hopkins University Press, 1991.

Winokur G, Clayton P, Reich T: Manic-Depressive Illness. St. Louis, C. V. Mosby, 1969.

CHAPTER 23

Anxiety Symptoms

CHARLES VAN VALKENBURG

Panic attacks are spells of intense anxiety, usually sudden and unexpected, lasting from a few minutes to 2 hours. Anxiety can be so intense that patients describe it as worse than the worst anxiety they could possibly have, a transcendental, unreal experience. Even those who have survived hundreds of panic attacks are often unable to calm themselves with this knowledge, nor to believe that this particular attack will not be the one that kills them. Many who have visited emergency departments during previous attacks without satisfaction feel compelled to do so again. They feel that something horrible is about to happen, that they are doomed. Their surroundings seem changed, menacing. They fear they will lose control of their bodies, perhaps urinating or defecating in front of everyone, perhaps fainting, perhaps running screaming and naked, or killing babies. They feel they are losing their minds, going crazy. They may feel that their bodies have become distorted, no longer theirs, or that they are floating outside their bodies. They feel their hearts pounding and feel that they may die of a heart attack or that they cannot get air despite hyperventilating. They sometimes feel that a lump or constriction in the throat is choking them. Their chests feel heavy, uncomfortable, painful. They feel waves of numbness or tingling in their arms and legs or around their mouths. They may feel that an electric shock has jolted through their bodies or feel hot or cold flashes. They feel as if they will faint, dizzy, unsteady, weakened, and tremulous. Some feel the need to escape from wherever they are. Others feel immobilized. Not all patients have all the symptoms. Sometimes the physical symptoms are present, but the fear is missing. (Kushner and Beitman, 1990, Russell et al., 1991).

Over the centuries, this syndrome has been called *anxiety hysteria* or *globus hystericus* (Sheehan et al., 1980); *neurasthenia* or *nervous exhaustion* (Beard, 1869); *irritable heart, soldier's heart,* or *Da Costa's syndrome* (DaCosta, 1871); *anxiety neurosis* (Freud, 1894); the *hyperventilation syndrome* (Ames, 1955); the *calamity syndrome;* the *phobic anxiety-depersonalization syndrome* (Roth, 1959); *endogenous anxiety* (Sheehan and Sheehan, 1982); and finally, *panic disorder* and *panic disorder with agarophobia* (American Psychiatric Association, 1980, 1992). Most new names have represented delineations of ever more discrete syndromes from earlier, broader categories.

Panic attacks are a common and serious problem. In the United States, 3 percent of the population have had panic attacks within the past 6 months, and 0.6 to 1 percent have current panic disorder (Von Korff et al., 1985). Panic patients are likely to need as much treatment as patients with schizophrenia, major affective disorders, or somatization disorder (Boyd, 1986). They are likely to have endocrine abnormalities (Roy-Byrne et al., 1986; Fishman et al., 1985; Fava et al., 1989), abnormal positron emission tomographic (PET) scans (Reiman et al., 1986), vestibular abnormalities (Jacob et al., 1985; Sklare et al., 1990), mitral valve prolapse and premature ventricular contractions (Crowe et al., 1979; Muskin, 1985), and disability (Noyes et al., 1980). They are at increased risk for suicide attempts. Susceptibility appears to be genetically transmitted (Crowe, 1990).

Panic patients are likely to have many phobias, including agoraphobia. They appear particularly susceptible to respiratory disease (Zandbergen et al., 1991). They are likely to become depressed.

Panic attacks constitute a syndrome, like fever, which can result from many illnesses. Panic disorder is diagnosed when all possible medical causes have been ruled out and when it is known that another, more serious psychiatric disorder does not cause panic attacks.

Patients who experience panic attacks typically go to primary-care specialists first. Those whose illnesses seem "functional" or not organic may be referred to psychiatrists, particularly if their symptoms do not respond to timid doses of benzodiazepines. However, a substantial portion of patients with panic symptoms come to psychiatrists first or are referred by nonmedical mental health workers. Before a psychiatric diagnosis can be established, organic causes of anxiety symptoms need to be ruled out.

ORGANIC ANXIETY SYNDROMES

Apart from anxiety, depersonalization, and derealization, most panic symptoms are physical (see Table 23-1). Some panic attacks consist of physical symptoms without anxiety (Kushner and Beitman, 1990; Russell et al., 1991). Most patients with panic attacks initially believe they have a physical illness. This is not an implausible assumption, considering the many physical illnesses that can cause such symptoms. Before categorizing symptoms as psychiatric, it must first be determined that physical illness is not their cause.

CARDIAC DISEASES

Myocardial Infarction

The predominant symptom of a heart attack is crushing chest pain. Shortness of breath, choking or smothering sensations, palpitations, heavy perspiration, and a feeling of impending death are secondary symptoms. Some heart attack patients experience out-of-body sensations and other forms of depersonalization or derealization. Many will have had previous attacks. Mild heart attacks could be misdiagnosed as panic attacks.

Fortunately, there are good diagnostic tests for heart attack. An electrocardiogram (ECG) can quickly establish the correct diagnosis, and assays of cardiac enzymes in the blood confirm it. Most clinicians and even untrained persons can recognize a serious heart attack. In anxiety syndromes, pain is rarely the worst symptom. If a heart attack feels like an elephant standing on your chest, with a panic attack, it's more like a large dog. The heart attack patient is in obvious physical pain, which is usually easy to discriminate from anxiety.

Angina Pectoris

Angina pectoris is characterized by episodes of chest pain or discomfort, heart palpitations, shortness of breath, trouble breathing, and, understandably, anxiety (Bass et al., 1983; Thompson et al., 1982).

TABLE 23-1. *Physical Illnesses Causing Anxiety Symptoms*

Cardiac	**Neurologic**
Myocardial infarction	Grand mal seizure
Angina pectoris	disorder
Microvascular angina	Partial complex seizures
Congestive heart failure	Transient ischemic attacks
Paradoxical atrial	Cerebrovascular
tachycardia	insufficiency
Cardiac dysrhythmia	Brain tumor, especially of
Anemia	third ventricle
Mitral insufficiency	Cerebral syphilis
Pulmonary	Encephalitis
Pulmonary emboli	Postencephalitic disorders
Asthma	Multiple sclerosis
Endocrine	Meniere's disease
Hyperthyroidism	Subclavian steal syndrome
Hypoparathyroidism	Posttraumatic,
Hypoglycemia	postconcussive cerebral
Pheochromocytoma	syndrome
Cushing's disease	Wilson's disease
Diabetes mellitus	Huntington's chorea
Pancreatic carcinoma	Combined system disease,
Hypopituitarism	posterolateral sclerosis
Eosinophilic pituitary	Myasthenia gravis
adenoma	Sleep apnea
Thyroiditis	Sleep terrors
Addison's disease	Dream anxiety attacks
Infections	**Drug-induced, intoxications**
Malaria	Caffeine, theophylline
Viral pneumonia	Amphetamine
Mononucleosis	Ephedrine,
Viral hepatitis	pseudoephedrine,
Rheumatic fever	phenylpropanolamine
Tuberculosis	Cocaine
Bacteremia	Cannabis
Viremia	LSD, psychotomimetic
Chronic fatigue syndrome	drugs, hallucinogens
Collagen-vascular diseases	Yohimbine
Systemic lupus	Beta-carboline
erythematosis	Cholecystokinin
Rheumatoid arthritis	tetrapeptide
Polyarteritis nodosa	Khat
Temporal arteritis	**Withdrawal states**
Raynaud's phenomenon	Alcohol
Metabolic	Sedative-hypnotic
Hypocalcemia	Beta blockers
Hypoglycemia	Antidepressant
Dieting or fasting	**Nondrug toxicities**
Malnutrition	Arsenic
Low weight	Mercury
Chronic vitamin deficiency	Lead
	Bisimuth
	Other heavy metals
	Carbon disulfide
	Organic solvents

The episodes are often precipitated by exertion or by typical anxiety-provoking stimuli, or they can appear to be spontaneous. Although there is general agreement that the symptoms of angina pectoris are caused by intermittent restrictions of blood flow to the heart muscle, this is often difficult to establish in individual cases (Banks and Shugoli, 1967). These patients can be mistakenly referred to psychiatrists (Ferrer, 1968). Laboratory tests will not necessarily differentiate angina from panic. An ECG exercise test can usually establish angina but often cannot. Arteriograms sometimes show narrowing of major coronary arteries, but the degree of narrowing correlates poorly with the severity of angina symptoms. Microvascular angina overlaps diagnostically with panic disorder (Roy-Byrne et al., 1989). Some difficult cases can be documented by 24-hour ambulatory ECG monitoring. To further complicate matters, many cases of cardiac ischemia are "silent" and present no symptoms. A patient may have symptomatic panic attacks and asymptomatic myocardial ischemia.

The diagnosis of angina rather than anxiety is suggested by later age of onset, presence of cardiac risk factors such as cigarette smoking or hypertension, and pain provoked mainly by exertion. Overanxious behavior and milder chest pain suggest anxiety disorder. The symptomatic overlap of angina and anxiety remains considerable. Both are relatively common, and an individual patient may have both diseases.

Cardiologists can diagnose angina pectoris about as well as psychiatrists can diagnose panic. The possibility of an anxiety disorder should not be ruled out just because someone has assessed the same symptoms as due to angina. However, many panic patients carry nitroglycerine they do not need and which might make their symptoms worse. Medications such as tricyclic antidepressants, often used to treat anxiety, can endanger an irregular heart (Taylor and Hayward, 1990). Benzodiazepines have proven useful in the management of angina and even silent ischemia (Williams, 1990). Patients treated for both angina and anxiety require clinicians familiar with both conditions or consultation between their specialists.

Hyperdynamic Beta-Adrenergic State

Hyperdynamic beta-adrenergic state (Frolich et al., 1969) is thought to be caused by increased sensitivity of the circulatory system to epinephrine or by elevated levels of catecholamines in the system. Its symptoms are not distinctly different from those of anxiety; indeed, some authorities consider that panic disorder is a hyperdynamic beta-adrenergic state (Charney et al., 1983). Isoproterenol can induce anxiety symptoms (Pohl et al., 1985), and panic patients are particularly sensitive to the effects of clonidine (Nutt, 1986). Except in extreme cases with left ventricular hypertrophy or a prominent murmur, the syndromes can be indistinguishable. Not all hyperadrenergic patients have increased anxiety, and not all panic patients have adrenergic abnormalities. Both syndromes can be improved by beta blockers, although for anxious patients they are typically inadequate (Munjack et al., 1989).

Mitral Valve Prolapse Syndrome

Mitral valve prolapse syndrome can cause panic attacks indistinguishable from panic disorder. Most instances of mitral valve prolapse are asymptomatic, however, and possibly not clinically important (Muskin, 1985).

There are at least two forms of mitral valve prolapse syndrome. In one form, the mitral valve itself is abnormal, thickened, and myxomatous, as in Marfan's syndrome. This disease can progress and is associated with cases of unexpected sudden death. Paradoxically, the patients with the physically threatening disease do not often have panic disorder. Patients with panic symptoms are often found to have "functional" mitral valve prolapse with anatomically normal valves. High beta-adrenergic activity or hyperthyroidism can be the cause. Inhalation of amyl nitrite will exacerbate mitral valve prolapse and can precipitate a panic attack. Beta blockers are useful in cases with physical symptoms. Physical signs include a midsystolic murmur or click, which is accentuated by having the patient squat or perform a Valsalva maneuver.

Some echocardiographers do not believe that "functional" mitral valve prolapse is important and will not diagnose it in cases where others will (Gorman et al., 1986). Those who do make the diagnosis in "soft" cases find it in up to half the patients with panic disorder.

Although many patients with panic attacks have mitral valve prolapse, most patients with prolapse do not have panic attacks (Devereux et al., 1989.)

Cardiac Dysrhythmias

Cardiac dysrhythmias can cause palpitations, chest pain or discomfort, dizziness, respiratory distress, fainting, and anxiety (Lynch, 1977). Patients with panic disorder often have dysrhythmias, including premature ventricular contractions. Not all dysrhythmias cause subjective symptoms, and not all dysrhythmic symptoms coincide with pulse and ECG changes.

Episodes of paradoxical atrial tachycardia (PAT) can be mistaken for panic attacks. Measured pulse rates in panic attacks are often normal (Barr et al., 1982–83) and seldom exceed 120 beats per minute. In contrast, PAT typically causes a pulse rate above 150 beats per minute.

Fortunately, most dysrhythmias can be documented and characterized by ECG and identified even by initial computer interpretations. Dysrhythmia can cause anxiety symptoms which may or may not resolve entirely with antiarrhythmic treatment. If residual anxiety is to be treated with medication, cardiac side effects are a serious consideration. Tricyclic antidepressants exert quinidine-like antidysrhythmic effects but exacerbate ventricular dysrhythmias. Beta blockers prescribed for anxiety will help some dysrhythmias and exacerbate others. Monoamine oxidase inhibitors may stress the heart by raising or lowering blood pressure and might preclude emergency treatment with catecholamines, anesthetics, narcotics, or other drugs heart patients are likely to need. Benzodiazepines have little effect on heart rhythm but can suppress respiration. Panic attacks cannot be dismissed as trivial and not worth the risk of treating in dysrhythmic patients, but neither should anxiety be treated without regard to potentially life-threatening side effects.

ENDOCRINE DISEASES

Hyperthyroidism

Like panic disorder, hyperthyroidism is associated with chronic and acute episodic anxiety (Pringuet et al., 1982). Thyrotoxicosis causes anxiety, palpitations, perspiration, hot skin, rapid pulse, active reflexes, diarrhea, weight loss, heat intolerance, proptosis, and lid lag. Severe cases are easy to recognize clinically. Early or mild cases can be discriminated from anxiety disorders by the serum levels of thyroid hormones. But many panic patients also have abnormal thyroid indices, particularly low thyroid-stimulating hormone (TSH) levels (Fishman et al., 1985). Chronic hyperthyroidism can cause permanent mitral valve prolapse syndrome.

Hypoparathyroidism

The symptoms of hypoparathyroidism are those of low serum calcium, and they vary considerably (Denko, 1962). Anxiety is the predominant symptom in 20 percent of cases. Other typical symptoms include paresthesias, muscle tension and cramps, spasm, and tetany. Most cases result from past surgical removal of the parathyroids during thyroidectomy. Diagnosis is suggested by low serum calcium and high phosphate levels and confirmed by parathormone assay. Any low serum calcium level requires immediate treatment.

Pheochromocytoma

Pheochromocytoma is uncommon but dangerous and treatable and so must always be borne in mind in the assessment of anxiety symptoms (Bravo and Gifford, 1984). Half of pheochromocytoma patients have acute attacks of anxiety, headache, sweating, flushing, and hypertension. Blood pressure is usually elevated between attacks as well. Pheochromocytoma attacks, like panic attacks, can be precipitated by emotional experiences. Pheochromocytoma attacks are more likely to cause crushing back pain, vomiting, and sweating of the whole body; the sweating in panic attacks is more likely to be confined to the hands, feet, and forehead. Pheochromocytoma can be established by measuring urinary or plasma catecholamines and metabolites. A single "spot" urine sample is often adequate to make the diagnosis (Kaplan et al., 1977), although to rule it out, a 24-hour sample is better.

Reactive Hypoglycemia

Many patients are convinced that they have reactive hypoglycemia, and a few actually do. Numerous medical and lay clinics support the rest in their belief system. Most patients who identify themselves as hypoglycemic actually have mental disorders, anxious, somatoform, or characterologic. Hypoglycemia can be ruled out as the exclusive cause of symptoms if a blood glucose level drawn during an attack is normal. True reactive hypoglycemia can be documented by a glucose tolerance test (Levine, 1974). Hypoglycemia secondary to insulinoma can be diagnosed by a 72-hour fast with frequent blood glucose levels. Patients with panic attacks are able to differentiate them from hypoglycemic attacks induced by insulin (Schweizer et al., 1986).

RESPIRATORY DISEASES

Respiratory symptoms are a central part of panic disorder. Although patients with panic tend to hyperventilate slightly between attacks (Salkovskis et al., 1986), their serious respiratory distress is episodic. Chronic obstructive pulmonary disease (COPD) and congestive heart failure (CHF) are seldom mistaken for panic disorder, although episodic respiratory diseases are. Panic patients are more likely than others to develop organic respiratory disease (Zandenberg et al., 1991).

Pulmonary Emboli

Small bits of clotted blood or debris released into the bloodstream usually come to rest in the lung. If a large enough area of blood flow is interrupted, impaired respiration results in shortness of breath, hyperventilation, and acute anxiety. Listening to the lungs will sometimes suggest pulmonary embolism, but in many cases there are no physical findings. A chest x-ray may not help either. Arterial blood gases may show decreased oxygen. Lung scan and pulmonary arteriogram can establish the diagnosis definitively. Recurrent pulmonary emboli are expected mainly in individuals with predisposing conditions, such as phlebitis or intravenous drug abuse.

Asthma

Like panic disorder, asthma is characterized by episodic attacks of cardiopulmonary symptoms and anxiety. Anxiety can precipitate and prolong asthma attacks (Thompson and Thompson, 1985). Asthma is easily differentiated from panic by listening to the chest, which is likely to be clear during a panic attack. Some of the more dramatically inclined panic patients make a lot of noise in their upper airways but not in their lungs. Although the diagnosis and treatment of asthma take precedence over that of panic disorder, management of anxiety is a part of treating asthma. Theophylline, used to treat asthma, can cause or exacerbate panic anxiety. Benzodiazepines can suppress respiration in asthmatics. It is possible for a patient to have both panic disorder and asthma (Bernstein et al., 1991).

NEUROLOGIC DISEASES

Seizure Disorders

In grand mal epilepsy, the primary illness is obvious. Seizure disorders can cause any psychiatric symptom, including any anxiety symptom (Bingley, 1958). Some temporal lobe seizures do not progress to generalized convulsions but present as episodes of anxiety, anger, or other affects. (Weil, 1959; Harper and Roth, 1962). Williams (1956) found fearfulness to be the predominant emotion in 61 percent of patients with partial complex seizures. The diagnosis can usually, but not always, be established by electroencephalography (EEG), particularly if nasopharyngeal leads are used with provocative stimuli such as hyperventilation. Additional cases can be detected by continuously monitored EEG and by characteristic EEG changes or an elevated serum prolactin level after partial complex seizures. Neuroleptic drugs also increase prolactin and give a false-positive result. Although often easy to establish, seizure disorders can be difficult to rule out. The most complete workups still leave an estimated 5 to 10 percent of cases undocumented. An extensive seizure workup is generally not indicated in panic patients unless there has been a serious head injury with loss of consciousness or symptoms strongly suggestive of partial complex seizures.

Transient Ischemic Attacks

Transient ischemic attacks (TIAs) include transient neurologic signs similar to those of stroke. Anxiety is often part of these episodes and may occur in discrete episodes or attacks for weeks or months before characteristic neurologic symptoms begin to appear. The attacks are caused by episodic arterial insufficiency, most often of the internal carotid or less often of the basilar artery. Patients with TIAs require prophylactic anticoagulant drugs or surgery. Stroke is a frequent outcome.

Combined Systemic Disease (Posterolateral Sclerosis)

Combined systemic disease, a vitamin B_{12} deficiency syndrome, can present as panic, even as a feeling of a need to escape. It frequently causes anxiety, paresthesias, weakness, hyperreflexia, and numerous "soft" symptoms easily misdiagnosed as anxious or hypochondriacal. In cases with severe pernicious anemia, the patients may hyperventilate and have other anxiety symptoms (Shulman, 1967), but mental symptoms can occur without anemia. Documentation of pernicious anemia or low serum B_{12} level with impaired absorption establishes the diagnosis. Posterolateral spinal tract degeneration occurs progressively, and the primary physical nature of the illness eventually becomes clear. Neurologic damage can be prevented by early diagnosis and treatment.

Huntington's Chorea

In a minority of cases, before choreiform movements and flaccid paralysis begin, the prodromal phase of this illness is dominated by panic anxiety (James and Mefferd, 1969). Other prodromal findings include antisocial personality change, suspiciousness, aggressiveness, and labile mood. Panic and anxiety symptoms may respond to antipsychotic or antianxiety drugs.

INTOXICATIONS

Caffeine and the Methylxanthines

Caffeine is a commonly consumed stimulant, and too much of it will provoke anxiety symptoms (Charney et al., 1985). While lower doses of caffeine can be pleasantly stimulating, higher doses cause hyperalertness, hypervigilence, motor tension and tremors, gastrointestinal distress, and anxiety. The acute symptoms of caffeine intoxication and generalized anxiety disorder are almost identical. In dosages of around 700 mg, about seven cups of American coffee, caffeine will provoke panic attacks in most persons with panic disorder and in many persons without prior panic attacks. Diagnostic evaluation of panic attacks must assess the possibility of caffeine intoxication. Caffeine appears to bind some of the same brain receptor sites as the benzodiazepines but to exert opposite effects. Not all of caffeine's effects are reversed by benzodiazepine (Mattila et al., 1988). Caffeine, theophylline, theobromine, and related methylxanthines are found in coffee, tea, cola and many other carbonated drinks, yerba maté, guarana, and other drinks derived from various plant leaves, fruits, and flowers. They are also ingredients in many medications, including analgesic combinations, diet pills, and nonprescription stimulants. Theophylline, the methylxanthine that predominates in tea, is prescribed for a variety of respiratory diseases and can cause the same generalized and panic anxiety as caffeine.

Most patients with panic disorder have already learned to avoid or limit caffeine. Patients who complain of anxiety and report heavy caffeine consumption should be advised to decrease or discontinue caffeine before other treatments are considered.

Amphetamines, Cocaine, and Sympathomimetic Abuse

Persons who use amphetamines or cocaine expect to become euphoric, energetic, confident, and accelerated. However, they can also become agitated, anxious, or panicky, particularly with higher doses or prolonged use. The anxiety can become so severe that abusers will take heroin to counteract it. Panic anxiety also can result from occasional use of cocaine (Geracioti and Post, 1991). Stimulant toxicity is relatively easy to diagnose. Dilated pupils, elevated blood pressure with slowed pulse, headache, dizziness, confusion, and aggressiveness suggest it, and a urine or blood test confirms it. The same symptoms can be caused by nonprescription diet pills containing phenylpropanolamine or by decongestants or hot drinks containing ephedrine or pseudoephedrine.

Yohimbine

Yohimbine is most often used as a stimulant or aphrodesiac, but it also can produce extreme anxiety (Holmberg and Gershon, 1961). It produces panic anxiety so reliably that it has been useful in experimental anxiety research. Intoxicated persons will show more overstimulation, irritability, and gastrointestinal distress than is typical of panic attacks. Few persons who have had yohimbine-induced panic are willing to try it again. Pharmacologically, yohimbine is an alpha-adrenergic blocker. It selectively blocks alpha$_2$ autoreceptors at lower dosages, but at higher dosages it blocks alpha$_1$ receptors as well (Charney et al., 1982, 1983). Clonidine does not block all its effects. (Mattila et al., 1988).

Khat

Khat is yet another botanical stimulant. Its stimulant effects are stronger than caffeine and weaker than amphetamine. Like other botanical stimulants, it produces extreme anxiety in higher doses.

Cannabis

Regular marijuana users typically believe the drug reduces their anxiety. There appears to be no perceived rebound of this anxiety when cannabis use is discontinued. For some persons, the depersonalization marijuana often causes is experienced as unpleasant and provokes anxiety, fearfulness, and agoraphobic symptoms (Moran, 1985).

LSD

LSD's occasional tendency to produce "bad trips" is legendary. These are often associated with severe anxiety, as anyone who has ever covered an emergency room near a rock concert can attest. Most persons who willingly ingest LSD know the risks of a "bad trip" in advance, although this foreknowledge often does not help them during the experience. At some rock concerts, well-meaning individuals with spray bottles mist LSD solutions onto the wrists of others or sometimes into their faces, giving them a "free trip" they may not want.

The effects of LSD are typically abolished within an hour by 50 mg chlorpromazine, given intramuscularly (Leiken et al., 1989). Contrary to the street lore of the 1960s, this use of chlorpromazine is usually quite safe.

Amyl Nitrite

Amyl nitrite is used medically as a short-acting vasodilator. It is abused primarily as a sexual stimulant, for prolonging and intensifying arousal, erection, and orgasm. It is used diagnostically to exacerbate mitral prolapse for echocardiograms. It can cause brief panic anxiety. Panic patients rarely experiment with it twice. Isobutyl nitrite, sold in drug and sex shops, has similar effects.

SEDATIVE WITHDRAWAL

Sedative-hypnotic drugs (e.g., benzodiazepines, barbiturates, meprobamate, methaqualone, chloral hydrate, paraldehyde, ethchlorvynol, and glutethamide) are taken to relieve anxiety or sleeplessness, but their discontinuation can cause rebound anxiety and worse. The severity of the withdrawal syndrome depends on the drug, dosage, duration of use, and speed of elimination. In general, the intermediate-acting (4 to 6 hours) drugs cause the worst withdrawal. Symptoms include hyperalertness, motor tension, muscle aches, agitation, anxiety, insomnia, hyperactive reflexes and startle response, postural hypotension, tremulousness, nausea, vomiting, convulsions, delirium, and death. The most dangerous barbiturates are now rarely prescribed, and methaqualone is no longer manufactured legally in the United States. Benzodiazepine withdrawal, though rarely fatal, can be very unpleasant. Withdrawal seizures can occur after prolonged use of diazepam in doses above 80 mg/day, alprazolam over 4 mg/day, or equivalent doses of other benzodiazepines. In anxious patients, severe rebound anxiety can occur after only a few weeks' use of recommended therapeutic doses. Lorazepam and alprazolam are short-acting agents, and their abrupt discontinuation is particularly likely to cause panic attacks. Anxious patients can have serious rebound anxiety the day after taking a single dose of a very short-acting hypnotic such as alprazolam or tybamate. Normal people may experience this rebound as stimulating.

Although antidepressants are rarely abused, their abrupt withdrawal can cause an abstinence syndrome of insomnia, vivid nightmares, and extreme anxiety (Gawin, 1981).

Sedative Abuse

Patients with primary panic disorder and no previous drug abuse are quite unlikely to abuse sedatives (Garvey, 1991). Although anxiety patients treated with sedative drugs typically become physically dependent, this dependence is not associated with the severe psychiatric and social problems typical of drug abusers. Drug abusers who like sedatives will tell doctors any lie to get them.

Most of the anxiety symptoms sedative abusers experience result from drug withdrawal. These anxiety states can be extreme. Sedative abusers report more muscle aches and vomiting than anxious patients experience. Patients with genuine anxiety disorders rarely take more medication than they need to control their symptoms and, in fact, are likely to take less than they need. The most distinguishing characteristic of sedative abusers is their rapid dose escalation. Physicians ideally should give genuine anxiety patients all the sedation they need and give the abusers none.

Alcoholism

Alcohol is pharmacologically an anesthetic. It reduces anxiety initially, but prolonged use increases anxiety. Anxious patients can experience severe rebound anxiety the day after moderate drinking. Their rebound following immoderate drinking is made worse by alcohol's toxicity. Patients with primary anxiety disorders often learn on their own to avoid alcohol.

In many patients who abuse alcohol and have panic attacks, alcohol is the primary problem and the principal cause of panic symptoms. However, anxiety disorders also seem to predispose certain persons to alcoholism. Alcohol abstainers with panic or agoraphobic disorders are more likely than others to have alcoholic relatives (Munjack and Moss, 1981; Leckman et al., 1983). The best way to determine whether alcoholism or panic is primary is to ask which began first. Often the anxiety is found to have preceeded alcohol problems and may have caused them (Cox et al., 1990). If panic attacks first occurred during periods of heavy drinking and the patient is still drinking heavily, it is best to first treat the primary alcoholism. Such patients' panic attacks and agoraphobic symptoms usually cease after alcohol withdrawal, and antipanic drugs are not needed (Blankfield, 1986).

If a patient has panic disorder that has clearly preceded alcohol abuse, it may have caused the alcohol abuse. If these patients are still drinking heavily, it is again necessary to treat the alcoholism first and to consider antipanic medications only if panic attacks persist several weeks after other alcohol withdrawal symptoms have resolved. Prescribing potentially addictive antipanic drugs to these patients poses an obvious risk, but sometimes no other treatment will help. Patients who have once met criteria for alcohol abuse or dependence are probably more likely than others to become addicted to sedative drugs. On the other hand, unabated panic attacks increase the risk of alcoholic relapse, and panic disorder or agoraphobia can be disabling. Anxiety disorders cannot be dismissed as negligible risks compared with chemical dependency. There is no uniform answer; each patient must be treated as an individual.

When interviewed comprehensively, many patients with primary panic disorder report past heavy drinking which, at one time, met the diagnostic criteria for alcohol abuse or dependence. They often report having decided that their drinking was making their anxiety worse and having stopped drinking without difficulty. Such patents also present a dilemma, one that less thorough physicians avoid by not adequately asking about alcohol to begin with. Most drugs marketed as antidepressants also have antipanic efficacy, and they are not much subject to abuse. If an antidepressant can be found that proves safe and effective for the panic patient who has abused alcohol, then it is the treatment of choice. However, many of these patients tolerate or respond only to the benzodiazepines. Many seem able to use them properly when they have been informed of the risks of dependence and when their prescriptions are monitored closely. Any evidence that patients are taking sedatives in an abusive manner, however, must be responded to immediately. Indications of abuse include increasing their own doses, seeking renewals early, reporting lost or stolen medication, using alcohol or other drugs to augment intoxication, or seeking drugs from additional physicians.

PANIC ATTACKS IN MENTAL DISORDERS

Even among the domain of mental illnesses, panic disorder is a diagnosis of exclusion. Several other mental illnesses cause panic attacks as secondary manifestations. The presence of panic attacks often has a bearing on the treatment and outcome of the primary illness.

Schizophrenia

Panic attacks are frequently a part of schizophrenia, especially early in its course. Schizophrenic panic attacks may be characterized by fearfulness, tension, agitation or immobility, disorganized thinking, dilated pupils, extreme insecurity and suspiciousness, and delusions of reference and persecution. Hallucinations often have derogatory accusative content. Voices may accuse the patient of being homosexual, a prostitute, or the Antichrist or of having AIDS.

Schizophrenia with panic attacks often proves in the long run to be a schizoaffective or psychotic affective disorder. Psychotic symptoms suggesting schizophrenia and panic attacks also occur transiently in patients meeting diagnostic criteria for "hysterical" conversion, somatization and borderline disorders, factitious states and malingering, brief reactive psychoses, bouffées délirantes, and similar conditions that will not progress to chronic schizophrenia.

Panic attacks in the course of a true schizophrenia may require different treatment from primary anxiety disorders. Antidepressants might make schizophrenia worse, particularly monoamine oxidase inhibitors, which augment dopamine function. Tricyclic antidepressants can relieve panic attacks in schizophrenia (Siris et al., 1989), but the first treatment may be to establish therapeutic levels of antipsychotic medication. Excessive dosage may provoke rather than eliminate anxiety (Argyle, 1990). If therapeutic levels are not adequate, a tricyclic antidepressant or benzodiazepine can be added.

Manic Disorder

Panic attacks can occur as part of manic-depressive disorder, in either the manic or depressed phase (Donnelly et al., 1978). In manic and hypomanic disorders, the predominant affect is usually cheerful and euphoric, but surprisingly, often it is dysphoric, with irritablity, extreme anxiety, or panic attacks. These panic attacks are best treated with antimanic medication. Antidepressants may make manic patients worse. Benzodiazepines such as clonazepam (Chouinard, 1987) or lorazepam (Bradwejn et al., 1990) have antimanic as well as antipanic properties.

Depressive Disorder

About half of patients with primary panic disorder develop major depression (a secondary depression), and almost all are bothered by some degree of depressed mood (Sheehan and Sheehan, 1982). At least a fifth of patients with major depression have panic attacks, and most of the rest have considerable anxiety. Depression with panic attacks responds less well to treatment (Overall et al., 1966; Paykel, 1972; VanValkenburg et al., 1984) and has a worse outcome (Clancy et al., 1978; Noyes et al., 1980; VanValkenburg et al., 1984; Nutzinger et al., 1985; Buller et al., 1986; Clayton et al., 1991). Agitated depression with anxiety and sometimes psychosis, sometimes called *involutional melancholia* (Brown et al., 1984), responds well to electroconvulsive therapy. Depression with anxiety and hostility responds well to antidepressant medication (Overall et al., 1966), although benzodiazepines can make these patients worse (Raskin et al., 1974).

Somatization Disorder

Hysteria has mimicked other disorders since antiquity. Some psychiatrists believe that endogenous anxiety and hysteria are indistinguishable (Sheehan and Sheehan, 1982), while neurologists often see little important difference between hysteria and malingering. However, conventional psychiatric wisdom holds that somatization disorder and anxiety disorders are separate (Guze, 1967; Guze and Perley, 1963). Patients with a single "hysterical conversion" or pseudoneurologic symptom often prove to have genuine and serious physical disease (Slater, 1965). Patients with somatization disorder report a wide variety of psychosomatic symptoms, including panic attacks, and claim to have most of the physical symptoms they are asked about. However, even patients with "pure" anxiety disorders tend to be hypochondriacal. Somatization patients are more likely to improve transiently on active medication or placebo but rarely to respond so well that they stop seeking unnecessary medical attention. Patients with panic disorder, however, seek at least as much psychiatric attention as those with somatization disorder (Boyd, 1986).

In family studies and within individual patients, somatic anxiety is associated with psychic anxiety and depression but also with antisocial personality disorder. Somatizers parasitize others the way antisocials prey on them. Since the term *hysteria* has rightly taken on derogatory connotations, the new term, *somatization disorder*, was adopted in 1980. Its use will probably persist until the hysterics learn what it means. It is hard to find a "nice" name for this condition. Patients usually accept being told their bodies are sensitive to their emotions.

Hypochondriasis

Briquet (1859), rejecting the notion that hysteria was caused by a wandering uterus, also dismissed the diagnosis of hypochondriasis as an artifact of clinicians' unwillingness to diagnose hysteria in any man, "for he has no uterus." Most severe hypochondriacs have a syndrome indistinguishable from somatization disorder. Kendell (1982) has pointed out that "no natural point of discontinuity between somatization disorder and other forms of somatic complaint has been demonstrated." Barsky and Klerman (1983) have suggested that the diagnosis of hypochondriasis be dropped.

Panic disorder and agoraphobia are associated with hypochondriasis, which is diminished when the panic attacks are treated (Noyes et al., 1986). A hypochondriacal patient with panic attacks should be considered to have panic disorder, unless the larger syndrome of somatization disorder is also present. Hypochondriasis is also likely to be seen during episodes of depression.

Mimicry

Mimicry abounds in nature, whenever it is to an organism's advantage to appear to be what it is not. Viceroy butterflies look like bad-tasting Monarchs, birds feign injury to draw predators away from the nest, nonvenomous hognose snakes behave like rattlesnakes when threatened, and baby cuckoos mimic chicks of the species whose nests they parasitize. Humans feign mental illness. An ancient example is the biblical David, who put on an act to escape possible execution: "And David . . . was much afraid of Achish the King of Gath. So he changed his behavior before them, and feigned himself mad in their hands, and made marks on the doors of the gate, and let his spittle run down his beard" (1 Samuel 21:12–13). Modern individuals exploit the human altruism that causes us to care for the sick by falsely reporting or mimicking the symptoms of illness. Those who mimic physical illness are often detected by better diagnostic tests than they know about. Those who specialize in mental symptoms are difficult to establish as fakes and may variously be diagnosed as having factitious illness such as Munchausen's syndrome, as "borderlines," or as malingerers. Malingering is diagnosed when the purpose of the mimicry seems quite obvious, such as to avoid responsibility or punishment or to get drugs. Clinicians must try to identify such individuals as best they can, particularly before prescribing potentially dangerous or addictive drugs, ordering hazardous diagnostic procedures, performing surgery, or directing society to pay expensive hospitalization or disability benefits. Unfortunately, identifying deceivers is often difficult. It remains impossible to prove that a person does not have panic attacks. Panic disorder is one of the easier psychiatric diseases to feign: Most of the symptoms can be duplicated by intentional hyperventilation. To further complicate matters, intentional hyperventilation provokes genuine panic attacks in patients with panic disorder (Bass et al., 1991). Presented with a patient who seems to be faking, the clinician should proceed with caution.

Posttraumatic Stress Disorder (PTSD)

PTSD is an anxiety disorder presumed to be caused by previous terrible experiences. The symptoms are closely related to the trauma and are made worse by reminders of the trauma. Some of these patients go to great lengths to avoid crowds or social situations; some camp for months in remote areas; others do farm work and avoid coming into town. These avoidance behaviors suggest agoraphobia. The "flashbacks" in which some of these patients reexperience the original trauma can have the same symptoms as panic attacks (Mellman and Davis, 1985). Antianxiety and antidepressant medications relieve the symptoms of PTSD; antipsychotic medications are less effective (Bleich et al., 1986).

Phobic Disorder

Phobias are the most common psychiatric disorders (Boyd et al., 1990) and are considered normal in children. The objects of fear tend to be things that would have been dangerous to children during the ice age: spiders, snakes, bats, cats (which could have been saber-toothed tigers), enclosed places (which could have caved in), the dark (night hunters) or wide-open spaces (those saber-toothed tigers were fast!). Naive chimpanzees have an instinctive and adaptive "snake phobia." Simple phobic disorders probably represent persistence into adult life of instincts that were once useful to survival. Phobia becomes a disorder when it interferes with an individual's life. Conventional wisdom holds that simple phobic disorders respond not to medication but to behavioral psychotherapy, in which patients progressively accustom themselves to the objects they fear. Patients with simple phobia may have panic symptoms when they are exposed to the specific thing they fear. Those who have spontaneous panic attacks should be considered to have panic disorder or agoraphobia with panic attacks.

Social Phobia

Social phobias were originally narrowly defined as fear of a single, specific social situation, such as public speaking, performing, visiting, using public showers or rest rooms, or eating in public places. These problems are typically treated behaviorally, like simple phobias, by instructing patients to gradually overcome the fear situation by exposing themselves to it. Benzodiazepines, beta blockers, and alcohol can ease the initial attempts, although behavioral purists denounce these.

Agoraphobic patients usually have multiple social phobias. The distinction between mild agoraphobia and severe social phobia can be difficult to make. Social phobias begin at younger ages, occur more in men and in higher social classes, and are less likely to be related to distance from home or to crowded surroundings (Amies et al., 1983). Social phobics are less generally fearful, less obsessive, and their symptoms are less likely to fluctuate over time, but their main phobic symptoms overlap considerably with those of agoraphobia (Solyom et al., 1986).

Social phobic symptoms mean a poorer prognosis in patients with panic disorder and secondary depression (Reiter et al., 1991). Surprisingly, in view of conventional wisdom, social phobias are as likely to be improved by the benzodiazepine alprazolam or the monoamine oxidase inhibitor phenelzine as by cognitive-behavioral therapy (Gelernter et al., 1991).

Spasmophilia

Spasmophilie, familiar to French psychiatrists, is characterized by anxiety, hyperventilation, hyperexcitability, visceral spasm, hyperreflexia, muscular shaking and contraction, and immobility (Manuila et al., 1981). In cases not caused by hypocalcemia, it may represent a cultural variant of panic disorder, in which the urge to escape is replaced by the alternate fear response of immobility.

Agoraphobia

Most simply, *agoraphobia* is a fear of leaving home, particularly alone. Most panic disorder patients have multiple phobias, including agoraphobia. Conventional wisdom (Klein, 1981) holds that clinical agoraphobia results from panic patients' increasing avoidance of places or situations in which their panic attacks would be particularly inconvenient or difficult to control. Agoraphobics most particularly avoid places from which escape would be difficult, such as bridges or crowded theaters. When they do go to theaters, they favor seats on the aisle and near the door. Panic attacks in agoraphobic patients are more likely to include fear of losing control, while those not associated with agoraphobia are more likely to include dyspnea and dizziness (Katerndahl et al., 1986).

Up to half of agoraphobics do not have panic attacks (Weissman et al., 1986). Those with panic attacks are more likely to seek treatment, while those with uncomplicated agoraphobia tend to stay home. Uncomplicated agoraphobia could resemble other phobias in being a residual childhood instinct, since leaving home alone was and is dangerous for a child. Agoraphobia without panic attacks may not differ fundamentally from simple phobias. It was previously thought that agoraphobic women were particularly likely to have unsatisfactory marriages. A controlled study has shown this not to be so (Arrindell et al., 1986).

Agoraphobia was long thought unamenable to psychotherapy, but recent studies have changed this view. Simple in vivo exposure can work as well for agoraphobia as for simple phobia (Chambless et al., 1990). Marks (1983, 1989) maintains that therapist-aided exposure is effective and medication ineffective in agoraphobia. Treating agoraphobia with panic attacks, Zitrin et al. (1978, 1980) have found medications effective and self-exposure homework superfluous, since once panic attacks are blocked by medication, agoraphobic patients are no longer afraid to leave home. In cases where imipramine is effective, psychotherapy has no immediate additional benefit (Mavissakalian and Michelson, 1986a). Each form of therapy appears effective as long at it is applied: imipramine (Mavissakalian and Michelson, 1986b), clonazepam (Pollack et al., 1986), in vivo exposure, or applied relaxation (Jansson et al, 1986). The advantage of the psychotherapies is that they can be continued by patients on their own (Lelliott et al., 1987).

Panic Disorder

When all the preceding exclusions have been ruled out, patients regularly troubled by panic attacks have *panic disorder*. Their symptoms are usually controlled by benzodiazepine anxiolytics, if given in adequate dosage (Ballenger, 1990). Imipramine and desipramine are equally effective (Kalus et al., 1991), though initially less easily tolerated. Many tricyclic side effects, such as increased pulse rate, perspiration, postural hypotension, and feelings of unreality, resemble those of the anxiety disorder they are meant to treat. Tricyclics appear to work by modifying the number of brain synaptic receptors. They take a couple of weeks to do this, which is also about the time it takes for panic attacks to come under control and side effects to diminish.

Recently, some behavioral psychotherapies have shown promise in panic disorder. Most of panic attacks' physical symptoms, and possibly the attacks themselves, result from hyperventilation (Zandbergen et al., 1989; Maddock and Carter, 1991). Thus panic patients can be helped by being taught to control their breathing (Salkovskis et al., 1986).

REFERENCES

American Psychiatric Association: Diagnostic and Statistical Manual of Mental Disorders, 3d ed. Washington, American Psychiatric Association, 1980.

American Psychiatric Association: Diagnostic and Statistical Manual of Mental Disorders, 4th ed. Washington, American Psychiatric Association, 1992.

Ames F: The hyperventilation syndrome. J Ment Sci 101:466–525, 1955.

Amies PL, Gelder MG, Shaw PM: Social phobia: A comparative clinical study. Br J Psychiatry 142:174–179, 1983.

Argyle N: Panic attacks in chronic schizophrenia. Br J Psychiatry 157:430–433, 1990.

Arrindell WA, Emmelkamp PM: Marital adjustment, intimacy and needs in female agoraphobics and their partners: A controlled study. Br J Psychiatry 149:592–602, 1986.

Ballenger JC: Efficacy of benzodiazepines in panic disorder and agoraphobia. J Psychiatr Res 24(suppl 2):15–25, 1990.

Banks T, Shugoli GI: Confirmatory physical findings in angina pectoris. JAMA 200:1031–1035, 1967.

Barr TC, Telch MJ, Hauvik D: Ambulatory heart rate changes during panic attacks. J Psychiatr Res 17:261–266, 1982–83.

Barsky AJ, Klerman GL: Overview: Hypochondriasis, bodily complaints, and somatic styles. Am J Psychiatry 140:273–283, 1983.

Bass C, Gardner WN, Jackson G: Unexplained breathlessness and psychiatric morbidity in patients with normal and abnormal coronary arteries (letter). Lancet 1:1282, 1983.

Bass C, Chambers JB, Gardner WN: Hyperventilation provocation in patients with chest pain and a negative treadmill exercise test. J Psychosom Res 35:83–89, 1991.

Beard CM: Neurasthenia or nervous exhaustion. Boston Med Surg J 3:217, 1869.

Bernstein JA, Sheridan E, Patterson R: Asthmatic patients with panic disorders: Report of three cases with management and outcome. Ann Allergy 66:311–314, 1991.

Bingley T: Mental symptoms in temporal lobe epilepsy. Acta Psychiatr Neurol 33(suppl 120):1–151, 1958.

Blankfield A: Psychiatric symptoms in alcohol dependence: diagnostic and treatment implications. J Subst Abuse Treat 3:275–278, 1986.

Bleich A, Siegel B, Garb R, Lerer B: Posttraumatic stress disorder following combat exposure: Clinical features and psychopharmacological treatment. Br J Psychiatry 149:365–369, 1986.

Boyd JH: Use of mental health services for the treatment of panic disorder. Am J Psychiatry 143:1569–1574, 1986.

Boyd JH, Rae DS, Thompson JW, et al: Phobia: Prevalence and risk factors. Soc Psychiatry Psychiatr Epidemiol 25:314–323, 1990.

Bowen RC, Kohut J: The relationship between agoraphobia and primary affective disorders. Can J Psychiatry 24:317–322, 1979.

Bradwejn J, Shriqui C, Koszycki D, Meterissian G: Double-blind comparison of the effects of clonazepam and lorazepam in acute mania. J Clin Psychopharmacol 10:403–408, 1990.

Bravo EL, Gifford KW: Pheochromocytoma: Diagnosis, localization and management. N Engl J Med 311:1298–1303, 1984.

Briquet P: Traité clinique et thérapeutique de l'hysterie. Paris, J.B. Ballière et Fils, 1859.

Brown RP, Sweeney J, Loutsch E, et al: Involuntional melancholia revisited. Am J Psychiatry 141:24–28, 1984.

Buller R, Maier W, Benkert O: Clinical subtypes in panic disorder: Their descriptive and prospective validity. J Affective Disord 11:105–114, 1986.

Chambless DL, Woody SR: Is agoraphobia harder to treat? A comparison of agoraphobics' and simple phobics' response to treatment. Behav Res Ther 28:305–312, 1990.

Charney DS, Heninger GR, Jatlow PI: Increased anxiogenic effects of caffeine in panic disorders. Arch Gen Psychiatry 42:233–243, 1985.

Charney DS, Heninger GR, Redmond DE Jr: Yohimbine induced anxiety and increased noradrenergic function in humans: Effects of diazepam and clonidine. Life Sci 40:19–29, 1983.

Charney DS, Heninger GR, Sternberg DE: Assessment of alpha-2 adrenergic autoreceptor function in humans: Effects of oral yohimbine. Life Sci 30:2033–2041, 1982.

Chouinard G. Clonazepam in acute and maintenance treatment of bipolar affective disorder. J Clin Psychiatry 48:29–37, 1987.

Clancy J, Noyes R, Hoenk PR, et al: Secondary depression in anxiety neurosis. J Nerv Ment Dis 166:846–850, 1978.

Clayton PJ, Grove WM, Coryell W, et al: Follow-up and family study of anxious depression. Am J Psychiatry 148:1512–1517, 1991.

Cox BJ, Norton GR, Swinson RP, Endler NS: Substance abuse and panic-related anxiety: A critical review. Behav Res Ther 28:385–393, 1990.

Crowe RR: Panic disorder: Genetic considerations. J Psychiatr Res 24(suppl 2):129–134, 1990.

Crowe RR, Pauls DL, Venkatesh A, et al: Exercise and anxiety neurosis: A comparison of patients with and without mitral valve prolapse. Arch Gen Psychiatry 36:652–663, 1979.

DaCosta JM: On irritable heart, a clinical form of functional cardiac disorder and its consequences. Am J Med Sci 61:17, 1871.

Denko JD, Kaelbling R: The psychiatric aspects of hypoparathyroidism. Acta Psychiatr Scand 38(suppl 164):1–70, 1962.

Devereux RB, Kramer-Fox R, Kligfield P: Mitral valve prolapse: Causes, clinical manifestations, and management. Ann Intern Med 111:305–317, 1989.

Donnelly EF, Murphy DL, Goodwin FK: Primary affective disorders: Anxiety in unipolar and bipolar depressed groups. J Clin Psychol 34:621–623, 1978.

Fava M, Rosenbaum JF, MacLaughlin RA, et al: Dehydroepiandrosterone sulfate/cortisol ratio in panic disorder. Psychiatry Res 28:345–350, 1989.

Feighner JP, Robins E, Guze S, et al: Diagnostic criteria for use in psychiatric research. Arch Gen Psychiatry 26:57–63, 1972.

Ferrer M: Mistaken psychiatric referral of occult serious cardiovascular disease. Arch Gen Psychiatry 18:112–113, 1968.

Fishman SM, Sheehan DV, Carr DB: Thyroid indices in panic disorder. J Clin Psychiatry 46:432–433, 1985.

Freud, S: The justification for detaching from neurasthenia a particular syndrome: The anxiety-neurosis (1894). In Jones E (ed): Collected Papers. New York, Basic Books, 1959, p 80.

Frolich ED, Tarazi RX, Dustan HP: Hyperdynamic beta-adrenergic circulatory state. Arch Intern Med 123:1–7, 1969.

Garvey M: Benzodiazepines for panic disorder. Are they safe? Postgrad Med 90:245–246, 249–252, 1991.

Gawin FH, Markoff RA: Panic anxiety after abrupt discontinuation of amitriptyline. Am J Psychiatry 138:117–118, 1981.

Gelernter CS, Uhde TW, Cimbolic P, et al: Cognitive-behavioral and pharmacological treatments of social phobia: A controlled study. Arch Gen Psychiatry 48:938–945, 1991.

Geracioti TD Jr, Post RM: Onset of panic disorder associated with rare use of cocaine. Biol Psychiatry 29:403–406, 1991.

Gorman JM, Shear MK, Devereaux RB: Prevalence of mitral valve prolapse in panic disorder: Effect of echocardiographic criteria. Psychosom Med 48:167–171, 1986.

Gurney C, Roth M, Garside RF, et al: Studies in the classification of affective disorders: The relationship between anxiety states and depressive illness. Br J Psychiatry 121:162–166, 1972.

Guze SB: The diagnosis of hysteria: What are we trying to do? Am J Psychiatry 124:491–498, 1967.

Guze SB, Perley MJ: Observations on the natural history of hysteria. Am J Psychiatry 119:960–965, 1963.

Guze SB, Woodruff RA, Clayton PJ: Hysteria and antisocial behavior: Further evidence of an association. Am J Psychiatry 127:957–960, 1971.

Harper M, Roth M: Temporal lobe epilepsy and the phobic anxiety-depersonalization syndrome. Compr Psychiatry 3:129–151, 1962.

Holmberg G, Gershon S: Automonic and psychiatric effects of yohimbine hydrochloride. Psychopharmacologia 2:93–106, 1961.

James WE, Mefferd RB, Kimball I: Early signs of Huntington's chorea. Dis Nerv Syst 30:556–559, 1969.

Jacob RG, Moller MB, Turner SM, Wall C III: Otoneurological examination in panic disorder and agoraphobia with panic attacks: A pilot study. Am J Psychiatry 142:715–720, 1985.

Jansson L, Jerremalm A, Ost LG: Follow-up of agoraphobic patients treated with exposure in vivo or applied relaxation. Br J Psychiatry 149:486–490, 1986.

Kahn RJ, McNair DM, Lipman RS, et al: Imipramine and chlordiazepoxide in depressive and anxiety disorders: II. Efficacy in anxious outpatients. Arch Gen Psychiatry 43:79–85, 1986.

Kalus O, Asnis GM, Rubinson E, et al: Desipramine treatment in panic disorder. J Affective Disord 21:239–244, 1991.

Kaplan NM, Kramer NJ, Holland BO, et al: Single-voided urine metanephrine assays in screening for pheochromocytoma. Arch Intern Med 137:190–193, 1977.

Katerndahl DA, Gabel LL, Monk JS: Comparative symptomatology of phobic and nonphobic panic attacks. Fam Pract Res J 6:106–113, 1986.

Kendell RE: The choice of diagnostic criteria for biological research. Arch Gen Psychiatry 39:1334–1339, 1982.

Klein DF: Anxiety reconceptualized. In Klein DF, Raskin J (eds): Anxiety: New Research and Changing Concepts. New York, Raven Press, 1981, pp 235–263.

Kushner MG, Beitman BD: Panic attacks without fear: An overview. Behav Res Ther 28:469–479, 1990.

Leckman JF, Weissman MM, Merikangas KR, et al: Panic disorder increases risk of major depression, alcoholism, panic, and phobic disorders in affectively ill families. Arch Gen Psychiatry 40:1055–1060, 1983.

Leikin JB, Krantz AJ, Zell-Kanter M, et al: Clinical features and management of intoxication due to hallucinogenic drugs. Med Toxicol Adverse Drug Exp 4:324–350, 1989.

Lelliott PT, Marks IM, Monteiro WO, et al: Agoraphobics 5 years after imipramine and exposure: Outcome and predictors. J Nerv Ment Dis 175:599–605, 1987.

Levine R: Hypoglycemia. JAMA 230:462–463, 1974.

Lynch JJ, Paskewitz DA, Gimbel KS, et al: Psychological aspects of cardiac arrhythmia. Am Heart J 93:645–657, 1977.

Maddock RJ, Carter CS: Hyperventilation-induced panic attacks in panic disorder with agoraphobia. Biol Psychiatry 29:843–854, 1991.

Manuila A, Manuila L, Nicole M, Lambert H: Dictionaire français de médecine et de biologie, vol 14. Paris, Masson, 1981, p 714.

Marks IM, Gray S, Cohen D, et al: Imipramine and brief therapist-aided exposure in agoraphobics having self-exposure homework. Arch Gen Psychiatry 40:153–162, 1983.

Marks IM, de Albuquerque A, Cottraux J, et al: The "efficacy" of alprazolam in panic disorder and agoraphobia: A critique of recent reports. Arch Gen Psychiatry 46:668–672, 1989.

Mattila M, Seppala T, Mattila MJ: Anxiogenic effect of yohimbine in healthy subjects: Comparison with caffeine and antagonism by clonidine and diazepam. Int Clin Psychopharmacol 3:215–229, 1988.

Mavissakalian M, Michelson L: Agoraphobia: Relative and combined effectiveness of therapist assisted in vivo exposure and imipramine. J Clin Psychiatry 47:117–122, 1986a.

Mavissakalian M, Michelson L: Two-year follow-up of exposure and imipramine treatment of agoraphobia. Am J Psychiatry 143:1106–1012, 1986b.

Mellman TA, Davis GC: Combat-related flashbacks in posttraumatic stress disorder: Phenomenology and similarity to panic attacks. J Clin Psychiatry 46:379–382, 1985.

Moran C: Depersonalization and agoraphobia associated with marijuana use. Br J Med Psychol 59:187–196, 1985.

Munjack DJ, Crocker B, Cabe D, et al: Alprazolam, propranolol, and placebo in the treatment of panic disorder and agoraphobia with panic attacks. J Clin Psychopharmacol 9:22–27, 1989.

Munjack DJ, Moss HB: Affective disorders and alcoholism in the families of agoraphobics. Arch Gen Psychiatry 38:869–871, 1981.

Muskin PR: Panics, prolapse, and PVCs. Gen Hosp Psychiatry 7:219–223, 1985.

Noyes DJ, Clancey J, Hoenk PR, et al: The prognosis of anxiety neurosis. Arch Gen Psychiatry 37:173–178, 1980.

Noyes R, Reich J, Clancey J, O'Gorman TW: Reduction in hypochondriasis with treatment of panic disorder. Br J Psychiatry 149:631–635, 1986.

Nutt DJ: Increased central alpha-2 adrenoceptor sensitivity in panic disorder. Psychopharmacology (Berlin) 90:268–269, 1986.

Nutzinger DO, Zapotoczky HG: The influence of depression on the outcome of cardiac phobia (panic disorder). Psychopathology 18:155–162, 1985.

Overall JE, Hollister LE, Johnson M, et al: Nosology of depression and differential response to drugs. JAMA 195:946–948, 1966.

Paykel ES: Depressive typologies and response to amitriptyline. Br J. Psychiatry 120:147–156, 1972.

Pohl R, Rainey J, Ortiz A, et al: Isoproterenol induced anxiety states. Psychopharmacol Bull 21:424–427, 1985.

Pollack MH, Tesar GE, Rosenbaum JF, Spier SA: Clonazepam in the treatment of panic disorder and agoraphobia: A one-year follow-up. J Clin Psychopharmacol 6:302–304, 1986.

Pringuet G, DePerson J: Death anxiety in thyrotoxicosis. Ann Med Psychol (Paris) 140:753–768, 1982.

Raskin A, Schulterbrandt JG, Reatig N, et al: Depression subtypes and response to phenelzine, diazepam, and placebo. Arch Gen Psychiatry 30:66–75, 1974.

Reiman EM, Raichle ME, Robins E, et al: The application of positron emission tomography to the study of panic disorder. Am J Psychiatry 143:469–477, 1986.

Reiter SR, Otto MW, Pollack MH, Rosenbaum JF: Major depression in panic disorder patients with comorbid social phobia. J Affective Disord 22:171–177, 1991.

Roth M: The phobic anxiety-depersonalization syndrome. Proc R Soc Med 52:587–595, 1959.

Roy-Byrne PP, Uhde TW, Rubinow DR, Post RM: Reduced TSH and prolactin responses to TRH in patients with panic disorder. Am J Psychiatry 143:503–507, 1986.

Roy-Byrne PP, Schmidt P, Cannon RO, et al: Microvascular angina and panic disorder. Int J Psychiatry Med 19:315–325, 1989.

Russell JL, Kushner MG, Beitman BD, Bartels KM: Nonfearful panic disorder in neurology patients validated by lactate challenge. Am J Psychiatry 148:361–364, 1991.

Salkovskis PM, Jones DR, Clark DM: Respiratory control in the treatment of panic attacks: Replication and extension with concurrent measurement of behaviour and pCO_2. Br J Psychiatry 148:526–532, 1986.

Schweizer E, Winokur A, Rickels K: Insulin induced hypoglycemia and panic attacks. Am J Psychiatry 143:654–655, 1986.

Sklare DA, Stein MB, Pikus AM, Uhde TW: Dysequilibrium and audiovestibular function in panic disorder: Symptom profiles and test findings. Am J Otol 11:338–341, 1990.

Sheehan DV, Ballenger J, Jacobsen G: Treatment of endogenous anxiety with phobic, hysterical and hypochondriacal symptoms. Arch Gen Psychiatry 37:51–59, 1980.

Sheehan DV, Sheehan KH: The classification of anxiety and hysterical states: I. Historical review and emirical delineation. J Clin Psychopharmacol 2:235–244, 1982.

Shulman R: Psychiatric aspects of pernicious anemia: A prospective study. Br Med J 3:266–269, 1967.

Siris SG, Aronson A, Sellew AP: Imipramine-responsive panic-like symptomatology in schizophrenia/schizoaffective disorder. Biol Psychiatry 25:485–488, 1989.

Slater E: Diagnosis of "hysteria." Br Med J 1:1395–1399, 1965.

Solyom L, Ledwidge B, Solyom C: Delineating social phobia. Br J Psychiatry 149:464–470, 1986.

Taylor CB, Hayward C: Cardiovascular considerations in selection of anti-panic pharmacotherapy. J Psychiatr Res 24(Suppl 2):43–49, 1990.

Thompson WL, Thompson TL Jr: Psychiatric aspects of asthma in adults. Adv Psychosom Med 14:33–47, 1985.

VanValkenburg C, Akiskal H, Puzantian V, et al: Anxious depressions: Clinical, family history, and naturalistic outcome comparisons with panic and major depressive disorders. J Affective Disord 6:67–82, 1984.

Von Korff MR, Eaton WW, Keyl PM: The epidemiology of panic attacks and panic disorder: Results of three community surveys. Am J Epidemiol 122:970–981, 1985.

Weil AA: Ictal emotions occurring in temporal lobe dysfunction. Arch Neurol 1:101–111, 1959.

Weissman MM, Leaf PJ, Blazer DG, et al: The relationship between panic disorder and agoraphobia: An epidemiological perspective. Psychopharmacol Bull 22:787–791, 1986.

Williams D: The structure of emotions reflected in epileptic experiences. Brain 79:29–67, 1956.

Williams RB Jr: Do benzodiazepines have a role in the prevention or treatment of coronary heart disease and other major medical disorders? J Psychiatr Res 24(Suppl 2):51–56, 1990.

Zandbergen J, Bright M, Pols H, et al: Higher lifetime prevalence of respiratory diseases in panic disorder? Am J Psychiatry 148:1583–1585, 1991.

Zandbergen J, Pols H, De Loof C, et al: Effect of hypercapnia and other disturbances in the acid–base balance on panic disorder. Hillside J Clin Psychiatry 11:185–197, 1989.

Zitrin CM, Klein DF, Woerner MG: Behavioral therapy, supportive therapy, imipramine and phobias. Arch Gen Psychiatry 35:307–316, 1978.

Zitrin CM, Klein DF, Woerner MG: Treatment of agorapohobia with group exposure in vivo and imipramine. Arch Gen Psychiatry 37:63–72, 1980.

CHAPTER 24

Thought Disorder

NANCY C. ANDREASEN

The term *thought disorder* is confusing to medical students, residents, and senior clinicians alike. The confusion arises because the term *thought disorder* has no universally agreed on definition, although some consensus has begun to emerge during the past 5 to 10 years. Some clinicians use the term very broadly to refer to such varied phenomena as disorganized speech, confusion, delusions, or even hallucinations. Others restrict the definition to a much narrower concept, sometimes referred to as *formal thought disorder*, or disorganized speech that is presumed to reflect disorganized thinking.

DEFINITION

Kraepelin and other great clinicians of the late nineteenth and early twentieth centuries frequently described abnormalities in language and cognition among the patients whom they observed (Kraepelin, 1919). The concept of *thought disorder* derives principally from Bleuler (1950), who defined it in terms of the association psychology that prevailed during his era and believed that it occurred only in schizophrenia:

Certain symptoms of schizophrenia are present in every case and at every period of illness even though, as with every other disease symptom, they must have attained a certain degree of intensity before they can be recognized with any certainty. . . . For example, the peculiar association disturbance is always present, but not each and every aspect of it. . . . Besides these specific or permanent symptoms, we can find a host of other, more accessory manifestations such as delusions, hallucinations, or catatonic symptoms. . . . As far as we know, the fundamental symptoms are characteristic of schizophrenia, while the accessory symptoms may also appear in other types of illness. . . .

It is not clear precisely what Bleuler means by "association disturbance," but he appears to be referring to many types of confused thinking, which are usually expressed in confused speech.

Bleuler's ideas have been very influential in modern psychiatry. Until recently, thought disorder was considered to be the pathognomonic symptom of schizophrenia. During past decades, clinicians and psychologists have developed many different methods for assessing this important symptom, including the use of proverb interpretation, IQ testing, perceptual tests such as the Rorschach or thematic apperception test, neuropsychological tests such as the Stroop or Continuous Performance Test, or even the use of physiologic techniques to measure attention, such as eye tracking, single photon emission computed tomography, or positron emission tomography (Goldstein, 1944; Kasanin, 1944; Chapman and McGhie, 1962; Cromwell and Dokeckie, 1968; Cameron, 1939; Payne and Friedlander, 1962; Harrow et al., 1965; Wynne and Singer, 1965; Andreasen, 1977; Holzman, 1983; Pardo et al., 1990; Buchsbaum, 1990; Andreasen et al., in press). Thought disorder is sometimes used as loosely equivalent to cognitive disorder, and cognition is an extremely broad concept.

In a clinical setting, it is probably useful to simplify the concept somewhat. In his classic text on psychopathology, Frank Fish (1962) outlined a logical system for categorizing abnormalities in cognition that is quite useful. He suggested dividing them into four main groups: disorders of perception, disorders of content of thought, disorders of process of thought, and disorders of form of thought. At its broadest, *thought disorder* is sometimes used to refer to all of these. At its narrowest, it refers only to "formal thought disorder" or disorders in process of thought.

Perceptual disorders are abnormalities in perceptual experiences. The most common perceptual abnormalities seen in psychiatric patients are hallucinations of various types. Hearing voices that are not really there, seeing forms that in fact do not exist, or experiencing a sensation of bugs crawling on one's skin when one is not infested are all types of perceptual disorders.

Disorders in content of thought are abnormalities in beliefs and in interpretation of experiences. The most common disorders in content of thought seen in psychiatric patients are delusions of various types. Typical delusions include beliefs such as that messages are being given over the radio or TV about the person, that people are conspiring against the person and trying to harm him or her, or that a person has some type of special or unusual ability.

Disorders in the process of thought involve abnormalities in the way ideas and language are formulated before they are expressed. Unlike hallucinations or delusions, which are usually determined to be present because the patient describes them, thought process disorders are usually inferred by observing what the patient says or does and only occasionally by self-report. One common manifestation of thought process disorder is *pressured speech*, in which the patient tends to speak loudly, intensely, and rapidly. Another common clinical manifestation is *blocking*, in which the patient stops suddenly in the middle of a sentence because he or she has lost the train of thought for some reason. Disordered thought processes also may be reflected by impaired attention, poor memory, or difficulty in formulating abstract concepts. These aspects of impaired thinking are assessed through observing the patient or through using simple mental status tests such as serial sevens or memory tests.

Disorders in the form of thought, or formal thought disorders, are abnormalities in the way thought is expressed in language, whether it be in speech or in writing. Clinically, this abnormality appears in various types of disorganized speech which are given a variety of different names (defined in more detail below), such as *incoherence*, *tangentiality*, or *derailment* (loose associations). This type of thought disorder is assessed simply by listening to the patient talk or by looking at his or her writing. The clinician observes the patient's verbal output and determines whether it is well connected, well organized, and seems to make sense or whether, on the other hand, it seems disconnected, disorganized, and bizarre.

The boundaries between these four types of cognitive abnormalities are not always clear. For example, when a patient feels a crawling sensation and then interprets it as due to an infestation of parasites living in his or her bed, is this a delusion, a hallucination, or both? (Probably both.) When a patient speaks very rapidly, skips from topic to topic, makes little sense, and admits that his or her thoughts seem to be occurring too rapidly to control, is this a disorder of thought process or thought form? (Again, probably both.) Further, some patients may clearly display all four classes of cognitive abnormality, while others may display one or two. The four types may, in theory, be mutually exclusive, but they may co-occur as symptoms in actual patients.

Other chapters in this book will focus in more detail on the first two types of cognitive abnormalities, disorders in perception (hallucinations) and disorders in content of thought (delusions). This chapter describes some common clinical manifestations of the last two types of cognitive abnormalities, disorders in the process of thought (dyslogias) and disorders in the form of thought (dysphasias).

WHAT ARE THE BOUNDARIES OF THOUGHT DISORDER?

Don't people who are otherwise normal sometimes speak in a disorganized manner? Doesn't everyone occasionally experience blocking or a rapid flood of ideas? How does one draw the line between "normal thinking" and "thought disorder"?

The following passage from James Joyce's last novel, *Finnegan's Wake*, illustrates the problem in an extreme case:

Oh, by the way, yes another thing occurs to me. You let me tell you, with the utmost politeness, where ordinarily designed, your birth wrong was, to fall in with the Plan, as out nationals should, as all nationalists must, and do a certain office (what, I will not tell you) in a certain holy office (nor will I say where) during certain agonizing office hours from such a year to such an hour on such and such a date at so and so much a week (which, May I remind, were just a gulp for you, failing in which you might have taken the scales off boilers like any boskp of Yorek) and do your little two bit and thus earn from the nation true thanks, right here in our place of burden, your bourne of travel and ville of tares [Joyce, 1939].

Joyce is using language in an idiosyncratic and confusing way, relying on punning, word play, and allusion. When this sample of speech was given to a group of clinicians to read blindly for severity of thought disorder and to assign a diagnosis, 95 percent of the clinicians thought it displayed thought disorder and 48 percent diagnosed its author as having schizophrenia (Andreasen et al., 1974). This result indicates that even clinicians are not clear on the boundaries of abnormal thinking, particularly when they must look at examples out of context and cannot rely on important clinical cues, such as the appearance of the individual, his or her manner of speech, the presence or absence of other symptoms, and past history. The boundaries of thought disorder are particularly blurred when language is used creatively, when it is used pedantically, or when it is used poorly because of low intelligence or inadequate education.

The difference between the creative use of language and thought disorder is largely a matter of intent and control rather than in the nature of the language actually produced. Writers depend on unusual associations to find fresh imagery and then enjoy playing with words and ideas, which may seem to represent "loose associations" or "derailment." However, writers and other creative individuals usually have their cognition under control, and they have a method in their madness. Because of this, an organization usually can be seen in the apparent disorganization, and the result is said to be "creative" or "original." On the other hand, patients who are psychotic are usually out of control, and their language and thinking are therefore perceived as disorganized rather than disciplined and as bizarre rather than creative.

Pedantic use of language also may resemble thought disorder. Verbose, pedantic, empty language is a hazard of some occupations or disciplines, such as politics, administration, philosophy, the ministry, and science. People in these occupations or disciplines may tend to speak verbosely, with excessive use of obscure or overly abstract terminology, and to say very little. Patients suffering from psychosis may have a similar problem, which is referred to as *poverty of content of speech*. Again, drawing the line between a "normal" thought disorder manifested by a government employee speaking bureaucratese and a psychotic patient with a thought disorder will depend heavily on contextual cues. Is the speaker in control? Can the speaker moderate his or her style if requested to be more specific or more concise? Can the speaker do better on another topic? Does the speaker have any other significant symptoms?

Finally, people who are mentally dull or uneducated also may show some characteristics similar to those patients with relatively severe psychopathology. The mentally handicapped or uneducated may be excessively concrete, may be unable to speak clearly and fluently in reply to a question, may use words idiosyncratically because they do not understand what they mean, or may use poor grammar. Unlike the creative individual or the bureaucrat, these individuals do not have conscious control and cannot shift their language patterns on request. In this instance, clinicians must evaluate their language and thinking in terms of norms adjusted for their intellectual and educational levels. They must take into account information concerning number of years of schooling, level of performance, and intelligence testing.

Thus *thought disorder* is probably not a phenomenon discontinuous from normality but rather is probably on a continuum with it. It may occur occasionally in the speech of normal people, particularly when they are fatigued or disinhibited, and it may occur more frequently in the conscious productions of artists. Whenever the clinician recognizes that he or she is reading or listening to unusual language and thinking, he or she must always evaluate it in terms of its context. He or she must ask questions such as the following: Is the abnormality under conscious control? Can it be varied and reversed to normal through prompting or through a change of subject? Does the patient have other symptoms? What is the patient's educational and intellectual background? Usually, intelligent use of context will help the clinician distinguish between normal thought disorder and thought disorder that has a pathologic significance.

WHAT ARE THE COMMON TYPES OF THOUGHT DISORDER?

Thought disorder is a heterogeneous phenomenon. During the past 50 years, clinicians have described many different manifestations of thought disorder, such as derailment, incoherence, tangentiality, poverty of speech, etc. The many different subtypes also have been a source of confusion, since they tend to be referred to by the global term *thought disorder*. During recent years, efforts have been made to define the various subtypes more carefully and precisely and to examine the relationship of the various subtypes to clinical diagnosis.

One recent approach has been to subdivide types of thought disorder into two main groups: *negative* and *positive* thought disorders. This distinction has been useful because some evidence suggests that negative thought disorders are more common in schizophrenia and also may predict a somewhat poorer prognosis, while positive thought disorders occur in both mania and schizophrenia and may predict a better outcome. Standard definitions of these types of thought disorder are as follows (Andreasen, 1979a).

Negative Thought Disorders

POVERTY OF SPEECH

This is a restriction in the *amount* of spontaneous speech so that replies to questions tend to be brief, concrete, and unelaborated. Unprompted additional information is rarely provided. For example, in answer to the question, "How many children do you have?" the patient replies, "Two. A girl and a boy. The girl is thirteen and the boy ten." "Two" is all that is required to answer the question, and the rest of the reply is additional information. Replies may be monosyllabic, and some questions may be left unanswered altogether. When confronted with this speech pattern, the interviewer may find himself or herself frequently prompting the patient in order to encourage elaboration of replies. Doing an interview to evaluate a patient with poverty of speech can be very hard work. To elicit this finding, the examiner must allow the patient adequate time to answer and to elaborate the answer.

EXAMPLE. Interviewer: "Do you think there's a lot of corruption in the government?" Patient: "Yeah, seems to be." Interviewer: "Do you think Oliver North was fairly treated?" Patient: "I don't know." Interviewer: "Were you working at all before you came to the hospital?" Patient: "No." Interviewer: "What kinds of jobs have you had in the past?" Patient: "Oh, some janitor jobs, painting." Interviewer: "What kind of work do you do?" Patient: "I don't." Interviewer: "How far did you go in school?" Patient: "Eleventh grade." Interviewer: "How old are you?" Patient: "Eighteen."

POVERTY OF CONTENT OF SPEECH

Although replies are long enough so that speech is adequate in amount, such replies convey little information in this disorder. Language tends to be vague, often overabstract or overconcrete, repetitive, and stereotyped. The interviewer may recognize this finding by observing that the patient has spoken at some length but has not given adequate information to answer the question. Alternatively, the patient may provide enough information but require many words to do so so that a lengthy reply can be summarized in a sentence or two. Sometimes the interviewer may characterize the speech as "empty philosophizing."

EXAMPLE. Interviewer: "Ok. Why, why is it, do you think, that people believe in God?" Patient: "Well, first of all because, he uh he are the person that is their personal savior. He walks with me and talks with me. And uh, the understanding that I have um, a lot of peoples, they don't really uh know they own personal self. Because, uh, they ain't they all, just don't know they personal self. They don't know that he uh, seems like to me a lot of em don't understand that he walks and talks with them. And uh, show them their way to go. I understand also that every man and every lady is just not pointed in the same direction. Some are pointed different. They go in their different ways. The way that uh Jesus Christ wanted em to go. Me myself I am pointed in the ways of uh knowing right from wrong and doing it. I can't do no more, or no less, than that."

BLOCKING

This is interruption of a train of speech before a thought or idea has been completed. After a period of silence which may last from a few seconds to minutes, the person indicates that he or she cannot recall what he or she had been saying or meant to say. Blocking should only be judged to be present either if a person voluntarily describes losing his or her thought or if upon questioning by the interviewer the person indicates that that was his or her reason for pausing.

PERSEVERATION

This involves persistent repetition of words, ideas, or subjects so that once a patient begins to refer to a particular subject or use a particular word, he or she continually returns to it in the process of speaking.

EXAMPLE. Interviewer: "Tell me what you are like, what kind of person you are." Patient: "I'm from Marshalltown, Iowa. That's sixty miles northwest, northeast of Des Moines, Iowa. And I'm married at the present time. I'm thirty-six years old. My wife is thirty-five. She lives in Garwin, Iowa. That's fifteen miles southeast of Marshalltown, Iowa. I'm getting a divorce at the present time. And I am presently in a mental institution in Iowa City, Iowa, which is a hundred miles southeast of Marshalltown, Iowa."

Positive Thought Disorders

DERAILMENT (LOOSE ASSOCIATIONS, FLIGHT OF IDEAS)

This is a pattern of spontaneous speech in which the ideas slip off the track onto another one which is clearly but obliquely related or onto one that is completely unrelated. Things may be said in juxtapositions that lack a meaningful relationship, or the patient may shift idiosyncratically from one frame of reference to another. At times there may be a vague connection between the idea, and at others none will be apparent. This pattern of speech is often characterized as sounding "disjointed." Perhaps the most common manifestation of this disorder is a slow, steady slippage, with no single derailment being particularly severe, so that the speaker gets farther and farther off the track with each derailment without showing an awareness that his or her reply no longer has a connection with the question that was asked. This abnormality is often characterized by lack of cohesion between clauses and sentences and by unclear pronoun references.

Although less severe derailments (i.e., those in which the relationship between juxtaposed ideas is oblique) have sometimes been referred to in the past as *tangentiality* or as *flight of ideas* when in the context of mania, such distinctions are not recommended because they tend to be unreliable. Flight of ideas is a derailment that occurs rapidly in the context of pressured speech. Tangentiality is defined as a different phenomenon in that it occurs as the immediate response to a question.

EXAMPLE. Interviewer: "Did you enjoy doing that?" Patient: "Um-hm. Oh hey well I, I oh I really enjoyed some communities I tried it, and the next day when I'd be going out you know, um I took control like uh, I put, um, bleach on my hair in, in California. My roommate was from Chicago, and she was going to the junior college. And we lived in the Y.M.C.A. so she wanted to put it, um, peroxide on my hair, and she did, and I got up and looked at the mirror and tears came to my eyes. Now do you understand it, I was fully aware of what was going on but why couldn't I, why the tears? I can't understand that, can you?'' Interviewer: ''No.'' Patient: ''Have you experienced anything like it?'' Interviewer: ''You just must be an emotional person that's all.'' Patient: ''Well, not very much, I mean, what if I were dead? It's funeral age. Well I um? Now I had my toenails, uh, operated on. They're uh, um got infected and I wasn't able to do it but they won't let me at my tools. Well.''

INCOHERENCE (WORD SALAD, JARGON APHASIA, PARAGRAMMATISM)

This is a pattern of speech which is essentially incomprehensible at times. The incoherence is due to several different mechanisms, which may sometimes all occur simultaneously. Sometimes portions of coherent sentences may be observed in the midst of a sentence that is incoherent as a whole. Sometimes the disturbance appears to be at a semantic level so that words are substituted in a phrase or sentence such that the meaning seems to be distorted or destroyed; the word choice may seem totally random or may appear to have some oblique connection with the context. Sometimes ''cementing words'' (coordinating and subordinating conjunctions such as *and* or *although*, adjectival pronouns such as *the, a*, and *an*) are deleted.

Incoherence is often accompanied by derailment. It differs from derailment in that in incoherence the abnormality occurs *within* the level of the sentence or clause that contains words or phrases that are joined incoherently. The abnormality in derailment involves unclear or confusing connections between larger units, such as sentences or clauses.

This type of language disorder is relatively rare. When it occurs, it tends to be severe or extreme, and mild forms are quite uncommon. It may sound quite similar to a Wernicke's aphasia or jargon aphasia, and in these cases the disorder should only be called incoherence (thereby implying a psychiatric disorder as opposed to a neurologic disorder) when history and laboratory data exclude the possibility of a known organic etiology and clinical testing for aphasia is negative.

EXAMPLES. Interviewer: ''Why do you think people believe in God?'' Patient: ''Um, because making a do in life. Isn't none of that stuff about evolution guiding isn't true any more now. It all happened a long time ago. It happened in eons and eons and stuff they wouldn't believe in him. The time that Jesus Christ people believed in their things people believed in, Jehovah God that they didn't believe in Jesus Christ that much.''

Interviewer: ''Um, what do you think about current political issues like the energy crisis?'' Patient: ''They're destroying too many cattle and oil just to make soap. If we need soap when you can jump into a pool of water, and then when you go to buy your gasoline, my folks always thought they should, get pop but the best thing to get is motor oil, and, money. May, may as well go there and, trade in some, pop caps and, uh, tires, and tractors to grup, car garage, so they can pull cars away from wrecks, is what I believed in. So I didn't go there to get no more pop when my folks said it. I just went there to get a ice cream cone, and some pop, in cans, or we can go over there and get a cigarette. And it was the largest thing you do to get cigarettes 'cause then you could trade off, what you owned, and go for something new, it was sentimental, and that's the only thing I needed was something sentimental, and there wasn't anything else more sentimental than that, except for knickknacks and most knickknacks, these cost thirty to forty dollars to get, a good billfold, or a little stand to put on your desk.''

TANGENTIALITY

This involves replying to a question in an oblique, tangential, or even irrelevant manner. The reply may be related to the question in some distant way. Or the reply may be unrelated and seem totally irrelevant. Tangentiality has sometimes been used as roughly equivalent to loose associations or derailment. The concept of tangentiality has been partially redefined so that it refers only to replies to questions and not to transitions in spontaneous speech.

EXAMPLE. Interviewer: ''What city are you from?'' Patient: ''Well, that's a hard question to answer because my parents . . . I was born in Iowa, but I know that I'm white instead of black so apparently I came from the North somewhere and I don't know where, you know. I really don't know where my ancestors came from. So I don't know whether I'm Irish or French or Scandinavian or I don't believe I'm Polish but I think I'm I think I might be German or Welsh. I'm not but that's all speculation and that that's one thing that I would like to know and is my ancestors you know where did I originate? But I never took the time to find out the answer to that question.''

ILLOGICALITY

This is a pattern of speech in which conclusions are reached that do not follow logically. This may take the form of non sequiturs (meaning ''it does not follow''), in which the patient makes a logical inference between two clauses that is unwarranted or illogical. It may take the form of faulty inductive inferences. It also may take the form of reaching conclusions based on a faulty premise without any actual delusional thinking.

EXAMPLE. ''Parents are the people that raise you. Any thing that raises you can be a parent. Parents can be anything, material, vegetable, or mineral, that has taught you something. Parents would be the world of things that are alive, that are there. Rocks, a person can look at a rock and learn something from it, so it could be a parent."

CLANGING

This is a pattern of speech in which sounds rather than meaningful relationships appear to govern word choice so that the intelligibility of the speech is impaired and redundant words are introduced. In addition to rhyming relationships, this pattern of speech also may include punning associations so that a word similar in sound brings in a new thought.

EXAMPLE. "I'm not trying to make noise. I'm trying to make sense. If you can make sense out of nonsense, well, have fun. I'm trying to make sense out of sense. I'm not making sense [cents] anymore. I have to make dollars."

NEOLOGISMS

This involves new word formations. A *neologism* is defined here as a completely new word or phrase whose derivation cannot be understood. Sometimes the term *neologism* also has been used to mean a word that has been incorrectly built up but with origins that are understandable as due to a misuse of the accepted methods of word formation. For purposes of clarity, these should be referred to as *word approximations*. Neologisms are quite uncommon.

EXAMPLE. "I got so angry I picked up a dish and threw it at the geshinker." "So I sort of bawked the whole thing up."

PRESSURED SPEECH

This is an increase in the amount of spontaneous speech as compared with what is considered ordinary or socially customary. The patient talks rapidly and is difficult to interrupt. Some sentences may be left uncompleted because of an eagerness to get on to a new idea. Simple questions that could be answered in only a few words or sentences are answered at great length so that the answer takes minutes rather than seconds and indeed may not stop at all if the speaker is not interrupted. Even when interrupted, the speaker often continues to talk. Speech tends to be loud and emphatic. Sometimes patients with severe pressure will talk without any social stimulation and even though no one is listening. When patients are receiving phenothiazines or lithium, their speech is often slowed down by the medication, and then it can be judged only on the basis of amount, volume, and social appropriateness. If a quantitative measure is applied to the rate of speech, then a rate greater than 150 words per minute is usually considered rapid or pressured. This disorder may be accompanied by derailment, tangentiality, or incoherence, but it is distinct from them.

DISTRACTIBLE SPEECH

During the course of a discussion or interview, the patient stops talking in the middle of a sentence or idea and changes the subject in response to a nearby stimulus, such as an object on a desk, the interviewer's clothing or appearance, etc.

EXAMPLE. "Then I left San Francisco and moved to . . . Where did you get that tie? It looks like it's left over from the 50's. I like the warm weather in San Diego. Is that a conch shell on your desk? Have you ever gone scuba diving?"

DIAGNOSTIC AND PROGNOSTIC SIGNIFICANCE OF THOUGHT DISORDER

Bleuler, the psychiatrist responsible for introducing the term *schizophrenia*, believed that thought disorder occurred only in schizophrenia. Recently, however, Bleuler's beliefs about the specificity of thought disorder have been questioned. A number of investigators have observed that thought disorder may occur in other diagnostic groups, such as manic patients, and that abnormalities in speech and thinking also occur in normal people. Finally, it has been observed that not all schizophrenic patients display thought disorder, thereby raising additional questions about its diagnostic specificity.

After the preceding definitions were developed, they were applied to consecutive admissions to the Iowa Psychiatric Hospital (Andreasen, 1979b, 1979c). The frequency with which various types of thought disorder could be found in various diagnostic groups was then determined. The results are shown in Table 24-1.

As the table indicates, manics have a great deal of formal thought disorder. Pressured speech, as might be expected, is their most prominent symptom, but they also have high rates of derailment, tangentiality, incoherence, and loss of goal. Incoherence does not occur with great frequency, but the frequency is equal to that found in schizophrenia. On the other hand, schizophrenic patients tend to have relatively more negative thought disorder than do the manics, but they also have relatively high rates of some types of positive thought disorder. The depressive patients have very little thought disorder. Their most prominent types are poverty of speech, poverty of content of speech, and circumstantiality.

These data have been replicated in several subsequent investigations (Andreasen et al., 1984). They confirm the fact that thought disorder is not pathognomonic of any particular type of psychosis. When thought disorder is divided into subtypes, such as positive versus negative, it may have somewhat more diagnostic significance. In particular, negative thought disorder in the absence of a full affective syndrome is highly suggestive of schizo-

TABLE 24-1. *Frequency of Types of Thought Disorder in Psychiatric Patients*

	Manics (n = 32)		Depressives (n = 36)		Schizophrenics (n = 45)	
	n	Percent	n	Percent	n	Percent
Negative thought disorder						
Poverty of speech	2	6	8	22	13	29
Poverty of content of speech	6	19	6	17	18	40
Blocking	1	3	2	6	2	4
Perseveration	11	34	2	6	11	24
Positive thought disorder						
Derailment	18	56	5	14	25	56
Incoherence	5	16	0	0	7	16
Tangentiality	11	34	9	25	16	36
Illogicality	8	25	0	0	12	27
Clanging	3	9	0	0	0	0
Neologisms	1	3	0	0	1	2
Pressured speech	23	72	2	6	12	27
Distractible speech	10	31	0	0	1	2

phrenia. These results also indicate the utility of subdividing thought disorder into various clinical subtypes.

Follow-up studies also have been conducted in order to determine the prognostic significance of thought disorder (Andreasen et al., 1984). When manics are evaluated 6 months after their index evaluation, most clinical manifestations of thought disorder (such as derailment or pressured speech) have fallen to normal levels. Thus manic thought disorder, while transiently as severe as that occurring in schizophrenia, tends to be reversible.

On the other hand, the thought disorder observed in schizophrenic patients is somewhat more complex. The negative thought disorders continue to persist for 6 months later and even to worsen. On the other hand, the positive thought disorders tend to diminish somewhat. When types of thought disorder are correlated with other measures of outcome, such as ability to work or to relate in normal social settings, then negative thought disorder is found to be a powerful predictor of outcome. Patients who had prominent negative thought disorder at index evaluation tended to perform poorly on measured social functioning 6 months later. Thus thought disorder, and particularly the type of thought disorder, has considerable clinical and prognostic significance.

RELATIONSHIP BETWEEN THOUGHT DISORDERS AND OTHER SYMPTOMS OF SCHIZOPHRENIA

Although we now recognize that various types of thought disorder may occur frequently in mood disorders as well as schizophrenia, the concept of thought disorder still remains quite central to the definition of schizophrenia. Because the symptoms of schizophrenia are varied and complex, during the past decade clinicians have developed a system for

simplifying and clarifying them by dividing them into two general groups: positive and negative. In general, *positive* symptoms are defined as a distortion or exaggeration of normal functions; conventionally, they include hallucinations (a disorder of perception), delusions (a disorder of inference), bizarre or disorganized behavior (a disorder of behavioral organization and control), positive formal thought disorder (disorganization of speech), and possibly inappropriate affect; *negative* symptoms represent a loss or diminution of function and include alogia (negative thought disorder such as poverty of speech), affective blunting, anhedonia and asociality, avolition, and possibly attentional impairment. (Andreasen, 1982a, 1982b, 1986, 1988, and 1990).

A large literature suggests that these two constellations of symptoms may identify important correlates of schizophrenia that have predictive value. Crow (1980) was the first to suggest that a syndrome characterized by negative symptoms typically manifests an early age of onset, poor premorbid adjustment, poor response to treatment with neuroleptics, indices of cognitive dysfunction ascertained with neuropsychological assessment, and evidence of structural brain abnormalities assessed with neuroimaging; the positive syndrome, on the other hand, may be characterized by better premorbid adjustment, later age of onset, good response to treatment, intact cognition, and absence of structural brain abnormalities. Crow hypothesized that the negative syndrome might represent a more "structural" and therefore irreversible form of schizophrenia, while the positive syndrome would represent a more neurochemical and reversible form.

Since Crow's original formulation, this distinction has been repeatedly evaluated in large numbers of research investigations. A consensus currently exists that the distinction between positive and negative symptoms is globally useful and that these symptoms are often correlated with other clinical features as originally described by Crow, although the relationship is by no means sufficiently strong to identify distinct subtypes of schizophrenia or to have consistent predictive validity. That is, prominent negative symptoms do typically suggest a worse outcome, but any individual patient with prominent negative symptoms may do well, respond to medication, and have normal indices of brain function. The same type of generalization can be made concerning the predictive validity of positive symptoms. Because this distinction has heuristic value, the definition of schizophrenia in DSM-IV will incorporate the concept of positive versus negative symptoms. Although an oversimplification, the distinction between positive and negative symptoms is a clinically useful oversimplification.

EDITORS' COMMENT

An alternative to the positive/negative distinction in schizophrenia is provided by the extremely complex clinical system of Leonhard (Fish F: Schizophrenia. Baltimore, Williams & Wilkins, 1962). Departing from Kraepelin's separation of schizophrenia, Leonhard presents 16 subtypes. There are 6 subtypes of catatonic schizophrenia, 4 subtypes of hebephrenic schizophrenia, and 6 subtypes of paranoid schizophrenia. Leonhard describes the number and quality of symptoms. For an end-state diagnosis of schizophrenia, an individual must fit into a specific combination. As an example of the difference, in parakinetic catatonia, a jerky choreiform set of involuntary movements appears, whereas in manneristic catatonia, posture and movement become stiff. Each of the subgroups is thought to be due to abnormalities in different neurologic systems. It would be very useful to investigate the varieties of thought disorder in the subtypes of schizophrenia that Leonhard presents. As it is, however, both the positive/negative distinction and the Leonhard classification are useful concepts in teaching about psychiatric patients.

One of the criticisms that has been launched against the distinction is that a simple subdivision of the symptoms of schizophrenia into positive and negative does not completely account for the complexity of thought disorder and its relationship to other positive symptoms. As described above, thought disorder is both positive and negative, with negative thought disorder encompassed in the concept of alogia and positive thought disorder encompassed in forms that manifest as very disorganized speech such as derailment and incoherence. Further, recent studies have examined the relationship between positive thought disorder and other positive symptoms and have consistently demonstrated, using factor analysis, that two symptom clusters tend to occur within the group of positive symptoms. (Bilder, 1985; Liddle, 1987; Arndt et al, 1991). While negative symptoms tend to be highly correlated with one another, positive symptoms subdivide themselves into two separate groups. One group tends to have high factor loading on

TABLE 24-2. *Factor Analysis of Symptom Scores from 207 Schizophrenic Patients*

Factor	1 Negative	2 Disorganized	3 Psychotic
Avolition	0.82	0.16	0.01
Anhedonia	0.81	−0.01	0.01
Affective flattening	0.79	0.07	0.18
Alogia	0.73	0.46	0.00
Attentional deficit	0.72	0.21	0.16
Positive thought disorder	0.07	0.86	0.12
Bizarre behavior	0.22	0.70	−0.01
Delusions	−0.03	0.11	0.83
Hallucinations	0.22	−0.02	0.78

From Arndt S, Alliger RJ, Andreasen NC: The positive and negative symptom distinction: The failure of a two-dimensional model. Br J Psychiatry 158:317–322, 1991; used with permission.

positive thought disorder and bizarre behavior; this group probably represents a "disorganization factor." In addition, inappropriate affect also tends to cluster with these two symptoms. The other major factor, with high loadings on delusions on hallucinations, may be considered a psychoticism factor. An example of a factor analysis of positive and negative symptoms appears in Table 24-2.

A consensus is emerging that the symptoms of schizophrenia might be best simplified through a division into three broad groups rather than two. One group consists of negative symptoms, while the remaining two dimensions are psychoticism and disorganization. These three dimensions of schizophrenia may represent a more useful conceptualization of its subtypes as well, although considerable work must still be done in order to evaluate this possibility.

REFERENCES

Andreasen NC: The reliability and validity of proverb interpretation to assess mental states. Compr Psychiatry 18:465–472, 1977.

Andreasen NC: Scales for the Assessment of Thought, Language, and Communication. Iowa City, University of Iowa, 1979a.

Andreasen NC: The clinical assessment of thought, language, and communication disorders: I. The definition of terms and evaluation of their reliability. Arch Gen Psychiatry 36:1315–1321, 1979b.

Andreasen NC: The clinical assessment of thought, language, and communication disorders: II. Diagnostic significance. Arch Gen Psychiatry 36:1325–1330, 1979c.

Andreasen NC: Negative symptoms in schizophrenia: Definition and reliability. Arch Gen Psychiatry 39:784–788, 1982a.

Andreasen NC: Negative versus positive schizophrenia: Definition and validation. Arch Gen Psychiatry 39:789–794, 1982b.

Andreasen NC: The Scale for the Assessment of Negative Symptoms *(SANS).* Iowa City, University of Iowa, 1983.

Andreasen NC: The Scale for the Assessment of Positive Symptoms (SAPS). Iowa City, University of Iowa, 1984.

Andreasen NC: Brain imaging: Applications in psychiatry. Science 239:1381–1388, 1988.

Andreasen NC, Hoffmann RE, Grove WM: Mapping abnormalities in language and cognition. In Alpert M (ed): Controversies in Schizophrenia, 1985. New York, Guilford Press, 1984, pp 199–226.

Andreasen NC, Tsuang MT, Canter A: The significance of thought disorder in diagnostic evaluation. Compr Psychiatry 15: 27–34, 1974.

Andreasen NC, Rezai K, Alliger R, et al: Hypofrontality in neuroleptic-naive and chronic schizophrenic patients: Assessment with xenon-133 single photon emission computed tomography and the tower of london. Arch Gen Psychiatry (in press).

Andreasen NC, Grove WM: Thought, language, and communication in schizophrenia: Diagnostic and prognostic significance. Schizophrenia Bulletin 12:348–359, 1986.

Andreasen NC, Flaum M, Swayze, VW, Tyrrell G: Positive and negative symptoms in schizophrenia: A critical reappraisal. Arch Gen Psychiatry 47:615–621, 1990.

Arndt S, Alliger RJ, Andreasen NC: The positive and negative symptom distinction: The failure of a two-dimensional model. Br J Psychiatry 158:317–322, 1991.

Bilder RM, Mukherjee S, Rieder RO, Pandurangi AK: Symptomatic and neuropsychological components of defect states. Schizophr Bull 11:409–419, 1985.

Bleuler E: Dementia Praecox or the Group of Schizophrenias, trans. J Zinkin. New York, International Universities Press, 1950.

Buchsbaum MS: The frontal lobes, basal ganglia, and temporal lobes as sites for schizophrenia. Arch Gen Psychiatry 16:379–384, 1990.

Cameron N: Deterioration and regression in schizophrenic thinking. J Abnorm Soc Psychol 34:265–270, 1939.

Chapman J, McGhie A: A comparative study of disordered attention in schizophrenia. J Ment Sci 108:487–500, 1962.

Cromwell RL, Dokeckie PR: Schizophrenic language: A disattention interpretation. In Rosenberg S, Koplin JH (eds): Developments in Applied Psycholinguistic Research. New York, Macmillan, 1968.

Crow TJ: Positive and negative schizophrenic symptoms and the role of dopamine. Br J Psychiatry 137:383–386, 1980.

Fish FJ: Schizophrenia. Bristol, England, Bright, 1962.

Goldstein K: Methodological approach to the study of schizophrenic thought disorder. In Kasanin JS (ed): Language and Thought in Schizophrenia. Los Angeles, University of California Press, 1944.

Harrow N, Tucker GH, Alder D: Concrete and idiosyncratic thinking in acute schizophrenic patients. Arch Gen Psychiatry 12:443–450, 1965.

Holtzman PS: Smooth pursuit eye movements in psychopathology. Schizophr Bull 9:33–72, 1983.

Joyce J: Finnegan's Wake. New York, Viking Press, 1939.

Kasanin JS: The disturbance of conceptual thinking in schizophrenia. In Kasanin JS (ed): Language and Thought in Schizophrenia. Los Angeles, University of California Press, 1944.

Kraepelin E: Dementia Praecox and Paraphrenia, fascimile 1919 edition, RM Barclay, GM Robertson (trans). Huntington, NY, Robert E. Krieger, 1971.

Liddle PF: The symptoms of chronic schizophrenia: A re-examination of the positive–negative dichotomy. Br J Psychiatry 151:145–151, 1987.

Pardo JV, Pardo PJ, Janer KW, Raichle ME: The anterior cingulate cortex mediates processing selection in the Stroop attentional conflict paradigm. Proc Natl Acad Sci USA 90: 256–259, 1990.

Payne RW, Friedlander D: A short battery of simple tests for measuring overinclusive thinking. J Ment Sci 108:362–367, 1962.

Wynne LC, Singer NT: Thought disorder and family relations of schizophrenics. Arch Gen Psychiatry 12:187–221, 1965.

CHAPTER 25

Phenomenology of Coarse Brain Disease

ROBERT G. ROBINSON

Organic mental disorders are mental and/or behavioral disturbances that are presumed to be etiologically related to permanent or temporary dysfunction of the brain. In DSM-IIIR, a distinction is made between organic mental *syndromes* and organic mental *disorders*. If there is no presumed etiologic relationship between the mental symptoms and the known brain dysfunction, the abnormality is termed an *organic mental syndrome*.

Even when used in the more restricted sense (i.e., a presumed etiologic relationship between brain dysfunction and mental disorder), organic mental disorders include a wide range of mental disorders and brain dysfunctions. The most common organic mental disorders include dementia, delirium, substance-induced disorders, psychotic disorders, mood disorders, anxiety disorders, and personality syndromes. Thus organic mental disorders include virtually all the emotional syndromes, which are not usually associated with brain dysfunction, as well as cognitive disorders (e.g., delirium and dementia), which are almost always associated with course brain disease.

An indepth discussion of all these disorders would require a textbook itself and is clearly beyond the scope of this chapter. However, since organic mental disorders may be associated with transient brain dysfunction as well as permanent brain damage, this chapter will focus primarily on brain disorders in which there is demonstrable structural change. This will provide more uniformity of clinical manifestation as well as temporal course. Even this more limited definition of organic disorders, however, includes a wide range of neuropathologic conditions from stroke and traumatic brain injury to Parkinson's disease, Alzheimer's disease, Huntington's disease, and other, less commonly occurring neurologic disorders. Although this chapter might

have been organized based on these underlying neurologic conditions, it is more clinically useful to the psychiatrist to have it organized by mental disorders. Differences in clinical manifestation based on different neuropathologic conditions will be discussed under each mental disorder. The cognitive disorders of dementia and delirium will be discussed first, followed by mood disorders, psychotic disorders, and anxiety disorders.

DEMENTIA

Dementia is defined as a deterioration in intellectual function. It is distinguished from mental retardation, in which impaired intellectual ability has been lifelong and may or may not be caused by brain injury, and from aphasia or Korsakoff's disorder, in which specific cognitive skills (i.e., language and memory, respectively) are impaired without a significant impairment in other cognitive functions.

The diagnosis of dementia is based on clinical criteria. There are two essential features of the dementia syndrome. The first is global impairment of intellectual function. Although the impairment in each cognitive domain need not be uniformly severe, there is, nevertheless, an impairment in all or nearly all aspects of cognitive function. The second essential feature of the dementia syndrome is that the deterioration of intellectual function occurs in a state of clear consciousness. This differentiates dementia from delirium, in which there is a decrease in the level of consciousness and usually a fluctuating cognitive impairment.

A wide variety of pathologic processes affecting either cortical or subcortical brain structures can lead to an impairment of intellectual capacity. The location, extent, and nature of the pathologic process may influence the nature and severity of the dementia syndrome. The challenge for the clinician is, first, to recognize the dementia in its earliest stages of manifestation and, second, to identify the neuropathologic process producing it.

Since there are both reversible and irreversible causes of dementia, recognition of the mental syndrome of dementia should evoke a clinical challenge to evaluate the nature and cause of the dementia with the expectation that some forms of dementia will be treatable. Once the diagnosis is established, disease-specific treatment and management can be initiated as well as a prognostic forecast made.

Differential Diagnosis

DEGENERATIVE DISORDERS

Degenerative dementia of the Alzheimer's type (DAT) is the single most common cause of dementia in the elderly. DAT accounts for 20 to 35 percent of all cases of dementia and up to 50 percent of cases of progressive chronic dementia (Evans et al., 1989). The onset of DAT usually occurs after age 55, and the disorder becomes increasingly prevalent with advancing age. It is estimated that 20 percent of those over age 85 are afflicted with DAT. The diagnosis of Alzheimer's disease is divided into definite, probable, and possible cases (McKhann et al., 1988). A definite diagnosis is based on excluding other potential causes of intellectual deterioration as well as identifying a clinical syndrome and course that are consistent with DAT and having histologic evidence from autopsy or biopsy of the characteristic neuronal plaques and tangles of Alzheimer's disease. Probable Alzheimer's disease requires all the above except the histologic evidence. Studies have found that 65 to 90 percent of patients with a diagnosis of probable Alzheimer's disease will have it confirmed at autopsy (Risse et al., 1990).

Clinical features of DAT include memory loss, visuospatial impairment, impaired abstraction and calculation, alteration in personality, and intact motor system function. The aphasia syndrome associated with DAT usually includes fluent verbal output with poor comprehension, anomia, intact repetition, poor reading comprehension, and impaired writing. Visuospatial abnormalities are evidenced by disorientation and inability to copy designs. The memory impairment involves difficulty both in learning new material and in recalling previously learned information. Personality changes may include indifference and agitation and catastrophic reactions (i.e., uncontrolled emotional outbursts usually provoked by stress) in the later stages of the illness. Psychosis with delusions of spousal infidelity, theft, or paranoid ideas occur in up to half of patients at some time during their illness (Cummings et al., 1987). Speech, articulation, muscular tone, posture, gait, and coordination are generally intact until the terminal stages of the illness. The clinical syndrome of visuospatial abnormalities, flu-

ent aphasia, cognitive impairment, and preserved motor functions reflect disproportionate involvement of the medial, temporal, parietal, and frontal convexity regions (Breen and Gustafson, 1976).

VASCULAR DEMENTIA SYNDROMES

Stroke-related dementia accounts for as many as 35 percent of cases of severe dementia and is second only to DAT as a cause of chronic progressive intellectual deterioration (Tomlinson et al., 1970). This dementia, produced by multiple areas of ischemic injury, is characterized by abrupt onset and stepwise deterioration associated with each subsequent infarct. In addition to this characteristic stepwise course, multiple-infarct dementia is also associated with a fluctuating course, since partial recovery occurs over time, but subsequent strokes lead to further deterioration. Multiple-infarct dementia is also characterized by relative preservation of personality, depression, a history of hypertension, and focal neurologic signs on examination. The features of the dementia and severity of intellectual impairment depend on the location and volume of the infarcted tissue.

Multiple-infarct dementia can result from multiple subcortical infarctions (i.e., a lacunar state), multiple cortical infarctions (primarily large-vessel disease with extensive areas of cortical infarction), ischemic injury to the deep white matter of the hemispheres (i.e., Binswanger's disease), or mixed vascular pathologies. Cortical infarctions of the dominant (usually left) hemisphere produce dementias similar to that seen with DAT, including aphasia, apraxia, verbal amnesia, and right-sided motor and sensory impairment. Right hemisphere infarctions, on the other hand, are frequently associated with disturbances in facial recognition, visuospatial impairment, nonverbal amnesia, aprosodia, and left motor and sensory deficit.

OTHER CAUSES

There are a large number of conditions associated with dementia that cannot be fully enumerated here. These conditions include demyelinating disorders, such as multiple sclerosis; degenerative disorders with motor symptoms, such as Huntington's or Parkinson's disease; traumatic conditions, such as subdural hematoma; and neoplastic conditions, such as angioma or glioma. In addition, dementias also may be associated with other conditions, such as hydrocephalus, inflammatory conditions, infectious conditions, toxic disorders, metabolic disorders, or psychiatric disorders (Cummings, 1984). The psychiatric disorders associated with dementia are typically depression, but other psychiatric disorders from schizophrenia to personality disorder also have been associated with cognitive impairment (Caine, 1981).

DELIRIUM

The other cognitive disorder commonly associated with structural brain disease is delirium. Although delirium is not usually associated with chronic brain disease, it can occur particularly in the acute period following traumatic brain injury, stroke, or other neuropathologic conditions or in the chronic stage of such conditions as subdural hematoma or neoplasms. The most common cause of delirium, however, is transient metabolic abnormality caused by drug intoxication, brain edema, infection, or drug withdrawal. The characteristic feature of delirium is a fluctuating but decreased level of consciousness. The patient is unable to maintain attention to external stimuli or to shift attention to new stimuli. Thinking is disorganized, and speech is rambling or incoherent. Patients are usually significantly cognitively impaired with disorientation to time, place, or person. Their ability to register and remember objects is impaired as well as their ability to follow lengthy commands. Patients with delirium are easily distracted by stimuli, and they may have difficulty attending to a conversation or providing coherent or consistent responses to questions. Thinking is disorganized, as revealed by incoherent speech, difficulty maintaining a topic, and difficulty drawing conclusions or reasoning (Wolff and Curran, 1935).

Sensory perceptions are commonly distorted in a patient with delirium, including illusions, misinterpretations, and hallucinations. Visual hallucinations are the most common type of hallucination, although other forms of hallucinations also may occur.

The sleep–wake cycle and level of consciousness are virtually always disturbed. The level of consciousness may range from a barely detectable level of drowsiness through stupor or semicoma. Some patients with delirium, however, appear to have an increased level of attention and seem to be hypervigilant. Restlessness and hyperactivity occur in many patients with delirium, while other patients may appear sommulant and sluggish in their psychomotor activities.

The course of delirium usually is abrupt in onset, e.g., after a head injury. At other times, however, it may be insidious in onset, particularly when a slow change in metabolic state or a progressive drug intoxication is leading to the delirium. Fluctuation in the severity of symptoms is one of the characteristics of delirium. Typically, patients are worse during the night but will have lucid intervals in which they appear more coherent. The duration of delirium is usually brief, lasting for a few days, but delirium may continue for weeks or months. Delirium occurs more commonly in the youngest and oldest patients, suggesting that the brain may be more susceptible to metabolic and toxic influences during its early stages of development and after a significant loss of neurons has occurred during the normal aging process.

One of the classic descriptions of delirium was published by Wolff and Curran (1935). This study was the first empirical study of delirium. It analyzed 106 cases of delirium and described the frequency of various symptoms, including hallucinations, which occurred in 72 patients, all of which were visual in nature. Delusions of being murdered were reported by 18 patients, while 45 patients reported belief that there plots being made against them. Wolff and Curran also noted the characteristic features of variability in clinical presentation based on fluctuating level of consciousness, clouding of consciousness, and restlessness with marked cognitive impairment.

MOOD DISORDERS

Depression

Investigators who have utilized structured psychiatric interviews and established diagnostic criteria have usually identified two forms of depressive disorder associated with brain disease. One type is *major depression*, which has generally been defined by DSM-III or DSM-IIIR symptom criteria (excluding the criterion that precludes an organic factor). The second type of depression is *dysthymic depression*, as defined by DSM-III or DSM-IIIR criteria (excluding the 2-year duration criterion and the exclusionary organic factor criterion).

The prevalence of these depressions varies depending on the duration of the underlying illness as well as the nature and location of the brain disorder. In a study of 103 consecutive patients admitted to the hospital with acute cerebral vascular lesion, Robinson et al. (1983) reported that 27 percent met symptom criteria for major depression, while 20 percent met symptom criteria for dysthymic (minor) depression (termed *minor depression* because the 2-year duration criterion was not met). Most other studies of patients with cerebrovascular lesions have reported similar frequencies of depression ranging from 25 to 50 percent of the population studied (Sinyor et al., 1986; Eastwood et al., 1989).

Similarly, in a study of a consecutive series of 105 patients with Parkinson's disease attending an outpatient follow-up clinic, Starkstein et al. (1990a) found that 21 percent met diagnostic criteria for major depression and 20 percent for minor depression. The highest frequency of depression was found in both the early and late stages of Parkinson's disease. Recent studies in another coarse brain disease (i.e., traumatic brain injury) found similar results. Fedoroff et al. (1992) found that 26 percent of 66 patients admitted to the hospital with closed head injury without significant spinal cord or other organ system injury met diagnostic criteria for major depression. In addition, 3 percent met criteria for minor (dysthymic) depressive disorder.

Thus, although the clinical correlates of depression may vary from one type of brain injury to another, the frequency of major depressive disorder appears to be relatively stable across disorders occurring in about one-quarter of the population.

PHENOMENOLOGY AND DIAGNOSIS

The clinical presentation of depressive disorder in patients with coarse brain injury is an important issue in diagnosis. The phenomenology of depression may be modified by the existence of brain injury or by differences in etiology of brain injury. This issue was examined in a recent study by Fedoroff et al. (1991) that evaluated the phenomenology of major depressive disorder in patients with stroke, recent myocardial infarction, or spinal cord injury. Although the existence of typical features of major depressive disorder were found in all three groups (decreased mood, feelings of self-blame, decreased energy, difficulty with concentration, loss of appetite, sleep disturbance), patients with major depression following acute stroke ($n = 44$) were found to have a significantly higher frequency of generalized anxiety and ideas of reference symptoms compared with patients with major depression following acute myocardial infarction ($n = 25$) or patients with major depression following acute spinal cord injury ($n = 12$). Consistent with this finding, significantly more of the patients with stroke met diagnostic criteria for generalized anxiety disorder (36 percent) compared with the other two groups (12 and 8 percent). These findings suggest that some aspects of the clinical presentation of depression are different from one associated disorder to the next. This clinical variability may reflect etiologic differences in these depressions.

In another study examining patients with stroke, Lipsey et al. (1986) compared 43 patients with major depression following stroke and 43 age-matched patients with functional (i.e., no known brain pathology) major depression. Results indicated that both groups showed almost identical profiles of symptoms (including symptoms that were not part of the diagnostic criteria). Over 50 percent of patients who met diagnostic criteria for post-stroke major depression had symptoms of sadness, anxiety, tension, loss of interest and concentration, sleep disturbance with early morning awakening, loss of appetite with weight loss, difficulty concentrating and thinking, and thoughts of death. Thus, although the clinical manifestations of major depression need to be investigated for all brain diseases, the available evidence suggests that the symptoms may be similar, if not identical, to those found in patients without brain injury.

An issue closely related to the question of phenomenology is the issue of specificity of depressive symptoms in patients with brain injury. For example, symptoms that are used for the diagnosis of depression, such as sleep disturbance or appetite disturbance, may occur as a nonspecific consequence of hospitalization or a serious medical illness and, therefore, may not be appropriate as a diagnostic criteria for depression. This issue also was examined by Fedoroff and colleagues (1991). A consecutive series of 85 patients with stroke who acknowledged the presence of a depressed mood were compared with 120 patients without a depressed mood. Groups were comparable in background characteristics such as age, duration of illness, and lesion location and size. The study found that except for early morning awakening, all affective and vegetative symptoms of depression were significantly more frequent among patients with a depressed mood than in patients without depressed mood (Table 25-1). Moreover, the mean number of nonspecific symptoms of depression (i.e., "depressive" symptoms in the nondepressed group) was one vegetative and one psychological symptom. This may have led to false-positive diagnoses in 3 percent of patients. There were, in addition, 5 percent of patients who had the symptoms necessary for a diagnosis of major depression except that they denied feelings of sadness (i.e., possible false-negative cases). Thus the use of DSM-III criteria in an acutely medically ill population did not appear to produce significant numbers of either false-positive or false-negative cases.

Similar studies have been conducted in patients with Parkinson's disease and in patients with traumatic brain injury (Starkstein et al., 1990b; Jorge et al., 1993). In Parkinson's disease, slowness and early morning awakening were nonspecific for depression. In traumatic brain injury, anxious foreboding, early morning awakening, and loss of libido were not significantly different between the depressed and nondepressed patients. Thus symptoms which may be associated with the underlying brain disease, such as slowness in Parkinson's disease, can produce nonspecific symptoms of depression. Therefore, each organic brain disorder needs to be examined separately for which symptoms of depression are specific or nonspecific to that disorder. Symptoms such as early morning awakening were nonspecific in all the neurologic disorders examined. Despite these nonspecific symptoms, however, DSM-III diagnostic criteria for depression do identify a coherent group of patients with relatively small numbers of false-positive or false-negative cases.

DURATION

The duration of depressive disorders without treatment is an important area for determining prognosis in patients with brain disease. This is another issue that appears to vary depending on the nature and location of the underlying neuropathology. In a 2-year follow-up study of 103 acute stroke patients, Robinson et al. (1987) found that most patients with major depression in the hospital had spontaneously recovered by the time of the 1-year follow-up. Patients with minor depression, however, had a

TABLE 25-1. *Autonomic and Psychological Symptoms in Acute Stroke Patients With and Without Depressed Mood*

Symptom	With depressed mood (n = 85)		Without depressed mood (n = 120)		p*
	n	Percent	n	Percent	
Autonomic					
Anxiety	42	49	12	10	<0.001
Anxious foreboding	34	40	11	9	<0.001
Morning depression	48	56	9	8	<0.001
Weight loss	33	39	19	22	<0.01
Delayed sleep	37	44	25	21	<0.01
Subjective anergia	48	56	29	24	<0.001
Early awakening	28	33	22	18	N.S.
Loss of libido	35	41	12	10	<0.001
Psychological					
Worrying	59	69	83	23	<0.001
Brooding	36	42	8	7	<0.001
Loss of interest	22	26	5	4	<0.001
Hopelessness	41	48	16	13	<0.001
Suicidal plans	15	18	1	1	<0.001
Social withdrawal	31	36	10	8	<0.001
Self-depreciation	23	27	7	6	<0.001
Guilty ideas of reference	23	27	8	7	<0.01
Pathological guilt	20	24	10	8	<0.05
Irritability	34	40	13	11	<0.001

*Bonferroni corrected.

less favorable prognosis, since only 30 percent were nondepressed at the 2-year follow-up. In addition, approximately 30 percent of patients who were not depressed in the hospital became depressed at some time during the 2-year follow-up.

Morris et al. (1990) found similar results among a group of 99 patients evaluated in a stroke rehabilitation hospital and followed for 15 months. The duration of major depression was 40 weeks, while patients with minor depression had a mean duration of only 12 weeks. House et al. (1990) reported that 2 of 10 patients with major depression at 1 month after a stroke continued to have depression at 1-year follow-up. Thus, of the studies that have examined the duration of depression following stroke, there is general agreement that the natural course of the disorder is somewhat less than 1 year. This is approximately the same duration of major depression that has been reported for patients with functional depression (Rennie, 1942).

Follow-up studies of depressive disorders associated with other structural brain disorders have revealed somewhat different findings for duration of illness. In a 1-year follow-up of patients with Parkinson's disease and major depression, Starkstein and colleagues (1992) found that 10 of 18 patients with major depression at the initial evaluation continued to have this diagnosis at 1-year follow-up, while 8 were no longer depressed. In contrast, however, the mean duration of the major depressive disorder in patients with traumatic brain injury was less than 6 months. Patients with traumatic injury involving the left dorsolateral frontal cortex or left basal ganglia had a mean duration of depression of 1.5 months. The overall group of patients with traumatic brain injury and major depression, however, had a mean duration of depression of 4.5 months. Thus the duration of major depression following traumatic brain injury does not appear to be as long as that associated with either stroke or Parkinson's disease.

These differences in duration of depression may be related to the nature of the underlying neuropathology. Injury produced by head trauma may be less extensive and provoke more processes of regeneration and neuronal compensation than degenerative disorders or large ischemic lesions, which may lead to more permanent neurophysiologic changes and longer duration depressions. This issue, however, needs to be examined in each of the conditions where brain disease is associated with depressive disorder.

EDITORS' COMMENT

All these relationships between stroke and dementia, delirium, and depression and the course of each need to be considered in the context of the overwhelming evidence of the strong relationship between heavy alcohol consumption, hypertension, and stroke (Kozarevic D, et al: Lancet 613–616, 1980; Taylor JR, et al: Am J Psychiatry 142:116–118, 1985; Kornhuber HH, et al: Eur Arch Psychiatr Neurol Sci 234:357–362, 1985; Donahue RP, et al: JAMA 255:2311–2314, 1986; Gill JS, et al: N Engl J Med 315:1041–1046, 1986; Saunders JB: Br Med J 294:1045–1046, 1987; Puddey IB, et al: Lancet 647–651, 1987).

CLINICOPATHOLOGIC CORRELATIONS

A statistically significant relationship between lesion location and severity of depressive symptoms or depressive disorder has been reported by every

investigator who has examined depression following stroke. The earliest study that evaluated this
issue examined patients admitted to a hospital after
an acute first-episode stroke (Robinson et al.,
1984). This study found that 14 of 22 patients with
a left hemisphere injury but only 2 of 14 patients
with a right hemisphere lesion ($\chi^2 = 9.4$, $df = 1$,
$p < 0.01$) had either major or minor depression.
This study also found that the intrahemispheric lesion location was important by demonstrating that
6 of 10 patients with left anterior lesions had depression compared with 1 of 8 patients with left posterior lesions ($\chi^2 = 4.4$, $df = 1$, $p < 0.05$). Finally, and
perhaps most important, there was a significant
correlation between the distance of the anterior border of the lesion from the frontal pole and the severity of depression ($r = -0.9$, $p < 0.05$). Although
the association of depressive disorders with left
hemisphere lesions compared with right hemisphere lesions has been confirmed by some but not
all studies, all investigators have found a significant
correlation between proximity of the lesion to the
frontal pole and the severity of depression. Sinyor et
al. (1986) found a significant correlation between
severity of depression and proximity of either right
or left hemisphere lesion to the frontal pole ($r =
-0.47$, $p < 0.05$). More recent studies by Eastwood
et al. (1989) and Morris et al. (1992) found that
after controlling for family history of mood disorders, patients with single left hemisphere lesions
(but not with right hemisphere lesions) showed
significant ($r = -0.74$ and $r = -0.87$, respectively) correlations between distance of the lesion

from the frontal pole and the severity of depression.
House et al. (1990) reported similar correlations,
although less robust than the other investigators.
    In another recent study of 45 patients with
stroke lesions restricted to either cortical or subcortical structures in the left or right hemisphere,
Starkstein et al. (1987a) found significant correlations between proximity of the lesion to the left
frontal pole and the severity of depression for both
cortical and subcortical lesions (Fig. 25-1). This
study also found that 44 percent of patients with left
cortical lesions ($n = 16$) were depressed, while 39
percent of patients with left subcortical lesions ($n =
13$), 11 percent of patients with right cortical lesions
($n = 9$), and 14 percent of patients with right subcortical lesions ($n = 7$) were depressed. Thus, although the frequencies of depression between patients with left cortical versus left subcortical lesions
were not significantly different, patients who had
lesions in the left hemisphere had significantly
higher rates of depression than patients with right
hemisphere lesions regardless of the cortical or subcortical location (χ^2 Yates $= 4.0$, $df = 1$, $p < 0.05$).
When patients were further divided into those with
anterior lesions and those with posterior lesions, all
patients with left cortical lesions involving the frontal lobe had depression ($n = 5$) as compared with
2 of 11 patients with left posterior cortical lesions
($p < 0.01$). Moreover, in a subsequent study,
Starkstein et al. (1988) found that 7 of 8 patients
with left basal ganglia lesions had major depression
following stroke compared with 1 of 7 patients with
comparable lesions of the right hemisphere and

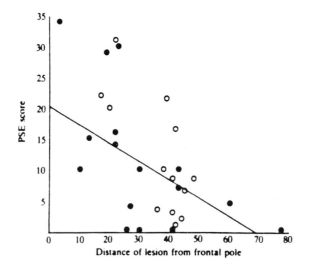

FIGURE 25-1.   *Relationship between PSE score and distance of the anterior border of the lesion from the frontal pole for
patients with either left hemisphere cortical lesions or left hemisphere subcortical lesions. The distance from the frontal pole is
expressed as a percentage of the total anteroposterior distance. The regression line on the graph is based on the overall patient
group. Filled circles = left cortical (*r* = −0.52); open circles = left subcortical (*r* = 0.68). Overall, *r* = 0.46.*

that none of the patients with left ($n = 6$) or right ($n = 4$) thalamic lesions had depressive disorder ($\chi^2 = 17.0$, $df = 3$, $p < 0.001$).

Although the issue of lesion location has not been studied extensively in patients with other brain disease, a recent study examined this issue in patients with traumatic brain injury. Nondepressed patients ($n = 41$) and patients with major depression ($n = 15$) who had abnormal CT scan findings following traumatic brain injury were compared for lesion location (Fedoroff et al., 1992). Using a logistic regression model, this study found a significant relationship between left dorsolateral or left basal ganglia and right parietal occipital lesions, lesion location, and the presence of major depression ($p = 0.0008$).

In summary, although the mechanism by which strategic lesions lead to the development of depressive disorder remains unknown, there appear to be similarities in clinicopathologic correlation among various forms of brain injury. Injury in the left dorsolateral frontal cortex and left basal ganglia are associated with the development of major depression. In addition, proximity of injury to frontal pole has been found in several studies to correlate significantly with the severity of depression.

RELATIONSHIP TO PHYSICAL AND COGNITIVE IMPAIRMENT

Although an empathic understanding of depression following brain injury would suggest that the severity of depression may have a relationship to the severity of the poststroke physical impairment, virtually all empirical studies have failed to show any more than a weak correlation between the severity of physical impairment and the severity of depression. The first investigators to examine this issue were Folstein et al. (1977), who compared 20 consecutively admitted stroke patients with 20 orthopedic patients. While the two groups were comparable in their severity of physical impairment, stroke patients had a significantly higher frequency of depression (45 versus 10 percent). This issue also was examined by Robinson et al. (1983), who found, in a consecutive series of 103 patients with acute stroke, that the correlation coefficient between Hamilton Depression Score and degree of impairment of activities of daily living was 0.37 ($p < 0.01$). Although this suggested a statistically significant relationship, the strength of the correlation suggested that severity of impairment would account for no more than 10 percent of the variance in severity of depression. Eastwood et al. (1989) examined 90 patients in a rehabilitation hospital following stroke. Results indicated a significant, although weak, correlation between severity of depression and severity of functional physical impairment. In another study of 99 patients in an Australian rehabilitation hospital following stroke, Morris et al. (1990) reported no statistically signifi-

cant difference between the activities of daily living scores of patients with and without depressive disorder.

Similar results were reported by Jorge et al. (1993), who examined the relationship between depression and activities of daily living (ADL) following traumatic brain injury. In hospital and at 3, 6, and 12 months of follow-up, 17 patients with major depressions were not significantly more impaired in their ADL than 47 nondepressed patients.

Although the nature of the relationship between severity of depression and severity of physical impairment may be construed as the physical impairment leading to depression, several recent studies have suggested that depression may influence physical impairment. For example, Parikh et al. (1990) compared recovery in ADL scores over a 2-year follow-up between 25 patients with poststroke major or minor depression and 38 nondepressed patients. Although both groups had similar impairments in ADL during the time they were hospitalized, the depressed patients had significantly less improvement by 2-year follow-up than the nondepressed patients ($p < 0.05$), even though the initially depressed patients had recovered from depression. This finding held true after controlling for important recovery variables such as the type and extent of in-hospital and rehabilitation treatment, the size and location of the lesion, the patient's demographic characteristics, the nature of the stroke, the occurrence of an intervening medical illness, recurrent stroke, and previous medical history.

In summary, the correlation between severity of depression and severity of physical impairment in patients with structural brain disease is weak. Physical impairment, however, may contribute to the development of depression, and if depression develops, it may have a significant effect on physical recovery. Moreover, the negative effect of depression on physical recovery may last even after the depression has subsided (i.e., the negative effect of depression on recovery lasts for at least 2 years, which is beyond the period of depression).

The relationship between severity of depression and severity of cognitive impairment also has been found to be relatively weak. As with physical impairment, however, although the severity of depression may be expected to reflect the level of intellectual impairment, several studies have suggested that depression may itself affect cognitive impairment. For example, Fogel and Sparadeo (1985) reported on a patient with severe depression following stroke associated with marked cognitive impairments. Both the depression and cognitive impairments, however, improved significantly after treatment with a tricyclic antidepressant. Robinson et al. (1986) reported that patients with major depression following left hemisphere cerebral infarction were significantly more impaired on the Mini-Mental State Examination (MMSE) (Folstein et al.,

1975) than a comparable group of nondepressed patients. Both the volume of the patients' strokes and their depression scores independently correlated with severity of cognitive impairment.

Starkstein et al. (1988) also examined this problem in a study comparing 13 pairs of patients matched for lesion size and location with one patient in each pair having major depression and the other having no mood disturbance. Ten of the 13 patients with major depression had lower (i.e., more impaired) MMSE scores than their matched controls. Two patients had the same score, and only 1 depressed patient had a higher score than his lesion-matched control ($\chi^2 = 14.7$, $df = 1$, $p < 0.001$). Thus, even when the effect of the lesion on cognitive impairment is controlled, depressed patients showed more cognitive impairment than nondepressed patients.

The relationship between cognitive impairment and depression also has been examined in patients with Parkinson's disease. Starkstein et al. (1989) examined 78 patients with Parkinson's disease who were attending an outpatient follow-up clinic. Patients with Parkinson's disease and major depression ($n = 15$) were compared with a group of nondepressed patients matched for age and stage of illness with Parkinson's disease ($n = 15$) using a neuropsychological battery. Major depressed patients were found to perform significantly worse on all neuropsychological tests, including the Wisconsin Card Sorting, Controlled Word Association, and Trial Making Tests. These results suggested that depression was associated with a significant cognitive impairment, particularly in tasks related to frontal lobe function. Mayeux et al. (1981) were the first to report a significant relationship between depression and intellectual impairment in patients with Parkinson's disease. Taylor et al. (1986), however, using neuropsychological instruments that assess short-term memory, found no significant differences between depressed and nondepressed Parkinson's disease patients who were matched for stage of illness. While these results showed no impairment in short-term memory related to depression, a structured psychiatric interview and diagnostic criteria for major depression were not used to determine the existence of depression. Patients were considered depressed if they scored above 7 on the Beck Depression Inventory. Thus the phenomenon of intellectual impairment related to depression may be a phenomenon of major depressive disorder. The findings of Starkstein et al. (1989) and Robinson et al. (1986) are consistent with this view, since patients with minor depression did not show intellectual impairment related to depression, as was found in patients with major depression.

In summary, the correlation between severity of depression and severity of cognitive impairment appears to be a weak, although a significant relationship exists in patients with structural brain disease. Intellectual impairment is related to both the size and location of the brain injury and the duration of Parkinson's disease, as well as to the existence of major depression. Anecdotal reports have demonstrated a significant improvement in neuropsychological function after treatment with tricyclic antidepressants. The effectiveness of antidepressant treatment on long-term recovery in cognitive deficits, however, has not been examined systematically.

TREATMENT

There have been relatively few studies that have examined the effectiveness of treatment of depression among patients with brain disease. There have been two randomized, double-blind treatment studies examining the efficacy of antidepressant treatment for depression following stroke. The first controlled treatment study was conducted by Lipsey et al. (1984), in which 39 patients who met diagnostic criteria for either major or minor depressive disorder were treated with nortriptyline or placebo. Eleven of the 17 active treatment patients completed the entire study. Of the 6 who did not complete the study, 3 experienced delirium, 1 had a syncopal episode, 1 complained of dizziness, and 1 complained of oversedation. Of the 22 patients receiving placebo, 15 completed the study; 1 noncompleted patient developed mania, 2 refused to be interviewed, 2 died (1 from a pulmonary embolism and 1 from a second stroke), and 2 were discharged from the hospital and lost to follow-up. Repeated-measure analysis of variance demonstrated that patients receiving nortriptyline showed a significantly greater improvement in depression, as measured by the Hamilton Depression Rating Scale (Fig. 25-2) and the Zung Self-Rating Depression Scale, than patients treated with placebo. Active and placebo groups, however, did not differ significantly in their mean Hamilton Depression Scores until weeks 4 and 6 of treatment.

The other double-blind treatment study of depression following stroke was conducted by Reding et al. (1986). In this study, 27 patients participating in a stroke rehabilitation program were randomly assigned to trazodone or placebo treatment. The major finding from this study was that patients who scored higher than 50 percent on the Zung Depression Scale ($n = 9$) or who had a "clinical diagnosis" of depression ($n = 8$) tended (though not statistically significantly) to have a greater improvement in their Barthel ADL scores when treated with trazodone than treated with placebo. When only patients with abnormal dexamethasone suppression tests (DST) were considered ($n = 16$), 7 patients treated with trazodone had a statistically significantly greater improvement in Barthel ADL scores than the 9 patients treated with placebo.

The effectiveness of tricyclic antidepressants in the treatment of depression in patients with Parkinson's disease has been demonstrated in several randomized, double-blind treatment studies (Strang,

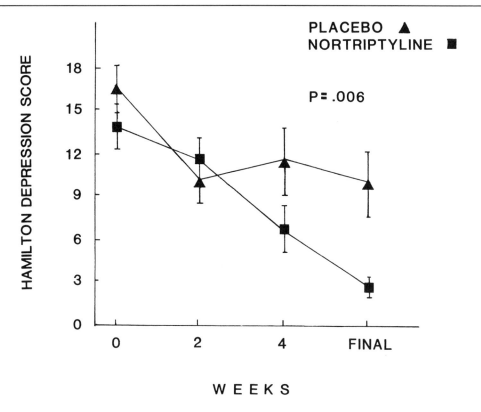

FIGURE 25-2.   *Hamilton Depression Scores during 6-week, double-blind treatment of poststroke depression with nortriptyline or placebo. p value is derived from repeated measures ANOVA. Bars indicate standard errors. The nortriptyline group had significantly lower Hamilton scores at weeks 4 and final compared with the placebo group.*

1965; Andersen et al., 1980). Thus far, there have been no double-blind treatment studies of depressive disorder following traumatic brain injury.

In summary, controlled treatment trials of depression in patients with stroke or Parkinson's disease have found significant improvement in depression associated with the use of antidepressant medications. Each treatment study, however, noted significant medication side effects in the active treatment group. Thus the selection of antidepressants and monitoring of their side effects require careful observation and management. None of the side effects, however, were irreversible, and there is at least anecdotal evidence that the use of antidepressants in patients with either stroke or Parkinson's disease may improve both their mood and their rate of recovery (or at least slow the rate of deterioration) in cognitive impairment.

Mania

Although mania occurs far less frequently than depression in patients with brain disease, mania is another mood disorder that may be associated with several neuropathologic conditions. Krauthammer

and Klerman (1978) reported several cases of mania which they referred to as "secondary" mania because they were associated with toxic, metabolic, or neurologic disorders. Although no epidemiologic studies have documented the incidence or prevalence of mania in patients with structural brain disease, Starkstein and Robinson (1992) reported that 3 of 300 consecutive patients examined with acute stroke had mania. Jorge et al. (1993) found that among 66 patients with acute traumatic brain injury, 6 patients met DSM-IIIR criteria for major affective disorder, manic episode. Thus, although additional systematic studies need to be conducted to determine the prevalence of mania following structural brain injury, the available evidence suggests that the frequency varies significantly depending on the nature of the underlying brain disorder.

Investigations of the relationship between lesion location and mania in patients with stroke have shown a consistent association between mania and right hemisphere lesion location. Cummings and Mendez (1984) reported 2 patients who developed mania following right thalamic strokes. Based on these cases and a review of the literature, they concluded that secondary mania is a disorder related to damage to the limbic areas of the right hemisphere.

Robinson et al. (1988) reported on 17 patients with secondary mania. All but 1 of these patients had a lesion involving the right hemisphere. Of the 9 patients with single stroke lesions, 8 had right hemisphere lesions and only 1 had a left hemisphere stroke. Lesions were found to involve either the orbital frontal cortex, the basal polar temporal cortex, the basal ganglia, or the thalamus. The frequency of right hemisphere lesions in patients with mania was significantly greater than that in patients with major depression following stroke or in patients with no mood disturbance ($p < 0.05$).

Analysis by Jorge et al. (in press) of 6 patients with mania following traumatic brain injury indicated a significant association between lesion location and the existence of mania. Logistic regression analysis demonstrated that basal polar temporal lesion location was significantly associated with secondary mania ($p = 0.0005$).

In order to examine why most patients with structural brain disease, even in the right temporal cortex, do not develop mania, Starkstein et al. (1987b) compared 11 patients with secondary mania with an equal number of patients without mood disorder who were matched for size, location, and etiology of brain lesion. Patients with secondary mania were found to have significantly more subcortical atrophy as measured by increased bifrontal and third ventricular to brain ratio than lesion-matched controls. In addition to this mild degree of subcortical atrophy (which probably preexisted the brain injury), genetic vulnerability also seemed to play a role in secondary mania. A family history of affective disorder was significantly more common among patients with poststroke mania (4 of 9) than among patients with post-stroke depression (3 of 31) ($p < 0.05$) (Robinson et al., 1988).

In summary, mania associated with structural brain disease appears to be clinically similar to mania not associated with known neuropathology (Starkstein et al., 1987b). Mania secondary to coarse brain disease, however, appears to be a consequence of injury to specific brain structures, particularly the right basal temporal cortex. There also appear to be risk factors for the development of mania which include subcortical atrophy, a family history of affective disorder, and the development of a seizure disorder (Shukla et al., 1987). These risk factors may explain why relatively small number of patients with right hemisphere lesions develop this mood disorder.

TREATMENT

Although there are no systematic studies examining the treatment of mania following brain injury, most of the cases of secondary mania reported in the literature were found to have a good response to the usual treatments with antimanic drugs (i.e., lithium and neuroleptics). Bakchine et al. (1989) carried out a double-blind, placebo-controlled study in a single patient with mania following brain injury. Clonidine (600 mg/day) (an alpha$_2$-adrenergic agonist used in the treatment of hypertension) rapidly reversed the manic symptoms, while carbamazepine (1200 mg/day) was associated with no mood change and levodopa (375 mg/day) produced an increase in manic symptoms. Shukla et al. (1987) reported that some patients with secondary mania may not respond to treatment with lithium (particularly those associated with a high frequency of seizure disorders). Successful treatments have been reported with anticonvulsant drugs, such as carbamazepine or valproate (Pope et al., 1988).

Bipolar Disorder

Among the group of patients with mania following brain injury, there is a subgroup which has a bipolar disorder. Among 19 patients with secondary mania, Starkstein et al. (1991) reported that 7 patients had a bipolar course, while the remaining 12 patients had a single episode or recurrent episodes of mania with no periods of depression. The follow-up period ranged from 6 months to 5 years. Although the "unipolar" mania and bipolar groups were not significantly different in background characteristics, handedness, personal or family history of psychiatric disorder, or neurologic findings, 6 of the 7 patients with bipolar disorder had subcortical lesions of the right hemisphere. In contrast, 10 of the 12 patients with mania had lesions of cortical regions ($p < 0.005$). All patients with bipolar disorder had depression prior to the onset of mania.

Although bipolar disorders have not been examined systematically in other brain diseases, the study by Jorge et al. (in press) of patients with mania following traumatic brain injury found that 1 patient of 6 had a bipolar course during the 1-year follow-up.

In summary, structural brain disease can lead to bipolar as well as unipolar mood disorders. Although the factors determining the nature of the mood disorder have not been studied extensively, bipolar disorder appears to be associated with subcortical lesions, while cortical lesions are associated with unipolar mania.

HALLUCINATORY AND DELUSIONAL DISORDERS

Historically, hallucinatory phenomena associated with brain disease are frequently related to sensory loss. Auditory hallucinations associated with deafness, for example, usually consist of simple words or phrases. Visual hallucinations following blindness are frequently visions of animals or faces that are not associated with delusions. These kinds of hallucinations have been reported with lesions of the midbrain, substantia nigra, subthalamic region, basal ganglia, thalamus, and limbic structures (Lanska et al., 1987). These kinds of hallucinations (sometimes termed *peduncular hallucinosis*) are usually recognized by the patient as being false perceptions (Starkstein et al., in press).

Psychotic disorders are not a common manifestation of coarse brain disease. Although the brain diseases usually associated with psychotic disorders are degenerative diseases (e.g., Alzheimer's disease and Parkinson's disease), these disorders also may be found in patients with focal brain lesions. Levine and Finkelstein (1982) reported on 8 patients who developed hallucinations with or without delusions following a cerebrovascular lesion. The most significant finding from this study was that all the patients had right hemisphere lesions involving partially or completely the temporal-parietal-occipital junction. In addition, 7 of the 8 patients had seizures following brain injury. Seizures preceded the onset of psychosis in 5 patients and followed the onset in the remaining 2. These psychotic episodes developed acutely and were present for days to months after brain injury.

Rabins et al. (1991) reported on 5 patients with hallucinations or delusions following stroke. All the patients had right hemisphere ischemic lesions. The 5 patients with delusions or hallucinations were then compared with a matched group of patients having the same size and location of stroke but without psychotic disorder. Although there were no significant differences between the psychotic and nonpsychotic patients in their background characteristics, personal or family history of psychiatric disorder, or neurologic examination, 3 of the 5 patients with secondary psychosis had developed seizures after the stroke lesions, while none of the nonpsychotic controls did. In addition, patients with psychotic symptoms had significantly more subcortical atrophy, as demonstrated by increased ventricular-to-brain ratios in the frontal horn and body of the lateral ventricle, as compared with the lesion-matched controls.

In summary, although the most common brain diseases associated with psychotic symptoms are degenerative brain diseases, such as Alzheimer's disease, studies of patients with focal brain injury and hallucinations or delusions have identified several factors that appear to play an important role in the development of these disorders. The first is a damage to the right hemisphere involving the temporal parietal occipital junction; the second is the presence of seizures some time after the brain lesion; and the third is the existence of subcortical atrophy in diencephalic brain regions. This subcortical atrophy probably preceded the brain injury and produced a "fertile" ground on which a brain lesion led to the development of hallucinations and delusions.

Treatment

There are two basic approaches that have been used in the treatment of secondary delusional or hallucinatory syndromes. One is the use of anticonvulsant therapies. This approach has its rationale in the frequent coexistence of seizure disorder with psychotic phenomena in patients with focal brain injury. In Levine and Finkelstein's series (1982), secondary psychotic symptoms did not usually respond to anticonvulsant treatment. Price and Mesulam (1985), on the other hand, reported a patient whose repeated psychotic episodes lasting from 1 day to 1 week were controlled with phenobarbital. The second approach to the treatment of hallucinations and delusions associated with brain injury is the use of neuroleptic medications. Although Levine and Finkelstein (1982) noted that some patients were resistant to neuroleptic medications, many of their patients showed significant improvement with neuroleptic medications. Unfortunately, there have been no systematically controlled studies of treatment of hallucinations and delusions in patients with focal brain disease.

ORGANIC ANXIETY DISORDERS

Anxiety disorders associated with brain injury have received relatively little attention in the medical literature. This situation is surprising because anxiety symptoms are so commonly found in patients with structural brain disease. In addition, studies of patients with functional (i.e., no known neuropathy) anxiety and depression have demonstrated that it is important to distinguish depression plus anxiety from depressions alone (Stravakaki and Vargo, 1986). Both the course and etiology of these disorders appear to be different (Stravakaki and Vargo, 1986).

Starkstein et al. (1990c) have recently examined a consecutive series of 98 patients with first-episode acute stroke lesions for the presence of both anxiety and depressive symptoms. The diagnosis of generalized anxiety disorder was based on the presence of anxious foreboding or excessive worry as well as motor tension, autonomic hyperactivity, vigilance, and scanning. Of the 98 patients with single stroke lesions, only 6 met the criteria for generalized anxiety disorder (GAD) in the absence of a mood disorder. On the other hand, 23 of the 47 patients with major depression met the criteria for GAD. The only clinical finding that distinguished the anxiety disorder (only) group from the depressed (only), depressed plus anxious, and no mood disorder groups was an increased frequency of alcohol abuse among the anxiety only group compared with the other three groups (4 of 6 patients versus 14 of 92 others; $p < 0.01$). Examination of patients with positive computed tomographic (CT) scans revealed that patients with anxiety plus depression had a significantly higher frequency of cortical lesions (16 of 19) compared with patients with major depression only (7 of 15) ($p < 0.02$) or with the no mood or anxiety disorder group (13 of 27) ($p < 0.02$). On the other hand, the major depression only group showed a significantly increased frequency of subcortical lesions (mainly involving the basal ganglia) (8 of 15) compared with the anxious depressed group (2 of 19) ($p < 0.01$).

Although anxiety disorder per se has not been examined in other groups of patients with structural brain disease, previous investigators have associated subcortical lesions with abulia, apathy, and indifference (i.e., nonanxious symptoms) (Graff-Radford et al., 1984), while lesions of the left frontal cortex have been associated with severe anxiety reactions (Gianotti, 1972).

There have been no systematic studies or even anecdotal reports of treatment of anxiety disorders in patients with structural brain disease. Price et al. (1992) suggested that anxiety symptoms associated with brain tumors should not be treated with neuroleptics unless psychotic features are present. Benzodiazepines are reported to be effective in treating anxiety and have the added benefit of possessing anticonvulsant properties. A potential problem with benzodiazepines is the increased likelihood of producing delirium. The potential for abuse of the benzodiazepines is another effect that needs to be monitored closely. Buspirone, which is free of these potentially negative effects, is an alternate to benzodiazepines as well as sedative tricyclic antidepressants (e.g., amitriptyline). These may be particularly useful if the anxiety disorder is accompanied by depression.

In summary, anxiety disorders are common following brain injury but are frequently accompanied by major depression. Anxiety disorder in the absence of depression is less common than anxiety disorder accompanying major depression. Studies examining patients with focal brain lesions have demonstrated that cortical lesions of the left hemisphere are associated with anxiety plus depression, while subcortical lesions of the left hemisphere are associated with depression and right hemisphere lesions are associated with anxiety alone (Castillo et al., 1993). Although there are no controlled treatment studies of anxiety disorder in patients with structural brain disorders, treatment with benzodiazepines or other anxiolytic agents appears to be effective.

SUMMARY

The psychiatric manifestations of structural brain disease include a wide range of mental disorders and a wide range of brain disorders. This chapter has focused on empirical studies that have examined the major psychiatric manifestations associated with structural brain disorders, such as stroke, traumatic injury, and Parkinson's disease. Cognitive disorders are the most common manifestation of brain injury and include both dementia, characterized by a global decline of intellectual function in the face of a normal level of consciousness, and delirium, in which the intellectual impairment is related to a fluctuating level of consciousness.

The most common emotional disorder associated with brain injury is depression. Major depression occurs in about 25 percent of patients with acute or chronic brain disease. The course of the disorder, however, depends on the type of depression (i.e., major versus minor depression) and the underlying neuropathology (e.g., traumatic brain injury produces shorter-duration depressions than stroke). Major depression has been associated with injury to strategic brain locations, such as the left dorsolateral frontal cortex or the left basal ganglia. Other factors, however, play a significant role in some of these depressive disorders, including a family history of psychiatric disorder, quality of social functioning, and the presence of subcortical atrophy before the brain injury.

Mania associated with brain injury appears to be phenomenologically similar to mania without structural brain disease. Secondary mania, however, is frequently a consequence of lesions of the right hemisphere involving either limbic cortical (i.e., orbitofrontal or basal polar temporal) or subcortical (i.e., basal ganglia or thalamus) regions. Bipolar disorder also may occur after coarse brain disease and has been shown to occur more frequently in patients with subcortical right hemisphere lesions than in patients with cortical lesions.

Delusions and hallucinations are a rare manifestation of focal brain disease. These disorders, however, occur more frequently with widespread degenerative disorders. They also may occur following lesions of the right parietal-temporal-occipital junction in patients with seizure disorder or in patients with a significant degree of subcortical atrophy.

Generalized anxiety disorder following structural brain disease occurs in approximately 50 percent of patients with major depression and in a significantly smaller percentage of patients without depressive disorder. Anxious depressions have been associated with left cortical brain injury and may respond to treatment with benzodiazepines or tricyclic antidepressants.

The investigation of psychiatric disorders associated with brain disease is in its early stages. Much empirical work needs to be done to detail the presentation, course, and response to treatment of psychiatric disorders associated with a wide variety of brain diseases. Each brain disease is likely to have differences in its associated psychiatric disorders. Furthermore, even in a single brain disease such as stroke and a single psychiatric disorder such as depression, there are likely to be multiple etiologies of depression.

One of the hopes in studying disorders where there is a known neuropathology is that investigation of the pathophysiology or biochemical consequences of these structural brain diseases will ultimately help to illuminate the mechanisms of the associated psychiatric disorder. This lesion method might, therefore, eventually lead to illumination of some of the mechanisms of these disorders in patients without structural brain disease and to treatment based on specific neurophysiologic abnormalities.

REFERENCES

Andersen J, Aabro E, Gulmann N, et al: Antidepressive treatment in Parkinson's disease. Acta Neurol Scand 62:210–219, 1980.

Bakchine S, Lacomblez L, Benoit N, et al: Manic-like state after orbitofrontal and right temporoparietal injury: Efficacy of clonidine. Neurology 39:777–781, 1989.

Breen A, Gustafson L: Distribution of cerebral degeneration in Alzheimer's disease. Arch Psychiatrie Nerv 223:15–33, 1976.

Caine ED: Pseudodementia. Arch Gen Psychiatry 38:1359–1364, 1981.

Castillo CS, Starkstein SE, Fedoroff JP, et al: Anxiety disorders following stroke. J Nerv Ment Dis 181:100–106, 1993.

Cummings J: Dementia: Definition, classification, and differential diagnoses. Psychiatr Ann 14:85–92, 1984.

Cummings JL, Mendez MF: Secondary mania with focal cerebrovascular lesions. Am J Psychiatry 141:1084–1087, 1984.

Cummings JL, Miller B, Hill MA, Neshkes R: Neuropsychiatric aspects of multi-infarct dementia and dementia of the Alzheimer's type. Arch Neurol 44:389–393, 1987.

Eastwood MR, Rifat SL, Nobbs H, Ruderman J: Mood disorder following cerebrovascular accident. Br J Psychiatry 154:195–200, 1989.

Evans DA, Funkenstein H, Albert MS, et al: Prevalence of Alzheimer's disease in a community population of older persons: Higher than previously reported. JAMA 262:2551–2556, 1989.

Fedoroff JP, Lipsey JR, Starkstein SE, et al: Phenomenological comparison of major depression following stroke, myocardial infarction or spinal cord lesion. J Affective Disord 22:83–89, 1991.

Fedoroff JP, Starkstein SE, Forrester AW, et al: Depression in patients with acute traumatic brain injury. Am J Psychiatry 149:918–923, 1992.

Fogel BS, Sparadeo FR: Focal cognitive deficits accentuated by depression. J Nerv Ment Dis 173:129–124, 1985.

Folstein MF, Folstein SE, McHugh PR: Mini-Mental State: A practical method for grading the cognitive state of patients for the clinician. J Psychiatr Res 12:189–298, 1975.

Folstein MF, Maiberger R, McHugh PR: Mood disorder as a specific complication of stroke. J Neurol Neurosurg Psychiatry 40:1018–1020, 1977.

Gainotti G: Emotional behavior and hemispheric side of the brain. Cortex 8:41–55, 1972.

Graff-Radford NR, Eslinger PJ, Damasio AR: Nonhemorrhagic infarction of the thalamus: Behavioral, anatomic, and physiologic correlates. Neurology 34:14–23, 1984.

House A, Dennis M, Mogridge L, et al: Mood disorders in the year after stroke. Br J Psychiatry 158:38–92, 1991.

House A, Dennis M, Warlow C, et al: Mood disorders after stroke and their relation to lesion location: A CT scan study. Brain 113:1113–1130, 1990.

Jorge RE, et al., Depression following traumatic brain injury; a one year longitudinal study. J Affective Dis 27:233–243, 1993.

Jorge RE, Robinson RG: Secondary mania following traumatic brain injury. Am J Psychiatry 150:916–921, 1993.

Jorge RE, Robinson RG, Arndt SV: Can a valid diagnosis of depression be made in patients with acute traumatic brain injury? J Nerv Ment Dis 181:91–99, 1993.

Krauthammer C, Klerman GL: Secondary mania: Manic symptoms associated with antecedent physical illness or drugs. Arch Gen Psychiatry 35:1333–1339, 1987.

Lanska DJ, Lanska MJ, Mendez MF: Brainstem auditory hallucinosis. Neurology 37:1685, 1987.

Levine DN, Finklestein S: Delayed psychosis after right temporoparietal stroke or trauma. Relation to epilepsy. Neurology 32:267–273, 1982.

Lipsey JR, Spencer WC, Rabins PV, Robinson RG: Phenomenological comparison of functional and poststroke depression. Am J Psychiatry 143:527–529, 1986.

Lipsey JR, Robinson RG, Pearlson GD, et al: Nortriptyline treatment of poststroke depression: A double-blind treatment trial. Lancet 1:297–300, 1984.

Mayeux R, Stern Y, Rosen J, Leventhal J: Depression, intellectual impairment, and Parkinson disease. Neurology 32:645–650, 1981.

McKhann G, Drackman D, Folstein MF, et al: Clinical diagnosis of Alzheimer's disease: Report of the NINCDS-ADRDA work group under the auspices of Department of Health and Human Services Task Force on Alzheimer's Disease. Neurology 34:939–944, 1984.

Morris PLP, Robinson RG, Raphael B: Prevalence and course of depressive disorders in hospitalized stroke patients. Int J Psychiatry Med 20:349–364, 1990.

Morris PLP, Robinson RG, Raphael B: Lesion location and depression in hospitalized stroke patients. Neuropsychiatry Neuropsychol Behav Neurol 3:75–82, 1992.

Parikh RM, Robinson RG, Lipsey JR, et al: The impact of poststroke depression on recovery in activities of daily living over two-year follow-up. Arch Neurol 47:785–789, 1990.

Pope HG, McElroy SL, Satlin A, et al: Head injury, bipolar disorder and response to valproate. Compr Psychiatry 29:34–38, 1988.

Price BH, Mesulam M: Psychiatric manifestations of right hemisphere infarctions. J Nerv Ment Dis 173:610–614, 1985.

Price TRP, Goetz KL, Lovell MR: Neuropsychiatric aspect of brain tumors. In Textbook of Neuropsychiatry, 2d ed. Washington, American Psychiatric Press, 1992.

Rabins PV, Starkstein SE, Robinson RG: Risk factors for developing atypical (schizophreniform) psychosis following stroke. J Neuropsychiatry Clin Neurosci 3:6–9, 1991.

Reding MJ, Orto LA, Winter SW: Antidepressant therapy after stroke: A double-blind trial. Arch Neurol 43:763–765, 1986.

Rennie TAC: Prognosis in manic-depressive psychoses. Am J Psychiatry 98:801–814, 1942.

Risse SC, Raskind MA, Nochlin D, et al: Neuropathological findings in patients with a clinical diagnoses of probable Alzheimer's disease. Am J Psychiatry 147:168–172, 1990.

Robinson RG, Bolduc P, Price TR: A two-year longitudinal study of poststroke depression: Diagnosis and outcome at one and two-year follow-up. Stroke 18:837–843, 1987.

Robinson RG, Boston JD, Starkstein SE, Price TR: Comparison of mania with depression following brain injury: Causal factors. Am J Psychiatry 145:172–178, 1988.

Robinson RG, Starr LB, Kubos KL, Price TR: A two-year longitudinal study of poststroke mood disorders: Findings during the initial evaluation. Stroke 14:736–744, 1983.

Robinson RG, Bolla-Wilson K, Kaplan E, et al: Depression influences intellectual impairment in stroke patients. Br J Psychiatry 148:541–547, 1986.

Robinson RG, Kubos KL, Starr LB, et al: Mood disorders in stroke patients: An importance of lesion location. Brain 197:81–93, 1984.

Sinyor D, Jacques P, Kaloupek DG: Poststroke depression and lesion location: An attempted replication. Brain 109:537–546, 1986.

Shukla S, Cook BL, Mukherjee S, et al: Mania following head trauma. Am J Psychiatry 144:93–96, 1987.

Starkstein SE, Robinson RG: Neuropsychiatric aspects of cerebral vascular disorders. In Textbook of Neuropsychiatry, 2d ed. Washington, American Psychiatric Press, 1992.

Starkstein SE, Robinson RG, Berthier ML: Poststroke hallucinatory delusional syndromes. J Neuropsychiatry Neuropsychol Behav Neurol (in press).

Starkstein SE, Robinson RG, Preziosi TJ: Depression in Parkinson's disease. J Nerv Ment Dis 178:27–31, 1990a.

Starkstein SE, Robinson RG, Berthier ML: Poststroke hallucinatory delusional syndromes. J Neuropsychiatry Neuropsychol Behav Neurol (in press).

Starkstein SE, Robinson RG, Preziosi TJ: Depression in Parkinson's disease. J Nerv Ment Dis 178:27–31, 1990a.

Starkstein SE, Robinson RG, Price TR: Comparison of cortical subcortical lesions in the production of poststroke mood disorders. Brain 110:1045–1059, 1987a.

Starkstein SE, Pearlson GD, Robinson RG: Mania after brain injury: A controlled study of etiological factors. Arch Neurol 44:1069–1073, 1987b.

Starkstein SE, Preziosi TJ, Forrester AW, Robinson RG: Specificity of affective and autonomic symptoms of depression in Parkinson's disease. J Neurol Neurosurg Psychiatry 53:869–873, 1990b.

Starkstein SE, Fedoroff JP, Berthier ML, Robinson RG: Manic depressive and pure manic states after brain lesions. Biol Psychiatry 29:149–158, 1991.

Starkstein SE, Cohen BS, Fedoroff P, et al: Relationship between anxiety disorders and depressive disorders in patients with cerebrovascular injury. Arch Gen Psychiatry 47:785–789, 1990c.

Starkstein SE, Mayberg HS, Leiguarda R, et al: A prospective longitudinal study of depression cognitive decline and physical impairments in patients with Parkinson's disease. J Neurol Neurosurg Psychiatr, 55:377–382, 1992.

Starkstein SE, Preziosi TJ, Berthier ML, et al: Depression and cognitive impairments in Parkinson's disease. Brain 112:1141–1153, 1989.

Starkstein SE, Robinson RG, Berthier ML, et al: Differential mood changes following basal ganglia versus thalamic lesions. Arch Neurol 45:727–730, 1988.

Strang RR: Imipramine in the treatment of Parkinsonism: A double-blind placebo study. Br Med J 2:33–34, 1965.

Stravakaki C, Vargo B: The relationship of anxiety and depression: A review of the literature. Br J Psychiatry 149:7–16, 1986.

Taylor AE, Saint-Cyr JA, Lang AE, Kenny FT: Parkinson's disease and depression: A critical re-evaluation. Brain 109:279–292, 1986.

Tomlinson BE, Blessed G, Roth M: Observations on the brains of demented old people. J Neurol Sci 11:205–242, 1970.

Wolff HG, Curran D: Nature of delirium and allied states. Arch Neurol Psychiatry 33:1175–1215, 1935.

CHAPTER 26

Motor Symptoms in Psychiatric Illnesses

KEITH L. ROGERS

The observation of motor behavior is an integral part of the psychiatric mental status examination, assuming an important role in both diagnosis and treatment. In diagnosis, for example, the finding of hyperactivity suggests that mania be included in the differential diagnosis. Motor behavior is important in treatment issues also. For example, stiffness in a patient on antipsychotics may indicate a need for alteration in the pharmacologic regimen. Not only do motor symptom clusters have an impact on diagnosis and treatment, motor behavior research also is widespread and overlaps anatomically and conceptually with other areas of neuroscience, e.g., cognitive research in the basal ganglia.

While classifying patients along axes of motor function has been used, as in the subgroup of catatonic schizophrenia, it is important to keep in mind that motor symptoms are nonspecific. Like most medical symptoms, they are not pathognomonic for any particular illness but rather signify a need for further investigation. This mistake was made when all patients exhibiting catatonia were assumed to have schizophrenia.

For this review, abnormal movements will be classified into idiopathic versus drug-induced categories, with the recognition that an individual can express both types. Conversely, many types of abnormal movements can fall into both categories. Parkinson's disease exists as an idiopathic syndrome, and parkinsonian-like movements are perhaps the most commonly seen side effect of antipsychotic drugs. The distinction of idiopathic versus iatrogenic is of great practical significance to the clinician who must often make the choice between investigating a "new" disorder or recognizing the need for alteration in the drug regimen. The designation *idiopathic* is not intended to exclude any etiology, especially genetic, but is used here to denote disorders that are not secondary to drug treatment.

IDIOPATHIC MOVEMENT ABNORMALITIES

The idiopathic movement abnormalities seen in disease states can be subdivided into those which are associated with primary psychiatric diseases such as schizophrenia and those motor diseases (e.g., Huntington's or Parkinson's disease) which manifest frequent psychiatric disturbances. The high rate of motor abnormalities in schizophrenia and the high rate of mental abnormalities in many "motor" diseases illustrate the artificial nature of our classification of illnesses into "psychiatric" and "neurologic." Nevertheless, the divergence persists, however artificial, and will be followed here for the sake of convention. When discussing these illnesses, the motor symptoms of the psychiatric illnesses and the mental symptoms of the motor illnesses will be emphasized because they may be the less familiar aspects to the psychiatrist.

Primary Psychiatric Diseases Exhibiting Movement Abnormalities

SCHIZOPHRENIA

Motor abnormalities are a current research focus in schizophrenia, as well as having been noted in the earliest descriptions of dementia praecox. Kraepelin noted echopraxia, catalepsy, negativism, and stupor in the catatonic subtype of dementia praecox but also noted choreiform movements and loss of coordination in hebephrenic and paranoid types (Kraeplin, 1971). Today, when motor symptoms predominate, the schizophrenia is subtyped *cata-*

tonic; when these symptoms are less obvious, then others such as thought disorder or paranoia have determined subtype assignment (DSM-IIIR).

The movement dysfunctions noted to occur in schizophrenia are varied and include generalized alterations in tone and coordination, neurologic "soft" signs, and neuro-ophthalmic abnormalities. The issue of idiopathic versus iatrogenic etiology is controversial, but schizophrenics exhibit greater than expected rates of all these abnormalities, probably regardless of prior drug treatment, although drug treatment may exacerbate or even precipitate the onset of the abnormal movements. This conclusion is based primarily on the observations of abnormal movements in schizophrenics in the preneuroleptic era.

Casey and Hansen (1984), in a review of spontaneous dyskinesia (i.e., non-neuroleptic-related), presented data from 24 studies involving 13,575 subjects. *Spontaneous (nontardive) dyskinesias* were defined as involuntary dystonic, athetoid, and/or choreiform movements of the face, trunk, or extremities. Spontaneous dyskinesia prevalence varied from 0 to 53 percent, with a weighted mean of 4.2 percent. However, Marsden et al. (1975) have claimed that true chorea or athetosis is rare in chronic psychiatric populations and, when found, is usually associated with neurologic disease (Mettler and Crandel, 1959).

Casey and Hansen (1984) excluded tremors, stereotypies (purposeless repetitive behaviors), and mannerisms (purposeful but odd behaviors) from spontaneous dyskinesia. The latter two types of movements are organized to a higher degree than, for example, choreiform movements and usually occur together. Stereotypies can vary from isolated ticlike movements to complex behaviors and can sometimes resemble orofacial dyskinesias with tongue protrusion, lip smacking, grimacing, and opening and closing of the eyes, for example. One can appreciate the difficulty of distinguishing between this and tardive or spontaneous dyskinesia. The lack of a uniform definition of terms, a familiar problem in psychiatric nosology, complicates the issue. There are few solid data upon which to base prevalence estimates for stereotypies and mannerisms, but Morrison (1973) reported that 26 and 14 percent of 250 catatonic schizophrenics exhibited stereotypies and mannerisms, respectively.

Neurologic "soft" signs (meaning nonlocalizing) also have been noted in schizophrenic populations with greater than expected frequency (Quitkin et al., 1976). Examples of such signs include clumsiness, articulatory imprecision, and poor performance of fine motor tasks. These signs, as well as the movements discussed above, are not generally found in all schizophrenics but may be more common in subsets of schizophrenics, e.g., those individuals suffering from more severe negative symptoms and increased ventricular/brain ratios on computed tomography (CT) (Andreasen and Olsen, 1982). However, King et al. (1991) found neurologic "soft" signs in 100 percent of examined chronic schizophrenic inpatients and found these to be associated with cognitive deficits, tardive dyskinesia, and severity of psychopathology, although *not* with ventricular/brain ratios.

A number of different extraocular movement abnormalities have been noted in schizophrenia. Staring is common in schizophrenia and is reminiscent of petite mal epilepsy, although the patient may be interrupted with no loss of memory or disorientation. Blink rates may be either increased, decreased, or occur in paroxysms in untreated schizophrenia (Stevens, 1978). Eye-tracking dysfunction in schizophrenia has been noted by many investigators (reviewed by Holzman, 1985). The disease specificity of this abnormality and its relationship to attention and drug treatment are not entirely clear. However, it seems that oculomotor disturbances occur frequently in schizophrenia, as do other types of motor symptoms.

From the preceding, one can readily appreciate the variety and frequency of motor disturbances in schizophrenia. Table 26-1 lists some of these observations, which are discussed in more detail in Manschreck (1986).

CATATONIA

It is acknowledged that catatonia is not a diagnostic entity. Catatonia is included as a separate category in this section to reinforce the idea that it is a nonspecific motor syndrome separate from any specific psychiatric illness. In other words, schizophrenia may occur with or without catatonia, bipolar illness may or may not present with catatonic symptoms, etc. Some of the typical clinical features of catatonia are presented in Table 26-2. In addition to exhibiting an association with psychiatric diseases, a catatonic presentation may occur secondary to focal central nervous system (CNS) lesions, intoxication, or metabolic derangements. Table 26-3 lists a variety of CNS and systemic dysfunctions that have been reported to exhibit catatonic signs and symptoms. It is important to remember that affective disorder (particularly bipolar affective disorder) is the psychiatric illness most likely to present with catatonia, and only 5 to 10 percent of catatonics have schizophrenia (Morrison, 1973; Abrams and Taylor, 1976; Taylor and Abrams, 1977). Catatonia,

TABLE 26-1. *Abnormal Movements Seen in Schizophrenia*

Location	Description
Head	Eyes open abnormally wide or squeezed shut, blinking, staring, grimacing, biting, chewing, tongue protrusion or licking, head nodding
Extremities	Picking, twisting, rubbing, tapping, stretching
Trunk	Shuffling, shrugging, rocking, hopping, turning

†Catatonic symptoms, listed in Table 26-2, are also seen in schizophrenia.
Adapted from Manschreck, 1986.

TABLE 26-2. *Typical Catatonic Motor Symptoms*

Symptoms	Description
Spontaneous	
Mutism	Verbally unresponsive
Stupor	Mutism with hypoactivity to the point of immobility; may be unresponsive to painful stimuli
Catalepsy	Prolonged maintenance of posture
Stereotypy	Non-goal-directed, repetitive actions; may be verbal or motor
Mannerisms	Goal-directed but odd, purposeful movements
Elicited by examination	
Echopraxia/echolalia	Copying of movements/speech
Waxy flexibility	Initial resistance to movement by the examiner, then catalepsy
Negativism	Failure to perform requested tasks; blends into akinesia and stupor if severe
Gegenhalten	A form of negativism; opposition of manipulation with force equal to that applied by the examiner
Automatic obedience	Obeying commands despite instructions not to; includes *mitgehen*—movement persists following light pressure

as a symptom of mania, generally predicts a good treatment response to lithium or electroconvulsive therapy (Abrams and Taylor, 1976). Other treatments for catatonia include benzodiazepines (Menza and Harris, 1989) and perhaps carbamazepine (Rankel and Rankel, 1988).

AFFECTIVE DISORDER

One of the hallmarks of the manic state is abnormal motor activity. Motor symptoms of hyperactivity,

TABLE 26-3. *Differential Diagnosis of Catatonia*

Central nervous system disorders
  Affective disorder (e.g., mania)
  Schizophrenia
  Dissociative states
  Basal ganglia disorders (e.g., globus pallidus lesions)
  Diencephalic disorders (e.g., third ventricle tumor/ hemorrhage, thalamic lesions)
  Limbic/temporal lobe disorders (e.g., encephalitis)
  Miscellaneous (e.g., frontal lobe tumors, tuberous sclerosis, Wernicke's encephalopathy, narcolepsy, postictal states)
Systemic disorders
  Ketoacidosis
  Hypercalcemia
  Systemic lupus erythematosus
  Acute intermittent porphyria
  Hepatic encephalopathy
  Homocystinuria
Pharmacologic/toxicologic
  Mescaline
  Phencyclidine
  Ethanol
  Amphetamine
  Aspirin overdose
  ACTH
  Antipsychotics
    Neuroleptic malignant syndrome and neuroleptic-induced catatonia

Data from Sours, 1962; Gelenberg, 1976; and Stoudemire, 1982.

pressured speech, distractability, and increased goal-directed activities are seen so commonly that they are included in DSM-IIIR as diagnositic criteria. As noted in the preceding section, catatonic symptoms are common in mania, and this diagnosis should be considered when such are noted. Corresponding to the low mood noted in depression, a generalized decrease in motor output is seen in association with this illness. Fatigue or loss of energy and psychomotor agitation or retardation appear in the diagnostic criteria. Monotonal speech with increased latency of response is noted frequently in depressives (Alpert, 1981).

EDITORS' COMMENT

Psychomotor retardation may be a hallmark of an endogenous depression, a depression that originates from bodily causes (Parker et al: Br J Psychiatry 157:55–65, 1990.)

ANXIETY DISORDERS

Patients with prominent anxiety may express tremors, rapid respiration, slight tachycardia, and brisk patellar and Achilles deep tendon reflexes (Cohen and White, 1949). A breathless, halting quality of speech also may be noted. Ritualistic motor behavior is prominent in obsessive-compulsive disorder, with repeated motor acts observed by the examiner or reported by the patient. Often the consequences of these sorts of behaviors are evident, such as the chapped, reddened hands of an individual with compulsive handwashing.

TIC DISORDERS

Motor tics alone (or vocal tics alone), such as Tourette syndrome (both motor and vocal tics), are often under some degree of voluntary control. Inhibition of the movements leads to a marked increase in the desire to move, with subsequent relief after the motor act. In this respect they are similar to compulsions and akathesia, although they are less complex and less "voluntary" than either. Tics are also exacerbated by stress. Tics usually begin in childhood in the facial musculature but may spread to other muscle groups. These are essentially motor psychiatric syndromes whose definition consists of motor symptoms alone, since there are no other psychopathologic or neuropathologic features. They may be primary idiopathic phenomenon or secondary to a variety of insults, including drugs (e.g., stimulants), other movement disorders (e.g., Huntington's disease, Wilson's disease), or the CNS lesions of stroke or multiple sclerosis.

ATTENTION DEFICIT HYPERACTIVITY DISORDER

As the name implies, hyperactivity, evidenced by difficulty in remaining seated, jumping or running inappropriately, and hypertalkativeness, is an integral part of this disorder.

Psychiatric Abnormalities Associated with Primary Movement Disorders

HUNTINGTON'S DISEASE

Presumably, degeneration of the caudate and putamen leads to the psychic as well as the motor disturbances seen in Huntington's disease. Dementia occurs in virtually every case of Huntington's chorea and may precede the appearance of the motor disturbance by years. Similarly, acute onset of psychiatric disturbance may herald the dementia (and the movement disorder). The mental abnormalities can take two forms, the first of these being an affective disturbance (either mania or depression) and the second being a delusional-hallucinatory state resembling acute schizophrenia (McHugh and Folstein, 1975). Dewhurst et al. (1970) found that a majority of Huntington's disease patients experienced affective disturbances at some time. Treatment for these types of secondary affective disturbances follows standard recommendations for the respective psychiatric illnesses.

PARKINSON'S DISEASE

The triad of bradykinesia (or akinesia), rigidity, and resting tremor is readily recognized as Parkinson's disease. However, before the triad is fully developed, low mood, lethargy, and anhedonia may suggest an affective disorder. Complicating the picture is the observation of high rates of depression in well-diagnosed Parkinson's disease patients—up to one-third may have an episode of depression (Celesia and Wanamaker, 1972). The depression may not resolve in the face of effective treatment of the motor disturbance, implying that the Parkinson's disease and the depression are not secondary to an identical pathophysiology, although their frequent co-occurence suggests some overlap in etiology (Mindham et al., 1976; Marsh and Markham, 1973).

Cognitive impairment occurs in a minority of patients with Parkinson's disease and may progress to dementia. Marttila and Rinne (1976) found that 29 percent of Parkinson's patients suffered dementia, with 20 percent of those being severely affected. Personality changes also have been noted in this population, typically an exaggeration of premorbid traits.

DYSTONIA

Idiopathic dystonia is a slow muscular contraction lasting seconds to hours of unknown etiology. These movements can be spontaneous or induced, e.g., "writers cramp." This induced dystonia has a gradual onset progressing from fatigue to difficulty holding the pen to complete inability to write. The temptation to attribute this disability to psychological conflicts is strong, but Sheehy and Marsden (1982) found no increase in psychiatric dysfunction in patients suffering this disorder. The finding that people are sometimes able to learn to write with the other hand and so carry on their work supports a nonpsychological etiology.

Meige's syndrome (blepharospasm–oromandibular dystonia) can be disabling, as can severe blepharospasm alone, due to functional blindness. Blepharospasm shows a good response to local botulinum toxin injection, whereas systemic treatments are generally ineffective (Elston, 1992). Torticollis is another focal dystonia in which the neck is pulled to one side by overactivity of the sternocleidomastoid muscle of the opposite side. This may occur as an independent symptom or may accompany other dystonias. Variants include retrocollis, involving the posterior cervical muscles, and anterocollis, involving both sternocleidomastoids.

Dystonia musculorum deformans, or torsion dystonia, occurs in both a hereditary and non-hereditary form, begins in childhood, and is progressive, affecting the limb and axial muscles. This gives a presentation of contorted postures, clumsiness, and dysarthric speech. These dystonias must be distinguished from tardive dyskinesia and chorea. No satisfactory treatments exist, but surgical lesions of the thalamus may be used as a last resort in torticollis and torsion dystonia.

WILSON'S DISEASE

Wilson's disease (hepatolenticular degeneration) is a rare, autosomal recessive inherited disorder involving abnormal copper metabolism. Varied psychiatric presentations are noted, including personality changes, affective disturbance, restricted affect, anxiety, and psychosis. Dementia is generally a late complication, but intellectual decline of a less severe nature is frequent. The neurologic manifestations are rigidity, tremor, spasticity, dysarthria, dysphagia, dystonia, and athetoid movements. Bearn (1972) has estimated that 40 percent of patients initially present with neurologic disturbance, 40 percent with hepatic abnormalities, and 20 percent with psychiatric symptoms.

The aim of treatment is to remove excess copper through the use of metal chelating agents such as penicillamine. The earlier treatment is initiated, the better is the response. Since the disorder is amenable to treatment and the presentation may be behavioral disturbance alone, this is an important illness to include in the psychiatric differential diagnosis and can be readily screened for by physical (e.g., Kayser-Fleischer corneal rings) and laboratory (e.g., decreased serum ceruloplasmin) examinations. Cartwright (1978) has shown that most patients with emotional disturbance secondary to Wilson's disease will have physical signs of the illness. It is an easy diagnosis to make if its presence is suspected. If it is missed, and psychopharmacologic treatment is initiated, then abnormal liver enzymes and extrapyramidal symptoms can be viewed as secondary phenomena preventing appropriate diagnosis and treatment.

PROGRESSIVE SUPRANUCLEAR PALSY (PSP)

Also called the *Steele-Richardson syndrome*, progressive supranuclear palsy is rare but may present as affective disturbance in the elderly. A subcortical dementia with profound latency of response and slowness of thinking is noted, along with gaze palsy (particularly in the vertical plane, for which the syndrome is named), rigidity, and pseudobulbar palsy.

Albert et al. (1974) noted an appearance of retarded depression or irritability/euphoria with rage outbursts in most patients with the syndrome. As noted earlier for Wilson's disease, thorough physical examination should lead the clinician to suspect PSP. Although treatment of PSP is not always satisfactory, levodopa may decrease the rigidity and gaze palsy. The treatment of the affective disorder is not clear at this time because of a lack of research in this area probably secondary to its rare occurrence.

SYDENHAM'S CHOREA

This disorder is a complication of rheumatic fever and largely affects children and adolescents. However, it may occur in adults for the first time, especially in the first half of pregnancy or following treatment with oral contraceptives. The choreiform movements may be accompanied by personality changes, anxiety, depression, or irritability/agitation/insomnia with hallucinations. This disorder is usually self-limiting and can be controlled with benzodiazepines and barbiturates. Retrospective study of children who had Syndenham's chorea shows an association with psychological stress prior to the chorea, with low achievement subsequently and personality disorder as adults (Freeman et al., 1965).

MYASTHENIA GRAVIS

Early in the course of the disorder, before obvious paresis is noted, these patients may be referred for psychiatric evaluation. A fluctuating course of weakness, blurred vision, labored breathing, and dysphagia is noted and may appear as part of a depressive episode or somatization disorder. The finding of progressive weakness of the involved muscles with improvement in strength following rest usually leads to the correct diagnosis. An increase in strength following anticholinergics is diagnostic, but these must sometimes be administered blindly to the patient when functional causes are suspected.

PERIODIC PARALYSIS

Recognition of this disorder is important for the psychiatrist because hypochondriasis might be suspected in a patient presenting with gradual onset of weakness occurring at rest. Neurologic examination may be normal or show decreased deep tendon reflexes and hypotonia. A family history positive for the disorder can be helpful, as is a history of vigorous exercise or heavy eating just prior to the onset of weakness. Treatment consists of careful monitoring of potassium intake, which has been linked to this inherited disorder (Adams and Victor, 1985).

IDIOPATHIC BASAL GANGLIA CALCIFICATION

Idiopathic basal ganglia calcification (sometimes called *Fahr's disease*) is probably most often noted as an incidental finding on CT scan, occurring in 0.3 to 0.6 percent of patients (Harrington et al., 1981). However, pathologic variants secondary to hypo- or hyperparathyroidism exist, as well as a familial variety that can masquerade as late-onset schizophrenia in the third or fourth decade. A parkinsonian syndrome with dysarthria is common, with seizures and ataxia noted less frequently. Eventually, the pathologic variety of the calcification progresses to a subcortical dementia with prominent motor symptoms. An awareness of the asymptomatic nature of basal ganglia calcification is important, but screening for parathyroid abnormalities is warranted. Imaging for basal ganglia calcification is indicated when treating a levodopa-resistant Parkinson's patient.

Psychiatric and Motoric Abnormalities Associated with Focal Lesions of the CNS

Dysfunction in the frontal or parietal lobe frequently leads to motoric as well as cognitive disturbances. Patients with lesions, sometimes unsuspected, in these areas can present to the psychiatrist for evaluation of behavioral problems. The physical examination may reveal motor findings that aid in diagnosis and indicate a need for further testing, usually an imaging procedure coupled with psychological testing to quantify the behavioral deficit.

Frontal lobe pathology due to trauma, tumors, infections, or vascular accident can have profound behavioral consequences. Disorders of personality include irritability with lowered inhibitions manifested by inappropriate lewd or erotic behavior. A "silly" attitude with apparent euphoria not consistent with the patient's reported inner mood can be seen. This appears as mania at times but usually exhibits a fluctuating course, occasionally alternating with periods of depressed mood (Hecaen and Albert, 1975).

A generalized decrease in motor output is common in frontal lobe disease, with impaired activities of daily living due to apathy rather than paralysis or confusion. So-called frontal release signs are evident, including the grasp, snout, and sucking reflexes. Bradykinesia, negativism, waxy flexibility, and abnormal gait and posture have been noted (Damasio, 1979). The similarity to catatonic states is obvious, and given the frequency of catatonia in manic states, frontal lobe disease is important to keep in mind when examining such a patient. The role of CNS lesions in affective disorder has been studied by Robinson et al. (1984), who have reported an association between severity of depression and a left anterior stroke location.

Parietal lobe pathology leads to subtle, but demonstrable, abnormalities in motor function. Sensory deficits, mild hemiparesis, neglect, and various types of dyspraxias are noted following parietal lesions. Gerstmann syndrome (right–left confusion, digital agnosia, agraphia, and acalculia), alexia, and astereognosis are associated with dominant parietal lobe lesions, while anosognosia and dressing apraxia are noted following lesions of the nondominant parietal lobe. These deficits reflect the parietal lobes' function in integrating somatosensory, visual, and auditory input into an awareness of the body in relation to outside space.

DRUG-INDUCED MOVEMENT ABNORMALITIES

Not only do antipsychotics exhibit prominent motoric side effects acutely and following chronic exposure, but monoamine oxidase inhibitors (MAOIs), tricyclic antidepressants, lithium, and benzodiazepines may cause motoric side effects. The antidepressants induce a fine resting tremor in a small percentage of patients, and lithium has been reported to induce tremor in one-half of patients on prophylactic doses (Vestergaard et al., 1980). Lithium also has been reported to produce rigidity and other parkinsonian symptoms similar to antipsychotics (Kane et al., 1978) and has been noted to reinduce tardive dyskinesia (Beitman, 1978). Course tremors, ataxia, myoclonus, and seizures can result from toxic levels of these agents. Benzodiazepines can induce mild ataxia and dysarthria in clinical doses, with profound effects at toxic doses. Despite these effects, by far the most frequent causes of motoric side effects are the antipsychotic drugs, with the exception of clozapine, and they will be the chief focus for the rest of this section. Drug-induced motor side effects are reviewed in Weiner and Lang (1989).

DYSTONIC REACTIONS

Drug-induced dystonia is identical in presentation to the idiopathic dystonias discussed earlier and can affect any voluntary muscle, although muscles of the head, face, and neck are involved most commonly. They occur within days of initiating or increasing the dosage of antipsychotic drugs and respond rapidly (within minutes) to intravenous anticholinergics. Young (<40 years) men are at greatest risk from this side effect, although the disorder can be seen in any patient on antipsychotics.

AKATHESIA

Akathesia is a subjective sensation of motor restlessness. The onset of this disturbance is within weeks of starting the antipsychotic and usually resolves within a week of stopping the drug. While anticholinergics are frequently prescribed for treatment of akathesia, they are less effective than they are for dystonia or parkinsonian symptoms. Benzodiazepines (primarily diazepam) and beta-adrenergic blockers (primarily propanolol) are employed occasionally to treat akathesia, usually after anticholinergics have been shown to be ineffective.

PARKINSONISM

Also called pseudoparkinsonism to distinguish it from idiopathic Parkinson's disease, this side effect is dose-related, increases with age, and generally has an onset within the first month of treatment. All the features of idiopathic Parkinson's disease may be present, with bradykinesia, rigidity, tremor, and gait and postural disturbances singly or in combination. However, Marsden et al. (1975) have noted important differences between drug-induced and idiopathic or postencephalitic Parkinson's symptoms. For example, these authors report that the drug-related symptoms are usually more symmetrical and are more likely to produce high-frequency postural or action tremors. These symptoms may subside with continued treatment as tolerance develops and are reversible following discontinuation of the offending agent. Caution must be exercised, however, since there is considerable variation in the presentation of all types of parkinsonian symptoms. Marsden and Jenner (1980) have suggested that susceptible individuals are predisposed to this side effect in a manner similar to a predisposition to idiopathic Parkinson's disease. This may account for the occasional persistence of drug-induced parkinsonism following drug discontinuation. Anticholinergic (or amantadine) therapy usually results in improvement in parkinsonian symptoms.

TARDIVE DYSKINESIA

This hyperkinetic involuntary movement syndrome affects primarily the mouth, lips, and tongue, but it can involve the extremities or trunk, producing choreiform or athetoid movements. Onset is after months to years of treatment and is often manifest following drug dosage reduction or discontinuation. This late-occurring dyskinesia is persistent and occasionally irreversible. Other than drug discontinuation, there is no effective treatment. Anticholinergic treatment may exacerbate tardive dyskinesia, although this is controversial, and may be a risk factor for the development of the disorder. However, the risk factor may actually be associated with the early manifestation of a need for anticholinergics, i.e., early severe parkinsonian side effects. Baclofen, benzodiazepines (especially clonazepam), and α-tocopherol have been reported to be effective in some patients, although none of these agents has been demonstrated consistently to be of benefit. Duration of treatment, female sex, and old age have been associated with the disorder.

NEUROLEPTIC MALIGNANT SYNDROME

Muscular rigidity, altered consciousness, hyperthermia, and autonomic dysfunction constitute this syndrome that has an onset either acutely or following chronic treatment with antipsychotics. Laboratory abnormalities include leukocytosis, elevated level of creatine phosphokinase, and electrolyte disturbances. Dantrolene, amantadine, and bromocriptine are clearly beneficial, and levodopa, electroconvulsive therapy, anticholinergics, and benzodiazepines may be of benefit in this disorder, although their use is less well defined (Addonizio and Susman, 1991).

CONCLUSIONS

The observation of motoric behavior is a critical part of the mental status examination, and if abnormalities are noted, the differential diagnosis is broad and follow-up examinations and studies may be indicated. Given the somewhat bizarre appearance of some movement disorders, it is not surprising that such patients are sometimes referred to psychiatrists for evaluation. Even in situations where the motor disorder diagnosis is clear, behavioral sequelae may necessitate psychiatric intervention. The psychiatric physician must be aware of the wide variety of abnormal movements seen in primary psychiatric illnesses and as side effects to psychotropic drugs. Furthermore, knowledge of the behavioral manifestations of primary motor disorders is essential for accurate psychiatric diagnosis and treatment. These reasons make understanding motor behavior important to the clinician. The frequent concurrence of motor and cognitive symptoms suggests common pathophysiologic processes at work. Research studies of subcortical "motor" structures are among the most encouraging for understanding the pathophysiology of mental illness.

REFERENCES

Abrams R, Taylor MA: Catatonia, a prospective clinical study. Arch Gen Psychiatry 33:579–581, 1976.

Adams RD, Victor M: Myasthenia gravis and episodic forms of muscular weakness. In Principles of Neurology, 3d ed. New York, McGraw-Hill, 1985, pp 1074–1089.

Addonizio G, Susman VL: Neuroleptic Malignant Syndrome: A Clinical Approach. St. Louis, Mosby–Year Book, 1991.

Alpert M: Speech and disturbances of affect. In Darby JK (ed): Speech Evaluation in Psychiatry. New York, Grune & Stratton, 1981, pp 359–367.

Albert ML, Feldman RG, Willis AL: The "subcortical dementia" of progressive supranuclear palsy. J Neurol Neurosurg Psychiatry 37:121–130, 1974.

Andreasen NC, Olson S: Negative versus positive schizophrenia. Arch Gen Psychiatry 39:789–794, 1982.

Bearn AG: Wilson's disease. In Stanbury JB, Wyngaarden JB, Fredrickson DS (eds): The Metabolic Basis of Inherited Disease, 3d ed. New York, McGraw-Hill, 1972.

Beitman BD: Tardive dyskinesia reinduced by lithium carbonate. Am J Psychiatry 135:1229–1230, 1978.

Cartwright GE: Diagnosis of treatable Wilson's disease. N Engl J Med 298:1347–1350, 1978.

Casey DE, Hansen TE: Spontaneous dyskinesias. In Jeste DW, Wyatt RJ (eds): Neuropsychiatric Movement Disorders. Washington, American Psychiatric Press, 1984, pp 68–95.

Celesia GG, Wanamaker WM: Psychiatric disturbances in parkinson's disease. Dis Nerv Syst 33:577–583, 1972.

Cohen ME, White PD: Life situations, emotions and neurocirculatory asthenia (anxiety neurosis, neuroasthenia, effort syndrome). Assoc Res Nerv Ment Dis Proc 29:832–869, 1949.

Damasio A: The frontal lobes. In Heilman KM, Valenstein E (eds): Clinical Neuropsychology. New York, Oxford University Press, 1979, pp 360–412.

Dewhurst K, Oliver JE, McKnight AL: Socio-psychiatric consequences of Huntington's disease. Br J Psychiatry 16:255–258, 1970.

Elston JS: The management of blepharospasm and hemifacial spasm. J Neurol 239:5–8, 1992.

Freeman JM, Aron AM, Collard JE, MacKay MC: The emotional correlates of Sydenham's chorea. Pediatrics 35:42–49, 1965.

Gelenberg AJ: The catatonic syndrome. Lancet 1:1339–1341, 1976.

Harrington MG, Macpherson P, Macintosh WB, et al: The significance of the incidental finding of basal ganglia calcification on computed tomography. J Neurol Neurosurg Psychiatry 44:1168–1170, 1981.

Hecaen H, Albert ML: Disorders of mental functioning related to frontal lobe pathology. In Benson DF, Blumer D (eds): Psychiatric Aspects of Neurological Disease. New York, Grune & Stratton, 1975, pp 137–149.

Holzman PS: Eye movement dysfunctions and psychosis. Int Rev Neurobiol 27:179–205, 1985.

Kane J, Rifkin A, Quitkin F, Klein DF: Extrapyramidal side effects with lithium treatment. Am J Psychiatry 135:851–853, 1978.

King DJ, Wilson A, Cooper SJ, Waddington JL: The clinical correlates of neurological soft signs in chronic schizophrenia. Br J Psychiatry 158:770–775, 1991.

Kraeplin E: Dementia praecox and paraphrenia, RM Barclay, GM Robertson (trans). Huntington, NY, Robert E. Krieger, 1971.

Manschreck TC: Motor abnormalities in schizophrenia. In Nasrallah HA, Weinberger DR (eds): The Neurology of Schizophrenia, vol 1. Amsterdam, Elsevier, 1986, pp 65–96.

Marsden CD, Jenner P: The pathophysiology of extrapyramidal side effects of neuroleptic drugs. Psychol Med 10:55–72, 1980.

Marsden CD, Tarsy D, Baldessarini RJ: Spontaneous and drug-induced movement disorders in psychotic patients. In Benson DF, Blumer D (eds): Psychiatric Aspects of Neurological Disease. New York, Grune & Stratton, 1975, pp 219–265.

Marsh GG, Markham CH: Does levodopa alter depression and psychopathology in parkinsonian patients? J Neurol Neurosurg Psychiatry 36:925–935, 1973.

Marttila RJ, Rinne UK: Dementia in Parkinson's disease. Acta Neurol Scand 54:431–441, 1976.

McHugh PR, Folstein MF: Psychiatric syndromes of Huntington's chorea: A clinical and phenomenologic study. In Bensen DF,

Blumer D (eds): Psychiatric Aspects of Neurological Disease. New York, Grune & Stratton, 1975, pp 267–286.

Menza MA, Harris D: Benzodiazepines and catatonia: An overview. Biol Psychiatry 26:842–846, 1989.

Mettler FA, Crandell A: Neurologic disorders in psychiatric institutions. J Nerv Ment Dis 128:148–159, 1959.

Mindham RHS, Marsden CD, Parkes JD: Psychiatric symptoms during L-dopa therapy for Parkinson's disease and their relationship to physical disability. Psychol Med 6:23–33, 1976.

Morrison JR: Catatonia, retarded and excited types. Arch Gen Psychiatry 28:39–41, 1973.

Quitkin F, Rifkin A, Klein DF: Neurologic soft signs in schizophrenia and character disorders. Arch Gen Psychiatry 33:845–853, 1976.

Rankel HW, Rankel LE: Carbamazepine in the treatment of catatonia. Am J Psychiatry 145:361–362, 1988.

Robinson RG, Kubos KL, Starr LB, et al: Mood disorders in stroke patients. Brain 107:81–93, 1984.

Sheehy MP, Marsden CD: Writer's cramp: A focal dystonia. Brain 105:461–480, 1982.

Sours JA: Akinetic mutism simulating catatonic schizophrenia. Am J Psychiatry 119:451–455, 1962.

Stevens JR: Disturbances of ocular movement and blinking in schizophrenia. J Neurol Neurosurg Psychiatry 40:1024–1031, 1978.

Stoudemire A: The differential diagnosis of catatonic states. Psychosomatics 23:245–251, 1982.

Taylor MA, Abrams R: Catatonia, prevalence and importance in the manic phase of manic-depressive illness. Arch Gen Psychiatry 34:1223–1225, 1977.

Vestergaard P, Amdisen A, Schou M: Clinically significant side effects of lithium treatment. Acta Psychiatr Scand 62:193–200, 1980.

Weiner WJ, Lang AE: Drug-induced movement disorders (not including tardive dyskinesia) and tardive dyskinesia. In Movement Disorders: A Comprehensive Survey. Mount Kisco, NY, Futura, 1989, pp 599–684.

CHAPTER 27

Personality Disorders

BRUCE PFOHL

DEFINITION

Personality traits are defined in the *Diagnostic and Statistical Manual of Mental Disorders*, third edition revised (DSM-IIIR), as "enduring patterns of perceiving, relating to, and thinking about the environment and oneself . . . [which] . . . are exhibited in a wide range of important social and personal contexts" (American Psychiatric Association, 1987). A personality disorder (PD) exists when personality traits form a syndrome that results in distress or disability. While this chapter will follow the DSM-IV convention of referring to *personality disorder* as a category that is present or absent, the clinician should recognize that problematic personality traits cover a wide range of severity, and the threshold for defining disorder is necessarily arbitrary.

DSM-IIIR codes personality disorders on Axis II of a multiaxial diagnostic system. Axis I includes the majority of clinical psychiatric syndromes. DSM-IIIR states, "The disorders listed in Axis II, Developmental Disorders and Personality Disorders, generally begin in childhood or adolescence and persist in a stable form (without periods of remission or exacerbation) into adult life. With only a few exceptions (e.g., the gender identity disorders and paraphilias), these features are not characteristic of the Axis I disorders." The distinction is more blurred than this statement suggests, since other disorders with an early onset may be no less stable (e.g., somatization disorder, social phobia, and obsessive-compulsive disorder), and many Axis II disorders show considerable instability of diagnosis and symptomatology over time (McGlashan, 1983; Paris, 1987; Karterud et al., 1992).

While the conceptual clarity of Axis II can be challenged, it is important to note those things which are not inherent in the definition of personality disorder. There is no assumption in the DSM system that Axis II disorders in general or personality disorders in particular are less likely than the Axis I disorders to be etiologically related to a variety of biologic and psychosocial risk factors. Nothing in the definition of Axis II precludes the possibility that a given personality disorder might be genetically related to one or more Axis I disorders, nor does it preclude the possibility that medications and psychotherapy may have a positive impact on personality traits or disorders.

To the extent that personality disorders can be demonstrated to significantly affect the implications of Axis I diagnoses, placement on a separate axis is conceptually meaningful. For example, a group of patients with major depression will differ considerably in course, response to treatment, compliance with treatment, and the way they interact with the clinician and others. If these individual differences relate to patterns of behavior that are consistent over time even when an Axis I disorder is not active, then, by definition, clinically significant personality traits are present.

CATEGORICAL PERSONALITY DIAGNOSIS

Personality theorists disagree about whether the series of discrete personality types described in DSM-III and DSM-IV represent the best approach to describing personality variables. Before considering some of these controversies, it is useful to review the types of prototypic personality types defined by the current Axis II criteria and how individuals who meet the criteria for these disorders typically present in a clinical setting.

DSM-III first described operational criteria for 11 personality disorders organized into three main clusters. The clusters are heuristically useful in thinking about and remembering the disorders; however, it is difficult to show more than a weak tendency for these disorders to cluster statistically (Fabrega et al., 1991). The disorders making up each cluster are described in Table 27-1. There is a trend for the clusters to be used by clinicians as a type of diagnostic shorthand. For example, a patient who is dramatic, with a tendency toward emotional outbursts and impulsive behavior, might be described as having "cluster B features."

Paranoid PD is characterized by distrust and suspiciousness of others such that their motives are interpreted as malevolent. Such individuals are not likely to see themselves as having mental difficulties. Presentation to the medical care system may result from some issue of litigation such as a disability or malpractice claim. Clinicians accustomed to developing a trusting relationship with their patients will find such patients very frustrating.

Schizoid PD is characterized by detachment from social relationships and a restricted range of expression of emotions in interpersonal settings. Individuals meeting criteria for this disorder are apparently rare in clinical populations. Since the social distance is not distressing to these patients, they will usually come to the clinician's attention for reasons completely unrelated to the personality disorder.

Schizotypal PD is characterized by social and interpersonal deficits marked by acute discomfort with and reduced capacity for close relationships as well as by cognitive or perceptual distortions and eccentricities of behavior. Despite social anxiety, these individuals are often sufficiently motivated to interact with others so as to be widely known as eccentric. Consultation with a mental health professional often stems from problems in occupational and social functioning and/or referral by concerned members of the community.

TABLE 27-1. *Personality Disorders Defined in the Current Draft of DSM-IV*

Cluster A (odd or eccentric)	
Paranoid	Schizotypal
Schizoid	

Cluster B (dramatic, emotional, or erratic)	
Narcissistic	Histrionic
Borderline	Antisocial

Cluster C (anxious or fearful)	
Avoidant	Obsessive-compulsive
Dependent	Passive-aggressive*

*The current draft of DSM-IV suggests that this diagnosis may be dropped.

Borderline PD is characterized by instability of interpersonal relationships, self-image, affects, and control over impulses. These individuals usually reach the attention of the medical care system after a crisis related to suicide threats or behavior, drug abuse, or angry outbursts. A physician who is inexperienced with such patients rapidly looses patience as the patient swings from dependent clinginess to hostile rejection. Early in treatment the patient may appear to be making rapid progress, which unravels in response to a seemingly minor stressor such as the clinician suggesting a switch from weekly sessions to bimonthly sessions.

Histrionic PD is characterized by excessive emotionality and attention seeking. These individuals may seek help for medical or emotional problems with a desperation that appears out of proportion to the actual size of the problem. They try to control and maintain attention from others by exaggerated compliments, bringing little gifts, requests for special treatment, flirtatiousness, and somatic complaints. The insecure clinician may be flattered by the patient's apparent devotion until it becomes clear that the demands for relief of emotional or medical problems are insatiable.

Narcissistic PD is characterized by grandiosity (in fantasy or behavior), need for admiration, and lack of empathy. These individuals will become frustrated and angry when someone does not give them the recognition they believe they deserve, but this is viewed as evidence that something is wrong with the other person. It is probably rare for such individuals to seek psychiatric help unless they receive a particularly severe challenge to their inflated self-concept. During a medical or psychiatric history, such patients will often describe the many important people they know and question whether the clinician is prestigious enough to treat them.

Antisocial PD is characterized by a history of irresponsible and antisocial behavior in which the rights of others are violated. This disorder is thoroughly described in a separate chapter.

Avoidant PD is characterized by social discomfort and reticence, low self-esteem, and hypersensitivity to negative evaluation. These individuals are often motivated to seek psychiatric help because their strong desire for social contact is frustrated by fear of rejection. Unlike the case with many other personality disorders, such patients often possess sufficient insight to spontaneously provide the clinician with all the criteria necessary for diagnosis. It is not clear how this disorder relates to the diagnosis of social phobia.

Dependent PD is characterized by need to be taken care of, which leads to submissive and clinging behavior and fears of separation. These individuals may come to medical attention when they are devastated by the exit of someone who formerly supported them or when that person becomes particularly emotionally and physically abusive. Such patients often reject suggestions that require more autonomous functioning due to lack of confidence in their ability. Alternatively, such patients may passively acquiesce to a plan to separate from a dominant and abusive partner only to go back to this person soon after discharge.

Obsessive-Compulsive PD is characterized by preoccupation with perfectionism, mental and interpersonal control, and orderliness at the expense of flexibility, openness, and efficiency. These personality traits may be difficult to detect by physicians, who depend on many of the same traits to get through medical school. Patients with this PD will often bring in a list of symptoms and questions, expect detailed explanations, and be frustrated by suggestions that the effective treatment may require a certain amount of trial and error. While such patients may be superficially polite, the clinician may come away from the encounter with the uneasy feeling that he or she somehow failed to measure up to the patient's expectations.

Passive-Aggressive PD is characterized by passive resistance and general obstructiveness in response to the expectations of others. Such individuals would rarely be assertive enough to openly disagree with a treatment plan but may express disagreement indirectly by "losing" a prescription or "forgetting" the psychotherapy homework assignment. The DSM-IV task force has proposed dropping this diagnosis from the manual because it may be better conceptualized as a trait present in several other personality disorders rather than as an independent disorder. The task force reportedly received several research reports suggesting that passive-aggressive PD is an extremely prevalent disorder, but these were somehow lost and never forwarded to the appropriate committee.

Several other personality disorders, including self-defeating PD (Fiester, 1991), sadistic PD (Spitzer et al., 1991; Fiester, 1991), depressive PD (Phillips, 1990), and negativistic PD (American Psychiatric Association, in press), have been proposed and may be included in an appendix of DSM-IV as disorders needing further study.

It is still unclear whether personality disorder is best conceptualized as a series of continuous dimensions or as discrete categories (Widiger, 1991). DSM-III used discrete categories, thus implying that personality traits tend to cluster in certain specific combinations or syndromes rather than varying independently from individual to individual. This may be true for patients with personality disorders even if it is not true for personality traits in the general population. For example, in cystic fibrosis, a single genetic abnormality results in a known pattern of symptoms reflecting changes across a variety of different organ systems. Theoretically, a single etiologic factor such as childhood sexual abuse or a gene related to risk for schizophrenia could lead to problems reflected across a variety of different components of personality functioning.

PERSONALITY TRAIT DIMENSIONS

The major limitation of the categorical approach is its failure to come to terms with the large body of research that describes a number of reproducible personality traits that are normally and independently distributed in the general populations (Digman, 1990). Most of these data are published in psychological rather than psychiatric journals, although there is growing interest among psychiatrists in determining whether a series of basic and independent personality trait dimensions can be detected in clinical populations (Cloninger, 1987; Heumann, 1990). Most such studies are based on self-administered questionnaires with a multiple-choice or true/false format.

The Eysenck Personality Inventory has been studied widely in both normal and clinical populations (Eysenck, 1970). It assesses three dimensions: neuroticism, extroversion, and psychoticism. The NEO Personality Inventory (Costa and McCrae, 1990) assesses five major dimensions, including neuroticism, extraversion, openness to experience, agreeableness, and constraint. The Tridimensional Personality Inventory (Clonninger, 1987) assesses novelty seeking, harm avoidance, and reward dependence, with scales to measure two or three additional dimensions still under development.

There is a developing concensus that these instruments represent slightly different approaches to measuring five or six basic dimensions of personality (Digman, 1992; Widiger, 1991). While this approach may eventually supplement or replace the categorical approach used for Axis II in the DSM system, several problems limit its immediate application. For many of these instruments, the majority of the data has been collected on relatively normal populations rather than those seen in a psychiatric setting. Several of the instruments fail to distinguish between episodic Axis I–related state symptoms and more stable Axis II traits. Even those instruments which do focus on Axis II traits have been shown to be influenced by episodic fluctuations of Axis I disorders (Hirschfeld, 1983; Reich, 1986). However, it also has been shown that scores on such dimensional measures of personality can predict worse outcome for the Axis I disorder independent of severity of Axis I at the time of index evaluation (Kerr et al., 1972; Weissman et al., 1978; Noyes et al., 1990; Pfohl et al., 1987).

THE SEARCH FOR RELIABLE AND VALID PERSONALITY DISORDER CRITERIA

In the case of Axis I disorders, committees developing operational criteria for DSM-III (American Psychiatric Association, 1980) often turned to previously published research criteria sets for which reliability and validity data were already available.

In the case of the Axis II personality disorders, the committees most often developed new criteria from scratch to identify personality types that had been historically described in more global and often psychoanalytic terms. Antisocial PD was the only clear exception to this. DSM-III provided criteria for 11 PDs. The level of inference necessary to rate Axis II criteria was often higher than that required for rating Axis I criteria, and diagnostic reliability often was low.

In 1987, revised criteria (DSM-IIIR) for PD were published. By this time, some limited data were available from structured interviews for PD that suggested that some of the criteria were too ambiguous to be interpreted consistently and that some of the PDs were defined by two few criteria to reliably identify the disorder. Criteria for two additional personality disorders, self-defeating PD (Fiester, 1991), and sadistic PD (Spitzer et al., 1991; Fiester, 1991), were defined but placed in the appendix because of controversy about their validity and potential for abuse.

While the final version of DSM-IV is due in 1994 and not available at the time of this writing, current drafts indicate few changes to the overall personality categories. As described in the *DSM-IV Source Book* (American Psychiatric Association, in press), data from more than half a dozen research centers were analyzed as part of the DSM-IV review process to identify criteria that performed poorly in discriminating between different personality disorders. For example, the DSM-IIIR criteria for histrionic PD—"constantly seeks or demands reassurance, approval, or praise"—was replaced because it was frequently present in patients with other personality disorders who did not meet criteria for histrionic PD. Other changes were based on evidence from self-rating inventories with respect to which traits tend to cluster together in the same individual (Pfohl, 1991a; Millon, 1985). DSM-IV also has attempted to improve reliability of diagnosis by providing more examples of how criteria should be rated in the text of the manual.

Other changes were made to provide for better agreement between DSM-IV and World Health Organization's *International Classification of Disease* (ICD-10) personality criteria. Ideally, data using external validators such as intrafamilial transmission of personality traits and association of traits with potential biologic and psychosocial etiologic factors should play a role in criteria selection. Data of this type were used in some of the decisions made about borderline, schizotypal, and antisocial PD (American Psychiatric Association, 1993).

Information on the effects of changes in criteria sets on interrater diagnostic agreement in different settings typically takes several years to acquire (Blashfield et al., 1992). Interrater agreement is most often measured using kappa. This statistic approaches 1.0 as interrater diagnostic agreement approaches perfection. For many of the better studied Axis I disorders, kappa values in the range of 0.7 to 0.8 are common. Using structured interview and carefully trained raters, it is possible to approach this level of reliability for many of the personality disorders (Zanarini et al., 1988; Pfohl, 1990; Loranger et al., 1991). However, most studies using unstructured clinical interview find rates of diagnostic agreement for personality (other than antisocial PD) poor (Mellsop et al., 1982; Spitzer et al., 1979).

While structured interviews may improve diagnostic reliability, such comprehensive assessments tend to highlight another challenge to diagnostic validity—the overlap of different personality diagnoses. Table 27-2 illustrates this problem with a series of 228 patients studied at the University of Iowa. Personality was assessed using Structured Interview for DSM-IIIR Personality Disorder (SIDP-R) (Stangl et al., 1985; Pfohl et al., 1991) in inpatients and outpatients. Many of the cases were assessed because the referring physician suspected personality problems; therefore, it is not surprising that 164 (72 percent) of the patients met criteria for a PD diagnosis. Among patients with at least one PD, 16 percent met criteria for two PD diagnoses, 20 percent met criteria for 3, and 30 percent met criteria for 4 or more.

A review of the row for histrionic PD in Table 27-2 illustrates the basic problem. It will be difficult to demonstrate that the distinctions between histrionic, dependent, and borderline PD are valid with respect to course, response to treatment, or biologic abnormality when 45 percent of histrionic PD cases met criteria for dependent PD and 48 percent met criteria for borderline PD. Similar rates of overlap have been documented by many investigators at other centers (Pfohl, 1991a).

COEXISTING AXIS I DISORDERS

The majority of patients with a personality diagnosis in the typical clinical setting have one or more Axis I diagnoses (Fyer et al., 1988). There are two fairly consistent findings from studies in which clinical samples with a defined Axis I disorder are assessed using a structured interview for personality disorder. First, roughly half the patients will have one or more Axis II PD diagnosis. Second, the patients with PD will show a poorer response to standard treatment for the Axis I disorder than patients with no PD. This has been demonstrated for major depression (Pfohl et al., 1987; Pilkonis and Ellen, 1989), panic disorder (Noyes et al., 1990), eating disorders (Gartner et al., 1989), and obsessive-compulsive disorder (Baer et al., 1990).

While clinical samples may be biased toward more severe cases, it is interesting that one study has found similar rates of PD among individuals with Axis I disorders who were identified through a family study rather than because of presentation to a

TABLE 27-2. *Numbers in Each Column Indicate the Percent of Cases with the Index Diagnosis (Indicated at the Top of the Column) Who also Met Criteria for the Row Diagnosis*

	Parnd	Szoid	Sztyp	Obcmp	Histr	Depnd	Antso	Narci	Avoid	Bordr
Cases (*n*)	42	5	16	60	67	64	9	20	95	63
Only one (%)	7	0	19	15	15	9	0	5	16	13
Paranoid (%)	100	60	50	40	25	25	44	40	27	29
Schizoid (%)	7	100	13	7	3	2	11	10	3	2
Schizotypal (%)	19	40	100	13	6	14	33	15	14	11
Obs/compulsive (%)	57	80	50	100	34	34	33	60	41	35
Histrionic (%)	40	40	25	38	100	47	56	70	40	51
Dependent (%)	38	20	56	37	45	100	33	45	52	57
Antisocial (%)	10	20	19	5	7	5	100	15	5	13
Narcissistic (%)	19	40	19	20	21	14	33	100	14	13
Avoidant (%)	62	60	81	65	57	77	56	65	100	54
Borderline (%)	43	20	44	37	48	56	89	40	36	100

Based on a sample of 228 nonpsychotic inpatients and outpatients who received the SIDP-R interview for DSM-IIIR personality disorders.

clinic. (Zimmerman and Coryell, 1989). These results suggest that failure to assess PD when making decisions about treatment and likely outcome of Axis I conditions is as ill-advised as failure to take Axis I disorders into account when diagnosing and treating PD.

Differences in sample selection and assessment make it difficult to compare across studies to determine if different PDs are more common among specific Axis I disorders. Among patients with depression, diagnoses such as histrionic, borderline, and avoidant PD tend to be the most common. Among patients with anxiety disorders, there is a trend in some studies for the cluster C diagnoses to be more common. While patients with obsessive-compulsive disorder may meet criteria for obsessive-compulsive PD, most do not, and other PD diagnoses tend to be even more common (Pfohl, 1991b).

The nature of the association between Axis I and Axis II disorders is not clear. It is possible that Axis II disorders predispose to Axis I disorders, or vice versa. Some third factor (biologic or psychosocial) could predispose to both disorders. Another possibility is that some Axis I–related symptoms could masquerade as an Axis II disorder. The complexity of the problem has been described by Gunderson and Phillips (1991) with respect to major depression and borderline PD. At least one prospective high-risk study suggests that personality abnormalities can be a risk factor for major depression in individuals with no history of major depression at the time of initial assessment (Hirschfeld, 1989).

ETIOLOGY

Psychosocial Factors

Some of the current PD categories have their roots in the psychoanalytic concepts of oral (dependent), anal (obsessive-compulsive), and phallic (histri-

onic) personality types. The anatomic references indicate the psychosexual stage of development during which a "fixation" might develop leading to the associated personality type (Auchincloss and Michels, 1983). Several studies using factor analysis have suggested that factors related to each of these types can be derived from clinical samples (Lazare et al., 1970; Torgersen, 1980). Attempts to verify the fixation hypothesis have not been as successful. Pollak (1979) reviewed more than a dozen studies that attempted to systematically assess anal character and childhood experience with toilet training without establishing any clear connection.

Analytic theories of etiology of borderline personality encompass seeming opposites from overprotective mothering (Levy, 1943; Masterson, 1976) to neglectful mothering (Guntrip, 1969; Gunderson and Englund, 1981). Some empirical studies are available that lend support to these explanations. Gunderson et al. (1980) abstracted family interview information from borderline patients and a like number of "neurotics" and paranoid schizophrenics. The diagnostic criteria for borderline were close to those in DSM-III. Blind ratings of more than 72 family characteristics showed families of borderline patients to be distinguishable by "the rigid tightness of the marital bond to the exclusion of the attention, support or protection of the children." The authors acknowledge methodologic problems. Similar results, however, were obtained by Frank and Paris (1981). Soloff and Millward (1983) present some empirical support for the presence of overinvolved mothers and underinvolved fathers in borderline PD.

An association between borderline PD and childhood sexual abuse has long been noted in the literature. More recently, systematic empirical studies generally relying on patient self-report of childhood emotional, physical, and sexual abuse support this association (Herman et al., 1989; Zanarini et al., 1989; Ludolph et al., 1990).

Studies such as these that investigate parenting behavior as it relates to personality diagnoses are few in number and hardly definitive. Even so, they do represent a willingness to investigate empirically what has too long been buried in layers of theory without recourse to scientific hypothesis testing. Future studies will need to take a number of issues into account, including retrospective falsification of reports of past behavior, the impact of the child's personality on the parents' behavior, and the possibility of genetic factors that might influence both parenting style and PD in the offspring. Because the concordance rate for PD among identical twins is not 100 percent, it makes sense to give some attention to psychosocial factors. What those psychosocial factors are or how much of the variance they might explain is not known.

Genetic Factors

The same questions about nature and nurture that surround research into Axis I disorders also apply to Axis II. Twin studies and adoption studies are the most useful research designs for separating out the effects of environment and heredity. With a few exceptions, these designs have not been applied to DSM-III personality disorders. Several studies have examined the relative contribution of nature versus nurture using dimensional measures of personality in series of twins and siblings. Virtually all of them find that genetic factors explain a substantial portion of the variance for personality, including such dimensions as extroversion, neuroticism and anxiety, "capacity to mobilize," and approach-withdrawal (Rutter et al., 1963; Young et al., 1971; Fuller and Thompson, 1978; Lochlin, 1982; Cattell et al., 1982). An association between blood group antigens and personality dimensions has been reported by several investigators as support for the presence of genetic factors (Angst and Maurer-Groeli, 1974; Eysenck, 1977, 1982; Jogawar, 1984).

Twin-study methodology has been applied to the Lazare et al. (1970) measure of oral (dependency), obsessive, and hysterical traits, described earlier. Torgersen (1980) examined correlations for these traits in a series of 50 monozygotic twins and 49 dizygotic twins. Some of the twins were identified by the fact that they had been previously hospitalized for a neurotic illness. Correlations between monozygotic female cotwins were above 0.5 for all three traits. Correlations for dizygotic female cotwins was low for oral and hysterical traits; the hereditability index reached statistical significance only for the other. Correlations between female dizygotic cotwins on obsessive traits was high (0.42), suggesting that a common childhood environment was influential in determining obsessionality in female cotwins. Correlations between monozygotic male cotwins was high only in the case of oral traits. The hereditability of this trait was statistically signif-

icant. The correlation for hysterical traits among male dyzygotic cotwins was sufficiently high (0.47), suggesting that a common childhood environment played an important role in this trait.

To what extent the dimensions examined in these studies represent components of Axis II disorders is not clear; nor is it clear whether these dimensions might be measuring symptoms of Axis I disorders. It is also possible that the hereditability estimates based on measurement of personality traits in normal individuals is not applicable to the more pathologic levels of traits seen in individuals labeled as having PD. For example, in the general population, parents' Wechsler Adult Intelligence Scale IQ scores show a significant correlation with their children's IQ scores. However, in a sample of parents and children where 20 percent of the children have Down syndrome, there would be a poor correlation between parents' and children's IQ scores. This results from the fact that risk for Down syndrome is not correlated with parental IQ.

A number of twin and adoption studies examine personality factors that may be genetically associated with schizophrenia in a family member. Before DSM-III, Kety et al. (1971) suggested that schizophrenia may be genetically related to a spectrum of PDs. Later, DSM-III criteria for both paranoid and schizotypal PD were retrospectively applied to the Kety et al. data. Schizotypal personality was found in 11 (10.5 percent) of 105 biologic relatives of schizophrenics, 0 of 48 adoptive relatives, and 2 (1.5 percent) of 138 controls (Kendler et al., 1981). Paranoid PD was found in 4 (3.8 percent) of 105 biologic relatives, in 1 of the adoptive relatives, and in none of the control relatives (Kendler and Gruenberg, 1981). The data were subsequently reanalyzed by applying DSM-III criteria for schizophrenia to the probands (Kendler and Gruenberg, 1984). Similar results for both schizotypal and paranoid PD were again obtained. In addition, biologic relatives of adoptees with schizophrenia were at higher risk for schizotypal personality than were relatives of adoptees with nonschizophrenic psychoses (14.3 versus 0 percent).

Torgersen (1984) studied a series of monozygotic and dizygotic twins in which at least one cotwin had either schizotypal personality or borderline personality, or both. Seven of 25 monozygotic twins versus 1 of 34 dizygotic twins were concordant for schizotypal personality. This suggests that heredity is strongly involved in this disorder.

EDITORS' COMMENT

A particularly compelling study of dimensional personality traits (Tellegen et al: J Pers Soc Psychol 54: 1031–1039, 1988) in monozygotic and dizygotic twins reared together and apart showed most scales to have a strong genetic component, with less attribution to shared environment.

FAMILIAL ASSOCIATIONS

Although adoption and twin studies can sort out familial from genetic factors in the etiology of PD, such studies are not available for most of the DSM-III PDs. Even so, there is a growing number of studies examining the rates of Axis I and Axis II disorders in families of patients with PD. A familial association of this type can result from the transmission of a relevant genetic factor. Another possibility is that the psychiatric illness diagnosed in one family member contributes to a family environment that predisposes to psychiatric illness in other family members.

There are several studies that examine the rate of Axis I disorders in first-degree relatives of borderlines using some type of control group. Loranger et al. (1982) used a chart review to study first-degree relatives of 83 borderline patients, 100 schizophrenics, and 100 bipolar patients. Morbidity risk for major depression among relatives of borderline patients (6 percent) differed significantly from that seen in relatives of schizophrenics (2 percent) but was similar to that seen in relatives of bipolar patients (7 percent). Morbidity risk for schizophrenia was 0, 3, and 0.3 percent among relatives of borderline, schizophrenic, and bipolar patients, respectively. Using rather broad family history criteria for diagnosing borderline personality, the morbidity risk for borderline personality was 12 percent among first-degree relatives of borderline patients and less than 2 percent in the other two groups. Pope et al. (1983) also found that borderline personality tended to run in families. In addition, both histrionic and antisocial PD were common among first-degree relatives of borderline probands.

The familial link between borderline personality and affective disorder described in the Loranger et al. (1982) study is still not clearly established. Soloff and Millward (1983) reported that families of borderlines were more likely to have depression than were families of schizophrenics, but interpretation of this study is confounded by several methodologic problems. Pope et al. (1983) found the prevalence for major affective disorder among relatives of borderline patients (6 percent) to be no different than that found among relatives of bipolar patients (8 percent) yet significantly higher than that found among relatives of schizophrenic patients (0.6 percent). However, when borderline probands without a concurrent major depression were examined separately, no familial association with affective disorder was observed. This suggests the possibility that there are two types of borderlines: one type that is related to affective disorder and one that is not. Despite the lack of clarity regarding affective disorders, these studies and several others form a strong consensus that there is no association between borderline personality disorder and schizophrenia (Akiskal, 1981; Andrulonis et al., 1981; Stone, 1979).

Several studies suggest that many borderline patients have first-degree relatives with alcoholism or substance abuse (Andrulonis et al., 1981; Akiskal, 1981; Soloff and Millward, 1983; Pope et al., 1983).

Neurobiologic Abnormalities

There are no neurobiologic tests ready for routine clinical use in detecting patients with PD. However, data accumulated over the past 10 years support the conclusion that neurobiologic abnormalities represent part of the puzzle that must be solved before PD is fully understood. Most researchers have followed the strategy of examining abnormalities detected in Axis I disorders as a means of determining the relationship between Axis I and Axis II.

Low platelet monamine oxidase (MAO) activity (Wyatt, 1979) and abnormalities in smooth-pursuit eye movement (SPEM) have been associated with the diagnosis of schizophrenia. Similar abnormalities have been reported in patients with schizotypal personality and no history of psychosis (Gattaz and Beckman, 1981; Siever et al., 1990). Even more intriguing, nonpatient volunteers categorized solely on the basis of these two laboratory tests show marked differences in rates of schizotypal traits (Siever, 1989; Baron et al., 1980).

Cerebrospinal fluid (CSF) 5-hydroxyindole-acetic acid (5-HIAA), a metabolite of serotonin, has been reported to be low in patients with affective disorders (Banki and Arato, 1983) and high in patients with obsessive-compulsive disorder (Insel, 1985). More recently, it has been suggested that low 5-HIAA may be more strongly associated with impulsiveness, risk taking, and suicidal behavior rather than any one diagnosis (Brown et al., 1982). Another index of serotonin activity, prolactin response to fenfluramine, has been found to be lower in patient with borderline PD (Coccaro et al., 1990).

Current work on neurobiologic correlates of personality tends to focus on associations with traits that may cross several Axis II or even Axis I diagnoses. Cloninger (1986, 1987) has proposed a system of three basic personality dimensions each of which may relate to a specific neurotransmitter system. The first dimension, novelty seeking, includes impulsiveness, excitability, and disorderliness. This dimension is theoretically associated with low basal dopaminergic activity. The second dimension is harm avoidance and is characterized by anticipatory worry, fear of uncertainty, shyness, and fatigability. This dimension is theoretically related to increased serotonin activity. Finally, reward dependence is defined by such traits as sentimentality, persistence, and dependence. This dimension is said to correlate with low basal noradrenergic activity.

Siever and Davis (1991) have proposed a slightly different scheme with four underlying traits that are said to be risk factors for both Axis I and Axis II disorders. Problems in cognitive and perceptual organization such as those seen in schizophrenia and schizotypal PD are said to be associated with abnormalities in eye movement, backward masking responses, and dopamine abnormalities. Impulsivity and aggression, as seen in several cluster B PDs and impulse disorders, are associated with serotonin abnormalities. Affective instability, as seen in major depression and some cluster B PDs, is associated with abnormalities in delayed onset of the rapid eye movement (REM) sleep stage and response to catecholaminergic challenges. Finally, it is postulated that anxiety and inhibition, as seen in anxiety disorders and avoidant PD, are associated with heart rate variability and responses to lactate infusion.

While these theories present an intriguing framework for further investigation, many of the predictions await further empirical support. While some of the findings are clearly reproducible in sufficiently large samples of patients, at the present time there is too much variability among individual patients to use these measures diagnostically.

DIFFERENTIAL DIAGNOSIS

Personality diagnoses generally should be considered only after a careful differential diagnosis of Axis I. An appreciation for Axis I problems allows the clinician to consider whether current or past examples of behavior reflect the patient's usual personality. Personality assessment becomes particularly difficult if the patient is currently suffering from an episode of major depression or the effects of some acute crisis, such as an adjustment disorder. Interviewing a knowledgeable informant or simply having repeated contact with the patient over time can help sort out these issues. In the case of schizophrenia, no personality diagnosis is made unless the PD clearly preceded the onset of schizophrenia. In the case of Axis I disorders, which are often chronic, such as dysthymia and agoraphobia, a concurrent PD is usually diagnosed if criteria are met.

Medical students and residents often have difficulty deciding what questions to ask to assess Axis II. The following questions are designed to screen for major personality problems. If the answer to a question is positive, the patient should be encouraged to elaborate or provide examples. Ideally, a knowledgeable informant should be asked many of the same questions about the patient if a personality disorder is suspected.

SOCIAL INTERACTION

Some people enjoy being the center of attention. Others prefer not to be noticed. How would you describe yourself? Can you think of any time that you did something risky or outrageous just to get noticed? Have you taken chances out of sheer boredom? Have you found that it is better not to let people get to know you too well? (*Remember to ask for elaboration or examples whenever the patient answers affirmatively.*)

CONFIDENCE

What is your usual level of self-confidence? Do you ever pretend to be something that you are not just to impress people? Do you find that your opinions keep changing so much that you are not sure what you believe anymore? Have you worried that others criticize you behind your back? Are your feelings easily hurt?

IRRITABILITY

What does it take to get you very angry? What are you like when you are angry? Do you let people know? Do you break things? Hit people? What kind of things make you jealous?

COMPULSIVITY

Are you perfectionistic? Do you often worry about details—want everything arranged just so? Do you get so caught up in your work that you have little time for friends or leisure activities?

FRIENDSHIPS

Do you have any close friends in whom you confide? Describe who they are. What do you admire about them? Do you dislike anything about them? Can you describe any situations in which friends let you down or betrayed you?

DEPENDENCY

When you have an important decision to make, is there someone you rely on to tell you what to do? Examples? Have you ever been physically or emotionally abused by someone that you depended on? Tell me about that.

MANIPULATION

If you are upset with someone, are you more likely to tell them or keep it bottled up inside? Can you think of situations in which you got even with someone by "forgetting" to do something they wanted you to do? . . . by dawdling or pretending to make mistakes? Can you describe any situations in which you decided that misleading people was necessary to get something important?

If the answers to these questions indicate problems, the specific criteria for Axis II disorders should be reviewed. It may then be necessary to return to the patient or a knowledgeable informant to clarify specific points required by the criteria.

In most cases, DSM-IV does not require a specific minimum age for a PD diagnosis; however, there is reason to believe that personality traits, as measured by some assessment tools, may not be stable or have the same implications in individuals less than about 25 years of age (Hirschfeld et al., 1989; Finn, 1986).

PSYCHOPHARMACOLOGIC TREATMENT

The majority of patients with PD probably never seek treatment. Many patients with schizotypal or compulsive personality, for example, are probably content with their lifestyle. PD is, by definition, a lifelong pattern of behavior. If an individual with PD disorder does seek treatment, the first step must be to investigate whether a more acute Axis I disorder, such as major depression, might not be responsible. As noted earlier, Axis I disorders are often more resistant to treatment when accompanied by a PD (Kerr et al., 1970; Weissman et al., 1978; Tyrer et al., 1983; Pope et al., 1983; Pfohl et al., 1984). On the other hand, patients with PD plus an Axis I disorder appear to have greater potential for improvement than do patients with PD alone (Akiskal et al., 1980; Pope et al., 1983; Cole et al., 1984). If a patient displays an Axis I disorder, such as major depression, panic disorder, agoraphobia, or so-called brief reactive psychosis, then the pharmacologic treatment generally recommended for those disorders should generally be considered.

The majority of drug treatment studies of PD involve either borderline or antisocial personality. Antisocial personality is considered in Chapter 13. Because many borderline patients have a history of drug abuse, such agents as amphetamines, barbiturates, and benzodiazepines should be avoided. Because suicide attempts also are common, it may be necessary to give prescriptions for shorter durations with weekly refills or admit the patient to the hospital for a drug trial. There is reason to believe that patients with borderline PD and major depression may be less likely to respond to tricyclic antidepressants (Soloff et al., 1990) and more likely to respond to monamine oxidase inhibitors (Parsons et al., 1989; Cowdry et al., 1988). Besides affective symptoms, symptoms such as impulsiveness and self-injury may respond to fluoxetine (Cornelius et al., 1991; Markovitz et al., 1991). Lithium has been reported to reduce impulsive behavior in some trials (Links, 1990), as has carbamazepine (Cowdry, 1988).

Low-dose neuroleptics also have been found to be efficacious in some studies (Leone, 1982; Cowdry et al., 1988). Before making the decision to put any patient on long-term neuroleptics, there should be clear evidence that significant symptoms recur if the medication is withdrawn or replaced with some other medication that is less likely to cause tardive dyskinesia. Soloff has reviewed pharmacologic approaches to borderline personality and related PDs (Soloff, 1990; Soloff et al., 1993).

PSYCHOTHERAPY

The issues and controversies surrounding the psychotherapy of PDs are the same as the issues and controversies surrounding psychotherapy in general. Opinions range from those who believe that PDs are the main indication for psychoanalysis (Auchincloss and Michels, 1983) to those who believe that psychotherapy can make some PDs worse (Stone, 1979). A review of psychotherapeutic approaches to PD is provided by Frosch (1983).

Patients with borderline, histrionic, antisocial, and passive-aggressive traits may be particularly likely to evoke frustration and anger in the therapist. Such irritation often results when the therapist becomes the victim of the manipulation and rapid shifts from overidealization to devaluation that characterize many PDs. The patients are frequently unaware of how their own behavior contributes to their problems.

It is often necessary to establish clear ground rules. The therapist may need to set up guidelines to limit telephone calls to the home or office. The skilled therapist learns simultaneously to reassure the patient that he or she will continue to be available but that this availability has certain constraints and limits that both patient and therapist must observe. Although the therapist may become angry with the patient, it is seldom appropriate to communicate this anger directly to the patient. On the other hand, it may be productive to point out specific behaviors and ask the patient to consider what types of reactions such behavior may be eliciting from those around them. It may be possible for the patient to recognize certain problem behaviors and rehearse alternatives.

Just as explicit diagnostic criteria for PD have encouraged better-designed psychopharmocolgic trials, new research is becoming available regarding psychotherapy of PDs. Beck and colleagues (1990) have developed a number of cognitive therapy techniques targeted at specific PD traits. Beck states that significant improvement in personality functioning can be detected with about 6 to 18 months of therapy. Compared with cognitive therapy for major depression, cognitive therapy for PD requires that greater time and attention be devoted to development of a therapeutic relationship with appropriate boundaries and modeling of healthy approaches to resolving conflict. Cognitive distortions regarding all-or-none thinking, catastrophizing about the consequences of the loss of a significant other, and the belief that impulses are hopelessly uncontrollable are major foci of therapy.

While more research is needed, there is good reason to believe that personality-related symptoms may show significant improvement in response to various types of psychotherapy (Stevenson and Meares, 1992; Tucker et al., 1987; Karterud et al., 1992) or simply the passage of sufficient time (McGlashan, 1986; Mehlum et al., 1991; Hoke et al., 1992). One study of borderline PD found that only 25 of 100 patients meeting diagnostic criteria for borderline PD at index still met criteria when followed up 15 years later (Paris et al., 1987).

The concept of *enduring patterns* is part of the definition of personality. The risk is that the definition may become a self-fulfilling prophecy if the clinician views *enduring* as a synonym for *intractable*. The single most important psychotherapeutic maneuver is to convey to patient and other staff the expectation that the identification of personality problems represents an opportunity to focus on specific behaviors that need to be replaced by more effective strategies. Psychotherapy as well as psychopharmacology may be useful in promoting this change.

REFERENCES

Akiskal HS: Subaffective disorders: Dysthymic, cyclothymic, and bipolar II disorders in the borderline realm. Psychiatr Clin North Am 4:25–46, 1981.

Akiskal HS, Rosenthal TL, Haykal RF, et al: Characterological depressions: Clinical and sleep EEG findings separating "subaffective dysthymias" from "character spectrum disorders." Arch Gen Psychiatry 37:777–783, 1980.

American Psychiatric Association: Diagnostic and Statistical Manual of Mental Disorders, 3d ed revised. Washington, American Psychiatric Association, 1987.

American Psychiatric Association: The DSM-IV Draft Criteria. Washington, American Psychiatric Association 1993.

Andrulonis PA, Glueck BC, Stroebel CF, et al: Organic brain dysfunction and the borderline syndrome. Psychiatr Clin North Am 4:47–66, 1981.

Angst J, Maurer-Groeli YA: Blutgruppen und personlichkeit. Arch Psychiatr Nervenkr 218:291–300, 1974.

Auchincloss EL, Michels R: Psychoanalytic theory of character. In Frosch JP (ed): Current Perspectives on Personality Disorders. Washington, American Psychiatric Press, 1983.

Baer L, Jenike MA, Ricciardi J: Standardized assessment of personality disorders in obsessive-compulsive disorder. Arch Gen Psychiatry 47:826–830, 1990.

Banki CM, Arato M: Relationship between cerebrospinal fluid amine metabolites, neuroendocrine findings and personality dimensions (Marke-Nyman scale factors) in psychiatric patients. Acta Psychiatr Scand 67:272–280, 1983.

Beck A: Cognitive Therapy of Personality Disorders. New York, Guilford Press, 1990.

Blashfield R, Blum N, Pfohl B: The effects of changing Axis II diagnostic criteria. Comprehensive Psychiatry 33:245–252, 1992.

Carroll BJ, Greden JF, Feinberg M, et al: Neuroendocrine evaluation of depression in borderline patients. Psychiatr Clin North Am 4:89–99, 1982.

Cattell RB, Vaughan DS, Schuerger JM, Rao DC: Heritabilities by the multiple abstract variance analysis (MAVA) model and objective test measures of personality traits. Behav Genet 12:361–378, 1982.

Cloninger CR: A systematic method for clinical description and classification of personality variants. Arch Gen Psychiatry 44:573–588, 1987.

Cloninger CR: A unified biosocial theory of personality and its role in the development of anxiety states. Psychiatr Dev 3:167–226, 1986.

Coccaro EF, Siever LJ, Klar HM, et al: Serotonergic studies in patients with affective and personality disorders: Correlates with suicidal and impulsive aggressive behavior. Arch Gen Psychiatry 46:587–599, 1989.

Cole JO, Salomon M, Gunderson J, et al: Drug therapy in borderline patients. Compr Psychiatry 25:249–254, 1984.

Cornelius JR, Soloff PH, Perel JM, Ulrich RF: A preliminary trial of fluoxetine in refractory borderline patients. J Clin Psychopharmacol 11:116–120, 1991.

Costa P, McCrae R: Personality disorders and the five-factor model of personality. J Pers Disord 4:362–371: 1990.

Cowdry RW, Gardner DL: Pharmacotherapy of borderline personality disorder: Alprazolam, carbamazepine, trifluoperazine, and tranylcypromine. Arch Gen Psychiatry 45:111–119, 1988.

Crowe R: An adoption study of antisocial personality. Arch Gen Psychiatry 31:785–791, 1974.

Digman J: Personality structure: Emergence of the five-factor model. Annu Rev Psychol 41:417–440, 1992.

Ellison JM, Adler DA: Psychopharmacologic approaches to borderline syndromes. Comprehensive Psychiatry 25:255–262, 1984.

Eysenck HJ: A dimensional system of psychodiagnosis. In Mahrer SR (ed): New Approaches to Personality Classification. New York, Columbia University Press, 1970, pp 169–208.

Eysenck HJ: National differences in personality as related to ABO blood group polymorphism. Psychol Rep 41:1257–1258, 1977.

Eysenck HJ: The biological basis of cross-cultural differences in personality: Blood group antigens. Psychol Rep 51:531–540, 1982.

Fabrega H, Ulrich R, Pilkonis P, Mezzich J: On the homogeneity of personality disorder clusters. Compr Psychiatry 32:373–386, 1991.

Fiester SJ: Sadistic personality disorder: A review of data and recommendations for DSM-IV. J Pers Disord 5:376–385, 1991.

Fiester SJ: Self-defeating personality disorder: A review of data and recommendations for DSM-IV. J Pers Disord 5:194–209, 1991.

Finn SE: Stability of personality self-ratings over 30 years: Evidence for an age/cohort interaction. J Pers Soc Psychol 50:813–818, 1986.

Frank H, Paris J: Recollections of family experience in borderline patients. Arch Gen Psychiatry 38:1031–1034, 1981.

Frosch JP: The psychosocial treatment of personality disorders. In Frosch JP (ed): Current perspectives on personality disorders. Washington, American Psychiatric Press, 1983.

Fuller JL, Thompson WR: Foundations of Behavioral Genetics. St. Louis, C.V. Mosby, 1978.

Fyer MR, Frances AJ, Sullivan T, et al: Comorbidity of borderline personality disorder. Arch Gen Psychiatry 45:348–352, 1988.

Gartner AF, Marcus RN, Halmi K, Loranger AW: DSM-III-R personality disorders in patients with eating disorders. Am J Psychiatry 146:1585–1591, 1989.

Gunderson JG, Englund DW: Characterizing the families of borderlines: A review of the literature. Psychiatr Clin North Am 4:159–168, 1981.

Gunderson JG, Kerr J, Woods D: The families of borderlines. Arch Gen Psychiatry 37:27–33, 1980.

Gunderson JG, Phillips KA: A current view of the interface between borderline personality disorder and depression. Am J Psychiatry 148:967–975, 1991.

Gunderson JG, Siever LJ, Spaulding E: The search for a schizotype. Arch Gen Psychiatry 40:15–22, 1983.

Guntrip H: Schizoid Phenomena, Object Relations, and the Self. New York, International Universities Press, 1969.

Herman JL, Perry JC, van der Kolk BA: Childhood trauma in borderline personality disorder. Am J Psychiatry 146:490–495, 1989.

Heumann KA, Morey LC: Reliability of categorical and dimensional judgments of personality disorder. Am J Psychiatry 147:498–500, 1990.

Hirschfeld RMA, Klerman GL, Clayton PJ, et al: Assessing personality: Effects of depressive state on trait measurement. Am J Psychiatry 140:695–699, 1983.

Hirschfeld RMA, Klerman GL, Clayton PJ, Keller MB, et al: Assessing personality: Effects of the depressive state on trait measurement. Am J Psychiatry 40:695–699, 1983.

Hirschfeld RMA, Klerman GL, Lavori P, et al: Premorbid personality assessments of first onset of major depression. Arch Gen Psychiatry 46:345–350, 1989.

Hoke LA, Lavori PW, Perry JC: Mood and global functioning in borderline personality disorder: Individual regression models for longitudinal measurements. J Psychiatr Res 26:1–16, 1992.

Insel TR, Mueller EA, Alterman I, et al: Obsessive-compulsive disorder and serotonin: Is there a connection? Biol Psychiatry 20:1174–1185, 1985.

Jogawar VV: Personality correlates of human blood groups. Personality and Individual Differences 4:215–216, 1984.

Karterud S, Vaglum S, Irion T, et al: Day hospital therapeutic community treatment for patients with personality disorders: An empirical evaluation of the containment of function. J Nerv Ment Dis 180:238–243, 1992.

Kendler KS, Gruenberg AM: Genetic relationship between paranoid personality disorder and the "schizophrenic spectrum" disorders. Am J Psychiatry 139:1185–1186, 1982.

Kendler KS, Gruenberg AM: An independent analysis of the Danish adoption study of schizophrenia: VI. The relationship between psychiatric disorders as defined by DSM-III in relatives and adoptees. Arch Gen Psychiatry 41:555–564, 1984.

Kendler KS, Gruenberg AM, Strauss JS: An independent analysis of the Copenhagen sample of the Danish adoption study of schizophrenia: II. Relationship between schizotypal personality disorder and schizophrenia. Arch Gen Psychiatry 38:982–984, 1981.

Kerr TA, Roth M, Schapira K, Gurney C: The assessment and prediction of outcome in affective disorders. Br J Psychiatry 121:167–174, 1972.

Kerr TA, Schapira K, Roth M, Garside RF: The relationship between the Maudsley Personality Inventory and the course of affective disorders. Br J Psychiatry 116:11–19, 1970.

Kety SS, Rosenthal D, Wender PH, Schulsinger F: Mental illness in the biologic and adoptive families of adopted schizophrenics. Am J Psychiatry 128:302–306, 1971.

Koenigsberg HW, Kernberg OF, Schomer J: Diagnosing borderline conditions in an outpatient setting. Arch Gen Psychiatry 40:49–53, 1983.

Lazare A, Klerman GL: Hysteria and depression: The frequency and significance of hysterical personality features in hospitalized depressed women. Am J Psychiatry 124:48–56, 1968.

Lazare A, Klerman G, Armor DJ: Oral, obsessive and hysterical personality patterns: Replication of factor analysis in an independent sample. J Psychol Res 7:275–279, 1970.

Leone NF: Response of borderline patients to loxapine and chlorpromazine. J Clinical Psychiatry 43:148–150, 1982.

Levy DM: Maternal Overprotection. New York, Columbia University Press, 1943.

Links PS, Steiner M, Boiago I, Irwin D: Lithium therapy for borderline patients: Preliminary findings. J Pers Disord 4:173–181; 1990.

Linnoila M, Virkkunen M, Scheinin M, et al: Low cerebrospinal fluid 5-hyroxyindoleacetic acid concentration differentiates impulsive from nonimpulsive violent behavior. Life Sci 33:2609–2614, 1983.

Lochlin JC: Are personality traits differentially heritable? Behav Genet 12:417–428, 1982.

Loranger AW, Hirschfeld RMA, Sartorius N, Regier DA: The WHO/ADAMHA international pilot study of personality disorders: Background and purpose. J Pers Disord 5:296–306, 1991.

Loranger AW, Oldham JM, Tulis EH: Familial transmission of DSM-III borderline personality disorder. Arch Gen Psychiatry 39:795–799, 1982.

Ludolph PS, Westen D, Misle B, et al: The borderline diagnosis in adolescents: Symptoms and developmental history. Am J Psychiatry 147(4):470–476, 1990.

Lumry AE, Gottesman II, Tuason VB: MMPI state dependency during the course of bipolar psychosis. Psychiatry Res 7:59–67, 1982.

Markovitz PJ, Calabrese JR, Schulz SC, Meltzer HY: Fluoxetine in the treatment of borderline and schizotypal personality disorders. Am J Psychiatry 148:1064–1067, 1991.

Masterson J: Psychotherapy of the Borderline Adult. New York, Brunner/Mazel, 1976.

McGlashan TH: The borderline syndrome: II. Is it a variant of schizophrenia or affective disorder? Arch Gen Psychiatry 40:1319–1323, 1983.

McGlashan TH: The Chestnut Lodge follow-up study: III. Long-term outcome of borderline personalities. Arch Gen Psychiatry 43:20–30, 1986.

Mehlum L, Friis S, Irion T, et al: Personality disorders 2 to 5 years after treatment: A prospective follow-up study. Acta Psychiatr Scand 84:72–77, 1991.

Mellsop G, Varghese F, Joshua S, Hicks A: The reliability of Axis II of DSM-III. Am J Psychiatry 139:1360–1361, 1982.

Millon T: The MCMI provides a good assessment of DSM-III disorders. J Pers Assess 49:379–391, 1985.

Noyes R, Reich J, Christiansen J, et al: Outcome of panic disorder: Relationship to diagnostic subtypes and comorbidity. Arch Gen Psychiatry 47:809–818, 1990.

Paris J, Brown R, Nowlis: Long-term follow-up of borderline patients in a general hospital. Compr Psychiatry 28:530–535, 1987.

Parsons B, Quitkin FM, McGrath PJ, et al: Phenelzine, imipramine, and placebo in borderline patients meeting criteria for atypical depression. Psychopharmacol Bull 25:524–535, 1989.

Pfohl B: Histrionic personality disorder: A review of available data and recommendations for DSM-IV. J Pers Disord 5:150–166, 1991a.

Pfohl B, Black DW, Noyes R, et al: Axis I/Axis II comorbidity findings: Implications for validity. In Oldham J (ed): Axis II: New Perspectives on Validity. Washington, American Psychiatric Association Press, 1990.

Pfohl B, Blum N: Obsessive-compulsive personality disorder: A review of available data and recommendations for DSM-IV. J Pers Disord 5:363–375, 1991b.

Pfohl B, Coryell W, Zimmerman M, Stangl D: DSM-III personality disorders: Diagnostic overlap and internal consistency of individual DSM-III criteria. Compr Psychiatry 27:21–34, 1986.

Pfohl B, Coryell W, Zimmerman M, Stangl D: Prognostic validity of self-report and interview measures of personality in depressed patients. J Clin Psychiatry 48:468–472, 1987.

Pfohl B, Stangl D, Zimmerman M: The Structured Interview for DSM-III Personality Disorders (SIDP). Dept of Psychiatry, University of Iowa, Iowa City, Iowa, 1982.

Pfohl B, Stangl D, Zimmerman M: Increasing Axis II reliability (letter). Am J Psychiatry 140:271–272, 1983.

Phillips KA, Gunderson JG, Hirschfeld RM, Smith LE: A review of the depressive personality. Am J Psychiatry 147:830–837, 1990.

Pilkonis PA, Frank E: Personality pathology in recurrent depression: Nature, prevalence, and relationship to treatment response. Am J Psychiatry 145:435–441, 1988.

Pope HG, Jonas J, Hudson J, et al: The validity of DSM-III borderline personality disorder. Arch Gen Psychiatry 40:23–30, 1983.

Reich JH, Noyes R, Coryell W, O'Gorman T: The effect of state anxiety of personality measurement. Am J Psychiatry 143:760–763, 1986.

Reveley MA, Glover V, Sandler M, Coppen A: Increased platelet monoamine oxidase activity in affective disorders. Psychopharmacology 73:257–260, 1981.

Rifkin A, Quitkin F, Carrillo C, Blumberg AG, Klein DF, Oaks G: Lithium carbonate in emotionally unstable character disorder. Arch Gen Psychiatry 27:519–523, 1972.

Rutter M, Korn S, Birch HG: Genetic and environmental factors in the development of "primary reaction patterns." Br J Soc Clin Psychol 2:161–178, 1963.

Schulsinger F: Psychopathy: Heredity and environment. Int J Ment Health 1:190–206, 1972.

Siever LJ, Coursey RD, Alterman IS, et al: Clinical, psychophysiological, and neurological characteristics of volunteers with impaired smooth pursuit eye movements. Biol Psychiatry 26:35–51, 1989.

Siever LJ, Davis KL: A psychobiological perspective on the personality disorders. Am J Psychiatry 148:1647–1658, 1991.

Siever LJ, Keefe R, Bernstein DP, et al: Eye tracking impairment in clinically identified patient with schizotypal personality disorder. Am J Psychiatry 147:740–745, 1990.

Soloff PH: What's new in personality disorders? An update on pharmacologic treatment. J Pers Disord 4:223–243, 1990.

Soloff PH, Anselm G, Nathan RS: The dexamethasone suppression test in patients with borderline personality disorders. Am J Psychiatry 139:1621–1623, 1982.

Soloff PH, Cornelius J, Anselm G et al: Efficacy of phenelzine and haloperidol in borderline personality disorder. Arch Gen Psychiatry 50:377–386, 1993.

Soloff PH, Millward JW: Developmental histories of borderline patients. Compr Psychiatry 24:574–588, 1983.

Soloff PH, Millward JW: Psychiatric disorders in the families of borderline patients. Arch Gen Psychiatry 40:37–44, 1983.

Spitzer RL, Endicott J, Gibbon M: Crossing the border into borderline personality and borderline schizophrenia. Arch Gen Psychiatry 36:17–24, 1979.

Spitzer RL, Feister SF, Gay M, Pfohl B: Results of a Survey of forensic psychiatrists on the validity of the sadistic personality disorder diagnoses. Am J Psychiatry 148:875–879, 1991.

Spitzer RL, Forman JBW, Nee J: DSM-III field trials. I. Initial interrater diagnostic reliability. Am J Psychiatry 136:815–817, 1979.

Stangl D, Pfohl B, Zimmerman M, Bowers W: A structured interview for DSM-III personality disorders. Arch Gen Psychiatry 42:591–596, 1985.

Stevenson J, Meares R: An outcome study of psychotherapy for patients with borderline personality disorder. Am J Psychiatry 149:358–362, 1992.

Stone MH: Contemporary shift of the borderline concept from subschizophrenic disorder to a subaffective disorder. Psychiatr Clin North Am 2:577–593, 1979.

Torgersen S: The oral, obsessive and hysterical personality syndromes: A study of hereditary and environmental factors by means of the twin method. Arch Gen Psychiatry 37:1272–1277, 1980.

Torgersen S: Genetic and nosological aspects of schizotypal and borderline personality disorders: A twin study. Arch Gen Psychiatry 41:546–554, 1984.

Tucker L, Bauer SF, Wagner S, et al: Long-term hospital treatment of borderline patients: A descriptive outcome study. Am J Psychiatry 144:1443–1448, 1987.

Tyrer P, Casey P, Gall J: Relationship between neurosis and personality disorder. Br J Psychiatry 142:404–408, 1983.

Van Valkenburg C, Lowry M, Winokur G, Cadoret R: Depression spectrum disease versus pure depressive disease. J Nerv Ment Dis 165:341–347, 1977.

Weissman MM, Prusoff BA, Klerman GL: Personality and the prediction of long-term outcome of depression. Am J Psychiatry 135:797–800, 1978.

Widiger TA: Personality disorder dimensional models proposed for DSM-IV. J Pers Disord, 5:386–398, 1991.

Winokur G: Depression spectrum disease: Description and family study. Compr Psychiatry 13:3–8, 1972.

Wyatt RJ, Steven GP, Murphy DL: Platelet monoamine oxidase activity in schizophrenia: A review of the data. Am J Psychiatry 136:377–385, 1979.

Yerevanian BI, Akiskal HS: "Neurotic," characterological, and dysthymic depressions. Psychiatr Clin North Am 2:595–617, 1979.

Young JPR, Fenton GW, Lader MH: The inheritance of neurotic traits: A twin study of the Middlesex Hospital Questionnaire. Br J Psychiatry 119:393–398, 1971.

Zanarini M, Frankenburg F, Chauncey D, Gunderson J: The diagnostic interview for personality disorders: Interrater and test-retest reliability. Compr Psychiatry 28:467–480, 1988.

Zanarini MC, Gunderson JC, Marino MF, et al: Childhood experiences of borderline patients. Comp Psychiatry 30:18–25, 1989.

Zimmerman M: The Positive and Negative Impact (PANI) Life Events Interview. Dept of Psychiatry, University of Iowa, Iowa City, Iowa, 1982.

Zimmerman M, Coryell W: DSM-III personality disorder diagnoses in a nonpatient sample. Arch Gen Psychiatry 46:682–689, 1989.

UNIT 4

Special Areas

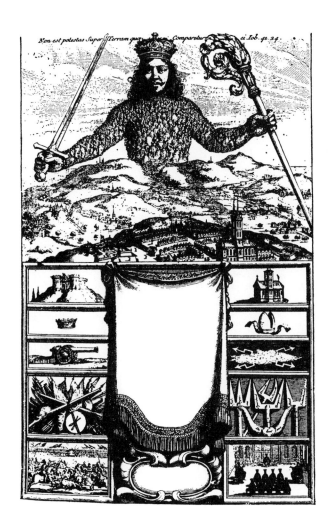

CHAPTER 28

The Neurobiologic Basis of Psychiatric Illnesses

FRITZ A. HENN

One of the central debates in psychiatry since the 1960s involves the question of nature versus nurture. Initially, this was a debate between those who held the view that behavior was the result of social and environmental influences and those who believed that behavior was programmed into the genetic makeup of an individual. The rise of modern neurosciences, which has as a principal tenet the view that all behavior is a result of brain function, appeared to support the latter view. More knowledge about the adaptability and plasticity of the nervous system has made it clear that the debate is fruitless. Brain clearly directs behavioral responses, but brain is also modified by environmental forces. Thus, regardless of one's bias, a clear understanding of brain structure and function is necessary to dissect the factors that lead to the behavioral malfunctions we call psychiatric syndromes. Our current biochemical theories of psychiatric illnesses are undoubtedly gross simplifications. A complete neurobiologic understanding requires precise specification of the nature of the genetic susceptibility, how this is acted on by environmental influences, and the alterations in the pathways controlling the behavior. Thus, in this chapter, we begin by looking at the neurobiologic foundations on which subsequent biochemical theories will be built; then the theories of specific illnesses are reviewed.

ORGANIZATIONAL ANATOMY

The brain, as the interpreter of the outside world and director of the musculoskeletal system, sits at the midpoint between the input of a variety of receptors bringing sensory information in and the output of a variety of tracts directing voluntary and involuntary responses to that information. Mal-functions in the analysis of the input lead to psychiatric symptomatology. Unfortunately, although we are beginning to have some understanding of how sensory information comes into the central nervous system (CNS) and how instructions flow out, we know relatively little about where and how they are analyzed. The brain (Fig. 28-1) monitors information coming in through the spinal cord and cranial nerves. The brain stem, a region comprising the medulla, the pons, and the midbrain, receives sensory input and relays it. Several collections of cells called *nuclei* in this region serve as the relay stations to higher centers. Among these are the neurons, using the monoamine transmitters that are of such interest in psychiatry. The cerebellum lies rostral and is important in regulating fine motor movement. Continuing upward from the midbrain leads to the diencephalon and the basal ganglia. The latter, consisting of caudate nucleus, putamen, and globus pallidus, are also involved in coordinating fine motor movements. These areas may be involved in behavioral responses as well. Many of the nuclei in the midbrain, using monoamines, appear to be adjuncts to the main information-carrying pathways and may serve as modulators. The main relay stations for information from the periphery is in the diencephalon. Here the thalamus contains a host of important relay nuclei related to sensation and movement. The hypothalamus integrates autonomic function and endocrine responses regulating homeostasis. Capping the CNS is the cerebral cortex, consisting of four lobes: frontal, parietal, temporal, and occipital. These structures are concerned with the integration of perceptual and motor functions, cognition, and elements of affect. Recent studies of language have clarified the role that the neocortex probably plays in integrating emotional responses with cognitive, perceptual, and motor

439

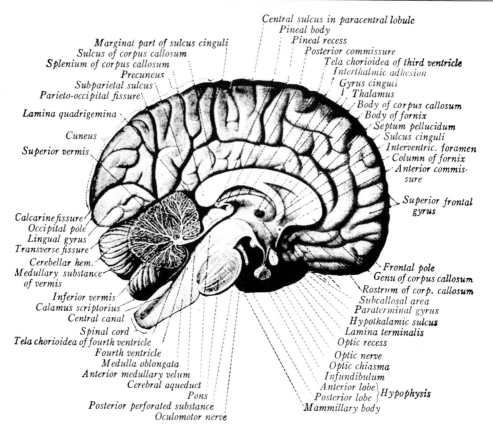

FIGURE 28-1. *Medial sagittal section of the human brain. (Sobotta-McMurrich.)* (From Ransom SW and Clark SL: The Anatomy of the Nervous System: Its Development and Function. Philadelphia, W.B. Saunders Company, 1959, with permission.)

functions. Heilman et al. (1975), among others, has shown that just as the comprehension of speech is localized in the left hemisphere, the comprehension of emotional gesturing and inflections in speech are localized in the right hemisphere. The new data complement our earlier understanding of the anatomic substrates of emotion, which arose from the work of Papez (1937). If the neocortex interprets and integrates emotions, it has been postulated that the limbic structures are the anatomic sites for their generation.

The idea of a limbic lobe was initially put forth by Broca to indicate the older cortical structures, which form a border (limbus) around the brain stem. These structures include the cingulate gyrus, fornix, septal nuclei, stria terminalis, amygdala, lateral striae, olfactory tubercle, medial striae, and hippocampus (see Fig. 28-1). In 1937, Papez published "A Proposed Mechanism of Emotion." In this contribution, Papez attempted to define the anatomic

basis for a connection between higher cortical centers and the hypothalamus. He believed that the hypothalamus had a central role in the production of emotion and that since emotions were part of consciousness, they also must be connected to higher cortical centers. He proposed a pathway that received cortical input by way of the cingulate gyrus. The cortical input was sent to the hippocampus, which processed the information, and relayed it through the fornix, to the mammillary bodies of the hypothalamus. It could then be sent back through the thalamus to the cingulate gyrus. The circuit is potentially a closed loop, allowing for the possibility of reverberatory activity. The theory was initially put forth with minimal hard evidence, but subsequent lesion studies have provided some support. Even today, however, we do not have convincing proof of these ideas. As we pass the fiftieth anniversary of Papez's contribution, it remains, nevertheless, the central hypothesis around which to structure an understanding of the anatomical localization of emotion.

In humans, bilateral temporal lobectomy results in a total loss of affect and emotional response. These studies interrupt the tracts connecting cortex to hypothalamus and so are consistent with the ideas of Papez. Modern neuroanatomy has provided evidence of extensive connections between the hippocampus and the neocortex and has demonstrated the relationship of other structures, such as the amygdala, the septum, the nucleus accumbens, and the subiculum. However, these details have not led to a much more refined picture than the notion that the neocortex receives and processes information, selecting those inputs that are significant. The material is relayed to structures in the limbic lobe and processed. The resulting emotions lead to motor and endocrine responses that are integrated when the information is passed to the hypothalamus. What we do now appreciate is the complexity of the responses that the hypothalamus can induce. This structure has a variety of peptides that may not only act as releasing factors for hormones but also may have a direct action on CNS receptors. Peptide neurotransmission and neuromodulation on brain sites unrelated to endocrine function vastly broaden the range of responses of the CNS to limbic stimulation. Although we have only the most general clues as to how the limbic circuitry may be involved with specific psychiatric syndromes, this material does provide a starting point for attempts to relate symptoms to anatomy. Such localizations may ultimately help us to define more precise points of neurochemical attack on psychiatric illnesses.

CNS CELLS—STRUCTURE AND FUNCTION

The unique properties of brain must arise from the particular cellular constituents that make it up. On the surface, the cellular composition of nervous tissue is surprisingly simple. It consists of neurons and glial cells. The remarkable complexity of output comes from the variety of neurons, their large numbers (10^{11}), the patterns of connections, and the mechanisms that modify output on the basis of experience. Any given neuron can receive thousands of inputs through its dendrites and send out thousands of outputs through branches from its axons.

Neurons contain the usual constituents found in cells: a nucleus (usually large), nucleoli, smooth and rough endoplasmic reticulum, Golgi complex, and mitochondria. What makes the cell unique is (1) its ability to transmit an electrical signal without decrement over relatively long distances—a property caused by the electrically active membrane—and (2) a mechanism to signal its neighbor. Signaling is usually accomplished through a specialized structure called the synapse. This structure is an area of specialized contact formed by the presynaptic terminal of one neuron and the specialized receptive area, the postsynaptic membrane region, of the second. Not surprisingly, the areas of contact are the regions implicated in the action of most psychopharmacologically active drugs, for by altering the nature of the communication between neurons, one most selectively can alter the behavioral output of the system.

In general, neuronal structure consists of a cell body or soma, a series of branched dendrites, an axon, and a region of presynaptic terminals. The cell body is often large, and the patterns of dendritic branches are varied. In general, there are multipolar cells with dendrites coming from all portions of the soma, bipolar cells with information coming in from one direction and flowing out through the axon in another, and unipolar cells with a short-fused axon that splits after leaving the soma. Larger cells with long axons often have them wrapped in a myelin sheath. This structure, formed by the oligodendroglia, acts as an insulator and is important to achieve high-speed conduction. The end of the axon that branches and forms regions of presynaptic fibers ends with little knoblike structures that form part of the synapse. These structures contain many mitochondria and dense granules, which can be viewed in the electron microscope. It is this region that must be examined in more detail, for most theories of biologic alterations in psychiatric disease suggest that it is at the point of transmission of information from one cell to another that alterations occur.

When one neuron signals another, the process begins with information going out through the axon. This occurs when the membrane is depolarized. All cells have a potential difference across their plasma membrane, the size of which is a function of the differences between the ion composition inside and outside and the resistance of the membrane itself. What is unique about neurons is that when they are depolarized sufficiently, they do not simply follow the imposed depolarization but rather undergo a spontaneous, rapid, self-limited depolarization that carries the membrane potential from the negative values usually seen to positive values of up to 30 mV. Then the potential returns to its initial value—this is the action potential and this electrical signal moves down the axon membrane to the presynaptic region. If a strong enough signal arrives at the presynaptic region, it causes the release of a transmitter substance. These substances are stored in the dense granules and are released in response to the action potential. The basis for the action potential is the transient opening of ion channels. Similarly, in the presynaptic area, ion channels are opened as a consequence of depolarization. However, here the important ion to enter is Ca^{2+}, which is central to the release of the transmitter. As the action potential arrives, Ca^{2+} permeability goes up, and subsequently, the transmitter is released. The transmitter diffuses through the region of the synaptic clef and reacts with a specific receptor of the postsynaptic membrane. This reaction often sets in motion a change in permeability that depolarizes the subsequent neuron. The transmitter is quickly removed from the synaptic region by reuptake into cells or metabolic destruction. It is the elements of this process—synthesis and degradation of transmitter, release, reuptake, and receptor activity—that are altered by most psychoactive drugs. We will consider the processes for several transmitters that appear to be related to psychiatric conditions.

First, a general word about transmitters. These substances include several classes of compounds: amines, amino acids, and peptides. Until recently, it appeared that transmitter candidates all acted to transmit information from one cell to an adjacent cell. Now complications have developed: Compounds do clearly carry out this transmission role, but they also may act as modulators in a variety of settings. These latter functions are still incompletely understood but may prove vital to an understanding of the pathophysiology of psychiatric diseases. In addition, such a role may be central to the action of a majority of CNS peptides. Such a modulating role may involve action on a variety of sites, not only communication with the next neuron.

RECEPTORS AND EFFECTORS

All modulators and neurotransmitters act by interacting with receptors. In the case of synaptic transmission, these receptors lie on the postsynaptic membrane, being the target of the transmitter in classic point-to-point neurotransmission. This we now know constitutes only a fraction of the receptor sites; we also can find presynaptic receptors, both autoreceptor and heteroreceptors, and even glial cell receptors. It turns out that a given transmitter may have a large number of different receptors which interact with it in different ways. Receptors can either act rapidly to open ion channels (class I receptors) or interact with a variety of G proteins to activate a second messenger system (class II receptors). Receptors with the exception of steriod and thyroid receptors appear to lie in the plasma membrane. The receptors can be thought of as floating in the lipid bilayer and after interaction with their appropriate ligand changing conformation so that they bind an effector molecule also floating in the membrane, either an ion channel or one of several G proteins. This complex then goes on to initiate the physiologic response which that receptor controls. The advantage of multiple receptors for a given transmitter is the ability of one signal to initiate several different responses at different sites. The current receptor families for various transmitters are

listed in Table 28-1. The growth of receptors using pharmacologic criteria has been rapid, and it is necessary to view this expansion of receptor subtypes critically. However, many members of receptor families have been cloned, giving unequivocal evidence of their existence. In general, the two classes of receptors have been shown to have similar structure, those coupling with G proteins having seven hydrophobic membrane regions and those coupling with ion receptors having four. Even these distinctions are not absolute in that some receptors have been suggested to gate ion channels at one site and activate second messenger systems at another.

The activation of receptors works through second messenger systems. The best known involves the generation of cyclic neucleotides, either cAMP or cGMP, and subsequent protein phosphorylation. A second system involves the breakdown of phosphoinositides. Here two messengers are formed, water-soluble inositol triphosphate and hydrophobic diacylglycerol. The inositol triphosphate increases intracellular free calcium and activates calmodulin to cause protein phosphorylation. Diacylglycerol also activates a protein kinase, leading to protein phosphorylation. This mechanism appears to be a ubiquitous pathway to activate and regulate a variety of cellular functions.

THE NEUROTRANSMITTER SYSTEMS

Norepinephrine

The catecholamines dopamine, norepinephrine, and epinephrine constitute the most studied class of neurotransmitters. Early studies showed that epinephrine and norepinephrine play a crucial role in the body's response to stress. This, plus an ability to measure and fairly early on an ability to localize these compounds histochemically, resulted in a great deal of information that provided the building blocks for several theories involving these compounds in the pathophysiology of psychiatric diseases.

NOREPINEPHRINE SYSTEM ANATOMY

The localization of norepinephrine neurons became possible with the discovery that formaldehyde reacted in situ with the catecholamines to produce a highly fluorescent product. This allowed Dahlstrom and Fuxe (1965) to begin mapping the CNS neurons containing norepinephrine. Subsequent advances using gloxylic acid and immunocytochemical techniques have refined the available mapping techniques. Basically, the norepinephrine system consists of two clusters of cell bodies sending widespread innervation throughout the CNS. The largest collection of cells is in the locus ceruleus, a small

TABLE 28-1. *Receptor Subtypes in CNS*

Norepinephrine	
Alpha$_1$	Postsynaptic localization; seen primarily in heart and brain; antagonist—prazosin
Alpha$_2$	Primarily presynaptic; seen in gastrointestinal tract and brain; antagonist—clonidine
Beta$_1$	Linked to adenylate cyclase; seen in heart, fat cells, and brain; antagonist—practolol
Beta$_2$	Linked to adenylate cyclase; seen in lung, blood vessels, and brain; antagonist—IPS-339
Dopaminergic	
D$_1$	Linked to adenylate cyclase; found in brain; antagonist—bromocriptine
D$_2$	Not linked to adenylate cyclase; found in brain; antagonist—spiroperidol
D$_3$	One of three recently cloned new dopamine receptors; limbic system distribution; appears coupled to K$^+$ ion channels
D$_4$	This receptor is related to the D$_2$ receptor but has 10-fold higher clozapine affinity; inhibits cAMP production seen in cortex and limbic region
D$_5$	More similar to the D$_1$ receptor; appears coupled to cAMP production; similar distribution to D$_1$
Cholinergic	
Muscarine benzilate (QNB)	All labeled by quinuclidinyl
M$_1$	Seen in striatum, sympathetic ganglia; selective antagonist—pirenzipine
M$_2$	Seen in cerebellum and heart; inhibits adenylate cyclase
Nicotinic	Very high affinity antagonist and bungarotoxin; seen at neuromuscular junction
Opiate	
Mu	Mediates analgesia, morphine; selective
Delta	Enkephalin-selective; seen in limbic region
Kappa	Dynorphin-sensitive, deep layers of cerebral cortex
Epsilon	Beta-endorphin–selective
Adenosine	
A$_1$	Labeled by ^{3}(H)-cyclohexyadenosine; inhibits adenylate cyclase
A$_2$	Labeled by 5^1-N(^{3}H)-ethylcarboxamide adenosine
Histamine	
H$_1$	Mediates bronchoconstriction; agonist—2-methylhistamine
H$_2$	Mediates gastric secretion; antagonist—cimetidine
Serotonergic	
5-HT$_{1a}$	Found in raphe and hippocampus; agonist is 8DH-DPAT; Opens K$^+$ channels
5-HT$_{1b}$	May regulate reuptake of serotonin; found concentrated in globus pallidus and substantia nigra
5-HT$_{1c}$	Found in choroid plexus; increases Cl$^-$ flux and interacts with LSD with high affinity
5-HT$_{1d}$	Also may be involved in serotonin reuptake; also found in basal ganglia in high concentration; agonist—methoxytroptamine
5-HT$_2$	Found in cortex; appears to interact through G proteins with phosphoinositol system
5-HT$_3$	Receptor that modulates Ca^{2+} flux and also may be coupled to phosphoinositol system in some sites; antagonist—Z acopride
GABAergic	
GABA A	Activated by muscimol; inhibited by bicuculline; increases CL$^-$ flux; found in highest concentration in hippocampus, striatum, and spinal cord; two subtypes have recently been cloned
GABA B	May act through G protein; presynaptic localization
Excitatory amino acid receptors	
NMDA (*N*-Methyl-D-aspartate)	Found in hippocampus and forebrain; selective antagonist—D-AP5
AMPA	Widespread distribution in CNS; may be receptor responsible for EPSP; specifically activated by glutamate; selective agonist—quisqualate
Kainic	Found concentrated in limbic system; selective agonist—kainic acid

nucleus consisting of a few thousand neurons located around the midline at the base of the pons. This nucleus takes its name from the blue color, owing to pigmented neurons, seen in primates and humans. Outflow from the locus goes along five major tracts and results in widespread innervation. Three tracts ascend to the cortical regions, following the major blood vessels and fascicular routes. These include (1) the central tegmental tract, (2) the central dorsal gray longitudinal fasciculus tracts, and (3) the ventral tegmental-medial forebrain tract. These pathways provide innervation to the thalamus and the hypothalamus as well as a relatively diffuse and even innervation of cortical areas. Another major outflow goes through the superior cerebellar peduncle to innervate the cerebellar cortex, while the final outflow pathway descends through the mesencephalon to the spinal cord. The other source of norepinephrine neurons is the lateral tegmental group. These cells are more diffuse than those located in the locus ceruleus. They are scattered throughout the lateral tegmental fields. The outflow from these cells mingles with the tracts from the locus. A major outflow goes to the spinal cord and another innervates the areas of the limbic system.

The fine structure of the anatomic innervation may provide an important clue to the functions of this system. There is a general pattern of innervation. The branches move into the cortical area by going through myelinated tracts up to cortical areas; then the axons form a characteristic T-shaped branch, with fine branches running parallel to the surface of the molecular layer. From these fine branches, nerve terminals come off at regular intervals. Studies suggest that not all these presynaptic boutons make contact with a postsynaptic membrane. Thus the fine structure points to a system that, at one level at least, is ideally structured to modulate the function of a wide area of cortex. This is not a system designed to deliver information from one nucleus directly to another (Descarries et al., 1977). The study of central norepinephrine pathways suggest that, at least in some instances, the transmitter acts to inhibit firing by way of a slow, hyperpolarizing response, which results in increased membrane resistance. The mechanism that appears responsible for this operates through the second messenger system by way of cyclic adenosine monophosphate (cAMP) formation. Pharmacologic studies suggest that a beta-adrenergic receptor mediates the response.

METABOLISM

All the catecholamines are derived from the amino acid tyrosine. The biosynthetic pathway is shown in Figure 28-2A. The first enzyme in the pathway is

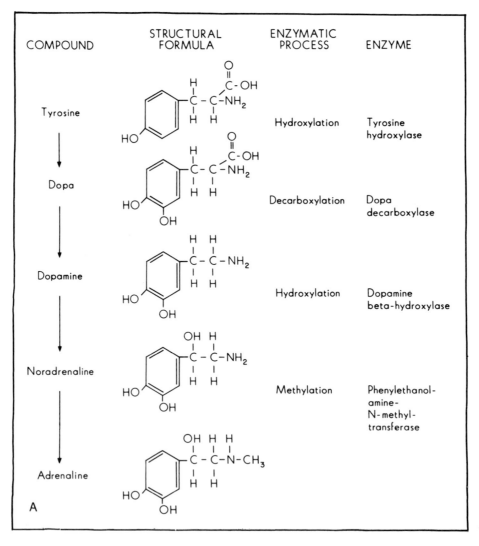

FIGURE 28-2A.   *The sequential synthesis of the catecholamines.* (From Gardiner, E: Fundamentals of Neurology. Philadelphia, W.B. Saunders Company, 1975, with permission.)

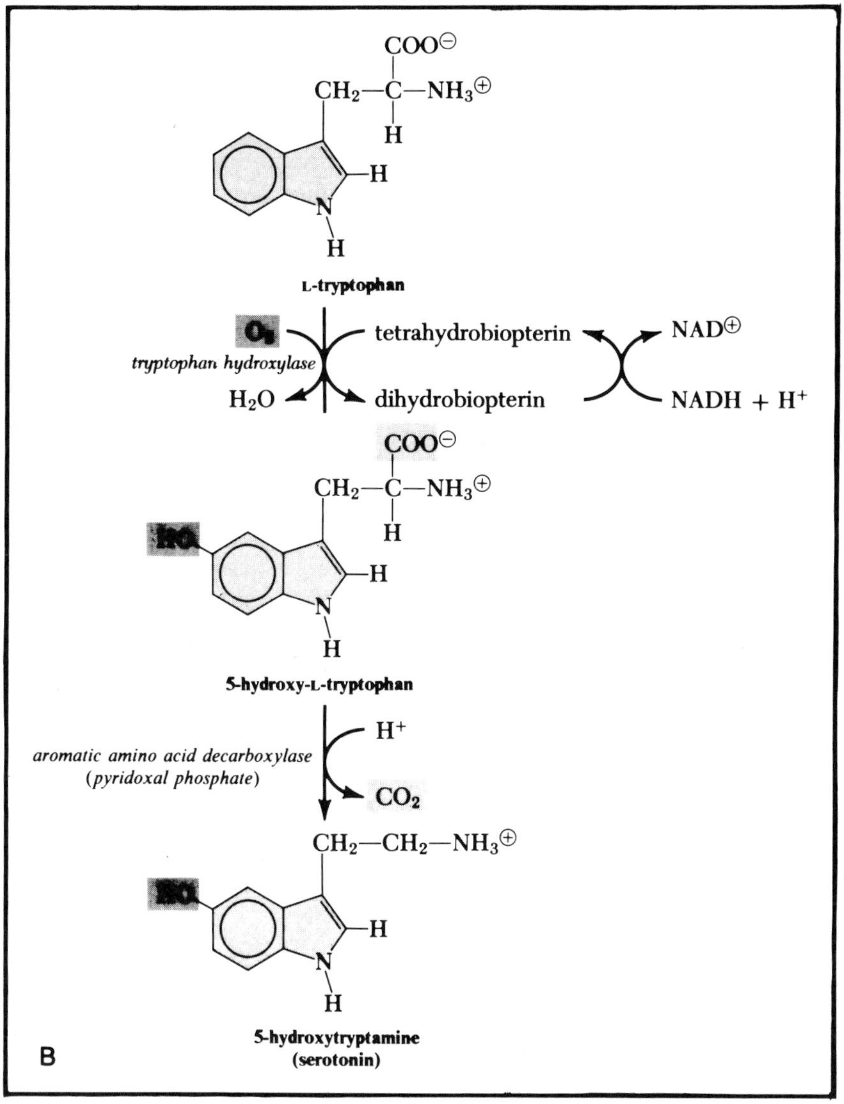

FIGURE 28-2B.   *The formation of serotonin from tryptophan.* (From McGilvery RW: Biochemistry: A functional approach. Philadelphia, W.B. Saunders Company, 1983.)

tyrosine hydroxylase, first described by Underfriend in 1966. This enzyme is specific to catecholamine-containing neurons in the CNS and the peripheral nervous system. It also controls the rate-limiting step in the synthesis of these compounds. The enzyme exhibits a high degree of stereospecificity, requires oxygen, Fe^{2+}, and a tetrahydropteridine cofactor, probably tetrahydrobiopterin. The K_m of the enzyme is in the range of 10^{-5}, while other enzymes in the biosynthetic pathway are 100- to 1000-fold more active. The next enzyme in this pathway is aromatic amino acid decarboxylase. The decarboxylase is not specific for DOPA, nor is its distribution restricted to nerve cells. It is an active

nonspecific decarboxylase that takes DOPA and converts it into dopamine. Inhibition of this enzyme has little effect on the concentration of norepinephrine available in tissue. The final enzyme used in the synthesis of norepinephrine is dopamine-β-hydroxylase. This enzyme is only present in adrenergic neurons but does not have a high degree of specificity. It will oxidize almost any phenylethylamine to the corresponding phenylethanolamine. The final enzyme that should be mentioned is phenylethanolamine-*N*-methyl transferase. This enzyme converts norepinephrine to epinephrine in the adrenal medulla and probably in the CNS as well.

The regulation of the synthesis of norepinephrine is complex and under a variety of controls. As mentioned, tyrosine hydroxylase is the rate-limiting enzyme. For example, when sympathetic nerves are repetitively stimulated, there is a marked increase in the synthesis of norepinephrine. The opposite effect is noted when tissues are exposed to monoamine oxidase inhibitors, compounds that prevent the breakdown of catecholamines and result in increased tissue levels of these compounds. This is evidence that a feedback loop controls the synthesis of norepinephrine. The studies aimed at defining this control mechanism have demonstrated a complex set of phenomena. Initially, studies on sympathetic nerve stimulation demonstrated that no new molecules of tyrosine hydroxylase were formed; rather, the enzyme showed greater activity per molecule under conditions of stimulation. This was explained by the demonstration that catechols could inhibit the enzyme; thus, when they were depleted, the enzyme was no longer inhibited, and synthesis increased. However, end-product inhibition did not explain all the changes seen. The enzyme appears to have altered affinities for cofactors and inhibitors after the period of active neuronal depolarization. Such alteration may be due to allosteric changes mediated by phosphorylation of the enzyme. This action could be mediated by way of calcium influx or cAMP and provides a second mechanism to regulate norepinephrine synthesis. If prolonged neuronal activity takes place, another mechanism comes into play. This involves the synthesis of new enzyme molecules. Even this brief consideration of the controls acting at the level of a rate-controlling enzyme suggests that this is an area in which both pharmacologic intervention and physiologic error can occur. The three mechanisms are general and can apply to most enzyme systems studied: (1) end-product inhibition, (2) allosteric alteration of activity (e.g., phosphorylation), and (3) new synthesis of enzyme. The signals for such regulatory steps can be varied as well. For example, hormonal signals can trigger such responses, as can signals from other neuromodulators. Thus the complexity and subtlety of the controls that regulate CNS activity can begin to be seen.

The breakdown of a neurotransmitter is another important step in controlling its activity. In general, the activity of released neurotransmitters is a function of how much is at an active receptor site. Thus the transport and metabolism of the transmitter directly affect its activity. The two enzymes that degrade the catecholamines are monoamine oxidase (MAO) and catechol-O-methyltransferase (COMT). The MAO enzymes oxidize amines to their corresponding aldehydes, while COMT adds a methyl group to the ring hydroxyl. There appear to be two forms of MAO, A and B. MAO A is inhibited by clorgyline and has a preference for norepinephrine and serotonin. MAO B is inhibited by deprenyl and prefers β-phenylethylamine as a substrate. Dopamine is equally metabolized by both forms. MAO is localized to the outer mitochondrial membrane. COMT appears to be, at least in part, extraneuronal and requires S-adenosinemethionine, a methyl donor, to function. Short-term inhibition of either of these enzymes does not appear to potentiate the effects of peripheral sympathetic nerve stimulation, suggesting that another mechanism must control the removal of the transmitter from the receptor site.

RELEASE AND UPTAKE

Once norepinephrine is synthesized, it is packaged and stored in granules. These subcellular particles occur in all tissues with catecholamines and serve to sequester the compounds, protect them from metabolism, and have them ready for release. The granules contain adenosine triphosphate (ATP) and dopamine-β-hydroxylase and may be the site for the final synthetic step converting dopamine to norepinephrine. These granules appear to be predominantly made in the cell body and transported down the axon to the nerve terminus. After nerve stimulation, norepinephrine is released at the synapse. This release is Ca^{2+} dependent. In the adrenal, it occurs by way of exocytosis, the contents of the granule being released as the granule fuses with the plasma membrane. It is unlikely that this occurs, at least exclusively, in the CNS. First, there is evidence that newly synthesized transmitters are preferentially released, and second, it is unlikely that the rate of synthesis of the granule proteins and ATP is sufficient to have them released with each nerve impulse. What is clear is that the permeability changes caused by the nerve impulse results in increased Ca^{2+} influx and release of norepinephrine into the synaptic clef.

After the transmitter is released, it reacts with the appropriate postsynaptic receptor. This action triggers the response in the postsynaptic cell. It is terminated by removal of the transmitter from the area of the membrane receptors. In the case of the catecholamines, the removal is accomplished by a high-affinity uptake system. This mechanism controls the immediate level of activity of norepinephrine at the receptor site. Iversen (1971) described a high-affinity uptake system with K_m values in the range of $10^{-8} M$. Although other cells in the CNS, notably glia, can transport catecholamines, their transport systems do not have the high affinity noted for the presynaptic system. Thus, after release, the transmitter is taken back up into the presynaptic neuron, where it can be stored in the storage granules and reused again. While this happens to a portion of the transmitter, some is metabolized. Not only does the norepinephrine neuron have sites for reuptake, but there are also presynaptic receptors, thought to be alpha$_2$ receptors, that regulate the rate of release. High levels of extracellular norepinephrine acting on these pre-synaptic receptors inhibit the release of more trans-mitter. An alternative control that does not involve presynaptic receptors uses prostaglandin E. This mechanism appears to limit the availability of Ca^{2+} and thus inhibit the release of norepinephrine.

Dopamine

The first neurotransmitter candidate to be formed in the biosynthetic reactions detailed earlier is dopa-mine. This catecholamine does not have a periph-eral system, such as the sympathetic nervous sys-tem; however, it is well defined because of its distinct role in the fine control of movement. It also is the transmitter implicated in psychotic processes owing to the pharmacology of the antipsychotic drugs.

DOPAMINE SYSTEM ANATOMY

The anatomy of the dopamine system is somewhat different than that of the adrenergic system. It in-volves discrete pathways and many more cells than the norepinephrine system. In general, there are three main projections of dopamine neurons and four minor systems. The major pathways include two long projections. First is the nigrostriatal path-way, linking the cells of the substantia nigra with those of the caudate and the putamen. This path-way, well known because of its role in Parkinson's disease, plays a role in the control of fine motor movements and has been well studied. The second pathway, now receiving more study because of its proposed role in psychotic illness, involves the pro-jections of cells in the ventral tegmental area to limbic and cortical areas. These are referred to as the *mesolimbic* and *mesocortical projections*. The final ma-jor pathway is the tuberohypophysial system, which has cells in the arcuate and periventricular nuclei projecting into the intermediate lobe of the pituitary. This short pathway plays a role in prolac-tin release.

The minor pathways are either short, such as the tuberohypophysial pathway, or intrinsic to cer-tain structures. The two intrinsic pathways include retinal cells linking the outer and inner plexiform layers and a group of cells in the olfactory bulb linking mitral cells from separate glomeruli. The short pathways involve cells in the dorsal posterior hypothalamus projecting to the dorsal anterior hy-pothalamus and septal nuclei and a group of cells around the dorsal motor nucleus of the vagal nerve.

METABOLISM

The metabolism of dopamine has been detailed under the discussion of norepinephrine. The bio-synthesis takes place through tyrosine hydroxylase and the degradation through MAO and COMT. The controls outlined earlier play a role in dopamine

regulation. The major antipsychotic drugs all inter-act with the dopamine system as either blockers or antagonists. Thus they cause increased dopamine synthesis. Chronic treatment results in differences in response between the long tracts for atypical drugs, such as thioridazine. The nigrostriatal tract appears not to go into depolarization block when atypical neuroleptics are used. Thus the increased rate of dopamine synthesis and release continues in cells of the substantia nigra. This results in a partial reversal of the dopamine blockage in this pathway. Thus less in the way of motor side effects is seen with these drugs.

RELEASE AND UPTAKE

The production and storage of dopamine are similar to those of norepinephrine. It is stored in granules and released in response to neuronal activity. The uptake system is also similar, having a high-affinity system located on the presynaptic membrane. The story of dopamine postsynaptic effects is not as clear, however. It is usually stated that dopamine is an inhibitory transmitter. However, the electro-physiologic data are ambiguous.

Serotonin

Serotonin (5-hydroxytryptamine, 5-HT) was first isolated by investigators as a possible hypertensive agent. It was a potent agent for the contraction of smooth muscle and only later was it identified in the CNS. After isolation of the hallucinogen LSD, it was found that serotonin and LSD apparently interacted at the same receptor in smooth muscle. This, plus the finding that reserpine depleted serotonin, soon led to a number of theories about its action in a variety of mental illnesses. Although some of these theories, such as those concerning psychotic illness, faded only to re-emerge, others, such as those con-cerned with affective disorders, are still very much under consideration.

SEROTONIN CELL ANATOMY IN THE CNS

Although 5-HT was shown to form fluorescent con-densation products when reacted with formal-dehyde vapors, it has been more difficult to get detailed anatomic data about this system. This is due to the short lifetime of the fluorescence and the inability to measure the nerve terminals using this technique. By applying immunocytochemical tech-niques, a fairly good picture of the anatomy has emerged. In general, 5-HT–containing neurons lie in clusters around the midline of the pons and up-per brain stem. These midline, or raphe, nuclei lie in nine distinct groups. In general, the lower or caudal nuclei project down to the medulla and the spinal cord, while the upper groups project to the limbic and cortical areas. The terminal fields of these neu-rons are diffuse and relatively formless. The fine structure of the 5-HT system has been the subject of a great deal of discussion. Descarries et al. (1975) have pointed out that the boutons of the 5-HT, as well as norepinephrine neurons, have widespread, relatively even distribution. Most important, the presynaptic boutons do not appear always to make contact with the postsynaptic membrane. This type of anatomy gives rise to the possibility that the 5-HT is functioning as a modulating system, regulating information flow in other transmitter systems.

METABOLISM

Peripherally, serotonin is predominantly found in cells, such as mast cells; however, peripheral serotonin cannot cross the blood–brain barrier. In the CNS, synthesis takes place in neurons. Tryptophan, another amino acid, is the precursor for 5-HT. The level of tryptophan intake in the diet controls the rate of serotonin synthesis in brain. Tryptophan is hydroxylated by the enzyme tryptophan decarboxyhydroxylase and then decarboxylated to form 5-HT. The rate-limiting step appears to be the hydroxylation, but this seems to be controlled by the amount of tryptophan available. In other words, the enzyme does not appear to be saturated under normal conditions. The decarboxylase is not the same general enzyme discussed under norepinephrine metabolism. Although its function is similar and the same enzyme operates peripherally, the CNS appears to have two separate and distinct decarboxylases. The synthesis of serotonin can be blocked with p-chlorophenylalanine, an inhibitor of tryptophan hydroxylase. This drug combines irreversibly with the enzyme, and the synthesis of more serotonin requires the synthesis of new enzyme molecules. The breakdown of 5-HT proceeds through MAO and the further oxidation of the aldehyde produced to form 5-hydroxyindoleacetic acid (5-HIAA). The control of serotonin synthesis does not appear to involve end-product inhibition. It may involve some feedback relating neuronal impulse flow to tryptophan hydroxylase activity; however, the nature of these controls is not clear.

RELEASE AND UPTAKE

Serotonin is stored in granules in nerve endings, just as the catecholamines. Release also appears to be Ca^{2+} dependent. The reuptake systems of serotonin are similar to those described for the catecholamines. The high-affinity uptake system is specific for serotonin and has been postulated to be the site of action of some antidepressant drugs. The drugs chlorimipramine and zimelidine are relatively specific inhibitors of 5-HT high-affinity transport systems, and recently available compounds such as the specific serotonin reuptake inhibitors (SSRIs) are quite specific. These drugs are used as antidepressants and antipanic/antiphobic agents.

PINEAL

The pineal gland, situated at the base of the brain outside the blood–brain barrier, is rich in serotonin. Here 5-HT may serve as a precursor for the synthesis of melatonin. Both melatonin and serotonin are under the control of environmental light, which entrains them in a cyclic daily rhythm. As such, melatonin is a marker of circadian rhythms, an area of active investigation in affective disorders. The control of melatonin is regulated directly by noradrenergic beta receptors, coupled to a second messenger system.

Acetylcholine

Acetylcholine (ACh) was the first neurotransmitter described and identified. It is used at the neuromuscular junction and by the parasympathetic nervous system. The exact nature of its central pathways has been difficult to determine, however, and although the study of this system's molecular details is fairly advanced, the system's functional aspects are by no means complete.

ANATOMY

The distribution of cholinergic neurons is widespread centrally. There are two groups of projecting nuclei as well as several sites in which cholinergic cells act as interneurons. Two areas of importance for psychiatry in which ACh neurons act as interneurons include the nucleus accumbens and the striatum. The cells in the basilar portion of the forebrain, especially the basal nucleus of Mynert, are also of increasing interest, having been implicated in dementias of the Alzheimer type. The fine structure of ACh systems suggest that many of the cells do project directly to a postsynaptic surface. Several features of ACh suggest that this compound also might have a hormonal role, as suggested earlier for the other amines. Among these is the stimulation of phosphate into phosphoinositol, the ability to release catecholamines, and a possible role in Na^+ transport in corneal epithelium.

METABOLISM

The synthesis of acetylcholine looks simple. It is a reaction in which acetylcoenzyme A (acetyl-CoA) and choline are joined to form ACh. The enzyme catalyzing this reaction is choline acetyltransferase. The two substrates appear to be common metabolities. Acetyl-CoA is the principal metabolite formed from the degradation of sugars or fats, while choline is a central constituent of lipids. It turns out that glucose is the preferred substrate for the formation of acetyl-CoA in the brain, while choline is not synthesized at all in the brain. Thus the choline must either be transported into the CNS or come from phospholipids, such as phosphatidylcholine.

This lipid is one of the main constituents of cell membranes; thus the synthesis of ACh is intimately tied to the metabolism of principal cell constituents glucose and phospholipid. The degradation of ACh is carried out by esterases, the most specific of which is acetylcholine esterase. Unlike the catecholamines and amino acid transmitters, ACh is not taken up to terminate its action after presynpatic release; rather, it is hydrolyzed. Acetylcholine esterase is well equipped to carry out the function, being one of the most rapid and efficient enzymes known. It is at this site that irreversible organophosphorous inhibitors bind. This binding results in the fatal buildup of ACh seen when these compounds were used as nerve gases. In addition to this enzyme, there are non-specific esterases, known as *butyrylcholinesterases*, which are less specific for ACh and not localized to neurons. They may, in fact, be associated with glial membranes and probably serve as a safety factor to ensure the destruction of all free ACh.

STORAGE, RELEASE, AND UPTAKE

Studies on the neuromuscular junction, the work of Katz (1966) and colleagues, demonstrated the quantal release of ACh. When ACh vesicles were discovered, an obvious interpretation was that the contents of a vesicle constituted a quanta of neuro-transmitter. This interpretation has been challenged in the CNS on the following grounds: (1) it is clear that newly synthesized ACh is preferentially re-leased, (2) in large axons of *Aplysia*, the injection of acetylcholinesterase inhibits release of ACh, sug-gesting that free, not bound, ACh is released, and (3) the speed of CNS transmission appears too fast for exocytotic release of vesicles to provide transmit-ter for each firing. Other facts in the discussion of the role of vesicles in transmitter release are the syn-apses, such as those using amino acids, which do not have vesicular storage. These fire as efficiently as those systems that do have storage granules. The release of ACh is a Ca^{2+}-mediated process. There is no high-affinity uptake system for ACh; rather, as mentioned earlier, the action of this transmitter is terminated by hydrolysis. There is, however, a high-affinity transport process to transport choline, one of the products of the hydrolysis. Choline is taken back up into the presynaptic neuron, where it is a valuable precursor for the resynthesis of ACh. The reuptake process is saturable and energy depend-ent, as are those described for the monoamines. The choline uptake system appears to be localized to regions of cholinergic innervation.

Amino Acid Transmitters

Although the amino acids are not as directly in-volved in the theories of psychiatric illnesses as the transmitters discussed thus far, they probably con-stitute the workhorses of both excitatory and inhibi-tory transmission. Dysfunction of these systems

may not be compatible with life; nonetheless, subtle changes in the transmission of these systems may play an important role in the control of mood and emotion. This is hinted at by the actions of the benzodiazepines, which probably affect the gamma-aminobutyric acid (GABA) system, which will be discussed when anxiety disorders are con-sidered. The principal excitatory amino acids are glutamic acid and aspartic acid, while the sulfur-containing amino acids are also being considered as reasonable neurotransmitter candidates. The pre-dominant inhibitory amino acids are GABA and glycine, with taurine being somewhat of a mystery candidate.

From the standpoint of neurotransmission, GABA is the most studied amino acid. This com-pound was found to be a major constituent of the CNS more than 30 years ago. A problem with at-tempts to define its anatomic distribution is its al-most ubiquitous distribution wherever neurons or nerve endings exist in the CNS. There is a gradient in the density of GABA between various cellular areas of the CNS, with the highest concentration found in the substantia nigra and globus pallidus and the lowest in the cerebellar cortex. The ratio between the concentration in these regions is less than 3, whereas the ratio between the cerebellar concentration, the area of cells with the lowest GABA concentrations, and regions of pure white matter exceeds 7. Any attempt to define GABA pathways suffers from an embarrassment of riches. It is safe to say that GABA plays a role in most CNS systems. One of the best ways to localize GABA is to examine the localization of glutamic acid decarbox-ylase (GAD), using immunocytochemical methods. This enzyme constitutes the biosynthetic pathway for the synthesis of GABA. Two forms of the enzyme exist—one primarily localized to GABAergic neu-rons and the other found in heart, glia, and kidney. These enzymes exhibit a differential sensitivity to Cl^- ion, with the neuronal enzyme showing inhibi-tion to the ion. The two forms of GAD are also immunologically distinct.

The synthesis of GABA takes place primarily in nerve endings. Although GABA does not appear to be stored in vesicles, it is estimated that high con-centrations of GABA are reached in the synaptic cleft; these have been calculated to be in the range of 100 mM. There is some evidence that GAD un-dergoes feedback inhibition; this must therefore take place at relatively high product concentrations. The cofactor used by the enzyme, pyridoxyl-5-phosphate, may be the other site of synthesis regu-lation. The enzyme may only be one-third saturated under some in vivo conditions.

The degradation of GABA involves two en-zymes that form a shunt pathway into the Krebs cycle. GABA transaminase (GABA-T) transfers an amine group from GABA to α-oxyglutamate—forming succinic semialdehyde. This can be further metabolized by a dehydrogenase to succinic acid, which then follows along the Krebs cycle. Its significance, metabolically, is unclear. For our purposes, it is important to note that GABA-T is widely distributed and rapidly metabolizes GABA. When released, GABA is rapidly taken up by high-affinity transport systems located both in the presynaptic neuron and on adjacent glial cells.

On release, GABA acts on a postsynaptic receptor that appears to be coupled to the Cl^- ion channel, thus inhibiting firing. This molecular receptor complex appears to be the site of action of the benzodiazepines, which act to increase the affinity of the GABA receptor for GABA. Bicuculline acts as an antagonist of the GABA receptor, while picrotoxin is a specific antagonist of the Cl^- ion channel.

The two other amino acids that appear to have inhibitory actions on neurons are glycine, which appears to act specifically on spinal cord neurons, and taurine, a sulfur-containing amino acid. Glycine has a high-affinity uptake system and asymmetrical distribution and mimics the inhibitory transmitter's actions on neurons in the spinal cord. Strychnine is a glycine antagonist. Taurine is found in high concentrations in mammalian brain; it has high-affinity uptake systems, is released in a Ca^{2+}-dependent process, and acts iontophoretically to inhibit neurons. This amino acid is crucial for the maintenance of photoreceptors, and the absence of taurine in the diet of kittens will cause photoreceptor degeneration. Because few drugs affect taurine, little is known about the CNS role this amino acid plays.

On the excitatory side of the spectrum, glutamate and aspartate appear as likely neurotransmitter candidates. Disassociating the metabolic pools of these amino acids from the putative transmitter pools has been difficult. The use of lesions in cerebellum and hippocampus supports the idea that glutamate is an excitatory neurotransmitter. Glutamate has a high and asymmetrical concentration in the CNS; possesses a high-affinity uptake system found in both neurons and glia, shows CA^{2+}-dependent release, and its biosynthesis is under feedback control. These are all properties that would be expected of a neurotransmitter.

NEUROPEPTIDES

The most rapidly emerging area of study in the neurosciences is that of peptides. To date, nearly 50 peptides have been proposed to be in the brain. Of these, at least 33 shown in Table 28-2 have been identified in mammalian neurons. Such a vast addition to the chemical messengers present in the CNS increases greatly the complexity of interactions possible. Several general features should be mentioned; first, there is probably no "typical" action for all peptides. True, they have been proposed to serve a modulatory role and to act over greater distances

TABLE 28-2. *Neuropeptides*

Pituitary peptides
 Corticotropin (ACTH)
 Growth hormone (GH)
 Lipotropin
 α-Melanocyte-stimulating hormone (alpha-MSH, three forms)
 Oxytocin
 Vasopressin
Hypothalamic-releasing hormones
 Corticotropin-releasing factor (CRF)
 Luteinizing hormone–releasing factor (LHRH)
 Somatostatin
 Thyrotropin-releasing hormone (TRH)
Circulating hormones
 Angiotensin
 Calcitonin
 Glucagon
 Insulin
Gut hormones
 Cholecystokinin (CCK)
 Gastrin
 Motilin
 Pancreatic polypeptide (PP)
 Secretin
 Substance P
 Vasoactive intestinal polypeptide (VIP)
 Opioid peptides
 Dynorphin
 β-Endorphin (three forms)
 Met-enkephalin
 Leu-enkephalin
 Kyotorphin
Miscellaneous peptides
 Bombesin
 Bradykinin
 Carnosine
 Neuropeptide Y
 Neurotensin
 Proctolin
 Substance K

and with a slower time course than normal transmitters. Undoubtedly some do, just as ACh, norepinephrine, and 5-HT may play such a modulatory role. An example of such an action is the role of luteinizing hormone–releasing hormone in the sympathetic ganglia of bullfrogs. This peptide probably exists in the same neurons as ACh but acts over much greater distances and has a much longer time course (Jan et al., 1980).

Other peptides, such as substance P, appear to act as classic synaptic neurotransmitters. In one respect, most larger peptides do share two unique properties for chemical messengers in the brain.

1. They are synthesized by way of the protein synthetic machinery of the cell, transcribed from DNA to messenger RNA, an energy- and time-consuming process.
2. The active portions are finally formed by the cleavage of larger peptides or prohormones, which usually contain a family of neuroactive peptides that are liberated by the action of cleavage enzymes.

These two features may at times operate together, since prohormones can give rise to multiple active peptides. The sequential release of peptides from a single precursor may govern a particular type of behavior. Many peptides are colocalized with other transmitters. Colocalization does not imply corelease, and in fact, it may be that the peptide is released only under certain conditions. For example, after a certain level of excitation is reached, peptides may be coreleased and alter the response to the classic transmitter.

An example of the multiple peptides of one family coming from one precursor is the story of pro-opiomelanocortin. This prohormone, identified and characterized from pituitary tissue, gives rise to the three forms of melanocyte-stimulating hormone, adrenocorticotropin hormone, and three forms of β-endorphin. Of particular interest is that various forms of β-endorphin are found in different proportions in different parts of the brain. For example, in the anterior pituitary, the full-length 1–31 amino acid form of β-endorphin predominates, while in the intermediate lobe, the shorter forms 1–26 and 1–27 β-endorphins constitute the major forms. This suggests that particular attention should be paid to the cleavage enzymes and the cleavage conditions, for they may alter the functions performed by the peptides.

A final example of how a family of peptides produced by closely related genes can regulate complex behavior comes from studies of the egg-laying behavior of *Aplysia*. This process, which involves a series of specific stereotypical behaviors, is induced by the extract of a group of cells known as *bag cells*. Actions in the bag cells and atrial gland of the animal appear to control this behavioral pattern, and it turns out that a related gene family differentially expressed in these tissues generates the peptides that control this behavior. Egg-laying hormone (ELH), a 36-amino-acid peptide, and α-BCP (bag cell peptide) are made in bag cells, while two closely related peptides, A and B, are made in the atrial gland. These peptides cause long-lasting activity in the CNS of *Aplysia*, which corresponds to the behavioral time course and results in egg laying. The genes encoding for these peptides appear to be different but are 90 percent homologous, and the peptides are quite different. These differences in structure are accomplished through selective cleavage of the precursor protein, in this case directed by the genes involved. ELH and α-BCP act together but in different ways. ELH causes long-lasting (hours) effects, while α-BCP causes effects that last for minutes. By coming from a common precursor, long- and short-term effects appear to be coordinated. Thus it may be that specific behavioral sequences are partially programmed into the peptide patterns produced in related families of genes. It is not known whether such a behavioral control exists in mammals, but it is probable that it does and that it can be modified by other factors acting on the CNS.

Summary

It is hoped that this overview of neurosciences will remind the student of psychiatry of both the promise of the biologic revolution and the incompleteness of our knowledge. Nervous system function can be regulated in a variety of ways. Some have been used by earlier workers to explain brain function; others await integration into our understanding of the CNS. Subtle dysfunctions of the brain that are represented by psychiatric illnesses are probably due to a breakdown of regulatory mechanisms. By finding ways to modulate the balance between competing neuronal systems, we hope to create a new generation of drugs that will help us to control psychiatric illness with fewer side effects and more precision.

AFFECTIVE DISORDERS

In considering the biochemical theories of affective disorders, two major lines of research must be considered: The first involves the monoamine hypothesis, and the second involves neuroendocrine studies. The serious study of amines began in 1958, when Strom-Olsen and Weil-Malherbe reported on the catecholamine content of the urine of depressed and manic patients. They found an increase in catecholamines in mania and a decrease in catecholamines during depression. This discovery was the start of an extensive investigation of blood, urine, and cerebrospinal fluid (CSF) of depressed patients, leading to the formalization of the catecholamine hypothesis in the mid-1960s. The initial theory put forth by numerous investigators, including Prange (1964), Schildkraut (1965), and Bunney and Davis (1965), suggested that there was a functional deficit of norepinephrine at synapses in depression and an excess in mania. Although some of the original impetus for this theory was from metabolic studies, the strongest support came from pharmacology.

Four drugs having an effect on mood disorders were brought into use in the 1950s: lithium salts, reserpine, monoamine oxidase inhibitors, and tricyclic antidepressants. Lithium salts were described by Cade in 1948 (see Cade, 1970) and were investigated heavily in the late 1950s. Reserpine was isolated in 1952 and used to treat both hypertension and psychosis. Although it was soon displaced from the psychiatrist's armamentarium, internists found that up to 15 percent of people treated for high blood pressure developed clinically severe depression. With the advent of iproniazid to treat tubercular patients, reports began to come back from the sanatoriums of inappropriately high spirits and increased energy and sexual drive among the patients. This drug was soon shown to be a monoamine oxidase inhibitor. Finally, in the late fifties, imipramine was discovered, and the era of effective antidepressant treatment was well under way. For each of these drugs, some connection to monoamines was found. For example, lithium is effective against mania and appears to inhibit the release of monoamines to some extent. Reserpine causes depletion of the monoamines chronically, and chronic usage can lead to depression. Iproniazid was shown to be an effective treatment for depression, and as an MAO inhibitor, it raises the concentration of amines. Finally, the tricyclic antidepressants were shown to be effective uptake inhibitors of the amines. Thus considerable support came from early pharmacologic studies, suggesting that functional decreases in monoamines could be correlated with depression, whereas functional increases in these compounds led to mania.

One problem with these studies is that they do not define which monoamines are causing changes in mood. Most drug effects can be shown to involve 5-HT, norepinephrine, and dopamine. Detailed pharmacologic and metabolic studies have not resolved the issue of the relative importance of these compounds in affective disorders. Two factors have complicated the studies. First, most drugs lack specificity and act on a number of systems. Second, the metabolites measured may not reflect the state of the relevant amine at the areas of important synaptic contact. For example, it is possible that only 10 percent of the norepinephrine synapses matter. Thus, when 3-methoxy-4-hydroxyphenylglycol (MHPG), the main norepinephrine metabolite, is measured in urine, probably about half comes from the peripheral nervous system, and changes in the central metabolite would be lost in the normal variance of the system. Another problem that cannot be controlled for is the possibility of biochemical (genetic) heterogeneity among affective disorders.

A summary of the physiologic data for depression produces somewhat inconsistent results. Looking at norepinephrine, urine studies in general have shown decreased MHPG in series of bipolar depressed patients (Schildkraut, 1982) and no real differences in MHPG levels of unipolar depressed patients and controls. Because of the variability in the results and limitations of MHPG as a marker of central norepinephrine levels, these results have been less than conclusive. MHPG does appear to be increased in mania, and while not decreased in all studies of depression, it may have a bimodal distribution. In fact, one series of studies suggest that those patients with low urinary MHPG respond better to drugs operating on the norepinephrine system, while those with normal MHPG do better with drugs active on the 5-HT system. In looking at 5-HT, Coppen (1967) and colleagues have consistently reported that the 5-HT metabolite 5-HIAA is decreased in the urine of a subgroup of depressed patients. Measurements on CSF have provided similar results. The serotonin metabolite 5-HIAA definitely appears to have a bimodal distribution, with a subgroup of depressives having lower 5-HIAA

levels. Thus urine metabolite studies suggest heterogeneity, rather than supporting one amine as causative of depression. Studies of the enzymes involved in amine metabolism also have been inconclusive. Analyses of postmortem material from suicide victims also have been carried out. These studies showed lower 5-HIAA levels in suicide brains, but no other striking findings emerged. In an effort to make sense of these data, depressions have been divided into a series of biochemically defined subgroups: those involving low norepinephrine, showing decreased MHPG, and those with normal MHPG and, by inference, low 5-HT. These divisions led to specific therapeutic recommendations. Those patients who had low MHPG should be more responsive to drugs acting on norepinephrine uptake, such as imipramine, whereas the normal MHPG group should be responsive to drugs with mixed or 5-HT activity, such as amitriptyline. These predictions have some support in the literature but have generally not been clinically useful. In part, this could be predicted, since antidepressants probably do not work by acting on uptake systems, as assumed in these formulations.

Precursor loading is also an approach that continues to be studied. This was first attempted by Pare and Sandler in 1959 using L-DOPA to increase dopamine and norepinephrine. Coppen and associates (1967) reported that tryptophan in high doses was an effective antidepressant for women. Currently, tyrosine is being suggested as a possible antidepressant. In general, the data suggest that substrate loading of the norepinephrine system is activating and that such loading of the 5-HT system helps to induce sleep, but neither approach results in clinically uniform antidepressant activity.

Thus, taken together, the physiologic data strongly suggest that amines are involved in depressive illness and that a unitary amine hypothesis is insufficient to account for the data. In other words, the general association between amine levels and mood appears to allow an understanding of the general biology of depression, but when a closer examination is made and the details are examined, no particular theory appears to hold up.

By examining the pharmacologic data, an analogous conclusion can be reached. The initial data suggested that all effective treatments for depression raised the concentration of amines. MAO inhibitors certainly operate this way by inhibiting the degradation of amines. The tricyclics are thought to inhibit reuptake of amines, and this is consistent. A closer look, however, poses the same problems seen with the physiologic studies. Tricyclics have widely varying ability to inhibit the uptake of norepinephrine and 5-HT, yet they are about equally effective in clinical situations if given in adequate dosage. Furthermore, their ability to inhibit amine reuptake is a rapid process, effective essentially as soon as effective concentrations are reached. Yet, clinically, these drugs sometimes take weeks to take effect. An even greater challenge to the reuptake theory is presented by newer anti-depressants. Mianserin and trazodone are effective antidepressants, yet they do not block the reuptake of either norepinephrine or 5-HT at clinically useful dosages. Thus the pharmacologic theories have had to undergo considerable revision.

New theories have been proposed that relate to receptor sensitivity changes. As mentioned earlier, a receptor is the mechanism by which a chemical transmitter signals its target cell. Receptors can undergo a variety of changes, analogous to those seen by enzymes, that alter the efficacy with which they translate a transmitter's message. For example, they can undergo conformational changes in response to the binding of small molecules that alter the affinity of their ligand, or the cell can change the absolute number of receptors in response to external conditions. These changes in functional receptors result in either up regulation or down regulation at the point of transmitter action. When antidepressant medications are given, the CNS receptors respond by down regulating. This was initially noted for beta-adrenergic receptors. All known treatments for depression, including electroconvulsive shock, result in the down-regulation of beta receptors. This down-regulation takes place over the same time course as the behavioral change caused by these medications. Thus one newer theory of antidepressant drug activity suggests that these compounds act to down-regulate beta receptors. Another receptor that has been proposed to play a role in antidepressant action is the alpha$_2$ receptor. These receptors sit on the presynaptic membrane and regulate the release of norepinephrine. When these receptors are stimulated, they inhibit the release of norepinephrine, forming a feedback loop to control adrenergic activity. There is evidence from basic and clinical studies that these receptors are down-regulated by antidepressants, thus allowing increased norepinephrine release.

The other neurotransmitter system discussed in depression, the 5-HT system, also has generated several receptor theories. Basically, data from antidepressant effects and CSF studies of 5-HIAA, the major metabolite of 5-HT, suggest that the efficacy of 5-HT is decreased in depression. This is supported by the action of fluoxetine and sertraline, two specific 5-HT uptake inhibitors that have proven to be effective antidepressants.

The result of all these pharmacologic studies has been a shift from the presynaptic neuron to the receptor field in theorizing about depression. Perhaps most important, a clear recognition that 5-HT and norepinephrine systems are related and in balance in the CNS is emerging (Janowsky et al., 1982). Thus no single transmitter can account for the changes seen in a complex behavioral phenomena such as depression. That the CNS is a complex interacting system with regard to mood is also seen looking at neuroendocrine variables. Norepineph-

rine inhibits the action of corticotropin-releasing factor and adrenocorticotropin. Thus it is no surprise that hypersecretion is seen in depressive states. This hypersecretion has become the basis of a laboratory test in which the potent corticosteroid dexamethasone is given and cortisol values are measured, usually at three intervals over the next 24 hours. In depressive states, there is an escape from the normal suppression seen after dexamethasone. In other words, continued cortisol is released. This test initially appeared to be relatively specific for depression; however, escape from dexamethasone suppression of cortisol production can be seen in a variety of other conditions, including conditions that involve decreased food intake. This test is a useful clinical correlate to the depressive state, and a reversion to normal suppression may be a good biochemical index of remission from depression. The levels of circulating cortisol in the blood of some depressives can reach levels seen in Cushing's disease. This is reminiscent of the levels of cortisol seen in a primate when it loses a dominance struggle. After this occurs, the animal is socially isolated and withdrawn, features often seen in human depression, and its cortisol levels go up. Thus it may be that cortisol secretion is a response to any stressor, and for humans, depression is such a stressor. Therefore, the question is whether cortisol secretion is a result of other more basic sites of pathology or a reflection of the pathology of depression directly.

A summary of the biochemical theories of affective disorders would not be complete without mention of the ACh system. Janowsky and colleagues (1972) have proposed that depression results from an imbalance between cholinergic and adrenergic systems. The data include the ability of physostigmine, an ACh agonist, to alleviate temporarily the symptoms of mania. Thus affective states involve all the neurotransmitter systems most studied. It will then be no surprise that a variety of biochemical defects have been proposed as markers of affective disorders. Unfortunately, none has been reliably reproduced in independent laboratories.

There has been enormous effort and some progress in understanding affective disorders since the 1950s. However, a clear concept of the anatomy, physiology, and biochemistry of such disorders has not yet occurred. This challenge for the new generation of biologic psychiatrists will undoubtedly involve coordination of the actions of various transmitter substances.

ALZHEIMER'S DEMENTIA

Until recently, little could be said about the biochemical concomitants of senile or presenile dementia. However, with the emergence of Alzheimer's dementia as one of the major problems in an increasingly aging population, more effort has gone into its study, and results are constantly being brought forth. An intriguing story is emerging that may put together many of the diverse findings in senile dementia of the Alzheimer's type (SDAT). Pathologically, the disease is characterized by widespread neuritic amyloid plaques and neurofibrillary tangles. These are the signs of damaged and dying neurons in this disorder. Early investigations showed that the degree of dementia is correlated with the number of plaques found. These plaques and tangles are widespread over the cortical surface and, until recently, did not appear to offer any clues concerning localization of a specific defect. Recent postmortem studies suggest that memory loss may be correlated specifically with pathology in the subiculum of the hippocampus. This is the outflow connecting the hippocampus with the cortex and hypothalamus (Hyman et al., 1985). The careful measurement of enzyme levels in dementia by several groups in the mid-70s suggested that there is a marked decrease in acetylcholine in SDAT. Choline acetyl transferase was found to be decreased by more than 50 percent in autopsy samples of patients with SDAT, suggesting that cholinergic neurons might be involved in the disease. Parallel to this work, researchers began to examine the physiology of the basal forebrain. It was discovered that the area is heavily cholinergic and responds to rewards and higher order behaviors. The area also was found to project into the cortical region. Autopsy studies of SDAT patients revealed almost total loss of nucleus basalis cells (Whitehouse et al., 1982). This particular nucleus in the basal forebrain is cholinergic and has a variety of cortical projections. Even more suggestive lesion studies of primates using a potent neurotoxin results in loss of ACh in the cortex. Could the slow loss of cholinergic neurons from the nucleus basalis result in plaques and tangles and account for the pathology seen in SDAT? It is possible, but some other facts have recently emerged that must be integrated into the story. First, other transmitter systems are also involved. The noradrenergic system has clear evidence of cell loss and lowered transmitter levels (Perry et al., 1981). In addition, recent suggestions point to diminished 5-HT function as well (Bowden et al., 1983). This correlates with measures of cell loss or volume loss in patients with SDAT. It is found that brains from patients who suffered from this disorder can have decreases corresponding to 25 percent of volume, while ACh neurons probably account for no more than 10 percent of the total volume of the CNS. Somatostatin is also found to be decreased in postmortem brain samples and may be more decreased in temporal lobes than in frontal lobes. Thus the disease appears in its ultimate expression to be much more complex than a single-transmitter, single-nucleus problem.

Considerable work, including family history studies, and an association between SDAT and Down syndrome support a genetic factor. Down syndrome results from an extra copy of chromosome 21, which suggests that this chromosome may be involved. Recently, the most exciting work in this area has resulted from a study of amyloid, the central constituent of the plaques. It appears that amyloid plaques are produced by the aggregation of a small protein. The gene for the control of this protein has recently been cloned by several groups and appears to encode several proteins. A gene for a large protein, termed *amyloid precursor protein* (APP), was found to be encoded on chromosome 21. Recently, studies of familial Alzheimer's disease suggest that at least some forms are due to a mutation in this gene. Does the APP gene play a role in all forms of Alzheimer's, and how does it produce cell death? The answers to these questions and an understanding of the etiology of Alzheimer's disease may well come from studies using the techniques of molecular neurobiology. Recent studies have pointed to the possibility of a posttranslational processing defect as being responsible for amyloid production. These rapid developments suggest that there is finally hope of understanding this difficult group of diseases.

EDITORS' COMMENT

A recent report (Schellenberg GD et al: Science 258: 668–671, 1992) provided evidence for a familial Alzheimer's disease locus on chromosome 14. Another locus reported has been on the amyloid precursor protein. Both studies used early-onset multiply-affected Alzheimer's families (in the first the disease, at least in number, was verified by autopsy) in which the disease has been reported to segregate as an autosomal dominant trait. These two loci may be related or distinct. A third locus on chromosome 19 has also recently been reported (Strittmatter WJ, Saunders AM, Schmechel D et al., Proc Natl Acad Sci USA 90 (1977–1981), 1993, and Pericak-Vance MA, Bebout JL, Gaskell PC, et al., Am Hum Genet 48:1034–1050, 1991). This suggests that there may be several different etiologies which all lead to amyloid deposition and cell death giving a similar clinical picture.

SCHIZOPHRENIA

Although the forms of schizophrenia are varied and the core concept has been elusive, the two major biochemical theories have been remarkably consistent. The initial idea was that some toxin might be involved. This originated from observations on hallucinogens and very early on was incorporated into the methylation hypothesis of Osmond and Smythies (1952). This hypothesis suggested that aberrant metabolic pathways might produce a toxin that caused the schizophrenic illness. This concept arose from the observation that methylated forms of catecholamine metabolites are hallucinogens. Unfortunately, hallucinogens do not mimic the psychotic symptoms seen in schizophrenia with any close correspondence, nor has a naturally occurring toxin been isolated, despite the analysis of many gallons of schizophrenic urine and blood. For these reasons, methylation theories have recently received less attention.

The second biochemical theory of schizophrenia, the dopamine hypothesis, arose somewhat later. The principal lines of support came from a study of toxic psychosis, namely, amphetamine psychosis, and from the pharmacology of antipsychotic drugs. This theory, the dopamine hypothesis of schizophrenia, has been of enormous value in directing research efforts and in understanding the pharmacology of antipsychotic drugs.

The dopamine theory of schizophrenia suggests that the illness is a result of the functional overactivity of DA at certain CNS synapses. Historically, the evidence on which this hypothesis is based began to appear in the late 1950s. Connell (1958) provided a careful review of amphetamine psychosis and noted that this condition could result in a paranoid psychosis with a clear sensorium. When the patient was first seen, this was difficult to distinguish from typical paranoid schizophrenia unless a history of drug ingestion was obtained. Thus it was felt that perhaps the action of amphetamine might be analogous to what spontaneously happens in schizophrenia. This rationale suggested that an understanding of the action of amphetamine action centrally would give some clues to the CNS abnormalities in schizophrenia. Amphetamine was shown to act at both norepinephrine and DA synapses in a variety of ways. Because both amphetamine and norepinephrine have stereoisometric forms, while DA does not, it should be possible to distinguish the site of action centrally. One example of how this distinction is used involved a study of the ability of amphetamine to block the reuptake of catecholamines. The L amphetamine isomer is the more potent norepinephrine inhibitor, while the D and L forms block DA reuptake about equally well. This suggests that if the isomers of amphetamine are equally effective, the action is on the DA system. Angrist and colleagues (1971) used this type of analysis to examine the potency of D or L isomers of amphetamine in causing a paranoid psychosis. They found that D or L amphetamines were about equally potent in causing paranoid psychosis, leading to the conclusion that dopamine systems were probably involved in the production of this psychosis and, by implication, involved in schizophrenia.

The greatest thrust for investigations into the biochemical basis of schizophrenia began with the discovery of antipsychotic drugs. These compounds were introduced in the late 1950s. Delay and Deniker (1957), who discovered the activity of chlorpromazine, coined the word *neuroleptic* to emphasize the similar actions of two drugs, reserpine and chlorpromazine. These drugs had effects on motor functions and psychosis. The motor effects were analogous to the symptoms seen in parkinsonism, so studies of this disorder had implications for schizophrenia. In 1960, Ehringer and Hornykiewicz were able to demonstrate that in autopsy samples from patients with parkinsonism, DA was almost entirely depleted from the striatum. Because it was well known that reserpine depleted amines centrally, the fact that DA was depleted in parkinsonism and neuroleptics caused Parkinson-like symptoms pointed to the possibility that neuroleptic drugs worked by depleting DA. Studies on chlorpromazine and haloperidol soon showed they did not deplete DA levels; thus alternative actions were sought. Carlsson and Lindqvist (1963) examined the effect of these drugs on the accumulation of catecholamine metabolites. Increased levels of metabolites were found, and the authors postulated that this could occur if the drugs in some way block the DA signal and caused increased synthesis, followed by increased degradation of these compounds. This was the first suggestion that DA blockade was a mechanism of action for neuroleptics. This work and the studies on amphetamine psychosis led to the formulation of the DA hypothesis by Van Rossen (1966), which, simply stated, suggests that schizophrenia is associated with an overactivity of DA synapses.

There has been enormous support of the idea that neuroleptic drugs act through the blockage of central DA receptors. The ability of these drugs to antagonize DA has been demonstrated in receptor studies, biochemical studies, electrophysiologic studies, and behavioral studies, leaving little doubt that this is the mechanism of action of these compounds. Some of the strongest support for this idea came from biochemical studies. Kebabian and Greengard (1971) described a DA-sensitive adenylate cyclase in striatal tissue. This is a specific enzyme and turned out to be sensitive to inhibition by a variety of neuroleptics. Unfortunately, when carefully measured, this inhibition did not correlate with the clinical potency of these compounds. Butyrophenones, potent drugs clinically proved to be weak inhibitors of the DA, stimulated adenylate cyclase. This discrepancy between the potency of drug dosages used to treat psychosis and inhibit the production of cAMP was resolved by the finding of multiple DA receptors. This concept was initially suggested from studies of DA turnover and supported by electrophysiologic studies. With the advent of receptor-binding studies, it was directly demonstrated. The direct measurement of DA receptors began when Seeman and coworkers developed a binding assay using butyrophenones as ligands (1975). Subsequent work with other ligands has identified at least two DA receptors—D_1, which stimulates adenylate cyclase, and D_2, which does not and appears to be the receptor responsible for antipsychotic and motor effects. The correlation of D_2 sites as measured by butyrophenone binding with the clinical potency of these drugs is excellent. Recent work cloning dopamine receptors has revealed at least six distinct molecular forms. The role of each of these in psychosis is the next step in understanding the role of dopamine.

The pharmacologic evidence established the site of action of antipsychotic drugs, but the question that remains is whether DA overactivity is etiologically involved in the production of schizophrenia. For that, pharmacology will not do, and evidence of DA overactivity must be looked for. One approach is to look at the metabolites of DA in CSF. If overproduction occurs, then perhaps an increased level of DA metabolites would be found. Multiple laboratories have done this study, and the results do not support increased metabolite levels; rather, there is a tendency for lowered levels of HVA, the principal DA metabolite. Another way to look at DA activity is to recall that prolactin release is, in part, regulated by DA. Thus several studies have attempted to find a difference between schizophrenic patients and controls in serum prolactin levels. Careful studies (Meltzer et al., 1981) have not demonstrated such a difference. A final way to examine this question is an examination of postmortem tissue of schizophrenic patients and controls. Studies of enzymatic activity are incomplete and difficult but have not resulted in any significant differences. Recently, however, a direct measurement of binding receptors has resulted in interesting data. In a variety of laboratories, postmortem binding studies have suggested that in both caudate and mesolimbic tissue, there are more receptors in the tissue from schizophrenic patients than in that from controls. The problem with these studies is that most of the patients had been on neuroleptic drugs before their deaths. The drugs appear to cause a supersensitivity reaction owing to prolonged DA blockade. Studies in animals support the idea that chronic neuroleptic use increases the number of DA receptors. Thus the role of increased DA is only partially supported by these studies.

What does DA blockage do in schizophrenia? Clearly, the drugs do not cure the illness. In fact, they only suppress one set of symptoms: the frankly psychotic symptoms that are not unique to schizophrenia. These are primarily symptoms such as hallucinations and delusions. The other group of symptoms that are an intrinsic part of the illness include the negative symptoms, such as lack of pleasure (anhedonia), lack of motivation, flat affect, and poverty of speech. These are unaffected, as shown by a summary of Crow et al.'s data (1982) in Figure 28-3. This dichotomy has prompted the suggestion that schizophrenia may consist of two main types: one in which psychotic features dominate and are responsive to neuroleptics and one in which negative symptoms are dominant and neuroleptics are not helpful. If this were to be the case, only the former type of patients would be expected to have DA overactivity.

In summary, it appears that all antipsychotic drugs used to date act by way of blockage of the dopamine system. This system appears central in the expression of psychotic symptoms such as hallucinations and delusions. The drugs are effective in suppressing these symptoms regardless of their cause, working well in psychotic forms of mania, depression, and organic brain syndromes, as well as in schizophrenic conditions. Thus it appears that dopamine overactivity is a final common pathway

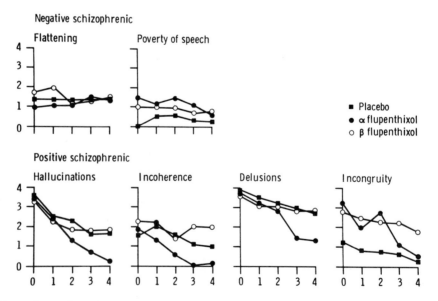

FIGURE 28-3. *Changes in positive and negative schizophrenic symptoms on* α- *and* β-*flupenthixol and placebo.* (From Henn, F., and Nasrallah, H.E.: Schizophrenia as a Brain Disease. Oxford, Oxford University Press, 1982.)

for psychotic processes, regardless of their origin. The evidence for DA overactivity playing an etiologic role in schizophrenia rests on the postmortem findings of increased DA receptor levels in schizophrenics opposed to controls. These findings, while suggestive, are less than conclusive because of the possible contribution of supersensitivity reactions and the fact that most patients sampled were end-stage patients. Thus it appears that a clear biochemical explanation of the schizophrenic illnesses is still lacking.

ANXIETY DISORDERS

One of the real difficulties in getting detailed biochemical information on various psychopathologic states has been the difficulty in finding valid models to study these conditions. The ability to induce psychopathologic states in patients under controlled conditions would be a real advantage. For only one condition has the possibility of laboratory-controlled study readily existed. This is the study of panic attacks. Pitts and McClure (1967) showed that if patients with a diagnosis of panic attacks were infused with sodium lactate, a large proportion ($>$ 90 percent) would experience typical panic attacks. This has been replicated numerous times and is accepted as a provocative research test for panic attacks with susceptible individuals. The mechanism behind lactate induction has not been fully explained. Pitts and McClure felt Ca^{2+} chelation played a role in the phenomena and showed that the addition of Ca^{2+} to the infusion mixture prevented the effect of lactate infusion. Adequate treatment of panic attacks with MAOIs or tricyclic antidepressants also prevents the initiation of panic attacks in susceptible individuals.

These findings suggest that drugs that act on the catecholamines can prevent anxiety attacks. Further studies with adrenergic agents showed that both isoproterenol, a beta agonist, and yohimbine, an alpha$_2$ antagonist could induce anxiety in patients. Thus the involvement of the adrenergic system has been postulated. This is not surprising; a basic description of the effects of stress include increases in blood pressure, heart rate, and plasma cortisol levels, all part of the activation of the peripheral sympathetic system, which uses norepinephrine. Questions of the origin of central anxiety and the role of peripheral factors have been debated without definite conclusions. The problem is, Can sensing of the peripheral features of anxiety, such as muscle tension, mediate the central perception of anxiety? Does lactate act peripherally or centrally? These questions have not been completely resolved. However, it is clear that there are central centers that mediate anxiety. Two basic models have come about through animal studies.

The first central pathway implicated in anxiety was the adrenergic pathway. Recently, this system

has been refined by Redmond and Huang (1979) to involve the alpha$_2$-adrenergic system as critical for the central expression of anxiety. Recall the central norepinephrine system is widely distributed and ideally situated to modulate a variety of CNS functions. More specifically, the locus ceruleus neurons may act to focus and enhance sensory stimulation. When signaled by this system, the organism reacts with an alarm state, which, if inappropriately activated, could result in pathologic anxiety. Redmond has recently shown that if the alpha$_2$ receptor is blocked in monkeys, causing increased norepinephrine release, an alarm state results. This is correlated with increased MHPG, a sign of increased norepinephrine activity. Very recently, similar studies have been carried out in humans, and it has been shown in several centers that the alpha$_2$ agonist clonidine is effective in alleviating panic attacks induced by lactate; therefore, one would predict that this drug also would protect susceptible patients against panic attacks. It appears that the alpha$_2$ system must mediate some of the effects of lactate-induced panic attacks and perhaps is the site of action for MAOIs and tricyclics in this disorder.

There is another central system for anxiety, however, but this system may not be related to the pathophysiology of panic attacks. This system has been elucidated through the pharmacology of the benzodiazepines. These compounds, with diazepam as a typical example, constitute the largest-selling drug group in the world. They clearly have some antianxiety properties but are not as effective against panic attacks as drugs that act on the amine system. The drugs all show four distinct activities. They are anxiolytic, sedative, cause muscle relaxation, and act as anticonvulsants. The interest in how these drugs work has been intense, and early electrophysiologic studies suggest that they work by way of an interaction with the GABA system. It was not until the demonstration of benzodiazepine receptors in 1977 that the localization and mechanistic study of their action advanced. It is now clear that this receptor is part of a multiprotein complex involving the GABA receptor, Cl^- channel protein, and the benzodiazepine receptor. The binding affinities of this receptor suggest that the drug effects of these compounds occur through the receptor. The antianxiety action of these compounds is not on the alarm or vigilance system, which appears to be mediated by the alpha$_2$ system, but rather works to reduce anxiety or fear in conflict situations.

Recently, the development of benzodiazepine antagonists such as carboline-3 carboxylic acid ethyl ester (beta-CCE) has allowed the development of another model of anxiety (Insel et al., 1984). This compound causes anxiety in primates, which also involves increases in blood pressure and heart rate without obvious increases in norepinephrine release. Cortisol is released after beta-CCE administration. These effects can be prevented by diazepam or clonidine. Thus it appears the benzodiazepine receptor is involved in an anxiety-controlling system that interacts with but is distinct from the adrenergic system. A clarification of the relationship between lactate-induced panic, generalized anxiety treated by benzodiazepines, and the $alpha_2$ system in the locus ceruleus is the next task for biologic psychiatrists who are interested in anxiety.

REFERENCES

Angrist B, Shopsin B, Gershon S: The comparative psychomimetic effects of stereoisomers of amphetamine. Nature 234:152–154, 1971.

Aprison MH, Hingtgen JN: Hypersensitive serotonin receptors: A new hypothesis for one subgroup of unipolar depression derived from an animal model. In Haber B, Gabay S, Alivisatos S, Issidorides M (eds): Serotonin—Current Aspects of Neurochemistry and Function. New York, Plenum Press, 1981, pp 627–656.

Bowden DM, Allen SJ, Benton JS, et al: Biochemical assessment of serotonergic and cholinergic dysfunction and cerebral atrophy in Alzheimer's disease. J Neurochem 41:266–272, 1983.

Bunney WE Jr, Davis M: Norepinephrine in depressive reactions. Arch Gen Psychiatry 13:483–494, 1965.

Cade JFJ: The story of lithium. In Ayd F, Blackwell B (eds): Discoveries in Biological Psychiatry. Philadelphia, JB Lippincott, 1970, pp 218–229.

Carlsson A, Lindqvist M: Effect of chlorpromazine or haloperidol on formation of 3-methyoxytyramine and normetanephrine in mouse brain. Acta Pharmacol 20:140–144, 1963.

Connell PH: Amphetamine Psychosis. London, Chapman & Hall, 1958.

Coppen A, Shaw DM, Herzberg B, Maggs R: Tryptophan in the treatment of depression. Lancet 2:1178–1180, 1967.

Coppen A: Depressed states and indolealkylamines. Adv Pharmacol 6:283–291, 1968.

Coyle J, Snyder SH: Catecholamine uptake by synaptosomes in homogenates of rat brain: Stereo-specificity in different areas. J Pharmacol Exp Ther 170:221–231, 1969.

Crow TJ, Cross AJ, Johnstone, Eve, Owen F: Two syndromes in schizophrenia and their pathogenesis. In Henn F, Nasrallah H (eds): Schizophrenia as a Brain Disease. New York, Oxford University Press, 1982, pp 196–234.

Dahlstrom A, Fuxe K: Evidence for the existence of monoamine containing neurons in the central nervous system—A demonstration of monoamines in cell bodies on brain stem neurons. Acta Physiol Scand Suppl 62:232:1, 1965.

Delay J, Deniker P: Caracteristiques psychophsiologiques des medicaments neuroleptiques. In Garattini S, Ghetti V (eds): The Psycotropic Drugs. Amsterdam, Elsevier, 1957, pp 485–501.

Descarries L, Watkins K, Lapierre Y: Noradrenergic axon terminals in the cerebral cortex of rat: III. Topometric structural analysis. Brain Res 133:197–222, 1977.

Descarries L, Beandet A, Watkins KC: Serotonin nerve terminals in adult rat neocortex. Brain Res 100:563–588, 1975.

Ehringer H, Hornykiewicz O: Distribution of noradrenaline and dopamine in the human brain and their behavior in diseases of the extrapyramidal system. Klin Wschr 38:1236–1239, 1960.

Heilman KM, Scholes R, Watson RT: Auditory affective agnosia—Disturbed comprehension of affective speech. J Neurol Neurosurg Psychol 38:69–72, 1975.

Hyman BT, Van Hoesen GW, Damasio AR, Barnes CL: Alzheimer's disease: Cell-specific pathology isolates the hippocampal formation. Science 225:1168–1170, 1985.

Insel T, Ninan P, Aloi J, et al: A benzodiazepine receptor mediated model of anxiety. Arch Gen Psychiatry 41:741–750, 1984.

Iverson L: Role of transmitter uptake mechanisms in synaptic neurotransmission. Br J Pharmacol 41:571–591, 1971.

Jan YN, Jan LY, Kuffler SW: Further evidence for peptidergic transmission in sympathetic ganglia. Proc Natl Acad Sci USA 77:5008–5012, 1980.

Janowsky A, Okada F, Manier DH, et al: Role of serotonergic input in the regulation of the beta-adrenergic receptor-coupled adenylate cyclase system. Science 218:900–901, 1982.

Janowsky D, El-Yousef K, Davis M, Sekerke HJ: A cholinergic-adrenergic hypothesis of mania and depression. Lancet 2:632–635, 1972.

Katz B: Nerve Muscle and Synapse. New York, McGraw-Hill, 1966.

Kebabian J, Greengard P: Dopamine sensitive adenyl cyclase: Possible role in synaptic transmission. Science 174:1346–1349, 1971.

Meltzer HY, Busch D, Fang US: Hormones, dopamine receptors and schizophrenia. Psychoneuroendocrinology 6:17–36, 1981.

Nadi SN, Nurnberger JI Jr, Gershon EG: Muscarinic cholinergic receptors on skin fibroblasts in familial affective disorder. N Engl J Med 311:225–230, 1984.

Osmond H, Smythies JR: Schizophrenia: A new approach. J Ment Sci 98:309–315, 1952.

Papez JW: A proposed mechanism of emotion. Arch Neurol Psychol 38:725–743, 1937.

Pare CMB, Sandler MJ: A clinical and biochemical study of a trial of iproniazid in the treatment of depression. J Neurol Neurosurg Psychol 22:247–251, 1959.

Perry EK, Blessed G, Tomlinson BE, et al: Neurochemical activities in the human temporal lobe related to aging and Alzheimer-type changes. Neurobiol Aging 2:251–256, 1981.

Pitts FN Jr, McClure JN Jr: Lactate metabolism in anxiety neurosis. N Engl J Med 277:1328–1336, 1967.

Prange AJ: The pharmacology and biochemistry of depression. Dis Nerv Syst 25:217–221, 1964.

Redmond DE, Huang YH: New evidence for a locus coeruleus-norepinephrine connection with anxiety. Life Sci 25:2149–2162, 1979.

Schildkraut JJ: The biochemical discrimination of subtype of depressive disorders: An outline of our studies on norepinephrine metabolism and psychoactive drugs in endogenous depression since 1976. Pharmakopsychiatry 15:121–127, 1982.

Schildkraut J: Catecholamine hypothesis of affective disorders. Am J Psychiatry 122:509–522, 1965.

Seeman PM, Chaw-Wong M, Tedesco J, Wong K: Brain receptors for antipsychotic drugs and dopamine: Direct loading assays. Proc Natl Acad Sci USA 72:4376–4380, 1975.

Strom-Olsen R, Weil-Malherbe H: Humoral changes in manic-depressive psychosis with particular reference to the excretion of catecholamines in urine. J Ment Sci 104:696–704, 1964.

Underfriend, S: Biosynthesis of the sympathetic neurotransmitter, norepinephrine. Harvey Lectures 60, pp 57–83, New York, Academic Press, 1966.

Van Rossen JM: The significance of dopamine receptor blockage for the mechanism of action of neuroleptic drugs. Arch Int Pharmacodyn Ther 160:492–494, 1966.

Whitehouse PJ, Price DL, Struble RG, et al: Alzheimer's disease and senile dementia: Loss of neurons in the basal forebrain. Science 215:1237–1239, 1982.

SUGGESTED READINGS

Copper JR, Bloom FE, Roth RH: The Biochemical Basis of Neuropharmacology. New York, Oxford University Press, 1982.

Kandel ER, Schwartz JH: Principles of Neural Science. New York, Elsevier/North-Holland, 1981.

CHAPTER 29

Genetics of Psychiatric Disorders

JOHN I. NURNBERGER, JR.
LYNN R. GOLDIN
ELLIOT S. GERSHON

INTRODUCTION

Since a major function of the human brain is to mediate the interaction of the person with his or her environment, and since learning is a significant component of the development of each of the intellectual and emotional capacities of a person, it is entirely reasonable to suppose that dysfunctions of these capacities which develop in the course of a normally progressing life and which are not due to a traumatic or toxic (infectious or chemical) insult to the brain result from the environmental interactional process gone awry. That is, one would naturally look for causes of mental and emotional illness in the input from the environment and in the processes a person employs in manipulation of his or her environment. This was the accepted wisdom in the mid-1960s, following a century of academic and political disputes over nature versus nurture in human behavior.

It is not surprising, then, that considerable intellectual discomfort was generated by publication in the late 1960s of evidence from studies (by Kety and colleagues, 1968; and by Heston, 1966) of adoption in schizophrenia; these studies showed conclusively that the vulnerability to the illness was transmitted *through the biologic parents and prior to the age of adoption*, which was less than 4 months in this series of studies.

By now, it is widely accepted that major psychiatric disorders, like many other medical conditions, appear to result partially from inherited predisposition. In psychiatric disorders, we are dealing with primary brain dysfunctions that, like those of other organ systems, result from abnormal microanatomy and physiology. The behavior of a person suffering an epileptic fit, harboring a brain tumor, intoxicated with a psychoactive drug, or undergoing a manic episode is behavior that is constrained by physical or chemical abnormalities—it is often behavior that may be regarded as stereotyped. In this sense, it is quite meaningful to think of the heritability of disorders that are manifested primarily in disordered human behavior.

What is the nature of the evidence that suggests heritability? What disorders are inherited? Is the genetic predisposition general or related to specific disorders? What is the mode of transmission? How does one apply this knowledge to the clinical situation? These questions are dealt with in this chapter.

Different strategies may be used to elucidate the genetics of a condition. Twin, family, and adoption studies may be used to provide evidence for or against heritability, to determine the mode of transmission, and to illuminate the spectrum of conditions that may result from a single genetic anomaly. Biologic markers can be used to give evidence about the nature of pathophysiologic processes or as tools in clinical genetic counseling. They may be tested in so-called high-risk studies that include offspring or other relatives of patients who are known empirically to have an increased chance of developing the disorder.

If we take as a fundamental goal of psychiatric genetic research the identification of any of the genetic mutations that predispose to a particular psychiatric illness, the scientific paradigms which may aid in reaching this goal are those listed in Table 29-1. Progress in each of these is reviewed in this chapter, with the conspicuous exception of inher-

TABLE 29-1. *Scientific Paradigms Leading to Detection of a Disease Susceptibility Gene*

Correlation of behaviors in relatives: twin, family, adoption studies

Genetic segregation models

Linkage to genetic markers

Association with specific genes, based on biologic or pharmacologic model systems (includes study of biologic markers in patients and relatives)

Inherited animal behaviors as model

---

ited animal behaviors as model. These have been developed successfully only for alcoholism (Li et al., 1987); a model corresponding to one of the other major psychiatric disorders would be a major accomplishment.

Twin Studies

A common initial strategy for assessing the genetic contribution to a disorder is the twin study. Identical (monozygotic, or MZ) twins have 100 percent identity of parental genes; fraternal (dizygotic, or DZ) twins, as other siblings, have 50 percent identity of parental genes. A trait that is under genetic control, therefore, should be more similar (or "concordant") in identical than in fraternal twins. The assumption is made that MZ and DZ pairs share environmental influences to the same extent. It may be argued that identical twins actually have more similar environments than do fraternal twins. This argument has been considered in detail by Kendler (1983), who argues that differential environments do not account for much of the MZ–DZ differences in concordance seen in many psychiatric disorders. A more definitive but difficult demonstration of genetic influence may be made on the basis of concordance in identical twins raised apart.

A comparison of the MZ and DZ twin concordance provides a broad estimate of heritability. Several functions have been suggested to quantitate heritability from the two types of twin data: an example is Holzinger's index (1929):

$$\text{Heritability} = \frac{\%\ \text{MZ concordance} - \%\ \text{DZ concordance}}{100 - \%\ \text{DZ concordance}}$$

Gottesman and Carey (1983), however, have argued that one may obtain a statistically more meaningful estimate of heritability by combining twin data with epidemiologic data on disease prevalence in the general population.

A deviation from 100 percent concordance in MZ twins implies a contribution of environmental influences to the onset of the condition. In the case of a single major gene, such a deviation is termed *variable penetrance.*

The ratio between MZ concordance and DZ concordance may give supplementary information

about the mode of inheritance. For a single gene trait, the ratio should be 2 to 4, whereas for traits requiring more than one locus, the ratio may be considerably larger. A ratio of less than 2 may result from significant environmental factors (although certain genetic conditions, such as heterogeneous illness with a high population prevalence, can produce this as well).

In the last few years, the twin method has been expanded to allow for more complex models of genetic and environmental components (Heath et al., 1989). It is possible to estimate a large number of genetic and environmental parameters from twin correlations. These models require large sample sizes and thus have usually been applied to study normal-range behavioral traits in large twin population registries. However, there also have been studies that have examined symptoms of anxiety and depression (Kendler et al., 1986, 1987).

Twins also may be used in the assessment of putative biologic markers. A common strategy is the comparison of illness-concordant versus illness-discordant MZ twins with regard to the measurement being considered. This strategy is useful in separating genetic from environmental influences on the biologic marker being tested, but it is not a useful demonstration that the marker is associated with inheritance of illness.

Adoption Studies

An adoption study may be performed in several ways. In one method, a group is identified of index probands who have the condition to be studied and who also happen to be adopted. A control group of adoptees without the illness is chosen. One then studies the adoptive and the biologic families of both groups. If the genetic hypothesis is correct, one sees an increased incidence of illness only in the biologic relatives of the index probands. The critical comparison is biologic relatives of index probands versus biologic relatives of controls (the comparison of biologic versus adoptive relatives is not meaningful because of selective factors in the adoption process). Variations on this strategy include (1) the study of adopted-away children of ill parents compared with adopted-away children of well parents and (2) the cross-fostering study—children of ill biologic parents raised by well adoptive parents compared with children of well biologic parents raised by ill adoptive parents. These strategies have been discussed at greater length by Rosenthal (1974).

For obvious reasons, these studies are difficult to carry out. The most successful adoption studies have been performed in the Scandinavian countries, where central registers of adoption and psychiatric hospitalization make identification of probands and relatives more straightforward.

Adoption studies offer no data regarding the mode of transmission of an illness. However, they do provide most definitive evidence that a prenatal or perinatal factor is at work. An adopted-away child sharing illness with his or her biologic parents is a relatively convincing argument for inheritance. One might still argue, however, that events in uterine life or in early infancy predispose a person to the illness in question, such as the possibility that a virus (e.g., a "slow virus") may be causing the illness.

Family Studies

Family studies are typically done by beginning with a patient having the illness under consideration (the proband) and examining that person's blood relatives. A family-history study is done without direct examination of relatives; in disorders in which there may be subtle manifestations and concealment because of social stigma, family history alone is sometimes inadequate (Gershon and Guroff, 1984).

Family studies may be used to assess whether individual disorders share a genetic vulnerability. If alcoholism and affective illness are related, for instance, then relatives of depressed probands ought to show an increased incidence of alcoholism and vice versa. Genetically related disorders are often referred to as part of a spectrum.

In the study of psychiatric disorders, as in the study of other disorders with variable age of onset, estimates of the prevalence of illness in relatives must be corrected for the proportion of the age of risk that each relative has yet to live through. During the last several years, it has been found that the probability of a person developing certain psychiatric disorders (such as major depression) is related to their birth cohort (see below). This needs to be taken into account in the analysis of family data.

Family-study data may be used to compute empirical risk figures for use in genetic counseling. Examples of such risk figures are given later in Table 29-7 and discussed in the appropriate section of this chapter.

Data from family studies also may be analyzed to detect mode of transmission. One may consider classes of relatives (e.g., a comparison of siblings of probands to offspring of probands to test for dominance effects). A more powerful approach is to examine the segregation of illness in families in terms of various genetic models and attempt to identify the most likely mode of transmission.

Reich and colleagues (1972) extended the multifactorial model proposed originally by Falconer (1965). This model assumes a large number of underlying liability factors that are normally distributed. The underlying factors can be modeled either as a polygenic mechanism or by a single major locus. A threshold point on the liability scale determines the expression of illness. Multiple threshold points can be added to account for illness of varying severity. A greater number of liability factors is associated with more transmission of illness. This model can test whether the transmission of different diagnostic entities fits a single dimension of liability factors, whether transmission is affected by sex, and whether single-locus is more likely than multifactorial transmission (Rice and Reich, 1985).

Elston and Stewart (1971) developed a likelihood approach for testing single-locus hypotheses in pedigree data. Briefly, one compares the likelihood of the observed familial data under various subhypotheses of the general model. This method is effective for ruling out possible modes of single-locus transmission. Morton and MacLean (1974) and Lalouel and Morton (1981) developed a likelihood method to test both a major-locus and a polygenic hypothesis under the same model (mixed model). This method is considered to be a powerful way of testing genetic hypotheses (see Lalouel et al., 1983). In the last several years, Bonney (1984, 1986) has developed regressive models that allow for tests of genetic hypotheses in family data while allowing for additional sources of correlation among relatives.

High-Risk Studies

Retrospective analysis of patients and controls is a poor strategy for determining predictors of illness. In clinical interviews of families, one often finds that there are as many hypotheses about the etiology and onset of a condition as there are informants. Even the temporal order of events is subject to unconscious falsification. Methodologic problems of such studies have been summarized elsewhere (Paykel, 1982). Cross-sectional studies of offspring of patients compared with offspring of controls answer these objections. However, such studies do not allow the investigator to differentiate between predictors of illness and nonspecific characteristics of life in a family with an ill person. High-risk studies allow this differentiation. The high-risk strategy is equally important in confirming putative genetic markers for vulnerability to an illness (Goldin et al., 1986). Examining markers in populations of ill patients versus controls lends itself to errors because of (1) the effects of the illness itself and (2) the effects of treatment. Such errors might be false-positive or false-negative results (treatment effects, for instance, may obscure real group differences). In our own previous work on affective illness we have attempted to avoid these errors by studying patients who are (1) euthymic and (2) removed from all medication for at least 2 weeks. It is clear, however, that in some instances these controls are not sufficient (Hanin et al., 1980; Nurnberger et al., 1983b; Shea et al., 1981). Studying genetically vulnerable individuals who have not yet manifested illness avoids these pitfalls.

In a typical high-risk study, offspring of patients with an illness are studied. The offspring should, ideally, just be entering the age of risk, although studies have been done even in infants. One may make two types of comparisons: (1) immediate results may be obtained by comparing off-spring of patients to offspring of controls; (2) a long-term result may be obtained by comparing offspring of patients who then become ill with those who do not. Both strategies are robust. The second has the added advantage of testing the ability of a patho-physiologic hypothesis to predict illness that has not yet occurred.

There are special statistical considerations in the choice of variables to be studied in a high-risk design; problems of possible heterogeneity are compounded by the fact that only some of the off-spring will in fact carry genetic vulnerability for the illness. These considerations are detailed by Goldin et al. (1986). One must essentially choose variables that show large mean differences between patients and controls (e.g., a two standard deviation difference in means) if one is to have a reasonable chance of differentiating vulnerable high-risk offspring from controls.

Studies of Biological Markers

One way to find an underlying genetic component for a complex disease is to find some biologic trait that is correlated with susceptibility to the illness. This may be, for example, an enzyme, a neuro-transmitter, or a receptor protein that is measured in psychiatric patients and controls. If a variant of such a trait can be shown to be associated with an illness in a population and to be genetically transmitted with the illness in families, then the trait may repre-sent a specific genetic susceptibility component (al-though other genetic and environmental compo-nents may exist).

DEFECTION OF SINGLE GENES
BY LINKAGE AND ASSOCIATION

Studies of populations of patients having both com-mon and uncommon diseases have revealed asso-ciations of certain diseases with genetic marker phe-notypes. For instance, blood group O has been consistently shown to be associated with an in-creased risk for duodenal ulcers (Mourant et al., 1978). The development of molecular genetic methods now allows for identification of a particu-lar (molecular) characteristic more frequent in pa-tients than in controls. This alternative is partic-ularly attractive for candidate-gene hypotheses. Association may be due to linkage disequilibrium or to the identity of the associated region with the disease gene. The chromosomal region of link-age disequilibrium will generally be considerably smaller than the region within which linkage is detectable in pedigrees (see Bodmer, 1986).

The statistical power of association studies (to detect an abnormality) is superior to that of linkage studies for very heterogeneous disorders (Gershon et al., 1989). For well-characterized candidate genes, particularly those with known genomic se-quences, association has become a preferred test for ruling in or out an etiologic role in illness.

Despite the statistical power of molecular asso-ciation methods, they have not yet been clearly successful in psychiatry. Some initial positive re-ports of associations of illness with restriction-frag-ment-length polymorphisms (RFLPs) (Blum et al., 1990; Leboyer et al., 1990) have not yet been con-firmed by others (Bolos et al., 1990; Korner et al., 1990). The base-pair-sequence differences that de-termine an RFLP represent only a small fraction of the possible molecular sequence differences, and it is desirable to have scanning of the base pairs of an entire expressed gene and flanking sequences in a series of patients and controls.

Recent developments do allow screening of ge-nomic sequences in a series of individuals much more efficiently than was previously possible. These methods include denaturing gradient gel electro-phoresis (DGGE) of amplified genomic fragments from different individuals (Sheffield et al., 1989; Kogan and Gitschier 1990; Traytsman et al., 1990) and genomic amplification with transcript sequenc-ing (GAWTS) (Stoflet et al., 1988; Bottema et al., 1989). We expect that these methods will be at-tempted with various neurotransmitter receptor molecules and other candidate genes in affective disorders.

Loci that are situated close to one another on the same chromosome do not assort independently and are said to be linked. However, rearrangement of alleles between pairs of homologous chromo-somes by crossing over (recombination) occurs dur-ing meiosis so that alleles at linked loci are not always transmitted together. The further apart two loci are situated, the more chances they have to recombine in this way. The distance between two loci is expressed as the percentage of recombination θ between them.

The lod score method developed by Morton (1955) is a means of testing the hypothesis of link-age between two loci when the mode of transmis-sion for each locus is known. The underlying assumptions are that (1) the parameters (gene fre-quency and genotypic penetrances) for the disease locus and marker locus are known, (2) there is no population association between the disease locus and marker locus, and (3) mating is random. Under these assumptions, one compares the probability of observing the pattern of segregation of the two traits in a family if there is linkage with the probability of observing the same pattern if there is no linkage. The probability of linkage is expressed as a function of the recombination fraction θ, where θ is some value between 0 and 0.5. The probability of no linkage is the probability that two loci are segregat-ing independently (i.e., $\theta = 0.5$). This odds ratio is expressed by a statistic called the *lod score* (or log of the odds ratio) and is defined as follows:

$$\text{lod score} = \log_{10} \frac{\text{probability of observed data given linkage } (\theta < 0.5)}{\text{probability of observed data given no linkage } (\theta = 0.5)}$$

A lod score of 3.0 (linkage is 1000 times more likely than nonlinkage) has traditionally been required to demonstrate linkage of two mendelian traits. However, for complex diseases, such as psychiatric disorders, the underlying parameters are unknown, and thus a larger lod score criterion is needed.

Linkage has traditionally been studied between a given marker locus and a disease locus. However, advances in molecular genetics have provided markers that are mapped and ordered throughout the genome. In addition, many of the markers available are highly polymorphic and thus very informative for linkage.

Thus it is now possible to test for linkage of a disease trait to a map of marker loci. The method for multipoint linkage analysis is simply an extension of the pairwise method described above, but it is considerably more powerful (Lander and Botstein, 1986). It is now common for investigators to attempt to map a disease gene using markers throughout the human genome.

Linkage also can be tested by collecting a sample of affected sib pairs. If a marker locus is linked to a disease locus, then affected pairs of siblings will have the same phenotype at the marker locus more often than expected by chance. This method has been mainly developed to apply to problems of detecting linkage to the human leukocyte antigen (HLA) loci (Suarez, 1978). Because there is so much polymorphism in the HLA region, each parental chromosome has a different set of HLA alleles (or haplotype). Thus it is usually possible to determine whether affected sib pairs share exactly 2, 1, or 0 haplotypes identical by descent (IBD) at the marker locus. If there is no linkage, then the proportion of affected sib pairs sharing 2, 1, and 0 haplotypes is $\frac{1}{4}$, $\frac{1}{2}$ and $\frac{1}{4}$, respectively. If linkage is present, then this distribution is skewed so that more than 25 percent of affected sib pairs have identical haplotypes. The simple hypothesis of linkage can be tested by comparing the observed IBD distribution in a sample of independent affected sib pairs with that expected when there is no linkage.

Recently, a method has been developed to test for nonrandom sharing of marker phenotypes among all affected individuals in pedigrees (Weeks and Lang, 1988). The advantage of methods that use only affected individuals is that it is not necessary to assume a genetic model for the disease. However, the power of these methods is generally much lower than the lod score method.

The power of linkage methods has been examined extensively under assumptions that a disease is complex and genetically heterogeneous. It has been shown that even under conditions of heterogeneity, linkage can be found in clinically feasible sample sizes (Martinez and Goldin, 1989).

AFFECTIVE DISORDERS

Twin Studies

Twin studies of affective disorder, as summarized over 50 years, show consistent evidence for heritability (Table 29-2). On average, monozygotic (MZ) twin pairs show concordance 65 percent of the time and dizygotic (DZ) twin pairs 19 percent of the time. Although the actual concordance figures vary widely (at least partially because of variation in diagnostic criteria), there is a consistent increased concordance in MZ as opposed to DZ twins. These figures are not age-corrected (although at least the Danish series reported by Bertelson have passed through most of the life span) and are reported as pairwise rather than probandwise concordance; thus they probably represent a conservative estimate of heritability. A representative statistic for heritability from twin studies is 59 percent by the method of Holzinger (1929). This is comparable

TABLE 29-2. *Concordance Rates for Affective Illness in Monozygotic and Dizygotic Twins**

Study	Monozygotic twins		Dizygotic twins	
	Concordant pairs/ total pairs	Concordance (%)	Concordant pairs/ total pairs	Concordance (%)
Luxenberger (1930)	3/4	75.0	0/13	0.0
Rosanoff et al. (1935)	16/23	69.6	11/67	16.4
Slater (1953)	4/7	57.1	4/17	23.5
Kallman (1954)	25/27	92.6	13/55	23.6
Harvald and Hauge (1965)	10/15	66.7	2/40	5.0
Allen et al. (1974)	5/15	33.3	0/34	0.0
Bertelsen (1979)	32/55	58.3	9/52	17.3
Torgersen (1986)	14/37	37.8	8/65	12.3
Totals	109/183	59.0	47/343	13.7

*Data not corrected for age. Diagnoses include both bipolar and unipolar illness.

with that for schizophrenia and with that for common diseases of other organ systems such as diabetes and hypertension. Environmental influences may be related to age of onset, timing of onset of episodes, and severity of course; however, the most important determinants of whether or not the disease is manifest appear to be genetic.

In the studies in Table 29-3 probands include bipolar (BP) as well as unipolar (UP) patients. Bertelson (1977) has shown that concordance in MZ twins increases with severity in this way: BP I probands, 80 percent concordance; BP II probands, 78 percent concordance, UP probands with 3 or more episodes, 59 percent concordance; and UP probands with less than 3 episodes, 33 percent concordance. This is consistent with family-study data,

TABLE 29-3. *Lifetime Prevalence of Affective Illness in First-Degree Relatives of Patients and Controls*

	Number at risk	Morbid risk %	
		Bipolar	Unipolar
Bipolar probands			
Perris (1966)	627	10.2	0.5
Winokur and Clayton (1967)	167	10.2	20.4
Goetzl et al. (1974)	212	2.8	13.7
Helzer and Winokur (1974)	151	4.6	10.6
Mendlewicz and Rainer (1974)	606	17.7	22.4
James and Chapman (1975)	239	6.4	13.2
Gershon et al. (1975b)	341	3.8	8.7
Smeraldi et al. (1977)	172	5.8	7.1
Johnson and Leeman (1977)	126	15.5	19.8
Pettersen (1977)	472	3.6	7.2
Angst et al. (1979, 1980)	401	2.5	7.0
Taylor et al. (1980)	601	4.8	4.2
Gershon et al. (1981b, 1982)	598 (572)*	8.0	14.9
Rice et al. (1987)	567	10.4	23.1
Unipolar probands			
Perris (1966)	684	0.3	6.4
Gershon et al. (1975b)	96	2.1	14.2
Smeraldi et al. (1977)	185	0.6	8.0
Angst et al. (1979, 1980)	766	0.1	5.9
Taylor et al. (1980)	96	4.1	8.3
Weissman et al. (1984) (Severe)	242 (234)	2.1	17.5
Weissman et al. (1984) (Mild)	414 (396)	3.4	16.7
Gershon et al. (1981b, 1982)	138 (133)	2.9	16.6
Rice et al. (1987)	1176	5.4	28.6
Normal probands			
Gershon et al. (1975b)	518 (411)	0.2	0.7
Weissman et al. (1984)	442 (427)	1.8	5.6
Gershon et al. (1981b, 1982)	217 (208)	0.5	5.8

*Number at risk (corrected for age) for bipolar illness appears first in at-risk column; in parenthesis is number at risk for unipolar illness when this is available separately.

which also show morbid risk of illness in relatives rising with the severity of the diagnosis of the proband. Heritability for minor depression or neurotic/reactive depression has not been consistently demonstrable in twin studies (Torgersen, 1986; Kendler et al., 1987; Andrews et al., 1990; Egeland and Klein, 1990; Torgersen, 1990).

Adoption Studies

Mendelwicz and Rainer (1977) reported on a study of BP adoptees. They found affective disorder in 31 percent of the biologic parents of these probands compared with 2 percent in biologic parents of normal adoptees. The morbid risk in biologic parents was comparable with the risk these investigators found in the parents of nonadopted bipolars (26 percent).

Schulsinger et al. (1979) and Kety (1979) reported preliminary data on an adoption study of suicide. The biologic relatives of 71 adopted persons with affective disorder had a disproportionate number of suicides (3.9 percent) in comparison with adoptive relatives of these persons (0.6 percent) or with adoptive relatives of control adoptees (0.3 and 0.6 percent, respectively). The difference between biologic relatives of affective patients and biologic relatives of controls is statistically significant at the 0.01 level. *Nonpsychiatric suicide*, defined as suicide with no preceding psychiatric hospitalization, also appeared to be genetically transmitted in this Danish adoption study. Whether this entity is independent of affective disorders is not clear from the published data.

Von Knorring and colleagues (1983) reported an adoption study from Sweden that included 56 probands with affective disorder and matched adopted and nonadopted controls. The proband diagnoses (following Perris's classification system) were BP or cycloid psychosis (similar to schizoaffective), 5; UP and other psychotic depression, 11; nonpsychotic depression, 40. Probands and relatives were diagnosed through medical records. The investigators found no general concordance of psychopathology between biologic parents and adoptees.

Wender and colleagues (1986) carried out an adoption study of affective disorders in Denmark. They ascertained adoptees who had been hospitalized for an affective disorder and then searched for hospitalization records for biologic relatives of these adoptees and those of a matched control group. They found an increase of affective disorders in the biologic relatives of the affectively ill patients as compared with controls if they considered as "ill" only relatives whose affective disorders were severe (bipolar, unipolar, and suicide) but not if they also included relatives with milder depressions. Both this study and the Swedish study indicated low heritability of "mild" depressions. The Danish study was able to detect heritability of more severe diagnoses, whereas the Swedish study did not have a large enough sample of severely ill probands or biologic relatives to be able to demonstrate heritability of severe affective disorder. The negative Swedish study also should not be seen as a failure to replicate the Danish adoption study of suicide. Suicide, the key outcome variable in the Danish study, could be entirely missed in the Swedish study. Some of these uncertainties could be resolved if patients and relatives were interviewed directly.

Family Studies

Family studies in affective disorder have consistently demonstrated aggregation of illness in relatives (Nurnberger and Gershon, 1984). In a recent study at the National Institute of Mental Health (NIMH), 25 percent of relatives of BP probands were found to have BP or UP illness themselves, compared with 20 percent of relatives of UP probands and 7 percent of relatives of controls. In the same study, 40 percent of the relatives of schizoaffective (SA) probands demonstrated affective illness at some point in their lives (age-corrected morbid risk data) (Gershon et al., 1982). These data demonstrate increased risk in relatives of patients; they also show that the various forms of affective illness appear to be related in a hierarchical way: Relatives of SA probands may have SA illness themselves but are more likely to have BP or UP illness; ill relatives of BP probands have either BP or (more likely) UP illness (see Table 29-3).

Heterogeneity is an emerging theme in consideration of the genetics of many psychiatric disorders. It is invoked to explain disparate results in schizophrenia and Alzheimer's disease as well as BP disorder. This seems consistent with our knowledge of the genetics of other common diseases such as coronary artery disease, hypertension, epilepsy, and diabetes. And it is consistent, also, with our knowledge of the multiple possible origins of the *syndromes* of the psychiatric disorders; that is, we know that many drugs and diseases may cause clinical manifestations identical to mania (Krauthammer and Klerman, 1978) or depression (Wood et al., 1988).

Age of onset may be useful in dividing affective illness into more genetically homogeneous subgroups. Early-onset probands have increased morbid risk of illness in relatives in some data sets (Weissman et al., 1988; Strober et al., 1988).

A birth-cohort effect has been observed in recent family studies; there is an increasing incidence of affective illness among persons born more recently (Klerman et al., 1985). This appears to be true for schizoaffective and BP illness as well as UP (Gershon et al., 1987b). It is true among relatives at risk to a greater degree than in the general population; this may be interpreted as a greater incidence of manifestation of illness among vulnerable persons or (if vulnerability is single locus) greater penetrance.

Mode of Transmission

The multiple threshold multifactorial model of Reich et al. (1972) has been applied to prevalences of affective illness in first-degree relatives (Gershon et al., 1976, 1982). The key question this model tests is whether there is shared or independent transmission of several disease entities under multifactorial inheritance. This model fit three of the four data sets to which is has been applied, including our own recent data in which the greatest transmissible vulnerability is found in schizoaffective (SA) disorder, followed by bipolar (BP) and then unipolar (UP) disorders (Table 29-4). Similarly, Tsuang et al. (1985) found that UP and BP disorder also fit a multifactorial model, with UP having less liability than BP disorder.

The biologic implications of the fit of the multifactorial model are that the BP vulnerability includes all the UP genetic vulnerability, plus transmissible factors that may be genetic or environmental. A similar statement can be made for SA as compared with BP, in the data of Gershon et al. (1982). In other words, the model predicts that there are vulnerability factors shared by all three diagnoses, and that there is more biologic abnormality to be found in BP and SA patients than in UP patients.

However, an analysis by Price et al. (1985) was unable to fit either a single-locus or multifactorial-threshold model to the combined data of Gershon et al. (1982) and Weissman et al. (1984) which had been collected collaboratively. In this analysis, the SA threshold was eliminated by reclassifying such individuals as either UP or BP. In both data sets, the prevalence of illness in offspring was much higher than the prevalence in parents. This is not predicted by the model but is presumably due to a cohort effect, since the offspring are generally from a younger cohort than are the parents. It is possible that some forms of UP disorder share common liability factors with BP but that UP is heterogeneous and more complicated by cohort effects.

Several studies have applied the likelihood method of Elston and Stewart (1971) to test single-locus transmission of affective disorders. Single-locus models have been rejected in most data sets in which they have been tested (see review in Nurnberger and Gershon, 1984). In one analysis (O'Rourke et al., 1983), a single-locus hypothesis was better than a hypothesis with no major locus. There have been some studies that have tested the single-locus and polygenic hypotheses under the general mixed model using the method of Lalouel et al. (1983). Rice et al. (1987) found no conclusive evidence for a major locus for BP disorder in a series of 187 BP families, even taking into account age of onset and cohort effects. Cox et al. (1989) analyzed 6 large multigenerational pedigrees with UP and BP illness, varying a large number of assumptions

TABLE 29-4. *Recent Genetic Analyses of Family Study and Pedigree Data in Affective Disorders*

Authors	Type of analysis	Results
Bucher & Elston (1981) and Bucher et al. (1981)	Pedigree analysis on 1969–1971 U.S. data [model of Elston and Stewart (1971) for single locus inheritance]	Not autosomal or X chromosome transmission
Smeraldi et al. (1981)	Segregation analysis	Could not distinguish single locus from polygenic transmission
Goldin et al. (1983)	Pedigree analysis of 1981 U.S. data [model of Elston and Stewart (1971)]	Not autosomal or X chromosome transmission in data set as a whole or in various subsets
Crowe et al. (1981)	Pedigree analysis of one UP family	Single gene not more likely than environmental transmission
Van Eerdewegh et al. (1980)	X chromosome multiple threshold model of prevalences in relatives	X chromosome transmission excluded in 2/3 data sets
Gershon et al. (1981b, 1982)	Autosomal multifactorial multiple threshold model of prevalences in relatives [Reich et al. (1972)]	Multifactorial inheritance with thresholds of liability defined by diagnosis fit 3 of 4 data sets analyzed
Tsuang et al. (1985)	Multifactorial threshold model	UP less liability than BP
Price et al. (1985)	Multifactorial threshold model to family study of Gershon et al. (1982) and Weissman et al. (1984)	Neither single locus nor multifactorial models fit the data
Rice et al. (1987)	Mixed model segregation analysis in a series of 187 BP families	No conclusive evidence for major locus
Cox et al. (1989)	Mixed model Segregation analysis in 6 multigenerational pedigress with BP and UP	Major locus supported only under a narrow range of assumptions

about diagnostic classification and population prevalence. They found that a major-locus hypothesis was supported only under a very narrow range of assumptions.

The conclusion from the many segregation analyses carried out is that single-locus transmission of BP and UP illness has not been demonstrated and that other methods will be needed to detect susceptibility loci for affective disorders.

Spectrum Disorders

The clinical genetic spectrum of affective disorders can be constructed by comparing the prevalence of illnesses in relatives of patients with the prevalence in relatives of controls.

SCHIZOAFFECTIVE DISORDER

We refer here to patients with episodic as opposed to chronic periods of schizophreniform psychosis along with affective symptoms and patients with some episodes that appear schizophrenic and some that appear affective in nature, again episodic over the lifetime. Most studies of first-degree relatives of patients with SA illness have shown more affective illness (particularly BP illness) and (to a lesser extent) schizophrenia in the relatives than SA illness (see review by Angst et al., 1979).

Although SA probands tend to have a high frequency of affective illness in relatives (and a low incidence of SA illness), the twin studies present a different picture. McCabe (1975) reviewed and combined the twin data of Kringlen (1967), Essen-Möller (1963), Tienari (1963), Fischer et al. (1969), and Cohen et al. (1972). Thirteen of 44 MZ twins

versus 1 of 45 same-sex DZ twins were concordant for type of illness. The twin studies thus show that the form of psychosis appears to be genetically transmitted, but this does not appear true in the family studies. Where the MZ twin concordance appears so much greater than the concordance among first-degree relatives, the data may be reflecting a complex (e.g., multifactorial) form of inheritance. The phenomenon may be produced by interaction among several loci, since MZ twins will be identical by descent at all loci, but the chances of two siblings (for example) being identical by descent at a given locus is one-half. The probability of being identical by descent at n loci is therefore 0.5^n, which becomes a vanishingly small number as the number of loci involved increases. An example of this type of inheritance appears to be found in the visual evoked response (Dustman and Beck, 1965).

As applied to SA disorder, this speculation suggests specific genetic factors that cause the psychosis to have an SA expression, since there is a high MZ twin concordance. But these factors in turn are superimposed on the genetic diathesis for affective illness, since this is the most common disorder found in relatives of SA patients.

ANOREXIA NERVOSA

Cantwell and colleagues (1977) reported in a family history study of anorectics that an excess of affective disorder was present in relatives. In a family study, Winokur and colleagues (1980) investigated 25 anorectic women and 192 of their first- and second-degree relatives. A group of 25 age-matched women with no history of anorexia or depression were used as controls. Of the relatives of the anorectics, 17.7 percent had UP illness and 4.7 percent had BP illness (not age corrected). The corresponding figures for controls' relatives were 9.2 and 0.6 percent. The difference in total incidence of affective illness was significant, suggesting a genetic relationship between the two disorders.

Gershon et al. (1983, 1984) have had similar findings, including a modest amount of anorexia in relatives of anorectics (2 percent) and as much affective disorder as in relatives of bipolars (8.3 percent BP and 13.3 percent UP). In relatives of bipolars, however, there is little anorexia (0.6 percent). Kassett et al. (1989) found increased affective illness in relatives of bulimics. However, a study in normal-weight bulimics did not find excess affective illness in relatives (Stern et al., 1984). It is difficult to assemble a population of eating-disorder probands who do not also have depression to test the relation of the two types of disorders further.

OTHER DIAGNOSES

Cyclothymic personality has been reviewed as a separate entity by Akiskal et al. (1977, 1979). Evidence from family studies (Gershon et al., 1975b, 1981b, 1982) suggests that it may be related to BP affective disorder. Attention deficit disorder children appear to have increased depression in their relatives (Biederman et al., 1987). The opposite has not been demonstrated (BP/UP probands have not been reported to have increased risk of attention deficit disorder in their offspring). Again, this suggests that the type of depression seen in relatives of those with other disorders may be distinct.

Alcoholism is probably not genetically related to BP illness. Winokur and colleagues (1971) have assembled evidence that UP depressive patients with alcoholic or sociopathic relatives are distinct from those without (see review in Nurnberger and Gershon, 1984). Nonpsychiatric suicide may belong in the clinical spectrum, as noted earlier.

Biologic Markers

LINKAGE AND ASSOCIATION STUDIES

Despite the effort devoted to gene mapping studies in BP illness, the studies to date have not yielded consistently reproducible linkages. With this perspective, we summarize the available reports of linkage and discuss the current state of genetic mapping methods relevant to these diseases.

Linkage has been reported to various loci, most notably on the X chromosome, where the first positive reports were of linkage to color blindness (Reich et al., 1969; Baron et al., 1987). However, nonreplications also have been reported in a sizable series of pedigrees (Gershon et al., 1979; Berrettini et al., 1990). Also, the reported linkage in some pedigrees to both color blindness *and* Xg (Mendlewicz and Fleiss, 1974) must be spurious, since Xg and color blindness are at opposite ends of the X

chromosome. Recent reanalysis of the marker genotypes in these pedigrees suggests a systematic genotyping error in the original analysis, since Xg and color blindness are linked *to each other* in these data (Gershon, 1991).

Risch and Baron (1982) reanalyzed all the published data using methods that allowed for multigenerational pedigrees and variable penetrance. They also tested for linkage in the presence of heterogeneity and concluded that if all the reported pedigrees were pooled together, they were consistent with linkage with heterogeneity of BP illness to color blindness and no linkage to Xg. Since then, the inconsistency among reports of linkage to the X chromosome has persisted. Baron et al. (1987) found linkage with no recombination of BP illness with color blindness and glucose-6-phosphate dehydrogenase deficiency (on chromosomal region Xq28) in four Sephardic pedigrees but not in one Ashkenazi pedigree in Israel. Mendlewicz et al. (1987) found loose linkage in Belgium of BP illness to factor IX (FIX), which is at Xq27, 30 to 35 cm from color blindness/G6PD deficiency. Berrettini et al. (1990) *excluded* linkage in nine new U.S. pedigrees to the Xq28 region using DNA probes of three loci (F8, DXS52, and DXS15). In the same pedigrees, Gejman et al. (1990) found no linkage to FIX and to two loci between FIX and Xq28 (DXS98 and DXS105).

Other linkages to BP illness have been reported, but the most recent evidence is not supportive. Egeland et al. (1987) reported that in an Amish pedigree in Pennsylvania, BP illness was linked to markers of 11p15. This has not been replicated in other pedigrees; furthermore, in extensions of the original Amish pedigree and in new cases in the original pedigree, the linkage did not hold up (Kelsoe et al., 1989).

Linkage of HLA to BP and UP illness has been reported, but several negative studies make this locus an unlikely candidate for affective disorder (reviewed by Gershon et al., 1987a).

Etiologic Markers

The quest for the physiologic basis of genetic vulnerability to mood disorder has led in multiple directions. Some of this work is summarized in Table 29-5. Most putative biologic vulnerability markers have not passed the tests of heritability and association with illness within pedigrees. A discussion of some of the more notable work in this area follows.

Platelet alpha$_2$-adrenoceptor density appears to be heritable and associated with illness but has not been studied in families (Kafka et al., 1980; Propping and Friedl, 1983). Beta-receptor density on lymphoblasts is reduced in BP patients in the work of Wright and colleagues (1984), but only a few ill relatives have been studied. These also had decreased density, whereas well relatives did not. Our group, however, was unable to replicate this finding (Berrettini et al., 1987).

TABLE 29-5. *Current Status of Proposed Genetic Vulnerability Markers for Major Affective Disorders*

Finding	Patient/control trait difference	Heritability	Pedigree study	High-risk study	Reference
Platelet MAO	Yes	Yes	Negative	No data	Rice et al., 1984
CSF-5-HIAA	Unclear	Possibly	No data	No data	vanPraag and deHaan, 1979; Oxenstierna et al., 1986
Platelet α-adrenoceptor	Possibly	Yes	Possibly	No data	Kafka et al., 1980; Propping and Friedl, 1983; Garcia-Sevilla et al., 1986, 1981
Lymphoblast β-receptor	Possibly	Yes	Possibly	No data	Wright et al., 1984; Berrettini et al., 1987
Lithium erythrocyte/ plasma ratio	Possibly	Yes	Negative	No data	Dorus et al., 1979, 1983; Nurnberger et al., 1983a
Platelet binding [³H]-IMI	No	Possibly	No data	No data	Berrettini et al., 1982; Mellerup et al., 1982; Suranyi-Cadotte et al., 1982; Friedl and Propping, 1984
Duarte PC 1 brain protein	Yes	Possibly	No data	No data	Comings, 1979
Melatonin suppression by light	Yes	Possibly	No data	Yes	Lewy et al., 1985; Nurnberger et al., 1988a
Cholinergic REM induction	Yes	Yes	Yes	No data	Sitaram et al., 1980, 1982; Nurnberger et al., 1983c
Urinary tyramine	Yes	No data	No data	No data	Bonham-Carter et al., 1980
Electrodermal response	Yes	Yes	No data	Negative	Zahn et al., 1989

LITHIUM TRANSPORT

Dorus et al. (1979, 1983) found that if erythrocyte/plasma lithium ratio and affective illness are considered as a single trait, no combination of single-locus and multifactorial inheritance could describe this trait, but that if the psychiatric criterion was changed to "ever hospitalized," a single-locus genetic model would fit. These data, however, have a modest number of ill relatives evaluated for lithium transport and no probands evaluated, so they cannot be accepted as a demonstration of segregation of lithium transport with illness in pedigrees.

Studying 73 individuals from 12 affective disorder families, Waters et al. (1983b) found no segregation of affective illness with inhibition of lithium efflux by phloretin, which is thought to measure the same Na–Li countertransport system as the Li erythrocyte/plasma ratio. Egeland et al. (1984) found no segregation of Li erythrocyte/plasma ratio with affective illness in a large Amish pedigree.

CHOLINERGIC REM INDUCTION

Sleep disturbance is common in depression; one of the most consistent observations is the shortening of REM latency. REM may be induced in volunteer subjects by an injection of a small dose of physostigmine or arecoline during sleep. In a series of studies, BP patients have been shown to be more sensitive than controls to the REM-inducing effects of arecoline, even when euthymic and off all medication. Further studies have shown that sensitivity to REM induction may be heritable and that it associates with affective disorder within pedigrees (see Table 29-5). These studies suggest central muscarinic cholinergic supersensitivity in brain stem

areas in BP illness. However, methodologic issues require resolution, and the precise neurochemical and anatomic interpretation of these studies remains to be elucidated.

LIGHT SUPPRESSION OF MELATONIN

Melatonin is secreted at high levels during the night and barely detectable levels during daytime. Nighttime melatonin secretion may be suppressed by 500 lx of light. In an initial study, BP patients were more sensitive to this effect of light, even when euthymic and medication-free (Lewy et al., 1985). However, two unsuccessful attempts at replication (with some methodologic differences) have been reported (Comings et al., 1991; Whalley et al., 1991). This issue awaits resolution. We found the supersensitivity to be true of young people with a BP parent also, prior to any manifestation of illness in that group (Nurnberger et al., 1988). The studies of light sensitivity appear to reflect changes in the multisynaptic pathway from the retina to the pineal, perhaps at the level of the suprachiasmatic nucleus. The secretion of melatonin is not demonstrated to have clear functional consequences in humans at this time. It may be related, however, to the timing of multiple circadian processes that are dysregulated in affective disorder.

High-Risk Studies

A number of investigators have examined offspring of manic-depressive patients in cross-sectional designs (Cytryn et al., 1984; Decina et al., 1983; Gaensbauer et al., 1984; Gershon et al., 1985; McNeil and Kaij, 1979; McNeil et al., 1983; Waters et al., 1983a, 1984; Winters et al., 1981; Zahn-Waxler et al., 1984).

We have begun a long-term follow-up study of adolescent and young adult offspring of BP parents. We studied 15- to 25-year-olds because this is the decade of greatest increase in new cases of BP illness in data from the NIMH family study (Gershon et al., 1982). Probands were specified as BP (or episodic SA). Excluding subjects with diagnoses that led to elimination of controls from the study, more off-spring of patients than controls had a diagnosed Axis I disorder (25 of 40 as compared with 12 of 39; $X^2 = 6.76$, $df = 2$, $p < 0.01$); this is consistent with previous reports (see above), although differences in ascertainment of the groups should be noted. The Sensation-Seeking Scale, in total score and in two subscales, differentiated the high-risk from the control group. The hypomania subscale on the General Behavior Inventory (GBI) (Depue et al., 1981) did likewise. Offspring of BP parents may be more prone to respond to dysphoric feeling states by "disinhibitory" behavior. During the course of a 4-year follow-up, nine high-risk offspring developed major affective disorders compared with none of the controls. Possible predictive markers are being tested.

SCHIZOPHRENIA

Twin Studies

Table 29-6 shows concordance rates for schizophrenia in MZ and DZ twins. Inouye (1972) has reported on nine pairs of MZ twins with schizophrenia reared apart during infancy. Three of nine (33 percent) were concordant using a "strict" definition, and 6 of 9 (67 percent) were concordant using a "broad" definition. The twin studies of

schizophrenia were recently reviewed by Kendler (1983). Using probandwise concordance, he found that estimates of heritability were fairly consistent and averaged about 70 percent. Kendler and Robinette (1983), studying the medical records of 15,924 pairs of twins in the National Academy of Sciences–National Research Council Twin Registry, found greater heritability for schizophrenia than for hypertension, diabetes, ischemic heart disease, ulcers, or chronic obstructive pulmonary disease. Abe (1969) utilized a twin-study paradigm to generate data regarding environmental effects in schizophrenia. Examining age of onset in the Maudsley Hospital twin series, he found that there was a high incidence of illness in the second of a pair of twins within 2 years of the onset in the first twin. Further categorizing the group on the basis of whether the twins lived together or lived apart, he found the excess to be primarily in those living together. That is, twins living together show concordance in age of onset, while twins living apart do not. This is an intriguing finding; it suggests an environmental factor. Crow (1982) has observed that this is consistent with the hypothesis of an infectious agent causing onset, although this theory has not been well substantiated thus far.

Adoption Studies

The adoption-study methodology was first applied to schizophrenia by Heston (1966), who found more schizophrenia in the adopted-away offspring of schizophrenic women than in control adoptees. A series of large, systematic studies was carried out by Kety et al. (1968, 1975, 1978) and Rosenthal et al. (1971), who made use of adoption and psychi-

TABLE 29-6. *Twin Studies of Schizophrenia*

Study	"Strict" schizophrenia					"Broad" schizophrenia				
	MZ con*		Same sex DZ con*		Heritability†	MZ con*		DZ con*		Heritability†
Luxenberger, 1928	10/17	59%	0/13	0%	0.59					
Rosanoff et al., 1934	18/41	44%	5/53	9%	0.38	13/17	76%	0/13	0%	0.76
Essen Möller, 1941	1/7	14%	2/24	8%	0.06	25/41	61%	7/53	13%	0.55
Kallmann, 1946						5/7	71%	4/24	17%	0.65
Slater, 1953						120/174	69%	34/296	11%	0.65
Inouye, 1963						23/37	65%	8/58	14%	0.59
Tienari, 1975	3/20	15%	3/42	7.5%	0.08	33/55	60%	2/11	18%	0.51
Kringlen, 1966	14/50	28%	6/94	6%	0.24	19/50	38%	13/94	14%	0.28
Fischer et al., 1969	5/21	24%	4/41	10%	0.16	10/21	48%	8/41	19%	0.36
Gottesman and Shields, 1972	8/20	40%	3/31	10%	0.33	11/22	50%	3/33	9%	0.45
Kendler and Robinette, 1983						30/164	18%	9/268	3%	0.15
Totals	59/176	33%	23/298	8%	0.27	289/588	49%	78/891	9%	0.44

If multiple publications have resulted from the same data, only the most definitive is included.
*Pairwise concordance figures, in general following the interpretation of Fischer et al. (1969).

$$\dagger \frac{(MZ - DZ)}{(1 - DZ)}$$

atric hospitalization registries in Denmark. In the later studies, subjects were directly interviewed. In all studies, adoptees were separated from their biologic parents at an early age and adopted by nonrelatives. In the original study design (Kety et al., 1968, 1975, 1978), it was found that there was more schizophrenia and schizophrenia spectrum disorders in the biologic relatives of schizophrenic adoptees than in the biologic relatives of psychiatrically normal adoptees. The prevalences of psychiatric illnesses in the adoptive relatives of the two groups were small and comparable.

In a second type of study (Rosenthal et al., 1971), the frequency of schizophrenia spectrum disorders was found to be higher in adopted-away offspring of schizophrenic parents than in the adopted-away offspring of normal parents. All these studies have been criticized for the selection of subjects, validity of diagnoses, and validity of comparisons (Lidz et al., 1981; Lidz and Blatt, 1983). This area has proved to be controversial, with comments written back and forth in the literature (Grove, 1983; Kety, 1983). However, the application of DSM-III (*Diagnostic and Statistical Manual of Mental Disorders*, third edition) criteria to subjects who were interviewed directly in these studies has confirmed the essential results; that is, biologic relatives of schizophrenics who have not shared the same environment have a significantly higher prevalence of schizophrenia and schizophrenic spectrum disorders than do biologic relatives of comparable control groups (Kendler et al., 1981b; Lowing et al., 1983).

Family Studies

Numerous studies have examined the rates of schizophrenia in various classes of relatives of schizophrenics. Gottesman and Shields (1982) have summarized the family data collected in Europe and Scandinavia. They have pooled these studies because the populations are relatively homogeneous and the definition of schizophrenia is comparable. Pooling the data also results in large sample sizes in most categories. They summarize the risk for schizophrenia to be 5.6 percent in parents, 10.1 percent in siblings, and 12.8 percent in children. The low rate in parents is thought to be a result of selection for mental health in individuals who marry and have children. The rate in siblings is probably not different from that in children because the children are not classified with respect to the disease status of the second parent. In fact, the risk for children of two schizophrenic parents is 46.3 percent.

As part of a large study in Iowa, Tsuang and colleagues (1980) found that 5.5 percent of first-degree relatives of 200 schizophrenic probands were diagnosed as schizophrenic either by direct interview or by family-history information. The corresponding rate in relatives of hospitalized controls was 0.6 percent. In a small study (128 relatives of 30 probands), Abrams and Taylor (1983) found only 1.6 percent of first-degree relatives affected. This is an extremely low rate. However, only 55 percent of relatives were personally interviewed, and no control population was studied. Guze and associates (1983) found that in ill relatives of 44 patients, 8.1 percent were diagnosed as schizophrenic. The corresponding rate in relatives of other psychiatric patients was 1.7 percent. It is hard to compare the familial risks for schizophrenia among these studies, since the diagnostic criteria vary. This stresses the necessity for each investigator to study a control population. None of these studies separates data on parents (who are expected to have lower rates) from that of sibs and offspring. Nonetheless, the rate of 8.1 percent in the Guze et al. (1983) study corresponds fairly well with the rate of roughly 10 percent in the pooled European data. The Tsuang et al. (1980) and Abrams and Taylor (1983) studies find much lower rates of illness. It would be useful for family studies to present data in ways that allow application of any of the commonly used diagnostic systems.

A more recent family study using modified research diagnostic criteria (Gershon et al., 1988) showed a risk of 3.1 versus 0.6 percent for chronic schizophrenia in relatives of patients versus controls and a risk of 6.2 versus 2.1 percent for all psychoses. For relatives of chronic SA probands, the risk for psychoses was 11.7 percent.

We would conclude that close relatives of schizophrenic patients suffer about a 5- to 10-fold excess risk for the illness and that the risk diminishes in more distant relatives. An additional group of first-degree relatives appears to develop "spectrum" disorders (see below). However, most relatives of schizophrenics are psychiatrically normal.

Two further questions may be approached using the family data: (1) Is there evidence for genetic determination of clinically defined schizophrenia subtypes? (2) Is there a clear genetic distinction between schizophrenia and affective disorder?

It is hard to make a strong case for genetic determination of the classical subtypes of schizophrenia (Kraepelin's hebephrenic, catatonic, and paranoid forms). Although there is significant concordance in MZ twins for subtype (see Gottesman and Shields, 1982), this does not hold true in family studies. The most comprehensive examination of this question was recently published by Kendler and colleagues (1988), again based on data from the Iowa 500 series. They studied 68 paranoid, 50 hebephrenic, 13 catatonic, and 121 undifferentiated probands. About three relatives per proband were assessed. No difference was found in morbid risk for schizophrenia, affective disorders, other psychoses, anxiety disorders, or alcoholism among the groups of relatives using any of three sets of diagnostic criteria. No difference was found if paranoid alone (arguably the most common and robust of the subtypes) was compared with nonparanoid. Moreover, there was no significant concordance in subtypes among relatives. One explanation suggested by the authors was that, in fact, clinical subtype often changes over time, with schizophrenic patients appearing to manifest classic syndromes early in the course of illness and appearing more "undifferentiated" in later years. Previous evidence from the same authors (Kendler et al., 1985) supports this view on the basis of long-term follow-up of Iowa 500 probands. This is similar to the type I–type II concept favored by Crow (1982), with "positive" symptoms tending to occur early in schizophrenia and "negative" or "defect state" symptoms tending to occur later. It would explain the difference between twin and family studies on subtypes, since twins are examined, generally, at the same time during the course of their illness, while probands and relatives often are not.

The question of the distinctness of schizophrenia and affective disorders is not easily settled. In a large family study using lifetime diagnoses and separately examining relatives of probands with schizophrenia, chronic SA disorder, acute SA disorder, BP affective disorder, UP affective disorder, and controls, Gershon et al. (1988) concluded that there was evidence for overlap in genetic liability. Specifically, an increase in UP disorder was seen in all groups of relatives of patients, and relatives of SA probands (both chronic and acute) showed both an excess of affective disorders and an excess of chronic psychoses. However, BP probands did not show an excess of schizophrenic relatives, nor did schizophrenic probands show an excess of BP relatives. The most parsimonious explanation of these data is that there is a "middle" group of disorders (SA) that is genetically related to both schizophrenia and affective illness and that it may not be possible at this time to completely separate the groups on clinical criteria. This still leaves the excess of UP disorder in relatives of schizophrenics to be explained, and one might postulate either genetic or environmental factors (or both) to be important here. Tsuang et al. (1980) found results in the same direction, though not significant. We should also note that Kendler (1980; 1982; Kendler et al., 1981b; Kendler and Hays, 1981) has argued for a separate entity characterized by paranoid delusions only (simple delusional disorder) with inheritance independent of schizophrenia and affective disorder.

Mode of Transmission

Almost every possible genetic mechanism has been proposed at one time or another to explain the familial transmission of schizophrenia. However, several studies have systematically tested these hypotheses, using current analytic methods. Elston and associates (1978) applied pedigree-analysis methods to Kallmann's family data and rejected single major locus inheritance. Debray and col-

leagues (1979) and Stewart and colleagues (1980) examined the relative likelihoods of several genetic models in a sample of 25 large French pedigrees. Although some models had lower likelihoods than others, it was not possible to distinguish models involving one, two, or four loci. Statistical testing of hypotheses was not performed, but the results suggest specific models to examine in future studies. Carter and Chung (1980) located records of all individuals hospitalized for schizophrenia in 1942 in Hawaii. They then ascertained all relatives of these individuals who had been hospitalized for schizophrenia and applied Morton's mixed model of analysis (Morton and MacLean, 1974) to their sample. Both a major-locus and a polygenic hypothesis were compatible with the data.

Tsuang et al. (1982, 1983) rejected major-locus transmission of schizophrenia in families of 200 probands collected in Iowa. They also rejected a multifactorial multiple-threshold model when various spectrum disorders were included as "mild" illness. Risch and Baron (1984) used the mixed model to test both polygenic and single-gene components in the transmission of schizophrenia and schizophrenia spectrum disorders. They concluded that the best-fitting model was a recessive locus with an additional polygenic component. However, a simple polygenic model could not be excluded.

A series of three studies have reanalyzed twin- and family-study data collected in Europe. The European data were used because of the greater clinical homogeneity of the studies. O'Rourke and colleagues (1982) examined the limits of familial prevalences and twin concordance rates based on a general single-locus model. They concluded that the majority of studies fell outside the expected limits, making a unitary single-locus etiology unlikely. Rao and associates (1981) and McGue and associates (1983) have estimated genetic and environmental variance components under a multifactorial liability threshold model using pooled familial and twin prevalence rates. In both analyses, the genetic heritability was 70 percent and the cultural heritability was 20 percent. Assortative mating and environment unique to twins also were found to be significant components.

Recently, Risch (1990) has demonstrated that overall twin concordances and recurrence risks in relatives for schizophrenia taken from the literature cannot be explained by either a single-locus model or by a pure polygenic model. He concluded that the data are most consistent with a small number of interacting loci but that such loci could still be detected using linkage methods.

From these analyses, one can conclude that the heritable component of schizophrenia is large but not consistent with a unitary single-locus hypothesis. This does not exclude the possibility that single, identifiable loci lead to susceptibility, but it suggests that there is no homogeneous single locus for schizophrenia. The problem may be the underlying assumption of the homogeneity of the schizophrenic population. As reviewed by Faraone and Tsuang (1985), this hypothesis has been tested, albeit indirectly, by Stewart and coworkers (1980). Pedigree simulation studies were performed in which the mechanism of transmission varied with the family. The results of segregation analyses of the simulated data were similar to actual analyses of collected family-study data. The simplifying assumption of homogeneity has been a reasonable place to begin analyzing mode of transmission in schizophrenia. It seems that it might be most parsimonious at this point, however, to assume that this syndrome is not genetically homogeneous. In fact, it is clear that multiple environmental and genetic factors will produce the clinical syndrome of schizophrenia. The essential difference between these conditions and what we call "schizophrenic illness" is that in the former case the cause is known and in the latter it is not. For enlightening summaries of these issues see Davison and Bagley (1969) and Propping (1983).

Spectrum Disorders

In the adoption studies of Wender and colleagues (1986), the concept of "borderline" schizophrenia was used to describe individuals with idiosyncratic experiences or communication styles that were similar to, but not as severe as, those of schizophrenic patients. Such individuals were more commonly found to be the biologic relatives of schizophrenic probands than they were to be the biologic relatives of controls.

The term *borderline* then underwent a decade of transition, during which it was widely and very imprecisely used. The present DSM-IIIR "borderline personality disorder" is probably more closely related to affective illness than to schizophrenia (Loranger et al., 1983). The concept of milder disorders related to schizophrenia, however, remains quite viable.

Several investigations in this area have been performed by Baron and coworkers (Baron et al., 1985). They have reported that up to 30 percent of first-degree relatives of schizophrenic patients have associated disorders. The particular DSM-IIIR diagnostic categories that seem to be implicated are paranoid personality and schizotypal personality. This area remains controversial.

It does seem most prudent to conclude that the genetic vulnerability to schizophrenia is manifest in a group of patients who meet operational criteria for that illness and in another group who are recognizably similar in some ways but not others. It is a testable hypothesis with some support that many members of that second group fall into the category of "paranoid personality" and "schizotypal personality."

Biologic Markers

ASSOCIATION AND LINKAGE

Numerous studies have compared ABO types in schizophrenic and control populations. A few early studies reported a higher frequency of type A in schizophrenics (reviewed in Mendlewicz et al., 1974). However, this association has not been consistently present. In a study of about 800 patients in Greece, Rinieris and colleagues (1982) found no differences between schizophrenics and controls. Gc types also have been reported to be associated with schizophrenia, but different alleles have been found to be significant in different studies (Böök et al., 1978; Pahina et al., 1982; Lange, 1982).

There have been studies of HLA types in schizophrenics since the mid-1970s. Although no specific antigen has been associated with schizophrenia, some trends have been seen. McGuffin et al. (1981) and Ivanyi et al. (1983) have compiled data on paranoid patients from several studies and have shown that, overall, there is significant association with HLA A9. We have pooled all the available data from the literature and find that the overall relative risk of A9 is about 1.25 in all patients and 1.61 for paranoid patients. Both these risks are significantly different from 1.0. These results suggest that the HLA region may play a small but significant role in susceptibility to schizophrenia.

A study by Turner (1979) suggested possible linkage of HLA to "atypical" schizophrenia. However, several subsequent studies were able to reject linkage of the HLA region under a wide range of assumptions [e.g., see McGuffin et al. (1983) and Goldin et al. (1987)].

Bassett et al. (1988) reported a single family with a translocation on chromosome 5 associated with schizophrenia. Subsequently, Sherrington et al. (1988) reported linkage to markers in the same area of chromosome 5 in five Icelandic families and two British families. However, the finding was not replicated by others or by the original group in further studies in the same populations (Mankoo, 1991).

Etiologic Markers

Among the multiplicity of neurochemical, neuroanatomic, and neurophysiologic theories of the etiology of schizophrenia, few have been tested using genetic methodologies. A hypothesis of considerable heuristic value since the 1960s has been the idea of dopaminergic overfunction in the CNS. Much data have accumulated on the presence of low platelet monoamine oxidase (MAO) levels in some schizophrenic patients [see, for instance, Wyatt et al. (1979)]. Platelet MAO is under genetic control, and the mode of inheritance appears to be codominant (Goldin et al., 1982; Rice et al., 1984). Wyatt et al. (1973) showed concordance of MAO activity in MZ twins discordant for schizophrenia, and Reveley and associates (1983) reported similar data. Recently, Baron and colleagues (1984) reported segregation of MAO activity with illness in schizophrenic families. However, a major problem in continuing to study this variable in schizophrenic patients is that it has become clear that neuroleptic medications lower platelet MAO activity (DeLisi et al., 1981; Chojnacki et al., 1981). Because almost all schizophrenics are today treated with neuroleptics at some point during their illness, it will be necessary to circumvent or control for this effect in some way. One possibility is to test MAO in a high-risk group and do follow-up studies.

Another finding in the dopamine system that is promising is the increase in spiroperidol binding in autopsy specimens of schizophrenic brain (Owen et al., 1978). This finding may not be simply a neuroleptic effect (Crow et al., 1980). However, it will need to be tied to a more accessible marker to be investigated genetically. Dopamine receptors in peripheral cells have been investigated. LeFur et al. (1980) originally reported success in measuring dopamine receptors on lymphocytes, and Bondy et al. (1984) have reported an association between schizophrenic illness and increased numbers of those receptors (as measured by ^{3}H-spiroperone binding). Dopamine receptors are not present on cultured fibroblasts (Berrettini et al., 1983). Amphetamine response (Schulz et al., 1981) and apomorphine response (Jeste et al., 1983) have been explored as a way of subtyping schizophrenic patients, but genetic studies remain to be done.

Other monoamine-related findings include elevation of 5-hydroxyindoleacetic acid (5-HIAA) and homovanillic acid (HVA) in CSF of schizophrenics with a positive family history of that illness. However, these measurements show similar concordances in MZ and DZ twins and therefore may not be significantly influenced by genetic factors (Sedvall et al., 1980; Sedvall and Oxenstierna, 1981). Increased alpha-adrenoceptor binding in platelets has been reported by Kafka et al. (1980). Recently, Propping and Friedl (1983) reported heritability of a similar measure. They used yohimbine rather than dihydroergocryptine as ligand. No pedigree studies have been done. Rotman et al. (1982) reported abnormal platelet serotonin uptake in schizophrenic patients and some of their relatives, but cosegregation of illness with the abnormality was not demonstrated.

The neuroanatomy of schizophrenia has been an area of renewed interest since the advent of new technologies for investigating brain conformation and gross activity. Computed tomography (CT) has consistently shown increased ventricular size in some schizophrenics (Johnstone et al., 1976; Weinberger et al., 1979). This can be found in untreated individuals suffering their first psychotic break (Weinberger et al., 1982). A study of schizophrenics and their siblings, however, did not demonstrate familial concordance in ventricular size (Weinberger et al., 1981). A recent twin study (Reveley et al., 1984) found increased ventricular size only in schizophrenics without a family history of the illness, and these authors hypothesized that some environmental factor, such as birth complications, probably was responsible for increased ventricular size in some schizophrenic patients. This is consistent with the results of Suddath et al. (1990), who found that in MZ twins discordant for schizophrenia, ill twins had larger ventricles than their well co-twins. However, another study (DeLisi et al., 1986) did find both familial and illness effects on ventricular size in schizophrenic siblings. A potential difficulty with ventricular size as a potential etiologic marker for schizophrenia is that it is found in a number of BP affective patients as well (Nasrallah et al., 1982). It is likely that this represents a nonspecific outcome with multiple possible etiologies.

Positron emission tomography (PET) has shown decreased activity in the frontal lobes of some schizophrenic patients (Buchsbaum et al., 1982), confirming previous studies of cerebral blood flow (Ingvar, 1980). A study, however, on patients assessed early in their course of illness and, for the most part, never medicated did not confirm this "hypofrontality" hypothesis (Sheppard et al., 1983). These "acute" schizophrenics may not have the same course as patients followed for a longer time, but it does raise the question of effects of neuroleptics and disease state in the "hypofrontality" findings. DeLisi et al. (1986) did not find a relationship between hypofrontality in schizophrenics and a family history of schizophrenia.

Attentional measures have been reported abnormal in schizophrenics and in several studies of high-risk offspring [a continuous-performance task deficit shown by Rutschmann et al. (1977) and a smaller auditory evoked potential augmentation in a study by Brecher and Begleiter (1983)]. Saitoh et al. (1984) reported evoked potential augmentation to be abnormal in schizophrenic patients and their well siblings.

Holzman et al. (1977, 1984) have reported extensive investigations of defects in smooth-pursuit eye movements (SPEMs). In this case, there is not a clear differentiation between ill relatives and well relatives—many well relatives have the SPEM abnormality as well. In response to this evidence, Holzman et al. (1988) have formulated what they call the "latent-trait" model to describe the relationship. In this model, a single-gene defect may manifest as schizophrenia in some individuals and eye movement dysfunction in others, for unknown reasons. Thus the genetic defect would be a necessary but not sufficient condition for the illness. Family studies employing SPEM measurements as well as clinical diagnosis regarding SPEM dysfunction as an alternate manifestation of the illness gene have been performed and are consistent with dominant inheritance.

A convincing demonstration of a genetic vulnerability marker for a significant proportion of schizophrenic patients has yet to be made.

ALCOHOLISM

Twin Studies

Twin studies have examined heritability of both drinking behavior in normal twins and alcohol abuse in twins ascertained through an alcoholic member. Large surveys of normal twins in Finland found significant heritability for frequency of drinking and total consumption (reviewed in Murray et al., 1983). In a study of a sample of normal twin pairs in England, it was found that 40 percent of the total variance of weekly alcohol consumption was due to additive genetic factors and 28 percent was due to common familial environments (Murray et al., 1983).

Data from a large twin study of alcohol abuse in Sweden carried out by Kaij have recently been reanalyzed by Gottesman and Carey (1983). In this study, alcohol abuse was defined by criteria of varying severity, including chronic alcoholism and multiple convictions for intoxication. Gottesman and Carey (1983) calculated heritability of the different severities of alcohol abuse, taking into account the population prevalence of these disorders. The heritability of chronic alcoholism itself was 98 percent. As the definition of alcohol abuse was widened to include convictions for intoxications, the genetic heritability decreased and the cultural heritability increased.

In a study of male twins serving in the U.S. armed forces, MZ twins were recorded to be significantly more concordant than DZ twins for alcohol-related disorders, as ascertained from the records of the Veterans Administration (Hrubec and Omenn, 1981).

Gurling et al. (1984) report a twin study using the Maudsley Hospital Twin Register. About 1000 twin probands were screened, locating 74 twin pairs with alcoholic probands. The pairwise concordance is 6 of 28 = 21.0 percent for MZ twins. The pairwise concordance for DZ twins is 7 of 28 = 25.0 percent. The authors suggested that the failure to replicate Kaij's results may have been because Kaij's sample tended to be more antisocial (reported by third parties) and the Maudsley alcoholics tended to

be more neurotic. They also note that 21 of 56 Maudsley twin pairs were women and that heritable factors have never been easy to demonstrate in women alcoholics. We also should note that traits with only moderate heritability are not likely to show significant MZ–DZ differences except in relatively large twin studies (i.e., 100 to 200 pairs of each zygosity). A more recent large twin study from Finland illustrates this (Kaprio et al., 1987).

EDITORS' COMMENT

A treatment sample of 50 MZ and 64 DZ men and 31 MZ and 24 DZ women found significantly higher concordance for DSM-III alcohol abuse and/or dependence in MZ male twins compared with DZ twins. For women twins, MZ twins showed significantly higher concordance than DZ twins for alcohol dependence only (Pickens et al: Arch Gen Psychiatry 48:19–28, 1991).

Adoption Studies

Adoption studies have generally shown a relationship between alcohol problems in an adoptee and such problems in biologic relatives. An exception to this is the small study by Roe (1945), in which 36 adopted-away children of alcoholics were compared with 25 adopted-away children of nonalcoholics. Two of the children of alcoholics and one of the children of nonalcoholics had alcohol-related problems during adolescence, but apparently none had problems when followed up during young adulthood.

Goodwin et al. (1973) compared 55 adopted-away male children of an alcoholic parent with 78 adoptees without an alcoholic parent. The groups were matched by age, sex, and time of adoption. The principal finding was that 18 percent of the proband group were alcoholic compared with 5 percent of the controls ($p < 0.02$). It is somewhat disconcerting that this pattern does not hold true for adoptees designated as "problem drinkers" or "heavy drinkers." There is no difference between groups if these categories are considered separately or if they are combined with the alcoholic group. It is only alcoholism itself that was heritable, alcoholism being defined as the presence of heavy drinking (1 year of daily drinking with six or more drinks at least twice a month or six or more drinks at least once a week for over a year) plus a problem in three of the following four groups: (1) disapproval of drinking by friends, parents, or wife, (2) trouble on the job because of drinking, traffic arrests, or other police problems, (3) frequent blackouts, tremor, or serious withdrawal symptoms, or (4) loss of control or repeated morning drinking. This result is consistent with Kaij's data that heritability increases with the severity of the disorder.

Goodwin and colleagues (1974) also compared adopted-away sons of alcoholics with sons of alcoholics raised by the alcoholic parent. There was no difference, a finding surely disturbing for those regarding "modeling" as important in the development of alcoholism. Twenty-five percent of the adopted sons became alcoholic, compared with 17 percent of nonadopted sons (however, the total numbers of subjects were only 20 and 30, respectively). Additional studies in daughters of alcoholics did not show evidence for a heritable predisposition to alcoholism in women (see also discussion below). They did show an increase in depression in daughters of alcoholic fathers, but only if raised by the alcoholic father and not if adopted away; this is an apparent demonstration of an environmental cause of depression (or a genetic–environmental interaction) (Goodwin et al., 1977).

Bohman (1978) used state registers in Stockholm to study 2324 adoptees born in that city between 1930 and 1949. Male adoptees whose fathers abused alcohol (excluding those who were also sociopathic) were more likely to be alcoholic themselves (39.4 versus 13.6 percent, $p < 0.01$) compared with adoptees without an alcoholic (or sociopathic) father. The findings were similar for male adoptees with an alcoholic biologic mother. A matching procedure was used in a smaller sample with similar though nonsignificant results (20 versus 6 percent).

Cloninger then collaborated with Bohman and Sigvardsson (1981) in a reanalysis of Bohman's data set. A cross-fostering analysis was done. This is a very powerful but difficult strategy that allows direct examination of both genetic effects and certain environmental effects in the same population. Adoptees with alcoholic biologic parents may sometimes be placed in homes with alcoholic adoptive parents as well. Are such young men more likely to develop alcoholism than adoptees with alcoholic biologic parents placed with nonalcoholic adoptive parents or adoptees with nonalcoholic biologic parents placed with alcoholic adoptive parents? The answer varies with the severity of the disorder studied in the adoptees. Those with mild alcohol abuse showed evidence for separate effects of both heredity and environment (and for adoptees with both biologic and adoptive parents who were alcoholic, the effects were more than additive). For those with moderate alcohol abuse, genetic effects were significant but environmental were not. For those adoptees with severe abuse, increases for both genetic and environmental factors were seen, but these were not statistically significant. The authors felt that the mild and moderate groups were differentiated by this analysis and that either could cross over into severe abuse.

These data formed the basis for a familial distinction of alcoholics that has been influential in modern alcohol research: the milieu-limited (type I) and male-limited (type II) groups of alcoholics. Type I alcoholics (as defined in Cloninger, 1987a) usually have onset after age 25, manifest problems with loss of control, and have a great deal of guilt and fear about alcohol use. Type II alcoholics have onset before age 25, are unable to abstain from alcohol and have fights and arrests when drinking, but less frequently show loss of control and guilt and fear about alcohol use. Cloninger reanalyzed the Stockholm adoption data using these specific categories. This analysis showed that type I alcoholics were significantly increased in prevalence only among those adoptees with both genetic and environmental risk factors (alcoholism in both biologic and adoptive parents). Type I was the most common type of alcoholism, however, being present in 4.3 percent of the controls with no risk factors. Type II alcoholism was present in only 1.9 percent of the controls but in 16.9 to 17.9 percent of adoptees with genetic risk factors, whereas the presence or absence of environmental risk factors (alcoholism in adoptive parents) did not appear to make a difference.

The Bohman–Cloninger analysis of the Stockholm sample is the largest adoption study in the field of alcoholism. However, the quality of the initial information (based on population registers) may not have been as complete as that gathered by Goodwin and colleagues, who performed personal interviews on the adoptees. Cloninger states that the population registers can identify about 70 percent of alcoholics without a bias for type I or type II; however, it is not clear that there might not be a bias for the unregistered 30 percent of alcoholics to be found preferentially in one or another of the adoptee groups. However, the two studies reach essentially the same conclusion: Heritable factors are important in the development of alcoholism in at least a subpopulation of heavy drinking men.

Bohman et al. (1981) extend this finding to women adoptees, identifying as particularly important the incidence of alcoholism in the biologic mothers of these adoptees. A variant on the usual adoption study format was reported by Schuckit et al. (1972), who studied a population of half-siblings of alcoholic probands. Half-siblings with an alcoholic biologic parent had a high risk for alcoholism (46 to 50 percent) whether or not they were raised with an alcoholic parent figure. Those without an alcoholic biologic parent had a lower risk, regardless of environmental variables considered.

Cadoret et al. (1980) reported an adoption study with a smaller number of probands than those of Goodwin et al. or Bohman and Cloninger; their conclusions are similar to those of the preceding authors.

Family Studies

Most family studies of primary alcoholism find that the prevalence of alcoholism in relatives of probands is severalfold higher than that in the population. Goodwin (1979) summarized the familial prevalences in the European studies and found the rates in the pooled studies to be about 25 percent in male relatives and 5 to 10 percent in female relatives. The corresponding population prevalences are 5 to 10 percent in males and 0.1 to 1 percent in females. As with other disorders, the prevalences will vary according to diagnostic criteria. For example, in a study in St. Louis, the familial prevalences were 34 percent in males and 6.4 percent in females, the population prevalences being 11.4 percent in males and 2.9 percent in females (Cloninger et al., 1978).

Mode of Transmission

There have not been many analyses of the mode of transmission of alcoholism, probably because of likely heterogeneity and the association of alcoholism with many other psychiatric disorders. Cloninger et al. (1978) have examined the fit of various multifactorial models to the familial data mentioned earlier. There are two ways to explain the observed sex difference in prevalence of alcoholism. In order to become ill, a female might require either more genetic susceptibility factors or more nonfamilial environmental factors. In the first case, since affected females should have more genetic liability factors than do males, their relatives should have more alcoholism than do relatives of males. In this study, the prevalence of alcoholism in relatives was *not* affected by sex of the proband. These data thus support the hypothesis that nonfamilial environmental factors cause the male–female differences (see discussion under Adoption Studies also).

SPECTRUM DISORDERS

Winokur et al. (1970) reported an increased prevalence of depression in female relatives of alcoholics roughly comparable with the increased prevalence of alcoholism in male relatives. This was not found in the adoption study of Goodwin et al. (1977), except in daughters brought up in the home of the alcoholic father; this may mean that the incidence of affective disorder and alcoholism in the same families may be related to environmental rather than genetic factors. A later study by Winokur and Coryell (1991) showing increased alcoholism in the relatives of female depressive probands but not male depressive probands is also compatible with this explanation. Some family studies in this area show an increase in risk for alcoholism in relatives of depressive probands, as well as an increase in depression in relatives of alcoholics; however, many other studies do not show this pattern (see review by Merikangas and Gelernter, 1990).

Bohman et al. (1984) and Cloninger et al. (1988) have observed that adopted-away daughters of type II (male-limited) alcoholics manifest no increase in alcoholism but do show an increase in somatization disorder.

It is not possible to conclude at this time that a single genetic predisposing factor may be manifest as either alcoholism or sociopathy. There does seem to be a genetic predisposition for a subtype of alcoholics (the male-limited type II alcoholics), who often manifest sociopathy as well; this may account for the increased prevalence noted in some family studies. Thus some sociopathic alcoholics may transmit both alcoholism and sociopathy but not independently, only as part of the same syndrome.

A series of studies has shown an increased prevalence of alcoholism in parents of children with hyperactivity (see Chap. 18). Earls et al. (1988) reported an increase in DSM-III behavior disorder in general (attention deficit disorder with hyperactivity, oppositional disorder, and conduct disorder) in offspring of alcoholic parents. The risk was greater for offspring of two alcoholic parents than of one alcoholic parent.

Cadoret et al. (1986) reported an adoption study of drug abuse. Drug abuse in adoptees is associated with alcohol problems in first-degree biologic relatives. The number of ill adoptees is not large in this study, and one may question the adequacy of information on biologic relatives (adoption records alone). Still, this association intuitively makes sense (alcohol not being unique among psychoactive drugs in its reinforcing and dependency-producing properties), and one looks for further tests of this hypothesis.

Biologic Markers

ASSOCIATION AND LINKAGE

Many studies have examined the distribution of red cell antigen types and other genetic markers in populations of alcoholics, although no consistent patterns have emerged (reviewed in Goodwin, 1982). However, HLA types may be associated with the development of liver cirrhosis in alcoholics [e.g., see Saunders et al. (1982) and Tait and Mackay (1982)].

Tanna et al. (1988) reported similar alleles at the esterase D locus in sib pairs concordant for alcoholism (lod = 1.64). This remains to be replicated; sib-pair analysis showed suggestive linkage to MNS in another study (Hill et al., 1988a).

An association between alcoholism and an allele at the D_2 receptor locus has been reported by Blum et al. (1990). This has not been replicated by Bolos et al. (1990) or by Gelernter et al. (1991). However, Parsian et al. (1991) and Comings et al. (1991) have results that are generally supportive. The evidence has recently been summarized by Conneally (1991) and Cloninger (1991), who find that the studies taken together tend to suggest a true association but not a linkage. This situation may result from a gene of minor effect. Within a given family (especially a multiplex family with presumably powerful determinants of illness), the associated allele may not be of great enough relative importance to result in a significant lod score. However, in a population study of a larger number of unrelated probands, the effect may be seen. It is very important to control for ethnic origin in such studies; clear diagnostic definition of control samples is also important, especially when studying the very common disorders we deal with in psychiatry; these factors should be carefully considered in the follow-up studies that are expected in the continuing assessment of the D_2 allele.

Etiologic Markers

Variants of enzymes of alcohol metabolism, alcohol dehydrogenase (ADH) and aldehyde dehydrogenase (ALDH), have been found to have altered biologic activities (reviewed in Goedde et al., 1983). For example, Asians have both a high rate of an atypical ADH enzyme and a high rate of deficiency of the ALDH type I. Presumably, these differences are related to the increased sensitivity to the adverse effects of alcohol in Asians. This is an example of a genetic variation that may *protect* against alcoholism.

One problem in attempting to identify biologic susceptibility factors in alcoholics is that differences found could be a result of chronic alcohol abuse. Alcoholics have been found to differ from controls in parameters such as levels of monoamine oxidase (Murphy et al., 1982), resting electroencephalographic (EEG) parameters (Propping et al., 1981), and levels of acetaldehyde after an ethanol dose (Korsten et al., 1975). An alternative approach to this problem is to study subjects who are not themselves alcoholic but who are at high risk for developing alcoholism by virtue of having an alcoholic first-degree relative. Schuckit and Rayses (1979) studied sons of alcoholics and sons of controls and found the high-risk subjects to have higher acetaldehyde levels than controls after an ethanol dose. This finding is somewhat controversial because of technical problems (Eriksson, 1980) and nonreplication (Behar et al., 1983). Behavioral and neuroendocrine responses to alcohol infusion have been studied in a series of high-risk populations by Schuckit. Offspring of alcoholics displayed less subjective intoxication, less muscle tension, and less body sway than controls (Schuckit, 1980, 1984a, 1985b). Cortisol levels following alcohol also were lower in family history–positive young men (Schuckit, 1984b), as were prolactin levels (Schuckit et al., 1983); these findings were not placebo-controlled, although Schuckit's more recent studies include a placebo comparison (Schuckit, 1988). Newlin (1985) has demonstrated that heart rate response to placebo (decrease) was greater in sons of alcoholics than in sons of controls. Newlin and Thompson (1990) have interpreted the alcohol challenge results of Schuckit and others as compatible with a model of greater initial alcohol effect but lesser effect on the falling curve of alcohol blood level (greater acute tolerance). More complete assessment of early response during alcohol challenge

would test this model. Evidence for heritability of the responses to alcohol in the challenge design is awaited; some evidence exists for heritability of body sway (a briefly described twin study by Martin, 1987).

A poorly synchronized resting EEG (lower alpha) has been proposed to be related to a predisposition for alcoholism (Naitoh, 1973). Change in alpha rhythm following alcohol is more concordant in MZ than in DZ twins (as are multiple other EEG parameters) (Propping, 1977, 1978). A relationship was found between resting EEG of the unselected twins and drinking behavior (less alpha in the twins who drank more). In subsequent work, Propping et al. (1981) found that relatives of alcoholics with poorly synchronized resting EEGs demonstrated the same characteristic themselves. Change in alpha following alcohol also was found to differentiate young adult subjects at high risk for alcoholism from controls (Pollock et al., 1983). Pollock et al., however, divide calculation of results into "slow alpha" and "fast alpha," which makes comparison with the results of other authors difficult.

Measurements of event-related potentials have shown smaller P_{300} waves following visual stimuli in high-risk offspring compared with controls (Begleiter et al., 1984). This study is remarkable in that the subjects ranged in age between 7 and 13 years, greatly lessening the likelihood of previous alcohol exposure. The findings themselves were not dependent on alcohol provocation. Similar findings using an auditory stimulus had been reported in an older group (aged 21 to 26) both before and after alcohol administration (Elmasian et al., 1982). This finding was essentially replicated by O'Connor et al. (1986) but not by Polich and Bloom (1986). Hill et al. (1988b) found a significant increase in P_{300} latency in adolescent and adult relatives of alcoholics compared with controls. Schmidt and Neville (1985) found a decreased amplitude in a later negative wave in young men at risk for alcoholism. The EEG/ERP area remains one of the more promising in the field of pathophysiologic markers for alcoholism. The genetic evidence has been summarized by Begleiter and Porjesz (1988).

Although there are no consistent biologic markers that predispose individuals to alcoholism, several promising findings have emerged that deserve further study. The high-risk approach may be the most powerful way to identify these traits.

ANTISOCIAL PERSONALITY

Twin Studies

In a large Danish twin series (Cloninger et al., 1978), the probandwise concordance for criminality in male MZ twins was 51.5 percent and in male DZ twins 26.2 percent (corresponding figures for females were 35.3 and 14.3 percent).

Adoption Studies

Adoption studies of criminality have provided evidence for important genetic *and* environmental factors in the development of antisocial personality. In the adoption study of Hutchings and Mednick (1975), for instance, both the adoptive and the biologic fathers of antisocial adoptees had an excess of criminal convictions.

Crowe (1974) studied adopted-away children of female criminals. Six of 46 were found to have antisocial personality by research criteria, while 0 of 46 controls received this diagnosis ($p < 0.01$). No other disorder was significantly increased in the probands. On the other hand, Bohman (1978) did not find an excess of criminality in adopted-away offspring of antisocial or alcoholic parents except among offspring with alcohol abuse themselves. This study was based on criminal and alcohol abuse records in Stockholm. Individual interviews of offspring were not performed. Bohman and colleagues (1982) and Cloninger and colleagues (1982) expanded this observation and demonstrated that in the absence of alcohol abuse, criminality in adopted-away offspring of criminals was likely to involve nonviolent property crime (petty criminality) and that this petty criminality could be best explained as a result of gene–environment interaction. The relative risk of an antisocial outcome in adoptees with criminality in both biologic and adoptive parents was nine times greater than in the population, as compared with a two times increased risk for those with criminal biologic parents alone or one and a half times for those with criminal adoptive parents alone. These authors noted that the threshold for antisocial behavior in women appears to be higher than that in men and that the women who actually do manifest antisocial behavior have a relatively greater genetic predisposition. Environmental influences that were implicated were multiple foster homes (for men) and extensive institutional care (in women).

Cadoret (Cadoret and Cain, 1981; Cadoret, 1982) also reported independent contributions of genetic predisposition and environmental variables (discontinuous mothering or the presence of a behavioral or psychiatric problem in a sibling or parent) in adoptees who subsequently showed antisocial behavior. There was evidence for a more than additive increase in vulnerability in persons with both genetic and environmental predisposing factors. These findings were essentially confirmed and additional environmental factors were identified in a second sample (Cadoret et al., 1987). In a combined analysis of two samples of adoptees, Cadoret et al. (1990) identified criminality in a biologic parent as a risk factor and criminality or alcoholism in an adoptive parent as an independent risk factor. Lower socioeconomic status in the adoptive home was a further risk factor for subjects with a criminal biologic parent.

Family Studies and Mode of Transmission

Cloninger and colleagues (1975) studied 227 first-degree relatives of sociopathic men or women and women with Briquet's syndrome (somatization disorder). The prevalence of Briquet's was increased in female relatives of sociopathic probands, and sociopathy was increased in male relatives of probands with Briquet's. Their data fit a multifactorial model of disease transmission in which the same genetic tendency might be expressed as sociopathy in men or as hysteria or (with a higher threshold) sociopathy in women. A follow-up study expanded the series of probands with Briquet's syndrome and confirmed the original results (Guze et al., 1986).

A similar clustering of illnesses was reported in family studies of hyperactive children by Morrison and Stewart (1971) and Cantwell (1972) and in a study of the biologic families of adopted hyperactive children by Morrison and Stewart (1973). These studies also noted an excess of alcoholism in fathers of hyperactive children.

Biologic Markers—The Y Chromosome

Jacobs et al. (1965, 1971) have noted that there is a 20-fold increased prevalence of the XYY karyotype in inmates of security hospitals for mentally disordered individuals who were violent or criminal or both. This karyotype also has been associated with increased height and decreased intelligence.

It has been difficult to evaluate the data that was based on surveys of institutionalized men because of the lack of adequate control groups from the rest of the population. This objection was overcome by a study from Denmark (Witkin et al., 1976) in which the group of men born to women living in Copenhagen between 1944 and 1947 was taken as a starting point. The tallest 15 percent of that population (4558) were asked to undergo chromosomal analysis, and the results were compared with data from penal records. Of 12 XYY males, 5 had a criminal conviction (41.7 percent), compared with 9.3 percent of the 4096 XY males ($p < 0.01$ by Fisher's exact test). Criminality appeared to be associated with decreased intelligence in the XYY males but not with height. The criminal acts involved in this study were not personally violent. Although the number of probands in the Danish study was quite small, it is the best-controlled assessment of the relationship of the XYY genotype to criminality. It does appear that there is a significantly increased risk of antisocial behavior in a male with this genotype. As for the societal impact of this increased risk, it is small. XYY males represent 0.5 to 3 percent of the institutionalized population (Shah and Roth, 1974). Other investigators have reported an increased length of the Y chromosome in persons with behavioral disturbance (Dorus, 1980; McConville et al., 1983). These two types of data suggest a possible role for the Y chromosome in the predisposition to socially disruptive behavior.

Other Biologic Markers

Low (to nondetectable) plasma dopamine β-hydroxylase (DBH) levels have been reported in a subpopulation of boys with conduct disorder (see review in Rogeness et al., 1988) but not in a recent group of juveniles from a detention center (Pliszka et al., 1988). Galvin et al. (1991) suggest that low DBH levels may be more closely related to childhood abuse or neglect. Low autonomic arousal has been implicated in a prospective study of psychophysiologic variables in male adolescents who later became criminal (Raine et al., 1990).

PANIC DISORDER AND OTHER ANXIETY DISORDERS

Studies of twins ascertained through population registers show a lack of specificity in genetic factors leading to mild to moderate anxiety and depressive disorders (Andrews et al., 1990, Torgersen, 1990). Twin studies focusing on severe anxiety disorders have not been done to our knowledge.

Crowe et al. (1980) reported a 31 percent risk of panic disorder in relatives of persons with anxiety neurosis. Among relatives personally interviewed, the incidence was 41 percent. The presence or absence of mitral valve prolapse in the proband did not affect the morbid risk in relatives. Alcoholism also was increased in relatives, but DSM-III major depression was not. In a pedigree study of these same families, Pauls and colleagues (1980) concluded that autosomal dominant transmission was likely. Crowe et al. (1983), in a follow-up including the data in their earlier study, reported a 25 percent incidence of definite or probable panic disorder in relatives of patients with panic. No excess of generalized anxiety disorder or major depressive disorder was found. A nonsignificant excess of alcoholism was present. Data were consistent with single-locus or polygenic transmission.

Twenty agoraphobic probands and their families were studied by Harris and associates (1983). An excess of "all-anxiety disorder" (agoraphobia, panic, generalized anxiety, atypical anxiety, social phobia, simple phobia, and obsessive-compulsive disorder) and alcoholism, but not affective disorders, was found in relatives of agoraphobic probands. In a larger study, Noyes et al. (1987) found a specificity of transmission for generalized anxiety disorder and panic disorder, with the relatives of probands of generalized anxiety disorder exhibiting characteristics of a mild adjustment disorder and relatives of panic disorder proband showing true panic disorder. Fyer et al. (1990) report specificity of transmission in a family study of simple phobia,

with relatives of phobic probands displaying phobias but not panic disorder.

However, Leckman et al. (1983) have studied probands with depression and panic disorder. Relatives of those persons show an increased risk of depression, anxiety disorder (phobias, panic disorder, and generalized anxiety), and alcoholism. Coryell et al. (1988) also found increased depression in relatives of depressed probands with depression plus panic attacks compared with probands with depression alone. Probands with a lifetime diagnosis of panic disorder and an index episode of secondary depression had less depression but increased rates of anxiety disorders. These data are compatible with a partially shared genetic predisposition to panic disorder and depression. Anxiety disorders themselves do clearly seem to be familially aggregated.

Crowe and colleagues (Crowe et al., 1987; 1990; Mutchler et al., 1990) report linkage studies in several series of multiple families with panic disorder. Initial studies suggested possible linkage to α-haptoglobin (lod score = 2.27), but this was not confirmed in a second series. Close linkage to tyrosine hydroxylase was excluded in 14 families. A general genomic screen is underway in these pedigrees.

OTHER GENETICALLY TRANSMITTED BEHAVIORAL/ COGNITIVE DISORDERS

Gilles de la Tourette's Syndrome

A rare syndrome of chronic vocal and motor tics, with a waxing and waning course, Gilles de la Tourette's syndrome is well known to be familial. Males are about three times more often affected than females. The prevalence has been found to be about tenfold less in adults than in school age children (0.5 per 10,000 compared with 5 per 10,000), suggesting either underdiagnosis in adults or resolution of symptoms during development (Burd et al., 1986a, 1986b). Tourette's appears to be highly concentrated in Ashkenazi Jews, a genetically homogeneous subgroup of Jews that includes nearly all European-origin Jews (Eldridge et al., 1979). A twin study is consistent with genetic transmission (Price et al., 1985). Analysis of the distribution of illness in families showed that chronic multiple tics were familially associated with Tourette's syndrome, apparently as a milder form of illness (Pauls et al., 1981; Kidd et al., 1980). A sex threshold effect in transmission appears present, with relatives of female probands having more Tourette's and more multiple tics than do relatives of male probands. Family study suggests also that obsessive-compulsive disorder may be an alternate expression of Tourette's (Pauls et al., 1986, 1991). An analysis of 250 families of Tourette's patients using the model of Lalouel and Morton (1981) concluded that a single semidominant major gene was likely to explain most of the variation in incidence of this condition (Comings et al., 1984). Pauls and Leckman (1986) and Price et al. (1988) also have published segregation analyses consistent with a single major gene effect. The Pauls et al. study is notable for the fact that the best fit assumed equal penetrance in both sexes and included mild phenotypes (e.g., ever having single tic) as affected.

A genomic search is now underway in independent samples of families from Holland and the United States. At last report, more than 50 percent of the genome had been excluded (Pakstis et al., 1991).

Specific Reading Disability

First described as "congenital word blindness" in 1896, the familial nature of this disorder has been known for most of this century. Males are more severely affected. Zerbin-Rudin (1967), in a review, found that MZ concordance was complete but that DZ concordance was 35 percent. Although not all cases fit a single mode of transmission (DeFries and Decker, 1982), a demonstration of autosomal dominant inheritance of at least a subtype of this disorder was provided by Smith et al. (1983), who found a significant linkage to a chromosomal banding polymorphism on chromosome 15 in a series of pedigrees. However, subsequent testing of additional families reduced the lod score to 1.56 (Smith et al., 1990). The authors suggest that heterogeneity may be present, but this hypothesis requires confirmation.

Male Homosexuality

Note: This category is included without the implication that it is a disorder. As reviewed by Pillard et al. (1981), the only large twin study was performed by Kallman more than 30 years earlier. MZ concordance was complete, and DZ concordance was much lower. Later authors have reported discordant MZ twins. The epidemiologic study of Pillard et al. (1982) consists of well-sampled homosexuals and controls and shows that in male, but not female, homosexuals, there is increase of homosexuality in relatives of the same sex.

A recent twin study of men based on responses to an ad in homophile publications (i.e., all the probands were male, homosexual, and a twin) showed 52 percent (29 of 56) concordance of homosexual orientation in MZ twins, 22 percent (12 of 54) in DZ twins, 11 percent (6 of 57) in adoptive brothers, and 9.2 percent (13 of 142) in nontwin brothers (Bailey et al., 1991). These data are puzzling; the difference between MZ and DZ twins is significant, as expected for a heritable trait, but the difference between DZ twins and brothers is also significant ($p = 0.02$, Fisher's exact test), which suggests that there is some nongenetic aspect of being a twin, as opposed to a brother, which leads to concordance for homosexuality.

Certain standard methodologic aspects of genetic epidemiologic diagnostic studies were lacking in this study: population-based sampling, use of validated measures of sexual orientation, direct study of all pertinent relatives, and an independent estimate of the population rate using the same methods as in the twins. Sexual preference is of considerable interest to our understanding of the biology of behavior and of current importance from a public health standpoint at this time, so the question of its heritability is worth solving.

Delusional Disorder

Kendler (1980), Kendler et al. (1981b), and Kendler and Hays (1981) argued that delusional disorder (paranoid psychosis without other signs and symptoms of schizophrenia) is genetically distinct from affective disorders and schizophrenia. The evidence does suggest that the persons with this uncommon disorder (about one-tenth as common as schizophrenia) have fewer schizophrenic relatives than otherwise defined schizophrenic probands.

GENETIC COUNSELING

Genetic counseling for psychiatric disorders should begin with the following general principles:

- The major psychiatric disorders appear to be inherited.
- The mode of transmission of these disorders is unknown.
- Biologic markers of genetic vulnerability are not sufficiently established to be of clinical use.
- Empirical risk estimates are available and should be used (see Table 29-7).
- A request for genetic counseling should be approached as a problem in short-term psychotherapy.

The most common questions that the psychiatric genetic counselor is asked are probably (1) "What is the chance of my child developing the same disorder that I/my spouse has?" and (2) "What are the chances of my developing the same disorder that my relative has?"

Consider the first of these questions. It is often asked in the context, "Should I have children?" The astute clinician will be aware of the concerns that are evident in this question—issues of self-esteem, competency, feelings of being damaged or impaired. These are concerns that should be addressed.

Practical issues regarding child bearing and child raising must be dealt with. Suppose the prospective mother has BP manic-depressive illness. Will she be able to manage the strains of pregnancy, birth, and dealing with a young child? Can she safely go off medication during pregnancy (lithium increases teratogenic risk; the data for antidepressants and neuroleptics are not as clear). If so, when should medication be restarted (most experts believe that the first trimester is the most dangerous). Most psychotropic agents are passed through breast milk, and therefore, if they are reinstituted after birth, the child should be bottle-fed. It is agreed that puerperium is a time of particular danger for mothers with affective illness.

If the prospective father has major psychiatric disorder, the issues are somewhat different. Psychodynamically, the major difficulty may be the shift in attention of his spouse, who now must devote her mothering energies to the new child rather than to an ill husband. Issues of medication-induced fetal damage do not appear to be a concern here.

If both mother and father have a psychiatric illness, all the previous issues apply as well as a new concern: The empirical risk of psychiatric illness in the child is then greatly increased, perhaps more than additively. For children of two parents with major affective illness, for instance, the risk is probably between 50 and 75 percent. The child of two schizophrenics has an observed risk of more than 40 percent to develop schizophrenia, whereas the child of one schizophrenic has a risk of approximately 10 percent (Gottesman and Shields, 1982). There is, in general, no advantage in amniocentesis for such couples because there is no marker to be found.

All this being said, the fact is that most prospective parents are not deterred from starting or enlarging a family by these concerns. Nor should they be. Most psychiatric illnesses are manageable and are likely to become more so. Exceptions might be the instance in which two persons with chronic schizophrenic or SA illness are prospective parents or in which the mother has poorly controlled rapid-cycling BP illness. The keynote of the discussion with parents concerned about their children developing a psychiatric illness should be in education about the nature of the condition and an inculcation of awareness, where it is indicated, that if such

symptoms develop, they should receive early professional attention. This is especially true for the affective disorders, for which early treatment can prevent major disruption of young adulthood.

Empirical risk figures for first-degree relatives are shown in Table 29-7. These are lifetime risks for the development of the indicated condition. In general, offspring of a person with one major psychiatric condition are not at increased risk for other illnesses (exceptions are noted in the spectrum sections). These figures should be used in conjunction with the population risk figures in the same table. These risk figures are for first-degree relatives: parents, siblings, children; the age of the subject should be taken into account when they are used (see below).

Second-degree relatives have in general a small increase in risk over the general population.

Special cases are (1) dual matings, considered earlier, and (2) identical twins, for whom lifetime risk is quite high (see summaries of twin studies in the individual sections of this chapter).

Consider the second common question posed to the counselor: "My [brother, mother, great aunt, ex-husband, roommate] has schizophenia. Will I also get it?" The last two examples are included not frivolously. The evidence for viral transmission of schizophrenia has been summarized by Crow (1983), and similar theories of affective illness are extant. One may specify, however, that, in general, the epidemiologic evidence for contagion rests on studies among relatives, i.e., among persons sharing both genetic *and* environmental factors.* Thus the family-study—derived figures, even if they included effects of a viral factor, would still be accurate; the danger of developing major psychiatric disorder by contact alone must be regarded as a hypothesis without evidence.

One should, of course, do a thorough diagnostic evaluation when presented with the second

---

* An exception is the study of Kazanetz, referred to by Crow, in which Moscow housing complexes were studied and propinquity alone found to be a risk factor for schizophrenic illness. The original report of this study was not available to us.

TABLE 29-7. *Empirical Data for Genetic Counselling*

Illness	Evidence for heritability	Mode of transmission	Risk first-degree relatives/ risk general population	Median age of onset
Affective disorder	Twin Family/adoption studies	Multifactorial?	20–25%/7%	25–30
Schizophrenia	Twin Family/adoption studies	Multifactorial?	6–10%/1%	20–25
Alcoholism	Twin Family/adoption studies	Unknown	25–35(males)/5–10% 5–10%(females)/1–3%	25–30
Antisocial personality	Twin Family/adoption studies	Multifactorial?	15–25%(males)/2–3% 2–11% (females)/0.5%	15–20
Panic disorder	Family studies	Autosomal Dominant?	40%/2%	20–25

References are found in the appropriate sections of the text.

question. It may be that the disorder has already been manifest but has been denied [e.g., the 35-year-old sister of a BP patient asks, "Will I become ill?" and under questioning reveals a major depressive episode 5 years previously; the answer is that she appears to be vulnerable to affective illness (Yes, she is ill), but the chances are that it will not be as severe as that of her brother (see Gershon et al., 1982)]. Or the son of an alcoholic patient who has already experienced blackouts from drinking—the real question in these and similar cases is, "Will my life be like that of [the sick relative]?" and the answer, in general, is "not with treatment."

Sometimes what may have been noted is a minor disorder of a type similar to that of the probands (for instance, cyclothymia or minor depression in the child of a BP patient). Here the answer is that we do not know what to expect—the major disorder *may* come, one should know the symptoms, and one should be aware of the difference that early treatment will make.

If the counselor is satisfied that a major disorder does not exist at present, then the question of the subject's age must be addressed (see Table 29-7 for median ages of onset for the various psychiatric disorders). For instance, a 25-year-old male with no history of antisocial behavior is highly unlikely to develop criminality, even if his family tree is loaded with criminals and he has the XYY genotype. However, a 25-year-old male with a BP sibling is just at the midpoint of his risk for affective disorder [i.e., his lifetime risk is $1/4$ (as the first-degree relative of a manic-depressive patient) $\times$ $1/2$ (since he has passed through half of the period of risk) $= 1/8$]. There is some evidence, although it is equivocal, of concordance in age of onset among relatives [for affective illness, Weissman et al. (submitted for publication); for schizophrenia, Abe (1969)]. This might confer an additional degree of safety on those well persons who have already passed considerably beyond the age at which their relative became ill.

The general attitude of the clinician in these circumstances should be reassuring but informing: reassuring because the news is usually more good than bad, but informing because, more than others, relatives of those with major psychiatric disorder need to know as much as possible about the signs, symptoms, and treatment of these conditions.

Two further observations on the meaning of inherited disorders for patients may be made. First, there is a widespread misapprehension that genetic illnesses are likely to be untreatable. Such is not the case. The prospects of cure for such illnesses are in the hands of the molecular biologists and may be available within the lifetimes of most of us. But more important, existing treatments for many genetic disorders are efficacious (e.g., dietary therapy for phenylketonuria). Second, the recognition of genetics as an important factor in etiology of these conditions may be a tremendous relief to families who have lived through an era when exaggerated claims were made for psychosocial causation and treatment. No credible evidence exists for specific psychosocial factors in the vulnerability for chronic schizophrenia, bipolar affective disorder, or panic disorder; such factors appear to play a role in antisocial personality and alcoholism, along with genetic factors. Life events may precipitate individual episodes of psychiatric disturbance (see review in Nurnberger et al., 1983a), but it is not clear that they contribute to the vulnerability of a person to develop the disorder at some point during his or her life. There is little evidence that drug abuse precipitates persistent psychiatric syndromes in unpredisposed persons (see review by Propping, 1983), although the possibility cannot be ruled out. For parents to realize that they have not caused a disorder in their children by something they did in their upbringing may often be liberating.

DISCUSSION

The points of significance for the clinician are summarized in the foregoing genetic counseling section and in Tables 29-7 and 29-8. What might be addressed at this point is the question, "What is needed in psychiatric genetics?" and the answer is,

TABLE 29-8. *Variable Expression of Vulnerability to Major Psychiatric Illness*

Illness	Spectrum disorders	Putative vulnerability markers
Affective disorder	BP, UP, schizoaffective, anorexia nervosa, bulimia, cyclothymic personality	REM induction; melatonin suppression; lithium ratio?
Schizophrenia	Schizotypal personality?	HLA-A$_9$; smooth pursuit eye movements; monoamine-related abnormalities in platelets; cognitive or attentional deficits
Alcoholism	—	Intoxication level; D$_2$ receptor allele A$_1$; P$_{300}$ after auditory stimulation
Antisocial personality	Briquet's syndrome Attention deficit disorder	XYY karyotype
Panic disorder	Agoraphobia Generalized anxiety disorder Obsessive compulsive disorder	—

References are found in the appropriate sections of the text.

essentially, "biologic markers." To assert that a disorder is heritable is to assert that an altered DNA produces an altered protein in persons having that disorder. We may make this assertion with regard to the major psychiatric disorders. There appear to be independent genetic vulnerability factors for affective illness, schizophrenia, alcoholism, anxiety, and sociopathy, although these diagnostic entities also show some overlap. There are, of course, many persons seeking psychiatric attention who do not fall neatly into one of these categories. What is necessary at this point is to identify the altered proteins that predispose a person to disrupted central nervous functioning. With a more specific biology of genetic vulnerability to psychiatric illness, the diagnostic schemes could be rewritten.

How should such markers be pursued? Perhaps a word is in order about how they should not be pursued. Biologic studies on acutely ill, medicated patients are not likely to be of value unless comparison groups of unmedicated, well patients are included. The definition of *unmedicated* may have to be revised from the previously accepted 3 days or 1 or even 2 weeks to months or *never medicated*. Of course, acute intake of alcohol or street drugs needs to be considered. Other factors that need to be considered for certain variables (besides the obvious ones of age, sex, and concurrent illnesses) include time of day, time of year, diet, and menstrual status of women.

One may argue that these kinds of restrictions make studies almost impossible to do. We would agree that the difficulties are extreme but would suggest that the field is in a state of maturity now such that it is worth taking the time to design appropriate, although difficult, studies.

Some methods that may get around the difficulties are the following:

1. *Linkage studies.* There are now DNA markers for nearly every interval on each human chromosome; these constitute the human genetic linkage map. Using these markers, if linkage is observed between a map location and a disease, this is proof that a gene for disease susceptibility exists at this location, and this information will eventually lead to the gene's complete characterization. To link an illness to a location on the map, one examines DNA markers in families in which the illness is distributed and observes if there are any markers that cosegregate with the disease. Enough family members are observed so that a chance cosegregation is unlikely. Despite several recent reports of linkage of manic-depressive illness to markers on chromosome 11 or on the X chromosome and of linkage of schizophrenia on chromosome 5, replication has not been forthcoming, and none of these mappings can be considered authoritative at this time (see above).

2. *Association studies.* Association is an alternative to linkage for testing a candidate gene hypothesis (a hypothesis that a particular gene, such as one of the muscarinic cholinergic receptor genes, is involved in disease susceptibility). Association exists when there is an allele that is more frequent in a series of unrelated patients as compared with population frequencies. When a linkage has been demonstrated, the disease mutation within the linkage region also will be associated with disease. Association, however, may be independent of observable linkage, as with genes whose effect on disease vulnerability is too small to detect through linkage. Association with an infrequent allele generally requires small sample sizes to be detected, in comparison with sample sizes needed to detect linkage in presence of heterogeneity (Thompson et al., 1988; Gershon et al., 1989). When its genomic structure is well elucidated, molecular scanning of the candidate gene for mutations in unrelated cases or in small families may be sufficient to demonstrate the disease mutation (Weinstein et al., 1990).

3. *High-risk studies.* Well offspring of patients or siblings of patients face increased risk of illness if they have not yet passed through the age of risk. Such persons are not yet biochemically influenced by the effects of illness or the treatments for it. Schuckit and Rayses (1979) used this method to study acetaldehyde as a marker for alcoholism. Similarly, Rutschman et al. (1977) have identified a psychomotor deficit in offspring of schizophrenics. Appropriate design and statistical considerations must be observed (Goldin et al., 1986). Follow-up studies of such populations are of value.

4. *Pharmacogenetic studies.* Pharmacologic responses in appropriate populations (well patients, twins, relatives) may be evaluated, similar to the use of a glucose tolerance test. The cholinergic REM induction test (Sitaram et al., 1980; Nurnberger et al., 1983c) is an example. We have found that an outpatient clinic in which selected patients are periodically asked to go off medication for testing is valuable. Such strategies also may be used to identify subgroups in the "normal" population that may be more sensitive to the effects of psychoactive drugs on a genetic basis (Nurnberger et al., 1982a).

5. *Comparison of familial risks in biologically characterized groups.* Schlesser and coworkers (1979, 1980) have pursued a variant of this strategy in studying familial correlates of the dexamethasone suppression test in affective illness. Reveley et al. (1984) have used this strategy in studying ventricular size in schizophrenia. An essential for such studies, however, is appropriate family study methodology (Gershon and Guroff, 1984).

6. *Preclinical studies.* If a biochemical abnormality predisposes to psychiatric illness in humans, one presumes that the same abnormality might be found in certain animal species. Appropriate animal models of psychiatric illness, however, are difficult to validate. Recently, Suomi (1983) described depression-like states in monkeys who were unusually sensitive to separation. There is some evidence

for a genetic predisposition to such states; they may be associated with dexamethasone nonsuppression; and they respond to imipramine. Biochemical hypotheses, such as increased D_2 receptors in schizophrenia (Owen et al., 1978) might be studied by examining inbred rodent populations. The physiologic and neuroanatomical "meaning" of these biochemical abnormalities might then become clearer. In a variant of this strategy, Murphy et al. (1982) have studied a strain of rats bred for alcohol-preferring behavior. These rats showed a difference in serotonin content in several brain areas, and this difference predates the exposure to alcohol.

The types of studies we have been discussing are possible now partly because of methodological advances in the laboratory, but more critically because of methodological advances in the clinic. A generation ago few basic researchers were interested in psychiatric problems. If clinicians could not agree on who had schizophrenia, how was one to inquire into the biology of it? The development of diagnostic criteria, while not eliminating differences of opinion, at least makes it clearer what sort of patients one is studying. A second major step has been the development of rigorous methodologies for making biologic measurements in intact humans. Only by adherence to such constraints may we hope to attract the interest and collaboration of the neurochemist, the molecular geneticist, the psycho-physiologist, and others who are essential to the enterprise of translating clinical genetic knowledge into a molecular understanding of brain dysfunction.

SUMMARY

Data from twin, family, and adoption studies suggest the following: a predisposition to affective illness is inherited. Elements of the affective spectrum include bipolar illness, unipolar illness, schizo-affective disorder, cyclothymic personality, and the eating disorders anorexia nervosa and bulimia. Schizophrenia, or at least some forms of it, appears to originate in genetic vulnerability. The spectrum of schizophrenic illness includes schizotypal personality. The development of antisocial personality is strongly influenced by both genetics and the home environment; XYY men are at increased risk for this disorder. Severe forms of alcoholism appear to be strongly heritable. Anxiety disorders are probably also heritable; the anxiety spectrum may include generalized anxiety, panic disorder, agoraphobia, and obsessive-compulsive disorder. Some forms of anxiety disorder may have overlapping vulnerability with depressive disorders.

The mode of transmission of these disorders is not yet clear; biologic markers of genetic vulnerability are not yet available for clinical use. Genetic counseling should be based on empirical risk

figures, some of which are presented herein. Strategies for the elucidation and testing of biologic markers are considered.

REFERENCES

Abe K: The morbidity rate and environmental influence in monozygotic cotwins of schizophrenics. Br J Psychiatry 115:519–531, 1969.

Abrams R, Taylor MA: The genetics of schizophrenia: A reassessment using modern criteria. Am J Psychiatry 140:171–175, 1983.

Akiskal HS, Djenderedjian AH, Rosenthal RH: Cyclothymic disorder: validating criteria for inclusion in the bipolar affective group. Am J Psychiatry 134:1227–1233, 1977.

Akiskal HS, Khan MK, Scott-Strauss A: Cyclothymic temperamental disorders. Psychiatr Clin North Am 2:527–554, 1979.

Allen MG, Cohen S, Pollin W, Greenspan SI: Affective illness in veteran twins. A diagnostic review. Am J Psychiatry 131:1234–1239, 1974.

Andrews G, Stewart G, Allen R, Henderson AS: The genetics of six neurotic disorders: A twin study. J Affective Disord 19:23–29, 1990.

Angst J, Felder W, Lohmeyer B: Schizoaffective disorders: results of a genetic investigation I. J Affect Disord 1:139–153, 1979.

Angst J, Frey R, Lohmeyer B, Zerbin-Rudin E: Bipolar manic depressive psychoses: results of a genetic investigation. Hum Genet 55:237–254, 1980.

Andreasen N, Endicott J, Spitzer R, et al: The family history method using diagnostic criteria: Reliability and validity. Arch Gen Psychiatry 34:1229–1235, 1977.

Bailey JM, Pillard RC: A genetic study of male sexual orientation. Arch Gen Psychiatry 48:1089–1096, 1991.

Baron M, Freimer NF, Risch N, Lever B, et al: Diminished support for linkage between manic depressive illness and X-chromosome markers in three Israeli pedigrees. Nature Genetics 3:49–55, 1993.

Baron M, Gruen R, Rainer JD, Kane J, et al: A family study of schizophrenia and normal control probands: Implications for the spectrum concept of schizophrenia. Am J Psychiatry 142:447–455, 1985.

Baron M, Levitt M, Gruen R, et al: Platelet monoamine oxidase activity and genetic vulnerability in schizophrenia. Am J Psychiatry 141:836–842, 1984.

Baron M, Risch N, Hamburger R, et al: Genetic linkage between X chromosome markers and bipolar affective illness. Nature 326(6110):289–292, 1987.

Bassett AS, McGillivray BC, Jones BD, Pantzar JT: Partial trisomy chromosome 5 cosegregating with schizophrenia. Lancet 1(8589):799–801, 1988.

Beckman L, Cedergren B, Perris C, Strandman E: Blood groups and affective disorders. Hum Hered 28:48–55, 1978.

Begleiter H, Porjesz B, Bihari B, Kissin B: Event-related brain potentials in boys at risk for alcoholism. Science 225:1493–1496, 1984.

Begleiter H, Porjesz B: Potential biological markers in individuals at high risk for developing alcoholism. Alcohol Clin Exp Res 12(4):488–493, 1988.

Behar D, Berg CJ, Rapoport JL, et al: Behavioral and physiological effects of ethanol in high risk and control children. A pilot study. Alcoholism 7:404–410, 1983.

Berrettini WH, Cappellari CB, Nurnberger JI Jr, Gershon ES: Beta-adrenergic receptors on lymphoblasts: A study of manic-depressive illness. Neuropsychobiology 17:(1–2)15–18, 1987.

Berrettini WH, Goldin LR, Gelernter J, et al: X chromosome markers and manic-depressive illness: Rejection of linkage to Xg28 in nine bipolar pedigrees. Arch Gen Psychiatry 47:366–373, 1990.

Berrettini WH, Nurnberger JI Jr, Hare T, et al: Plasma and CSF GABA in affective illness. Br J Psychiatry 141:483–488, 1982.

Berrettini WH, Nurnberger JI Jr, Hare TA, et al: Reduced plasma and CSF GABA in affective illness: Effect of lithium carbonate. Biol Psychiatry 18:185–194, 1983.

Bertelsen A: A Danish twin study of manic-depressive disorders. In Schou M, Stromgren E (eds): Origin, Prevention and Treatment of Affective Disorders. London, Academic Press, 1979, pp 227–239.

Bertelsen A, Harvald B, Hauge M: A danish twin study of manic-depressive disorders. Br J Psychiatry 130:330–351, 1977.

Biederman J, Munir K, Knee D, et al: A family study of patients with attention deficit disorder and normal controls. J Psychiatr Res 20:263–274, 1987.

Blum K, Noble EP, Sheridan PJ, et al: Allelic association of human dopamine D₂ receptor gene in alcoholism. JAMA 263(15): 2055–2060, 1990.

Bodmer WF: Human genetics: The molecular challenge. In Cold Spring Harbor Symposium on Quantitative Biology, vol 51. Cold Spring Harbor, NY, Cold Spring Harbor Laboratory, 1986, pp 1–13.

Bohman M: Some genetic aspects of alcoholism and criminality. Arch Gen Psychiatry 35:269–276, 1978.

Bohman M, Cloninger CR, Sigvardsson S, Von Knorring AL: Predisposition to petty criminality in Swedish adoptees: I. Genetic and environmental heterogeneity. Arch Gen Psychiatry 39:1233–1241, 1982.

Bohman M, Cloninger C, von Knorring AL, Sigvardsson S: An adoption study of somatoform disorders. Arch Gen Psychiatry 41:872–878, 1984.

Bohman M, Sigvardsson S, Cloninger CR: Maternal inheritance of alcohol abuse. Cross-fostering analysis of adopted women. Arch Gen Psychiatry 38:965–969, 1981.

Bolos AM, Dean M, Brown GL, Goldman D: Population and pedigree studies rule out a widespread association between the dopamine D₂ receptor gene and alcoholism. Am J Hum Genet 47(3):(0187)A49, 1990.

Bondy B, Ackenheil M, Birzle W, et al: Catecholamines and their receptors in blood: Evidence for alterations in schizophrenia. Biol Psychiatry 19:1377–1393, 1984.

Bonham-Carter SM, Reveley MA, Sandler M, et al: Decreased urinary output of conjugated tyramine is associated with lifetime vulnerability to depressive illness. Psychiatry Res 3:13–22, 1980.

Bonney GE: On the statistical determination of major gene mechanisms in continuous human traits: Regressive models. Am J Med Genet 18:731–749, 1984.

Bonney GE: Regressive logistic models for familial disease and other binary traits. Biometrics 42:611–625, 1986.

Böök JA, Wetterberg L, Modrzewska K: Schizophrenia in a North Swedish geographical isolate, 1900–1977. Epidemiology, genetics and biochemistry. Clin Genet 14:373–394, 1978.

Bottema CD, Koeberl DD, Sommer SS: Direct carrier testing in 14 families with haemophilia B. Lancet 2(8662):526–529, 1989.

Brecher M, Begleiter H: Event-related brain potentials to high-incentive stimuli in unmedicated schizophrenic patients. Biol Psychiatry 18:661–674, 1983.

Bucher KD, Elston RC: The transmission of manic depressive illness: I. Theory, description of the model, and summary of results. J Psychiatr Res 16:53–63, 1981.

Bucher KD, Elston RC, Green R, et al: The transmission of manic depressive illness: II. Segregation analysis of three sets of family data. J Psychiatr Res 16:65–78, 1981.

Buchsbaum MS, Ingvar DH, Kessler R, et al: Cerebral glucography with positron tomography. Use in normal subjects and in patients with schizophrenia. Arch Gen Psychiatry 39:251–259, 1982.

Burd L, Kerbeshian J, Wikenheiser M, Fisher W: Prevalence of Gilles de la Tourette's syndrome in North Dakota adults. Am J Psychiatry 143:6, 1986a.

Burd L, Kerbeshian J, Wikenheiser M, Fisher W: A prevalence study of Gilles de la Tourette syndrome in North Dakota school-age children. J Am Acad Child Adolesc Psychiatry 25(4):552–553, 1986b.

Cadoret RJ, Cain CA: Genetic-environmental interaction in adoption studies of antisocial behavior. Presented at the World Congress of Biological Psychiatry, Stockholm, Sweden, June 1981.

Cadoret RJ: Genotype-environment interaction in antisocial behavior. Psychol Med 12:235–239, 1982.

Cadoret RJ, Cain C, Grove W: Development of alcoholism in adoptees raised apart from alcoholic biologic relatives. Arch Gen Psychiatry 37:561–563, 1980.

Cadoret RJ, Troughton E, O'Gorman TW, Heywood E: An adoption study of genetic and environmental factors in drug abuse. Arch Gen Psychiatry 43:1131–1136, 1986.

Cadoret RJ, Troughton E, O'Gorman TW: Genetic and environmental factors in alcohol abuse and antisocial personality. J Stud Alcohol 48(1):1–8, 1987.

Cadoret RJ, Troughton E, Bagford J, Woodworth G: Genetic and environmental factors in adoptee antisocial personality. Eur Arch Psychiatr Neurol Sci 239:231–240, 1990.

Cantwell DP: Psychiatric illness in the families of hyperactive children. Arch Gen Psychiatry 27:414–417, 1972.

Cantwell DP, Sturzenberger S, Burroughs J, et al: Anorexia nervosa: an affective disorder. Arch Gen Psychiatry 34:1087–1093, 1977.

Carter CL, Chung CS: Segregation analysis of schizophrenia under a mixed genetic model. Hum Hered 30:350–356, 1980.

Chojnacki M, Kralik P, Allen RH, et al: Neuroleptic induced decrease in platelet MAO activity of schizophrenic patients. Am J Psychiatry 138:838–840, 1981.

Cloninger C: Neurogenetic adaptive mechanisms in alcoholism. Science 236:410–416, 1987a.

Cloninger CR: D₂ dopamine receptor gene is associated but not linked with alcoholism. JAMA 266(13):1833–1834, 1991.

Cloninger CR, Sigvardsson S, Gilligan SB, et al: Genetic heterogeneity and the classification of alcoholism. Adv Alcohol Subst Abuse 7(3–4):3–16, 1988.

Cloninger CR, Bohman M, Sigvardsson S: Inheritance of alcohol abuse. Cross-fostering analysis of adopted men. Arch Gen Psychiatry 38:861–868, 1981.

Cloninger CR, Christiansen KD, Reich T, Gottesman II: Implications of sex differences in the prevalences of antisocial personality, alcoholism, and criminality for familial transmission. Arch Gen Psychiatry 35:941–951, 1978.

Cloninger CR, Lavis G, Rice J, Reich T: Strategies for resolution of cultural and biological inheritance. In Gershon ES, Matthyse S, Breakefield XO, Ciaranello RD (eds): Genetic Research Strategies in Psychobiology and Psychiatry. Pacific Grove, CA, Boxwood Press, 1981, pp 319–332.

Cloninger CR, Reich T, Guze SB: The multifactorial model of disease transmission: III. Familial relationship between sociopathy and hysteria (Briquet's syndrome). Br J Psychiatry 127:23–32, 1975.

Cloninger CR, Reich T, Wetzel R: Alcoholism and affective disorders: familial associations and genetic models. In Goodwin DW, Erickson CK (eds): Alcoholism and Affective Disorders: Clinical, Genetic and Biochemical Studies. New York, Spectrum Publications, 1979, pp 57–86.

Cloninger CR, Sigvardsson S, Bohman M, Von-Knorring AL: Predisposition to petty criminality in Swedish adoptees: III. Cross fostering analysis of gene-environment interaction. Arch Gen Psychiatry 39:1242–1253, 1982.

Cohen SM, Allen MG, Pollin W, Hrubec Z: Relationship of schizo-affective psychosis to manic-depressive psychosis and schizophrenia. Arch Gen Psychiatry 26:539–551, 1972.

Comings DE: Pc 1 Duarte, a common polymorphism of a human brain protein, and its relationship to depressive disease and multiple sclerosis. Nature 277:28–32, 1979.

Comings DE, Comings BG, Devor EJ, Cloninger CR: Detection of major gene for Gilles de la Tourette Syndrome. Am J Hum Genet 36:586–600, 1984.

Comings DE, Comings BG, Muhleman D, et al: The dopamine D₂ receptor locus as a modifying gene in neuropsychiatric disorders. JAMA 266(13):1793–1800, 1991.

Conneally MP: Association between the D₂ dopamine receptor gene and alcoholism. Arch Gen Psychiatry 48:664–666, 1991.

Coryell W, Endicott J, Andreasen NC, et al: Depression and panic attacks: the significance of overlap as reflected in follow-up and family study data. Am J Psychiatry 145(3):293–300, 1988.

Cox N, Reich T, Rice J, et al: Segregation and linkage analyses of bipolar and major depressive illnesses in multigenerational pedigrees. J Psychiatr Res 23:109–123, 1989.

Crow TJ: The biology of schizophrenia. Experimentia 38:1275–1282, 1982.

Crow TJ: Is schizophrenia an infectious disease? Lancet 1:173–175, 1983.

Crow TJ, Cross AJ, Johnstone EC, et al: Time course of the antipsychotic effect in schizophrenia and some changes in postmortem brain and their relation to neuroleptic medication. Adv Biochem Pharmacol 24:495–503, 1980.

Crowe RR: An adoption study of antisocial personality. Arch Gen Psychiatry 31:785–791, 1974.

Crowe RR, Namboodiri KK, Ashby HB, Elston RC: Segregation and linkage analysis of a large kindred of unipolar depression. Neuropsychobiology 7:20–25, 1981.

Crowe RR, Noyes R, Pauls DL, Slymen D: A family study of panic disorder. Arch Gen Psychiatry 40:1065–1069, 1983.

Crowe RR, Noyes R, Samuelson S, et al: Close linkage between panic disorder and α-haptoglobin excluded in 10 families. Arch Gen Psychiatry 47:377–380, 1990.

Crowe RR, Noyes R, Wilson AF, et al: A linkage study of panic disorder. Arch Gen Psychiatry 44:933–937, 1987.

Crowe RR, Pauls DL, Slymen DJ, Noyes R: A family study of anxiety neurosis. Morbidity risk in families of patients with and without mitral valve prolapse. Arch Gen Psychiatry 37:77–79, 1980.

Cytryn L, McKnew DH, Zahn-Waxler C, et al: A developmental view of affective disturbances in the children of affectively ill parents. Am J Psychiatry 141(2):219–222, 1984.

Daiguji M, Meltzer HY, Tong C, et al: Alpha-2-adrenergic receptors in platelet membranes of depressed patients: No change in number of ³H-yohimbine affinity. Life Sci 29(20):2059–2064, 1981.

Davison K, Bagley CR: Schizophrenia-like psychoses associated with organic disorders in the central nervous system: A review of the literature. In Herrington RN (ed): Current Problems in Neuropsychiatry. Kent, Ashford Headley Brothers, Ltd., 1969, pp 113–183.

Debray Q, Caillard V, Stewart J: Schizophrenia: A study of genetic models. Hum Hered 29:27–36, 1979.

Decina P, Kestenbaum CJ, Farber S, et al: Clinical and psychological assessment of children of bipolar probands. Am J Psychiatry 140:548–553, 1983.

DeFries JC, Decker SN: Genetic aspects of reading disability: a family study. In Malatesha RN, Aaron PG (eds): Reading Disorders: Varieties and Treatments. New York, Academic Press, 1982, pp 255–279.

DeLisi LE, Goldin LR, Hamovit JR, et al: A family study of the association of increased ventricular size with schizophrenia. Arch Gen Psychiatry 43:148–153, 1986.

DeLisi LE, Wise CD, Bridge TP, et al: A probable effect of neuroleptic medication on platelet monoamine oxidase activity. Psychiatry Res 4:95–107, 1981.

Depue RA, Slater JF, Wolfstetter-Kausch H, et al: A behavioral paradigm for identifying persons at risk for bipolar depressive disorder: A conceptual framework and five validation studies. J Abnorm Psychol 90:381–437, 1981.

Dorus E: Variability in the Y chromosome and variability of human behavior. Arch Gen Psychiatry 37:587–594, 1980.

Dorus E, Cox NJ, Gibbon RD, et al: Lithium ion transport and affective disorders within families of bipolar patients. Arch Gen Psychiatry 40:545–552, 1983.

Dorus E, Pandey GN, Shaughnessey R, et al: Lithium transport across the red cell membrane: a cell membrane abnormality in manic depressive illness. Science 205:932–934, 1979.

Dustman RE, Beckbeg EC: The visually evoked potential in twins. Electrocephalogr Clin Neurophysiol 19:570–575, 1965.

Earls F, Reich W, Jung KG, Cloninger CR: Psychopathology in children of alcoholic and antisocial parents. Alcohol Clin Exp Res 12(4):481–487, 1988.

Egeland J, Frazer A, Kidd K: Affective disorders among the Amish: III. Na–Li counterflow and COMT in bipolar pedigrees. Am J Psychiatry 141:1049–1054, 1984.

Egeland JA, Gerhard DS, Pauls DL, et al: Bipolar affective disorders linked to DNA markers on chromosome II. Nature 325:783–787, 1987.

Egeland JA, Klein DN: The genetics of neurotic-reactive depression: A reanalysis of Shapiro's (1970) twin study using diagnostic criteria. J Affective Disord 18:247–252, 1990.

Eldridge R, Wassman ER, Nee L, Koerber T: Gilles de la Tourette Syndrome. In Goodman RM, Motulsky AG (eds): Genetic Diseases Among Ashkenazi Jews. New York, Raven Press, 1979, pp 171–185.

Elmasian R, Neville H, Woods D, et al: Event-related brain potentials are different in individuals at high and low risk for developing alcoholism. Proc Natl Acad Sci USA 79:7900–7903, 1982.

Elston RC, Namboodiri KK, Spence MA, Rainer JD: A genetic study of schizophrenia pedigrees. II. One locus hypothesis. Neuropsychobiology 4:193–206, 1978.

Elston RC, Stewart J: A general method for the genetic analysis of pedigree data. Hum Hered 21:523–542, 1971.

Eriksson CPJ: Elevated blood acetaldehyde levels in alcoholics and their relatives: A re-evaluation. Science 207:1383–1394, 1980.

Essen-Möller E: Twin research and psychiatry. Acta Psychiatr Scand 39:65–77, 1963.

Essen-Möller E: Psychiatrische untersuchungen an einen serie von zwillingen. Acta Psychiatr Neurol Suppl 23:1–200, 1941.

Falconer DS: The inheritance of liability to certain diseases, estimated from the incidence among relatives. Ann Hum Genet 29:51–76, 1965.

Faraone SV, Tsuang MT: Quantitative models of the genetic transmission of schizophrenia. Psychol Bull 98(1):41–66, 1985.

Fischer M, Harvald B, Hauge M: A Danish twin study of schizophrenia. Br J Psychiatry 115:981–990, 1969.

Flemenbau A, Larson JW: ABO-Rh blood groups and psychiatric diagnosis: A critical review. Dis Nerv Sys 37:581–583, 1976.

Foch TT, DeFries JC, McClearn GE, Singer SM: Familial patterns of impairment in reading disability. J Educational Psychol 69:316–329, 1977.

Friedl W, Propping P: ³H-imipramine binding in human platelets: A study in normal twins. Psychiatry Res 11:279–285, 1984.

Fyer AJ, Mannuzza S, Gallops MS, et al: Familial transmission of simple phobias and fears. Arch Gen Psychiatry 47:252–256, 1990.

Gaensbauer TJ, Harmon RJ, Cytryn L, McKnew DH: Social and affective development in infants with manic-depressive parent. Am J Psychiatry 141(2):223–229, 1984.

Galvin M, Shekhar A, Simon J, et al: Low dopamine-beta-hydroxylase: A biological sequela of abuse and neglect. Psychiatry Res 39(1):1–13, 1991.

Garcia-Sevilla JA, Zis AP, Hollingsworth PJ, et al: Platelet alpha-2-adrenergic receptors in major depressive disorder: Binding of tritiated clonidine before and after tricyclic antidepressant drug treatment. Arch Gen Psychiatry 38(12):1327–1333, 1981.

Garcia-Sevilla JA, Guimon J, Garcia-Vallejo P, Fuster MJ: Biochemical and functional evidence of supersensitive platelet alpha-2-adrenoceptors in major affective disorder: Effect of long-term lithium carbonate treatment. Arch Gen Psychiatry 43(1):51–57, 1986.

Gejman PV, Detera-Wadleigh S, Martinez MM, et al: Manic depressive illness not linked to factor IX region in an independent series of pedigrees. Genomics 8(4):648–655, 1990.

Gelernter J, O'Malley S, Risch N, et al: No association between an allele at the D₂ dopamine receptor gene (DRD₂) and alcoholism. JAMA 266(13):1801–1807, 1991.

Gershon ES: Marker genotyping errors in old data on X-linkage in bipolar illness. Biol Psychiatry 29(7):721–729, 1991.

Gershon ES, Berrettini W, Nurnberger JI Jr, Goldin LR: Genetics of affective illness. In Meltzer HY (ed): Psychopharmacology: A Third Generation of Progress. New York, Raven Press, 1987a, pp 481–491.

Gershon ES, Bunney WE Jr, Leckman JF, et al: The inheritance of affective disorders: A review of data and of hypotheses. Behav Genet 6:227–261, 1976.

Gershon ES, DeLisi LE, Hamovit J, et al: A controlled family study of chronic psychoses. Arch Gen Psychiatry 45:328–336, 1988.

Gershon ES, Goldin LR, Lake CR, et al: Genetics of plasma dopamine-beta-hydroxylase (DBH), erythrocyte catechol-O-methyltransferase (COMT), and platelet monoamine oxidase (MAO) in pedigree of patients with affective disorders. In Usdin E, Sourkes P, Youdim MBH (eds): Enzymes and Neurotransmitters in Mental Disease. London, John Wiley & Sons Ltd, 1980, pp 281–299.

Gershon ES, Goldin LR, Weissman MM, Nurnberger JI Jr: Family and genetic studies of affective disorders in the Eastern United States: A provisional summary. In Perris C, Struwe G, Jansson B (eds): Biological Psychiatry. Amsterdam, Elsevier, 1981, pp 157–162.

Gershon ES, Guroff JJ: Information from relatives: diagnosis of affective disorders. Arch Gen Psychiatry 41:173–180, 1984.

Gershon ES, Hamovit J, Guroff JJ, et al: A family study of schizoaffective, bipolar I, bipolar II, unipolar and normal control probands. Arch Gen Psychiatry 39:1157–1167, 1982.

Gershon ES, Hamovit JH, Guroff JJ, Nurnberger JI Jr: Birth cohort changes in manic and depressive disorders in relatives of bipolar and schizoaffective patients. Arch Gen Psychiatry 44:314–319, 1987b.

Gershon ES, Hamovit JR, Schreiber JL, et al: Anorexia nervosa and major affective disorders associated in families: a preliminary report. In Guze SB, Earls FJ, Barrett JE (eds): Childhood Psychopathology and Development. New York, Raven Press, 1983, pp 279–286.

Gershon ES, Mark A, Cohen N, et al: Transmitted factors in the morbidity of affective disorders: A controlled study. J Psychiatr Res 12:283–299, 1975b.

Gershon ES, Martinez M, Goldin L, et al: Detection of marker associations with a dominant disease gene in genetically complex and heterogeneous diseases. Am J Hum Genet 45:578–585, 1989.

Gershon ES, McKnew D, Cytryn L, et al: Diagnosis in school-age children of bipolar affective disorder patients and normal controls. J Affective Disord 8(3):283–291, 1985.

Gershon ES, Nurnberger JI Jr: Genetics of major psychoses. In Kety SS, Rowland LP, Sidman RL, Matthysses (eds): Genetics of Neurological and Psychiatric Disorders. New York, Raven Press, 1983, pp 121–144.

Gershon ES, Targum SD, Matthysse S, Bunney WE Jr: Color blindness not closely linked to bipolar illness. Arch Gen Psychiatry 36:1423–1434, 1979.

Goedde HW, Agarwal DP, Harada S: The role of alcohol dehydrogenase and aldehyde dehydrogenase isozymes in alcohol metabolism, alcohol sensitivity, and alcoholism. In Isozymes: Current Topics in Biological and Medical Research, vol 8. New York, Alan R. Liss, 1983, pp 175–193.

Goetzl V, Green R, Whybrow P, et al: X-linkage revisited: A further family study of manic depressive illness. Arch Gen Psychiatry 31:665–673, 1974.

Goldin LR, Clerget-Darpoux F, Gershon ES: Relationship of HLA to major affective disorder not supported. Psychiatry Res 7:29–45, 1982.

Goldin LR, DeLisi LE, Gershon ES: The relationship of HLA to schizophrenia in 10 nuclear families. Psychiatry Res 20:69–77, 1987.

Goldin LR, Gershon ES, Targum SD, et al: Segregation and linkage analyses in families of patients with bipolar, unipolar and schizoaffective mood disorders. Am J Hum Genet 35:274–287, 1983.

Goldin LR, Nurnberger JI Jr, Gershon ES: Clinical methods in psychiatric genetics: II. The high risk approach. Acta Psychiatr Scand 74:119–128, 1986.

Goodwin DW: Alcoholism and heredity. A review and hypotheses. Arch Gen Psychiatry 36:57–61, 1979.

Goodwin DW: The genetics of alcoholism. In Usdin E, Hanin I (eds): Biological Markers in Psychiatry and Neurology. Oxford, Pergamon Press, 1982, pp 433–443.

Goodwin DW, Schulsinger F, Hermansen L, et al: Alcohol problems in adoptees raised apart from alcoholic biological parents. Arch Gen Psychiatry 28:238–243, 1973.

Goodwin DW, Schulsinger F, Knop J, et al: Alcoholism and depression in adopted-out daughters of alcoholics. Arch Gen Psychiatry 34:751–755, 1977.

Goodwin DW, Schulsinger F, Moller N, et al: Drinking problems in adopted and non-adopted sons of alcoholics. Arch Gen Psychiatry 31:164–169, 1974.

Gottesman II, Carey G: Extracting meaning and direction from twin data. Psychiatr Dev 1:35–50, 1983.

Gottesman II, Shields J: Schizophrenia and Genetics: A Twin Study Vantage Point. New York, Academic Press, 1972.

Gottesman II, Shields J: Schizophrenia: The Epigenetic Puzzle. New York, Cambridge University Press, 1982.

Grove WM: Comment on Lidz and associate's critique of the Danish-American studies of the offspring of schizophrenic parents. Am J Psychiatry 140:998–1002, 1983.

Gurling H, Oppenheim B, Murray R: Depression, criminality and psychopathology associated with alcoholism: Evidence from a twin study. Acta Genet Med Gemellol (Roma) 33:333–339, 1984.

Guze SB, Cloninger CR, Martin RL, Clayton PJ: A follow-up and family study of schizophrenia. Arch Gen Psychiatry 40:1273–1276, 1983.

Guze SB, Cloninger CR, Martin RL, Clayton PJ: A follow-up and family study of Briquet's syndrome. Br J Psychiatry 149:17–23, 1986.

Hanin I, Mallinger AG, Kopp U, et al: Mechanism of lithium-induced elevation in red blood cell choline content: An in vitro analysis. Commun Psychopharmacol 4(5):345–355, 1980.

Harris EL, Noyes R, Crowe RR, Chaudhry DR: Family study of agoraphobia. Report of a pilot study. Arch Gen Psychiatry 40:1061–1064, 1983.

Harvald B, Hauge M: Hereditary factors elucidated by twin studies. In Neal JV, Shaw MW, Shull WJ (eds): Genetics and the Epidemiology of Chronic Diseases. Washington, DC, PHS Publication 1163, 1965, pp 61–76.

Heath AC, Neale MC, Hewitt JK, et al: Testing structural equation models for twin data using LISREL. Behav Genet 19:9–36, 1989.

Helzer JE, Winokur G: A family interview study of male manic-depressives. Arch Gen Psychiatry 31:73–77, 1974.

Heston LL: Psychiatric disorders in foster home reared children of schizophrenic mothers. Br J Psychiatry 112:819–825, 1966.

Hill SY, Aston C, Rabin B: Suggestive evidence of genetic linkage between alcoholism and the MNS blood group. Alcohol Clin Exp Res 12(6):811–814, 1988a.

Hill SY, Steinhauer SR, Zubin J, Baughman T: Event-related potentials as markers for alcoholism risk in high density families. Alcohol Clin Exp Res 12(4):545–554, 1988b.

Holzinger KJ: The relative effect of nature and nurture influences on twin differences. J Educational Psychol 20:241, 1929.

Holzman PS, Kringlen E, Levy DL, et al: Abnormal-pursuit eye movements in schizophrenia. Arch Gen Psychiatry 34:802–805, 1977.

Holzman PS, Kringlen E, Matthysse S, et al: A single dominant gene can account for eye tracking dysfunctions and schizophrenia in offspring of discordant twins. Arch Gen Psychiatry 45:641–647, 1988.

Holzman PS, Solomon CM, Levin S, Waternaux CS: Pursuit eye movement dysfunctions in schizophrenia. Arch Gen Psychiatry 41:136–139, 1984.

Hrubec Z, Omenn GS: Evidence of a genetic predisposition to alcoholic cirrhosis and psychosis. Alcoholism 5:207–215, 1981.

Hutchings B and Mednick SA: Registered criminality in the adoptive and biological parents of registered male criminal adoptees. In Fieve RR, Rosenthal D, Brill H (eds): Genetic Research in Psychiatry. Baltimore, Hopkins, 1975, pp 105–116.

Ingvar DH: Abnormal distribution of cerebral activity in chronic schizophrenia: A neurophysiological interpretation. In Baxter CF, Melnechuk T (eds): Current Perspectives in Schizophrenia Research. New York, Raven Press, 1980, pp 107–125.

Inouye E: Similarity and dissimilarity of schizophrenia in twins. In Proceedings Third International Congress of Psychiatry, 1961. Montreal, University of Toronto Press, 1963, pp 524–530.

Inouye E: Monozygotic twins with schizophrenia reared apart in infancy. J Hum Genet 16:182–190, 1972.

Ivanyi P, Droes J, Schreuder GMT, et al: A search for association of HLA antigens with paranoid schizophrenia. Tissue Antigens 22:186–193, 1983.

Jacobs PA, Brunton M, Melville MM, et al: Aggressive behaviour, mental subnormality and the XYY male. Nature 208:1351–1352, 1965.

Jacobs PA, Price WH, Richmond S, Ratcliff RAW: Chromosome surveys in penal institutions and approved schools. J Med Genet 8:49–53, 1971.

James NM, Chapman CJ: A genetic study of bipolar affective disorder. Br J Psychiatry 126:449–456, 1975.

Janowsky DS, El-Yousef MK, Davis JM: Cholinergic-adrenergic hypothesis of mania and depression. Lancet 2:632, 1972.

Jeste DV, Zalcman S, Weinberger DR, et al: Apomorphine response and subtyping of schizophrenia. Prog Neuropsychopharmacol Biol Psychiatry 7:83–88, 1983.

Johnson GFS, Leeman MM: Analysis of familial factors in bipolar affective illness. Arch Gen Psychiatry 34:1074–1083, 1977.

Johnstone EC, Crow TJ, Frith CD, et al: Cerebral ventricular size and cognitive impairment in chronic schizophrenia. Lancet 2:924–926, 1976.

Kafka MS, van Kammen DP, Kleinman JE, et al: Alpha-adrenergic receptor function in schizophrenia, affective disorders and some neurological diseases. Commun Psychopharmacol 4:477–486, 1980.

Kallman F: Genetic principles in manic depressive psychosis. In Hoch PH, Zubin J (eds): Depression, New York, Grune & Stratton, 1954, pp 1–24.

Kallman FJ: The genetic theory of schizophrenia. An analysis of 691 schizophrenic twin index families. Am J Psychiatry 103:309–322, 1946.

Kan YW, Dozy AM: Polymorphism of DNA sequence adjacent to human beta-globin structural gene: relation to sickle mutation. Proc Natl Acad Sci 75:5631, 1978.

Kaprio J, Koskenvuo M, Langinvainio H, et al: Genetic influences on use and abuse of alcohol: A study of 5638 adult Finnish twin brothers. Alcohol Clin Exp Res 11(4):349–355, 1987.

Kassett JA, Gershon ES, Maxwell ME, et al: Psychiatric disorders in the first-degree relatives of probands with bulimia nervosa. Am J Psychiatry 146:1468–1471, 1989.

Kelsoe JR, Gillin C, Janowsky DS, Brown JH, et al: Letter to the editor. N Engl J Med 312:861–862, 1985.

Kelsoe JR, Ginns EI, Egeland JA, et al: Re-evaluation of the linkage relationship between chromosome 11p loci and the gene for bipolar affective disorder in the Old Order Amish. Nature 342:238–243, 1989.

Kendler KS: The nosologic validity of paranoia (simple delusional disorder). A review. Arch Gen Psychiatry 37:699–706, 1980.

Kendler KS: Demography of paranoid psychosis (delusional disorder): A review and comparison with schizophrenia and affective illness. Arch Gen Psychiatry 39:890–902, 1982.

Kendler KS: Overview: A current perspective on twin studies of schizophrenia. Am J Psychiatry 140:1413–1425, 1983.

Kendler KS, Gruenberg AM, Strauss JS: An independent analysis of the Copenhagen sample of the Danish adoption study of schizophrenia: II. The relationship between schizotypal personality disorder and schizophrenia. Arch Gen Psychiatry 38:982–984, 1981a.

Kendler KS, Gruenberg AM, Strauss JS: An independent analysis of the Copenhagen sample of the Danish adoption study of schizophrenia: IV. The relationship between paranoid psychosis (delusional disorder) and the schizophrenia spectrum disorders. Arch Gen Psychiatry 38:985–987, 1981.

Kendler KS, Gruenberg AM, Tsuang MT: Subtype stability in schizophrenia. Am J Psychiatry 142:827–832, 1985.

Kendler KS, Gruenberg AM, Tsuang MT: A family study of the subtypes of schizophrenia. Am J Psychiatry 145:57–62, 1988.

Kendler KS, Hays P: Paranoid psychosis (delusional disorder) and schizophrenia. A family history study. Arch Gen Psychiatry 38:547–551, 1981.

Kendler KS, Robinette RD: Schizophrenia in the National Academy of Sciences—National Research Council Twin Registry: A 16-year update. Am J Psychiatry 140:1551–1563, 1983.

Kendler KS, Heath A, Martin NG, Eaves LG: Symptoms of anxiety and depression in a volunteer twin population: The etiologic role of genetic and environmental factors. Arch Gen Psychiatry 43:213–221, 1986.

Kendler KS, Heath A, Martin NG, Eaves LJ: Symptoms of anxiety and symptoms of depression: same genes, different environments? Arch Gen Psychiatry 44:451–457, 1987.

Kety SS: Disorders of the human brain. Sci Am 241:202–218, 1979.

Kety SS: Mental illness in the biological and adoptive relatives of schizophrenia adoptees: findings relevant to genetic and environmental factors in etiology. Am J Psychiatry 140:720–727, 1983.

Kety SS, Rosenthal D, Wender PH, Schulsinger F: The types and prevalence of mental illness in the biological and adoptive families of adopted schizophrenics. In Rosenthal D, Kety SS (eds): The Transmission of Schizophrenia. Oxford, Pergamon Press, 1968, pp 159–166.

Kety SS, Rosenthal D, Wender PH, et al: Mental illness in the biological and adoptive families of adopted individuals who have become schizophrenic: A preliminary report based upon psychiatric interviews. In Fieve R, Rosenthal D, Brill H (eds): Genetic Research in Psychiatry. Baltimore, Johns Hopkins University Press, 1975, pp 147–165.

Kety SS, Wender PH, Rosenthal D: Genetic relationships within the schizophrenia spectrum: evidence from adoption studies. In Spitzer RL, Klein DF (eds): Critical Issues in Psychiatric Diagnosis. New York, Raven Press, 1978, pp 213–223.

Kidd KK, Prusoff BA, Cohen DJ: The familial pattern of Gilles de la Tourette's Syndrome. Arch Gen Psychiatry 37:1336–1339, 1980.

Klerman GL, Lavori PW, Rice J, et al: Birth-cohort trends in rates of major depressive disorder among relatives of patients with affective disorder. Arch Gen Psychiatry 42:689–693, 1985.

Kogan S, Gitschier J: Mutations and a polymorphism in the factor VIII gene discovered by denaturing gradient gel electrophoresis. Proc Natl Acad Sci USA 87:2092–2096, 1990.

Korner J, Fritze J, Propping P: RFLP alleles at the tyrosine hydroxylase locus: No association found to affective disorders. Psychiatry Res 32:275–280, 1990.

Korsten MA, Matsuzaki S, Feinman L, Lieber CS: High blood acetaldehyde levels after ethanol administration: differences between alcoholic and nonalcoholic subjects. N Engl J Med 292:386–389, 1975.

Krauthammer C, Klerman GL: Secondary mania: Manic syndromes associated with antecedent physical illness or drugs. Arch Gen Psychiatry 35:1333–1339, 1978.

Kringlen E: Schizophrenia in twins. An epidemiological-clinical study. Psychiatry 29:172–184, 1966.

Kringlen E: Heredity and Environment in the Functional Psychoses. London, Heinemann, 1967.

Lalouel JM, Morton NE: Complex segregation analysis with pointers. Hum Hered 31:312–321, 1981.

Lalouel JM, Rao DC, Morton NE, Elston RC: A unified model for complex segregation analysis. Am J Hum Genet 35:816–826, 1983.

Lam RW, Berkowitz AL, Berga SL, et al: Melatonin suppression in bipolar and unipolar mood disorders. Psychiatry Res 33:129–134, 1990.

Lander ES, Botstein D: Strategies for studying heterogeneous genetic traits in humans by using a linkage map of restriction fragment length polymorphisms. Proc Natl Acad Sci USA 83:7353–7357, 1986.

Lange V: Genetic markers for schizophrenic subgroups. Psychiatr Clin 15:133–144, 1982.

Leboyer M, Malafosse A, Boularand S, et al: Tyrosine hydroxylase polymorphisms associated with manic-depressive illness. Lancet 335:1219, 1990.

Leckman JF, Weissman MM, Merikangas KR, et al: Panic disorders and major depression. Increased risk of depression, alcoholism, panic and phobic disorders in families of depressed probands with panic disorders. Arch Gen Psychiatry 40:1055–1060, 1983.

Le Fur G, Meininger V, Phair T, et al: Decrease in lymphocyte [³H] spiroperidol binding sites in Parkinsonism. Life Sci 27:1587–1591, 1980.

Lewy AJ, Nurnberger JI Jr, Wehr TA, et al: Supersensitivity to light: Possible trait marker for manic-depressive illness. Am J Psychiatry 142:725–727, 1985.

Li T-K, Lumeng L, McBride WJ, Murphy JM: Rodent lines selected for factors affecting alcohol consumption. Alcohol Alcoholism Suppl 1:91–96, 1987.

Lidz T, Blatt S: Critique of the Danish-American studies of the biological and adoptive relatives of adoptees who became schizophrenic. Am J Psychiatry 140:426–435, 1983.

Lidz T, Blatt S, Cook B: Critique of the Danish American studies of the adopted away offspring of schizophrenic parents. Am J Psychiatry 138:1063–1068, 1981.

Lowing PA, Mirsky AF, Pereira R: The inheritance of schizophrenic spectrum disorders: a reanalysis of the Danish adoptee study data. Am J Psychiatry 140:1167–1171, 1983.

Luxenberger H: Vorländiger bericht über psychiatrische serienuntersuchungen an Zwillengen. Zentralbl Gesamte Neurol Psychiatrie 116:297–326, 1928.

Luxenberger H: Psychiatrisch-neurologische zwillings-pathologie. Zentral Diagesamte Neurol Psychiatrie 14:56–57, 145–180, 1930.

Mankoo B, Sherrington R, Brynjolfsson J, et al: New microsatellite polymorphisms provide a highly polymorphic map of chromosome 5 bands q11.2–113.3 for linkage analysis of Icelandic and English families affected by schizophrenia. Presented at Second World Congress on Psychiatric Genetics, Regents College, London, August 14–16, 1991.

Martin NG: Genetic differences in drinking habits, alcohol metabolism and sensitivity in unselected samples of twins. In Genetics and Alcoholism. New York, Alan R. Liss, 1987, pp. 109–119.

Martinez MM, Goldin LR: The detection of linkage and heterogeneity of nuclear families for complex disorders: One versus two marker loci. Am J Hum Genet 44:552–559, 1989.

McCabe MS: Reactive psychoses. Acta Psychiatr Scand Suppl 259:1–33, 1975.

McConville BJ, Soudek D, Sroka H, et al: Length of the Y chromosome and chromosomal variants in inpatient children with psychiatric disorders: two studies. Can J Psychiatry 28:8–13, 1983.

McGue M, Gottesman II, Rao DC: The transmission of schizophrenia under a multifactorial threshold model. Am J Hum Genet 35:1161–1178, 1983.

McGuffin P, Farmer AE, Yonace AH: HLA antigens and subtypes of schizophrenia. Psychiatry Res 5:115–122, 1981.

McGuffin P, Festenstein H, Murray R: A family study of HLA antigens and other genetic markers in schizophrenia. Psychol Med 13:31–43, 1983.

McNeil TJ, Kaij L: Etiological relevance of comparisons of high-risk and low-risk groups. Acta Psychiatr Scand 59:545–560, 1979.

McNeil TF, Kaij L, Malmquist-Larsson A, et al: Offspring of women with nonorganic psychoses: Development of a longitudinal study of children at high risk. Acta Psychiatr Scand 68:234–250, 1983.

Mellerup ET, Plenge P, Rosenberg R: H-imipramine binding sites in platelets from psychiatric patients. Psychiatry Res 7:221–227, 1982.

Mendlewicz J, Fleiss JL: Linkage studies with X chromosome markers in bipolar (manic-depressive) and unipolar (depressive) illness. Biol Psychiatry 9:261–294, 1974.

Mendlewicz J, Massart-Guiot T, Wilmotte J, Fleiss JL: Blood groups in manic-depressive illness and schizophrenia. Dis Nerv Sys 35:39–41, 1974.

Mendlewicz J, Rainer JD: Morbidity risk and genetic transmission in manic depressive illness. Am J Hum Genet 26:692–701, 1974.

Mendlewicz J, Rainer JD: Adoption study supporting genetic transmission in manic depressive illness. Nature 268:327–329, 1977.

Mendlewicz J, Simon P, Sevy S, et al: Polymorphic DNA marker on X chromosome and manic depression. Lancet 1:1230–1232, 1987.

Merikangas K, Gelernter C: Comorbidity for alcoholism and depression. Psychiatr Clin North Am 13(4):613–632, 1990.

Morrison JR, Stewart MA: A family study of the hyperactive child syndrome. Biol Psychiatry 3:189–195, 1971.

Morrison JR, Stewart MA: The psychiatric status of the legal families of adopted hyperactive children. Arch Gen Psychiatry 28:888–891, 1973.

Morton NE: Sequential tests for the detection of linkage. Am J Hum Genet 7:277–318, 1955.

Morton NE, MacLean CJ: Analysis of familial resemblance: II. Complex segregation analysis of quantitative traits. Am J Hum Genet 26:489–503, 1974.

Mourant AE, Kopac AC, Domaniewska-Sobczak K: Blood Groups and Disease: A Study of Associations of Diseases with Blood Groups and Other Polymorphisms. Oxford, Oxford University Press, 1978.

Murphy DL, Coursey RD, Haenel T, et al: Platelet monoamine oxidase as a biological marker in the affective disorders and alcoholism. In Usdin E, Hanin I (eds): Biological Markers in Psychiatry and Neurology. Oxford, Pergamon Press, 1982, pp 123–134.

Murphy JM, McBride WJ, Lumeng L, Li TK: Regional brain levels of monoamines in alcohol-preferring and non-preferring lines of rats. Pharmacol Biochem Behav 16:145–149, 1982.

Murray RM, Clifford C, Gurling HMD, et al: Current genetic and biological approaches to alcoholism. Psychiatr Dev 1:179–192, 1983.

Mutchler K, Crowe RR, Noyes R Jr, Wesner RW: Exclusion of the tyrosine hydroxylase gene in 14 panic disorder pedigrees. Am J Psychiatry 147(10):1367–1369, 1990.

Naitoh P: The value of electroencephalography in alcoholism. Ann NY Acad Sci 215:303–320, 1973.

Nasrallah HA: Neurodevelopmental aspects of bipolar affective disorder [Editorial]. Biol Psychiatry 29:1–2, 1991.

Newlin D: Offspring of alcoholics have enhanced antagonistic placebo response. J Stud Alcohol 46:490–494, 1985.

Newlin DB, Thomson JB: Alcohol challenge with sons of alcoholics: A critical review and analysis. Psychol Bull 108(3):383–402, 1990.

Noyes R Jr, Clarkson C, Crowe RR, et al: A family study of generalized anxiety disorder. Am J Psychiatry 144(8):1019–1024, 1987.

Nurnberger JI Jr, Berrettini W, Tamarkin L, et al: Supersensitivity to melatonin suppression by light in young people at high risk for affective disorder: A preliminary report. Neuropsychopharmacology 1:217–223, 1988.

Nurnberger JI Jr, Gershon ES: Genetics of affective disorders. In Post RM, Ballenger J (eds): Neurobiology of Mood Disorders. Baltimore, Williams & Wilkins, 1984, pp 76–101.

Nurnberger JI Jr, Gershon ES, Simmons S, et al: Behavioral, biochemical and neuroendocrine response to amphetamine in normal twins and "well state" bipolar patients. Psychoneuroendocrinology 7:163–176, 1982a.

Nurnberger JI Jr, Jimerson DC, Bunney WE Jr: A risk factor strategy for investigating affective illness. Biol Psychiatry 18:903–909, 1983a.

Nurnberger JI Jr, Pandey G, Gershon ES, Davis JM: Lithium ratio in psychiatric patients: a caveat. Psychiatry Res 9:201–206, 1983b.

Nurnberger JI Jr, Sitaram N, Gershon ES, Gillin JC: A twin study of cholinergic REM induction. Biol Psychiatry 18:1161–1173, 1983c.

O'Connor S, Resselbrock V, Tasman A: Correlates of increased risk for alcoholism in young men. Prog Neuropsychopharmacol Biol Psychiatry 10:211–218, 1986.

O'Rouke DH, Gottesman II, Suarez BK, et al: Refutation of the general single locus model for the etiology of schizophrenia. Am J Hum Genet 34:630–649, 1982.

O'Rourke DH, McGuffin P, Reich T: Genetic analysis of manic-depressive illness. Am J Phys Anthropol 62:51–59, 1983.

Orvaschel H, Thompson W, Belanger A, et al: Comparison of the family history method to direct interview: Factors affecting the diagnosis of depression. J Affective Disord 4:49–59, 1982.

Ott J: Estimation of the recombination fraction in human pedigree: Efficient computation of the likelihood for human linkage. Am J Hum Genet 26:588–597, 1974.

Owen F, Cross AJ, Crow TJ, et al: Increased dopamine-receptor sensitivity in schizophrenia. Lancet ii: 223–226, 1978.

Oxenstierna G, Edman G, Iselius L, et al: Concentrations of monoamine metabolites in the cerebrospinal fluid of twins and unrelated individuals—A genetic study. J Psychiatr Res 20(1):19–29, 1986.

Pahina SS, Roberts DF, McLeish L: Group-specific component (Gc) subtypes and schizophrenia. Clin Genet 22:321–326, 1982.

Pakstis AJ, Heutink P, Pauls DL, et al: Progress in the search for genetic linkage with Tourette Syndrome: an exclusion map covering more than 50% of the autosomal genome. Am J Genet 48:281–294, 1991.

Parsian A, Todd RD, Devor EJ, et al: Alcoholism and alleles of the human D_2 dopamine receptor locus: Studies of association and linkage. Arch Gen Psychiatry 48(7):655–663, 1991.

Pauls DL, Bucher KD, Crowe RR, Noyes R Jr: A genetic study of panic disorder pedigrees. Am J Hum Genet 32:639–644, 1980.

Pauls DL, Cohen DJ, Heimbuch R, et al: Familial pattern and transmission of Gilles de la Tourette Syndrome and multiple tics. Arch Gen Psychiatry 38:1091–1093, 1981.

Pauls DL, Leckman JF: The inheritance of Gilles De La Tourette's syndrome and associated behaviors. N Engl J Med 315(16): 993–997, 1986.

Pauls DL, Raymond CL, Stevenson JM, Leckman JF: A family study of Gilles de la Tourette syndrome. Am J Hum Genet 48:154–163, 1991.

Pauls DL, Towbin KE, Leckman JF, et al: Gilles de la Tourette's syndrome and obsessive-compulsive disorder. Arch Gen Psychiatry 43:1180–1182, 1986.

Paykel ES: Life events and early environment. In Paykel ES (ed.): Handbook of Affective Disorders. New York, Churchill Livingstone, 1982, pp 146–161.

Perris C: A study of bipolar (manic-depressive) and unipolar recurrent depressive psychoses. Acta Psychiatr Scand Suppl 194:15–44, 1966.

Pettersen U: Manic depressive illness: a clinical social and genetic study. Acta Psychiatr Scand Suppl 269:1–93, 1977.

Pillard RC, Poumadere J, Caretta RA: Is homosexuality familial? A review, some data, and a suggestion. Arch Sex Behav 10: 465–475, 1981.

Pillard RC, Poumadere J, Caretta RA: A family study of sexual orientation. Arch Sex Behav 11:511–520, 1982.

Pliszka SR, Rogeness GA, Renner P, et al: Plasma neurochemistry in juvenile offenders. J Am Acad Child Adolesc Psychiatry 27(5):588–594, 1988.

Polich J, Bloom F: P_{300} and alcohol consumption in normals and individuals at risk for alcoholism. Prog Neuropsychopharmacol Biol Psychiatry 10:201–210, 1986.

Pollack VE, Volavka J, Goodwin DW, et al: The EEG after alcohol administration in men at high risk for alcoholism. Arch Gen Psychiatry 40:857–861, 1983.

Price RA, Kidd KK, Pauls DL, et al: Multiple threshold models for the affective disorders: The Yale-NIMH collaborative family study. J Psychiatr Res 19:533–546, 1985.

Price RA, Pauls DL, Kruger SD, Caine ED: Family data support a dominant major gene for Tourette syndrome. Psychiatry Res 24:251–261, 1988.

Propping P: Genetic control of ethanol action on the central nervous system: An EEG study in twins. Hum Genet 35: 309–334, 1977.

Propping P: Alcohol and alcoholism. Hum Genet 1:91–99, 1978.

Propping P: Genetic disorders presenting as "Schizophrenia." Karl Bonhoeffer's early view of the psychoses in the light of medical genetics. Hum Genet 65:1–10, 1983.

Propping P, Friedl W: Genetic control of adrenergic receptors on human platelets. A twin study. Hum Genet 64:105–109, 1983.

Propping P, Krüger J, Mark N: Genetic disposition to alcoholism. An EEG study in alcoholics and their relatives. Hum Genet 59:51–59, 1981.

Rao DC, Morton NE, Gottesman II, Lew R: Path analysis of qualitative data on pairs of relatives: application to schizophrenia. Hum Hered 31:325–333, 1981.

Reich T, Clayton PJ, Winokur G: Family history studies: V. The genetics of mania. Am J Psychiatry 125:1358–1369, 1969.

Reich T, James JW, Morris CA: The use of multiple thresholds in determining the mode of transmission of semi-continuous traits. Ann Hum Genet 36:163–184, 1972.

Reveley MA, Reveley AM, Clifford CA, Murray RM: Genetics of platelet MAO activity in discordant schizophrenia and normal twins. Br J Psychiatry 142:560–565, 1983.

Reveley AM, Reveley MA, Murray RM: Cerebral ventricular enlargement in non genetic schizophrenia: A controlled twin study. Br J Psychiatry 144:89–93, 1984.

Rice J, Reich T: Familial analysis of qualitative traits under mutlifactorial inheritance. Genet Epidemiol 2:301–315, 1985.

Rice J, Reich T, Andreasen NC, et al: The familial transmission of bipolar illness. Arch Gen Psychiatry 44:441–447, 1987.

Rice J, McGuffin P, Goldin LR, et al: Platelet monoamine oxidase (MAO) activity: evidence for a single major locus. Am J Hum Genet 36:36–43, 1984.

Rinieris P, Stefanis C, Lykouras E, Varsou E: Subtypes of schizophrenia and ABO blood types. Neuropsychobiology 8:57–59, 1982.

Risch N: Linkage strategies for genetically complex traits: I. Multilocus models. Am J Hum Genet 46:222–228, 1990.

Risch N, Baron M: X-linkage and genetic heterogeneity in bipolar-related major affective illness: re-analysis of linkage data. Ann Hum Genet 46:153–166, 1982.

Risch N, Baron M: Segregation analysis of schizophrenia and related disorders. Am J Hum Genet 36:1039–1059, 1984.

Roe A: The adult adjustment of children of alcoholic parents raised in foster-homes. Q J Stud Alcohol 5:378–393, 1945.

Rogeness GA, Maas JW, Javors MA, et al: Diagnoses, catecholamine metabolism, and plasma dopamine-β-hydroxylase. J Am Acad Child Adolesc Psychiatry 27(1):121–125, 1988.

Rosanoff JA, Handy L, Plesset IR: The etiology of manic-depressive syndromes with special reference to their occurrence in twins. Am J Psychiatry 91:724–762, 1935.

Rosanoff JA, Handy LM, Plesset IR, Brush S: The etiology of so-called schizophrenic psychoses with special reference to their occurrence in twins. Am J Psychiatry 91:247–286, 1934.

Rosenthal D: A program of research on heredity in schizophrenia. In Mednick SA, Schulsinger F, Higgins J, Bell B (eds): Genetics, Environment, and Psychopathology, American Elsevier Publishing Company, Inc., 1974, pp. 19–35.

Rosenthal D, Wender PH, Kety SS, et al: The adopted-away offspring of schizophrenics. Am J Psychiatry 128:307–311, 1971.

Rotman A, Zemishlany Z, Munitz H, Wijsenbeek H: The active uptake of serotonin by platelets of schizophrenic patients and their families: possibility of a genetic marker. Psychopharmacology 77:171–174, 1982.

Rutschman J, Cornblatt B, Erlenmeyer-Kimling L: Sustained attention in children at risk for schizophrenia. Arch Gen Psychiatry 34:571–575, 1977.

Saitoh O, Niwa S, Hiramatsu K, et al: Abnormalities in late positive components of event-related potentials may reflect a genetic predisposition to schizophrenia. Biol Psychiatry 19(3):293–303, 1984.

Saunders JB, Wodak AD, Haines A, et al: Accelerated development of alcoholic cirrhosis in patients with HLA B8. Lancet 1:1381–1384, 1982.

Schlesser MA, Winokur G, Elston RC: Hypothalamic-pituitary-adrenal axis activity in depressive illness: its relationship to classification. Arch Gen Psychiatry 37:737–743, 1980.

Schlesser MA, Winokur G, Sherman BM: Genetic subtypes of unipolar primary depressive illness distinguished by hypothalmic-pituitary-adrenal axis activity. Lancet 1:739–741, 1979.

Schmidt AL, Neville HJ: Language processing in men at risk for alcoholism: An event-related potential study. Alcohol 2: 529–533, 1985.

Schuckit M: Biological markers: Metabolism and acute reactions to alcohol in sons of alcoholics. Pharmacol Biochem Behav 13:9–16, 1980.

Schuckit M: Subjective responses to alcohol in sons of alcoholics and control subjects. Arch Gen Psychiatry 41:879–884, 1984a.

Schuckit M: Differences in plasma cortisol after ingestion of ethanol in relatives of alcoholics and controls: Preliminary results. Clin Psychiatry 45:374–376, 1984b.

Schuckit M: Genetics and the risk for alcoholism. JAMA 254:2614–2617, 1985.

Schuckit MA: Reactions to alcohol in sons of alcoholics and controls. Alcohol Clin Exp Res 12(4):465–470, 1988.

Schuckit M, Goodwin D, Winokur G: Brief communications: A study of alcoholism in half siblings. Am J Psychiatry 128: 1132–1136, 1972.

Schuckit MA, Parker DC, Rossman LR: Ethanol-related prolactin responses and risk for alcoholism. Biol Psychiatry 18:1153–1159, 1983.

Schuckit M, Rayses V: Ethanol ingestion: differences in blood acetaldehyde concentrations in relatives of alcoholics and controls. Science 203:54–55, 1979.

Schulsinger F, Kety SS, Rosenthal D, Wender PH: A family study of suicide. In Schou M, Stromgren E (eds): Origin, Prevention and Treatment of Affective Disorders. London, Academic Press, 1979, pp 277–287.

Schulz SC, van Kammen DP, Rogol AD, et al: Amphetamine increases prolactin but not growth hormone nor beta-endorphin immunoreactivity in schizophrenic patients. Psychopharmacol Bull 17:193–195, 1981.

Sedvall G, Fyro B, Gullberg B, et al: Relationships in healthy volunteers between concentrations of monoamine metabolites in cerebrospinal fluid and family history of psychiatric morbidity. Br J Psychiatry 136:366–374, 1980.

Shah SA, Roth LH: Biological and psychophysiological factors in criminality. In Glaser D (ed): Handbook of Criminology. Rand McNally College Publishing, 1974, pp 101–173.

Shea PA, Small JG, Hendrie HC: Elevation of choline and glycine in red blood cells of psychiatric patients due to lithium treatment. Biol Psychiatry 16(9):825–830, 1981.

Sheffield VC, Cox DR, Lerman LS, Myers RM: Attachment of a 40-base-pair g + c-rich sequence (gc-clamp) to genomic DNA fragments by the polymerase chain reaction results in improved detection of single-base changes. Proc Natl Acad Sci USA 86:232–236, 1989.

Sheppard G, Gruzelier J, Manchanda R, et al: 15° Positron emission tomographic scanning in predominantly never-treated acute schizophrenic patients. Lancet 2:1448–1452, 1983.

Sherrington R, Brynjolfsson J, Petursson H, et al: Localization of a susceptability locus for schizophrenia on chromosome 5. Nature 336:164–167, 1988.

Sitaram N, Nurnberger JI Jr, Gershon ES, Gillin JC: Faster cholinergic REM sleep induction in euthymic patients with primary affective illness. Science 208:200–202, 1980.

Sitaram N, Nurnberger JI Jr, Gershon ES, Gillin JC: Cholinergic regulation of mood and REM sleep: potential model and marker of vulnerability to affective disorder. Am J Psychiatry 139:571–576, 1982.

Slater E: Psychotic and neurotic illnesses in twins. Medical Research Council of Great Britain, Special Report Series, Her Majesty's Stationery Office, London, 1953.

Smeraldi E, Negri R, Heimbuch RC, Kidd KK: Familial patterns and possible modes of inheritance of primary affective disorder. J Affect Disord 3:173–182, 1981.

Smeraldi E, Negri F, Melica AM: A genetic study of affective disorder. Acta Psychiatr Scand 56:382–398, 1977.

Smith SD, Kimberling WJ, Pennington BF, Lubs HA: Specific reading disability: Identification of an inherited form through linkage analysis. Science 219:1345–1347, 1983.

Smith SD, Pennington BF, Kimberling WJ, Ing PS: Familial dyslexia: Use of genetic linkage data to define subtypes. J Am Acad Child Adolesc Psychiatry 29(2):204–213, 1990.

Stern SL, Dixon KN, Nemzer E, et al: Affective disorder in the families of women with normal weight bulimia. Am J Psychiatry 141(10):1224–1227, 1984.

Stewart J, Debray Q, Caillard V: Schizophrenia: the testing of genetic models by pedigree analysis. Am J Hum Genet 32:55–63, 1980.

Stoflet ES, Koeberl DD, Sarkar G, Sommer SS: Genomic amplification with transcript sequencing. Science 239(4839):491–494, 1988.

Strober M, Morrell W, Burroughs J, et al: A family study of bipolar I disorder in adolescence: Early onset of symptoms linked to increased familial loading and lithium resistance. J Affective Disord 15(3):255–268, 1988.

Suarez BK: The affected sib-pair IBD distribution for HLA linked disease susceptibility loci. Tissue Antigens 12:87–93, 1978.

Suddath RL, Christison GW, Torrey EF, et al: Anatomical abnormalities in the brains of monozygotic twins discordant for schizophrenia. N Engl J Med 332(12):789–794, 1990.

Suomi S: Models of depression in primates. Psychol Med 13:465–468, 1983.

Suranyi-Cadotte BE, Wood PL, Nair NPV, Schwartz G: Normalization of platelet ³H-imipramine binding in depressed patients during remission. Eur J Pharmacol 85:357–358, 1982.

Tait BD, Mackay IR: HLA and alcoholic cirrhosis. Tissue Antigens 19:6–10, 1982.

Tanna VL, Wilson AF, Winokur G, Elston RC: Possible linkage between alcoholism and esterase-D. J Stud Alcohol 49(5):472–476, 1988.

Taylor MA, Abrams R, Hayman MA: The classification of affective disorders: a reassessment of the bipolar-unipolar dichotomy. J Affect Dis 2:95–109, 1980.

Thompson EA, Deeb S, Walker D, Motulsky AG: The detection of linkage disequilibrium between closely linked markers: RFLPs at the AI-CIII apolipoprotein genes. Am J Hum Genet 42(1):113–124, 1988.

Tienari P: Psychiatric illnesses in identical twins. Acta Psychiatr Scand (Suppl):171, 1963.

Tienari P: Schizophrenia in Finnish male twins. Br J Psychiatry, Special Publication No. 10:29–35, 1975.

Torgersen S: Genetic factors in moderately severe and mild affective disorders. Arch Gen Psychiatry 43:222–226, 1986.

Torgersen S: Comorbidity of major depression and anxiety disorders in twin pairs. Am J Psychiatry 147(9):1199–1202, 1990.

Traystman MD, Higuchi M, Kasper CK, et al: Use of denaturing gradient gel electrophoresis to detect point mutations in the factor VIII gene. Genomics 6:293–301, 1990.

Tsuang MT, Bucher KD, Fleming JA: Testing the monogenic theory of schizophrenia: An application of segregation analysis to blind family study data. Br J Psychiatry 140:595–599, 1982.

Tsuang MT, Bucher KD, Fleming JA: A search for schizophrenic spectrum disorders: An application of a multiple threshold model to blind family study data. Br J Psychiatry 143:572–577, 1983.

Tsuang MT, Faraone SV, Fleming JA: Familial transmission of major affective disorder: Is there evidence supporting the distinction between unipolar and bipolar disorders? Br J Psychiatry 146:268–271, 1985.

Tsuang MT, Winokur G, Crowe RR: Morbidity risks of schizophrenia and affective disorders among first degree relatives and patients with schizophrenia, mania, depression and surgical conditions. Br J Psychiatry 137:497–504, 1980.

Turner WJ: Genetic markers for schizotaxia. Biol Psychiatry 14:177–206, 1979.

van Eerdewegh MM, Gershon ES, van Eerdewegh PM: X-chromosome threshold models of bipolar manic depressive illness. J Psychiatr Res 15:215–238, 1980.

vanPraag HM, deHaan S: Depression vulnerability and 5-hydroxytryptophan prophylaxis. Psychiatry Res 3:75–83, 1980.

von Knorring A-L, Cloninger CR, Bohman M, Sigvardsson A: An adoption study of depressive disorders and substance abuse. Arch Gen Psychiatry 40:943–950, 1983.

Waters B, Marchenko I, Smiley D: Affective disorder, paranatal and educational factors in the offspring of bipolar manic-depressives. Can J Psychiatry 28:527–531, 1983a.

Waters B, Thakkar J, Lapierre Y: Erythrocyte lithium transport variables as a marker for manic-depressive disorder. Neuropsychobiology 9:94–98, 1983b.

Weeks DE, Lange K: The affected-pedigree-member method of linkage analysis. Am J Hum Genet 42:315–326, 1988.

Weinberger DR, DeLisi LE, Neophytides AN, Wyatt RJ: Familial aspects of CT scan abnormalities in chronic schizophrenia patients. Psychiatry Res 4:65–71, 1981.

Weinberger DR, DeLisi LE, Perman GP, et al: Computed tomography in schizophreniform disorder and other acute psychiatric disorders. Arch Gen Psychiatry 39:778–783, 1982.

Weinberger DR, Torrey EF, Neophytides AN, Wyatt RJ: Lateral cerebral ventricular enlargement in chronic schizophrenia. Arch Gen Psychiatry 36:735–739, 1979.

Weinstein LS, Gejman PV, Friedman E, et al: Gsα gene mutations in Albright's hereditary osteodystrophy detected by denaturing gradient gel electrophoresis. Proc Natl Acad Sci USA 87:8287–8290, 1990.

Weissman MM, Gershon ES, Kidd KK, et al: Psychiatric disorders in the relatives of probands with affective disorder. Arch Gen Psychiatry 41:13–21, 1984.

Weissman MM, Warner V, Wickramaratne P, Prusoff BA: Early-onset major depression in parents and their children. J Affective Disord 15:269–277, 1988.

Weissman MM, Merikangas KR, Wickramaratne P, et al: Understanding the clinical heterogeneity of major depression using family data. Arch Gen Psychiatry 43:430–434, 1986.

Weitkamp LR, Stancer HC, Persad E, et al: Depressive disorders and HLA: A gene on chromosome 6 that can affect behavior. N Engl J Med 305:1301–1306, 1981.

Wender PH, Kety SS, Rosenthal D, et al: Psychiatric disorders in the biological and adoptive families of adopted individuals with affective disorders. Arch Gen Psychiatry 43:923–929, 1986.

Whalley LJ, Perini T, Shering A, Bennie J: Melatonin response to bright light in recovered, drug-free, bipolar patients. Psychiatry Res 38:13–19, 1991.

Winokur G: Depression spectrum disease: description and family study. Compr Psychiatry 13:3–8, 1972.

Winokur G, Clayton P: in Wortis J (ed): Recent Advances in Biological Psychiatry, vol 9. New York, Plenum Press, 1967.

Winokur G, Coryell W: Familial alcoholism in primary unipolar major depressive disorder. Am J Psychiatry, 148(2):184–188, 1991.

Winokur G, Cadoret R, Dorzab J, Baker M: Depressive disease: A genetic study. Arch Gen Psychiatry 24:135–144, 1971.

Winokur G, March V, Mendels J: Primary affective disorder in relatives of patients with anorexia nervosa. Am J Psychiatry 137:695–698, 1980.

Winokur G, Reich T, Rimmer J, Pitts F Jr: Alcoholism: III. Diagnosis and familial psychiatric illness in 259 alcoholic probands. Arch Gen Psychiatry 23:104–111, 1970.

Winters KC, Stone AA, Weintraub S, et al: Cognitive and attentional deficits in children vulnerable to psychopathology. J Abnorm Child Psychol 94(4):435–453, 1981.

Witkin HA, Mednick SA, Schulsinger F, et al: Criminality in XYY and XXY in men. Science 193:547–554, 1976.

Wood KA, Harris MJ, Morreale A, Rizos AL: Drug-induced psychosis and depression in the elderly. Psychiatr Clin North Am 11:167–193, 1988.

Wright AF, Condon JB, Hampson ME, et al: Beta adrenoceptor binding defects in lymphoblastoid cell lines from manic depressive patients. In Proceedings of the 14th Collegium Internationale Neuropsychopharmacology Congress. New York, Raven Press, 1984, pp 194–195.

Wyatt RJ, Murphy DL, Belmaker R, et al: Reduced monoamine oxidase activity in platelets: A possible genetic marker for vulnerability to schizophrenia. Science 173:916–918, 1973.

Wyatt RJ, Potkin SG, Murphy DL: Platelet monoamine oxidase activity in schizophrenia: A review of the data. Am J Psychiatry 136:377–385, 1979.

Zahn-Waxler C, McKnew DH, Cummings EM, et al: Problem behaviors and peer interactions of young children with a manic-depressive parent. Am J Psychiatry 141(2):236–240, 1984.

Zerbin-Rudin E: Congenital word-blindness. In PE Becker (ed): Humangenetik. Stuttgart, Germany, Thieme, 1967 (Bulletin of the Orton Society 17:47–54, 1967).

CHAPTER 30

Use of the Laboratory in Psychiatry

RONALD L. MARTIN

SHELDON H. PRESKORN

INTRODUCTION

During this century, medicine, as a scientific discipline, has progressed dramatically. This advance is attributable, in part, to the development of *standardized and reliable procedures of assessing physical parameters yielding data of demonstrated validity*, i.e., useful laboratory procedure(s).

As the other chapters of this book attest, during the past four decades, psychiatry has reawakened as a scientifically oriented branch of medicine. Although the role of the laboratory in psychiatry is at a more rudimentary stage than in medicine generally, it is becoming increasingly important.

The laboratory is used in three major ways in psychiatry. The first, and most widely applied, use is in the identification of an underlying pharmacologic affect, or a medical, neurologic, or surgical conditions in patients presenting psychiatrically. Traditionally, such factors have been designated *organic* or *physical*. As will be discussed below, this chapter utilizes the DSM-IV (Task Force on DSM-IV, 1993) designation *direct effects of a substance or a general medical condition*. A second use is in monitoring plasma levels of psychotropic drugs. A third use is the identification of biologic markers for the diagnosis, treatment, monitoring, and, ultimately, the pathophysiologic understanding of psychiatric disorders. The three sections of this chapter reflect these divisions.

The less inferential *general medical condition* was adopted in DSM-IV to emphasize that psychiatric conditions are still medical and to avoid the obsolete dichotomy between *organic* and *functional* psychiatric disorders, which implied that some disorders have organic or biologic causes, while others have nonorganic, nonbiologic or purely psychologi-

cal causes. Today, few would argue that schizophrenia, affective disorder, and anxiety disorder, for example, do not involve organic changes.

This chapter should be seen as an overview. The reader is directed to basic texts and laboratory guides for more detailed discussion and data. A particularly useful source is the *Concise Guide to Laboratory Diagnostic Testing in Psychiatry* (Bosse et al, 1989).

IDENTIFICATION OF UNDERLYING GENERAL MEDICAL CONDITIONS

Rationale for Electing Laboratory Evaluations

Normal central nervous system (CNS) functioning is intimately dependent on metabolic homeostasis. Thus CNS function can be disrupted by a variety of endogenous and exogenous factors. Not surprisingly, psychiatric symptoms may occur in association with many medical conditions.

Because laboratory evaluations are a major tool in diagnosing such conditions, a complete description of the use of the laboratory in this regard would be encyclopedic. Rather than provide such a review, this section is designed as a guide for deciding when laboratory procedures are indicated and how to proceed generally.

Considering the large numbers of patients consulting a psychiatrist each year, a routine screening battery of laboratory tests would be a misallocation of resources. The yield in detected pathology would not justify such a policy. Thus a rationale for requesting laboratory evaluations should be followed. The following strategy is suggested:

1. In general, laboratory tests are indicated when there is a reasonable possibility of an underlying general medical condition. This possibility is increased by any of the following: (a) a history of a medical condition known to cause psychiatric symptoms, (b) the presence of physical as well as psychiatric complaints, (c) abnormalities in the physical examination, (d) aspects of the psychiatric history or mental status examination that are not typical of a specific psychiatric disorder.
2. The morbidity, discomfort, and cost of the contemplated test should be weighed against its potential diagnostic value and the relative probability of yielding useful information.
3. Less specific screening tests should be done before a more elaborate and specific workup is initiated.
4. If an evaluation requires special expertise, consultants should be utilized to prevent the initiation of extensive, yet unneccessary, testing.

The first step in assessment is obtaining a thorough medical history. Certain historical information, such as a past history of liver disease or of hypothyroidism, mandates certain laboratory tests whatever the psychiatric presentation. Enquiry regarding current medications and use of psychoactive substances (especially caffeine, alcohol, drugs of abuse) should be made. Realizing that an anxious, restless patient with a tachycardia is suffering from caffeinism may prevent unneccessary testing of thyroid functions.

Generally, physical complaints make the probability of a general medical condition more likely. However, such complaints are common in a variety of psychiatric disorders. Patients with anxiety disorders may have symptoms such as chest pain and palpitations, suggesting heart disease. Depressed patients may present primarily with fatigue, loss of weight, and other "vegetative" signs, suggesting an underlying medical condition. In addition, they may have somatic delusions, such as "my heart has stopped beating" or "my blood has turned solid." Schizophrenic patients also may have somatic delusions, often of a bizarre nature; "half my brain was removed last week in my sleep," "I have been pregnant for the past 12 years."

In addition, physical complaints are the essential feature of the somatoform and factitious disorders as described in DSM-IIIR (American Psychiatric Association, 1987) and the proposed DSM-IV (Task Force for DSM-IV, 1993). The somatoform disorders include somatization (hysteria or Briquet's syndrome), conversion, hypochondriasis, body dysmorphic, and pain disorders, as well as undifferentiated somatoform disorder and somatoform disorder not otherwise specified. Patients with each of these disorders are characterized, in one way or another, by nonintentional and medically unexplained somatic complaints. In the facti-

tious disorders, medical illness is purposely feigned. The severest form of this class of disorders has been traditionally called Munchausen's syndrome. Patients with this disorder show a chronic pattern of gaining admission to hospitals by mimicking various illnesses, receiving extensive workups, medical treatments, and even surgeries.

The judgment of whether a physical complaint is attributable to an underlying general medical condition or not is a difficult one. It should be based on all sources of information available, including the patient's past history, current presentation, and a physical examination. The cost of possible negative laboratory tests must be balanced in each case against the risk of not identifying a potentially reversible underlying general medical condition.

The physical examination should not be neglected. Clinicians sometimes opt to order a laboratory evaluation rather than thoroughly examining a patient. If an underlying general medical condition is being considered, a physical examination is mandatory, whether performed by the treating psychiatrist or by a consultant.

Although details may vary, there is enough consistency within psychiatric syndromes such that the appearance of atypical features in either the mental status examination or the history should alert the clinician to the possibility of an underlying general medical condition.

For example, schizophrenia is typically characterized by an insidious onset, an absence of disorientation and memory impairment, and auditory rather than visual hallucinations. A precipitous development of psychosis, disorientation, or profound memory impairment or reports of visual hallucinations indicate an underlying general medical condition until proved otherwise. The investigative procedure should continue until an explanation is identified or efforts to detect an underlying general medical etiology are exhausted.

Selection of laboratory tests should be individualized, based on the specifics of the particular case. Indications will be affected not only by the particular symptomatic picture but also by demographic factors. For example, the diagnostic and laboratory approach to an agitated, uncooperative, and disoriented patient would differ for a 44-year-old, recently divorced, unemployed bartender; a 65-year-old, married Mennonite pastor from a rural community with no history of psychiatric illness; or a 23-year-old with a 4-year history of recurrent episodes of psychosis with multiple state hospital admissions.

Identification of General Medical Conditions in Particular Psychiatric Syndromes

Whatever the insult, the CNS has a rather limited repertoire of possible symptom clusters. Thus the same psychiatric symptoms may result from a number of disparate medical conditions.

The remainder of this section reviews the major psychiatric syndromes resulting from such conditions. These include (1) delirium and dementias, (2) psychoses, and (3) anxiety and affective disturbances.

DELIRIUM AND DEMENTIA

The diagnosis of these disorders is at two levels. The first consideration concerns the likelihood that the syndrome is attributable to an underlying general medical condition. Dissociative or catatonic syndromes, the so-called pseudodementia syndrome of depression, and other psychiatric syndromes can mimic such disorders. The second consideration regards the identification of specific causes.

Delirium

In general, delirium presents acutely. The diagnostic process must begin immediately. Any delay increases the risk of irreversible brain damage, other serious complications, or death. Varied clinical pictures are seen. Symptomatic pictures vary from (and often fluctuate between) agitation/hyperactivity to somnolence/lethargy, inattentiveness to hypervigilance, and from total unresponsiveness to moments of lucidity. However, whatever the specific picture, some generalizations about the use of the laboratory can be made.

A careful plan should be instituted, a subject that has been well reviewed (Plum and Posner, 1980). Electroencephalography (EEG) may be useful. Delirium with a metabolic cause for impaired cognition generally shows high-voltage slow activity in stupor or low-voltage fast activity in excitement, whereas in psychiatric cases, good background alpha activity with response to visual and auditory stimuli is typical. Unfortunately, the EEG is often not expedient in an emergency situation, and determination on this basis may not be feasible.

A myriad of specific factors are possible. In one review (Plum and Posner, 1980), 99 are listed. To focus the diagnostic process, these can be grouped into a number of more general categories (see Table 30-1). The most common on medical or surgical wards are hypoxia, ischemia, hypoglycemia, and sedative-hypnotic or other drug intoxication or withdrawal. In most emergency department settings, drug intoxication and withdrawal are the most frequent.

Fortunately, the laboratory evaluations necessary to evaluate these possibilities are readily available at most medical facilities, often in the form of screening profiles. A careful history and thorough physical examination, followed by serum glucose, electrolytes, enzymes, and urea nitrogen (BUN) determinations and a complete blood count (CBC), will screen for most of the suspected causes. Adequate evaluation will improve substantially when additional procedures are done as clinically indicated: arterial blood gas analysis, lumbar puncture,

TABLE 30-1. *Causes of Delirium*

Deprivation of oxygen, substrate, or metabolic cofactors
Diseases of organs other than brain
Exogenous drugs or toxins
Drug withdrawal
Abnormalities of ionic or acid-base CNS environment
Disordered temperature regulation
Infections or inflammation of CNS
Primary neuronal or glial disorders
Seizures or postictal states
Head injury or concussion
Postoperative or intensive care unit delirium

Adapted from Plum F, Posner J: The Diagnosis of Stupor and Coma, ed 3. Philadelphia, FA Davis, 1980, pp. 177–303.

serum and/or urine alcohol and drug screening (see Table 30-2).

Patients with a known psychiatric history present a special problem. A tragic error is to not recognize delirium as an additional syndrome and to attribute changes in cognition to the preexisting psychiatric disorder. It must be remembered that, if anything, psychiatric patients are at increased risk of delirium. Many will be on psychotropic medications. Toxicity from these medications, either from overdose or from toxic plasma levels on prescribed doses, is not infrequent. Patients on tricyclic antidepressants (TCAs) should be observed for anticholinergic symptoms. Plasma drug levels should be drawn. Patients with TCA toxicity may suffer cardiotoxic death (especially if plasma levels are greater than 1000 ng/ml) even as the mental status is clearing. Patients on neuroleptics may be suffering from the neuroleptic malignant syndrome, consisting of stupor or coma, muscle rigidity and fasciculations, and hyperthermia. Elevated levels of serum creatinine phosphokinase (CPK) are a hallmark of this potentially fatal syndrome. Elevation of urinary myoglobin, and a leukocytosis may aid in the diagnosis also.

Psychiatric patients are subject to other factors that place them at increased risk of delirium. Inattention to or neglect of nutritional, hygienic, or medical problems is frequent. Psychotic patients may do unusual things, such as drink excessive

TABLE 30-2. *Laboratory Studies for Dementia in Absence of Specific Indications*

Blood tests: Complete blood count; 12-parameter metabolic screen; test for syphilis; thyroid function tests; vitamin B_{12} and folate levels
Urinalysis
Electrocardiogram
Chest x-ray

Adapted from National Institutes of Health Consensus Development Panel: Differential Diagnosis of Dementing Disease. National Institutes of Health Consensus Development Conference Statement, Washington, 1987.

amounts of water (e.g., to "flush out" poison believed to have been placed in food), resulting in overhydration and hyponatremia. In such a case, if fluid and electrolyte balance is not properly restored, agitation and confusion may progress to intractable seizures and death.

Patients with delirium resulting from alcohol or sedative-hypnotic withdrawal deserve special attention. Abstinence syndromes may be accompanied by hypoglycemia, ketosis, and acid–base, fluid and electrolyte imbalances. These parameters should be carefully assessed with serum and urine testing. Intravenous glucose can be both diagnostic and lifesaving. In addition, such patients often fall or sustain other traumatic injuries, resulting in intracranial bleeds. If there is a suggestion of such injury, a skull x-ray or cranial computed tomographic (CT) scan is indicated.

Dementia

In dementia, the need for an explanation is not as acute as in delirium, so more protracted laboratory procedures are possible. It must be remembered, however, that dementia and delirium often coexist. In fact, demented patients have a lower threshold for becoming delirious. Delirium superimposed on dementia demands the same rapid assessment as delirium itself.

The first diagnostic discrimination, again, is whether or not an underlying general medical or toxic condition is present. Reviews of the clinical, nonlaboratory methods of approaching this differentiation are available (e.g., Wells and Duncan, 1980).

Diagnosis can be aided by a relatively simple battery of tests recommended by an NIH Consensus Development Panel (1987), as shown in Table 30-2. The serum free treponemal antibody absorption (FTA-ABS) test is recommended for screening for syphilis. The commonly performed VDRL test is insufficiently sensitive. It will be nonreactive in many cases of late neurosyphilis (Simon, 1985).

Recommended supplemental studies are shown in Table 30-3. Note that human immunodeficiency virus (HIV) testing is included. HIV-induced impairment (the so-called AIDS dementia complex) can occur even before immunosuppression and its sequelae are evident (Perry, 1990). Any suggestion of risk should be considered an indication for HIV testing.

The major importance of making as specific a diagnosis as possible in dementia is the possibility of identifying a treatable cause. The screening battery with supplements will identify most treatable dementias—those associated with chronic anemia, neurosyphilis, major organ failure (e.g., hepatic, renal), hypothyroidism, vitamin B_{12} (pernicious anemia, subacute combined lateral sclerosis) or folate deficiency, metastases to lung or brain, and other space-occupying intracranial lesions.

Laboratory evaluations will not necessarily offer a definitive answer, at least not early in the course of a dementia. The majority of demented patients will suffer from dementia of the Alzheimer's type (DAT). Chemistries will be generally normal. The EEG is not necessarily abnormal, although some DAT patients will show some diffuse slowing. Cranial tomography (CT) cannot be entirely relied on. In many cases of DAT, cerebral atrophy is not observed. In addition, some intellectually intact elderly will show cerebral atrophy. See the brain imaging techniques section of this chapter for a discussion of the potential use of these more sophisticated procedures.

Certain specific neurologic disorders may present with dementia and yet not be evident on routine laboratory testing. Some (such as Parkinson's disease and Huntington's disease) are primarily diagnosed on the basis of history and neurologic examination. The laboratory may be of more specific value in others. If Wilson's disease (hepatolenticular degeneration) is suspected on the basis of the neurologic examination, hepatic dysfunction, or a Kayser-Fleischer ring, serum should be examined

TABLE 30-3. *Additional Studies for Dementia as Specifically Indicated*

Tests	Indications
Tests with established indications	
Human immunodeficiency virus (HIV) antibodies	History suggests risk of HIV exposure; evidence of immuno suppression
Lumbar puncture (LP)	Suggestion of CNS infection (e.g., meningitis) or of vasculitis
Electroencephalogram (EEG)	Altered consciousness (e.g., delirium); suspected seizures
Computed tomography (CT)	History suggests CNS mass lesion; focal neurologic signs; dementia of brief duration
Magnetic resonance imaging (MRI)	Ambiguous CT findings: MRI more sensitive to small infarcts, mass lesions, atrophy of brainstem and other subcortical structures
Carotid ultrasound	Localize source of infarcts
Brain biopsy	Differential diagnosis by tissue sample
Experimental tests	
Event-related potentials (EP); computerized electroencephalographic topography (CET) or brain electrical activity mapping (BEAM); regional cerebral blood flow (rCBF); positron-emission tomography (PET); single-photon-emission tomography (SPECT)	

Adapted from National Institutes of Health Consensus Development Panel: Differential Diagnosis of Dementing Disease. National Institutes of Health Consensus Development Conference Statement, Washington, 1987.

for increased copper and decreased ceruloplasmin, and urine tested for increased copper. If detected early, appropriate treatment may allay progression of the cognitive impairment. If Creutzfeldt-Jakob (subacute spongiform encephalopathy) is suspected, an EEG may be indicated. While EEG will show slowing early in the course, later periodic biphasic or triphasic slow bursts, often accompanied by characteristic myoclonic jerks of the extremities, are seen in most (90 percent) cases but are seldom seen in other types of dementia (Wilson et al., 1977).

PSYCHOSES

Patients presenting with psychotic symptoms in the absence of disruption of attention, memory, or orientation represent a somewhat different situation diagnostically. In cases of recent origin, with no prior history of psychosis, the approach would be similar to that outlined for delirium. The assumption would be that, although cognitive impairment was not evident, the psychosis was still attributable to disruption of brain functioning on a metabolic or toxic basis.

Particular attention should be paid to the possibility of a drug intoxication, particularly from hallucinogens and stimulants (including cocaine). Important diagnostic tools are urine and serum drug screens. Although more susceptible to tampering, urine samples are generally preferable to serum screens because most drugs and drug metabolites remain detectable longer in urine than in blood. The accuracy of these screens varies greatly among laboratories, especially at low concentrations. Moreover, they are often sensitive to interference from multiple other substances. Many of the drugs, particularly the hallucinogens, exert their effects at low serum concentrations. Some, such as phencyclidine (PCP), may have a prolonged psychotomimetic effect, even after measurable levels of the drug have disappeared from serum and even urine.

Psychoses of a more long-standing nature require a diagnostic approach resembling that for dementia (Tables 30-2 and 30-3). It must be remembered, in fact, that dementias may initially present with psychosis rather than with cognitive impairment.

Careful attention must be paid to the history and physical examination as well as to the initial screening laboratory values in determining additional testing.

ANXIETY AND AFFECTIVE DISTURBANCES

Delirium, dementia, and psychosis are remarkable events. They occur with rarity in the general population, and when they occur, they are rather easily recognizable, since they are discontinuous in the course of the person's life.

Anxiety and affective syndromes are more subtle. Minor fluctuations in level of anxiety or mood are part and parcel of everyday life for most people. Even if the degree of disturbance reaches the point that medical attention is sought, anxiety and affective disorders are so commonplace that diagnosis is often made and treatment initiated without careful medical scrutiny.

A number of medical illnesses may present with anxiety and affective symptoms. These diseases can be subsumed under several categories: endocrinopathies, neurologic disorders, neoplasms, metabolic and toxic disorders, hematologic disorders, chronic systemic disorders, and infections.

Endocrinopathies
The nervous and endocrine systems are intimately interrelated (Brown and Seggie, 1980; Haskett and Rose, 1981). The control center of the endocrine system, the hypothalamus, is considered part of the limbic system, a functional part of the CNS that is thought to specifically modulate emotions. Anatomically, the hypothalamus is richly innervated by the limbic system. It also receives inputs from the frontal cortex and ascending reticular activating system. The hypothalamus is reactive to many neurotransmitters, including monoamines such as dopamine, norepinephrine, and serotonin—substances implicated in the pathophysiology of schizophrenia and affective disorders.

The relationship of endocrine imbalance and mood is perhaps most direct with disturbances in thyroid hormones and adrenocortical steroids. Psychiatric symptoms are a relatively consistent and striking aspect in the clinical picture in such imbalances. In fact, they are often the presenting complaint. In both cases, psychiatric syndromes occur with both hormone deficiency and excess.

THYROID. Thyroid hormone has perhaps the most general metabolic effect of any of the endocrine hormones. Deficiency in thyroid hormone results in hypometabolism; excess results in hypermetabolism.

Hypothyroidism (myxedema) may have profound psychiatric effects. These effects vary with the age at onset of the deficiency. Neonatal hypothyroidism, if untreated, results in retardation of physical and mental development (cretinism). This disorder is observed in about 1 of every 5000 births, and measurement of serum or cord thyroxine (T_4) or thyroid-stimulating hormone (TSH) is required at birth in most states as a screening procedure.

In older children, failure to continue on growth or development curves should raise suspicion of hypothyroidism, particularly if x-rays reveal failure of expected epiphyseal closures.

In adults, hypothyroidism often presents insidiously with nonspecific symptoms such as lethargy, anergia, and fatigability. If the deficiency state continues, these symptoms, as well as the classic physical signs of myxedema, will progress. Classically, myxedematous patients are apathetic, withdrawn, and psychomotor retarded and show impaired memory and difficulty in concentrating. Profound dysphoria with suicidal thoughts may occur—a picture not unlike melancholic depression. The affective disturbance may reach psychotic proportions, hence "myxedema madness."

Diagnosis, first of all, depends on a careful history and examination for the classic physical signs of myxedema. A profoundly depressed patient with no prior history of such, or of a syndrome in which apathy-lethargy type symptoms predominate over dysphoria, should make one suspicious.

Concern should be raised in the presence of certain other laboratory abnormalities. Increased serum cholesterol, CPK, serum glutamic-oxaloacetic transferase (SGOT), and lactate dehydrogenase (LDH) often, but not invariably, occur.

The crux of the diagnosis is thyroid testing. Recent American Thyroid Association guidelines suggest that most cases of hypo- or hyperthyroidism will be ascertained by determination of free serum thyroxine (free $3,5,3',5'$-tetraiodothyronine or free T_4) and serum thyrotropin (thyroid-stimulating hormone, or TSH) (Surks et al., 1990). Different laboratories use various specific assay techniques. The accuracy and standardization of these measures have improved greatly in the past decade. Metabolic indices, such as determination of the basal metabolism rate (BMR), are seldom done today because of their inconvenience and because they are affected by many nonthyroidal factors.

The typical picture in hypothyroidism is a decreased level of free T_4 and an elevated TSH. Although free T_4 and TSH levels are affected less than many other thyroid function tests, levels may still be altered by severe medical illnesses and certain drugs, including phenytoin and carbamazepine. Faced with confusing laboratory findings, appropriate consultation should be obtained.

The same psychiatric manifestations may be seen whether hypothyroidism results from lesions of the thyroid itself, the pituitary, or the hypothalamus. Once having determined hypothyroidism by initial testing, appropriate consultation should be obtained for more specific testing. Psychiatric symptoms may persist after a euthyroid state is reestablished, necessitating the usual treatments for depression.

As with hypothyroidism, the psychiatric manifestations of thyroid excess often develop insidiously. Common early symptoms of hyperthyroidism include emotional instability, nervousness, hyperactivity, a fine tremor, loss of weight and strength, and, at times, palpitations. Generally, if the syndrome has developed rapidly, the patient complains of anxiety; if more gradually, depression. Occasionally, a patient may become hyperactive and grandiose such that a manic-like state is observed. Syndromes resembling anxiety or depressive disorders are more common, however.

Again, diagnosis depends, first of all, on a good history and examination of the patient. In addition to the psychiatric symptoms mentioned, hyperthyroid patients characteristically have heat intolerance. On physical examination, they may (if suffering from Graves' disease) demonstrate a characteristic ophthalmopathy (exophthalmos), a diffuse goiter (sometimes accompanied by a bruit), and a dermopathy.

Laboratory evaluation should, again, start with a basic screen (e.g., free T_4 and TSH). Typically, an elevated free T_4 and a depressed TSH are observed in hyperthyroidism. However, exceptions do occur, such as in triiodothyronine (T_3) thyrotoxicosis. Hyperthyroidism indicates a disturbance in either the thyroid itself or the hypothalamic–pituitary axis. The exact etiology must be found and corrected. Thus appropriate consultation should be obtained.

ADRENAL CORTEX. Both insufficiency and excess in adrenocortical hormones may be associated with psychiatric syndromes of highly variable presentation but with a predominance of affective or anxiety symptoms.

Adrenocortical insufficiency (Addison's disease) most often presents psychiatrically with depressive symptoms, particularly of an apathetic, negativistic nature and with fatigue and poverty of thought. In extreme cases, a delirium-like picture can develop with disorientation and memory loss. Addison's disease should be suspected in patients who, at one time, were receiving steroids as a medical treatment. Suspicion also should be raised in cases of depression in which the degree of weakness and lethargy appear to be out of step with the rest of the picture and in which *hypo*tension is notable. Blood pressure changes occur consequent to lowered levels of aldosterone, a mineralocorticoid, which may be affected as well as the glucocorticoids, such as cortisol. A characteristic form of hyperpigmentation [attributable to elevated levels of adrenocorticotropin hormone (ACTH)] is the hallmark of the syndrome. Its absence, however, does not exclude hypoadrenocortisolism.

In milder cases, routine laboratory values may be normal, but in advanced stages, hyponatremia, paired with hyperkalemia, may occur. Documentation of adrenal insufficiency is essential and includes 24-hour urine collections for 17-hydroxy and 17-ketosteroids. Plasma cortisol and ACTH levels are also helpful. Stimulation with the synthetic ACTH cosyntropin can demonstrate whether the insufficiency is associated with adrenal failure or is of hypothalamic–pituitary origin.

Excess levels of cortisol, whether of adrenal or exogenous (iatrogenic) origin, result in the classic picture of Cushing's syndrome. Psychiatrically, patients with hyperadrenocortisolism may present with a syndrome resembling an anxiety or depressive disorder with fatigue and weakness. In some cases, especially with exogenous corticoids, manic-like syndromes may be seen with euphoria, but this is uncommon and generally transient, with depression ensuing. The psychiatric syndrome may progress to include psychotic features. Hypertension is nearly always present. The diagnosis of hypercortisolism should be considered in depressed patients on exogenous steroids. Once the classic physical signs of Cushing's syndrome appear (altered habitus with round facies and truncal obesity, hirsutism and amenorrhea in women, and cutaneous striae), the diagnosis is fairly obvious, but it must be remembered that the psychiatric syndrome may antedate the other signs.

The laboratory diagnosis of Cushing's syndrome hinges on the demonstration of increased cortisol levels. This is most easily demonstrated by high plasma and urinary 17-hydroxycorticoid levels. Individual plasma levels are not especially meaningful because of diurnal variation and the fact that cortisol is released in pulselike, rather than continuous, fashion. The diagnosis can be refined with various modifications of the dexamethasone suppression test (DST), a test that is discussed in detail later in this chapter.

PHEOCHROMOCYTOMA. Catecholamine-producing tumors of the adrenal medulla and other chromaffin-staining tissues frequently present with anxiety symptoms or, in more chronic cases, depression. Symptoms of autonomic hyperexcitability such as tremulousness, sweatiness, heat intolerance, palpitations, and chest pains are particularly common. Labile hypertension is a prominent feature. Diagnosis should be suspected when paroxysms of such symptoms begin to occur in someone without such a history, especially if they also have labile hypertension.

Laboratory evaluation involves the measurement of norepinephrine, epinephrine, and the metabolites metanephrine and vanillylmandelic acid (VMA) in 24-hour urine. Many dietary factors and concomitant medications can influence the assay. If pheochromocytoma is suspected, appropriate consultation is indicated. Even if this tumor is not found, control of the patient's labile hypertension is indicated.

PARATHYROID. Both hypoparathyroidism and hyperparathyroidism are associated with psychiatric manifestations. The mechanism differs from that of thyroid or adrenocortical dysfunction in that the symptoms appear to be a function of alteration in calcium levels rather than direct effects of parathormone on the CNS. Psychiatric symptoms are rather nonspecific but correlate with the magnitude of deviation in serum calcium. With mild hypocalcemia, anxiety symptoms and paresthesias are common. As hypocalcemia becomes more marked, tetany may occur; at lower levels yet, seizures. Permanent brain damage may result. With hypercalcemia, depressive symptoms (fatigue, lethargy, or irritability) may be seen at mild elevations (11 to 16 mg/dl). At elevations greater than 16 mg/dl, delirium often occurs.

These syndromes are often detected from serum calcium levels in a routine chemical profile.

Hypoparathyroidism (or pseudohypoparathyroidism) should be suspected in patients with anxiety symptoms and paresthesias are common. As hypocalcemia becomes more marked, tetany may occur; at lower levels yet, seizures. Permanent brain damage may result. With hypercalcemia, depressive symptoms (fatigue, lethargy, or irritability) may be seen at mild elevations (11 to 16 mg/dl). At elevations greater than 16 mg/dl, delerium often occurs.

These syndromes are often detected from serum calcium levels in a routine chemical profile. Hypoparathyroidism (or pseudohypoparathyroidism) should be suspected in patients with tetany or in patients with a history of neck surgery; hyperparathyroidism (or pseudohyperparathyroidism) should be suspected in patients with repeated nephrolithiasis or with the bone disease osteitis fibrosa cystica.

Laboratory evaluation should start with serum calcium determination. Radioimmunoassay (RIA) of parathormone also should be considered. After such basic testing, the diagnostic workup should probably be continued by a consultant. The differential diagnosis gets complicated, considering the possibilities of primary, secondary, "pseudo," and even "pseudopseudo" hypoparathyroidism. A prompt, definitive diagnosis is advisable, considering the potential complications and the fact that some of the "pseudo" cases may be associated with a malignancy.

ESTROGEN. Two syndromes have been postulated as directly or indirectly related to estrogen deficiency: the premenstrual syndrome and the menopausal syndrome. In the premenstrual syndrome ("premenstrual dysphoric disorder" in the DSM-IV Appendix), women report increased anxiety or depressive symptoms, somatic complaints, and behavioral changes during the 7 to 10 days before menses. In the menopausal syndrome, these same symptoms plus hot flashes are reported. A symptomatically similar posthysterectomy syndrome has been proposed as well. Hot flashes do appear to be related to luteinizing hormone (LH) surges. Otherwise, efforts to delineate these syndromes endocrinologically have not been successful. Thus laboratory tests have not, as yet, been found to be useful in delineating these syndromes (Abplanalp et al., 1980).

HYPOGLYCEMIA. When of gradual onset and long duration, hypoglycemia is often associated with CNS symptoms such as apathy, dizziness, confusion, and intellectual decline and is to be considered in the differential diagnosis of dementia. A rapid drop in blood glucose, on the other hand, more often results in anxiety, tremulousness, sweatiness, tachycardia, and palpitations—a syndrome reminiscent of panic disorder. Serum glucose levels below 50 mg/dl are usually necessary for such symptoms to develop. The mechanism is thought to involve excessive secretion of epinephrine in response to the fall in blood sugar.

The differential diagnosis of hypoglycemia is broad, ranging from excessive insulin administration by diabetics to various causes of excessive insulin production. When symptoms continue and appear to be temporally related to meals or in response to certain types of foods, yet no organic illness can be identified, postprandial hypoglycemia should be considered. This syndrome has been observed in patients with a history of gastrointestinal surgery.

Because the symptomatic picture of hypoglycemia overlaps with that of panic or anxiety disorders, the diagnosis should be verified by laboratory evaluations before it is accepted. Glucose tolerance tests are difficult to interpret and may have little bearing on the syndrome. The definitive diagnostic procedure is serum glucose determination during a symptomatic attack. Patients with panic disorder will not show a low serum glucose level and may actually show an elevated serum glucose because of the hyperglycemic effects of epinephrine and cortisol.

Neurologic Disorders

PARKINSONISM. Affective symptoms may occur in relation to the disease itself. Pathologic changes similar to those seen in the substantia nigra have been observed in the locus ceruleus of parkinsonian patients. Because this locus is the main norepinephrine nucleus in the brain, the affective symptoms may be neurochemically mediated. Affective syndromes also may occur in association with certain treatments, particularly L-dopa. Depressive, as well as manic-like syndromes, sometimes of psychotic proportions, have been reported with L-dopa use. Thus L-dopa plasma levels may be useful in adjusting dosage. Lowering levels into the therapeutic range may alleviate these symptoms. Nonetheless, some patients will develop psychiatric symptoms even within the therapeutic range.

HUNTINGTON'S DISEASE AND WILSON'S DISEASE. Affective syndromes or psychotic syndromes resembling schizophrenia may be the first presentation of these two disorders. Laboratory tests involved in their diagnosis were discussed previously in reference to dementia.

MULTIPLE SCLEROSIS (MS). This disorder may present with personality changes and lability of mood, which, together with the frequent vagueness of the neurologic picture at least early in the course of the disorder, may suggest a psychiatric rather than a neurologic disorder. Certain laboratory evaluations can be helpful. Cerebrospinal fluid (CSF) studies will often reveal elevation in gamma globulins and the presence of oligoclonal bands and myelin basic protein. Such changes are not specific for MS, however. Evoked potential studies will demonstrate demyelination, particularly of the optic nerve, but the diagnosis of MS is dependent on the distribution of lesions. Perhaps the best laboratory evidence is the demonstration of disseminated white matter lesions by CT or by magnetic resonance imaging (MRI) which provides better resolution of small lesions.

Neoplasms

Anxiety and depression in the context of malignancies have been the object of a great deal of recent interest (Petty and Noyes, 1981). A certain amount of depressive symptomatology can be attributed to a reaction to incapacitation, pain, and the anticipation of death. Depression is also associated with irradiation and several of the antineoplastic drugs. Some studies, however, have shown that depression can occur before the detection of the malignancy. This has been reported with pancreatic carcinoma, for example.

An occult malignancy should be suspected in cases of depression in which weight loss and debility outstep the degree of mood or cognitive symptoms. Testing should begin with a routine chemical profile, CBC, chest x-ray, and any tests that are symptomatically or demographically indicated.

Metabolic and Toxic Disorders

A wide variety of metabolic illnesses are probably associated with depressive symptoms, if not a full depressive syndrome. Similarly, many drugs appear to induce affective symptoms both in toxic and therapeutic plasma concentration ranges. Laboratory testing in these situations would be indicated according to historical and symptomatic information. One syndrome (acute intermittent porphyria) deserves special mention, since it is often diagnosed only after unnecessary delay.

ACUTE INTERMITTENT PORPHYRIA. Acute intermittent porphyria, associated with an inborn error of heme metabolism, is characterized by acute attacks often precipitated by the ingestion of one of a number of substances, including barbiturates, anticonvulsants, alcohol, and hormones. These attacks can resemble panic attacks. The one feature of such attacks that is not typical of panic attacks is excruciating abdominal pain, which often heralds the onset of an attack. The abdomen is often surprisingly (considering the degree of complaint) soft and nontender, and a confusing admixture of neurologic signs are often present. Thus a somatoform disorder is sometimes suggested. The syndrome may be life-threatening, with the development of hyponatremia (attributable, in part, to vomiting) and with resulting delirium, coma, and seizures. Thus prompt diagnosis is crucial so that supportive measures are not delayed. Medications such as barbiturates and anticonvulsants, which may aggravate or prolong attacks, are to be avoided.

Diagnosis in a previously unidentified case is made by documenting excessive excretion of the heme precursors porphobilinogen (PBG) and δ-aminolerulinic acid (ALA) in urine preferably during an acute attack. Between attacks, it may be necessary to measure the level of the porphyrin synthesizing enzyme erythrocyte uroporphrinogen-L-synthetase.

Chronic Systemic Disorders

As with metabolic disorders, depressive symptoms are common in the course of many chronic systemic disorders. In most cases, the underlying disorder and need for laboratory testing are evident.

SYSTEMIC LUPUS ERYTHEMATOSUS (SLE). The diagnosis of SLE generally becomes evident with the occurrence of the typical physical changes in the renal, cardiopulmonary, and musculoskeletal systems and the skin. Early in the course of the illness, complaints may be vague and include anorexia, vomiting, and depression, thus resembling an affective disorder.

Routine laboratory tests may show nonspecific abnormalities, such as anemia, leukopenia, an elevated sedimentation rate (ESR), and mild proteinuria and microscopic hematuria. Given such a picture, a more specific evaluation is indicated and should include determination of autoantibodies [e.g., serum antinuclear antibodies (ANA), anti-DNA, and perhaps a lupus erythematosus cell test (LE prep)]. Many medications, including neuroleptics, can lead to false-positive determinations. Definitive diagnosis, especially at early stages, is problematic, and consultation with an internist or rheumatologist may be indicated.

Infections

NEUROSYPHILIS. As reviewed by Simon (1985), secondary syphilis with meningitis (within 2 years of initial infection) or cerebrovascular involvement (from months to 12 years of infection) typically presents with varying confusion, headache, and neurologic signs. Tertiary syphilis of the tabetic type (incubation 10 to 20 years) has notable neurologic symptoms. However, tertiary syphilis of the paretic type (incubation again from 10 to 20 years) may present without neurologic signs and, in early stages, an absence of cognitive impairment, but a mimickry of virtually any psychiatric illness, including affective disorders. A classic grandiose delusional state can resemble mania. With the advent of penicillin, such syndromes had become relatively rare. However, a worldwide rise in the incidence of early syphilis has been documented. This suggests that there will be an increase in neurosyphilis as well, making detection of increasing importance so that treatment can be initiated immediately to prevent progression. It appears that the commonly performed serum VDRL test is insufficiently specific and is relatively insensitive (false-negative rate of 25 percent) in late neurosyphilis (Simon, 1985). The serum fluorescent treponemal antibody absorption (FTA-ABS) test remains reactive in more than 95 percent of late syphilis cases, making it the test of choice and other testing (including of the CSF) virtually unnecessary.

LYME DISEASE. Patients with infection with the spirochete *Borrelia burgdorferi* can present with a variety of psychiatric complaints, including chronic fatigue and depression, these occurring months to years after the initial tick bite, which may have gone unnoticed. At this point, tests for infection (generally involving detection of serum antibodies) are improving, but diagnosis is ultimately on the basis of clinical symptoms and history.

CHRONIC HERPESVIRUS INFECTIONS. A great deal of interest has been directed to a proposed relationship between chronic infection with Ebstein-Barr virus (EBV) and cytomegalovirus (CMV). Acute infections cause infectious mononucleosis and similarly presenting syndromes which may have associated depression, personality change, and even psychosis. Whether or not chronic syndrome may result is controversial. Examinations for elevated titers of antibodies have yielded inconsistent results (Bosse et al., 1989).

ACUTE IMMUNODEFICIENCY SYNDROME (AIDS). As discussed under dementia in this chapter, human immunodeficiency virus (HIV) infection often presents with psychiatric symptoms. Again, any suggestion of risk should prompt HIV testing.

THERAPEUTIC DRUG MONITORING (TDM)

Monitoring of plasma concentration levels of certain nonpsychiatric drugs, such as anticonvulsants and cardiac glycosides, is commonplace, especially when the therapeutic range is well established and the therapeutic index (the mean toxic dose divided by the mean therapeutic dose) is low. In such cases, the determination of proper dosage is critical to ensure that a patient achieves a therapeutic but not a toxic (or even lethal) level. Certain psychiatric drugs, such as lithium carbonate, carbamazepine, and the tricyclic antidepressants (TCAs), also have low therapeutic indices.

Plasma levels are an aspect of the pharmacokinetics (the time course) rather than the pharmacodynamics (the physiologic effects and mechanisms of action) of a given drug and its metabolites. The time course of a drug is a function of its absorption, distribution, metabolism, and excretion. These determine the plasma and brain levels of the drug and its metabolites.

Important pharmacokinetic parameters are plasma half-life and steady state. The *plasma half-life* is the time after the administration of a single dose of a drug at which half has been eliminated from the plasma compartment. A *steady state* exists when the amount of the drug ingested per dosing interval equals the amount eliminated. At steady state, an equilibrium exists between drug levels in plasma and the other body compartments. Thus the amount of drug at the effector site (CNS neurons) is in equilibrium with the free concentration in plasma. Generally, steady state occurs after 5 half-lives, given that the patient remains on the same dose and dosing schedule.

Principles of pharmacokinetics and pharmaco-dynamics are merged in consideration of concentration–response relationships. *Response* here refers to the therapeutic effects of a drug, but it can refer to side effects as well. It is assumed that a critical drug concentration must be achieved at the site of action before an effect is observed.

Lithium Carbonate

Lithium's therapeutic effects in treating mania were discovered in 1949, making it the first specifically effective psychotropic drug (Fieve, 1980). However, its toxicity and potential lethality also were known, causing it to be banned in the United States until 1970. It was used cautiously but effectively elsewhere. Given its narrow therapeutic index, it is unlikely that it would have been approved for use without TDM.

The plasma concentration of lithium is easily measured by several relatively simple analytical techniques such as atomic absorption or flame emission photometry.

The mean half-life of lithium for healthy adults is 24 hours, ranging from 18 hours in some adolescents to 30 to 36 hours in the elderly. Thus steady-state plasma levels are obtainable after approximately 5 days on a constant dosage. Levels are often determined more frequently during the early phases of treatment, especially if higher concentrations are sought in an attempt to terminate a manic episode.

Three- or four-times-a-day dosage regimens are generally followed; a twice-a-day schedule is followed when slow-release formulations are used. With standard preparations, peak concentrations are observed within 2 hours—within 5 hours for the slow-release drug. Plasma samples are best drawn at 10 to 12 hours after the last dose to ensure that the patient is in the elimination rather than the absorption or distribution phase.

Therapeutic effects occur at concentrations between approximately 0.7 and 1.5 mEq/liter. Acute side effects occur in some patients within the therapeutic range but in most at levels above 1.5 mEq/liter. Mild side effects include polyuria/polydipsia, nausea or diarrhea, sedation, and a fine tremor. At higher levels, these effects are exacerbated. With moderate toxicity, generally at levels from 2.0 to 2.5 mEq/liter, a coarse tremor, along with muscle weakness or hyperirritability with fasciculations, may occur. At high levels (greater than 2.5 mEq/liter), muscular hypertonicity, hyperactive deep tendon reflexes, and choreiform–athetoid movements may appear. Consciousness may be grossly impaired. With severe toxicity, coma and death may ensue.

This schema of concentration–side effect correlations is a general guideline. There is a great deal of individual variation in sensitivity to toxic effects. Because there is also individual variation in steady-state concentration on the same dosage, TDM of

lithium is invaluable in maintaining a patient within a desired therapeutic range and in avoiding inadvertent toxicity.

CARBAMAZEPINE. Also used in the acute and maintenance treatment of bipolar illness, carbamazepine also has a narrow therapeutic window. It is recommended that the therapeutic serum anticonvulsant range of 4 to 12 μg/ml during the steady-state elimination phase also be used for psychiatric indications. In addition to CNS effects, toxic levels of carbamazepine can result in malignant cardiac arrhythmias and heart block. One problem with maintaining this range is that carbamazepine induces its own hepatic enzymes. Thus, after several weeks, its half-life may decrease from 30 to 40 hours to 6 to 20 hours. Maintenance therapy in the 'herapeutic range is associated with bone marrow suppression (leukopenia, thrombocytopenia, anemia, and even aplastic anemia) and hepatotoxicity. Thus, after careful pretreatment screening, laboratory monitoring of the CBC and liver function tests is required.

VALPROIC ACID. Also useful in the acute and maintenance treatment of bipolar illness, it is recommended that serum elimination-phase steady-state levels be maintained in the anticonvulsant range of 30 to 100 μg/ml. Toxic hematologic and hepatic effects similar to those described with carbamazepine require TDM. Unlike carbamazepine, valproate does not induce its own metabolic enzymes.

Tricyclic Antidepressant Drugs (TCAs)

Like lithium, TCAs have a narrow therapeutic index with potentially serious and even lethal side effects. Also, large interindividual pharmacokinetic variability is observed. Thus, with ready availability of commercial testing, TDM is now a standard aspect of the clinical use of TCAs (Preskorn et al, 1988; Preskorn and Fast, 1991).

Assays are generally done by chromatographic techniques, with gas chromatography–mass spectrophotometry (GC–MS) the most accurate from the standpoint of sensitivity and specificity. It is also the most expensive and time-consuming. Hence it is used mainly to standardize more convenient assays. Gas chromatography (GC) and high-performance liquid chromatography (HPLC) are reasonably accurate and are the most commonly used techniques (Preskorn and Mac, 1984). Over the past decade, as assays have become more routine, they have become more standardized. Yet it is still advisable to use a laboratory that performs assays in high volume on a regular basis.

To date, plasma levels of amitriptyline, nortriptyline, imipramine, and desipramine have been studied most extensively. Of these, therapeutic ranges for nortriptyline and imipramine are the most widely accepted. Laboratories can now measure most of the antidepressants, including new nontricyclics such as trazodone, bupropion, fluoxetine, sertraline, and paroxetine (Preskorn, 1993). Among these drugs, bupropion has a narrow therapeutic index with potentially serious toxicity (risk of seizures) and interindividual pharmacokinetic variability (Preskorn, 1991). This suggests a clinical utility of TDM for bupropion but not necessarily the others.

The mean half-life of the TCAs varies from 17 hours for doxepin to 78 hours for protriptyline (Richardson and Richelson, 1984). For practical purposes, a half-life of 24 to 36 hours is a reasonable approximation for amitriptyline, nortriptyline, imipramine, and desipramine. Thus steady-state levels can be determined after approximately 7 days.

Samples should be drawn 10 to 12 hours after the last dose to ensure measurement in the elimination phase. Hemolysis should be avoided because red blood cells have a higher TCA concentration than plasma.

TDM can be useful in several ways: checking compliance, adjusting dosage to achieve a level in the therapeutic range, minimizing the risk of toxicity, and assessing danger with overdose (Preskorn and Fast, 1991).

Patients frequently do not take medications as prescribed. An unusually low plasma level on a particular dosage of TCA may indicate noncompliance. On the other hand, since there is as much as a 36-fold interindividual variation in metabolism rates of TCAs, the patient may simply be a "fast" metabolizer. However, failure of the concentration to increase with an increase in dose would strongly suggest noncompliance. Knowledge that the level will be "checked" may encourage compliance.

Unlike many drugs in which linear or sigmoidal relationships exist, a nonlinear concentration–antidepressant response curve has been reported with certain TCAs, particularly nortriptyline. A "therapeutic window" appears to exist in which antidepressant effects occur only between certain minimum and maximum levels (Asberg et al., 1971). Above the maximum threshold, not only will side effects be more frequent but the antidepressant effect itself also will be diminished.

In the case of nortriptyline, the antidepressant therapeutic window is estimated between 50 and 175 ng/ml; for amitriptyline, a combined concentration of it and its active metabolite nortriptyline, the optimal therapeutic range is between 150 and 250 ng/ml.

The concentration–response curve for imipramine appears to be linear (Perry et al., 1987). The minimum effective level is approximately 150 ng/ml. However, increasing the concentration above 300 ng/ml in nonresponsive patients is not generally recommended. Above 450 ng/ml the risks of toxicity are so great that any potential increase in efficacy is clearly outweighed.

The adverse side effects of TCAs are many. TCAs affect multiple neurotransmitter systems, most of which may have nothing to do with antidepressant effects. Some side effects are mainly a nuisance (e.g., dry mouth) or may even be useful in some patients (e.g., sedation). Others can be incapacitating (e.g., memory impairment) or life-threatening (e.g., cardiotoxicity). Although wide interindividual variations in sensitivity to side effects exist, they are usually concentration-dependent. With the wide variation in the metabolism of TCAs, some patients may develop toxic plasma concentrations on routine dosages. Without TDM, it would not be possible to detect these "slow metabolizers" until signs of toxicity developed.

Recently, it has been noted that patients concomitantly on the antidepressant fluoxetine may develop unusually high levels of TCAs on doses ordinarily leading to therapeutic plasma concentrations (Preskorn et al., 1990). This has been shown to occur because of fluoxetine inhibition of P450 cytochrome oxidase. Thus such patients should be routinely monitored. With the long half-life of fluoxetine, such an effect may occur as long as several weeks after its discontinuation.

TCAs have a serious overdose potential, with major CNS and cardiotoxic effects. Both CNS and cardiac toxicities are concentration-dependent but are not always correlated with each other. Thus a patient whose mental status is clearing may still have toxic plasma levels and suffer a fatal cardiac arrhythmia. All patients with plasma levels of total TCAs greater than 1000 ng/ml show impaired intracardiac conduction with QRS prolongation. Death from cardiac arrhythmias has occurred at concentrations as low as 500 ng/ml (Preskorn and Irwin, 1982). During the first 24 hours, all TCA overdose patients with a QRS longer than 160 μs should be monitored by electrocardiography (ECG) until the duration falls below this. In overdose cases, TCA plasma levels are not a foolproof method of screening for potentially dangerous overdoses, since absorption may not be complete. In addition, prompt assays may not be available. Monitoring the ECG and other physical signs is still the best method for assessing risk in an overdose patient.

Neuroleptics

Delineation of the clinical utility of TDM for neuroleptics has lagged far behind that for TCAs. Results of concentration–response studies have been contradictory.

A number of assay techniques exist. As with the TCAs, chromatographic methods are generally used, particularly HPLC and GC (Friedel, 1984). They are fairly accurate and are much less expensive and time-consuming than GC/MS, which is, again, used mainly for standardization. RIAs require development of a specific antibody for each drug assayed (Friedel, 1984). A radioligand dopamine receptor–binding displacement assay is also available. This technique measures the amount of parent neuroleptic drug and any of its metabolites that displace a radiolabeled ligand from the dopamine (DA) receptor. Thus, theoretically, the assay measures the actual antidopaminergic effects of a neuroleptic drug and its metabolites. This would address problems in establishing concentration–response relationships resulting from the fact that most neuroleptics, particularly the phenothiazines, have multiple metabolites that differ from the parent compound in binding affinity for dopamine receptors, the presumed site of antipsychotic action. The fact that a neuroleptic and its metabolites may differ in plasma/brain concentration gradient would remain.

In addition, many of the existing studies of neuroleptic therapy suffer from serious methodologic problems. As argued by Van Putten (1984), fixed-dose design is necessary. Thus far, only chlorpromazine, fluphenazine, haloperidol, and thiothixene have been studied in this way. As interpreted by Van Putten, these studies suggest that among these drugs, a linear relationship may exist only for thiothixene. Thus it may be possible to continue increasing the dosage of thiothixene, as tolerated in terms of side effects, without diminution of antipsychotic effects. In contrast, higher dose levels of the other drugs may cause "psychotoxicity" (i.e., aggravation of the psychosis). It may be hypothesized that at low concentrations the postsynaptic dopamine receptor is minimally blocked and the presynaptic dopamine reuptake is unaffected; hence there is no antipsychotic effect. In the therapeutic range, blockade occurs at both sites, leading to an antipsychotic effect. At higher concentrations, there may be little additional postsynaptic blockade and an enhancement of presynaptic dopamine release, leading to dopaminergic activation and an increase in psychotic symptoms.

DIAGNOSING AND MONITORING PSYCHIATRIC DISORDERS

Such use of the laboratory in psychiatry is in its infancy. The purpose of this section is to review some promising developments.

Neuroendocrine Strategies

The CNS and endocrine systems are so interrelated that, for many purposes, the two can be referred to as one—the *neuroendocrine system*. Ramifications of this unity are discussed in detail in several excellent reviews, including those of Brown and Seggie (1980) and Haskett and Rose (1981).

As reviewed earlier, endocrine dysfunction has long been known to result in serious disruption in CNS function, leading to psychiatric symptoms. Likewise, it appears that CNS dysfunction is accompanied by changes in endocrine function. Some

changes have been long reported (e.g., hypercortisolemia in melancholic depressions and gonadotropin changes in anorexia nervosa). The changes observed, however, have lacked sufficient specificity to be useful clinically. From a theoretical or research point of view, it is not clear that such changes are related to a process basic to the pathophysiology of the psychiatric disorder or are merely epiphenomena.

In recent years, some neuroendocrine strategies made possible, in part, by technologic advances such as RIA have allowed more exacting and clinically feasible assessment of neuroendocrine functioning during the course of psychiatric disturbance. Thus subtle alterations in the responsivity of specific neuroendocrine systems to various challenges may be detected. Such alterations may prove useful as biologic markers for certain major psychiatric disorders. With this in mind, various techniques currently in use in clinical and research settings will be reviewed.

Affective Disorders

DEXAMETHASONE SUPPRESSION TEST (DST)

"Normally," ingestion of dexamethasone, a potent synthetic corticosteroid-like compound, leads to temporary suppression of adrenocortical secretion of corticosteroids, of which cortisol constitutes 75 to 95 percent. The mechanism is thought to involve a feedback loop, inhibiting hypothalamic secretion of corticotropin-releasing factor (CRF) and resulting in a fall in the pituitary secretion of ACTH. This, in turn, results in a fall in cortisol secretion by the adrenal glands. Nonsuppression occurs with pathology in the hypothalamic–pituitary–adrenal axis and also with various medical conditions, medications, and certain psychiatric disorders.

As standardized by Carroll et al. (1981), the overnight DST test involves 1 mg of dexamethasone in tablet form at 11 P.M., just before sleep. Plasma levels are then drawn at 8 A.M., 4 P.M., and 11 P.M. the next day. In outpatients, the 4 P.M. level is often the only level obtained. Any serum plasma level greater than 5 μg/dl is defined as nonsuppression.

Extensively studied, the DST is now seen to have major limitations in its clinical utility. As discussed in an APA Task Force on Laboratory Tests in Psychiatry report (1987), it is not particularly useful when the likelihood of a major affective disorder is either very high or very low. Furthermore, because of its low specificity, it is not useful in patients on one of a host of medications or with major medical illness. It may be useful in certain specific situations, such as distinguishing a depression with psychotic features from a schizophrenic illness. Also, there is some indication that failure of a nonsuppressor to "convert" to suppression with apparent recovery from depression suggests an increased risk of relapse and suicide.

THYROID-RELEASING HORMONE STIMULATION

As reviewed earlier, hypothyroidism is often accompanied by depression. Conversely, most depressed patients are euthyroid, at least by the usual parameters. It has been suggested, however, that subtler dysregulation exists in the form of blunted thyrotropin (TSH) response to thyrotropin-releasing hormone (TRH).

In this test, TRH is administered in the morning after an overnight fast. A baseline TSH level is obtained. Then, 500 μg of TRH is infused over 30 seconds. Serial TSH collections are taken 15, 30, and 45 minutes after infusion. An increase in plasma TSH of 10 to 20 μU/ml above baseline is expected. An increase of less than 7 μU/ml is considered a blunted response (Targum, 1983). In the absence of a primary pituitary disorder, a blunted response is reported in 25 to 35 percent of endogenously depressed patients but rarely in others. Although highly specific, the relatively low sensitivity of the TRH stimulation test to endogenous depression limits its value when used by itself. Some have argued that the test is more useful when used in conjunction with other neuroendocrine tests, such as the DST (Targum et al., 1982).

DOPAMINE AGONIST STUDIES

Preliminary work in studying the effects of DA agonists on plasma levels of various pituitary hormones known to be affected by these compounds suggests another area of dysregulation (Jimerson and Post, 1984). Certain depressed patients show increased pituitary sensitivity to DA and its agonists. A dramatic fall in plasma prolactin levels has been observed in depressed patients in comparison with controls. However, growth hormone (GH) secretion stimulated by DA agonists did not distinguish depressed from nondepressed patients. This prolactin effect is of theoretical interest, suggesting that antidepressant response may be mediated, in part, by dopaminergic mechanisms. The antidepressant action of bupropion may be related to such effects.

Anorexia Nervosa

Anorexia nervosa is virtually always accompanied by endocrine changes (Vande Wiele, 1977; Garfinkel and Garner, 1984). Affected women typically present with breast atrophy and amenorrhea and low plasma concentrations of 17B-estradiol, LH, and follicle-stimulating hormone (FSH). Plasma cortisol is usually high or normal, with free T_4 usually low-normal and FSH high-normal. The relative preservation of pituitary–adrenal and pituitary–thyroid axes differentiates the hypogonadotropism of anorexia nervosa from that seen in panhypopituitarism. Yet some alteration in these pathways is observed in response to challenge. In anorexia nervosa, LH and FSH response to luteinizing hormone–releasing hormone (LHRH) infusion is quantitatively normal but delayed, as is FSH response to TRH infusion.

However, it is not clear whether these changes are related to the basic pathophysiology of anorexia nervosa or are epiphenomena representing nonspecific responses to starvation, weight loss, or even emotional stresses that precede the lowering of caloric absorption and the resultant weight loss. No single explanation is consistent with all of the information. Some patients (perhaps 25 percent) become amenorrheic and have lowered plasma LH months before any weight loss or *detectable* dieting (Vande Wiele, 1977). In some, resumption of menstruation and rise in LH will occur simply with weight gain even while preoccupation with dieting and a distorted body image continue.

NEUROTRANSMITTER STUDIES

The pathogenesis and pathophysiology of the major psychiatric disorders remain unknown. Yet suggestive evidence has implicated various neurotransmitters: the catecholamines and serotonin in affective disorders and dopamine in schizophrenia. Intensive research efforts are under way to test postulated neurochemical bases. Conceivably, such efforts will lead to laboratory procedures to aid in the diagnosis of psychiatric disorders in a manner analogous to the use of such tests in general medicine.

Affective Disorders

A durable, if not proven, biochemical hypothesis is that affective disorders result from a deficit (in the case of depression) or an excess (in mania) in certain amine neurotransmitters (Preskorn et al., 1991). This "catecholamine" (pertaining primarily to norepinephrine) or "monoamine" (including serotonin as well) hypothesis derived from certain clinical observations. Drugs such as reserpine, which are known to deplete the brain of these monoamines, produce, in some patients, a depressive syndrome. In addition, the first two classes of drugs known to alleviate depression, the monoamine oxidase inhibitors (MAOIs) and the TCAs, are known to increase monoamine availability to the postsynaptic receptor.

Some laboratory findings have supported the monoamine hypothesis. Low urinary levels of the norepinephrine metabolite 3-methoxy-4-hydroxyphenylglycol (MHPG) have been observed in some depressed patients. Another subgroup of depressed patients appears to have low cerebrospinal fluid (CSF) levels of the serotonin metabolite 5-hydroxyindoleacetic acid (5-HIAA). Low levels of these metabolites suggest a decrease in the synthesis or release of the respective neurotransmitter.

Based on these findings, it has been suggested that it may be possible to tailor pharmacologic intervention on the basis of whether a patient was norepinephrine-deficient or serotonin-deficient.

Presumably, drugs that are relatively selective for enhancing norepinephrine activity (e.g., desipramine and nortriptyline) versus serotonin (e.g., trazodone, chlorimipramine, fluoxetine, sertraline or paroxetine) could be differentially prescribed. Of interest, up to 65 percent of depressed patients who fail to respond to one class will respond to the other (Preskorn, 1991). Furthermore, low 5-HIAA levels in CSF predict differential responses to selective serotonin reuptake blockers. Such observations suggest the existence of biologically different subtypes of major depressive disorders.

A modification of the monoamine hypothesis is that rather than a deficit in the availability of specific monoamines, the pathophysiology of depression involves altered monoamine receptor function. For example, in depression, alpha$_2$- or beta-adrenergic supersensitivity has been postulated. This supersensitivity would result in attenuated CNS adrenergic function, since alpha$_2$-adrenergic stimulation inhibits release of norepinephrine from the presynaptic nerve terminal. It appears that antidepressant drugs, as well as nonpharmacologic treatments such as electroconvulsive therapy and rapid eye movement sleep deprivation, reduce these supersensitivities.

Supersensitivity in platelet alpha$_2$- and leukocyte beta-adrenergic receptors has been reported in depressed patients. The advantages of having such biologic markers for depression so readily available in the peripheral blood are obvious. However, these reports are preliminary.

Schizophrenia

The DA hypothesis proposes that DA hyperactivity in the mesolimbic or mesocortical region is involved in the pathogenesis of schizophrenia. This hypothesis has proved to be the most durable biologic hypothesis in psychiatry and perhaps the most heuristically stimulating, having led to a great body of research about the role of DA in the CNS.

As with the monoamine hypothesis of affective disorders, the DA hypothesis was generated from clinical observations. Amphetamine-induced psychoses were noted to resemble closely acute schizophrenic episodes. In addition, a characteristic common to all early antipsychotic drugs was potent DA-blocking effects.

The DA hypothesis has been useful. In addition to the stimulation of basic research, it suggested an effective method of screening drugs for potential antipsychotic effects. The ability of drugs to block DA agonist activity in animals (amphetamine-induced stereotypic behavior in rats and apomorphine-induced vomiting in cats) has resulted in the identification of a number of chemically unrelated classes of neuroleptics in addition to the original reserpine and phenothiazines.

Laboratory studies on schizophrenics have been less supportive of the DA hypothesis, at least as simplistically formulated (Henn, 1982). DA is known to be a potent inhibitor of prolactin release. Patients on neuroleptics show increased prolactin levels (evidence of DA blockade with such drugs), yet untreated schizophrenics do not differ from controls on this parameter.

Neurotransmitter and enzymatic studies have not consistently shown abnormalities in the DA system (Hughes et al., 1985). Homovanillic acid (HVA), the principal metabolite of CNS DA, has not been shown to be abnormal in the CSF of schizophrenic patients. Autopsy studies also have not shown evidence of increased brain DA activity, such as increased levels of DA and HVA, or defects in MAO activity. The search for something to measure peripherally led to the observation of reduced platelet MAO activity in schizophrenic patients.

Some investigations have shown increased density of the D$_2$ DA receptor in postmortem brains of schizophrenics compared with controls. However, the confounding effects of long-term neuroleptic exposure have not been adequately accounted for.

In summary, the DA hypothesis has been useful in predicting the psychotomimetic effects of DA agonists and amelioration of psychosis by DA antagonists. Yet laboratory measurements have not demonstrated definitive abnormalities in schizophrenic patients. Conceivably, DA may be related more closely to certain "positive symptoms," such as hallucinations and delusions than to a core defect in schizophrenia. This postulate is consistent with the clinical observation that dopamine-blocking neuroleptics are more effective in treating "positive symptoms" than "negative" or "deficit" symptoms, such as apathy, social withdrawal, and vague peculiarities in thought and action. If this hypothesis proves correct, it may lead to neurochemical procedures to validate this clinical distinction. Already, clozapine, which shows little direct effect on dopamine activity, shows promise in better alleviating negative symptoms than traditional dopamine-blocking neuroleptics (Martin, 1991).

BRAIN IMAGING TECHNIQUES

Technologic advances, including applications of computer science, allow visualization of the brain to an extent only dreamed of previously (Andreasen, 1988). In the past, psychiatrists were limited to information from skull x-rays, invasive techniques such as pneumoencephalography and angiography, radioisotope brain scans, and multilead but nonintegrated conventional electroencephalography (EEG) evoked potential (EP) studies. Now, computed tomography (CT) and magnetic resonance imaging (MRI) provide structural views only available previously at autopsy and then not on live tissues. Other techniques, including computerized electroencephalographic tomography (CET) and regional cerebral blood flow (rCBF) studies, especially utilizing single-photon-emission computed tomography (SPECT), and positron-emission tomography (PET), delineate regional physiologic activities in the living brain at rest and while performing various functions. At present, the major utility of such structural and physiologic imagery is the exclusion of general medical conditions. However, increasing attention has been turned to the study of changes with psychiatric conditions per se. The newly organized International Society for Neuroimaging in Psychiatry (ISNIP) has published *Neuroimaging* since 1990 as a forum for such advances.

Computed Tomography (CT)
CT of the head provides cross-sectional images of the brain at various axial (transverse) levels (Weinberger and Wyatt, 1983). With radiation exposure comparable with that of a skull x-ray series, CT images differentiate densities of CSF, blood, bone, and various brain tissues. Without contrast material, CT can demonstrate anatomic changes such as atrophy, midline shifts, certain tumors, and calcifications. Contrast (or "enhanced") studies involving the injection of radiopaque dies are useful in visualizing lesions such as recent stroke, infections and abscesses, and tumors in which the blood–brain barrier integrity is disrupted (Bosse et al., 1989). Use of contrast material involves risk of allergic reactions, so it should not be done routinely.

Apart from the evaluation of dementia and other cognitive impairment, the major psychiatric focus with CT has been on schizophrenia, where ventricular enlargement has been found with some consistency. It has been posited that such enlargement is associated with type II schizophrenia (characterized by negative symptoms, neurologic signs, poor premorbid adjustment, and poor response to neuroleptics).

Magnetic Resonance Imaging (MRI)
MRI is based on the detection of radio frequencies emitted by hydrogen nuclei (particularly of water) in an applied magnetic field (Garber et al., 1980). The varying water content of tissues allows differentiation, producing remarkable visualization of anatomic structures and pathologic changes. MRI is very good at visualizing subcortical and white matter lesions such as demyelinization and dead or necrotic tissue as in strokes. MRI allows sagittal (side) and frontal (coronal) views, in addition to the transverse plane, as obtained with CT. Certain areas, such as the posterior fossa, not well visualized with CT can be superbly examined with MRI.

Two imaging modes can be obtained in each study. T_1-*weighted images* visualize brain anatomy generally, while T_2-*weighted images* are particularly useful in demonstrating white matter lesions. MRI can be used in patients who will not tolerate the contrast material for enhanced CT studies. MRI cannot be done on patients with pacemakers or any embedded metallic objects or who are pregnant.

Procedures combining MRI with measurement of metabolic function or the localization of psychotropic drug activity are under development (Keshaven et al., 1991).

Positron-Emission Tomography (PET)
PET utilizes detection of positrons emitted by intravenously injected compounds labeled with radioactive nuclides such as ^{18}F, ^{15}O, and ^{11}C. When these radioactive atoms decay, a positron is emitted and detected regionally by the PET scanner. The localization of the emission identifies the distribution of the radioisotope (Bench et al., 1990; AAN Therapeutics and Technology Subcommittee, 1991). To date, most studies have used ^{18}F-fluro-2-deoxy-D-glucose (FDG), an analogue of glucose. This compound follows the distribution of glucose, is not metabolized, and accumulates in various locations at levels proportional to glucose metabolism at that point.

PET studies have suggested parietal–temporal hypometabolism in Alzheimer's disease (distinct from other dementias), frontal hypo- and basal ganglia hypermetabolism in schizophrenia, inferior frontal hypometabolism in depression, orbital cortex and caudate hypermetabolism in obsessive-compulsive disorder, and parahippocampal hyperactivity during lactate-induced panic attacks.

Other potential uses include studies of psychotropic drugs to localize sites of concentration and action. One factor that will probably hamper the widespread clinical usage of PET scanning is the high cost and the availability of a nearby cyclotron, since the radioisotopes utilized have an extremely short half-life (roughly 2 minutes for ^{15}O, 20 minutes for ^{11}C, and almost 2 hours for ^{18}F (Bench et al., 1990).

Single-Photon-Emission
Computed Tomography (SPECT)
Regional cerebral blood flow (rCBF) determination using inhaled ^{133}Xe has been available for many years (Andreasen, 1988). Such techniques gave quantitative estimates of regional blood flow. SPECT, a newer technique, in addition to ^{133}Xe, utilizes radioisotopes such as ^{123}I-iodoamphetamine, ^{99m}Tc hexamethylpropyllamine oxime (^{99m}TcHMPAO), and labeled dopamine and acetylcholine. Thus far, studies have produced findings in parallel with those of PET in terms of brain activity. One exception is an "uncoupling" in cerebral ischemia in which blood flow may be decreased, but oxygen extraction is increased (Trzepacz, 1992). A disadvantage of SPECT is in resolution. Even with maximal technical advances, inherent limitations to the technique will never allow the resolving power of PET. Advantages include the ability to use isotopes with longer half lives, which can be used remote from a cyclotron at substantial savings in cost.

Computerized Electroencephalographic
Topography (CET)

Also designated *brain electrical activity mapping*
(BEAM), a topographic look at brain activity can be
obtained with computerized analysis of electroencephalogram (EEG) and evoked potential (EP) data
(Bunney et al., 1983; Morihisa, 1985). Topographic
color maps showing sequential changes in brain
activity can be obtained. It appears that brain activity detected by CET parallels characterization of
activity by PET and SPECT. Thus far, evidence for
increased slow (delta) wave activity in frontal brain
areas has been reported in schizophrenic patients.
Currently, clinical utilization of CET for diagnostic
purposes is premature. However, efforts are underway to standardize techniques between products
and to obtain normative data so that comparisons
can be made.

In summary, while CT and MRI can visualize
structural changes and abnormalities, regional
brain activity can potentially be localized on the
basis of metabolic activity (PET), blood flow
(SPECT), and electrical activity (CET). Generally,
the three measures are correlated. What this means
to the pathophysiologic understanding of the various psychiatric disorders remains to be seen.

CONCLUSIONS

The use of the laboratory in psychiatry parallels, in
many ways, the state of knowledge in psychiatry.
The diagnosis of psychiatric disorders requires, first
of all, the identification of underlying general medical conditions or the direct effects of a substance
(also referred to as organic or physical factors). At
present, the principal use of the laboratory is to aid
in this process. Increasingly, laboratory investigations are used in monitoring therapy (as in TDM). In
the future, the laboratory will be useful in delineating psychiatric disorders per se and will lead to
better pathophysiologic and pathogenetic understanding of normal and abnormal brain processes.

REFERENCES

AAN Therapeutic and Technology Assessment Subcommittee: Assessment: Positron emission tomography. Neurology 41:
163–167, 1991.
Abplanalp J, Haskett R, Rose R: The premenstrual syndrome.
Psychiatr Clin North Am 3:327–347, 1980.
American Psychiatric Association: Diagnostic and Statistical Manual of Mental Disorders, 3d ed revised. Washington, American Psychiatric Association, 1987.
Andreasen NC: Evaluation of brain imaging techniques in mental
illness. Annu Rev Med 39:335–345, 1988.
APA Task Force on Laboratory Tests in Psychiatry: The dexamethasone suppression test: An overview of its current
status in psychiatry. Am J Psychiatry 144:1253–1262, 1987.
Asberg M, Cronholm B, Sjoqvist F, Tuck D: Relationship between
plasma level and therapeutic effect of nortriptyline. Br Med J
3:331–334, 1971.

Bench CJ, Dolan RJ, Friston KJ, Frackowiak RST: Position emission tomography in the study of brain metabolism in psychiatric and neuropsychiatric disorders. Br J Psychiatry 157
(suppl 9):82–95, 1990.
Bosse RB, Giese AA, Deutsch SI, Morihisa JM: Concise Guide to
Laboratory and Diagnostic Testing in Psychiatry. Washington, American Psychiatric Association, 1989.
Brown G, Seggie J: Neuroendocrine mechanisms and their implications for psychiatric research. Psychiatr Clin North Am
3:205–221, 1980.
Carroll B, Feinberg M, Greden J, et al: A specific laboratory test for
the diagnosis of melancholia. Arch Gen Psychiatry 38:
15–22, 1981.
Fieve R: Lithium therapy. In Kaplin H, Freedman A, Sadock B
(eds): Comprehensive Textbook of Psychiatry, 3d ed. Baltimore, Williams & Wilkins, 1980, pp 2348–2352.
Friedel R: An overview of neuroleptic plasma levels: Pharmacokinetics and assay methodology. J Clin Psychiatry Monogr
2:8–12, 1984.
Garber HJ, Weilburg JB, Buonanno FS, et al: Use of magnetic
resonance imaging in psychiatry. Am J Psychiatry 145:
164–171, 1988.
Garfinkel P, Garner D: Menstrual disorders and anorexia nervosa.
Psychiatr Ann 14:436–441, 1984.
Haskett R, Rose R: Neuroendocrine disorders and psychopathol-
ogy. Psychiatr Clin North Am 4:239–252, 1981.
Henn F: Dopamine: A role in psychosis or schizophrenia. In Henn
F, Nasrallah H (eds): Schizophrenia as a Brain Disease. New
York, Oxford University Press, 1982, pp 176–195.
Hughes C, Preskorn S, Adams R, Kent T: Neurobiological etiology
of schizophrenia and affective disorders. In Cavenar J (ed):
Psychiatry. Philadelphia, JB Lippincott, 1985, ch. 64, pp
1–16.
Jimerson D, Post R: Psychomotor stimulants and dopamine ago-
nists in depression. In Post R, Ballenger J (eds): Neurobiol-
ogy of Mood Disorders, Baltimore, William & Wilkins, 1984,
pp 619–628.
Keshavan MS, Kapur S, Pettegrew JW: Magnetic resonance spec-
troscopy in psychiatry: Potential, pitfalls, and promise. Am J
Psychiatry 148:976–984, 1991.
Martin RL: Outpatient management of schizophrenia. Am Fam
Physician 43:921–933, 1991.
Morihisa JM: Computerized topographic mapping of electrophysiologic data in psychiatry. Psychiatr Ann 15:250–253,
1985.
National Institutes of Health Consensus Development Panel: Differential diagnosis of dementing diseases. National Institutes
of Health Consensus Development Conference Statement
6:1–10, 1987.
Perry PJ, Pfohl BM, Holstad SG: The relationship between antidepressant response and tricyclic antidepressant plasma
concentrations. Clin Pharmacokinet 13:381–392, 1987.
Perry SW: Organic mental disorders caused by HIV: Update on
early diagnosis and treatment. Am J Psychiatry 147:
696–710, 1990.
Petty F, Noyes R: Depression secondary to cancer. Biol Psychiatry
16:1203–1220, 1981.
Plum F, Posner J: The Diagnosis of Stupor and Coma, 3d ed.
Philadelphia, FA Davis, 1980.
Preskorn SH: Should bupropion dosage be adjusted based upon
therapeutic drug monitoring? Psychopharmacol Bull 27:
637–643, 1991.
Preskorn SH: Dose-effect and concentration-effect relationships
with new antidepressants. In Graham LF, Balant LP, Meltzer
HY, et al. (eds): Clinical Pharmacology in Psychiatry.
Heidelberg, Springer-Verlag, pp. 174–189, 1993.
Preskorn SH, Beber JM, Faul JC, Hirschfeld RM: Serious adverse
effects of combining fluoxetine and tricyclic antidepressants.
Am J Psychiatry 147:532, 1990.
Preskorn SH, Dorey RC, Jerkovich GS: Therapeutic drug monitor-
ing of tricyclic antidepressants. Clin Chem 34:822–828,
1988.
Preskorn SH, Fast GA: Therapeutic drug monitoring for antidepres-
sants: Efficacy, safety, and cost-effectiveness. J Clin Psychia-
try 52:23–33, 1991.
Preskorn S, Irwin H: Toxicity of tricyclic antidepressants—Ki-

netics, mechanism, intervention: A review. J Clin Psychiatry 4:151–156, 1982.

Preskorn S, Mac D: The implication of concentration: Response studies of tricyclic antidepressants for psychiatric research and practice. Psychiatr Dev 3:201–222, 1984.

Richardson J, Richelson E: Antidepressants: A clinical update for medical practitioners. Mayo Clin Proc 59:330–337, 1984.

Simon RP: Neurosyphilis. Arch Neurol 42:606–613, 1985.

Surks MI, Chopra IJ, Mariash CN, et al: American Thyroid Association guidelines for use of laboratory tests in thyroid disorders. JAMA 11:1529–1532, 1990.

Targum SD: Neuroendocrine challenge studies in clinical psychiatry. Psychiatr Ann 13:385–395, 1983.

Targum SD, Sullivan AC, Byrnes SM: Neuroendocrine interrelationships in major depressive disorder. Am J Psychiatry 193:282–286, 1982.

Task Force on DSM-IV: DSM-IV Draft Criteria (3/1/93). Washington, American Psychiatric Association, 1993.

Trzepacz P, Herweck M, Starratt C, et al: The relationship of SPECT scans to behavioral dysfunction in neuropsychiatric patients. Psychosomatics 33:62–71, 1992.

Vande Wiele R: Anorexia nervosa and the hypothalamus. Hosp Pract 12:45–50, 1977.

Van Putten T: Guidelines to the use of plasma levels: A clinical perspective. J Clin Psychiatry Monogr 2:28–32, 1984.

Weinberger D, Wyatt R: Enlarged cerebral ventricles in schizophrenia. Psychiatr Ann 13:412–418, 1983.

Wells C, Duncan G: Neurology for Psychiatrists. Philadelphia, FA Davis, 1980.

Wilson W. Musella L, Short M: The electroencephalogram in dementia. In Wells C (ed): Dementia. Philadelphia, FA Davis, 1977.

CHAPTER 31

Epidemiology of Psychiatric Illness

THOMAS J. CRAIG

DEFINITION

Epidemiology (literally *epi* = "upon" and *demos* = "the people") is the study of the distribution and dynamics of health and illness in space and time in a given population and of the factors that influence this distribution. Thus epidemiology differs from clinical research primarily in its focus on defined populations as the denominator and clinical cases as the numerator from which it calculates rates of illness occurrence.

APPLICATIONS OF EPIDEMIOLOGY IN PSYCHIATRY

Epidemiologic methods have been applied in four general ways to the study of psychiatric illness:

1. *Descriptive epidemiology.* Clues to the etiology of psychiatric illness have been sought through the study of the incidence and prevalence rates of disease in the community and the association of variations in those rates with variations in community characteristics (e.g., age, sex, social class).
2. *Analytic epidemiology.* Once etiologic hypotheses have been identified, they can be tested using a variety of analytic strategies comparing the relative frequency with which persons with a given risk factor (e.g., a positive family history) or set of risk factors for a specific disorder develop that disorder as compared with persons without such a risk factor.
3. *Experimental epidemiology.* Once a suspected etiologic risk factor has been identified, experiments may be carried out in which the investigator artificially manipulates this risk factor while holding all other variables constant. Because of the current

state of knowledge regarding risk factors in psychiatry, the use of this experimental approach has, for the most part, been limited to clinical therapeutic trials. However, psychiatric epidemiologists have capitalized on naturally occurring quasi-experimental situations, such as disasters (e.g., the Three Mile Island accident; Bromet, Schulberg, Dunn, 1982) or the adoption of children (e.g., the Danish adoption studies of schizophrenia), to study the effects of a specific risk factor on the subsequent development of psychiatric illness or condition.
4. *Program planning and evaluation.* Descriptive epidemiologic methods have been widely used to estimate the need for mental health services in defined populations (Goodman and Craig, 1982) and determine the extent to which available services are meeting these needs. Studies such as these have been used to develop more effective and efficient approaches to the delivery of mental health services.

METHODOLOGIC ISSUES IN PSYCHIATRIC EPIDEMIOLOGY

A critical understanding of the findings of the epidemiologic studies of psychiatric illness requires an appreciation of the methodologic problems inherent in the epidemiologic method.

PRIMARY MEASUREMENTS

The primary measurements of epidemiology (incidence and prevalence) require a numerator (cases), a denominator (population at risk), and a time frame. (See below.)

Numerator Data

The accurate enumeration of cases requires a specific definition of a case and the detection of all cases in the study population. In terms of case ascertainment, most studies have used either treatment source information or community surveys to estimate the number of cases present in the population. Both sources have potential drawbacks, which are more serious for those studies using treatment source data only. For example, the use of mental health services is known to be influenced by a variety of demographic variables (including age, sex, race, and, especially, the distance one lives from the treatment facility) as well as characteristics of the facility itself (e.g., number of beds available, accessibility, reputation in the community, admission policies) and public policy (e.g., legislation discouraging the admission of the elderly). Although attempts have been made to establish more comprehensive sources of treatment data through the use of psychiatric case registers covering all mental health providers in a geographically defined area, the use of these data will seriously underestimate the numerator of incidence and prevalence rates in ways that are not uniformly distributed across different population subgroups.

$$\text{Incidence} = \frac{\text{number of new cases per unit time}}{\text{average population at risk during time period}}$$

$$\text{Prevalence (point)} = \frac{\text{number of existing cases at one point in time}}{\text{average population at risk at that point in time}}$$

$$\text{Prevalence (period)} = \frac{\text{number of existing cases during a period of time}}{\text{average population at risk during that time period}}$$

The other major source of numerator data—community survey data—has advantages and disadvantages that mirror those of treatment source data. Surveys are generally much more expensive and time-consuming to carry out. Therefore, most surveys cannot assess the total population to ascertain the total number of cases and must rely on a sampling of the population. In order to ensure that the findings of the survey are representative of the population surveyed, probability sampling techniques must be used in which the investigator can specify the probability that each person in the population will be included in the survey sample. Community surveys also require a method to determine the presence of a psychiatric disorder. Because diagnosis of every respondent by a clinician is prohibitively expensive, most recent surveys have relied on either questionnaires completed by respondents or

structured interviews by nonclinician interviewers. In either case, the survey instruments must meet tests of reliability and validity to ensure that those identified as cases would be diagnosed as such if a clinician examined them. The major advantage of the community survey is its ability to ascertain in a relatively unbiased way the proportion of persons in the study population with definable disorders.

Denominator Data

An estimate of the population at risk is usually obtained from census data. Thus the main problems with these data involve the extent to which the true population size might be underestimated by the census and the proximity in time between the collection of numerator and denominator data. As regards underestimation, for example, young minority men are known to be seriously undercounted in the U.S. census. Thus incidence and prevalence rates based on this denominator will generally tend to be overestimates of the true prevalence of disorder in these subgroups, since numerator data may be more accurately ascertained. These biases are more pronounced when treatment source data are used to estimate the number of cases, since surveys will ascertain both numerator and denominator information directly. However, with survey data, the response rate becomes crucial, since persons who refuse to participate in surveys or who cannot be located are likely to have a higher rate of psychiatric disorder than those who do participate. Thus surveys with response rates less than 70 percent are generally considered potentially biased toward underestimation of true prevalence.

Time Perspective

In general, for episodic conditions, prevalence = incidence × duration. For etiologic investigations, incidence rates are more useful than prevalence rates, since factors that affect the duration of the condition but that are unrelated to its cause will be associated with prevalence, whereas only factors causative of the illness will be associated with incidence. However, for rarely occurring disorders, in which the exact time of onset of the illness cannot be accurately ascertained (characteristic of many psychiatric disorders), incidence data may be either impossible or inordinately expensive to collect. To compensate partially for this situation, psychiatric epidemiologic studies have used the concept of lifetime prevalence (i.e., the probability of a respondent ever having experienced a specific condition up to the date of assessment). This risk will be influenced by the proportion of the population who have passed through the age of risk for the disorder as well as by possible biases owing to disorder-associated mortality or an unwillingness to report or failure to recall disorders that had occurred many years earlier (Robins et al., 1984).

Definition of a Case

The most crucial variable in any epidemiologic study, and the one that accounts for the greatest amount of variation in the findings of psychiatric epidemiology to date, is case definition.

Historically, psychiatric epidemiologic studies have used different concepts of case definition and, consequently, have obtained different rates of illness occurrence. In studies carried out in Europe and in the United States before World War II, mental illness was considered to be not a unitary concept, but one in which could be defined discrete, categorically distinct disorders with different etiologies and differing treatments. Cases were defined according to diagnostic criteria current at the time, and rates of illness were calculated separately for these disorders (Lin and Standley, 1962).

In contrast, after World War II, in the predominant psychiatric epidemiologic studies in the United States, mental disorder was seen as unitary and on a continuum, rather than as a set of diagnostically distinct conditions. In addition, health was defined as the absence of symptoms or functional impairment and was categorized according to intensity or severity of symptomatology or impairment, despite the fact that most of the population is not totally asymptomatic or totally functional at any point in time (Weissman and Klerman, 1978). Thus these studies reported high rates of mental impairment (e.g., the Midtown Manhattan study found only 19 percent of the population to be free of significant symptoms, while 23 percent were significantly impaired) (Srole et al., 1962). However, these studies substantially advanced survey methodology in the areas of sampling, instrument development, and statistical analysis but could not generate rates of specific psychiatric disorders.

As noted by Weissman and Klerman (1978), beginning in the 1960s, several events occurred that significantly influenced psychiatric epidemiology. Research strategies in genetic psychiatry—chiefly twin studies, family studies, and adoption and cross-fostering techniques, as well as the development of sophisticated methods of statistical analysis (described in an earlier chapter)—strengthened the evidence for the existence of discrete psychiatric disorders with different patterns of heritability. In addition, advances in the biologic treatment of psychiatric disorders, including the use of electroconvulsive therapies, as well as the development of psychopharmacologic agents with specific clinical effectiveness for specific disorders, supported the concept of specific psychiatric disorders as opposed to the unitary concept of mental illness.

Both these sets of developments highlighted the need for valid and reliable diagnostic criteria. The epidemiologic observation of markedly different treated prevalence rates for schizophrenia and affective disorders between the United States (where schizophrenia was about one-third more prevalent) and the United Kingdom (where the

prevalence of affective disorders was several times greater) led to a series of studies (Kramer, 1969; Zubin, 1969) that demonstrated that these differences were largely attributable to the different diagnostic practices of British and American psychiatrists rather than to differences in the actual prevalence of the two disorders. When structured interviewing techniques and specified diagnostic criteria were used, good reliability among clinicians and researchers could be obtained. In the United States, the first published, specified criteria for a subset of mental disorders were the Feighner criteria (Feighner et al., 1972). Subsequently, a set of Research Diagnostic Criteria (RDC) was developed (Spitzer et al., 1978). These developments provided impetus for a third revision of the *Diagnostic and Statistical Manual of Mental Disorders* (DSM-III) of the American Psychiatric Association, which became the official U.S. psychiatric nosology in 1980, the most recent revision of which (DSM-IIIR) was published in 1987.

The impact of these diagnostic developments on psychiatric epidemiology in the United States has been recent and far-reaching. As noted earlier, most U.S. epidemiologic studies from World War II to the mid-1970s defined illness in terms of symptom frequency or intensity or functional impairment. Dohrenwend et al. (1980) have described these measures as indicators of nonspecific psychological distress or demoralization (Frank, 1973). Although many, if not most, psychiatrically ill individuals will score highly (as "cases") on such instruments, many persons with no diagnosable mental illness will also score in the "case" range. In addition, these measures do not permit the identification of persons with diagnosable conditions (true positive) from those without diagnoses (false positive) or the division of the mentally ill into specific diagnostic categories. Thus these nonspecific measures do not permit the calculation of incidence and prevalence rates by specific diagnoses, a prerequisite for the development or testing of specific etiologic hypotheses.

The first study in the United States that applied these specified diagnostic criteria to a community sample was carried out by Weissman and colleagues (1978), using the RDC in a pilot study of 500 persons.

After the conclusion of this study, the Division of Biometry and Epidemiology of the National Institute of Mental Health initiated the development of a new instrument, the Diagnostic Interview Schedule (DIS), which could be conducted by lay interviewers, thus permitting its use in large-scale studies (Robins et al., 1984). The DIS was constructed to elicit diagnoses according to Feighner, RDC, and DSM-III criteria for a subset of adult DSM-III diagnoses selected on the basis of prevalence, clinical significance, and scientific validity based on treatment response, family studies, and follow-up studies (Myers et al., 1984). This instrument was then used in the largest series of community surveys to date—the Epidemiologic Catchment Area (ECA) Study—conducted in five locations (New Haven, Baltimore, St. Louis, Los Angeles, and North Carolina), each site including approximately 3000 community respondents.

DIAGNOSTIC INSTRUMENTS

Even given the availability of valid diagnostic criteria such as those provided by DSM-III, the instruments used to gather these data must meet tests of reliability and validity in their construction and administration. If constructed and administered properly, it would be expected that scores on the instrument would always reflect true differences in the characteristic being measured (e.g., a person reporting symptoms of schizophrenia should "truly" have a schizophrenic diagnosis). However, a number of other factors may cause spurious variations or lack of variations in scores. For example, differences in transient personal factors (e.g., fatigue, mental set), situational factors (e.g., another person present during the interview), administration of the interview (e.g., nonuniform methods of administration), lack of clarity of the instrument (e.g., ambiguous questions or language barrier), mechanical factors (e.g., checking wrong boxes), and factors in the analysis all may produce invalid data. In addition, the administration of the instrument may be subject to error introduced by some factor that systematically affects the characteristic being measured or the interview process (e.g., sex or race of interviewer and respondent). In order to minimize these spurious sources of variation, instruments must meet tests of validity and reliability.

Validity is the extent to which differences in scores reflect true differences in the characteristic that the test measures and the degree to which the instrument measures what is intended. Measures of validity include

- *Predictive validity:* The ability to predict a future event by knowledge of the test score (e.g., a diagnosis of depression should predict responsiveness to antidepressant treatment).
- *Concurrent validity:* The ability to predict the presence or absence of an event when compared with a known criterion (e.g., a diagnosis of depression should correlate with biologic measures indicative of depression).
- *Content validity:* A measure of the pertinence of the instrument to the characteristic tested and the extent to which all aspects of the characteristic are tested (e.g., a depression scale should contain symptoms characteristic of depression).
- *Construct validity:* The relation of the score to other related aspects of the condition (e.g., a depression scale should show higher scores in

depressed patients than in nondepressed individuals).

Reliability is the amount of variation in scores among individuals that is due to inconsistencies in measurement (Helzer et al., 1977). In epidemiologic surveys, reliability is generally tested in terms of:

- *Test-retest reliability:* The same test is administered at different times and the results are correlated. However, if the two tests are repeated too closely in time, there may be a spurious inflation of reliability owing to memory of the earlier test, while if clinical change occurs between administration, the reliability will be artificially lowered.
- *Interrater reliability:* The observation of the same interview by two or more raters, each of whom independently scores the results.

Sensitivity and Specificity

In evaluating the utility of an instrument designed to provide diagnostic information, results are compared with a standard criterion to determine the instrument's sensitivity (i.e., ability to detect true positives) and specificity (i.e., ability to detect true negatives) (Earls, 1980a). In the case of psychiatric diagnoses, since no "objective" diagnostic tests are available, the instrument results are usually compared with diagnoses made by experienced clinicians, as shown below.

Instrument		Clinician diagnosis	
		Positive	Negative
Diagnosis	Positive	TP	FP
	Negative	FN	TN

TP, true positive; TN, true negative; FP, false positive; FN, false negative.

From this analysis, the following dimensions can be generated:

$$\text{Sensitivity} = \frac{TP}{TP + FN} \quad \text{Specificity} = \frac{TN}{TN + FN}$$

$$\text{Positive predictive value} = \frac{TP}{TP + FP}$$

$$\text{Negative predictive value} = \frac{TN}{TN + FN}$$

$$\text{False-positive rate} = \frac{FP}{TN + FP}$$

$$\text{False-negative rate} = \frac{FN}{TP + FN}$$

For an instrument to be useful in epidemiologic investigations, it should demonstrate high sensitivity and at least moderately high specificity, since the more crucial characteristic is its ability to detect cases, especially in view of the relatively low prevalence of most specific psychiatric disorders. In this regard, the DIS is one of the first diagnostic instruments used in psychiatric epidemiology to have been exposed to rigorous tests of sensitivity and specificity before its field application. Most earlier studies have merely demonstrated evidence of satisfactory reliability with little attention to validity issues.

However, even in the presence of adequate levels of sensitivity and specificity, the population prevalence of a given condition will have a major influence on the utility of the instrument. For example, if a specific disorder has a 1 percent "true" prevalence and the interview instrument has a 1 percent "false" positive rate, then almost half the identified "cases" will be false positives (Baldessarini et al., 1983).

DESCRIPTIVE EPIDEMIOLOGY

Incidence Studies

Because of the relatively infrequent occurrence of specific psychiatric disorders, their tendency to recurrence, and the difficulty of attempting to date the onset of the illness accurately, large-scale epidemiologic surveys of the incidence of mental disorders are virtually nonexistent. A few incidence studies have been carried out in small, isolated communities, chiefly in Europe, but the ECA study, which has as one of its goals a follow-up of previously examined respondents, represents one of the first attempts at determining the incidence of specific disorders in a large, representative sample of a demographically diverse population.

Table 31-1 lists incidence rates calculated from the ECA initial and 1-year follow-up interviews for selected diagnoses (Eaton et al., 1989; Tien and Eaton, 1992). The numerators of these are all new cases of each diagnosis reported to have occurred in the year between interviews in persons who never had this diagnosis in the past. The denominators are the total survey population with no lifetime history of the diagnosis at the first interview who were interviewed for a second time at 1 year. Because of methodologic differences, data from only four sites were used for these analyses, New Haven data being excluded. In general, these incidence rates indicate a substantial generation of new cases in a 1-year period of a magnitude reaching almost half the 1-year prevalence for some diagnoses (e.g., phobia and cognitive impairment). Conversely, Eaton et al. (1989a) report that most 1-year prevalence rates declined between the two interviews, suggesting considerable diagnostic flux in the initiation and

TABLE 31-1. *Incidence (per 100 Person-Years) and Prevalence (% 1 year and lifetime) Rates of DIS/DSM-III Disorders Among Persons 18 Years and Older in Five ECA Sites*

Disorder	Incidence*	Prevalence†	
		1 year	Lifetime
Any disorders		20	32
Substance use disorder			
Alcohol abuse/ dependence	1.8	6.3	13.8
Drug abuse/ dependence	1.1	2.5	6.2
Schizophrenia/ schizophreniform	0.2	1.0	1.5
Affective disorders			
Mania	—	0.6	0.8
Major depression	1.6	3.7	6.4
Dysthymia‡	—	—	3.3
Anxiety disorders			
Phobia	4.0	8.8	14.3
Panic	0.6	0.9	1.6
Obsessive compulsive	0.7	1.7	2.6
Generalized anxiety	—	3.8	8.5
Somatization disorders	—	0.1	0.1
Antisocial personality disorder	—	1.2	2.6
Cognitive impairment‡ (severe)	1.2	—	0.9

*All incidence rate data from Eaton et al. (1989), except schizophrenia, which is from Tien and Eaton (1992)—standardized for age, gender, and race. Only four sites were studied; New Haven was not included.
†Prevalence rate data from Robins et al. (1991).
‡Dysthymia and cognitive impairment have no recent information; therefore, prevalence rates are the same.

remission of active disease. As they note, a complete picture of the population dynamics of these disorders would require not only reliable incidence and prevalence (1-year and lifetime) rates but mortality data as well. As Tien and Eaton (1992) note, the ECA-generated incidence rates for schizophrenia exceed rates previously reported from clinical sources and registries by 3- to 30-fold (0.08 to 0.70 per 1000 persons per year). They cite a number of possible explanations, including the fact that up to half the persons with active schizophrenia in the ECA study were found not to be receiving treatment and the relatively unreliable performance of the DIS-generated diagnoses of schizophrenia when compared with clinician examinations (Eaton et al., 1989b). For these reasons, the listed rates must be considered preliminary until confirmed elsewhere.

Even given the size of the ECA population, which is unprecedented in psychiatric epidemiology, the number of new cases in most diagnostic categories is relatively small on which to base the multivariate analyses needed to determine etiologic causal inferences. However, this study is a major step forward in this direction.

Prevalence Studies

ADULT MENTAL ILLNESS

As summarized by Plunkett and Gordon (1960) and Lin (1953), surveys of mental illness among the adult general population from the United States, Europe, and Asia, which were carried out before 1950 and used specific diagnostic criteria for case definition, cited prevalence rates of 0.7 to 6.9 percent for total mental disorders and rates of 0.2 to 1.4 percent for psychoses. In contrast, studies carried out after 1950 using diagnostic criteria yielded total mental illness prevalence rates of 10.9 to 13.8 percent, while those using nondiagnostic criteria of symptom frequency or intensity or functional impairment found total mental illness prevalence rates in excess of 20 percent.

Because of these factors, rather than cataloging the varying rates of disorder found in earlier studies of treated and untreated prevalence, this chapter describes the prevalence rates reported from the most recent study (the ECA study), which incorporates the superior design features noted earlier and promises to be the "gold standard" against which future estimates of prevalence will be compared. These rates have been reported (Robins and Regier, 1991) for the assessments conducted at the five study sites. The use of multiple sites for this study is especially advantageous in permitting the study of a broad range of demographic variables in relation to prevalence rates. It also permits replication of the findings using relatively standardized diagnostic criteria in large population samples—a major test of the reliability and robustness of the rates obtained.

ECA STUDY DESCRIPTION

Briefly, the ECA study reported on 15 DIS/DSM-III diagnoses without exclusion because of the presence of other diagnoses. At each study site, representative samples were drawn from official community mental health catchment areas with populations of 200,000 or more. All sites used lay interviewers, who received a 2-week training program. Adults 18 or older were surveyed at each site with similar completion rates (75 to 80 percent).

Despite these major methodologic advances, the prevalence rates reported must be recognized as most likely a minimum estimate of both total and specific psychiatric illness in the surveyed populations. First of all, only 15 of the large number of DSM-III diagnostic categories were studied. While these represent the great bulk of common disorders, the exclusion of other diagnostic categories ensures an underestimate of total prevalence of psychiatric illness. Second, because 20 to 25 percent of the samples were nonrespondents, who generally have higher rates of mental disorder, this may contribute to an underestimate of the "true" prevalence. Finally, because some of the disorders examined (especially mania and alcohol/substance abuse/dependence) are notoriously underreported when instruments such as the DIS are used, it is to be anticipated that the rates obtained for these disorders (in the absence of corroborating information from a third party) may represent underestimates.

Table 31-1 presents the 1-year and lifetime prevalence rates for the major DIS/DSM-III disorders reported for the ECA study (Robins et al., 1991). The 1-year prevalence is a period prevalence that indicates current (or recent) psychopathology, whereas lifetime prevalence indicates current and past history of a diagnosable disorder.

Approximately 20 percent of the samples of both sexes reported having a current diagnosable disorder, a rate similar to those reported in recent studies using diagnostic criteria. In addition, however, almost as many additional respondents reported having had a diagnosable condition in the past, resulting in a lifetime prevalence of approximately 32 percent.

Two studies using methodology derived from the ECA study, including translations of the DIS, have been reported from Puerto Rico (Canino et al., 1987) and Taiwan (Compton et al., 1991). Prevalence rates from these cross-cultural studies were remarkably similar to those for the original ECA populations. In the Puerto Rico study, prevalence of somatization disorder differed from that in the ECA study both in rate (0.7 versus 0.1 percent for 6 months and lifetime) and gender (equal prevalence in men and women in Puerto Rico versus marked female preponderance in the ECA). Interestingly, prevalence rates of the disorder in the Mexican-American subsample at the Los Angeles site were lower than those for the Anglo population (Burnham et al., 1987). In the Taiwan study, lifetime prevalence rates were generally lower than those in the ECA study both for overall prevalence (22 versus 36 percent) and for most specific disorders, none of which was higher in Taiwan. Finally, a comparison of ECA prevalence rates with those obtained using another structured interview, the Present State Exam (PSE) in Europe, Australia, and Africa (Regier et al., 1988) revealed similar prevalence rates for specific affective and anxiety disorders as those obtained in the ECA program. The exceptions to this observation were increased prevalence of both anxiety disorders and affective disorders among women in Athens and markedly increased rates of affective disorder (both major depression and manic disorder) for both sexes in Uganda. Thus the available data suggest that ECA data may represent relatively generalizable estimates of the prevalence of mental disorders, accepting the likelihood that culturally specific differences may exist for one or more specific disorders. The identification of such exceptions to the general pattern may point toward possible etiologic inferences. An example of this use of epidemiologic differences is given by Helzer et al. (1990), who compared DIS/

DSM-III alcohol abuse/dependence rates in two North American (U.S. and Canada) populations, Puerto Rico, and two Asian (Taiwan and Korea) populations.

Lifetime prevalence rates for abuse were similar for males in the United States, Canada, and rural Taiwan, whereas the Puerto Rican and urban Taiwan rates were lower and the Korean rates were markedly higher. In contrast, alcohol dependence among males showed similar prevalence across all populations except Taiwan, which had rates one-eighth of the other sites. Among women, the North American and Korean rates were similar for both abuse and dependence, while the Puerto Rican and Taiwan rates were substantially lower. Risk factors for alcoholism were generally similar across all sites, but the authors suggest that a different physiologic response to alcohol among Koreans as compared with Taiwanese (slower onset and less intense flush on exposure to alcohol) might explain the differences in observed prevalence rates.

INSTITUTIONAL PREVALENCE

One major strength of the ECA study over earlier surveys was the determination of prevalence rates of mental illness among the major institutionalized populations in the study catchment areas (prisons and residences, mental hospitals, and nursing homes). Overall, the lifetime and 1-year prevalence rates were two to three times those in the general population, with no difference across institutions (e.g., lifetime prevalence 65 versus 32 percent;

1-year prevalence 51 versus 20 percent). However, rates for specific disorders varied significantly by type of institution. Thus prison and community residence populations showed significantly higher prevalence rates than the general population for affective disorder, alcohol and drug abuse/dependence, panic and phobic disorders, obsessive-compulsive disorder, and antisocial personality disorder. Increased prevalence rates for affective disorder, somatization disorder, and cognitive impairment were found among nursing home residents, while mental hospital patients had increased rates for alcohol and drug abuse/dependence, obsessive-compulsive disorder, and panic and phobic disorders (Robins et al., 1991).

REMISSION

Table 31-2 indicates the proportion of persons with a lifetime diagnosis of a specific disorder who were in remission, as indicated by the absence of a current (1-year) diagnosis of that disorder (Robins et al., 1991). In general, over half of those with lifetime alcohol/drug disorder, generalized anxiety disorder, and antisocial personality disorder were currently in remission, with lower rates for the other diagnoses, especially somatization disorder. While these findings must be interpreted in light of possible methodologic effects (e.g., memory variation, overreporting certain symptoms, etc.), these data suggest a substantial ongoing morbidity due to these illnesses. For patients in remission, the average duration of illness prior to remission varied from

TABLE 31-2. *Percent Remission, Comorbidity, and Use of Mental Health Services for DIS/DSM-III Disorders Among Persons 18 Years and Older in Five ECA Sites* *

Disorder	Remission†	Comorbidity‡	Use of MH services§
Substance abuse			
Alcohol abuse/			
dependence	54	52	10
Drug abuse/			
dependence	59	75	10
Schizophrenia/			
schizophreniform	36	91	40
Affective disorder			
Mania	28	—	34
Major depression	42	75	36
Dysthymia	—	86	—
Anxiety disorder			
Phobia	38	84	12
Panic	42	91	47
Obsessive-compulsive	33	79	20
Somatization disorder	8	100	67
Antisocial personality			
disorder	53	93	4
Cognitive impairment			
(Severe)	—	38	5

*All rate data from Robins et al. (1991).
†Remission indicates percent with lifetime diagnosis who have had no symptoms in the past year.
‡Comorbidity indicates percent with at least one other lifetime diagnosis among those positive for the latest diagnosis.
§Use of mental health services for those reporting only one DIS/DSM-III disorder—outpatient use in last 6 months, inpatient in last year.

2.7 years for drug abuse/dependence to 19.7 years for antisocial personality disorder. Phobic disorder (15.4 years), alcohol abuse/dependence (8.7 years), panic disorder (7.1 years), and major depression and obsessive-compulsive disorder (both 6.4 years) also had relatively long durations prior to remission. Antisocial personality disorder revealed a pattern that closely corroborated clinical observation in having a long duration but high likelihood of remission with aging. Thus 40 percent of those under 30 years of age with this lifetime diagnosis are symptom-free for 1 year compared with virtually all respondents over age 45. Thus this disorder seems to remit in the 40-year age group.

COMORBIDITY

As indicated in Table 31-2, all categories except cognitive impairment had prevalence rates of at least one additional diagnosis of over 50 percent, with four categories (somatization, antisocial personality disorder, panic disorder, and schizophrenia/schizophreniform) having over 90 percent comorbidity (Robins et al., 1991). The strongest statistical associations included schizophrenia with mania and panic disorder; depression with mania, panic disorder, and somatoform disorder; mania with panic disorder, obsessive-compulsive disorder, and somatoform disorder; somatoform disorder with panic, phobic, and obsessive-compulsive disorders; and antisocial personality disorder with alcohol and drug abuse/dependence. Robins et al. (1991) suggest that since relatively few disorders share symptoms as diagnostic criteria or risk factors, the most likely reason for this co-occurrence is that having one disorder increases the risk of developing a second disorder, which may imply a causal relationship. Further investigation of age of onset of each disorder is needed to determine the direction of causation.

USE OF MENTAL HEALTH SERVICES

As indicated in Table 31-2, relatively few persons suffering from most specific current diagnoses have used mental health services (Robins et al., 1991). While the percentage in Table 31-2 correspond only to persons with a single diagnosis and the majority of persons with most diagnoses have comorbidity, it is unlikely that the latter persons would be markedly different in their utilization of services, since the overall rate of utilization of mental health services for all disorders is 13 percent for those with a single diagnosis and 19 percent for all respondents with one or more diagnoses. These findings confirm the calculations of Regier et al. (1978) that only about one-fifth of all persons in the community with an active disorder receive specific mental health services. Of particular note is the fact that the majority of even those respondents with major disorders such as mania and schizophrenia fail to receive treatment, reinforcing the notion that treated prevalence rates seriously underestimate the magnitude of the prevalence of mental illness in nonrandom ways. For example, only 40 percent of all persons meeting a lifetime diagnosis of schizophrenia were ever hospitalized, and only 57 percent with a current schizophrenic illness (including those with comorbidity) had received mental health treatment. Clearly, these data indicate a vast untreated population which may in part explain the long average duration and low lifetime remission rates noted earlier.

DISORDERS OF CHILDHOOD AND ADOLESCENCE

Studies of the incidence and prevalence of psychiatric illness among children and adolescents have been rare and have suffered to a great extent from problems similar to those described earlier. In the 1980s, several community surveys using DSM-III criteria and methodology similar to the ECA study were undertaken. While no incidence rates have as yet been reported, overall current prevalence rates have been remarkably similar to the ECA findings. Kashani et al. (1987) reported an overall prevalence of 18.7 percent for 150 adolescents aged 14 to 16 years of age of DSM-III diagnoses, of whom 75 percent had more than one disorder. The most common disorders were drug and alcohol dependence (rates 11.3 and 9.3 percent, respectively), followed by anxiety disorder and conduct disorder (each 8.7 percent) and depression (major depression and dysthymia combined rate 8.0 percent). Less frequent diagnoses were attention deficit disorder (2.0 percent) and somatization disorder (1.3 percent) and mania (0.7 percent). While, as with ECA data, both anxiety disorder and affective disorder were three times more prevalent among girls, there were no significant gender differences for alcohol/drug abuse/dependence, suggesting a major change in female rates for these disorders.

Offord et al. (1987), using DSM-III criteria for four disorders among 4- to 16-year-olds in Ontario, found an 18.7 percent overall prevalence of disorders (19.2 percent for boys, 16.9 percent for girls). Boys showed a two- to threefold increase in prevalence of conduct disorder (8.1 versus 3.3 percent), while girls had higher rates of "emotional disorders" (overanxious, affective, and obsessive-compulsive disorder combined rates of 11.9 versus 7.9 percent) and somatization disorder (10.7 versus 4.5 percent).

In another study of 4- to 16-year-old children in Puerto Rico, Bird et al. (1988), using DSM-III criteria and a structured interview (the DISC), found an overall prevalence of 17.9 percent, with specific prevalences of oppositional disorder (9.9 percent), attention deficit disorder (9.5 percent), depression/dysthymia (5.9 percent), separation anxiety and enuresis (4.7 percent each), adjustment disorder (4.2 percent), and simple phobia (2.7 percent). The only significant gender differences were for oppositional and attention deficit disorders, both more prevalent in boys. Similar findings were reported by Anderson et al. (1987) in a DSM-III study of 11-year-old children that found a 17.6 percent overall rate and 55 percent comorbidity. Again, attention deficit disorder (6.7 percent) and oppositional disorder (5.7 percent) were most frequent diagnoses and more likely in boys, as was conduct disorder (3.4 percent), whereas separation anxiety (3.5 percent), simple phobia (2.4 percent), and social phobia (0.9 percent) were more common in girls. Unusual was the finding that depression/dysthymia (1.8 percent) was more common in boys.

Finally, Whitaker et al. (1990) found rates of major depression (4.0 percent), dysthymia (4.9 percent), and obsessive-compulsive disorder (1.9 percent) similar in an adolescent population to ECA data but a lower rate of panic disorder (0.6 percent). Only 41 percent of this population had received mental health services.

In searching for risk factors predisposing to mental illness in children and adolescents, Offord et al. (1986) reported a significantly increased risk for indices of low social class (welfare, subsidized housing, low income, unemployment, overcrowding, and low maternal education) plus being raised by a single parent. Kashani et al. (1987) cited high-risk variables for adolescent psychopathology including history of physical abuse, behavior disorder, sexual activity, use of aggression, lower self-concept, and less caring parents. However, many of these factors could be the result rather than the cause of the disorders. Hammen et al. (1987) reported that maternal affective disorder, illness, and stress increased the risk for childhood psychopathology, similar to conclusions drawn by Cantwell and Baker (1984). Parental death was observed to precede the development of major depressive symptoms in 37 percent of bereaved children (Weller et al., 1991), while Maziade et al. (1985) reported that a "difficult" temperament at age 7 predicted a DSM-III diagnosis in 50 percent of these children at age 12 as compared with only 7 percent of "easy" children meeting DSM-III criteria. Finally, Garmezy (1983) reported some characteristics that seem to be protective against childhood psychopathology, including the child's disposition (flexible, positive mood and self-esteem, interpersonal skills), family cohesion and warmth, support from one or more individuals in the environment and school (role models), and female gender. Clearly, more longitudinal studies are needed to identify the course of mental disorders from childhood to adulthood and the extent to which there is continuity of disability. However, the data cited above are particularly disquieting in their demonstration that children and adolescents have already attained a prevalence rate for significant DSM-III disorders equal to that in the adult population before having even reached the age of risk for adult disorders. These findings plus the ECA findings of birth-cohort effect (described below) for several adult disorders suggest that the prevalence rates of future cohorts in the population may well exceed those found in the ECA data.

ANALYTIC EPIDEMIOLOGY

Descriptive epidemiologic studies, such as the ECA study, through their ability to generate prevalence rates of disorders in population subgroups, provide data for the generation of hypotheses related to the etiology of these disorders. Analytic studies can then be carried out to test these hypotheses, using both the data of the descriptive studies as well as data derived from subsequent studies designed specifically to examine these questions.

Analytic Strategies

In psychiatric epidemiology, two analytic strategies have been generally used: retrospective (or case-control) and prospective (or longitudinal). The basic concept of these strategies can be illustrated from the following table:

| | Retrospective | | |
Prospective	With disorder	Without disorder	Total
With risk factor	a	b	$a + b$
Without risk factor	c	d	$c + d$
Total	$a + c$	$b + d$	N

Retrospective studies use as their index the presence or absence of illness and attempt to determine whether a suspected risk factor is more common among those with the disorder than among those without the disorder. Thus, if the rate $a/a + c$ is significantly greater than $b/b + d$, a statistical association is said to exist between the disorder and the risk factor.

Basic assumptions underlying this strategy are (1) the risk factor predated the onset of disease, (2) the controls (without disease) will not subsequently develop the disease, (3) cases (with the disease) are representative of all persons with the disease, and (4) controls (without the disease) give an unbiased estimate of the prevalence of the risk factor among the entire nondiseased population. Unfortunately, these assumptions are rarely fulfilled completely, the major problem being the difficulty in determining the temporal sequence of risk factor and disease. The advantages of this approach are its inexpensiveness and the ability to carry out such studies quickly with smaller samples. With rarely occurring disorders, the retrospective approach may be the only feasible strategy. Because most discrete psychiatric disorders are relatively uncommon, most analytic studies in psychiatric epidemiology have been retrospective.

Prospective studies select a population sample before the onset of disease and follow them over time after the presence or absence of the presumed risk factor has been established. The subsequent development of disease is then ascertained either by periodic reexamination or by checking records. The analysis then compares incidence rates of the disease among those with and without the risk factor. If $a/a + b$ is significantly greater than $c/c + d$, a statistically significant association between the risk factor and the disease is said to exist.

The basic assumptions of this strategy are (1) that the initial sample does not include diseased individuals and (2) that follow-up is complete or nearly so. This strategy permits a direct estimate of the risk of disease given the presence of the risk factor and eliminates the problem of retrospective studies regarding the temporal relationship of risk factor and disease and subjective bias owing to selective memory. However, it is a much more expensive and time-consuming strategy that is inefficient for studying uncommon diseases. (For example, given a lifetime prevalence for schizophrenia of 1 to 2 percent, a prospective study of 10,000 persons would be expected to yield only 100 to 200 cases.) Also, even modest levels of attrition may seriously bias the results, since persons lost to follow-up tend to have disproportionately high rates of mental illness. In addition, the follow-up procedures themselves may influence the rate of disease development.

Multifactorial Causation

Whichever analytic strategy is used, it is generally accepted that most psychiatric disorders are the result of an interaction of a variety of risk factors, including genetic, biologic, and psychosocial variables. Thus the straightforward analysis of the statistical association between a risk factor and a disorder becomes a complex procedure in which sophisticated statistical techniques are required both to control for potentially confounding variables and to identify potentially significant interactions between variables and classes of variables.

Because of this multifactorial causation, the logic of testing hypotheses regarding causal relationships becomes more complex in psychiatric epidemiology when compared with the epidemiology of infectious diseases (Bebbington, 1980). In the latter category, there is usually a *necessary condition* (one that must occur if the disease is to occur, e.g., an infectious agent) and often a *sufficient condition* (one that is always followed by the disease). With the exception of substance abuse, in which the presence of the drug or alcohol is a necessary condition, psychiatric disorders in general have not been shown to have either necessary or sufficient conditions resulting in disease onset. Rather, there appear to be a variety of *contributing conditions* that increase the likelihood of the disease occurrence but do not guarantee it. Thus the task of analytic epidemiology is to determine which sets of contributory conditions become necessary and sufficient conditions for the occurrence of specific diseases.

Evidence relevant to this causal inference include the following:

1. *Concomitant variation:* the assumed causal factor (independent variable) should be associated with the disease (dependent variable) in a way consistent with the hypothesis.
2. *Time sequence:* the cause should precede the effect.
3. Evidence ruling out other possible factors should be present.
4. The statistical association between cause and disorder should be assessed for
   a. Strength of association (usually by significance testing).
   b. Specificity of association (the extent to which the occurrence of the cause can be used to predict the occurrence of the effect; e.g., some "causes," such as life stress, may nonspecifically increase the risk for several psychiatric disorders in genetically susceptible individuals).
   c. Dose–response relationship (the risk of developing the disease is related to the degree of exposure to the presumed cause).
   d. Consistency of the association.
5. Scientific plausibility of the relationship between presumed cause and effect.

ETIOLOGY OF PSYCHIATRIC DISORDERS

The remainder of this chapter discusses epidemiologic findings relevant to the etiology of psychiatric disorders. The most successful investigations into the etiology of mental disorder are those in the area of genetics and the heritability of specific disorders, which are discussed in Chapter 30. This chapter discusses epidemiologic findings in the demographic and psychosocial areas.

Psychosocial Factors

Stress is defined as that state of an organism in which energy is used in continuously dealing with problems over and above the energy required if the problems had been resolved. In recent years, a body of sociologic literature has suggested a variety of models through which stressful events might cause physical or mental illness (Dohrenwend and Dohrenwend, 1981). Most of these models postulate that the occurrence of a stressful event interacts with the individual's personal predisposition, coping abilities, and social support such that the individual either masters the stress, seeks help through which the problem is resolved, or develops physical or mental symptoms.

The types of stressful circumstances that may lead to stress in the individual include

- *Background stressors* inherent in the individual's social position, role, etc.
- *Strain of chronic stressors*, which are enduring problems related to frustrations of daily living, including role conflict, goal/means discrepancies, and perceived inequities or excessive demands.
- *Changes in the pace of daily living* owing to the occurrence of life events.
- *Traumatic life events*, which are usually single-episode events with overwhelming and long-lasting effects (e.g., posttraumatic stress disorder).

The assessment of the association of stressful events with psychiatric illness has been hampered by differences across studies in the types of events measured and their quantification. In addition, Brown (1973) has described several potential sources of error in the reporting of events owing to *direct contamination* (i.e., the subject with a psychiatric disorder retrospectively reports more events than a control subject out of an attempt to explain the illness); *indirect contamination*, in which a subject's condition (e.g., the presence of anxiety) may prospectively increase both the tendency to report a life event and the subsequent development of the illness; and *spuriousness*, in which accurate report of life events has been made, but the association with the psychiatric disorder is due to a third factor causing both the life event and the illness. An additional methodologic issue has been the need to separate life events that may be either prodromal to the illness or the result of the illness (e.g., job loss) from those which are independent of and antecedent to the illness. Also, as noted by Hirschfeld and Cross (1983), specific causality for a psychiatric disorder must be demonstrated. Finally, Kessler (1979) has presented data suggesting that the impact of the event on the individual rather than the mere fact of the occurrence of a life event may be more crucial to the development of emotional distress. Also, reliability of reporting life events may vary by diagnosis (Neugebauer, 1983) and whether patient self-reports are corroborated by relatives and friends (Yager et al., 1981; Schless and Mendels, 1978).

Two studies (Jacobs and Myers, 1976; Brown and Birley, 1968) have shown that the number of life events reported by schizophrenics before the onset of a psychotic episode was significantly greater than the number reported by controls during a comparable period, but most of these events could be related to patients' mental status. However, Brown and Birley also found that events independent of the patient's psychiatric condition occurred more frequently during the 3 weeks before the onset of psychosis, leading Brown to suggest that life stress may trigger schizophrenic episodes but not be causative of schizophrenia per se.

As regards depressive illness, several studies have suggested that "markedly threatening" life events (Brown et al., 1973), "exit" events (Jacobs et al., 1974), and "undesirable" events (Paykel et al., 1969) occurred more frequently to persons who subsequently suffered depression than to normal controls or schizophrenic patients. The association between severe life events and depression has been replicated in geriatric patients (Murphy, 1982). The presence of medical or psychiatric illness also has been associated with increased risk for depression. Brown (1978) has interpreted these data as indicating that life events are causative of subsequent depression, and Paykel (1978) has estimated that 9 to 10 percent of all exits are followed by depression. However, the presence of these events accounted for a relatively small amount of the variance (1 to 9 percent) in the onset of depression, suggesting that stress, while contributing as a cause in some depressive disorders, is a relatively weak predictor of depression. A recent report (Kennedy et al., 1983) also has suggested a role for life events in the precipitation of mania, while Finlay-Jones and Brown (1981) have suggested that loss events may be causal for depressive disorders, severe danger may be causal for anxiety states, and both types of events may result in mixed anxiety/depressive disorders. However, most of these findings have been based on retrospectively collected data, whereas a review of prospective studies of life events and psychological morbidity concluded that these findings do not seem to show that life events have a substantial causal role in "neurotic illness" (Tennant, 1983).

Several studies have found an association between life events and anxiety disorders. Faravelli and Pallanti (1989) found more life events in the year before the onset of panic disorder, especially uncontrolled and loss events in the months before onset, suggesting a precipitating role. Likewise, Roy-Byrne et al. (1986) found more life events with adverse impact but not more total events preceding the onset of panic disorder, concluding that the effect of the events rather than mere occurrence is most important. Similarly, Rapee et al. (1990) found anxious subjects (panic, agoraphobia, and other anxiety disorders) to rate life events as having a greater negative impact than nonanxious controls. They, too, postulated a triggering role for life events in a predisposed individual. Finally, Blazer et al. (1987), using data from the Durham ECA site, found patients with generalized anxiety disorder to be associated with life events according to demographic subgroups and type of life event. Males (but not females) with four or more life events had an increased risk of 8.5 times for generalized anxiety disorder over those with three or fewer events, while both males and females with one or more unexpected, negative, very important life event had a threefold increased risk for generalized anxiety disorder.

A specific life event reported to be associated with the onset of psychiatric disorder is childbirth. Several studies using case registers (Nott, 1982) have shown a marked increase in rates of psychoses (primarily affective) during the postpartum period as compared with rates during pregnancy, with little or no difference in rates of other diagnostic categories.

TRAUMATIC LIFE EVENTS

Trauma in childhood has been linked to an increased risk for adult mental illness in a number of retrospective case-control studies. Parental loss through death or separation has been associated with depression (Lloyd, 1980; Nelson, 1982; Roy, 1981; Pfohl et al., 1983), agoraphobia with panic attacks (Faravelli, 1985), and generalized anxiety disorder (Torgerson, 1986). However, other studies have questioned this association (Ragan and McGlashan, 1986). Breier et al. (1988) suggested that it is not the loss itself but the quality of childhood adjustment to the loss that determines the ultimate impact on adult pathology. They found an increased risk for subsequent illness under circumstances where there was a nonsupportive relationship with the surviving parent. Incest and physical or sexual abuse in childhood also have been found associated with adult disorders such as borderline personality disorder (Ogata et al., 1990; Herman et al., 1989), somatization disorder (Morrison, 1989), anxiety disorders (panic disorder, agoraphobia, and social phobia), major depression, and alcohol abuse/dependence (Pribas and Dinwiddie, 1992). Due to the limitations of retrospective studies noted earlier, especially with regard to the reliability and validity of long-term memory of childhood trauma, prospective studies are needed to clarify the specificity and magnitude of these factors' contribution to the prevalence of these disorders. Of interest is the fact that several of these disorders have shown a birth-cohort effect of increasing lifetime prevalence at younger ages. If childhood trauma is a significant etiologic factor in their genesis, this observation may indicate an increased prevalence of such trauma, suggesting the need for vigorous preventive intervention to reduce both the prevalence of the trauma and its impact on its victims.

Severe external trauma in adulthood has been associated with the development of psychopathology in general and has been required etiologically for the development of an anxiety disorder first identified nosologically in DSM-III—namely, posttraumatic stress disorder (PTSD). Environmental disasters such as the Three Mile Island (TMI) nuclear accident (Bromet et al., 1982) and the Mount St. Helens volcanic eruption (Shore et al., 1986) have been followed by an increased prevalence of both affective (e.g., major depression) and anxiety (e.g., generalized anxiety) disorders among exposed individuals. In the case of TMI, mothers of young children showed a twofold increase in the rate of both conditions in the year after the accident. Vulnerability factors increasing this risk included living closer to the plant, a prior history of psychiatric problems, and less adequate social support from friends, relatives, and/or spouse. At Mount St. Helens, people with high exposure experienced rates of depression, generalized anxiety disorder, and PTSD over three times those of people with low exposure and more than ten times those of controls over the year after the eruption.

Sexual assault also has been found to be a risk factor for a two- to threefold increase in prevalence of major depression, alcohol and drug abuse/dependence, PTSD, and obsessive-compulsive disorder (Winfield et al., 1990).

In the 1970s, the specific syndrome of PTSD was identified as a sequel to a variety of overwhelming traumatic experiences. Diagnostic criteria for this disorder include a triad of symptoms: intrusive reexperiencing of the traumatic event (e.g., nightmares), numbing avoidance of interpersonal contact, and physiologic arousal and hypervigilence. PTSD has been reported in diverse populations such as Vietnam veterans exposed to combat stressors and/or atrocities (Breslau and Davis, 1987; Green et al., 1990), Israeli soldiers (Solomon et al., 1987), victims of sexual assault (Winfield et al., 1990), Southeast Asian refugees (Kroll et al., 1989; Kinzie et al., 1990), and children exposed to a school shooting (Schwartz and Kowalski, 1990). Helzer et al. (1987) reported an ECA prevalence from the St. Louis site for PTSD of 1 percent for the general population, 3.5 percent for civilians exposed to physical attacks, and 20 percent among veterans wounded in Vietnam. Prevalence rates of PTSD among Vietnam veterans not seeking treatment of 15 to 17 percent have been reported in other studies as well (Green et al., 1990; Kulka et al., 1988). Comorbidity with other psychiatric disorders was present for 80 percent of those with PTSD in the Helzer et al. (1987) study, especially obsessive-compulsive disorder and dysthymic and major affective disorders. Risk factors for PTSD included behavior problems before age 15 (which predicted both adult exposure to physical attack and to combat in Vietnam as well as the development of PTSD) (Helzer et al., 1987). However, the war stressors were found to be specifically linked to the development of PTSD symptoms (Breslau and Davis, 1987; Green et al., 1990).

Personal resources, including both the individual's coping skills and personal behavior as well as family ties, social networks, and support systems, have been hypothesized as providing buffering in time of stress. However, studies of these variables have suffered from difficulties in quantifying these measures and have primarily suggested that deficiency of some of these resources may be related to nonspecific psychological distress. A major obstacle to this research has been the problem of whether a deficiency in personal resources is the cause or the result of psychiatric impairment. Two recent studies have suggested protective effects of the presence of personal resources and social support. Green et al. (1990) found that Vietnam veterans who reported both having support from family/friends at their homecoming and having current social support had a decreased risk for PTSD. In addition, Tienari et al. (1989) reported that among adopted-away offspring of schizophrenic mothers, no seriously disturbed offspring was found to have been reared in a healthy or mildly disturbed adoptive family, suggesting that the support of such a family environment may protect against the expression of a biologic predisposition to schizophrenia. This finding supports Fish's (1987) clinical impression that the major protective factor for some subjects at high risk for schizophrenia through genetic liability was the consistent support and stimulation provided by one parent capable of responding to their changing needs. However, Erlenmeyer-Kimling and Cornblatt (1987) reported that a healthy nonpatient parent in their high-risk group did not relate to the study children's current functional status. In addition, in this latter study, the absence of a personal resource, namely, a lower IQ, was found to be a potentiator of early emergence of psychiatric illness.

However the mechanisms by which social support may exert its protective effect are as yet unclear, as indicated by Parry and Shapiro (1986), who reviewed the extensive literature for and against the prevalent concept that support serves to buffer against the adverse effect of stress. Likewise, Starker (1986) has cited a number of concerns regarding current knowledge in this area, including problems with clear definitions of support, the reliability of the assessment instrument, failure to consider negative and conflictual aspects of support, and individual differences in needs and environmental factors.

Demographic Factors

SEX

While the overall ECA lifetime prevalence rates for all disorders was higher for males (36 percent) than for females (30 percent), 1-year rates were virtually identical across the sexes (Robins and Regier, 1991). These findings suggest that the excess rates reported for females in earlier surveys were probably due to the mix of disorders included, which generally excluded diagnoses with male excess (e.g., alcohol and drug abuse/dependence and antisocial personality disorder). While there were no differences in overall rates for schizophrenia by sex, females tend to have a later onset and briefer course, which probably explains the treatment source finding of an excess of male schizophrenics. Other diagnoses with relatively equal sex ratios are bipolar disorder, cognitive impairment, and obsessive-compulsive disorder (after controlling for other demographic variables). Females had rates exceeding males for major depression (three times), dysthymia (two times), generalized anxiety disorder (two times), and somatization disorder (ten times). Of those disorders with male excess noted above, the widest sex ratio was for antisocial personality disorder, which was five times more prevalent in males. However, rates in these categories tended to be closer in males and females in the younger age groups.

As Weissman and Klerman (1977) have pointed out for depressive disorders, a variety of genetic, biologic, and psychosocial hypotheses have been proposed to explain these differences, but as yet no definitive conclusions have been forthcoming. However, since the ECA findings are based on a community survey, many of the explanations based on differential treatment utilization (e.g., women are more likely to seek psychiatric care, while men tend to enter correctional facilities) are clearly not operative.

AGE

One-year prevalence data from the ECA study (Robins et al., 1991) show an overall prevalence of mental disorder to be about twice as high for adults less than 45 years of age when compared with those 45 years and older. By specific disorder, affective disorders, substance abuse/dependency, and antisocial personality disorders are disorders of the young, while panic, obsessive-compulsive, and phobic disorders are more evenly distributed across all ages, and cognitive impairment shows a linear increase with age, reaching rates of 12 to 18 percent for mild impairment and 4 to 6 percent for severe impairment in the age group 65 and older.

Age of onset among patients with affective disorders is somewhat earlier for bipolar disorders (mean age in late 20s) compared with nonbipolar disorders (mean mid to late 30s) (Hirschfeld and Cross, 1983). Among schizophrenics, Loranger (1984) commented on a significant sex difference in age of onset, with males having an average age at onset about 5 years earlier than females and paranoid patients showing a significantly later age of onset for both sexes than patients with other subtypes of schizophrenia. Again, as with the sex differences, these age variations have been explained as being due to differential patterns of treatment utilization, to different exposure to and impact of stressful circumstances, and to biologic (e.g., hormonal) differences. However, no definitive explanation has yet been established.

Comparisons of age at onset for several ECA diagnostic categories revealed evidence suggesting a shift toward increased rates for major depression and drug abuse/dependence between the ages of 15 and 19 years (Burke et al., 1991). Similar but less pronounced shifts were seen for alcohol abuse/dependence and obsessive-compulsive disorder but not for bipolar disorder, panic disorder, or phobias. Prospective studies are now needed both to replicate these findings and to explore the possible genetic and/or environmental factors responsible for these changes.

ETHNICITY

In general, studies of symptomatology and prevalence of specific psychiatric disorders within a culture have shown little, if any, evidence of major ethnic differences when similar assessment techniques have been applied and social class is controlled (Simon et al., 1973). For example, ECA data (Robins and Regier, 1991) show an increased prevalence of total mental disorders among blacks (38 percent lifetime, 26 percent 1 year) which was most prominent in the population over 45 years of age. However, when controlled for age, gender, marital status, and socioeconomic status, there were virtually no significant differences in ethnicity by specific diagnostic categories.

In a critique of epidemiologic study methodology (including that of the ECA program), Williams (1986) asserted that past surveys have consistently undersampled both middle-class Afro-Americans and poor, unemployed young urban Afro-American males, leading to misleading prevalence rates and a biased representation of mental illness in Afro-Americans.

Eaton (1983) cites evidence that Irish, Croats, Russians, and native-born Israelis have higher risks for schizophrenia (2:1), while Ashkenazic Jews have higher risks for affective disorders and American blacks have higher risks for antisocial personality disorders. Also, studies of isolated populations (e.g., Hutterites and Amish) have suggested extremely low prevalence of schizophrenia (Egeland and Hostetter, 1983) as compared with affective disorders. However, high or low prevalence rates in highly inbred populations may represent a predominantly genetic influence rather than the effect of cultural characteristics.

SOCIAL CLASS

Social class has been defined using indices of occupation, education, and income that are often not well correlated, thus contributing to problems of interpretation. In addition, current social class may be the result of the presence of a psychiatric illness and its effect on social and occupational function, making causal inferences invalid.

Studies of treated prevalence (Faris and Dunham, 1939; Hollingshead and Redlich, 1958) have consistently found an inverse correlation between indices of social class and the overall risk for mental disorder. However, in part, this finding has been a function of the less adequate treatment accorded lower-class patients with resultant prolonged duration of illness. Community surveys also have shown an increased prevalence of psychiatric symptomatology (Craig and Van Natta, 1979) and overall mental disorder (Leaf et al., 1984) in the lower social classes.

In view of these findings, two major theories have evolved to explain the predominance of pathology in the lowest social class: social causation (i.e., stresses, etc. inherent in being a member of the lower social class cause these disorders) versus social selection or drift (individuals with mental disorders tend to move into lower-class areas as a result of social and vocational impairment).

Perhaps the most thoroughly studied psychiatric disorder with regard to social class influence is schizophrenia, in which the vast majority of studies have shown a relative risk of 3:1 to 10:1 between lowest and highest social class (Dohrenwend and Dohrenwend, 1969). In this condition, evidence from several sources suggests that the major factor is most likely social selection/drift (Wiersma et al., 1983, Wender et al., 1973). Treated incidence studies have shown the lower-class predominance of schizophrenia to be largely a phenomenon of large cities (Kohn, 1972; Goodman et al., 1983), which is much less apparent in smaller communities. Also, Eaton and Lasry (1978) had shown evidence for downward social mobility among schizophrenics after the onset of the disorder.

Nonbipolar affective disorders show an inverse association with social class, which is most evident in minor depressive disorders and depressive symptomatology (Craig and Van Natta, 1979). In this case, there are treated incidence data (Goodman et al., 1983) to suggest a possible social causation effect, which is consistent with Brown's (1979) findings regarding social stress. Lower-class individuals appear to be more vulnerable to social stressors, at least in part because of their limited personal resources. In contrast, bipolar disorders have been reported to show a modest positive relationship with social class, with higher rates among professional persons (Hirschfeld and Cross, 1983).

From the ECA data, Holzer et al. (1986), using an index of socioeconomic status from the U.S. Census (education, occupation, and household income), confirmed earlier data (Hollingshead and Redlich, 1958) suggesting an inverse relationship between socioeconomic status and prevalence of several specific disorders which was strongest for schizophrenia and cognitive impairment, intermediate for alcohol abuse/dependence, and weakest but still significant for major depression. In a longitudinal study, Murphy et al. (1991) also found a higher prevalence of depression in persons with lower socioeconomic status and saw a nonsignificant trend for downward social mobility and increased incidence of depression in lower social status groups, suggesting both selection and causation factors. In this study there was less clarity in the relation between anxiety disorders and social class.

ECA findings regarding education (Robins and Regier, 1991) showed an overall increased prevalence of mental disorders among those with less than a high school education which was particularly significant for the specific diagnostic categories of bipolar disorder, somatization disorder, and cognitive impairment. For several specific categories, however, the failure to complete the last level of education (grade school, high school, or college) was associated with increased prevalence rates rather than the absolute level of schooling. This finding was significant for alcohol and drug abuse/dependence, antisocial personality disorder, and obsessive-compulsive disorder (except at the college level) and showed a nonsignificant trend for schizophrenia. Panic disorder, phobic disorder, and generalized anxiety disorder showed no relation to educational level.

OCCUPATION

Occupation has rarely been linked as a specific risk factor for a specific diagnostic category. Welner et al. (1979) have reported an increased prevalence of primary affective disorder, chiefly depression, among professional women (51 percent among M.D.s and 32 percent among Ph.D.s). However, the explanation for this finding is unclear and may suggest a selection phenomenon rather than an etiologic role for occupation. In addition, a form of traumatic dementia has been reported in professional prizefighters (Brody and White, 1982).

From the ECA study (Robins and Regier, 1988), overall prevalence rates were highest in unemployed (48 percent lifetime, 29 percent active). This finding held true for the specific diagnoses of schizophrenia and major depression, while prevalence rates for alcohol abuse/dependence, obsessive-compulsive disorder, somatization disorder, and antisocial personality disorder were increased among the underemployed. There was an inverse correlation between occupational level and prevalence rates for respondents with alcohol and drug abuse/dependence and generalized anxiety disorder. In a review, Catalano (1991) cites evidence for a clear effect of economic insecurity on increased symptoms of psychiatric disorder and seeking help for psychiatric disorder which was also fairly strong for suicide rates. In addition, Penkower et al. (1988) cite evidence that a husband's layoff is associated with increased psychiatric symptomatology among their wives which manifested after some period of time and was associated with risk factors of a familial history of psychiatric illness, financial difficulties, and low social support from relatives, suggesting an interaction between stress of layoff and preexisting vulnerabilities.

MARITAL STATUS

Marital status has been linked with the presence of mental illness in a variety of ways. Leaf et al. (1984), using ECA findings, found total mental disorders to be highest among the separated (26.7 percent) and divorced (25.8 percent), followed by the never married (21.5 percent). However, by sex, men's rates were highest among widowed, separated, and divorced (30.4 percent), while female rates were highest among singles (21.4 percent). Relationship with spouse, however, showed a strong correlation with prevalence. Those who reported a poor marital relationship had a prevalence rate of 51.2 versus 20.1 percent (fairly good relationship) and 12.0 percent (very good relationship). There was also a linear inverse relationship between reported ability to confide in spouse and overall prevalence of mental disorder.

For specific diagnoses, the risk for schizophrenia is about four times higher among the never married (greater among males) as compared with the married, probably largely owing to the early age of onset and adverse premorbid personality of many schizophrenics, making marriage unlikely (Eaton, 1983). Among the affective disorders, nonbipolar prevalence rates are lower in the married than in the unmarried, consistent with Brown's (1979) findings of a protective effect conferred by a close, confiding relationship. However, no significant relationship has been demonstrated between marital status and bipolar disorders except for the high prevalence of marital conflict seen among these patients (Hirschfeld and Cross, 1983).

MIGRATION

Rosenthal et al. (1974) report that virtually all treated prevalence studies of migration and schizophrenia reveal increased prevalence rates among migrants, although in many cases, the differences noted are trivial. As with social class, these findings have raised questions as to causation versus social selection. In summarizing these findings, Rosenthal et al. (1974) present data suggesting that the major factor to be studied is the motivation for migration, a social selection factor. Thus, in most earlier studies, preschizophrenics were seen to be more likely to migrate because of adverse economic circumstances in their countries of origin, whereas in Denmark in the 1950s, schizophrenics were only one-fifth as likely to migrate as matched controls. Data on migration as a factor in other psychiatric disorders are scanty.

A recent study using DSM-III criteria found a markedly increased rate of migration among bipolar patients and their parents but not among schizophrenic patients, suggesting that earlier studies that found increased migration among schizophrenic patients may have included substantial numbers of bipolar patients misdiagnosed as schizophrenic and accounting for their findings (Pope et al., 1983).

SEASON OF BIRTH

A number of studies have found a relative excess of schizophrenic births during the winter and spring months on the order of 5 to 15 percent (Torrey et al., 1977). In general, this finding has been more striking in countries with more marked seasonal variations, with a few exceptions, and has been reproduced in both hemispheres. A number of hypotheses have been proposed to explain this phenomenon, including nutritional (e.g., first-trimester protein deficiency), environmental (e.g., exposure to pesticides in first trimester), climatologic effects on ovum maturation, genetic (e.g., heat damage or exaggerated resistance to infectious diseases in the prenatal period), infectious (e.g., exposure to infectious agents with seasonal patterns), or reproductive patterns of mothers of schizophrenics. Kinney and Jacobsen (1978) cited evidence for seasonally related prenatal brain injury among patients with low genetic liability to schizophrenia using adoption techniques. Watson et al. (1984) found greater seasonality in years directly following those with high levels of infectious diseases (especially diphtheria, pneumonia, and influenza) in unmarried, but not married, patients, and no association with temperature extremes. They interpreted these data as consistent with prenatal influence chiefly affecting poor outcome patients and suggested that these effects may hold for only a portion of the total schizophrenic population. Studies in Finland (Mednick et al., 1988) and Denmark (Barr et al., 1990) have reported an association between possible fetal exposure to the influenza virus during the second trimester and subsequent excess of schizophrenic births, leading the authors to postulate a virus-induced adverse effect on fetal neurodevelopment specific to this stage of pregnancy.

URBANIZATION

Overall, the ECA study (Robins and Regier, 1991) showed little urban/rural differences in prevalence of mental illness in the two sites with both types of populations (Durham and St. Louis). However, within diagnostic categories, bipolar disorder and antisocial personality disorder were significantly more prevalent in urban areas in both sites. Site-specific findings included increased urban rates for major depression and agoraphobia and panic disorder (George et al., 1986) in Durham and rural increases in major depression (St. Louis) and alcohol-related problems among blacks (Durham) (Blazer et al., 1987).

INTEGRATION OF ETIOLOGIC THEORIES

Unfortunately, to date there has been relatively little integration of the findings from genetic, biologic, and psychosocial studies of etiologic factors related to psychiatric illness. As regards schizophrenia, Pol-

lin (1972) proposed a model in which a biologic factor (hyperactivity of the CNS catecholamine system), which may have both genetic or biologic/environmental origins (e.g., prenatal injury), may predispose an individual to react to psychosocial factors (e.g., stressors) with hyperarousal, which, if not moderated by the availability of personal resources and social support, can result in a psychotic episode. Although this approach is intuitively logical, future prospective studies, including structured assessment of all sets of variables (genetic, biologic, and psychosocial), in both high-risk and general population samples are now needed to begin to integrate these theoretical models and to specify their relevance to specific diagnostic entities if psychiatric epidemiology is to achieve its full potential.

REFERENCES

Anderson JC, Williams S, McGee R, Silva PA: DSM-III disorders in preadolescent children: Prevalence in a large sample from the general population. Arch Gen Psychiatry 44:69–76, 1987.

Baldessarini RJ, Finkelstein S, Arana GW: The predictive power of diagnostic tests and the effect of prevalence of illness. Arch Gen Psychiatry 40:569–573, 1983.

Barr CE, Mednick SA, Munk-Jorgensen P: Exposure to influenza epidemics during gestation and adult schizophrenia. Arch Gen Psychiatry 47:869–874, 1990.

Bebbington P: Causal models and logical inference in epidemiologic psychiatry. Br J Psychiatry 136:317–325, 1980.

Bird HR, Canino G, Rubio-Stipec M, et al: Estimates of the prevalence of childhood maladjustment in a community survey in Puerto Rico: The use of combined measures. Arch Gen Psychiatry 45:1120–1126, 1988.

Blazer D, Crowell BA, George LK: Alcohol abuse and dependence in the rural south. Arch Gen Psychiatry 44:736–740, 1987a.

Blazer D, Hughes D, George LK: Stressful life events and onset of generalized anxiety syndrome. Am J Psychiatry 144:1178–1183, 1987b.

Breier A, Kelsoe JR Jr, Kerwin PD, et al: Early parental loss and development of adult psychopathology. Arch Gen Psychiatry 45:987–993, 1988.

Breslau N, Davis GC: Posttraumatic stress disorder: The etiologic specificity of wartime stressors. Am J Psychiatry 144:578–583, 1987.

Brody JA, White LR: An epidemiologic perspective on senile dementia—Facts and fragments. Psychopharmacol Bull 18:222–224, 1982.

Bromet E, Parkinson D, Shulberg H: Mental health of residents near the Three Mile Island reactor: A comparative study of selected groups. J Prev Psychiatry 2:275–301, 1984.

Bromet E, Schulberg HC, Dunn L: Reactions of psychiatric patients to the Three Mile Island nuclear accident. Arch Gen Psychiatry 39:725–730, 1982.

Brown GW, Birley JLT: Crises and life changes and the onset of schizophrenia. J Health Soc Behav 9:203–214, 1968.

Brown GW, Skain F, Harris TO, Birley JLT: Life events and psychiatric disorder: I. Some methodological issues. Psychol Med 3:74–87, 1973.

Burke KC, Burke JD Jr, Rae DS, Regier DA: Comparing age at onset of major depression and other psychiatric disorders by birth cohorts in five US community populations. Arch Gen Psychiatry 48:789–795, 1991.

Burnham MA, Hough RL, Escobar JI, et al: Six-month prevalence of specific psychiatric disorders among Mexican-Americans and non-Hispanic whites in Los Angeles. Arch Gen Psychiatry 44:687–694, 1987.

Canino GJ, Bird HR, Shrout PE, et al: The prevalence of specific psychiatric disorders in Puerto Rico. Arch Gen Psychiatry 44:727–735, 1987.

Cantwell D, Baker L: Parental mental illness and psychiatric disorders in "at risk" children. J Clin Psychiatry 45:503–507, 1991.

Catalano R: The health effects of economic insecurity. Am J Public Health 81:1148–1152, 1991.

Compton WM III, Helzer JE, Hwu H-G, et al: New methods in cross cultural psychiatry: Psychiatric illness in Taiwan and the United States. Am J Psychiatry 148:1697–1704, 1991.

Craig TJ, Van Natta PA: Effect of demographic variables on symptoms of depression. Arch Gen Psychiatry 36:149–154, 1979.

Dohrenwend BS, Dohrenwend BP: Social Status and Psychological Disorder. New York, John Wiley & Sons, 1969.

Dohrenwend BS, Dohrenwend BP: Life stress and illness: Formulation of the issues. In Dohrenwend BS, Dohrenwend BP (eds): Stressful Life Events and Their Contexts (Monographs in Psychosocial Epidemiology 2). New York, Prodist, 1981, pp 1–27.

Dohrenwend BS, Dohrenwend BP: Life stress and psychopathology. In Regier DA, Allen G (eds): Risk Factor Research in the Major Mental Disorders (National Institute of Mental Health, DHHS Pub. No. (ADM) 83-1068). Rockville, MD, The Institute, 1983, pp 55–67.

Dohrenwend BP, Shrout PE, Egri G, Mendelsohn FS: Nonspecific psychological distress and other dimensions of psychopathology: Measures for use in the general population. Arch Gen Psychiatry 37:1229–1236, 1980.

Eaton WW: Demographic and social ecologic risk factors for mental disorders. In Regier DA, Allen G (eds): Risk Factor Research in the Major Mental Disorders (National Institute of Mental Health, DHHS Pub. No. (ADM) 83-1068). Rockville, MD, The Institute, 1983, pp 111–129.

Eaton WW, Lasry JC: Mental health and occupational mobility in a group of immigrants. Soc Sci Med 12:53–58, 1978.

Eaton WW Jr, Kramer M, Anthony JC, et al: The incidence of specific DIS/DSM-III mental disorders: Data from the Epidemiologic Catchment Area Program. Acta Psychiatr Scand 79:163–178, 1989a.

Eaton WW, Kramer M, Anthony JC, et al: Conceptual and methodological problems in estimation of the incidence of mental disorders from survey data. In Cooper JB, Helgason T (eds): Epidemiology and the Prevention of Mental Disorders. London, Routledge, 1989b, pp 108–127.

Egeland JA, Hostetter AM: Amish study: I. Affective disorders among the Amish, 1976–1980. Am J Psychiatry 140:56–61, 1983.

Erlenmeyer-Kimling L, Cornblatt B: The New York high-risk project: A follow-up report. Schizophr Bull 13:451–461, 1987.

Faravelli C, Webb T, Ambonetti A, et al: Prevalence of traumatic early life events in 31 agoraphobic patients with panic attacks. Am J Psychiatry 142:1493–1494, 1985.

Faravelli C, Pallanti S: Recent life events and panic disorder. Am J Psychiatry 146:622–626, 1989.

Faris REL, Dunham HW: Mental Disorders in Urban Areas: An Ecological Study of Schizophrenia and Other Psychoses. Chicago, University of Chicago Press, 1939.

Feighner JP, Robins E, Guze SB, et al: Diagnostic criteria for use in psychiatric research. Arch Gen Psychiatry 26:57–63, 1972.

Finlay-Jones R, Brown G: Types of stressful life event and the onset of anxiety and depressive disorders. Psychol Med 11:803–815, 1981.

Fish B: Infant predictors of the longitudinal course of schizophrenic development. Schizophr Bull 13:395–409, 1987.

Frank JD: Persuasion and Healing. Baltimore, Johns Hopkins University Press, 1973, pp 312–318.

Garmezy N: Stressors of childhood. In Garmezy N, Rutter M (eds): Stress, Coping and Development of Children. New York, McGraw-Hill, 1983.

George LK, Hughes DC, Blazer DG: Urban/rural differences in the prevalence of anxiety disorders. Am J Soc Psychiatry 6:249–258, 1986.

Goodman AB, Craig TJ: A needs assessment strategy for an era of limited resources. Am J Epidemiol 115:624–632, 1982.

Goodman AB, Siegel C, Craig TJ, Lin SP: The relationship between socioeconomic class and prevalence of schizophrenia, alcoholism and affective disorders treated by inpatient care in a suburban area. Am J Psychiatry 140:166–170, 1983.

Green BL, Grace MC, Lindy JD, et al: Risk factors for PTSD and other diagnoses in a general sample of Vietnam veterans. Am J Psychiatry 147:729–733, 1990.

Hammen C, Gordon D, Burge D, et al: Maternal affective disorders, illness and stress: Risk for children's psychopathology. Am J Psychiatry 144:736–741, 1987.

Helzer JE, Robins LN, Taibleson M, et al: Reliability of psychiatric diagnosis. Arch Gen Psychiatry 34:129–133, 1977.

Helzer JE, Robins LN, McEvoy L: Posttraumatic stress disorder in the general population. N Engl J Med 317:1630–1634, 1987.

Helzer JE, Canino GJ, Yeh E-K, et al: Alcoholism—North America and Asia: A comparison of population surveys with the Diagnostic Interview Schedule. Arch Gen Psychiatry 47:313–319, 1990.

Herman JL, Perry JC, van der Kolk BA: Childhood trauma in borderline personality disorder. Am J Psychiatry 146:490–495, 1989.

Hirschfeld RMA, Cross CK: Psychosocial risk factors for depression. In Regier DA, Allen G (eds): Risk Factor Research in the Major Mental Disorders (National Institute of Mental Health, DHHS Pub. No. (ADM) 131–143). Rockville, MD, The Institute, 1983.

Hollingshead AB, Redlich FC: Social Class and Mental Illness. New York, John Wiley & Sons, 1958.

Holzer CE, Shea BM, Swanson JW, et al: The increased risk for specific psychiatric disorders among persons of low socioeconomic status. Am J Soc Pschiatry 6:259–270, 1986.

Jacobs S, Myers J: Recent life events and acute schizophrenic psychosis: A controlled study. J Nerv Ment Dis 162:75–87, 1976.

Jacobs S, Prusoff BA, Paykel ES: Recent life events in schizophrenia and depression. Psychol Med 4:444–453, 1974.

Kashani JH, Beck NC, Hoeper EW, et al: Psychiatric disorders in a community sample of adolescents. Am J Psychiatry 144:584–589, 1987.

Kennedy S, Thompson R, Stancer HC, et al: Life events precipitating mania. Br J Psychiatry 142:398–403, 1983.

Kessler RC: A strategy for studying differential vulnerability to the psychological consequences of stress. J Health Soc Behav 20:100–108, 1979.

Kinney DK, Jacobsen B: Environmental factors in schizophrenia: New adoption study evidence. In Wynne LC, Cromwell RL, Matthysse S (eds): The Nature of Schizophrenia. New York, John Wiley & Sons, 1978.

Kinzie JD, Boehnlein JK, Leung PK, et al: The prevalence of posttraumatic stress disorder and its clinical significance among Southeast Asian refugees. Am J Psychiatry 147:913–917, 1990.

Kohn MLK: Class, family and schizophrenia: A reformulation. Soc Forces 50:295–304, 1972.

Kramer M: Cross-national study of diagnosis of the mental disorders: Origin of the problem. Am J Psychiatry 125(suppl):1–4, 1969.

Kroll J, Halbernicht M, Mackenzie T, et al: Depression and posttraumatic stress disorder in Southeast Asian refugees. Am J Psychiatry 146:1592–1597, 1989.

Kulka RA, Schlenger WE, Fairbank JA: National Vietnam Veterans Readjustment Study (NVVRS): Description, Current Status, and Initial PTSD Prevalence Rates. Research Triangle Park, NC, Research Triangle Institute, 1988.

Leaf PJ, Weissman MM, Myers JK, et al: Social factors related to psychiatric disorder: The Yale Epidemiologic Catchment Area Study. Soc Psychiatry 19:53–61, 1984.

Lin T: A study of incidence of mental disorder in Chinese and other cultures. Psychiatry 16:313, 1953.

Lin T-Y, Standley CC: The Scope of Epidemiology in Psychiatry. Geneva, World Health Organization, 1962.

Lloyd C: Life events and depressive disorders reviewed. Arch Gen Psychiatry 37:529–535, 1980.

Loranger AW: Sex difference in age at onset of schizophrenia. Arch Gen Psychiatry 41:157–161, 1984.

Maziade M, Caperaa P, Laplante B, et al: Value of difficult temperament among 7 year olds in the general population for predicting psychiatric diagnosis at age 12. Am J Psychiatry 142:943–946, 1985.

Mednick SA, Machon RA, Huttunen MO, Bonett D: Adult schizophrenia following prenatal exposure to an influenza epidemic. Arch Gen Psychiatry 45:189–192, 1988.

Morrison J: Childhood sexual histories of women with somatization disorder. Am J Psychiatry 146:239–241, 1989.

Murphy JM, Olivier DC, Monson RR, et al: Depression and anxiety in relation to social status. Arch Gen Psychiatry 48:223–229, 1991.

Myers JK, Lindenthal JJ, Pepper MP: Life events and mental status: A longitudinal study. J Health Soc Behav 13:398–406, 1972.

Nelson G: Parental death during childhood and adult depression: Some additional data. Soc Psychiatry 17:37–42, 1982.

Neugebauer R: Reliability of life-event interviews with outpatient schizophrenics. Arch Gen Psychiatry 40:378–383, 1983.

Nott PN: Psychiatric illness following childbirth in Southampton: A case register study. Psychol Med 12:557–561, 1982.

Offord DR, Alder RJ, Boyle MH: Prevalence and sociodemographic correlates of conduct disorder. Am J Soc Psychiatry 6:272–278, 1986.

Ogata SN, Silk KR, Goodrich S, et al: Childhood sexual and physical abuse in adult patients with borderline personality disorder. Am J Psychiatry 147:1008–1013, 1990.

Parry A, Shapiro D: Social support and life events in working class women. Arch Gen Psychiatry 43:315–323, 1986.

Paykel ES: Contribution of life events to causation of psychiatric illness. Psychol Med 8:245–254, 1978.

Paykel ES, Myers JK, Dieralt MN, et al: Life events and depression: A controlled study. Arch Gen Psychiatry 21:753–760, 1969.

Penkower L, Bromet EJ, Dew MA: Husbands' layoff and wives' mental health. Arch Gen Psychiatry 45:994–1000, 1988.

Pfohl B, Stangl D, Tsuang MT: The association between early parental loss and diagnosis in the Iowa 500. Arch Gen Psychiatry 40:965–967, 1983.

Plunkett R, Gordon J: Epidemiology and Mental Illness. New York, Basic Books, 1960.

Pollin W: The pathogenesis of schizophrenia: Possible relationships between genetic, biochemical, and experimental factors. Arch Gen Psychiatry 27:29–37, 1972.

Pope HG Jr, Ionescu-Pioggia M, Yurgelun-Todd D: Migration and manic-depressive illness. Compr Psychiatry 24:158–165, 1983.

Pribor EF, Dinwiddie SH: Psychiatric correlates of incest in childhood. Am J Psychiatry 149:52–56, 1992.

Ragan PV, McGlashan TA: Childhood parental death and adult psychopathology. Am J Psychiatry 143:153–157, 1986.

Rapee RM, Litwin EM, Barlow DH: Impact of life events on subjects with panic disorder and on comparison subjects. Am J Psychiatry 147:640–644, 1990.

Regier DA, Boyd JH, Burke JD Jr, et al: One-month prevalence of mental disorders in the US: Based on five epidemiologic catchment area sites. Arch Gen Psychiatry 45:977–986, 1988.

Regier DA, Goldberg ID, Taube CA: The de facto US mental health services system: A public health perspective. Arch Gen Psychiatry 35:685–693, 1978.

Robins LN, Helzer JE, Croughan J, Ratcliff, KS: National Institute of Mental Health diagnostic interview schedule. Arch Gen Psychiatry 34:129–133, 1977.

Robins LN: Longitudinal methods in the study of normal and pathological development. In Earls F (ed): Studies of Children: Monographs in Psychosocial Epidemiology. New York, Prodist, 1980, pp 34–83.

Robins LN, Locke BZ, Regier DA: An overview of psychiatric disorders in America. In Robins LN, Regier DA (eds): Psychiatric Disorders in America: The Epidemiologic Catchment Area Study. New York, Free Press, 1991, Chap 13, pp 328–366.

Robins LN, Regier DA (eds): Psychiatric Disorders in America: The Epidemiologic Catchment Area Study. New York, Free Press, 1991.

Rosenthal D, Goldberg I, Jacobsen B, et al: Migration, heredity, and schizophrenia. Psychiatry 37:321–339, 1974.

Roy A: Role of past loss in depression. Arch Gen Psychiatry 38:301–302, 1981.

Roy-Byrne PP, Geraci M, Uhde TW: Life events and the onset of panic disorder. Am J Psychiatry 143:1424–1427, 1986.

Schless AP, Mendels J: The value of interviewing family and friends in assessing life stressors. Arch Gen Psychiatry 35:565–567, 1978.

Schwartz ED, Kowalski JM: Posttraumatic stress disorder after a school shooting: Effects of symptom threshold selection and diagnosis by DSM-III, DSM-IIIR, and proposed DSM-IV. Am J Psychiatry 148:592–597, 1991.

Shore J, Tatum E, Vollmer W: Evaluation of mental effects of disaster, Mount St. Helens eruption. Am J Public Health 76(suppl):76–83, 1986.

Simon RJ, Fleiss JL, Gurland BJ, et al: Depression and schizophrenia in hospitalized black and white mental patients. Arch Gen Psychiatry 28:509–512, 1973.

Solomon Z, Weisenberg M, Schwartzwald J, Mikulincer M: Posttraumatic stress disorder among frontline soldiers with combat stress reaction: The 1982 Israeli experience. Am J Psychiatry 144:448–454, 1987.

Spitzer RL, Endicott J, Robins E: Research diagnostic criteria: Rationale and reliability. Arch Gen Psychiatry 35:773–782, 1978.

Srole L, Langner TS, Michael ST, et al: Mental Health in the Metropolis: The Midtown Manhattan Study. New York, McGraw-Hill, 1962.

Starker J: Methodological and conceptual issues in research on social support. Hosp Commun Psychiatry 37:485–490, 1986.

Task Force on DSM-IV: DSM-IV Options Book: Work in Progress 9/1/91. Washington, American Psychiatric Association, 1991.

Tennant C: Life events and psychological morbidity: The evidence from prospective studies. Psychol Med 13:483–486, 1983.

Tien AY, Eaton WW: Psychopathologic precursors and sociodemographic risk factors for the schizophrenic syndrome. Arch Gen Psychiatry 49:37–46, 1992.

Tienari P, Sorri A, Lahti I, et al: Genetic and psychosocial factors in schizophrenia: The Finnish adoptive family study. Schizophr Bull 13:477–484, 1987.

Torgersen S: Childhood and family characteristics in panic and generalized anxiety disorders. Am J Psychiatry 143:630–632, 1986.

Torrey EF, Torrey BB, Peterson MR: Seasonality of schizophrenic births in the United States. Arch Gen Psychiatry 34:1065–1070, 1977.

Watson CG, Keecala T, Tilleskjor C, Jacobs L: Schizophrenic birth seasonality in relation to the incidence of the infectious diseases and temperature extreme. Arch Gen Psychiatry 41:85–90, 1984.

Weissman MM, Klerman GL: Epidemiology of mental disorders: Emerging trends in the United States. Arch Gen Psychiatry 35:705–712, 1978.

Weissman MM, Klerman GL: Sex differences and the epidemiology of depression. Arch Gen Psychiatry 34:98–111, 1977.

Weissman MM, Myers JK, Harding PS: Psychiatric disorders in a US urban community: 1975–1976. Am J Psychiatry 135:459–462, 1978.

Weller RA, Weller EB, Fristad MA, Bower JM: Depression in recently bereaved prepubertal children. Am J Psychiatry 148:1536–1540, 1991.

Welner A, Welner Z, Fishman R: The group of schizoaffective and related psychoses: IV. A family study. Compr. Psychiatry 20:21–26, 1979.

Wender PH, Rosenthal D, Katz SS, et al: Social class and psychopathology in adopters. Arch Gen Psychiatry 28:318–325, 1973.

Whitaker A, Johnson J, Shaffer D, et al: Uncommon troubles of young people: Prevalence estimates in a nonreferred adolescent population. Arch Gen Psychiatry 47:487–496, 1990.

Wiersma D, Giel R, DeJong A, Slooff CJ: Social class and schizophrenia in a Dutch cohort. Psychol Med 13:141–150, 1983.

Williams DH: The epidemiology of mental illness in Afro-Americans. Hosp Commun Psychiatry 37:42–54, 1986.

Winfield I, George LK, Swartz M, Blazer DG: Sexual assault and psychiatric disorders among a community sample of women. Am J Psychiatry 147:335–341, 1990.

Yager J, Grant I, Sweetwood HL, Gerst M: Life event reports by psychiatric patients, nonpatients and their partners. Arch Gen Psychiatry 38:343–347, 1981.

Zubin J: Cross-national study of diagnosis of the mental disorders: Methodology and planning. Am J Psychiatry 125(suppl):12–20, 1969.

CHAPTER 32

Suicide and Attempted Suicide

GEORGE E. MURPHY

Suicide is not a diagnosis or a disorder but a behavior; a mode or manner of death, as opposed to a method or cause. The determination of that manner is the responsibility of the coroner or medical examiner of the district in which the death occurs. Such an official must draw an inference from physical circumstances (e.g., victim hanging or still holding a personally owned firearm) and from psychosocial information obtained from survivors that the death was neither a homicide nor an accident. Non-medically-trained and untrained coroners may require overwhelming evidence (beyond reasonable doubt) for the decision, while medical examiners commonly decide on a "more likely than not" (balance of probabilities) basis, the same way they decide on medical diagnoses. Cause of death has a bearing on the verdict, being more likely to be judged a suicide in the case of hanging and less likely when poisoning (excepting carbon monoxide asphyxia) is the means (Ovenstone, 1973). Social factors such as protecting the family from embarrassment or from hassles over life insurance sometimes enter the picture. As a consequence, suicide figures are underestimated both here and abroad.

Opinions differ as to the magnitude of the underestimation. Available evidence suggests a range between 24 percent (Brent et al., 1987) and 33 percent (Ovenstone, 1973), while undocumented opinion may claim misclassification rates two to three times higher. Most of the missed cases of suicide are hidden in the category of cause undetermined. The preceding investigators, as well as Holding and Barraclough (1978), have presented evidence that missed cases are descriptively more like suicides than like accident victims. The achievement of uniformly high-quality ascertainment practices would increase the number of suicides identified but would not be likely to change the nature of the findings. Studies based on coroners' verdicts will therefore not mislead us.

DEMOGRAPHICS

In the United States, men are more than three times as likely as women to take their lives. Whites of both sexes have overall suicide rates twice as high as their black counterparts. The age structure of the suicide rate curves differs both between the sexes and between races. That for males has changed dramatically over the last 40 years. Formerly, the rate for white males rose linearly with age (Fig. 32-1). Now it rises very steeply between ages 15 and 24, dips slightly, and then remains essentially flat until age 65, when it trends steeply upward for the remaining years (Fig. 32-2). A similar early rise in the rate has developed among black men. It peaks at age 35 and then declines with only a modest increase in later years. The curves for women have changed little. The peak for white women now occurs slightly earlier, at around age 50. The very low suicide rate for black women is highest from age 35 to 40. A satisfactory explanation of these changes continues to elude us.

The single, the widowed, and the divorced all have higher suicide rates than the married. Socioeconomic status does not appear to play a major role. Suicide rates by occupational group do not differ as much as is commonly believed. A widely quoted publication (Blachly et al., 1963) reported high rates for physicians, dentists, and attorneys compared with all males over age 19. The population base was that of a single western state, and the number of cases was small. More recent nationwide studies of physicians' deaths have substantially revised the conclusion for the medical profession.

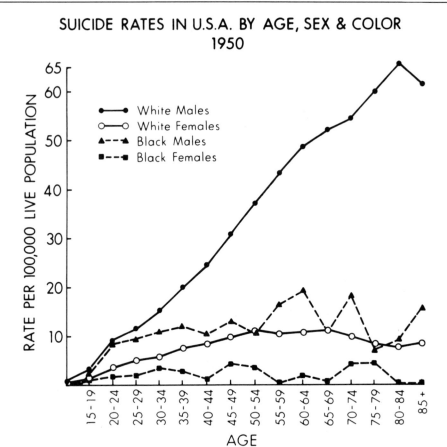

SUICIDE RATES IN U.S.A. BY AGE, SEX & COLOR
1950

Calculated from Vital Statistics of the United States for 1950.

FIGURE 32-1. *Suicide rates in the U.S.A. by age, sex, and color (1950).* (From Vital Statistics of the United States for 1950).

Among male physicians, the age-specific suicide rates are mildly (1.15 times expected) but significantly greater than those for the age-matched general male population. This relationship has not changed in 30 years.

Surprisingly, women physicians exhibit a suicide rate slightly higher than that of male physicians and more than three times that of women in general (Steppacher and Mausner, 1974; Pitts et al., 1979). This phenomenon is not unique to women physicians. Li (1969) reported that the age-adjusted suicide rate among female members of the American Chemical Society was five times that of the general U.S. population of white women in 1959 and nearly three times that of male chemists. Mausner and Steppacher (1973) found that almost three times as many female psychologists committed suicide as expected between 1960 and 1969. The rate for male psychologists was slightly less than expected. For female physicians, Pitts et al. (1979) postulate an excess of affective disorders as responsible for their findings. Whatever the actual causes, it seems clear that women in the professions carry a risk of suicide equal to or greater than that of their male counterparts.

Method of Suicide

Firearms rank first as a cause of suicidal death in both males and females (Table 32-1). Sixty-five percent of male and 56 percent of female adolescents chose firearms in 1988. Fewer women nowadays than formerly resort to poisoning, a method chosen by few men. Hanging, strangulation, and suffocation together rank second for men and third for women, followed by carbon monoxide asphyxia. Suicide by jumping from a high place, drowning, or cutting and piercing is infrequent. Asphyxiation by

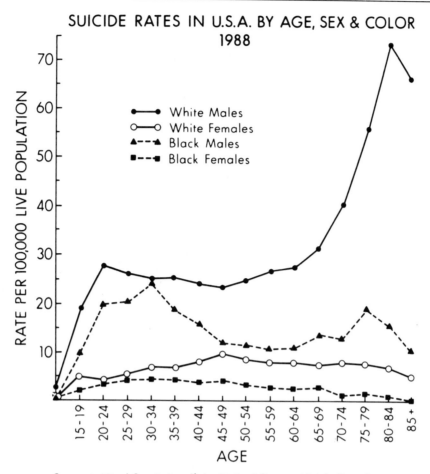

SUICIDE RATES IN U.S.A. BY AGE, SEX & COLOR
1988

Source: Vital Statistics of the United States, Vol 2, Part A,
Mortality

FIGURE 32-2.   *Suicide rates in the U.S.A. by age, sex, and color (1988).* (From Vital Statistics of the United States, vol. 2, part A, Mortality.)

domestic gas is rarely used in the United States. Determinants of the choice of method are complex and include physical availability, familiarity, psychological acceptability, suggestion or contagion, symbolic, and perhaps other factors.

Poisonings are usually with psychotropic or hypnotic medications. Only seldom nowadays are classic poisons, such as household disinfectants, caustics, or pesticides, used in the United States. Specific agents used in self-poisoning deaths are not detailed in the vital statistics system. Poison-control reporting by the Drug Enforcement Administration's Drug Abuse Warning Network (DAWN) comes from reports of 135 medical examiners located in 27 metropolitan areas. Antidepressant medications have ranked first for at least the past 8 years, being mentioned in 21 percent of suicides by overdose. Narcotic analgesics rank second in the

suicide category at 12.9 percent, with tranquilizers (essentially benzodiazepines) third, being mentioned in 11.5 percent of these deaths. Barbiturate sedatives dropped from second in 1982 (10.4 percent) to fifth (5.3 percent) in 1990 (DAWN, 1983, Table 3.11; DAWN, 1991, Table 2.11), being replaced by the much safer benzodiazepines in the hypnotic-sedative market. A mean of two drugs per suicide is mentioned. All these figures on agents of suicide are provisional. As many deaths from drug overdose are ruled accidental in a year as are ruled suicide *from all causes* in the United States.

Hanging, strangulation, and suffocation are available to all, as are jumping from high places, submersion or drowning, and cutting or piercing. The means are readily at hand if there is matching motivation. Unlike the cartoon version involving an overturned chair, the hanging victim typically se-

TABLE 32-1. *Proportion of Suicides by Method and Sex, 1988*

	Males (%)	Females (%)	Total (%)
Firearms	65.0	39.7	59.7
Hanging, strangulation, etc.	14.9	12.4	14.4
Poisoning	5.9	27.0	10.3
Carbon monoxide asphyxiation	8.4	11.0	8.7
Jumping from high places	1.8	2.9	2.1
Cutting and piercing	1.5	1.7	1.5
Submersion (drowning)	1.0	2.5	1.3
Other and unspecified	1.6	2.7	1.9

From Vital Statistics of the United States, 1988, vol II: Mortality, part A. Washington, U.S. Dept. of Health and Human Services, 1989.

cures some sort of loop around the neck and then around a stationary object. Relaxing bodily support results in death within 5 to 7 minutes by interrupting blood return from the brain. The means are as simple as a piece of rope, a belt, or even a wire coat hanger and a doorknob. Multiple methods are sometimes used. Simultaneous ingestion of two or more drugs is the most common. Significant alcohol consumption attends 30 to 40 percent of cases. Some suicides ingest an overdose of medication before asphyxiation, hanging, drowning, leaping, cutting, or gunshot. All attest to a determination to do "a good job."

Motor vehicle fatalities are seldom investigated as possible suicides. Pokorny and colleagues (1972) systematically investigated 28 consecutive automobile crash fatalities of drivers. In addition to physical autopsy, they performed a "psychological autopsy" and "automobile autopsy." They concluded that 4 (14 percent) of the 28 were suicides. Prior communication of suicidal intent had occurred in each of these cases. In a larger study, Schmidt and associates (1972) identified only 3

suicides among 111 single-vehicle fatalities, a rate of 2.7 percent. The truth probably lies toward the lower end of the range. With about 55,000 motor vehicle fatalities annually in the United States, this would represent around 1000 to 2000 vehicular suicides in a year. It is unlikely that medical examiners and coroners will soon change their investigational procedures to search more diligently for suicides among vehicular fatalities when the probability is below 5 percent.

PATHOGENESIS OF SUICIDE

Suicide is a rare event, occurring only slightly more than once among 10,000 persons annually in the United States. Prospective studies of the phenomenon are thus substantially out of the question because of the huge sample size needed for a statistically meaningful result. An alternative strategy is that of retrospective study of persons adjudicated to have died by their own hand. This type of investigation, carried out by interviewing family members, attending physicians, and others, as well as by reviewing hospital and other official records, has come to be called the *psychological autopsy* (Litman et al., 1963). To avoid selection bias, it is customary to look into a consecutive and therefore unselected series of cases.

Since preparation of the first edition of this chapter, the number of community studies of suicide available to us has doubled and includes reports from three additional countries (Table 32-2). The overall conclusions have not changed, but some details have. Studies up to 1980 reported a single leading diagnosis for each case (hierarchical diagnosis). With but one exception (Åsgård, 1990), more recent studies have given multiple and overlapping diagnoses per subject. The hierarchical method clearly identifies psychiatric illness as the nearly universal antecedent to self-destruction, but

TABLE 32-2. *Selected Diagnoses in Community Samples of Suicide*

	n	Affective disorder (%)	Alcoholism (%)	Schizophrenia (%)	Substance abuse/ dependency (%)	No psychiatric illness (%)
Robins et al., U.S.A. (1959a)	134	45	24 (30)*	2	25	6
Dorpat and Ripley, U.S.A. (1960)	114	30	27	12	31	0
Barraclough et al., U.K. (1974)	100	70	15	3	19	7
Beskow, Sweden (1979)	270	28 (45)*	31	3	37	4
Hagnell and Rorsman, Sweden (1979)	28	50	19	7	39	7
Chynoweth et al., Australia (1980)	135	33 (55)*	20	4	22 (34)*	2
Mitterauer, Austria (1981)	94	63*	30	5	45*	0
Kapamadzija et al., Yugoslavia (1982)	100	61*	41*	3*	44*	0?
Rich et al., U.S.A. (1986)	283	44*	29 (54)*	3*	60*	5
Arato et al., Hungary (1988)	200	51*	20*	8*	—	14
Åsgård, Sweden (1990)	104	59	7	3	12*	<5

*Diagnoses inclusive, not heirarchical.

it obscures potentially important detail. Multiple diagnoses bring comorbidity to the fore and add richness of texture through subanalyses of the data. Comparison with earlier studies is more difficult, however, and the assignment of etiologic responsibility becomes more complex.

Few suicides (less than 5 percent) have been found lacking in psychiatric symptoms. Most have been diagnosable. When a psychiatric diagnosis has not been made, it usually has been because of unavailability of knowledgeable informants, not because there was a clear lack of symptoms. An apparent exception to the low frequency of undiagnosed cases is found in a very brief report from Hungary (Arató et al., 1988), where 20 percent of the suicides received no psychiatric diagnosis and 14 percent had neither psychiatric nor medical illness. Hungary has long held the dubious distinction of having much the highest suicide rate of any reporting country: 41.6 per 100,000 population in 1990 (World Health Organization, 1991). It is possible that this high rate reflects a cultural tradition that somehow lowers the personal threshold for self-destruction. The Hungarian data to the contrary notwithstanding, psychiatric illness is virtually a necessary, albeit not a sufficient, condition for suicide. Certain psychiatric illnesses are more contributory than others.

Affective Disorder

Major depressive disorder plays the dominant role in all the systematic studies of suicide (see Table 32-2). Both differing diagnostic styles and personal preferences for assigning first diagnoses, as well as the nature of the base populations, affect the absolute figures. These range from 28 percent in a sample of males only (Beskow, 1979) to 70 percent in an older population base (Barraclough et al., 1974). The mean for studies in which a primary diagnosis can be established is 41 percent; with multiple diagnoses, major depression is diagnosed in 53 percent of cases. By either method, it is the most common diagnosis encountered. Subsyndromal depressive features are found in a further fraction of the whole. Dorpat and Ripley (1962) commented that "symptoms of depression were elicited in every completed suicide . . . where adequate information was available."

Some controversy exists in the general affective disorder literature as to whether the bipolar form has a greater or lesser propensity to suicide. Dorpat and Ripley (1960) reported that their category of psychotic depression "included six with manic-depressive psychosis." Under the official nomenclature of that time, the diagnosis of manic-depressive illness, depressed type "consists exclusively of depressive episodes" (American Psychiatric Association, 1968). This diagnosis was to be made when the disorder was thought to be endogenous rather than reactive. Nothing can be concluded from their

report, since history of an episode of mania was not required for the diagnosis. Barraclough et al. (1974) found 11 (17 percent) of 64 uncomplicated depressives to have had a prior history of mania. Åsgård (1990) found 5 bipolar women (10 percent) among 52 suffering from periodic affective disorders. One subject with a lifetime diagnosis of schizoaffective disorder, manic type, was further diagnosed as having manic disorder in the final month. Robins (1981), on the other hand, reported that "as far as could be determined, none of the 63 subjects with affective disorder had ever had a manic episode" (p. 48). None of the other studies cited comments on bipolarity. Clearly, the systematic studies are of little help in resolving the question. However, among the more than 1550 suicides systematically studied with attention given to clinical diagnosis, *only one case of terminal mania was reported*. It may be concluded that the manic state itself does not constitute a risk factor for suicide. It must be kept in mind, however, that mania can give way abruptly to depression, in which case protection is lost.

Psychoactive Substance Abuse Disorder

In earlier studies, alcoholism was always the second most frequent psychiatric diagnosis made. Psychoactive substance abuse today includes a considerably broader range of intoxicants than simply ethanol. Substance abuse disorder was identified in 23 percent of the hierarchically diagnosed suicides and 39 percent of the multiply diagnosed suicides in Table 32-2. Psychoactive substance abuse beyond alcohol was more prominent in the young. In the San Diego study of Rich and colleagues (1989), the overall rate of substance abuse in suicides under age 30 was 54 percent compared with 37 percent in those older. Of substance-abusing suicides under age 30, only 2 percent abused alcohol alone, compared with 39 percent of those age 30 and older. Furthermore, among the young, "the typical drug and alcohol use disorder was . . . usually characterized by multiple drug abuse for many years" (Fowler et al., 1986). Marijuana was abused by three-quarters of both pure drug abusers and mixed alcohol and drug abusers. Cocaine was abused by 45 percent, amphetamines by one-third, and opiates by one-quarter of the young suicides. The polydrug phenomenon and its relationship to suicide are now widespread among the young (Brent et al., 1988). Alcohol abuse alone is still the second most frequent diagnosis in suicides in the fourth and later decades of life. Together, affective disorder and psychoactive substance abuse disorder account for two-thirds of self-inflicted deaths.

Schizophrenia

Schizophrenia has been found in 5.6 percent (mean) of suicides (Table 32-2). Being about one-tenth as common as major depressive disorder, its *proportionate* risk seems to be about the same. Its representation in studies of clinical populations is higher than in community samples (Morrison, 1982), since it is a chronic, disruptive disorder, more likely than others to come to treatment. Its relative infrequency in the community contributes to the variability in its proportionate representation from study to study. Small numbers generate unstable statistics. Differing diagnostic practices may play a role as well.

Schizoaffective disorder, characterized by a mixture of affective and schizophrenic features, typically follows a phasic course. Clinically, prognostically, and familially, it falls between the two major diagnoses. It was not diagnosed in any of the studies published prior to 1986, most of which followed the hierarchical diagnostic strategy. Rich and colleagues (1986) reported seven instances of schizoaffective disorder (3 percent) under the rubric of "other psychoses." Arató et al. (1988) made the diagnosis twice (1 percent). It was not possible to tell if in any case it was regarded as primary. Åsgård (1990) found it in 11 cases, considering it the primary diagnosis in 2 (2 percent). In the absence of a known base rate, its risk level for a suicidal outcome cannot be assessed. If the lifetime risk of suicide in schizophrenia is about the same as that for major affective disorder, it will be impossible to judge whether the motivation for suicide in persons with this mixed disorder stems more from one than from the other. At the least, schizoaffective disorder cannot be assumed to be protective from this outcome.

Organic Brain Disorders

As a first diagnosis, organic brain disorders (dementia and delirium) make a small contribution to self-destruction: 4 percent (Dorpat and Ripley, 1960; Achté and Vauhkonen, 1971; Robins, 1981). In multiply diagnosed cases, it has been reported to be as high as 28 percent (Kapamadžija et al., 1982). Much depends on the criteria employed in making the assessment. The phenomenon of poststroke depression is by now well recognized and may be considered to be a major factor in this infrequent outcome.

Personality Disorders

Perhaps the biggest change in the described psychopathology antecedent to suicide is in the emerging emphasis on personality disorders. Robins et al. (1959), Barraclough et al. (1974), Robins (1981), Arató et al. (1988), and Åsgård (1991) do not mention it. Dorpat and Ripley (1960) diagnosed 9.3 percent of 108 suicides as having "personality and sociopathic disorders" and did not further discuss that group. Beskow (1979) found "personality disorders" in 4 percent of 270 Swedish male suicides. The figure was 3 percent in Chynoweth and associates' (1980) study. Rich et al. (1986) diagnosed

antisocial personality disorder in 5 percent of 283 suicides and mixed personality disorder in 1 additional case. "Of the 15 cases with personality disorders (14 antisocial, 1 mixed), 14 had histories of SA [substance abuse]" (Rich et al., 1989). Runeson (1989) diagnosed borderline personality disorder in 19 (33 percent) of 58 multiply diagnosed Swedish suicides aged 15 to 29 years.

We are currently in an inflationary period regarding personality disorder diagnoses, particularly that of the borderline variety. Two fundamental problems argue for a skeptical view of the proceedings. One is the rather ad hoc nature of the diagnostic criteria, with insufficient attention being given to a clear separation from better established diagnoses. The other is a paucity of follow-up and family studies to show whether these are stable entities with a familial element or simply variants of disorders already described and delimited. To emphasize the point, all but two of the suicides diagnosed by Runeson as having borderline personality disorder had another, better-established psychiatric diagnosis as well (Runeson and Beskow, 1991). Half were associated with antisocial personality disorder, which has a clear diagnostic pattern, a stable, if unfortunate, prognosis, and a strong familial background as the male counterpart of Briquet's hysteria (Guze et al., 1986).

Panic Disorder

A recent literature of impressive unanimity has identified panic disorder (PD) as having a statistically significant excess mortality from suicide (Coryell, 1988; Allgulander and Lavori, 1991). Follow-up studies of both inpatients and outpatients produce similar results. While one does not doubt the association, it seems highly unlikely that PD provides the impetus to suicide. As Coryell (1988) points out, "other psychiatric syndromes—substance abuse, alcoholism, major depression, or combinations thereof—may be a necessary prelude to suicide in panic disorder." The fact that it has never been identified in more than 1550 suicides studied retrospectively may be traced to limitations of the inquiry in some instances, but not in all. There is not a hint of it in these studies as a late antemortem problem. Åsgård (1990) diagnosed *generalized* anxiety disorder in four cases, one in association with alcoholism and three on a lifetime and current basis. I conclude that panic disorder is not itself a meaningful contributor to suicide but simply keeps bad company.

Terminal Medical Illness

Terminal medical illness (cancer) accounted for 4 percent of suicides in one series (Robins et al., 1959; Robins, 1981). In light of its unpleasant nature, as well as its prevalence, this seems like a rather small proportion. The finding attests to the fact that suicide is not everyone's cup of hemlock. At the same time, it must be borne in mind that substantially all patients dying of cancer are under a physician's care. Their deaths do not automatically become a matter for the medical examiner. The attending physician completes the death certificate as he or she chooses. Some suicides among the terminally ill are certainly concealed in this way. The magnitude of this concealment will probably never be known. The *belief* that one has cancer, coupled with avoidance of medical consultation, may contribute equally to suicide. It is usually a symptom of a major depressive episode, sometimes in association with alcoholism (Conwell et al., 1990; Murphy, 1992).

Suicide in the absence of clinical illness, whether medical or psychiatric, is rare—representing little more than 5 percent of cases (see Table 32-2). In any event, persons who are not ill are unlikely to be under medical care. Thus they are not a part of the clinical problem.

Suicide in Adolescence

The suicide rate among adolescents has tripled over the past 30 years (Murphy and Wetzel, 1980). The overall numbers are small, but the trend seems to be continuing, albeit at a slower pace. This change has provided impetus for several systematic studies of adolescent suicide. Only a small number have been reported as yet. The still low frequency of the phenomenon makes for slow data collection. Suicides younger than 20 years of age comprised 7.6 percent of the total in the United States in 1988. Adolescent suicide remains infrequent, despite its greater than threefold increase.

In an unusually thorough postmortem investigation of 21 adolescent suicides, Shafii and colleagues (1988) made at least one Axis I diagnosis in all but 1 case. This was double the frequency of psychiatric disorders found in closely matched living friends of the victims. The diagnostic distribution was much like that found in adults: 43 percent with a primary or secondary major depression (76 percent if dysthymic disorder is included) and 62 percent with a primary or secondary diagnosis of substance abuse disorder. Overall, 81 percent had two or more psychiatric diagnoses. Six victims (29 percent) received an "underlying" Axis II diagnosis. Only one youth was under psychiatric care at the time of his suicide.

Brent et al. (1988) studied 27 suicides aged 13 to 19 years in Allegheny County (Pittsburgh), Pennsylvania, in 1984–1986. Twenty-five (92.6 percent) had at least one psychiatric diagnosis. Major depressive disorder was diagnosed in 41 percent and dysthymic disorder in 22 percent. There seem to have been 6 subjects (22 percent) with bipolar disorder, 2 of them dying in "mixed states" and 4 in the depressed phase. Substance abuse disorder was found in 37 percent, conduct disorder in 22 percent,

and attention deficit disorder in 26 percent. Neither schizophrenia nor panic disorder was found. The diagnostic distribution was rather similar among 56 adolescents hospitalized for suicide attempts or ideation. Only one-third of the suicides had had as much as one lifetime mental health contact, 2 (7 percent) were in active treatment, and only 1 was receiving appropriate psychotropic medication. One can hardly escape the conclusion that active treatment was the difference between those alive and those dead by their own hand.

In contrast to the above, Rich et al. (1990) made no diagnosis of major depressive disorder among the 14 adolescent suicides (13 males) in the San Diego study. Substance abuse was recognized in half the cases. Only one subject was known to be in active treatment at the time of the suicide. "Eleven subjects were found to have sustained an interpersonal loss or rejection as a recent stressor. In nine subjects, the stressors were believed by the investigator to have precipitated the suicide" (Rich et al., 1990). Almost all their adolescent subjects "had long histories of adaptational difficulties, which included such behavioral manifestations as frequent threats of suicide, running away, arson, assault, and theft."

Preliminary data from 114 cases in Shaffer's large adolescent suicide study (Shaffer et al., 1988) show 21 percent of the 97 males and 50 percent of the 17 females to have a diagnosis of major depression. Substance abuse was found in 37 percent of the males and 5 percent of the females. Antisocial behavior was identified in 67 percent of the males and 30 percent of the females. How these figures regarding behaviors will compare with formal diagnoses in the final report remains to be seen.

Marttunen et al. (1991) have recently reported on the adolescents in a massive interview study encompassing all suicides in Finland over a 1-year period. Fifty-three (3.8 percent) of this epochal cohort were between the ages of 13 and 19 years. Fifty of them received a psychiatric diagnosis, with 51 percent having a depressive disorder and 30 percent an alcohol/substance abuse disorder. Personality disorder was diagnosed in 17 cases (32 percent) and was considered the principal diagnosis in 11 (21 percent). Borderline personality disorder was diagnosed in 6 cases (1.7 percent). Of 9 with a diagnosis of antisocial personality disorder or conduct disorder, 7 had alcohol/substance abuse as well, 6 had a comorbid depressive disorder, and 5 had both. Adjustment disorder was diagnosed in 11 cases (21 percent) and was thought to be the disorder most relevant to the suicidal process in 8 (15 percent). (This diagnosis has been found to be prodromal to an Axis I disorder in half or more of cases; Andreasen and Hoenk, 1982). No instance of bipolar affective disorder was encountered. The authors recognize that conduct disorder and antisocial personality disorders are sometimes diagnosed crosssectionally though a bipolar illness might emerge on follow-up.

Suicide in the Elderly

Over the past decade there has been a steady rise in the suicide rate of persons aged 65 years and older (Meehan et al., 1991). Males account for 80 percent of these deaths and for the bulk of the increase (see Fig. 32-1). This change parallels growth in the proportion of elderly persons in the U.S. population, accompanied by a steadily deteriorating economic picture for them. While critical data are lacking, it seems likely that major depression, rather than substance abuse disorder, would be the central psychiatric variable.

THE GENETICS OF SUICIDE

Haberlandt (1967) reviewed the world literature on suicide in twins. Among 51 sets of monozygotic twin pairs with a suicide in one, he found 9 concordant for self-destruction. There was no concordance for suicide among 98 dizygotic twin pairs. One must be aware of the likelihood of bias in collecting published case studies. Those supporting a favored hypothesis or presenting a striking contrast are more likely to be submitted for publication. Although the direction of the trend is likely to be correct, its magnitude is uncertain.

In a large Danish adoption study, 57 adoptee probands had committed suicide. Eleven came from biologic families containing 12 other suicides. In a matched control sample of equal size, there were 2 suicides, both in one biologic family. The difference has a probability of 0.06 by Fisher's exact test. There were no suicides among adoptive parents (Schulsinger et al., 1979). Because the psychiatric illnesses that contribute most to suicide are known to be familial, it is of interest that concordance for psychiatric diagnosis between probands and families was small. The history of their biologic families was officially shielded from the probands, so family tradition appears to be ruled out in these cases. These findings suggest not simply a familial (i.e., modeling) explanation but possibly *a genetic predisposition to suicide independent of the disposition to psychiatric disorder.* This conclusion is strongly supported by studies conducted by Mitterauer (1990). Independent transmission is not always the case, however. A recent family pedigree study shows tight linkage between suicide and major affective disorder in the Old Order Amish, a society where there is almost no alcohol or drug abuse, no unemployment, and no poverty. It is characterized by strong social cohesion, veneration of the elderly, and religious sanctions against self-destruction. Suicide was found to cluster in a small number of pedigrees with unipolar and bipolar affective disorder (Egeland and Sussex, 1985).

EDITORS' COMMENT

A study by Tsuang (J Clin Psychiatry 44:396–400, 1983) evaluated family members of 195 schizophrenics and 315 patients with bipolar illness and unipolar depression. There was clear evidence of predisposition to suicide independent of the disposition to psychiatric disorder. Of the 458 relatives of bipolar index cases who were investigated, there was a tenfold increase in suicide in the relatives of those bipolar patients who committed suicide themselves over the relatives of those bipolar patients who did not commit suicide. For the 1144 relatives of depressive patients, there was a 3.4 time increase in suicides of the relatives of the depressive patients who themselves committed suicide. No such differential was true of the 746 relatives of schizophrenics or of the 672 relatives of controls. This finding involved a 30- to 40-year follow-up of probands, a personal examination of all live family members, and a search of records of hospitalizations and suicides. It shows evidence of a familial transmission of suicide but does not prove that such a transmission is genetic. An adoption study does have the capacity to separate a genetic from a social type of familial transmission.

PREDICTING SUICIDE

Suicide is a rare event. Moreover, there are no pathognomonic signs or symptoms of impending suicide. All of its identified associations are distributed widely in the population. Granting that nearly all suicides are psychiatrically ill, the lifetime prevalence of the three psychiatric disorders most commonly associated with it sum to about 25 percent of the adult U.S. population (Regier et al., 1988), so diagnosis alone is not strongly distinguishing. Around two-thirds of suicides communicate their intentions in advance (Robins et al., 1959). One way of doing so is by a suicide attempt. There are 10 to 20 times as many suicide attempts as suicides. Verbal communication of intent is three times more common. Warnings, therefore, do not translate strongly into predictions.

A number of investigators have reported that hopelessness correlates more strongly with suicidal intent in suicide attempters than does depression. Beck and associates (1990) have shown that an elevated score on a hopelessness scale (Beck et al., 1974) "predicts" suicide on long follow-up, but a level of hopelessness that identified 91 percent of the future suicides had an 88 percent false-positive prediction rate. Fawcett et al. (1990) found hopelessness to be a long-term but not a short-term predictor of suicide in a 10-year follow-up of patients with major affective disorder. Undermining the likelihood of their finding being meaningful is the fact that all the subjects were under psychiatric care. Before the short-term significance of hopelessness is dismissed, proof will be required that the manifestations of hopelessness did not activate more vigorous or protective intervention on the part of the treating psychiatrists.

What is the utility to the clinician of the knowledge that his or her patient may, at some future time, take his or her life? As Pokorny (1983) has pointed out, "In each case, the decision is not what to do for all time, but rather what to do next, for the near future." Rather than pursue the chimera of prediction, we must focus on identifying those factors which signal heightened *risk* of suicide. Given that certain psychiatric illnesses confer the primary risk, one must next be aware of how further risk factors differ between diagnoses.

ASSESSMENT OF RISK OF SUICIDE

Suicide is a volitional act, one that is nearly always preceded by planning. As Beskow (1979) has said, "Suicide does not just happen. It has a history." Discovering that history at the clinical level provides useful tools for the identification of those persons with a substantially increased likelihood of taking their lives. This is the assessment of suicidal risk.

Communication of Suicidal Intent

Two-thirds (Robins et al., 1959) to four-fifths (Beskow, 1979) of suicides have communicated their thoughts of death or their suicidal intent to others. They characteristically do so to more than one person, on more than one occasion, and in more than one way. The most common means is the direct statement of intent, e.g., "I'm going to kill myself" or "I'm going to jump in the river." Around 40 percent of suicides are reported to have given such clear notice (Robins et al., 1959; Dorpat and Ripley, 1960).

Other ways of communicating intent include assertions of a desire to die, of belief that one's self or one's family would be better off for the death, reference to methods of suicide, and dire predictions. Examples of the last category are such statements as, "You'll find a dead man in the street" and "This is your last kiss." A history of one or more suicide attempts is found in one-third of cases, but more often in women. The suicide attempt might have been recent or remote, belonging to an earlier episode. Suicidal ideas may have been expressed for years or only more recently. Where the communication was of long-standing, there had been an increase in such behavior in the past year. As common as suicidal communication may be among the psychiatrically ill, the physician must always ask if self-destructive thoughts are present. If present, the clinical status and other risk factors must be assessed.

The starting point is identification of the presence of certain psychiatric illnesses. Failure to diagnose leaves the patient untreated and vulnerable to suicide (Murphy, 1975). A diagnosis of major depressive disorder, of alcohol/substance abuse, or of schizophrenia already places the patient at a many-fold increase in risk, since the three-fourths of the population that are free of psychiatric disorders are also virtually free of the likelihood of suicide. One-quarter of the adult population represents a huge pool of false-positive results. This is not the serious problem that *false-positive* seems to imply, since it is never inappropriate to treat these disorders.

Risk Factors for Suicide in Affective Disorders

There is little evidence of external precipitation in the suicides of persons with a primary diagnosis of major depressive disorder. Recent loss or disruption of a close interpersonal relationship is infrequent (Murphy and Robins, 1967; Rich et al., 1988). Thoughts of death and of suicide are a hallmark of depression. They are so ubiquitous as to form one of the criterion symptoms for the diagnosis of the disorder. Being so common, however, limits their predictive value. It is unclear what else must be present to transform the thought into action, except a mental state of hopelessness (Beck et al., 1990). Living alone may be a risk factor, having been found to be twice as frequent in suicides with this disorder as in the general population (Murphy and Robins, 1967). Duration of the depression does not correlate strongly. Usually it is well established, having lasted for months or even years. Occasionally it may have been present for only a few days or weeks. Persons with uncomplicated affective disorder have not been shown to be at risk when manic or between episodes (Robins et al., 1959; Robins, 1981). No other risk factors have been identified. The depressive's internal state seems to be critical.

One sometimes hears it said that there is little to fear from suicide in patients with a severely retarded depression. "They just can't get up the energy." The statement betrays a lack of knowledge. Such patients can and do commit suicide. A more frequently heard statement is that risk is greatest when the depression starts to lift. It has not been shown that the suicidal urge increases with symptomatic improvement. More likely, opportunity for suicide increases as protective measures are relaxed.

Alcohol/Substance Abuse

Alcoholism is a chronic disorder in which a variety of risk factors play a role. Unlike depressives, alcoholics tend to be highly reactive to environmental cues. Loss of a close interpersonal relationship within 6 weeks of self-inflicted deaths of alcoholic suicides is both significantly greater than chance ($p < 0.01$) and different from the experience of depressives (Murphy and Robins, 1967; Rich et al., 1988). The finding regarding recent loss has been replicated in two other series of alcoholic suicides (Murphy et al., 1979; Rich et al., 1988). Recent loss characterizes suicide among abusers of other psychoactive substances to an equal extent (Rich et al., 1988). This very strongly replicated finding has considerable standing as a predictor of risk of suicide in psychoactive substance abusers. Nevertheless, it can be held accountable for no more than one-fourth to two-fifths of such deaths. What gives loss such potency? In 19 of 20 cases, the loss occurred on a background of progressively diminished social support. Often, what was lost was the last remaining relationship (Murphy, 1992).

Certain subacute and chronic features have recently been shown to have a cumulative relationship to risk of suicide. They include continued drinking up to the time of the act, communication of suicidal thoughts, lack of social support, the development of a comorbid major depression, serious medical illness, unemployment, and living alone. Their frequency in the 82 subjects of two combined series of alcoholic suicides (Robins, 1981; Murphy et al., 1979) is shown in Table 32-3. Nearly four-fifths of the suicides had accumulated four or more of these seven factors and 9 of 10 had at least three of them (Table 32-4) (Murphy et al., 1992). Living alcoholics have opposite frequency distributions of these features, as do primarily depressed suicides. This suggests the desirability of monitoring the level of risk as these factors accumulate. Active intervention becomes increasingly urgent with each new development. Securing a patient's abstinence will arrest the downhill slide, but is not easily or often achieved. Treating the comorbid depression is often more to the point (Murphy, et al., 1992).

TABLE 32-3. *Risk Factors for Suicide in Alcoholics, Based on 82 Unselected Cases*

Factors	Frequency of occurrence (%)
Current heavy drinking	98
Talk or threat of suicide	84
Major depression	60
Little social support	70
Serious medical problem	51
Unemployed	56
Living alone	43
Recent loss of relationship	38

From Murphy GE: Suicide in Alcoholism. New York, Oxford University Press, 1992.

TABLE 32-4. *Distribution of Seven Subacute Risk Factors* in 82 Alcoholic Suicides*

Number of risk factors per subject	Number of subjects
0	0
1	1
2	5
3	11
4	19
5	27
6	11
7	8

*The risk factors are current heavy drinking, talk of suicide, little or no social support, major depressive episode, unemployment, serious medical disorder, and living alone.
From Murphy GE: Suicide in Alcoholism. New York, Oxford University Press, 1992, Table 9.8, p 223.

Age and number of years of drinking are additional risk factors. Age is related in a curvilinear way. The greatest numbers of alcoholic suicides are in their 40s and 50s. Few are past age 60. The ranks of alcoholics become thinned through premature deaths from other causes as well as late-developing abstinence. The mean duration of abusive drinking approaches 20 years, but the range is wide. Treatment is also relevant. The lifetime risk of suicide in alcoholics not previously hospitalized is around 2 percent; for those with a history of inpatient treatment, it is about 3.4 percent (Murphy and Wetzel, 1990). The reason for this seeming reversal is that mainly the more severely afflicted receive hospitalization.

Abuse of other psychoactive substances is found predominantly in younger suicides, those under age 40, mostly 30 and younger. Alcohol is usually abused as well. The duration of psychoactive substance abuse leading to suicide is shorter than that for alcohol, with a median around 12 years (Rich et al., 1989). The fact that nonalcoholic substance abusers show the identical rate of recent interpersonal loss as alcoholics (Rich et al., 1988) suggests that the other risk factors just described will prove to be similarly predictive.

Schizophrenia

Suicide in schizophrenia appears to be more often impulsive than in other psychiatric disorders. The data base is not robust, but several identifying features have been noted. Among these are chronic course of the disorder, severe social/vocational disability, nonpsychotic awareness of the limitations imposed by that disability, and a history of one or more previous suicide attempts (Drake et al., 1985; Nyman and Jonsson, 1986). It is not the case, however, that suicide is confined to the young with this disorder or that all the characteristics just mentioned are necessarily present. Opinions differ as to the importance of a complicating depression. There is little support for indicting command hallucinations, as likely as that might seem. Rather, the suicide seems usually to occur in a quiescent period, when psychotic manifestations have ebbed. These finding are of little clinical utility from a prediction standpoint, as they are commonly encountered features of the disorder. A suicide attempt or other communication of suicidal thoughts must be taken seriously and responded to with emotional support to help the patient adjust to a more limited future.

Organic Brain Disorders

Little has been found to predict suicide risk in the presence of delirium or dementia. Impulse is more likely than planning and is difficult to guard against. Complicating depression is a danger signal. Restricting opportunity for defenestration is advised.

Personality Disorders

Suicides given borderline and unspecified personality disorder diagnoses will have additional diagnoses of antisocial personality disorder (ASPD), affective disorder, substance abuse disorder, or more than one of these. Suicide is rarely encountered in ASPD unless it is complicated by psychoactive substance abuse and/or a major depression. The risk inheres in the affective or substance abuse component. Suicide attempts are common in persons diagnosed with personality disorder. The acts may be multiple and sometimes end in a completed suicide. The frankly manipulative behavior that either characterizes or incites the diagnosis makes both treatment and protection difficult.

PREVENTING SUICIDES

Suicide is an infrequent event in anyone's clinical practice, so the danger is easily forgotten. About half of all suicides have consulted a physician within a month or less of the fatal act, although not often for treatment of the psychiatric illness giving rise to their self-destructive bent. Typically, that illness has gone unrecognized, untreated, or undertreated (Barraclough et al., 1974; Murphy, 1975; Brent et al., 1988; Åsgård, 1990). Interviews with physicians who had lost a patient to suicide showed that they readily recognized depressed mood, but they had often failed to identify the syndrome of depression (Murphy, 1975). As a consequence, they failed to treat it. Some recognized the syndrome but viewed it as a psychosocial phenomenon rather than as an illness. Having an explanation in terms of the patient's life situation, they did not treat. It is well to keep in mind Fawcett's (1972) pithy aphorism: "The presence of a 'reason' for depression does not constitute a reason for ignoring its presence." Those patients who take their lives have fallen through the diagnostic net. Much larger numbers of sufferers from these same disorders do receive better treatment. This is the best general evidence that psychiatric treatment is preventive. The fundamental rule of suicide prevention is to treat the underlying psychiatric disorder.

Despite the prevalence of antemortem communication of suicidal thoughts, few physicians attending suicides—only about one in six—seem to have been aware of it (Murphy, 1975). Because there is some evidence that suicidal patients will tell a physician if asked (DeLong and Robins, 1961), it seems likely that such patients often were not asked. In a few cases, patients denied to a physician the intention they carried out. The old wives' tale that "those who talk about it won't do it" is just that. Those who talk about it may indeed do it. It is important to ask each depressed or alcoholic patient about suicidal thoughts. The fear of implanting an idea that may be acted on is unjustified. Most depressed or alcoholic patients have already thought of it. Many are relieved to be asked. Ask family members as well whether there has been talk of suicide. The patient who has a fully formulated plan and the means available to carry it out requires close surveillance. Admission to the closed ward of a psychiatric unit is the safest measure.

Affective Disorders

External precipitants are found to play a very minor role in suicide in these disorders. Rather, it is the internal state, particularly a sense of hopelessness, that gives rise to fatal action. Suicide risk runs with the disorder, remitting when the depression remits. Antidepressants act slowly on the roots of the disorder, dispelling hopelessness only uncertainly. Psychotherapy is slower yet. Suicide can occur at any stage of the episode, so one's first thought must be of protection. Hospitalization will not always prevent a suicide, but the risk is greatly reduced when vigorous treatment is provided in a well-designed facility with a well-trained staff. For the seriously suicidal, electroconvulsive therapy (ECT) is the treatment of choice. Suicides occur with increased frequency in the weeks immediately following hospital discharge (Temoche et al., 1964; Ettlinger, 1975). Discharge sometimes occurs too early. In addition, on discharge, many patients are given a next appointment weeks away. After seeing the doctor daily during the hospital stay, this may be experienced as abandonment. A modest downturn in mood may then more readily give rise to renewed feelings of hopelessness.

It is better to treat depression before it evolves to a seriously suicidal state. Rutz et al. (1989) have shown that increased physician awareness of depression and its treatment can actually reduce suicides. On the Swedish island of Gotland (population 56,000), they carried out a 2-year project designed "to increase GPs' knowledge of diagnosis and treatment of depressive disorders . . . " and to evaluate the outcome. Ninety percent of permanently employed general practitioners attended, and copies of the educational materials were distributed to the remainder. The suicide rate on Gotland declined during the second year of the program and dropped very significantly ($p < 0.01$) the following year, while remaining stable in Sweden as a whole. Early recognition and treatment of the underlying disorder are clearly both effective and lifesaving.

Substance Abuse Disorder

In principle, we should be able to devise preventive strategies for psychoactive substance abuse. In practice, we lack the necessary understanding of their mechanism(s). Our treatment interventions are no more effective today than they were 50 years ago (Murphy, 1992, Chap. 10). Perhaps that is so because we are practicing the wrong interventions

(Miller and Hester, 1986). Nevertheless, as disappointing as the results may be, they are not negligible and should not be neglected. More readily amenable is the depression that supervenes.

The effectiveness of antidepressants in the treatment of alcoholism has been little studied. A number of disappointing treatment trials have addressed the ability of tricyclic antidepressants to reduce *drinking behavior*, not depression. One recent study assessed the impact of such treatment on depression. Keeping in mind the need for higher medication dosage in substance abusers, it was favorable (Mason and Kocsis, 1991). Since it is never inappropriate to treat an identifiable depression, this will be the treatment of choice when depression is present. The incidence of depression accompanying alcoholism in the community may be as low as 5 percent (Regier et al., 1990). It is substantially more frequent in studies of hospitalized alcoholics, where it plays a role in bringing the alcoholic to treatment (Mason and Kocsis, 1991). Most suicidal crises do not end in death. At the same time, a miscalculation is irretrievable. Overtreatment is not the mistake it might be with other conditions. Undertreatment is. Whether or not the depressed or alcoholic patient is as suicidal as he or she appears, there is considerable suffering from the illness. The likelihood of a favorable response to treatment is good.

Others

The apparent impulsiveness of suicide in schizophrenia and in organic brain disorders offers scant promise of specific preventive measures. However, a majority of these deaths take place in hospitals, so attention to physical aspects of the building can be protective. Limitation of the extent to which windows can be opened and barring patient access to elevated balconies and rooftops are obvious steps. At another level, unbreakable window glass, recessed shower heads, and breakaway ventilator grilles, clothing rods, and shower curtains add a measure of safety.

It is not possible in every case to prevent suicide. A few give no warning. Some individuals hide not only the depth of their despair but also their suicidal thoughts and plans from even those closest to them. This has been called the *executive suicide* because of the self-contained, decisive way in which it is accomplished. The symptoms of depression may not even be recognized in retrospect. Physicians and other professionals who kill themselves often fit this description. Much more commonly, however, suicides communicate both their distress and their suicidal thoughts to others. Some patients are chronically suicidal despite all efforts. When failure of prevention occurs, it should be in spite of the appropriate treatment rather than on account of its absence.

ATTEMPTED SUICIDE

Definition

Attempted suicide is any *act*, including overdose, cutting, or otherwise producing tissue injury, that is so labeled by the person undertaking it or by those involved in that person's care. It does not include threats, however dangerous, such as standing on a ledge of a high building. There is no utility, other than a pejorative one, in characterizing one act as a "gesture" and another as "genuine." They share the same background, purpose, and prognosis.

Journal articles and books continue to be published with titles identifying the subject matter as suicide but in which the population reported on was all still living. The persistent confusion of suicide attempt with suicide in this literature is both frustrating and misleading. Incautious statements about suicide that have only, or principally, to do with suicide attempters are one result.

There is more reason than semantics to distinguish between these two phenomena. Suicides are three times as likely to be men as women. They are about equally frequent before and after age 40. They are most commonly suffering from one of two major psychiatric illnesses. They usually plan the act, choose rapidly effective means, and use them in isolation or with provisions made to forestall interruption. The purpose is to die. In contrast, suicide attempters are predominantly women (2:1). They are mostly under age 40 and are less likely to be suffering from one of the psychiatric illnesses most commonly associated with suicide. They usually act impulsively and use ineffective or slowly effective means. They carry out the act in the presence of others or notify others of what they are about to do or have just done; i.e., they make provisions for rescue. The purpose is to survive. The principal feature that the two behaviors have in common is the terminology. Attempted suicide is not failed suicide.

Etiology and Pathogenesis

Maris (1981), in an extensive study of 266 suicides controlled by 64 suicide attempters and 71 natural deaths, explored the concept of "suicidal careers." He hoped to be able to characterize the life course of individuals dying by suicide and to produce a general theory of suicide. As it turned out, a number of historical and clinical variables he had expected to be strongly correlated with suicide were more strikingly associated with attempted suicide. These included early separation from a parent, early traumatic experiences, coming from a multiproblem family, heavy drinking, heavy drug use, "sexual deviation," negative interaction, and history of suicide attempt. These features were not altogether lacking among suicides, but they were generally lowest among those dying natural deaths. Characteristics most often associated with suicide were hardly surprises: older age, male sex, hopelessness, and view of death as escape from pain. The supposed pathogenetic features that Maris identified among suicides were more strongly characteristic of his only living group: suicide attempters. Few of this group will become suicides.

Who may attempt suicide? Diagnostically, there is an overlap with suicide. Around one fourth to one third of attempters are clinically depressed. About an equal proportion are alcoholics or abusers of other substances. Diagnoses that are uncommon among suicides, such as somatization disorder (Briquet's syndrome) and antisocial personality disorder, are seen with considerable frequency among suicide attempters. These and other personality disorders together may constitute upward of 40 percent of a suicide attempt population (Murphy and Wetzel, 1982). In some studies, all the attempters have been judged psychiatrically ill (Schmidt et al., 1954). In others, from 5 percent (Ettlinger and Flordh, 1955; Murphy and Wetzel, 1982) to 20 percent (Dahlgren, 1945) were thought not to be ill. Although the depressed patient who makes a suicide attempt may not, at the moment, be bent on self-destruction, the potential is there. To a somewhat lesser extent, the same may be said for the alcoholic.

Follow-up studies of attempters show that 1 to 2 percent will take their lives within 1 year of the index event and 1 percent annually thereafter (Ettlinger, 1975, p. 100). The few follow-up studies that exceed 10 years suggest that the incidence may flatten off later—it does not go up endlessly. Much the longest such study (Dahlgren, 1977) found that 10.9 percent (14 percent of men and 8.8 percent of women) had taken their lives over 31 to 45 years following a suicide attempt. The lifetime risk of suicide among suicide attempters is perhaps a bit above 10 percent. Such grave morbidity as there is in attempted suicide (social impairment, subsequent hospitalization, suicide) is generally attributable to the underlying psychiatric condition and not to the attempt itself.

There is a familial aspect to suicide attempt. In my series of 127 cases (Murphy and Wetzel, 1982), 34 percent reported a family history of suicide attempt and 20 percent a history of suicide in the family. Others have reported lower frequencies, but it is not always clear how diligently the information had been sought.

Responses to inquiry as to motivation tend to be highly idiosyncratic. They lend themselves poorly to tabulation. One strategy for constraining the free-form response is to offer a series of likely responses for endorsement. Using this method with 128 attempters, Bancroft and colleagues (1976) obtained the following frequencies: seeking help, 33 percent; relief from a state of mind, 52 percent; influence someone, 19 percent; "wanting to die,"

38 percent; don't care if live or die, 34 percent; none of these, 18 percent. Responses overlap and often conflict. Bancroft et al. caution that the endorsement of "wanting to die" should not be taken at face value. Respondents often feel a need to save face—to make the act appear more socially acceptable. The same may be said for a number of other responses. Wanting to influence someone (19 percent) is surely a gross underestimate.

When asked, attempters will cite more than one problem. Yet the purpose of the act is mostly the same. Behind the great majority of attempts lies a wish to make an impact on another person's awareness. The act generally takes place in a social context. It is literally a cry for help. A specific recipient of the message is readily identifiable in most instances. Some change is sought, whether in the recipient's attitude or behavior or in the relationship. The distress is genuine, although the method of communication is unconventional. Often it follows a period of failure of more customary efforts at communication. The final straw that triggers the behavior may in itself have been trivial. To the uninformed observer, the act may appear petulant and capricious, when in fact it expresses desperation. For some, it reaches the stage of "I don't care if I live or die"; for a few, the genuine hope is to die.

Epidemiology

Attempted suicide is not a reportable act, so there are no national or local statistics. Sampling is likely to be strongly biased according to the catchment area chosen. Where most admissions are to a single facility, as in Edinburgh (Kreitman, 1977), it appears that the lower socioeconomic classes are overrepresented. Despite law or custom, those with more means may circumvent the established treatment program.

Attempted suicide is many times more frequent than suicide. Just how much more has been the subject of much opinion and a little research. Estimates range from 5 to 100 times as frequent. Parkin and Stengel (1965) conducted the most methodologically rigorous study. In the city of Sheffield, England, they found attempted suicides to outnumber suicides by 9.7:1 over a 2-year period. A later careful study by Kreitman (1977, p. 160) in Edinburgh gave a ratio of about 7:1. Studies of comparable quality have not been reported from the United States.

Jacobziner (1965) compared suicides with attempts by poisoning in adolescents aged 12 to 20 years in New York City during 1960–1961. He found a surprising ratio of about 100:1 for this restricted age-group. It may be this figure that has been cited by others without specification of the age group examined, since there is no other documentation for it. The suicide rate among the young has tripled in the intervening time. Whether the incidence of suicide attempts has increased proportionately is unknown. For the population as a whole, there is no clear evidence for an attempted suicide/suicide ratio greater than 10:1.

Clinical Picture

A large minority of suicide attempters come from families in which suicide or attempted suicide has occurred. There is frequently a background of a broken home or social deprivation. Nearly all attempters suffer from chronic low self-esteem. Their interpersonal skills are poor. While desiring the company and support of others, they have not learned to develop and maintain such relationships. Those they do have tend to be formed with exploitative, insensitive individuals. The social class structure of the suicide attempt population is skewed toward the low end. Many of these individuals live unsatisfying, frustrated lives marred by their own social ineptitude. A specific problem is often engrafted on a chronically frustrating life situation. Partly because of poor communication skills, partly because of a nonreciprocal relationship, problems seem insurmountable. Hopelessness is commonly reported (Dyer and Kreitman, 1984). The final straw may be quite small. Alcohol consumption is a frequent releaser of the act.

Attempters tend to use what is at hand. Eighty to 90 percent of suicide attempts are by overdose. Aspirin is found in nearly every medicine cabinet. It is favored by the youngest segment of the attempter population—adolescents. More often, hypnotics, sedatives, and pain killers are swallowed. In the midst of an argument, the attempter may angrily or tearfully run to the medicine cabinet and start gulping pills. More often she (more than two-thirds are women) sits brooding and then starts to swallow her medication, one or a few capsules at a time until she becomes sleepy or alarmed. She may do this in a place where others are sure to come soon. Otherwise, she will call someone and let it be known what she has just done. The message may be direct or by means of slurred or incoherent speech. The rescue has been arranged.

About 10 percent of suicide attempts are by cutting or piercing. Most of this is lateral laceration of the wrist. An older literature describes wrist cutters as attractive, intelligent young women who repeat the act endlessly. While such persons exist, two-thirds as many wrist cutters are male as female. Proportional to the number of attempters of each sex, more males than females cut. Repetition is not particularly characteristic of them (Clendenin and Murphy, 1971; Weissman, 1975). There is a tendency for persons making more medically serious attempts to have a poorer prognosis, both psychiatrically and with respect to subsequent repetition. The patient who gives a self-oriented reason for the act (depressed, guilty, want to die) is at higher risk than the one whose behavior is in reaction to external circumstances. It is also the case that the more

closely the suicide attempter resembles suicides (in age, sex, motivation, psychiatric diagnosis, evidence of planning), the greater is the risk of subsequent suicide (Pallis et al., 1984).

Clinical Management

The majority of overdoses present little danger to life. The management of acute poisonings is best left to the clinical toxicologist. I recommend hospital admission for all attempters. Both the medical and the psychiatric seriousness of the act must be evaluated. Experts agree that the apparent triviality of the act is no guide to the overall risk. A minor overdose may result from the unexpected interruption of a serious effort to end life. Minor lacerations of the wrist may be a trial run before a more determined effort. Without careful psychiatric assessment, the patient's potential for suicide must not be assumed. One-third of suicides are preceded by a suicide attempt. Denial of suicidal intent cannot—indeed must not—be taken at face value. The patient may be seeking early release in order to complete an abortive attempt. Patients with depression, alcoholism, schizophrenia, or an organic brain syndrome are at increased risk. Treatment of the underlying psychiatric condition is central to suicide prevention.

In addition to clinical evaluation, the hospital admission provides an ideal opportunity to bring the patient and others concerned together for a frank discussion of the issues that led to the act. If each person in turn is allowed to voice his or her version of the issues, the stage is set for negotiation. The psychiatrist's role is to ensure that each person has an opportunity to express his or her views without interruption and to facilitate discussion. A resolution need not be reached. Opening the communication will usually suffice. Further psychotherapy may be offered if indicated. The great majority of attempters do not repeat the act.

The attention-seeking aspect of the attempt and the attempter should be reinforced only within clinically indicated limits. The patient should not be allowed to exploit the hospital admission for social purposes. To this end, I recommend no personal telephone or television, strict limitation of visiting privileges, and no off-unit privileges during a stay that is as short as feasible to accomplish the clinical goals. This restrictive program does not include aloofness on the part of the physician. Warmth, acceptance, and understanding are appropriate attitudes for the therapist to exhibit. Medical and nursing staff attitudes, particularly in the emergency and intensive care units, tend to be somewhat harsh and distant toward the suicide attempter. Because these people are involved in acute life-preserving activities, they tend to view the suicide attempter's voluntary endangering of his or her life as antithetical to their values. It is possible to soften this attitude by interpreting the personal distress that is the background for the behavior. Attempted suicide is a desperate act and necessitates understanding.

REFERENCES

Achté KA, Vauhkonen ML: Suicides committed in general hospitals. Psychiatr Fenn 221–228, 1971.

Allgulander C, Lavori PW: Excess mortality among 3302 patients with 'pure' anxiety neurosis. Arch Gen Psychiatry 48: 599–602, 1991.

American Psychiatric Association Committee on Nomenclature and Statistics: Diagnostic and Statistical Manual of Mental Disorders, 2d ed (DSM-II). Washington, American Psychiatric Association, 1968.

American Psychiatric Association: Diagnostic and Statistical Manual of Mental Disorders, 3d ed revised (DSM-IIIR). Washington, American Psychiatric Association, 1987.

Andreasen NC, Hoenk PR: The predictive value of adjustment disorders: A follow-up study. Am J Psychiatry 139:584–590, 1982.

Arató M, Demeter E, Rihmer Z, Somogyi E: Retrospective psychiatric assessment of 200 suicides in Budapest. Acta Psychiatr Scand 77:454–456, 1988.

Åsgård U: A psychiatric study of suicide among urban Swedish women. Acta Psychiatr Scand 82:115–124, 1990.

Bancroft JHJ, Skrimshire AM, Simkin S: The reasons people give for taking overdoses. Br J Psychiatry 128:538–548, 1976.

Barraclough B, Bunch J, Nelson B, Sainsbury P: A hundred cases of suicide: Clinical aspects. Br J Psychiatry 125:355–373, 1974.

Beck AT, Brown G, Berchick RJ, et al: Relationship between hopelessness and ultimate suicide: A replication with psychiatric outpatients. Am J Psychiatry 147:190–195, 1990.

Beck AT, Weissman A, Lester D, Trexler L: The measurement of pessimism: The hopelessness scale. J Consult Clin Psychol 42:861–865, 1974.

Beskow J: Suicide and mental disorder in Swedish men. Acta Psychiatr Scand Suppl. 277:1–138, 1979.

Blachly PH, Osterud HT, Josslin R: Suicide in professional groups. N Engl J Med 268:1278–1281, 1963.

Brent DA, Perper JA, Allman CJ: Alcohol, firearms and suicide among youth: Temporal trends in Allegheny County, Pennsylvania, 1960 to 1963. JAMA 267:3369–3372, 1987.

Brent DA, Perper JA, Goldstein CE, et al: Risk factors for adolescent suicide. Arch Gen Psychiatry 45:581–588, 1988.

Chynoweth R, Tonge JI, Armstrong J: Suicide in Brisbane: A retrospective psychosocial study. Aust NZ J Psychiatry 14: 37–45, 1980.

Clendenin WW, Murphy GE: Wrist cutting: New epidemiological findings. Arch Gen Psychiatry 25:465–469, 1971.

Conwell Y, Caine ED, Olsen K: Suicide and cancer in late life. Hosp Commun Psychiatry 41:1334–1339, 1990.

Coryell W: Panic disorder and mortality. Psychiatr Clin North Am 11:433–440, 1988.

Dahlgren KG: On Suicide and Attempted Suicide: A Psychiatrical and Statistical Investigation. Lund, Linstedts Univ. Bokhandel, 1945.

Dahlgren KG: Attempted suicide: 35 years afterward. Suicide Life Threat Behav 7:75–79, 1977.

Delong WB, Robins E: The communication of suicidal intent prior to psychiatric hospitalization: A study of 87 patients. Am J Psychiatry 117:695–705, 1961.

Dorpat TL, Ripley HS: A study of suicide in the Seattle area. Compr Psychiatry 1:349–359, 1960.

Drake RE, Gates C, Whitaker A, Cotton PG: Suicide among schizophrenics: A review. Compr Psychiatry 26:90–100, 1985.

DAWN (Drug Abuse Warning Newwork), United States Department of Justice, Drug Enforcement Administration, 1982.

DAWN (Drug Abuse Warning Newwork), United States Department of Justice, Drug Enforcement Administration, 1991.

Dyer JAT, Kreitman N: Hopelessness, depression and suicidal intent in parasuicide. Br J Psychiatry 144:127–133, 1984.

Egeland JA, Sussex JN: Suicide and family loading for affective disorders. JAMA 254:915–918, 1985.

Ettlinger R: Evaluation of suicide prevention after attempted suicide. Acta Psychiatr Scand Suppl 260:135, 1975.

Ettlinger RW, Flordh P: Attempted suicide: Experience of five hundred cases at a general hospital. Acta Psychiatr Neurol Scand Suppl 103:1–45, 1955.

Fawcett J: Suicidal depression and physician illness. JAMA 219:1303–1306, 1972.

Fawcett J, Scheftner WA, Fogg L, et al: Time-related predictors of suicide in major affective disorder. Am J Psychiatry 147:1189–1194, 1990.

Fowler RC, Rich CL, Young D: San Diego suicide study: II. Substance abuse in young cases. Arch Gen Psychiatry 43:962–965, 1986.

Guze SB, Cloninger CR, Martin RL, Clayton PJ: A follow-up and family study of Briquet's syndrome. Br J Psychiatry 149:17–23, 1986.

Haberlandt W: Aportacion a la genetica del suicido. Folia Clin Int 17:319–322, 1967.

Hagnell O, Rorsman B: Suicide in the Lundby study: A comparative investigation of clinical aspects. Neuropsychobiology 5:61–73, 1979.

Holding TA, Barraclough BM: Undetermined deaths: Suicide or accident? Br J Psychiatry 133:542–549, 1978.

Jacobziner H: Attempted suicides in adolescence. JAMA 191:7–11, 1965.

Kapamadžija B, Biro M, Sovljanski M: Socio-Psihijatrijska: I. Patomorfoloska Analiza 100 Izvrsenih Samoubistava. Soc Psihijat 10:35–56, 1982.

Kreitman N: Parasuicide. New York; John Wiley & Sons, 1977.

Li FP: Suicide among chemists. Arch Environ Health 19:518–520, 1969.

Litman RE, Curphey T, Shneidman ES, et al: Investigations of equivocal suicides. JAMA 184:924–929, 1963.

Maris RW: Pathways to Suicide: A Survey of Self-Destructive Behaviors. Baltimore: Johns Hopkins University Press, 1981.

Marttunen MJ, Aro H, Henriksson MM, Lonnqvist JK: Mental disorders in adolescent suicide: DSM-IIIR axes I and II diagnoses in suicides among 13- to 19-year-olds in Finland. Arch Gen Psychiatry 48:834–839, 1991.

Mason BJ, Kocsis JH: Desipramine treatment of alcoholism. Psychopharmacol Bull 27:155–161, 1991.

Mausner JS, Steppacher RC: Suicide in professionals: A study of male and female psychologists. Am J Epidemiol 98: 436–445, 1973.

Meehan PJ, Saltzman LE, Sattin RW: Suicide among older United States residents: Epidemiologic characteristics and trends. Am J Public Health 81:1198–1200, 1991.

Miller WR, Hester RK: The effectiveness of alcoholism treatment: What research shows. In Miller WR, Heather NH (eds): Treating Addictive Behaviors. New York, Plenum Press, 1986.

Mitterauer B: Mehrdimensionale Diagnostik von 121 Suiziden im Bundesland Salzburg im Jahre 1978. Wien Med Wochenschr 9:229–234, 1981.

Mitterauer B: A contribution to the discussion of the role of the genetic factor in suicide, based on five studies in an epidemiologically defined area (province of Salzburg, Austria). Compr Psychiatry 31:557–565, 1990.

Morrison JR: Suicide in a psychiatric practice population. J Clin Psychiatry 43:348–352, 1982.

Murphy GE: The physician's responsibility for suicide: II. Errors of omission. Ann Intern Med 82:305–309, 1975.

Murphy GE: Suicide in Alcoholism. New York, Oxford University Press, 1992.

Murphy GE, Robins E: Social factors in suicide. JAMA 199: 303–308, 1967.

Murphy GE, Wetzel RD: Suicide risk by birth cohort in the United States, 1949 to 1974. Arch Gen Psychiatry 37:519–523, 1980.

Murphy GE, Wetzel RD: Family history of suicidal behavior among suicide attempters. J Nerv Ment Dis 170:86–90, 1982.

Murphy GE, Wetzel RD: The lifetime risk of suicide in alcoholism. Arch Gen Psychiatry 47:383–392, 1990.

Murphy GE, Wetzel RD, Robins E, McEvoy L: Multiple risk factors predict suicide in alcoholism. Arch Gen Psychiatry 49: 459–463, 1992.

Murphy GE, Armstrong JW, Hermele SL, et al: Suicide and alcoholism: Interpersonal loss confirmed as a predictor. Arch Gen Psychiatry 36:65–69, 1979.

Nyman AK, Jonsson H: Patterns of self-destructive behaviour in schizophrenia. Acta Psychiatr Scand 73:252–262, 1986.

Ovenstone IMK: A psychiatric approach to the diagnosis of suicide and its effect upon the Edinburgh statistics. Br J Psychiatry 123:15–21, 1973.

Pallis DJ, Gibbons JS, Pierce DW: Estimating suicide risk among attempted suicides: II. Efficiency of predictive scales after the attempt. Br J Psychiatry 144:139–148, 1984.

Parkin D, Stengel E: Incidence of suicidal attempts in an urban community. Br Med J 2:133–138, 1965.

Pitts FN, Schuller AB, Rich CL, Pitts AF: Suicide among U.S. women physicians, 1967–1972. Am J Psychiatry 136: 694–696, 1979.

Pokorny AD: Prediction of suicide in psychiatric patients. Arch Gen Psychiatry 40:249–257, 1983.

Pokorny AD, Smith JP, Finch JR: Vehicular suicides. Life-Threat Behav 2:105–119, 1972.

Regier DA, Boyd JH, Burke JD Jr, et al: One-month prevalence of mental disorders in the United States: Based on five epidemiologic catchment area sites. Arch Gen Psychiatry 45: 977–986, 1988.

Regier DA, Farmer ME, Rae DS, et al: Comorbidity of mental disorders with alcohol and other drug abuse: Results from the epidemiologic catchment area (ECA) study. JAMA 264:2511–2518, 1990.

Rich CL, Fowler RC, Fogarty LA, Young D: San Diego suicide study: III. Relationships between diagnoses and stressors. Arch Gen Psychiatry 45:589–592, 1988.

Rich CL, Fowler RC, Young D: Substance abuse and suicide: The San Diego study. Ann Clin Psychiatry 1:79–85, 1989.

Rich CL, Sherman M, Fowler RC: San Diego suicide study: The adolescents. Adolescence 25:855–865, 1990.

Rich CL, Young D, Fowler RC: San Diego suicide study: I. Young vs old subjects. Arch Gen Psychiatry 43:577–582, 1986.

Robins E: The Final Months: A Study of the Lives of 134 Persons Who Committed Suicide. New York, Oxford University Press, 1981.

Robins E, Gassner S, Kayes J, et al: The communication of suicidal intent: A study of 134 consecutive cases of successful (completed) suicide. Am J Psychiatry 115:724–733, 1959.

Robins E, Murphy GE, Wilkinson RH, et al: Some clinical considerations in the prevention of suicide based on a study of 134 successful suicides. Am J Public Health 49:888–899, 1959.

Runeson B: Mental disorder in youth suicides: DSM-IIIR axes I and II. Acta Psychiatr Scand 79:490–497, 1989.

Runeson B, Beskow J: Borderline personality disorder in young Swedish suicides. J Nerv Ment Dis 179:153–156, 1991.

Rutz W, von Knorring L, Walinder J: Frequency of suicide on Gotland after systematic postgraduate education of general practitioners. Acta Psychiatr Scand 80:151–154, 1989.

Schmidt CW Jr, Perlin S, Townes W, et al: Characteristics of drivers involved in single-car accidents: A comparative study. Arch Gen Psychiatry 27:800–803, 1972.

Schmidt EH, O'Neal P, Robins E: Evaluation of suicide attempts as guide to therapy: Clinical and follow-up study of one hundred nine patients. JAMA 155:549–557, 1954.

Schulsinger F, Kety SS, Rosenthal D, Wender PH: A family study of suicide. In Schou M, Stromgren E (eds): Origin, Prevention and Treatment of Affective Disorder. New York, Academic Press, 1979, pp 278–287.

Shaffer D, Garland A, Gould M, et al: Preventing teenage suicide: A critical review. J Am Acad Child Adolesc Psychiatry 27: 675–687, 1988.

Shafii M, Stelz-Lenarsky J, Derrick AM, et al: Comorbidity of mental disorders in the post mortem diagnosis of completed suicide in children and adolescents. J Affective Disord 15:227–233, 1988.

Steppacher RC, Mausner JS: Suicide in male and female physicians. JAMA 228:323–328, 1974.

Temoche A, Pugh RF, MacMahon B: Suicide rates among current and former mental institution patients. J Nerv Ment Disord 138:124–130, 1964.

Vital Statistics of the United States, 1988, vol II: Mortality, part A. Washington, United States Department of Health and Human Services.

Weissman MM: Wrist cutting: Relationship between clinical observations and epidemiological findings. Arch Gen Psychiatry 32:1166–1171, 1975.

World Health Statistics Annual, 1990. Geneva: World Health Organization, 1991.

CHAPTER 33

Clinical Psychopharmacology and Other Somatic Therapies

PAUL J. PERRY
BRUCE ALEXANDER
MICHAEL J. GARVEY

SCHIZOPHRENIA AND OTHER PSYCHOSES

Members of antipsychotic classes (e.g., phenothiazine, butyrophenone, thioxanthene, dihydroindolone, and dibenzoxazepine) introduced in the United States between 1954 and 1979 are referred to as *typical antipsychotics*. The only *atypical* antipsychotic is clozapine.

Typical Antipsychotics

EFFICACY

The primary use of antipsychotics is in the management of schizophrenia. Improvement rates range from 40 to 75 percent. All antipsychotics are equally efficacious (Black et al., 1985; Kane, 1989; Davis, 1977; Remington, 1989).

Attempts to predict a response to a specific antipsychotic or to predict a response based on a patient's demographics (e.g., sex, socioeconomic or marital status), psychiatric history (e.g., age of onset, duration of illness, family history, premorbid characteristics), or clinical characteristics (e.g., specific symptoms, positive or negative symptoms) have not been successful (Kane, 1989; Remington, 1989; Ortiz et al., 1986; Awad, 1989).

The major therapeutic effect of antipsychotics is to ameliorate psychotic symptoms. There is a reduction but rarely elimination of such fundamental "core" target symptoms (i.e., "positive symptoms") as thought disorders (i.e., loose associations, conceptual disorganization), hallucinations, and delusions (Chandler and Winokur, 1989). Early studies reported that "negative symptoms" (e.g., emotional and social withdrawal, poverty of thought, flat affect, ambivalence, poor self-care) usually do not respond as well as positive symptoms. However, more recent literature indicates equal improvement between positive and negative symptoms (Awad, 1989; Breier et al., 1987; Kay et al., 1989; Remington, 1989; Tandon et al., 1989).

The rate of improvement varies among patients. Some improve within several days of the start of antipsychotic therapy. However, most early literature suggests that the greatest degree of therapeutic improvement usually occurs within the first 4 to 6 weeks of antipsychotic treatment, although 12 to 18 weeks of treatment was occasionally needed (Davis et al., 1977; Keck et al., 1989a). If a patient does not respond to an adequate trial of an antipsychotic of one chemical class, a drug in another class may be tried (Kane, 1989; Alexander, 1988; Marder et al., 1988).

The first acute episode of schizophrenia requires continuous antipsychotic treatment for at least 12 months. Unfortunately, there are no reliable predictors that can distinguish between patients who will maintain remission and those who will relapse (Davis et al., 1977; Johnson, 1985). Maintenance antipsychotic treatment in patients who have had two or more relapses is effective in reducing the morbidity associated with schizophrenia. Sixty-eight percent of patients with schizophrenia treated with placebo relapsed within 1 year after hospitalization. An additional 65 percent of the patients surviving the first year on placebo relapsed the next year. Patients treated with maintenance antipsychotics for 2 years relapsed at rates of only 41 and 15 percent at the end of 1 and 2 years, respectively. Thus maintenance antipsychotic treatment controls psychotic symptoms without altering the natural history of schizophrenia (Johnson, 1985).

A review of five studies reported noncompliance with oral antipsychotics to average 33 percent (Kane et al., 1985). Because constant drug intake is important in preventing relapse of symptoms and rehospitalization, long-acting parenteral antipsychotics (LAPA) are indicated for patients who are repeatedly noncompliant with oral medication (Kane, 1984; Johnson, 1984; Del Giudice et al., 1975). The high percentage of patients on drug treatment who do relapse suggests that nonpharmacologic factors (e.g., social and family environment) is also important.

A small number of studies support the efficacy of antipsychotics in the older person with schizophrenia; however, these patients deserve a dose-reduction or drug-discontinuation trial to determine a continuing need for maintenance antipsychotic treatment.

As a result of diagnostic ambiguity, the role of antipsychotics in the treatment of schizoaffective disorder is unclear. Most studies report improvement in psychotic symptoms in these patients. The exact response rate is unknown because of diagnostic heterogenicity between studies and, generally, small sample size (Delva et al., 1982). Schizophreniform illness is treated the same as schizophrenia, except that the patients receive antipsychotics for 6 months to 1 year after a psychotic episode (Davis et al., 1977).

Assuming equivalent doses, there are no data to support the practice of antipsychotic drug polypharmacy.

DOSING

All antipsychotics are equally effective in treating psychotic disorders when given in equipotent doses. For example, chlorpromazine 100 mg is approximately equal in therapeutic use to trifluoperazine 4 mg, thioridazine 100 mg, fluphenazine 2 mg, thiothixene 5 mg, or haloperidol 2 mg (Davis et al., 1977; McIntyre et al., 1985). Antipsychotics can be divided into low- or high-potency compounds based on their relative oral potency (Black et al., 1985; Rhoades et al., 1984).

A dose of chlorpromazine 300 mg/d PO or its equivalent is considered a minimal therapeutic dose for the treatment of acute psychosis. Dose–response studies in schizophrenic patients indicated that the peak response occurred at approximately chlorpromazine 600 mg/d or its equivalent (Baldessarini et al., 1988). Doses of chlorpromazine >1200 mg/d or its equivalent do not produce substantially greater improvement than smaller doses (Davis

et al., 1977; McIntyre et al., 1985; Baldessarini et al., 1988). However, patients do respond to widely differing dosages. Although the Food and Drug Administration (FDA) has set the maximum daily dose of thioridazine at 800 mg, there is no absolute daily maximum dose for any antipsychotic drug except thioridazine.

An acutely psychotic patient who is not uncontrollably agitated can be started on chlorpromazine 100 mg or its equivalent on a q8–12h schedule. The dose is gradually increased at a rate of chlorpromazine 100 to 200 mg/d or its equivalent until clinical response occurs, until the upper limit of the recommended dose range is reached, or until intolerable adverse effects occur. The medication should be administered at bedtime beginning a week after a stable dose is achieved.

Studies have demonstrated no significant difference in the degree of improvement or speed of improvement when oral loading doses of chlorpromazine >800 mg/d or its equivalent were compared with <800 mg/d (Baldessarini et al., 1988). Patients should initially receive chlorpromazine <800 mg/d or its equivalent, unless higher doses are known to be effective in the past (Baldessarini et al., 1988).

The immediate goal of treatment of an agitated, acutely psychotic patient is to reduce the agitation, irritability, and/or hostility so the patient is not a physical danger to himself or herself or others. Alleviation of the delusions and/or hallucinations, which are assumed to be the basis of the agitated behavior, is the ultimate goal.

The technique of titrating the antipsychotic dosage against psychotic symptomatology by administering a series of closely spaced parenteral doses over a period of hours is termed *rapid neuroleptization* (Ortiz et al., 1986). Due to the likelihood of impaired mental status and significant extrapyramidal side effects (EPSEs) that occur with high-dose antipsychotic treatment, this technique should be reserved for patients who are agitated and do not respond to conventional doses of antipsychotics. The patient receives chlorpromazine or its equivalent 100 mg PO or 25 mg IM q1–2h until agitation and psychosis are under control. Seldom is chlorpromazine >800 mg or its equivalent recommended or required in a 24-hour period (Baldessarini et al., 1988). As the result of chlorpromazine's cardiovascular adverse effects (e.g., hypotension), haloperidol 2 to 10 mg PO or IM q1/2–2 h has been recommended. Although haloperidol has been used extensively, there is evidence suggesting that other high-potency antipsychotics are equally safe and effective (Ortiz et al., 1986). After IM treatment, the dose of the antipsychotic administered PO should be equivalent to the preceding 24 hours of parenteral treatment corrected for bioavailability differences.

Uncontrolled trials have recommended benzodiazepines (BZDs) as a sole treatment or as an adjunct to antipsychotics for control of an agitated psychotic patient (Baldessarini et al., 1988; Gelenberg, 1986). Antipsychotics are the preferred treatment for controlling psychotic symptoms in the agitated patient. However, BZDs may play a role in the early (i.e., ≤1 week) control of agitation if recommended doses of antipsychotics have been ineffective for this symptom.

Uncontrolled trials using supranormal doses of antipsychotics have suggested that some patients respond better to high than to low doses of antipsychotics. Daily doses of chlorpromazine 5000 mg, fluphenazine 1500 mg, and haloperidol 100 mg and depot injections of fluphenazine enanthate starting at 250 mg have been used. However, a review of 11 double-blind studies failed to demonstrate a significant superiority of megadosing versus conventional dosing. Seven of these studies reported that EPSEs were more common in the high-dose groups. The review recommended that patients be considered refractory to conventional doses only after 4 to 6 months of treatment (Aubree et al., 1980). A more recent review of 33 studies agreed with the earlier recommendations (Baldessarini et al., 1988).

Maintenance doses must be individually determined based on patients' responses and their tolerance of adverse effects. Reviews of this literature suggest that high doses of antipsychotics are usually not necessary. Therefore, the majority of patients can be maintained on chlorpromazine 300 to 600 mg/d or its equivalent (Baldessarini et al., 1988). Once the patient enters outpatient treatment, a reasonable goal is to achieve a maintenance dose over the next 1 to 3 years. Because relapse of the symptoms may not occur for 3 months or longer after a dose reduction, dose changes should not be made more frequently (Johnson, 1985). Several antipsychotic discontinuation studies note that approximately 50 percent of the patients will relapse within 6 months after drug discontinuation (Davis et al., 1977).

A patient with an organic mental disorder may be unusually sensitive to the therapeutic and adverse effects of antipsychotics; therefore, chlorpromazine ≤300 mg/d or its equivalent is initially used. Dose titration then depends on therapeutic response and adverse effects (Raskind et al., 1986; Whalley, 1989).

Some antipsychotics are available for IM use; therefore, it is important to know the bioavailability of the PO versus IM dosage forms for proper dosing. For example, the IM form of chlorpromazine HCl is four times more bioavailable than an equivalent PO dose, so ≤25 mg IM would be required to yield the same blood concentration as chlorpromazine 100 mg PO (Hollister et al., 1963).

Long-acting parenteral antipsychotics (LAPA) available in the United States include the fluphenazine esters (e.g., decanoate, enanthate) and haloperidol decanoate. Fluphenazine decanoate is preferred to fluphenazine enanthate because of a lower incidence of adverse effects and a longer duration of action (Groves et al., 1975; Van Pragg et al., 1973). Only the decanoate ester of fluphenazine and haloperidol will be discussed.

Most clinicians recommend that patients being considered for a decanoate dosage form have their treatment initiated with a PO antipsychotic (Nair et al., 1986; Yadalam et al., 1988). Patients receiving PO antipsychotics other than fluphenazine or haloperidol should have their antipsychotic converted to the respective drug using relative oral potency. The rationale is that the PO form allows flexibility in daily dosing and the ability to quickly withdraw the drug if "significant" adverse effects occur. However, this practice requires the patient to be converted from PO to decanoate dosage form after clinical improvement. Typically, the patient who responds to an oral drug will be administered one or two injections of the decanoate as an inpatient with plans to taper the PO dose as an outpatient over a variable time period. However, once discharged, the patient may be noncompliant with the oral drug. This may significantly affect the total serum concentration of the antipsychotic, potentially leading to relapse. Likewise, noncompliance with the PO drug may lead to confusion about the required maintenance dose if the patient is continuously prescribed both the oral and depot antipsychotic (Johnson, 1985). Therefore, long-term use of this combination of dosage forms is not recommended.

The literature on conversion of PO fluphenazine to decanoate indicates a wide variability in recommended doses (Yadalam et al., 1988; Ereshefsky et al., 1984). Due to assay technical difficulties and significant interpatient variability in PO fluphenazine first-pass metabolism, serum concentration data comparing PO with decanoate doses indicate a poor relationship (Yadalam et al., 1988; Ereshefsky et al., 1984). Typical starting doses for fluphenazine decanoate range from 6.25 to 25 mg q2 wk (Yadalam et al., 1988).

Although loading doses of fluphenazine decanoate might alleviate the need for continuing PO fluphenazine during the conversion, this approach has not been investigated.

A review of four studies concluded that fluphenazine decanoate 10 to 30 mg q2wk provides the greatest protection against relapse. Interestingly, 45 mg q2wk was associated with a worse outcome (Baldessarini et al., 1988).

Fluphenazine decanoate has typically been administered on a weekly or biweekly schedule. One study reported that 30 percent of the patients could be maintained successfully when the drug was given at 3-week intervals, and 30 percent were maintained on monthly injections up to 1 year (Johnson, 1975). Another report indicated that 76 percent of the patients could be maintained on monthly injections for as long as 2 years (Marriott et al., 1984). In a more recent study, 30 percent of the patients were managed with monthly injections over an 8-month period (Chouinard et al., 1989). Patients stabilized on fluphenazine decanoate should be considered for an increased interval between injections as a dose reduction strategy.

Haloperidol PO to decanoate conversion presents similar concerns as fluphenazine. However, the metabolic pattern of haloperidol is less complicated (Beresford et al., 1987; Kane, 1986). Conversion recommendations based on haloperidol PO doses with and without a loading dose of the decanoate have been reported.

A review of U.S. studies indicated that a decanoate (mg/mo) to PO (mg/d) dose ratio of 10 to 15 was more reasonable than the European literature ratio of 20 (Kane, 1986). For example, using the U.S. studies' recommendations, if the patient was stabilized on 20 mg/d PO, then the decanoate dose would be 200 mg each month.

Like fluphenazine, no guidelines are available for initiating haloperidol decanoate and tapering the PO dose. Because steady-state haloperidol concentrations are not reached for 3 months with the decanoate, a tapering schedule of PO haloperidol similar to that of fluphenazine's is recommended. If adverse effects occur during this period, acceleration of the PO tapering might be considered.

Loading doses have been investigated to obviate the need for continuing PO drug therapy. A retrospective study reported stabilizing patients on haloperidol 16 ± 5 mg/d PO over 1 to 2 weeks. The patients received a haloperidol decanoate loading dose 20 to 25 times (370 ± 92 mg) the stabilized PO dose. The calculated loading dose was divided into three doses and administered every 3 to 7 days (e.g., 100 to 150 mg q3–7d). Oral haloperidol was immediately discontinued at the start of the loading dose. No increase in adverse effects nor loss of antipsychotic effect occurred during the first month after the loading dose. No information was available on subsequent decanoate maintenance doses. However, a conversion factor of 10 would yield a maintenance dose of approximately 150 mg every month in their patients (Ereshefsky et al., 1989a).

The usual haloperidol decanoate doses are 75 to 300 mg/mo, but 500 mg/mo has been used. A review of six studies indicated that the haloperidol decanoate maintenance dose ranged from 50 to 150 mg/mo (Beresford et al., 1987). One study reported average doses of 225 mg/mo (Chouinard et al., 1989).

One difficulty in determining the lowest effective maintenance dose for depot antipsychotics is the delay in symptom relapse after dose reduction. Several studies have demonstrated that after drug discontinuation, significant concentrations of the drug remain in the tissues for weeks to months (Gitlin et al., 1988; Wistedt et al., 1981; Nayak et al., 1987). A decrease in serum prolactin concentrations may take longer (Gitlin et al., 1988; Wistedt et

al., 1981). A recent undocumented recommendation suggested that a dose reduction of fluphenazine or haloperidol should not exceed 10 percent every 3 months (Chouinard et al., 1989). This recommendation might produce a better correlation between dose and onset of relapse symptoms.

Six of seven haloperidol decanoate maintenance studies used monthly intervals (Beresford et al., 1987). One study reported that their patients were divided equally into three groups and were administered the drug at 2- , 3- , and 4-week intervals (Chouinard et al., 1989).

Three studies report haloperidol to fluphenazine decanoate dose ratios of 1.4:1, 3:1, and 7:1 (Chouinard et al., 1989; Wistedt et al., 1984; Kissling et al., 1985). However, the use of supplemental PO antipsychotics in these reports make direct comparisons difficult. The 3:1 ratio would be a reasonable starting point. Subsequent dose adjustment should be based on therapeutic response and adverse effects.

Maintenance treatment with antipsychotic drugs is associated with a risk of long-term adverse effects, such as tardive dyskinesia. To reduce total drug exposure and possibly the risk of adverse effects, the use of drug holidays has been recommended. A decade ago, literature suggested that patients would not relapse with drug holidays of 2- or 3-day per week (Davis et al., 1977). In one study, no patients relapsed after having their fluphenazine decanoate discontinued for 6 weeks (Shenoy et al., 1981). However, there are reports that suggest that drug holidays increase the risk of tardive dyskinesia (Degivity, 1969; Jester et al., 1979; McGreadie et al., 1980).

Recently, "targeted" or "intermittent" antipsychotic treatment has been suggested as a method of reducing total drug exposure during maintenance treatment (Herz, 1984; Carpenter et al., 1987; Jolly et al., 1989). This strategy is based on the observation that some patients can remain off their medication for several months to 1 year without relapse of their symptoms. The patients are treated only when they have active symptoms. After they respond the antipsychotic is discontinued and they are closely followed. Once the patient demonstrates the prodromal symptoms of an acute psychotic relapse, the antipsychotic is restarted. Although this method is reportedly successful, there are no direct studies comparing targeted treatment and low-dose continuous dosing strategies (Kane, 1988). Continuous, low-dose antipsychotics still are recommended.

ADVERSE EFFECTS

The adverse effects of antipsychotics can be classified as allergic, autonomic, cardiovascular, dermatologic, endocrine, hematologic, hepatotoxic, metabolic, neurologic, ophthalmologic, overdosage, sexual dysfunction, and teratogenic. Common adverse effects involve the autonomic (i.e., hypotension) and neurologic (i.e., sedation, extrapyramidal) systems. Relatively more sedative and vascular effects are seen with low-potency antipsychotics (i.e., chlorpromazine, thioridazine, mesoridazine, chlorprothixene) compared with more extrapyramidal side effects (EPSEs) with high-potency compounds (i.e., haloperidol, perphenazine, fluphenazine, thiothixene) (Rhoades et al., 1984).

CARDIAC. Postural hypotension usually occurs during the first few hours or days of treatment. Patients receiving low-potency antipsychotics should be given the following cautionary instructions: Rise from bed gradually, sit at first with legs dangling, wait for a minute, and then rise only if there is no feeling of dizziness or faintness (Simpson et al., 1981; Shader et al., 1970).

Electrocardiogram (ECG) changes have been reported. Phenothiazines, in particular chlorpromazine and thioridazine, have been commonly reported to produce broadened, flattened T waves and an increase in the QR interval; this is of uncertain clinical significance. Similar reports with chlorprothixene, loxapine, molindone, and thiothixene also have appeared.

DERMATOLOGIC. Simple allergic skin reactions are manifested in three forms. The most common, a maculopapular rash on the face, neck, or upper chest and extremities, occurs in 5 to 10 percent of patients taking chlorpromazine within 14 to 60 days after the start of therapy. Other reactions include erythema multiforme and localized or generalized urticaria. The reactions may be treated with antihistamines as well as steroids in the more serious cases. Interruption of treatment usually is unnecessary, but if required, the drug may be resumed as the rash subsides. Recurrence of the rash is uncommon. If a patient develops angioneurotic edema or exfoliative dermatitis, treatment is discontinued (Simpson et al., 1981; Shader et al., 1970).

Photosensitivity reactions have been reported to occur in 3 percent of patients taking antipsychotics, with most cases related to chlorpromazine (Simpson et al., 1981; Shader et al., 1970). Patients should wear protective clothing and/or sun screen of SPF ≥15.

Long-term skin effects include pigmentary skin changes. Pigmentary changes include a tan color that progresses to a slate gray, metallic blue, or purple color over the areas of the skin exposed to sunlight. Skin biopsy has demonstrated golden-brown pigment granules similar, but not identical, to melanin. The frequency of bluish pigmentation is approximately 1 percent with all antipsychotics. These skin disorders are thought to occur less frequently today than in the 1950s, possibly because of the utilization of lower doses and the preferential use of high-potency antipsychotics. Haloperidol reportedly does not cause this adverse effect (Simpson et al., 1981; Shader et al., 1970).

ENDOCRINE. Adverse effects include amenorrhea, galactorrhea, and gynecomastia (Simpson et al., 1981; Shader et al., 1970). Amenorrhea is reported to occur in 18 to 95 percent of women receiving antipsychotics compared with 3 to 5 percent of the general female population (Zito et al., 1990). Galactorrhea occurs in women and is frequently accompanied by some degree of breast enlargement or engorgement. One study reported an incidence of 57 percent (Inoué et al., 1980). Gynecomastia (breast enlargement) from any cause is uncommon; therefore, other medical causes should be considered. Gynecomastia in males has rarely been reported (Overall et al., 1978).

Weight gain has been frequently reported in patients receiving antipsychotics. Management includes exercise and dietary restriction. Molindone and loxapine have been associated with weight loss during treatment but this has not been conclusively demonstrated. Prescribing amphetamine or amphetamine-like appetite suppressants is unwarranted because of their potential to exacerbate psychosis (Parent et al., 1986; Shader et al., 1970).

NEUROLOGIC. *Neuroleptic malignant syndrome* (NMS), which is characterized by muscular rigidity, hyperthermia, altered consciousness, and autonomic dysfunction, has been reported in patients primarily receiving typical antipsychotics (O'Brien et al., 1989). The reported incidence varies from 0.5 to 2.4 percent (Keck et al., 1989b). Ninety percent of the patients who developed NMS did so within 10 days of drug initiation (Rosenberg et al., 1989; Susman et al., 1988; Shalev et al., 1986). The overall mortality rate for cases reported between 1959 and 1987 was 18.8 percent. Since 1984, the rate has decreased to 11.6 percent (Shalev et al., 1989). Patients with myoglobinemia and renal failure have a mortality rate of 47 and 56 percent, respectively. Other complications, such as seizures, pulmonary embolus, or disseminated intravascular coagulation, may lead to death. When NMS is suspected, the antipsychotic should be discontinued and supportive care instituted immediately. Intubation, mechanical ventilation, fever reduction, and other supportive measures may be required until the muscular rigidity and fever begin to resolve (Rosenberg et al., 1989). The exact pharmacologic treatment of NMS has not been established. The rationale for drug treatment is relieving the primary target symptom of rigidity. This subject has recently been reviewed (Rosenberg et al., 1989; Shalev et al., 1989; Guerrero et al., 1988). Muscle relaxants, dopamine agonists, anticholinergics, calcium-channel blockers, and electroconvulsive therapy (ECT) have been used. Antipsychotics should not be reinstituted until 2 weeks after complete resolution of symptoms and the patient has completed treatment for NMS (Wells et al., 1988). If the patient developed NMS on a high-potency drug, a low-potency antipsychotic trial is recommended. If the same or similar potency antipsychotic is started, low doses should be used. Although the literature does not support the conclusion that lithium increases the risk of NMS, close monitoring is recommended if lithium is used.

Extrapyramidal side effects (EPSEs) are divided into early- and late-onset types. Early-onset symptoms usually occur within the first 4 weeks of treatment and include dystonia, akathisia, and pseudoparkinsonism. Late-onset types occurring after 6 months of treatment are represented by tardive dyskinesia, tardive dystonia, and tardive akathisia. Estimates of the incidence of EPSEs with antipsychotics vary widely, ranging from 2.2 to 95 percent. Much of the variation in the reported percentages may be explained by differences in the antipsychotic prescribed (low versus high potency), length of treatment, dosage, individual sensitivity, and definitions of EPSEs. All antipsychotics have been associated with tardive dyskinesia, but real differences in incidences among antipsychotics, if they exist, have not been demonstrated. These syndromes wax and wane over time, disappear during sleep, and are exacerbated by emotionally disturbing experiences (Simpson et al., 1981; Shader et al., 1970). Dystonic reactions consist of involuntary tonic contraction of skeletal muscles of virtually any striated muscle group (Simpson et al., 1981; Shader et al., 1970). The most common dystonias involve the muscles of the head and face, producing buccal spasms, oculogyric crisis, facial grimacing, tics, or trismus. Involvement of the neck musculature produces torticollis or retrocollis. If the trunk is involved, shoulder shrugging, tortipelvis, opisthotonos, or scoliosis may occur. Carpopedal spasms, dorsiflexion of the toes, contraction of muscle groups of arms or legs, or a dystonic gait may be seen if the limbs are involved. Ninety percent of dystonic reactions occur by day 4 of antipsychotic treatment. They may occur after one dose of an antipsychotic regardless of the route of administration. They usually occur once but occasionally recur when there is an increase in dosage.

The reported incidence of dystonia ranges from 2.3 to 64 percent depending on the antipsychotic studied. Although a dystonic reaction may occur at any age, it is more common in patients <35 years of age and is twice as likely to occur in men. Dystonias usually are benign and disappear without treatment. However, because of the extreme discomfort to the patient and the possibility of serious sequelae, dystonic reactions are treated as soon after their appearance as possible. Many agents have been recommended to treat dystonias, but IV diphenhydramine (Benadryl) 50 mg or benztropine (Cogentin) 2 mg will reverse the dystonia, usually within 2 minutes. If no relief occurs within 5 minutes, the dose should be repeated. The IM route has been used successfully, but resolution of the dystonia may take 20 to 40 minutes (Lee, 1979).

Akathisia refers to a subjective experience of motor restlessness. Patients may complain of an inability to sit or stand still or a compulsion to pace (Van Putten et al., 1984). They also may complain of being restless and having to be in constant motion. While standing, they may rock to and fro or shift their weight from one leg to another. Patients also may suffer from initial insomnia because they cannot lie motionless in bed long enough to fall asleep. Typically, akathisia occurs within 2 to 3 weeks of initiation of the antipsychotic. Ninety percent of the cases develop within the first 73 days of treatment. However, some patients may develop this within hours of the first antipsychotic dose. Estimates of the incidence of akathisias range from 21 to 71 percent. Akathisia tends to occur more frequently in the middle-aged, with women twice as likely to experience it. An accurate diagnosis is important because misdiagnosis may lead to an unnecessary increase in antipsychotic medication with worsening of the akathisia. Dose reduction or a change to an agent less prone to cause EPSEs (i.e., a low-potency drug) may alleviate the need to add a pharmacologic agent. Upon discontinuation of the antipsychotic, akathisia symptoms generally resolve in 7 days but may take several weeks. Propranolol may be useful in antipsychotic-induced akathisia (Fleischhacker et al., 1990). Anticholinergics often are ineffective in the management of akathisia. Diazepam 5 mg IV has been shown to be as effective as diphenhydramine 50 mg IV. Limited experience indicates that PO BZDs may be beneficial.

The pseudoparkinsonian adverse effects manifest themselves as tremor, rigidity, and akinesia, individually or in combination (Simpson et al., 1981; Shader et al., 1970). Drooling, an accelerating gait, oily skin, dysarthria, and dysphagia may accompany the symptoms. Akinesia may present early as slowness in initiating motor tasks and fatigue when performing activities requiring repetitive movements (bradykinesia). Affected persons appear apathetic with little facial expression, have difficulty walking, and their handwriting may take on a cramped appearance (micrographia). This drug-induced condition should not be misinterpreted as depressive symptomatology. The typical antipsychotic-induced pseudoparkinsonian tremor may be present during movement as well as at rest. Tremor usually begins in one or both upper extremities and in severe cases may involve the tongue, jaw, and lower extremities. The tremor may involve the mouth, chin, and lips, which has been termed the *rabbit syndrome*. Cogwheel rigidity, in which a ratchet-like phenomenon can be elicited upon passive movement of a limb, is the result of the presence of both rigidity and tremor. As with all drug-induced EPSEs, there is a wide variance in the reported incidence. The range is from 2.2 to 56 percent. Pseudoparkinsonism occurs at varying intervals after the initiation of antipsychotic drug therapy but usually occurs within 4 weeks. Like akathisia, pseudoparkinsonism's occurrence is usually dose- and patient-related. Drug-induced pseudoparkinsonism tends to occur most often in the elderly, with women twice as likely to develop it as men. Treatment of antipsychotic-induced pseudo-parkinsonism includes dose reduction, changing to an agent less likely to produce EPSEs (i.e., low-potency drug), addition of conventional anticholinergics such as benztropine, or addition of amantadine. The condition disappears upon discontinuation of drug therapy, but this may take several weeks to months depending upon the dosage and individual patient.

Tardive dyskinesia is a complex syndrome of hyperkinetic involuntary movements (Simpson et al., 1981; Shader et al., 1970). The most widely described symptoms make up the buccolinguo-masticatory triad, which consists of (1) sucking and smacking movements of the lips, (2) lateral jaw movements, and (3) puffing of the cheeks, with the tongue thrusting, rolling, or making fly-catching movements. Such movements may be carried on with the mouth closed with bites of the tongue and inside of the cheek as well as a chewing movement. The extremities may show choreiform movements that are variable, purposeless, involuntary, and quick. Frequently associated with these symptoms are athetoid movements, which are continuous, arrhythmic, wavelike slow movements in the distal parts of the limbs. Axial hyperkinesia (i.e., to and fro clonic movement of the spine in an antero-posterior direction) and ballistic movements (i.e., rhythmical side to side swaying) also may be present. All involuntary movements disappear during sleep and are exacerbated by emotionally upsetting situations. Drug-induced parkinsonism is present in 30 to 40 percent of patients with tardive dyskinesia (Wirshing et al., 1989).

Although tardive dyskinesia usually is recognized after more than a year of treatment, onset within 6 months of initiation of antipsychotics has been reported. Tardive dyskinesia has been reported in patients exposed to virtually all classes of antipsychotics. The prevalence of tardive dyskinesia, corrected for spontaneous dyskinesia, averages 15 to 20 percent. The incidence is estimated at 2 to 5 percent per year over 5 to 6 years of treatment (Kane, 1989). Evidence of an association between tardive dyskinesia and women is conflicting; however, there appears to be an association between this condition and advanced age.

Dyskinesia usually has an insidious onset while the patients are still receiving antipsychotics, although abnormal movements often appear for the first time or increase dramatically following a reduction in dose or discontinuation of the drug. Despite discontinuation of the antipsychotic, the dyskinesia is potentially irreversible. It is reversible in approximately 50 percent of patients in whom all antipsychotics are discontinued for 1 year. Complete recovery usually is observed in children and recovery appears to be likely in young adults as well. Several studies indicated that although antipsychotics are continued, tardive dyskinetic movements are not generally progressive and may improve (Kane, 1989; Bergen et al., 1989).

Many agents have been utilized in attempting to treat tardive dyskinesia, but these agents have produced only inconsistent and temporary improvement (Remington et al., 1989).

A form of tardive dyskinesia, termed *tardive dystonia*, which is characterized by sustained or slow involuntary twisting movements of the face, neck, trunk, or limbs, has been described (Remington et al., 1989). This condition may coexist with tardive dyskinesia and has been estimated to occur in 2 percent of patients who receive long-term antipsychotic treatment. It reportedly does not respond to anticholinergics. Tardive akathisia, a late-onset effect that resembles the clinical presentation of the early-onset form, has been described.

The prolonged use of antipsychotics should be restricted to situations in which there are compelling indications, (e.g., schizophrenia). Long-term antipsychotic treatment in the management of anxiety disorders, depression, mania, and personality disorders should be avoided, except in unusual clinical situations. Whether to discontinue antipsychotics in patients with schizophrenia is a matter of clinical judgment.

There is a growing clinical impression that the earlier tardive dyskinesia is recognized and the drug withdrawn, the better is the prognosis for recovery. Drug holidays have been advocated to decrease the total dose of drug received over time in hope of delaying or eliminating tardive dyskinesia. However, recent studies do not support the use of drug holidays for the prevention of tardive dyskinesia.

The use of antipsychotics should be supported with a proper indication, demonstrated response (preferably with drug discontinuation), dose minimization, informed consent, and a structured assessment (e.g., Abnormal Movement Inventory Scale) performed at least yearly for tardive dyskinesia (Bergen et al., 1989; Munetz et al., 1988; Davis, 1983).

Sedation occurs in the first few days of treatment, and patients may develop tolerance to this effect within several weeks. All available antipsychotics can cause sedation; however, they differ in their tendency to do so. This effect can be minimized by administering the total dose of antipsychotic at bedtime (Simpson et al., 1981; Shader et al., 1970).

All available antipsychotics reduce the *seizure* threshold. Generalized and focal motor seizures have been reported, but the incidence is <1 percent. In general, antipsychotic-induced seizures do not pose a management problem. Patients develop tolerance to this effect, and seizures will continue to occur only if higher doses are used. Seizure activity usually occurs as an early complication in treatment (Simpson et al., 1981; Shader et al., 1970).

Sexual disturbances in males include ejaculatory dysfunction, impotence, reduced libido, and priapism. An incidence of 25 to 60 percent has been reported for ejaculatory disturbance, reduced libido, and impotence. No incidence rate is available for priapism. Ejaculatory disturbances have been attributed to thioridazine, chlorpromazine, mesoridazine, and chlorprothixene. At lower antipsychotic doses, ejaculation may be delayed or completely blocked without interfering with erection. Patients report absence of ejaculation on masturbation or sexual intercourse and, occasionally, suprapubic pain on orgasm. This effect may be dose-related, so dose reduction might be tried. If this fails, a high-potency nonphenothiazine (i.e., thiothixene, haloperidol) may be substituted (Segraves, 1989).

Impotence and decreased libido have been associated with chlorpromazine, fluphenazine decanoate, haloperidol, pimozide, thioridazine, and thiothixene. Management might include dose reduction and drug substitution, as indicated for ejaculatory disturbances (Segraves, 1989). Antipsychotic-induced priapism (a prolonged, painful erection) has been reported with chlorpromazine, fluphenazine, haloperidol, mesoridazine, molindone, perphenazine, thioridazine, and thiothixene in a total of 17 cases (Chan et al., 1990). It does not appear to be dose-related. Priapism is considered a medical emergency. Prompt discontinuation of the antipsychotic is absolutely necessary, although reversal may not occur with antipsychotic discontinuation. Without resolution of the erection, it is reported that 18 to 80 percent of patients will become impotent. Treatment may include intracavernosal injection of an alpha-adrenergic agonist (e.g., metaraminol, ephedrine, or epinephrine), aspiration of the corpora cavernosa, or placement of a corpora cavernosa to corpus spongiosum shunt. Management includes substitution of an antipsychotic of a different chemical class and close monitoring.

OPHTHALMOLOGIC. Cornea and lens changes have been noted with chlorpromazine, trifluoperazine, perphenazine, fluphenazine, chlorprothixene, and thiothixene (Simpson et al., 1981; Shader et al., 1970). Chlorpromazine is most clearly associated with these changes, which are related to a total lifetime dose of 1 to 3 kg. The eye changes are described as whitish brown granular deposits concentrated in the anterior subcapsular area, which, in more severe cases, also may be found in the anterior and posterior lens cortex. Generally, these changes are visible only by slit-lamp examination. They progress to opaque-white or yellow-brown granules, often stellate in shape. In some patients, the conjunctiva is discolored by a brown pigment. Vision usually is not impaired. These lens changes differ from those of senile cataracts and are not related to them, since these are depositions in the lens and are not loss of transparency of the lens. Overall, incidences range from 27 to 90 percent. If skin pigmentation is present, simultaneous deposition in the eye almost certainly occurs. Cornea and lens changes appear to be positively correlated with severe photosensitivity response to chlorprom-

azine; thus patients who develop photosensitivity reactions should have eye examinations if exposed to high doses of chlorpromazine for many years. Treatment of skin, corneal, and lens changes includes lowering the dose of the antipsychotic, assigning drug holidays, or changing to an antipsychotic that has not been reported to cause these reactions.

Pigmentary retinopathy is primarily associated with thioridazine, although it has been reported with chlorpromazine (Simpson et al., 1981; Shader et al., 1970). Pigment deposits start in the middle zone of the retina, and over a 3 to 4-week period, the deposits coalesce and edema appears. Retinal changes have occurred after thioridazine 1200 mg/d has been given for a period of 4 to 8 weeks. The relationship appears to be a function of time and dose rather than dose accumulation. Thioridazine ≤800 mg/d has been defined as safe. When thioridazine causes retinal pigmentation, a drastic reduction in visual acuity and even blindness may result. It is believed that the retinal pigment deposition is irreversible, but occasionally, the pigment recedes when the drug is stopped. Visual acuity returns when thioridazine is discontinued, but some reports have indicated progression of the retinopathy after discontinuation of the drug. Treatment is discontinuation and substitution of another antipsychotic.

Although *supersensitivity psychosis* after long-term antipsychotics and rebound psychoses after drug discontinuation have been suggested, conclusive evidence that this is related primarily to drug treatment is lacking (Kahne 1989).

TERATOGENIC. Antipsychotics have not been clearly documented to cause congenital anomalies (Simpson et al., 1981; Shader et al., 1970; Calabrese et al., 1985; Marken et al., 1989). However, they should not be prescribed during the first trimester of pregnancy if they can be avoided. Low-dose, high-potency antipsychotics (i.e., haloperidol, fluphenazine) might be preferred because low-potency drugs might produce maternal hypotension and uteroplacental insufficiency.

The clinical significance of antipsychotic concentrations in breast milk is unclear (Calabrese et al., 1985). Chlorpromazine, trifluoperazine, prochlorperazine, thioridazine, and mesoridazine have been detected in breast milk. Breast feeding is not recommended.

Clozapine

EFFICACY

Synthesized in 1960, clozapine is a member of the dibenzodiazepine class of atypical antipsychotics. The drug has a pharmacologic profile unlike typical antipsychotics.

As a result of its potential adverse hematologic effects, the FDA has restricted clozapine to patients who are refractory to typical antipsychotics or to those with severe intolerable adverse effects (Ereshefsky et al., 1989b). Although not specified in the manufacturer's literature, the adverse effects related to typical antipsychotics that might indicate clozapine include treatment-resistant, early-onset (e.g., pseudoparkinsonism, akathisia) or late-onset (e.g., tardive dyskinesia, tardive dystonia) EPSEs.

Of drugs available in the United States, clozapine has been compared with chlorpromazine, haloperidol, perphenazine, and trifluoperazine. In acutely psychotic or chronically ill patients with schizophrenia, clozapine was equal to or more effective than the reference typical antipsychotic (Ereshefsky et al., 1989b).

Approval of clozapine for U.S. marketing was based on the results of a 16-center trial of clozapine in treatment-resistant schizophrenia (Kane et al., 1988). These patients had not responded to three different antipsychotic trials at doses of chlorpromazine >1000 mg/d or its equivalent administered for at least 6 weeks. Subsequently, the nonresponders were treated with chlorpromazine 600 to 1800 mg/d plus benztropine 6 mg/d or clozapine 50 to 900 mg/d plus placebo for 6 weeks. Five (3.5 percent) of the chlorpromazine patients responded and 38 (30 percent) of the clozapine patients responded. Clozapine was more effective than chlorpromazine in the treatment of positive and negative symptoms. Significant improvement with clozapine as compared with chlorpromazine occurred within 1 to 2 weeks.

Clozapine's long-term effects (e.g., >6 weeks) in treatment-resistant patients were reported in a nonblind study (Meltzer et al., 1990). Of 51 patients, 31 were considered responders at a median time of 8.9 months. This finding has led authors to suggest that a clozapine trial should last at least 6 to 9 months.

A retrospective study reported that about 40 percent of patients were able to return to part-time or full-time employment after treatment with clozapine (Lindstrom, 1988). Another retrospective report on 87 treatment-resistant patients indicated that clozapine provided an average savings of $9000 to $14000 in "mental health services" after 2 years of treatment (Honigfeld et al., 1990).

ADVERSE EFFECTS

The attention paid to clozapine's hematologic effects and the lack of early-onset (i.e., dystonia, akathisia, pseudo-parkinsonism) and late-onset EPSEs (i.e., tardive dyskinesia) has overshadowed its other common and troublesome adverse effects. Besides hematologic effects, these primarily include central nervous system, cardiovascular, gastrointestinal, and metabolic effects. Adverse effects of clozapine and their management has been reviewed (Lieberman et al., 1989).

AUTONOMIC. Constipation may be a significant problem in some patients due to the anticholinergic properties of clozapine. Some 6 to 31 percent of clozapine-treated patients will experience some degree of excessive salivation. They especially may complain of significant drooling at night.

Sudden loss of muscle tone without a loss of consciousness has been infrequently reported. This may affect the whole body or be limited to a specific muscle group. It has not been associated with auras, incontinence, or other signs of a seizure. However, a workup to rule out a seizure is recommended. There is no specific treatment.

CARDIAC. Hypotension and dizziness are primarily observed during the initiation of treatment and/or after dose escalation. Orthostatic blood pressure should be monitored, especially during the start of treatment and during dosage increases. The rate of dosage increase may be slowed if blood pressure reductions are noted. Patients should be warned of potential dizziness and instructed how to arise from a lying or sitting position. A liberal sodium diet and support stockings have been recommended.

An increase in heart rate occurs in >90 percent of patients and may approach 120 beats per minute. The effect is dose-related. If the patient experiences palpitations, then clozapine's dose may be reduced and/or a beta-blocker with low central nervous system penetrability (i.e., atenolol 25 to 50 mg/d) might be added. The blood pressure should be monitored because of possible additive hypotensive effects of combined clozapine and atenolol.

ENDOCRINE. No evidence of amenorrhea, galactorrhea, or gynecomastia has been reported in several large studies that used doses >600 mg/d.

Similar to typical antipsychotics, clozapine has been associated with significant weight gain. A recent case series reported that seven patients gained 6 to 69 lb during 4 to 9 months of treatment (Cohen et al., 1990). Caloric restriction and/or increased activity should be considered.

HEMATOLOGIC. In 1975, 16 cases of granulocytopenia were reported in Finland. Thirteen patients developed agranulocytosis, and eight died from a secondary infection. The remaining five patients recovered with drug discontinuation. In the U.S. studies, a cumulative incidence of 2 percent was reported. Overall, estimates indicate that this adverse effect is 10 times higher than with typical antipsychotics. Although the mechanism is unknown, the time course and complete reversibility with drug discontinuation suggests an immune-mediated reaction.

The majority of cases occur between 6 and 18 weeks. Typically, the decrease in the white blood cell (WBC) count is gradual. The risk of granulocytopenia is not related to the dose, nor to the patient's sex or age. With drug discontinuation, the granulocytopenia reverses within 2 weeks. As the granulocytopenia is reversible and agranulocytosis is potentially fatal, the manufacturer and the FDA require weekly complete blood counts (CBCs).

To ensure that the CBCs will be obtained, clozapine will be available only through registered distributors, prescribers, and pharmacies. Information on this program may be obtained from the manufacturer's representative.

Current guidelines indicate that clozapine should be immediately discontinued if the total WBC count falls to <3000 cells/mm^3 or the absolute number of polymorphonuclear leukocytes falls to <1000 cells/mm^3. The patient should not receive clozapine again, since the hematologic reaction may be immune-mediated. Reexposure may result in a rapidly progressive course.

HEPATIC. Mild increases in liver enzymes have been observed with routine monitoring; however, significant clinical consequences (i.e., jaundice) have not been reported. Routine laboratory monitoring does not appear necessary.

NEUROLOGIC. Cases of neuroleptic malignant syndrome have been reported with clozapine. Short-term administration of clozapine produces a 10 percent incidence of early-onset EPSEs (e.g., rigidity, tremor, and akathisia). This rate is less than that reported with typical antipsychotics. In the U.S. studies, neither dystonia nor the parkinsonian symptom of hypokinesia were observed.

Tardive dyskinesia has not been conclusively associated with clozapine, but long-term treatment in a large number of patients has not been reported. Overall, in patients with tardive dyskinesia, clozapine has produced improvement but has rarely completely suppressed dyskinetic movements. However, typical antipsychotics also produce short-term improvement in tardive dyskinesia. More research on clozapine in tardive dyskinesia is required.

A number of case reports have documented clozapine-induced seizures. The seizure rate is related to dose and rate of dose increase. Daily doses and seizure incidences based on experience with 1700 patients treated in the United States are <300 mg/d, 1 percent; 300 to <600 mg/d, 1.4 percent; and 600 to 900 mg/d, 14 percent. Patients with a history of epilepsy or brain damage may be at an increased risk of seizures. If a seizure occurs, clozapine should be discontinued. If the neurology workup is abnormal and an anticonvulsant is started, clozapine may be reinstituted after therapeutic concentrations of the anticonvulsant are achieved. If the seizure workup is unremarkable, then clozapine may be reintroduced and increased to 50 percent of the dose at which the seizure occurred.

Sedation is a dose-related adverse effect. Some degree of tolerance may develop in most patients and complete tolerance may be achieved in some. To minimize this effect, initiate treatment with doses of 12.5 mg once or twice daily. Doses should be increased by 25 to 50 mg/d as tolerated. Administering most or all of the dose at bedtime may help.

Return of psychotic and negative symptoms within several days of clozapine discontinuation has been described. Abrupt discontinuation was necessary because of adverse hematologic effects. Patients should be instructed not to abruptly discontinue clozapine, unless directed by a prescriber.

A benign temperature elevation of 1 to 2°F has been noted within the first 5 to 20 days of treatment. It is estimated to occur in 7 to 14 percent of patients. The temperature increase might indicate a possible infection secondary to leukopenia or, possibly, NMS. Patients with hyperthermia should have a CBC and sedimentation rate done to rule out infection and should be followed for signs of NMS. Typically, this resolves without treatment or clozapine discontinuation. Antipyretics (i.e., acetaminophen) effectively lower the temperature.

Clozapine's effect on sexual function has not been specifically evaluated. There have been several case reports of priapism.

DEPRESSION

Tricyclic Antidepressants (TCAs)

EFFICACY

Patients with major depressive disorders with symptoms that include an insidious onset, anorexia, weight loss, middle or terminal insomnia, diurnal variation in mood, psychomotor retardation, or agitation are more likely to experience a positive response to a TCA (Bielski and Friedel, 1976; Schneider et al., 1986). However, the presence of delusions in conjunction with major depressive disorder is a predictor of a negative response to TCAs (Spiker et al., 1986). In controlled studies in which the TCAs were compared with each other, it is consistently observed that overall no single TCA is superior to any other (Morris and Beck, 1974). Thus the choice of the TCA to be utilized is dependent on the drugs' adverse effect profiles, the probability of response to an individual TCA based on blood levels, and the patient's past response to a particular agent.

MAJOR DEPRESSIVE EPISODE. TCA efficacy in the treatment of acute depressions is well established. A 1965 review calculated the imipramine response rates in controlled studies to be 65 percent compared with 32 percent in placebo-treated patients (Klerman and Cole, 1965). Despite changes in depression diagnostic criteria, this figure remains remarkably stable. A 66 percent initial response rate for antidepressant drug treatment was calculated for a series of studies published between 1974 and 1985 (Feinberg and Halbreich, 1986). Because 35 percent of patients with major depression will not respond to TCAs, the management of these treatment resistant patients is an appropriate question. Of the numerous treatment options suggested, two are justifiable: (1) electroconvulsive therapy (ECT) and (2) lithium carbonate augmentation of TCA treatment. ECT was estimated to be effective in 72 percent of TCA treatment failures (Avery and Lubrano, 1979). The augmentation of TCA therapy with lithium carbonate has been shown to be effective in 63 percent of treated patients versus a 12 percent rate in controls (Perry et al., 1991). Some patients respond quickly, relapse within a few days, and then respond with continued lithium treatment. Most responders will respond within 21 days. Usually, lithium doses of 600 to 1200 mg/d producing concentrations in excess of 0.3 mEq/liter are sufficient. TCA augmentation with liothyronine is commonly suggested as a treatment alternative for refractory patients. The most recent controlled study that examined its effectiveness found the treatment no more effective than 4 additional weeks of TCA treatment (Gitlin et al., 1987). Thus the therapeutic options of ECT and lithium augmentation are the first alternatives considered in the treatment of nonresponding patients.

MAJOR DEPRESSIVE EPISODE WITH PSYCHOTIC FEATURES. Depressed patients who are delusional normally require ECT. The literature estimates that 82 percent of psychotic depressives who fail to respond to TCA will respond to ECT (Spiker et al., 1986). While 66 percent of nondelusional depressed patients respond to TCAs, only 34 percent of delusional depressed patients respond to a three week trial of TCAs. If ECT is not a viable alternative, the possibly less effective combination treatment of a TCA with an antipsychotic is recommended. Combination drug treatment can be optimized by prescribing a TCA dose that falls within the higher end of the recommended therapeutic plasma ranges for the TCAs. As an example, a nortriptyline concentration of 140 to 150 ng/ml would be a reasonable initial target concentration. If the patient does not respond, higher doses may be utilized. Antipsychotic drugs interact with TCAs to increase their concentrations. Thus it is hypothesized that the ineffectiveness of TCAs in treating delusional depression may be the result of utilizing subtherapeutic doses. Only 41 percent of delusional depressives treated with amitriptyline responded, whereas the antipsychotic/antidepressant combination of perphenazine/amitriptyline was, as expected, effective in 78 percent of patients (Spiker et al., 1985). However, after the data considered the effect of the drug's serum concentration, it was found that the 64 percent of the amitriptyline patients with total levels greater than 250 ng/ml responded, which was a similar response produced by the combination drug treatment of a TCA and an antipsychotic. Even more important than the TCA dosage is the duration of TCA treatment. A 9-week trial of primarily amitriptyline or imipramine (200 to 250 mg/d) in delusional depressives resulted in response rates of only 32 percent after 3 weeks but 62 percent after 9 weeks (Howarth and Grace, 1985). Thus TCAs are effective in the treatment of delusional depression, but probably only at high therapeutic blood levels, given for up to 9 weeks.

GRIEF REACTIONS. Few data are available concerning the role of TCAs in the treatment of bereavement reactions. Fifteen percent of bereaved spouses meet criteria for depression 12 months after their loss. A 10-patient, uncontrolled study concluded that 4 weeks of desipramine produced moderate to marked improvement in 70 percent of the bereaved spouses (Jacobs et al., 1987). In a study of 13 bereaved spouses, nortriptyline at an average dose of 49 mg/d (mean nortriptyline concentration 68 ng/ml) produced a 68 percent decrease in the depressive symptoms after a median treatment interval of 6.4 weeks (Pasternak et al., 1991). A controlled clinical trial to determine the placebo response rate and the relapse rate after discontinuation of medication is needed.

RECURRENT MAJOR DEPRESSIVE EPISODES. Between 50 and 85 percent of patients with major depression will experience at least one additional episode in their lifetime. Nearly 50 percent of these patients will relapse within 2 years, with the greatest risk of relapse occurring within 4 to 6 months of the initial remission. Finally, 15 to 20 percent of patients with recurrent depression do not fully recover from any given episode (Prien and Kupfer, 1986). Thus a significant number of depressed patients require preventative maintenance treatment with either lithium or a tricyclic antidepressant. Both agents are equally effective in preventing recurrent unipolar illness, whereas lithium is more effective in recurrent bipolar illness (Consensus Development Panel, 1985). Prophylactic treatment is indicated in unipolar depressed patients if they have had three prior episodes, particularly if one episode has occurred within the last 5 years. In bipolar depressed patients, prophylactic treatment should be begun after the second episode (Angst, 1981). Factors associated with an increased risk of recurrence in patients with unipolar illness include the presence of another mental disorder, a chronic medical disorder, chronic affective symptoms, an older age of onset for the first episode, psychotic affective episodes, a serious suicide attempt, serious functional impairment while depressed, and a positive family history for either suicide and/or bipolar illness (Consensus Development Panel, 1985). Clinicians should be quite conservative in their timeframe of discontinuing medication in patients who have a majority of these risk factors.

DOSING

EMPIRICAL DOSING. When empirically dosing patients with TCAs, treatment with either drug is initiated at a dose of 25, 50, or 75 mg/d administered as a single dose at bedtime because of the TCAs' long half-lives. The dose should then be increased by 25 to 50 mg every 1 to 2 days until a dosage of 150 mg/d is reached. If a response is going to occur, the patient should show significant clinical improvement in anxiety, physical expression of distress, cognitive impairment, and depressed mood within the first week at this dose. If these symptoms have not improved and if there are no medical contraindications or manifestations of toxicity, the dosage should be titrated upward at a rate of 25 mg/d, normally to a maximum dose of 300 mg/d or until the patient begins to show improvement or intolerable side effects occur. This dosing schedule is appropriate not only for imipramine and amitriptyline but also for doxepin, desipramine, and trimipramine. However, the dose must be adjusted downward for nortriptyline, which is approximately two times more potent than imipramine, and protriptyline, which is five times more potent than imipramine.

THERAPEUTIC TRIAL. Commonly, 10 to 20 days of therapy are required before improvement in mood and affect become apparent to the physician, the family, and the patient. This delay must be explained to patients and their families to increase compliance. Maximum tolerable doses should be maintained for at least 3 weeks before it is concluded that the medication is of no benefit. Of nondelusional depressed patients who respond to TCAs, it has been reported that 88 percent do so within 3 weeks, whereas a similar percentage, 90 percent, of delusional depressives require up to 7 weeks to respond (Howarth and Grace, 1985).

EDITORS' COMMENT

The speed with which antidepressant therapy becomes effective is open to debate. Most psychiatrists believe that it takes 3 weeks of treatment before improvement in mood and affect become apparent. However, in a study using nortriptyline and amitriptyline (Ziegler et al. Arch Gen Psychiatry 34:607–612, 1977), the steepest gradient of improvement occurred between the beginning of treatment and the first 7 days. The second steepest gradient of improvement occurred between the first and second week of treatment. By the third week of treatment, most of the improvement had taken place. Thus the onset of action of the antidepressants occurred within the first week, and there was apparent improvement in the depression during that time.

The acutely depressed patient must remain on the TCA until asymptomatic for at least 16 weeks. If this therapeutic axiom is not adhered to, the patient has a 50 percent risk of experiencing a relapse within the next 4 to 6 months following the initial remission (Prien and Kupfer, 1986). At the end of this period, the outpatient should be tapered off the TCA at the rate of approximately 50 mg per week for amitriptyline, imipramine, desipramine, doxepin, and trimipramine; 25 mg per week for nortriptyline; and 10 mg per week for protriptyline. Inpatients can be tapered at a faster rate (every third day) since they are being monitored on a daily basis. If

the TCA is abruptly discontinued, a withdrawal syndrome includes nausea, headache, malaise, vomiting, dizziness, chills, cold sweats, abdominal cramps, diarrhea, insomnia, anxiety, restlessness, and irritability can occur. If the immediate discontinuation of a TCA is imperative and the patient subsequently experiences TCA withdrawal symptoms, the administration of an anticholinergic medication such as diphenhydramine will usually reverse the symptoms (Perry et al., 1991).

BLOOD LEVELS. A review of the studies examining the relationship between the antidepressant effect of TCAs and their plasma concentrations concluded that imipramine, nortriptyline, and desipramine blood level measurements generate information that can increase patient response rates (Perry et al., 1987). For nortriptyline, the traditional "therapeutic window" of 60 to 150 ng/ml demonstrated a 68 percent response rate within the range, whereas the response rate outside the "window" was only 29 percent. Thus utilization of nortriptyline plasma concentration measurements can more than double the probability of response. For desipramine, a therapeutic window of 108 to 158 ng/ml demonstrated a 59 percent response rate within the range, whereas the response rate outside the window was only 29 percent. If the patient is unresponsive, the dose should then be adjusted to the high-level "therapeutic threshold" to attain a concentration of greater than 290 ng/ml, where the response rate was 63 percent but based on very little data. The therapeutic threshold plasma concentration for a total imipramine (imipramine + desipramine) is apparent at 244 ng/ml. At concentrations of greater than 243 ng/ml, the probability of response to imipramine was increased nearly threefold by utilizing plasma concentration measurements. For the remaining TCAs there is not enough data available in the literature to come to any firm conclusion as to the validity of plasma concentrations measurements. Since absorption and tissue distribution of a TCA may take as long as 5 to 8 hours, it is recommended that steady-state plasma sampling be carried out at approximately 12 hours after the last dose. A 12-hour sampling time guarantees that plasma levels are being measured during the elimination phase, which in contrast to the absorption and distribution phase demonstrates much less flux in the levels. The plasma sample should be drawn after steady state (when the amount of drug ingested daily equals the amount of drug excreted daily) has been reached (usually 1 week).

RETROSPECTIVE DOSING. Since TCAs follow first-order linear kinetics as the dose increases or decreases, the steady-state TCA concentration must increase or decrease proportionately. Thus a patient with a steady-state nortriptyline concentration of 50 ng/ml, at 75 mg/d, will have a steady-state level of 100 ng/ml if the dose is increased to 150 mg/d, whereas if the dose is decreased to 50 mg/d, the steady-state level should be 33 ng/ml. It must be remembered that the steady-state TCA level in this mathematical relationship is the mean plasma concentration, not the peak or 12-hour or trough plasma level. However, clinically, this method can be utilized as a reasonable approximation of the 12-hour steady-state level (Perry et al., 1991).

PROSPECTIVE DOSING—SINGLE-POINT METHOD. The nortriptyline dosing nomogram in Fig. 33-1 can be utilized to prospectively dose patients. The only data required to predict steady-state doses for maintenance doses between 50 and 150 mg/d using the nomogram is a plasma nortriptyline concentration measured 24 hours following the administration of a 100-mg test dose of nortriptyline. The only caveat regarding the use of the nomogram is that a dose of 150 mg/d should not be exceeded because of the potential for the relationship of nortriptyline plasma concentrations and maintenance doses not being linear at higher doses (Perry et al., 1984).

ADVERSE EFFECTS

From a practical standpoint, the TCAs are classified as either dimethylated TCAs (amitriptyline, imipramine, doxepin, and trimipramine) or monomethylated TCAs (nortriptyline, desipramine, and protrip-

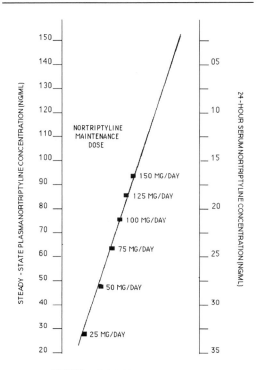

NORTRIPTYLINE SINGLE POINT DOSING NOMOGRAM

FIGURE 33-1. *Nortriptyline single-point-dosing-nomogram.*

tyline). The dimethylated amine TCAs primarily block serotonin reuptake, while the monomethylated amine TCAs primarily block norepinephrine reuptake. Dimethylated TCAs are clinically considered to be more sedating, more potent as anticholinergic agents, and cause greater weight gain than the monomethylated TCAs. Monomethylated TCAs cause less postural hypotension than does the dimethylated class (Richelson and Nelson, 1984).

ANTICHOLINERGIC EFFECTS. Anticholinergic side effects are not necessarily dose-related and usually mild and remit after a few weeks. *Blurred vision*, noticed when the patient focuses on close objects, is rarely serious and usually lasts about 1 week. Dose reduction may be helpful if the problem is persistent or serious. Patients should be cautioned against operating motor vehicles if the problem is marked. *Urinary retention* is most commonly manifested as micturition difficulty or hesitancy because of the increase in bladder sphincter tone and volume of fluid necessary to trigger detrusor contraction. It is related to dose, patient age, and duration of treatment. It may be helped by bethanechol. The true prevalence of *dry mouth* is 40 percent of the depressed patients taking imipramine. It is relieved symptomatically by increased fluid intake and by agents that stimulate salivation, such as hard (sugarless) candy. A therapeutic mouthwash, Xerolube, has been developed that not only relieves the painful soft-tissue problem but also remineralizes tooth surfaces damaged as a result of salivary deprivation. TCA-induced constipation occurs in 15 percent of patients. It is best treated with a bulk laxative such as Metamucil, hydration, and/or exercise. TCAs can increase intraocular pressure in patients with closed-angle but not open-angle *glaucoma*. An in vitro estimation of the anticholinergic potency of the TCAs that considered the potency of the individual agents yielded the following order of anticholinergic activity: amitriptyline > trimipramine > doxepin > imipramine > protriptyline > desipramine > nortriptyline. If anticholinergic adverse effects are a perceived either prospectively or retrospectively as a problem, the use of a less anticholinergic TCA such as desipramine or nortriptyline is indicated (Perry et al., 1991).

CARDIOVASCULAR. The most common cardiovascular problem precipitated by TCA use is *orthostatic hypotension*. The problem can be reduced by utilizing nortriptyline. In addition, patients should be instructed to always rise slowly from a lying or sitting position, avoid excessive bed rest, tilt the head of their bed upward, maintain adequate fluid intake, self-monitor their blood pressure, increase dietary salt unless contraindicated, and wear support hose. The TCA do not cause any further impairment of the left ventricular ejection fraction in patients with *congestive heart failure*. However, imipramine but not nortriptyline does cause a worsening of orthostatic hypotension. TCA-induced *sinus tachycardia* (rate > 100/min) is uncommon at therapeutic doses, and symptomatic sinus tachycardia is rare. Should the latter occur, a less anticholinergic TCA such as nortriptyline is indicated. In patients with *prolonged PR intervals*, TCAs are not contraindicated. However, these patients require ECG monitoring until maximal TCA doses are reached. Patients having *bundle-branch blocks* require blood pressure, TCA plasma concentration, and ECG monitoring. These extraordinary measures suggest that ECT or second-generation antidepressants such as fluoxetine or bupropion are more appropriate treatment alternatives.

DERMATOLOGIC. Cutaneous vasculitis, urticaria, and photosensitivity are the dermatologic adverse effects that have been reported. Usually occurring within the first 2 months of therapy, the skin reactions usually are harmless and rarely require discontinuation of therapy (Perry et al., 1991).

HEMATOLOGIC. Hematologic adverse effects secondary to the TCAs are usually neither a serious nor a common problem. Eosinophilia can occur in the first few weeks of therapy, but it is of no clinical significance. Leukopenia is also an apparently benign and transient effect of the TCAs. Agranulocytosis, although quite rare, has a 10 to 20 percent mortality rate. It occurs most often in the second month of therapy, usually in elderly, female patients. Routine periodic white blood cell counts are not recommended (Perry et al., 1991).

HEPATIC. Jaundice associated with cholestasis has been described with the TCAs. Elevations of transaminases and alkaline phosphatase are common during TCA treatment. However, discontinuation is only indicated if the patients become symptomatic. Patients should become cognizant of the symptoms of jaundice and contact their physicians at the first hint of symptoms. A potentially fatal liver necrosis is thought to be an allergic hypersensitivity reaction (Perry et al., 1991).

METABOLIC/ENDOCRINE. *Galactorrhea* and *amenorrhea* in women, and excessive *weight gain* in both sexes have been reported. The galactorrhea and amenorrhea are often successfully managed by dose reduction. The weight gain is not always reversible on TCA discontinuation. Since weight gain can result in potentially serious compliance problems, it is appropriate to avoid use of the TCAs in these patients. Fluoxetine and bupropion are reasonable alternative antidepressants (Perry et al., 1991).

NEUROLOGIC/PSYCHIATRIC. The acute organic brain syndrome or *delirium* secondary to the anticholinergic activity of the TCAs is characterized by recent memory loss, disorientation, flushed, dry skin, ataxia, dysarthria, and hallucinations. It is estimated that 8 percent of patients receiving TCAs experience anticholinergic delirium. Generally, the sensorium clears in 35 percent in less than 24 hours. Thus the use of physostigmine is only rarely necessary. A fine resting tremor caused by the TCAs is of a faster frequency than the pseudoparkinsonian

tremor observed with antipsychotics. It does not respond to antiparkinsonian drug therapy but does respond to propranolol. TCAs can lower the *seizure* threshold. However, this usually occurs only at high therapeutic doses or in overdoses. Thus the presence of a seizure disorder would not contraindicate the use of a TCA. *Erectile dysfunction* associated with imipramine, desipramine, clomipramine, amitriptyline, and protriptyline (in descending order of potency) are usually the TCAs responsible for causing a disturbance in sexual function. The problems are reversible upon decreasing the dose or discontinuing the drug. Drugs with cholinergic action such as bethanecol 20 mg PO 1 to 2 hours before sexual activity appear to correct erectile and ejaculatory impairment (Perry et al., 1991).

TCA/MAOI COMBINATION THERAPY. The concomitant use of a TCA and an MAOI has been utilized occasionally for the patient unresponsive to a TCA and a MAOI used separately and sequentially. Reports of hyperpyrexia, seizures, and cardiorespiratory collapse with the combination have been limited to scattered reports when overdoses and other drugs were involved. Although rarely utilized any more, if this combination is used, it is recommended that all antidepressants be discontinued, 5 to 10 days for TCA and 14 days for MAOI, before the combination is started and that preferably amitriptyline 150 mg/d and isocarboxazid 10 to 20 mg/d be administered simultaneously at conservative doses (Perry et al., 1991).

TERATOGENICITY AND EXCRETION INTO BREAST MILK. The use of these drugs during pregnancy is safe. However, common sense dictates that they should be avoided in pregnant women, especially in the first trimester, unless the need for the drug is absolutely necessary for the treatment of the patient's depression. Despite receiving relatively small quantities of TCA in breast milk neonates can be exposed to potentially hazardous TCA concentrations due to the immaturity of their liver. Thus it is appropriate that the drug be discontinued close to parturition and the mother should not expect to breast-feed while receiving a TCA. Children born to mothers exposed to TCAs have occasionally been reported to have experienced some of the following symptoms at birth: urinary retention, nonspecific respiratory distress, peripheral cyanosis, hypertonia with tremor, clonus, and spasm (Perry et al., 1991).

Monoamine Oxidase Inhibitors (MAOIs)

EFFICACY

It has been suggested since the late 1950s that the MAOIs are indicated for "atypical" or "hysterical" depressions. The responders were symptomatically characterized as presenting most commonly with somatic preoccupations, diurnal mood variation characterized by evening rather than morning dysphoria, hypersomnia, and weight gain. Improvement following the start of MAOI therapy appeared sooner than expected in the atypical group (usually within 5 to 8 days), while improvement in the typical endogenous group was rarely as quick or complete. A body of evidence has developed suggesting that there is a diagnostically definable subgroup of depressed patients who are likely to respond to MAOIs. Thus these atypical depressions may be defined according to the following criteria: (1) presence of frequent and persisting depressions with retained emotional reactivity to outside stimuli and absence of fixed lowering of mood, (2) features which might be particularly MAOI responsive include either "reverse" vegetative symptoms (evening worsening of mood, initial insomnia, increased appetite or weight gain, and hypersomnia), the presence of features of dysthymic disorder, and/or the presence of preexisting anxiety, particularly agoraphobia, (3) absence of delusional guilt or manic episodes, and (4) absence of alcoholism, organic brain syndromes, schizophrenia, or longstanding characterologic depression (Nies, 1984).

MAOIs are usually considered not as effective as TCAs in the treatment of depression. However, this perception was based on early efficacy studies that often utilized subtherapeutic or borderline therapeutic MAOI doses. Additionally, their onset of action is slower than the TCAs, and short therapeutic trials were often utilized in contrasting their effectiveness to the TCAs. Based on earlier controlled studies conducted prior to 1974, it was usually assumed that MAOIs were probably less effective than TCAs (Morris and Beck, 1974). More recent studies, using larger phenelzine doses (60 to 75 mg/d), produced more impressive results as to the efficacy of the MAOIs in depression. Phenelzine is as effective as the TCA in the treatment of *melancholic depression*, more effective than the TCA in the treatment of *dysthymia* (Vallejo et al., 1987), and in-

effective in the treatment of *delusional depression* (Janicak et al., 1988).

DOSING

The target dose of phenelzine is 1.0 mg/kg per day. Because of the variability between patients experiencing stimulation or sedation from phenelzine, the dose schedule should be adjusted appropriately to avoid drug-induced insomnia or daytime sedation, which is often seen in patients receiving MAOI. Usually, the drug is administered on a twice-daily dosage schedule. An adequate *therapeutic trial* of an MAOI is 4 to 6 weeks. Two weeks are required before the maximum monoamine oxidase inhibitory effect of phenelzine 30 mg/d is reached, while 4 weeks are required for a 60 mg/d dose. It is estimated that tranylcypromine 0.7 mg/kg per day equals phenelzine 1.0 mg/kg per day. When switching a patient from one MAOI to another, especially tranylcypromine, at least a 10-day "washout" period is advisable because of the potential risk of a hypertensive crisis (Perry et al., 1991).

ADVERSE EFFECTS

Table 33-1 contrasts the adverse drug reaction prevalences for phenelzine and tranylcypromine with imipramine and placebo. Most of the adverse effects occurred with phenelzine, although they did not result in more frequent discontinuation of the drug than with tranylcypromine. Additionally, the adverse reactions could not be accounted for by patient differences in age, sex, diagnosis, or duration of treatment. The mean maximum doses were 269 mg/d for imipramine, 69 mg/d for phenelzine, and 50 mg/d for tranylcypromine (Rabkin et al., 1984).

CARDIOVASCULAR. Phenelzine at a 60 mg/d dose can be expected to significantly decrease the QTc interval of the ECG but not affect the PR interval or

TABLE 33-1. *Prevalence (%) of MAOI Adverse Effects*

Adverse effect	Placebo	Imipramine	Phenelzine	Tranylcypromine
Hypomania	0	0	10	7
Hypertensive crisis	0	0	8	2
Convulsion	0	2	0	0
Syncope	0	9	11	17
Disorientation	0	3	5	2
Edema*	0	0	4	0
Rash*	2	2	1	2
Weight gain* (>15 lb)	0	0	8	0
Urinary retention	0	3	5	2
Paresthesias	0	3	5	2
Drowsiness*	0	0	3	0
Anorgasmia/impotence	0	5	22	2
None	96	71	40	56

*Drug discontinued
Source: From Sheehan DV, Claycomb JB, Kauretos N: Monoamine oxidase inhibitors: Prescription and patient management. Int J Psychiatry Med 10:99–109, 1980–81, with permission.

the QRS complex. Orthostatic hypotension also can be seen. The *blood pressure* effects of phenelzine differ from the TCAs in that (1) phenelzine affects both lying systolic blood pressure as well as orthostatic and (2) the orthostatic hypotensive effects of phenelzine have a slower onset, maximize at 4 weeks, and then appear to decrease in intensity. Patients over 50 years of age are more likely to experience declines in standing and sitting blood pressure than younger patients. Initially during the first 6 weeks of treatment, phenelzine will produce a decrease in systolic and diastolic pressure. However, patients on chronic MAOI therapy for months to years will have their sitting diastolic and systolic pressures increase significantly during the first 2 hours after ingestion of the dose, after which they return to normal (Perry et al., 1991).

The concomitant ingestion of MAOI and substances containing certain pressor amines has been associated with potentially serious *hypertensive crisis*. The primary reactions are headache and increased blood pressure resulting from sympathetic overstimulation. *Tyramine* is the dietary pressor amine usually associated with these reactions. The reactions also can be precipitated by food containing phenylethylamine or dopamine. Normally, MAO found in the gastrointestinal tract inactivates tyramine. However, when MAOIs block this reaction, exogenous tyramine is absorbed, and it exerts its indirect pressor action by releasing norepinephrine from the presynaptic storage sites. Additionally, indirect-acting sympathomimetics such as amphetamines, methylphenidate, ephedrine, pseudoephedrine, phenylpropanolamine, and phenylephrine have been reported to interact with MAOIs. *Cheeses* are the foodstuff most often reported to precipitate hypertensive crisis with MAOIs. However, not all types of cheese contain significant amounts of tyramine to cause this adverse reaction. As a general rule, any protein-containing food that has undergone degradation may present a hazard. Therefore, nonmatured cheeses such as cottage cheese, cream cheese, as well as milk and yogurt are safe, since these contain little or no tyramine. New evidence suggests that all *alcoholic beverages* and even their nonalcoholic counterparts (alcohol-free beer) ought to be restricted to guarantee the safety of the MAOI-treated patient. *Yeast/protein extracts* sometimes found in packet soups as well as yeast vitamin supplements (brewer's yeast, marmite) are to be avoided, whereas the baker's yeast contained in baked goods is safe. Unacceptable *meats and fish* include smoked or pickled fish (herring) and shrimp paste, caviar, beef or chicken liver, and fermented sausages (bologna, pepperoni, salami, summer sausage). Restricted *fruits and vegetables* include avocados, canned or overripe figs, and stewed whole bananas/banana peel, although small amounts of banana pulp are allowed. Products containing fermented bean curd (soya beans, soya paste, soy sauce) contain large amounts of tyramine. The time course of normalization of oral tyramine sensitivity after stopping MAOI treatment demands that patients stay on their tyramine-free diet for 3 to 4 weeks after the drug is discontinued. There are a number of *non-tyramine-containing foods* that are not permitted. *Fava* or broad beans, which contain dopamine, are not allowed, while the other shelled beans or legumes are permitted. Large amounts of *caffeine* can have enough pressor activity to cause problems. *Chocolate* contains phenylethylamine, a weak pressor agent, if ingested in large amounts. Some ginseng-containing products have caused headache, tremors, and manic-like symptoms. Monosodium glutamate (MSG) has been associated with complaints of headaches and palpitations (Perry et al., 1991).

NEUROLOGIC. These side effects occur rarely but usually include ataxia, tremor, hyperreflexia, paresthesias, and seizures possibly as a result of a pyridoxine deficiency. Pyridoxine 150 to 300 mg/d for several weeks reverses the paresthesias (Stewart et al., 1984).

WITHDRAWAL REACTIONS

The abrupt discontinuation of a MAOI can result in withdrawal symptoms but only rarely. Of the four cases reported, they are characterized by REM rebound producing disturbed sleep and nightmares, hallucinations and delirium. We do not recommend routine tapering MAOIs because of the infrequency of the withdrawal reactions.

Second-Generation Antidepressants

EFFICACY

Of the numerous efficacy studies that compared the effectiveness of the second-generation antidepressants amoxapine, maprotiline, trazodone, fluoxetine, and bupropion with the TCAs and placebo, one consistent theme is obvious. These drugs are equal in efficacy to the TCAs and more effective than placebo. If they did not meet these minimal criteria, they would not be accepted as a treatment for depression by the FDA. The finding that *amoxapine* has a faster onset of action than the TCAs is not a consistent finding. Additionally, there are reports of a premature loss of efficacy after 6 to 12 weeks of therapy. *Maprotiline* as well does not have a faster onset of action than the TCAs, whereas *fluoxetine* has a slower onset of action than the TCAs. Fluoxetine has been found to be more effective than imipramine in the treatment of 86 percent of bipolar depressed patients, while bupropion was effective in the treatment of 63 percent of TCA-refractory patients (Perry et al., 1991). The benzodiazepine alprazolam may have antidepressant activity despite this not being an FDA-approved indication. A review of the efficacy has led to the conclusion that alprazolam may be an effective antidepressant in mild to moderately ill depressed patients. However, in moderate to severely depressed patients it appears less effective than the TCAs (Perry et al., 1991).

DOSING

The dosage usually recommended for *amoxapine* is 200 to 300 mg/d as a single dose at bedtime. Elderly patients should be started on an initial dose of 75 mg/d. A single daily dose of *maprotiline* 150 mg at bedtime is considered the threshold level for treating acute depressions, with the dose being increased to a maximum level of 300 mg/d. The dose can be given once daily, preferably at bedtime. Additionally, it is recommended that the initial dosage and titration in the elderly be conservative, since hallucinations with or without delirium have been reported in patients over 60 years old taking daily doses of 200 mg or more. The initial dose of *trazodone* is 150 mg/d, being increased to a maximum inpatient dose of 600 mg/d at a rate of 50 mg/d every third day. It is the authors' clinical impression that many of the nonresponders to trazodone are a result of patients being unable to tolerate the drug's sedation, thereby leading to the prescribing of subtherapeutic doses of the medication. Despite the drug's short half-life, it is preferable to give the entire dose at bedtime in order to take advantage of the strong sedative action of the drug. The initial dose of *fluoxetine* is 20 mg/d for 4 weeks. A fixed-dose study of fluoxetine 20, 40, and 60 mg/d reported no differences in effectiveness between the three strengths. There are data that suggest that a dose of 5 mg/d is as effective as higher doses and produces fewer adverse effects. *Bupropion* dosing is instituted at 100 mg b.i.d. or 75 mg t.i.d., with doses taken at least 6 hours apart. The dose can be increased at a rate of 75 to 100 mg every 3 days to a maximum daily dose of 150 mg t.i.d. (Perry et al., 1991).

ADVERSE EFFECTS

AMOXAPINE. The *anticholinergic* adverse effects of dry mouth, constipation, blurred vision, and urinary retention are the most common adverse effects reported for amoxapine. The 28 percent incidence rate is similar to amitriptyline and imipramine. Orthostatic drops in both systolic and diastolic *blood pressure* occurred as commonly with amoxapine as with imipramine and amitriptyline. No serious ECG abnormalities have been observed; atrial flutter and fibrillation and conduction defects similar to those associated with the TCA have been reported. *Sedation* occurs at a rate similar to the sedating TCAs amitriptyline and imipramine. *Seizures* have been reported in patients receiving therapeutic doses of amoxapine. In overdoses, the drug seems to have the ability to produce unusual neurologic alterations, as well as a tendency to produce severe and

frequent, i.e., 36 percent, generalized seizures or status epilepticus, which are difficult to treat, as evidenced by a 15 percent fatality rate associated with the overdoses. The estimated prevalence of seizures and fatalities in TCA overdoses is 4 and 0.7 percent, respectively. *Extrapyramidal side effects (EPSE)* secondary to amoxapine's dopamine blocking metabolite include pseudoparkinsonism, akathisia, and tardive dyskinesia. Amoxapine-induced withdrawal dyskinesias account for one-third of all antidepressant-associated dyskinesias. Thus maintenance therapy with this agent is discouraged. A *neuroleptic malignant syndrome* has been reported. More pronounced in women, *hyperprolactinemia* can result in delayed menses, breast engorgement, loss of libido, galactorrhea, and fluid retention. The teratogenic potential of amoxapine is unknown at this time. The drug is excreted in breast milk, and thus breast feeding is discouraged (Perry et al., 1991).

MAPROTILINE. Since this antidepressant is a molecular manipulation of the TCA, it is not surprising that its adverse effect profile is similar to the TCAs with a few notable exceptions. The *anticholinergic* adverse effects of dry mouth, constipation, and blurred vision occur with similar frequencies for maprotiline when compared with amitriptyline and imipramine. *ECG abnormalities* are similar to those seen with amitriptyline. T-wave changes, sinus tachycardia, or incomplete bundle-branch block are usually only seen with doses of maprotiline of 300 mg/d or more. Like TCAs, maprotiline produces a quinidine-like membrane stabilization effect. *Postural hypotension* is less common with maprotiline than with amitriptyline. *Rashes* occur twice as frequently with maprotiline than with amitriptyline or imipramine. They are described as usually small, localized, and nonpruritic. Of the less common effects, maprotiline-induced *seizures* have received the most attention. The prevalence of seizures in patients receiving maprotiline was observed to be 16 versus 2 percent in TCA-treated patients. Maprotiline appears in breast milk such that breast feeding is not recommended in women receiving the drug for postpartum depressions. Dysmorphogenic studies performed in animals suggest no potential problems (Perry et al., 1991).

TRAZODONE. The most common adverse effect with trazodone is *sedation*. *Anticholinergic* adverse effects are not associated with trazodone. Initially trazodone was considered to be a noncardiotoxic drug because it did not increase ventricular conduction. However, it has been shown to exacerbate preexisting myocardial irritability, which potentially has resulted in *ventricular tachycardia*. Patients with cardiac arrhythmias and/or mitral valve prolapse should be carefully monitored when administered trazodone. *Orthostatic hypotension* differs from the TCAs in that it is transient, lasting for approximately 4 to 6 hours after the dose. The problem can be avoided by administering the drug at bedtime. It also can cause *bradycardia*. *Drowsiness* is the most commonly reported adverse effect and has been reported in up to 45 percent of patients. Many of the central nervous system adverse effects noted by the manufacturer can originate from sedation or disinhibition effects produced by the drug. There are reports of hepatoxicity within the first few weeks of trazodone therapy that are reversible after drug discontinuation. A total of 123 cases of trazodone-associated *priapism* have been reported in the United States to the manufacturer, who estimates the incidence at a conservative 1 in 6000 male patients due to the voluntary reporting nature of the system. It is most likely to occur within the first 4 weeks of treatment at doses of ≤150 mg/d. Half the patients experienced spontaneous detumescence after discontinuing the drug. Dysmorphogenic studies in animals do not indicate a *teratogenic* potential for trazodone. As is the case with the other antidepressants, it is best to advise women with postpartum depressions not to breast feed their newborns (Perry et al., 1991).

FLUOXETINE. Clinical trials conclude that fluoxetine causes fewer adverse effects than the TCAs. This finding is due primarily to less anticholinergic and sedative adverse effects. Overall, nausea (25 percent), nervousness (21 percent), and insomnia (19 percent) were reported significantly more often with fluoxetine than with the reference antidepressants. These effects resulted in fluoxetine being discontinued in 2 to 4 percent of patients, with nausea being the most common reason. The restlessness resembles akathisia from the antipsychotic. It can be managed by the administration of propranolol 40 mg/d. Additionally, there is no basis for the reports in the lay press suggesting that fluoxetine causes patients to become violent, homicidal, and suicidal. In comparison studies in patients without cardiovascular disease, fluoxetine has been shown to produce a modest but significant decrease in heart rate, although the drug has no effect on PR interval or QRS complex. It does not cause orthostatic hypotension. The drug has not been studied in patients with cardiovascular disease, and therefore, caution, i.e., blood pressure measurements and ECG monitoring, is recommended if fluoxetine is prescribed for this depressed population (Perry et al., 1991).

BUPROPION. In contrast to amitriptyline, adverse effects that occur more often with bupropion include headache, decreased appetite, nausea, vomiting, agitation, insomnia, and decreased libido. *Maculopapular lesions* and/or pruritus occur at doses of 300 to 900 mg/d. The maculopapular rashes clear in 3 to 4 days following drug discontinuation. Pruritus alone usually will clear with a reduction in dosage. A transient *weight loss* of at least 5 lb has been found to occur over a 3- to 6-week treatment period in up to 30 percent of patients on bupropion. The weight returns to baseline within 6 months. The relationship between *seizure* occur-

rence and bupropion use at therapeutic doses is 0.80 percent (37 of 4259). The incidence is 0.44 percent (15 of 3395) in patients receiving doses no greater than 450 mg/d, while the rate for doses greater than 450 mg/d demonstrated a fivefold increase, 2.2 percent (19 of 864). Seizure risk factors included a history of bulimia, doses greater than 450 mg/d, and a past history of seizures. Because bupropion has dopamine agonist activity, it is advisable not to utilize the drug in the treatment of delusion or hallucinating patients (Perry et al., 1991).

CNS Stimulants

A rather substantial anecdotal literature exists suggesting that CNS stimulants may have some utility in depression. The inflated response rate to stimulants in the treatment of depression reported in uncontrolled studies has not been replicated in 9 of the 10 placebo-controlled trials. All but one of the studies were reported between 1958 and 1972. Of similarly designed controlled studies involving the TCA imipramine, 14 of 23 showed the TCA to be clearly superior to placebo. However, according to the findings of controlled studies, stimulant use may have more validity in the treatment of apathetic "senile" geriatric patients who do not have a primary depression. Partial responses but not remissions are observed in these patients. Although some anecdotal or uncontrolled data suggest that stimulants may be useful in medically ill patients with depression, confirmation of this finding in controlled studies is still lacking. Finally, the stimulants are reported in uncontrolled studies to be effective in the treatment of TCA-refractory patients. However, controlled studies have reported placebo response rates in this patient population ranging from 57 to 78 percent (Satel and Nelson, 1989).

Overall, fewer adverse effects are reported with the stimulants than the TCAs. Habituation is commonly described as a risk, but it has not been confirmed in control trials. Side effects in decreasing order of frequency include insomnia, nausea, tremor, appetite change, palpitations, blurred vision, dry mouth, constipation, and dizziness. Signs in their decreasing order of frequency include blood pressure changes in either direction, dysrhythmias, and tremor.

MANIA

Lithium

EFFICACY

The primary clinical indications for lithium in psychiatry are the treatment of acute mania and the prophylactic treatment of patients with recurrent unipolar or bipolar affective illness. In placebo-controlled studies of acute manics, 76 percent of all lithium-treated patients improved. More relevant pharmacotherapy comparisons of the treatment of acute mania involve lithium versus the antipsychotics. They demonstrate several distinct differences in the effectiveness of the two in the treatment of mania. In appropriate doses ($\geq$1800 mg/d or $\geq$0.8 mEq/liter), lithium produces marked improvement or remission in $\geq$70 percent of patients. The probability of patients showing remission or marked improvement of manic symptoms is greater with lithium than with antipsychotics. Lithium is particularly effective in ameliorating the affective and ideational symptoms associated with mania, whereas antipsychotics are superior to lithium in controlling, at least initially, the increased psychomotor activity associated with mania. The antipsychotic haloperidol more quickly reduces the severity of hostility, excitement, grandiosity, and suspiciousness than either lithium or chlorpromazine. Hospitalized manics treated with lithium rather than an antipsychotic are discharged sooner. Because of the 6- to 10-day delay of onset of action of lithium, the extremely hyperactive manic patient is best treated with lithium and an antipsychotic (Goodwin and Zis, 1979). The antipsychotic is discontinued once the patient's behavior normalizes. This is an important consideration, since affectively ill patients are more likely to develop tardive dyskinesia. Manic patients refractory to lithium or the lithium/antipsychotic combination therapy may respond to ECT in addition to the second-line pharmacotherapeutic alternatives of carbamazepine, verapamil, or valproic acid. One study found that all manic patients refractory to chlorpromazine did respond to ECT, although 39 percent relapsed shortly thereafter (McCabe and Norris, 1977). Thus prophylactic lithium is indicated following a course of ECT in the acutely manic patient.

Lithium is extremely effective in preventing relapses in patients with recurrent bipolar or unipolar affective illness. For bipolar patients, in most studies the annualized rate of relapse was reduced by 50 percent compared with placebo, and the recurrences were less severe (Consensus Development Panel, 1985). As an example a 24-month NIMH follow-up study found that the overall relapse rate was 67 percent for placebo, 67 percent for imipramine, but only 17 percent for lithium (Prien et al., 1973). For unipolar patients, numerous controlled studies using follow-up periods ranging from 5 months to 3 years have shown that either lithium or the TCAs amitriptyline or imipramine were equally effective in significantly reducing recurrences of depressive episodes. In the above-mentioned NIMH study, the pooled rate of unipolar patients relapsing was 85 percent for placebo, which was significantly greater than the 29 percent for imipramine and 41 percent for lithium (Prien et al., 1973). Additionally, the combination of a TCA and lithium is superior to lithium in the prevention of any relapse, mania or depression, and the combi-

nation is superior to imipramine in the prevention of depressive relapses (Kim et al., 1990). Thus lithium is a significantly more effective prophylactic drug than antidepressants in bipolar patients and equal to the TCAs in unipolar patients. Additionally, if a unipolar patient fails a prophylactic trial of either lithium or a TCA, then it is appropriate to treat the patient with a combination of the two agents. Patients receiving prophylactic lithium suggest that responders are more likely to be bipolar patients with a positive family history of either unipolar or bipolar illness or unipolar patients with endogenous illness and familial pure depressive disease (no alcoholism or sociopathy in first-degree relatives). Also, they are less likely to have personality disorders than fair to poor responders. Finally, a beneficial long-term response is most likely in bipolar patients who responded within 6 months and unipolar patients who responded within the first year (Abou-Saleh and Coppen, 1986).

One of the most important decisions a clinician is confronted with in treating patients with recurrent affective illness is at what point in time should prophylactic therapy be initiated. Apart from the present episode, in bipolar depressed patients, prophylactic treatment should begin after the two past episodes, whereas unipolar depressed patients should be treated prophylactically following three previous episodes (Angst, 1981).

There is minimal information concerning the use of lithium in acute *schizoaffective* patients. The available data indicate that lithium is effective in the initial treatment of schizoaffective mania, whereas antidepressants and antipsychotics either alone or in combination are effective in the treatment of schizoaffective depression. The onset of response for lithium is slower in schizoaffective mania than bipolar mania (Goodnick and Meltzer, 1984). Prophylactic administration of lithium can decrease the number of relapses and hospitalizations in schizoaffective patients. A past history of bipolar illness is a positive predictor of lithium response in these patients while a diagnosis of schizodepressive is a negative response predictor (Maj, 1988).

DOSING

ACUTE MANIA. The generally recommended therapeutic range for lithium is 0.9 to 1.4 mEq/liter. The data suggest that patients with levels greater than 1.4 mEq/liter experience no greater improvement in their manic symptoms than patients with lower serum lithium concentrations. Patients with concentrations less than 0.9 mEq/liter usually do not experience complete remission of manic symptoms. Control of the attack usually occurs within 4 to 10 days after the start of treatment depending on how quickly the lithium dose reaches the therapeutic range. Acutely manic patients tolerate and require higher lithium doses due to their increased lithium clearances. The initial doses may not be tolerated once the manic episode begins to abate. Thus lithium levels ought to be drawn twice weekly when treating an acutely manic patient because of the predictable but potentially toxic paroxysmal increase in the lithium level as the manic hyperactivity begins to resolve.

PROPHYLAXIS. The ideal prophylactic serum lithium concentration is debatable based on findings of considerable variance between several English and one American study. Overall, these data have led us to conclude that a serum lithium concentration of 0.45 to 0.59 mEq/liter on a single daily dose schedule is appropriate in the prophylactic treatment of affectively ill patients, although higher concentrations are required in the elderly. However, patients should increase their dose by 1.5 times at the first signs of any manic or depressive symptoms and then slowly taper downward to the lower concentration as the symptoms resolve (Perry et al., 1991).

SERUM LITHIUM CONCENTRATION SAMPLING. Lithium levels are usually obtained 12 hours after the last dose to guarantee that the lithium was in the elimination phase of the concentration versus time disposition curve, i.e., the least dynamic component of the drug's absorption–distribution–elimination curve. The half-life of lithium in psychiatric patients has been estimated to range from 15 to 55 hours (Thornhill and Field, 1982). Assuming an individual patient's lithium half-life is unknown and that lithium half-lives range from 15 to 55 hours for patients with normal renal function, approximately 220 hours (4 half-lives) may need to elapse before a true steady-state lithium concentration is apparent. Lithium levels in outpatients are usually checked monthly for 3 months and then every 3 months thereafter.

Often a patient on a divided daily dosing schedule, because of significant polyuria, requires a single daily dosing schedule. If the clinician assumes a 24-hour half-life for the patient, then an approximate 20 percent increase in the 12-hour steady-state serum lithium concentration ought to be anticipated. However, an even more reasonable and conservative estimate of the increase in the steady-state level would be to expect a 0.2 mEq/liter increase (Perry et al., 1991).

PRODUCT FORMULATIONS. Slow-absorption lithium product formulations were developed in an attempt to decrease the adverse effects associated with peak and rapidly rising serum lithium concentrations as well as to increase compliance. The only comparison study of regular-release lithium with the slow-release lithium product available in the United States did not demonstrate a difference in the adverse effect profile of the two formulations (Lyskowski and Nasrallah, 1981).

RETROSPECTIVE DOSING—STEADY-STATE CONCENTRATION MONITORING. As lithium dose increases or decreases, the steady-state serum lithium concentration increases or decreases in direct proportion to the change. A patient with a steady-state concentration of 1.0 mEq/liter at 1200 mg/d will have a steady-state concentration of 1.50 mEq/liter if the dose is increased to 1800 mg/d, whereas if the dose is decreased to 600 mg/d, the steady-state concentration should be 0.50 mEq/liter.

PROSPECTIVE DOSING—SINGLE-POINT METHOD. The lithium dosing nomogram in Fig. 33-2 can be utilized as an efficient means to prospectively dose patients. The only data that are required to predict steady-state doses for maintenance dose between 900 and 2400 mg/d using the nomogram is a serum lithium concentration measured 24 hours following the administration of a 1200-mg test dose of lithium carbonate to a lithium-naive patient. Since acute manic patients' lithium requirements decrease once they start sleeping more because their clearance decreases in a prone position, the clinician should anticipate reducing the lithium maintenance dose in acute manics as they cycle into a euthymic state.

ADVERSE EFFECTS

During the first week of lithium treatment, there are numerous adverse effect complaints by patients receiving the drug that include primarily gastrointestinal irritation, tremor, muscle weakness, and polydipsia/polyuria. Direct questioning concerning adverse effects in patients receiving lithium prophylactically found the following incidences: polyuria and polydipsia, 79 percent; tremor, 45 percent;

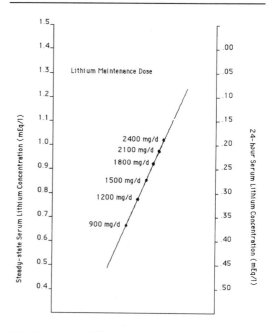

FIGURE 33-2. *Lithium single-point dosing nomogram.*

loose stools, 20 percent; weight gain greater than 10 kg, 20 percent; edema, 10 percent; dermatitides, 3 percent; and muscle weakness, 1.6 percent (Vestergaard et al., 1980). These adverse effects can be managed quite often by single daily dosing and maintaining the prophylactic serum lithium concentration between 0.45 to 0.60 mEq/liter.

CENTRAL NERVOUS SYSTEM. Delirium manifested by distractibility, poor memory, disorientation, incoherence, poor concentration, and impaired judgment occurs predictably at supratherapeutic and rarely at therapeutic lithium levels. The organic symptoms may be accompanied by involuntary movements, ataxia, and dysarthria. The symptoms often appear insidiously and may be unrecognized as lithium-related. CNS-compromised patients (e.g., seizure disorders, schizophrenics) may be predisposed to this adverse effect. Thus in this latter patient population lithium should be dosed conservatively. Usually, however, the symptoms of a lithium intoxication do not begin to exhibit themselves until the serum concentration exceeds 1.5 mEq/liter. As mentioned above, clinical manifestations are primarily neurologic (i.e., confusion, poor concentration, clouding of consciousness, delirium, and coma). Cerebellar disturbances are manifested by dysarthria, nystagmus, and ataxia (El-Mallakh, 1986). A 2-liter normal saline infusion has been shown to increase the lithium clearance to 40 ml/min and should be considered the cornerstone of therapy for intoxications with levels <3 mEq/liter (Holstad et al., 1986). Hemodialysis is normally indicated only when the concentration exceeds 3 mEq/liter.

DERMATOLOGIC. Lithium has been associated with a wide range of dermatologic problems of varying clinical significance. Transient maculopapular eruptions and follicular eruptions which often remit spontaneously are usually not significant problems. However, exacerbations of acne and psoriasis may be severe enough that compliance may become a problem. In this case, a second-line bipolar illness drug such as carbamazepine is indicated (Perry et al., 1991).

GASTROINTESTINAL. Gastrointestinal complaints include epigastric bloating, slight abdominal pain, nausea, vomiting, and anorexia. Fortunately, these adverse effects are transient. They are minimized by administering the lithium with food and by dividing the total daily dose into small divided doses and possibly by utilizing a slow-release dosage form of lithium. Loose stools, diarrhea, and occasional bloody stools are a far more serious problem because the sodium and water loss predisposes the patient to lithium retention and potential intoxication. The diarrhea results from the unabsorbed lithium in the colon acting as an osmotic cathartic. However, this problem can be circumvented by utilizing the more quickly absorbed liquid lithium citrate product formulation (Perry et al., 1991).

HEMATOLOGIC. Both leukocytosis and thrombocytosis occur in the majority of patients receiving lithium. However, both are regarded as innocuous adverse effects. The leukocytosis is not marked by a "shift to the left." The peak elevation typically occurs within 1 week and is reversible within 1 to 2 weeks. The elevated platelet counts may require 2 to 4 months to normalize (Perry et al., 1991).

ENDOCRINE. *Weight gains* of greater than 10 lb are estimated to occur in 11 to 64 percent of patients taking lithium. The gain is minimized and reversed by caloric restriction and restriction of intake of glucose containing fluids. It is important to inform patients of the potential for weight gain and to avoid high-calorie soft drinks in replacement of fluid loss secondary to polyuria. Hypothyroidism and other endocrine abnormalities are associated with lithium. Approximately 15 percent of the patients had elevated thyroid-stimulating hormone (TSH) values in the range of 8 to 20 mU/ml. Patients developing hypothyroidism are most commonly women over 40 years of age. Treatment may not be necessary as the majority of cases of lithium-induced thyroid abnormalities are transient and often without clinical symptoms. Despite the lack of a dose–response relationship, some clinicians report that lowering the dose may reverse the hypothyroid symptoms. Goiter and the hypothyroid state can be reversed with thyroid supplementation. Preexisting hypothyroidism is not an absolute contraindication to lithium treatment. Lithium can increase serum calcium, reduce serum phosphorous, and increase *parathyroid hormone* (PTH) in about 10 to 15 percent of patients. Complications of primary hyperparathyroidism do not occur, though osteopenia has been reported. Hypercalcemic patients taking lithium can appear either dysphoric, apathetic, or ataxic. Thus patients appearing psychomotor retarded or depressed ought to have their calcium checked before antidepressant therapy is started (Perry et al., 1991).

NEUROMUSCULAR. Lithium-induced *tremor* is reported to occur in 10 to 65 percent of patients. It may occur at rest and during purposeful movements. An exacerbation or worsening of the tremor or extension to other parts of the body can be regarded as a prodromal symptom of impending lithium toxicity. Additionally, emotional stress and excessive caffeine intake also may worsen the tremor. However, because of its diuretic effect, reducing caffeine intake may increase lithium levels and worsen tremor. Decreasing the dose is an effective means of management. If this is not effective, the beta blocker, propranolol 30 to 80 mg/d is an alternative. *Muscle weakness*, a transient side effect, appears to be dose-related and disappears with reduction of discontinuation of lithium (Perry et al., 1991).

RENAL. Although lithium-induced polyuria and polydipsia are common, they are usually reasonably well tolerated by the patients and completely or partially reversible upon the discontinuation of the lithium therapy. Nevertheless, we have observed serious polyuria cases where as much as 18 liter/d of urine has been excreted by a patient. Thus the severe cases can result in serious fluid and electrolyte disturbances which could result in toxicity. Since significant polyuria is a predisposing factor toward potential future renal dysfunction, it is imperative to minimize the degree of this adverse effect. We have found that the use of single daily dosing or the diuretics hydrochlorothiazide 50 mg/d or amiloride 10 to 20 mg/d are equally effective in reducing the polyuria. Additionally, renal function in these patients should be monitored closely. The most practical method available to routinely monitor the glomerular filtration rate is the use of the Cockcroft-Gault method (Cockcroft and Gault, 1976) for estimating creatinine clearance (Cl_{Cr}), where

$$Cl_{Cr} = \frac{(140 - \text{age}) \ (\text{kg body weight})}{(72) \ (\text{fasting serum creatinine})}$$

There are three important points to remember about the use of this equation to ensure its accuracy: (1) the calculated Cl_{Cr} should be reduced by 15 percent in women, (2) a correction to lean or ideal body weight is necessary in excessively obese, edematous patients, and (3) the serum creatinine value should be drawn in the fasting state. The Cl_{Cr} ought to be estimated by this method ideally every 6 to 12 months (Perry et al., 1991).

TERATOGENICITY AND EXCRETION INTO BREAST MILK. Lithium is associated with an increased number of cardiovascular anomalies such as Ebstein's anomaly, atrial septal defect, and tricuspid valve malformation in children exposed to lithium in the first trimester of pregnancy. Thus it is recommended that lithium be avoided, unless strongly indicated, in pregnant women, especially during the first trimester. Verapamil is the only antimanic drug that is an acceptable alternative (Perry et al., 1991). Lithium is excreted in breast milk at a concentration about 30 to 100 percent that of the mother's serum. Therefore, bottle feeding of newborns is recommended in women concomitantly receiving lithium (Perry et al., 1991).

Carbamazepine (CBZ)

EFFICACY

Three double-blind, controlled trials directly compared the effectiveness of CBZ with that of lithium in the treatment of acute mania (Lusznat et al., 1988; Okuma et al., 1990; Small et al., 1991). Moderate to marked improvement was noted in 52 percent of patients treated with CBZ ($n = 90$), while 46 percent of the lithium-treated patients demonstrated similar improvement. Four investigations (Okuma et al., 1979; Grossi et al., 1984; Placidi et al., 1986; Lerer et al., 1987) included lithium-naive patients being treated with either lithium, CBZ, or chlorpromazine, whereas one

study (Post and Uhde, 1985) included patients refractory to lithium. Among the lithium-naive patients, the overall response rates were 71 percent for lithium ($n = 41$), 61 percent for CBZ ($n = 103$), and 59 percent for chlorpromazine ($n = 38$). Among the lithium-refractory patients, the overall response rate was 60 percent for CBZ ($n = 17$).

Overall, it is estimated that in the prophylactic treatment of affective illness, CBZ prevents the recurrence of manic episodes in 70 percent and depressive episodes in 65 percent of patients studied. In a series of 24 bipolar and unipolar patients who were either lithium-intolerant or lithium-refractory, CBZ prevented recurrences in 63 percent of the population (Stuppaeck et al., 1990).

DOSING

The initial dose is 200 mg given twice daily with meals and increased in 200-mg increments every other day. Acutely ill patients generally require doses ranging from 600 to 1600 mg/d, while "rapid cyclers" or lithium-refractory patients usually require higher doses ranging between 1000 and 2000 mg/d. Patients being treated prophylactically require smaller doses. Effective carbamazepine plasma concentrations in the treatment of acute mania ranged from 4.7 to 14.0 mg/ml (mean 8.8 mg/ml), while effective prophylactic concentrations ranged from 4 to 7 mg/ml (mean 5.7 mg/ml) (Post, 1988). However, it must be kept in mind that no significant correlation has ever been demonstrated between carbamazepine concentrations and the antimanic therapeutic response. Thus these recommendations are nothing more than initial target serum concentrations. Plasma sampling is best accomplished just prior to the next dose to estimate a trough level of the drug. Because carbamazepine stimulates its own hepatic metabolism, steady-state plasma concentrations may be 50 percent below the expected values. Maximal hepatic enzyme induction reportedly occurs within 3 to 5 weeks. A serum sample drawn at this time should reflect a true steady-state concentration. After this time, any further changes in the carbamazepine dosage will require approximately 1 week for concentrations to reflect the new steady-state concentration (Bertilsson and Tomson, 1986).

ADVERSE EFFECTS

Carbamazepine's chemical structure resembles a tricyclic antidepressant. Thus much of its adverse effect profile resembles that of a tricyclic antidepressant.

CARDIAC. Carbamazepine can suppress both atrioventricular conduction and ventricular automaticity. However, significant ECG changes have only been reported in patients with preexisting conduction disturbances. The drug is contraindicated in patients with bundle-branch blocks (Perry et al., 1991).

CENTRAL NERVOUS SYSTEM. CNS adverse effects of dizziness (29 percent), ataxia (21 percent), clumsiness (17 percent), and drowsiness (13 percent) usually occur at the start of therapy (Ballenger and Post, 1980). Delirium and hallucinations are a result of central anticholinergic activity. Dystonic reactions and dopamine blockade can occur 2 to 3 weeks after the start of therapy (Perry et al., 1991).

DERMATOLOGIC. Carbamazepine-induced dermatologic reactions occur in 3 to 8 percent of patients (Livingston et al., 1974; Ballenger and Post, 1980). The reactions occur within the first 5 months of treatment. They include rashes with or without edema, systemic lupus erythematosus, dermatomyositis, erythema multiforme, and Stevens-Johnson syndrome. Resolution of the rash occurs on discontinuation of the drug, although concomitant antihistamines allow some patients to continue treatment. Erythematous rashes can resolve without discontinuation of the therapy (Perry et al., 1991).

ENDOCRINE/METABOLIC. Carbamazepine is a vasopressin agonist and can cause hyponatremia and water intoxication. When administered with lithium, the hyponatremia has precipitated lithium intoxication reactions (Perry et al., 1991).

GASTROINTESTINAL. Nausea (8 percent) is the most frequent adverse effect that occurs during the initiation of carbamazepine therapy (Ballenger and Post, 1980).

HEMATOLOGIC. A transient mild leukopenia occurs in approximately 10 percent of patients following the start of therapy, but it normally resolves within the first 4 months of treatment. Although relatively rarely reported, aplastic anemia (27 cases) and agranulocytosis (23 cases) are associated with carbamazepine. The following conservative approach to the monitoring of possible bone marrow function is suggested: (1) if baseline complete blood count (CBC) is in the middle to upper range, no further monitoring is recommended; (2) if baseline CBC is in the low-normal or below-normal range, the CBC should be measured every 2 weeks for the next 1 to 3 months; and (3) if the white count falls below 3000/mm^3, the dose should be decreased or the drug discontinued. Because of the rapid onset of aplastic anemia, agranulocytosis, and thrombocytopenia, the patient must be educated to immediately contact his or her physician at the first sign of an infection, fever, fatigue, ecchymosis, and/or mucous membrane bleeding (Sobotka et al., 1990).

HEPATIC. Cholestatic jaundice, hepatic necrosis, and granulomatous hepatitis have been associated with carbamazepine use (Perry et al., 1991).

TERATOGENICITY AND EXCRETION INTO BREAST MILK. A recent study utilizing retrospective and prospective data has demonstrated that carbamazepine is a teratogenic agent. The anomaly incidence was 11 percent for craniofacial defects, 26 percent for fingernail hypoplasia, and 20 percent for developmental delay (Jones et al., 1989). This presentation is similar to fetal hydantoin syndrome. As with the TCAs and lithium, it is not recommended that women ingesting carbamazepine breast feed their newborn children.

Verapamil

EFFICACY

Sixteen manic patients were treated with verapamil versus placebo in three reports (Dubovsky et al., 1986, 1982; Dose et al., 1986). An 81 percent response rate was observed in the patients who received verapamil 160 to 480 mg/d. Twelve acutely ill manic patients were treated with 30-day trials of lithium 0.84 to 1.26 mEq/liter and verapamil 320 mg/d, separated by 10 days of placebo, in a crossover design. The drugs were equally effective and more effective, respectively, than was the placebo (Giannini et al., 1984). A 20-day crossover trial of verapamil 320 mg/d was found to be more effective than clonidine in the treatment of 20 lithium nonresponders (Giannini et al., 1985).

Twenty patients considered lithium responders were prophylactically treated with lithium 0.8 to 1.0 mEq/liter and verapamil 320 mg/d in a crossover study of 180 days for each drug. Verapamil was therapeutically superior to lithium, though both drugs were effective (Giannini et al., 1987).

DOSING

Effective antimanic dosages of verapamil range from 160 to 480 mg/d with a median dose of 320 mg/d (80 mg qid). Patients usually can be started on this dose without having to titrate the dose. In noncompliant patients, the 240-mg sustained-release dosage formulation can be given as a single dose in the morning with breakfast, followed by an 80-mg regular release dose at dinner.

ADVERSE EFFECTS

Verapamil is generally well tolerated and rarely requires discontinuation because of adverse effects.

CARDIAC. The estimated incidence of bradycardia (<50 beats/min) is 0.33 percent, while palpitations are reported in 0.37 percent of patients.

CENTRAL NERVOUS SYSTEM. The most common CNS adverse effects are fatigue (1.1 percent), headache (1.6 percent), and dizziness (3.6 percent). Normally, they are mild and transient. They rarely require discontinuation (Perry et al., 1991).

DERMATOLOGIC. The dermatitides (0.55 percent) associated with verapamil include urticaria, itching, and exanthema (Perry et al., 1991).

GASTROINTESTINAL. Mild to moderate constipation is the most common side effect (5.2 percent) associated with verapamil. Nausea and vomiting (0.99 percent) are far less common. Abdominal discomfort is relieved by taking the medication with food (Perry et al., 1991).

TERATOGENICITY AND EXCRETION INTO BREAST MILK. Currently available data suggest that verapamil is not teratogenic. Thus it is the only antimanic agent that appears to be safe for patients to take in the first trimester of pregnancy. Since it is excreted in the breast milk, it is recommended to bottle feed newborns whose mothers are receiving verapamil (Perry et al., 1991).

Valproic Acid

EFFICACY

Valproic acid is indicated either by itself or in combination with other anticonvulsants in the prophylactic management of simple and complex (petit mal) seizures. There is a limited amount of controlled trial data suggesting that it may be of some use in the treatment of acute mania. The four published controlled studies of valproic acid in acutely manic patients demonstrated a 64 percent (28 of 44) response rate at doses ranging from 900 to 3600 mg/d (50 to 100 μg/ml) (Brennan et al., 1984; Emrich et al., 1985; Pope et al., 1991; Freeman et al., 1992). The controlled trial that directly compared valproic acid with lithium found a 64 percent (9 of 14) response rate in the valproic acid patients. However, this was a modest response when contrasted with the 92 percent (12 of 13) response rate in the lithium-treated patients (Freeman et al., 1992). Among valproic acid responders, most responded within 1 to 4 days of reaching a valproic acid serum concentration of 50 μg/ml. Its role as a prophylactic agent in the treatment of affective illness remains to be defined, since a controlled trial contrasting the prophylactic effectiveness of valproic acid with lithium has not been conducted.

DOSING

The use of the enteric-coated formulation of valproic acid, divalproex sodium, may minimize gastrointestinal complaints. All valproic acid formulations are rapidly absorbed after oral ingestion with the exception of the enteric-coated divalproex sodium, whose absorption is delayed by about 2 to 4 hours. Valproic acid is administered initially at a dose of 500 to 1000 mg/d in 2 to 4 divided doses. Blood levels are drawn 12 hours after the last dose and adjusted to achieve a steady-state concentration between 50 and 100 μg/ml. A response should be anticipated usually within a few days of attaining a therapeutic blood level, although a therapeutic trial is a minimum of 3 weeks (Perry et al., 1991).

ADVERSE EFFECTS

CENTRAL NERVOUS SYSTEM. The most common CNS effect of valproic acid is sedation, which is observed in 4 percent of patients (Perry et al., 1991).

DERMATOLOGIC. Transient alopecia has been reported in three studies in 3.6 percent of patients.

ENDOCRINE. Weight gain and increased appetite are commonly observed in patients receiving val-

proic acid. Idiosyncratic pancreatitis occurring within the first 6 months of treatment is a potentially fatal but rare adverse reaction associated with valproic acid. Abdominal pain associated with an increased amylase level demands that the drug be discontinued immediately (Perry et al., 1991).

GASTROINTESTINAL. By far these are the most commonly reported adverse effects associated with valproic acid. They present as either anorexia (11.6 percent); indigestion, heartburn, and nausea (13.8 percent); vomiting (19.2 percent); and/or transient diarrhea (1.7 percent). It is approximated that 85 percent of the patients unable to tolerate the standard formulation can be successfully switched to the enteric-coated form of the drug (Perry et al., 1991).

HEMATOLOGIC. In a series of 45 children followed over a period of 1 year, neutropenia and thrombocytopenia were observed in 27 and 33 percent of the population, respectively. Both were transient and self-limiting in all cases, with no data being presented on rate of clearing (Perry et al., 1991).

HEPATIC. Potentially fatal, idiosyncratic, but rare (1 per 37,000) hepatotoxicity is associated with valproic acid. However, fatalities have only occurred in children less than 10 years old (Perry et al., 1991).

NEUROLOGIC. An essential tremor occurred within 1 month of the start of treatment in 7 of 10 adult patients receiving valproic acid (Perry et al., 1991).

TERATOGENICITY AND EXCRETION INTO BREAST MILK. There is an increased risk (1 to 2 percent) of neural tube defects in children exposed to valproic acid with or without other antiepileptic drugs in the first trimester of pregnancy (Jeavons, 1982). Since valproic acid is excreted in the breast milk, breast feeding is not recommended.

ANXIETY DISORDERS

Benzodiazepines

The following benzodiazepines (BZDs) have anxiety as an approved indication: chlordiazepoxide (Librium, other names), diazepam (Valium, other names), oxazepam (Serax, other names), clorazepate (Tranxene, other names), lorazepam (Ativan, other names), prazepam (Centrax), halazepam (Paxipam), and alprazolam (Xanax). Five BZDs are approved for the management of insomnia: flurazepam (Dalmane, other names), temazepam (Restoril, other names), quazepam (Doral), estazolam (ProSom), and triazolam (Halcion). A given BZD, with the dosage adjusted upward or downward, can serve both as a hypnotic and as an anxiolytic, respectively (Dubovsky, 1990).

EFFICACY

A review of 17 recent controlled studies noted numerous problems that make determination of an overall conclusion about BZD efficacy in *generalized anxiety disorder* (GAD) difficult (Perry et al., 1990). Fifty-six percent of the reviewed studies found BZDs to be much better, and 33 percent considered BZDs to be slightly better than placebo for the treatment of anxiety. However, 18 percent found no difference between the two, and 1 percent found placebo better than diazepam. About 35 percent of GAD patients treated with BZDs experience marked improvement, 40 percent are moderately improved but still symptomatic, and 25 percent are unresponsive (Dubovsky, 1990). There is some evidence that BZDs are of greater benefit when used to treat patients with moderate to high levels of anxiety (Shapiro et al., 1983).

Response to BZDs may be noted within 1 to 2 weeks of initiation of treatment. It is estimated that only half of patients with GAD have a return of symptoms after the discontinuation of diazepam after either 6, 14, or 22 weeks of treatment (Rickels et al., 1983). BZDs should be tapered and discontinued after a 2-month treatment course after the initial diagnosis (Dubovsky, 1990). The long-term efficacy of BZDs and other anxiolytics is still being investigated (Rickels et al., 1988; Murphy et al., 1989).

Although most reviews indicate no significant difference in overall efficacy in the management of generalized anxiety when comparing one BZD with another (Dubovsky, 1990), some authors challenge this (Baskin et al., 1982; Butler et al., 1987).

BZDs are the preferred class of antianxiety agents for the management of GAD compared with barbiturates and meprobamate because of their high therapeutic index, low abuse potential, and relative lack of drug interactions as compared with the other classes of anxiolytics. The least expensive agent should be utilized. Chlordiazepoxide, lorazepam, prazepam, oxazepam, and diazepam are generically available.

Early experience with BZDs found them only partially effective for the treatment of *panic disorder* (Ballenger, 1986). However, recent short-term trials indicate that BZDs are effective when taken regularly and in sufficient doses (Jann et al., 1987).

Diazepam was rated to be effective in 86 percent of patients in one controlled trial (Noyes et al., 1984). Four double-blind, placebo-controlled trials have suggested that alprazolam is more effective than placebo. Reported response rates varied from 55 to 88 percent (Chouinard et al., 1982; Sheehan et al., 1984; Taylor et al., 1990; Munjack et al., 1989). A more recent study reported similar results (Ballenger et al., 1988). Alprazolam has been compared with lorazepam, clonazepam, and diazepam in three controlled studies (Tesar et al., 1987; Dunner et al., 1986; Schweizer et al., 1988). No efficacy differences between drugs were noted.

Although one uncontrolled report found clonazepam to be effective in patients nonresponsive to other BZDs and antidepressants, differences in efficacy, if they exist, await the results of ongoing investigations (Ballenger, 1986).

Uncontrolled reports of long-term treatment with clonazepam (1 year) and alprazolam (2½ years) reported that the drugs maintained their efficacy and were well tolerated (Pollack, 1990). Studies of the relative efficacy of BZDs and antidepressants in panic disorder indicate no difference (Taylor et al., 1990; Pollack, 1990).

Data have suggested that patients continue to improve for up to 6 months of treatment. Newly diagnosed patients who respond should be treated for a year before a trial discontinuation is considered to determine continuing pharmacologic need (Noyes et al., 1984).

The use of BZDs in the treatment of simple phobia has not been extensively researched (Dommisse et al., 1987).

BZDs are reported to be of limited value in the treatment of social phobia, but this has not been extensively researched (Dommisse et al., 1987). However, a recent open trial of clonazepam 1 to 6 mg/d (average 2.75 mg) produced significant improvement in symptoms of social phobia (Munjack et al., 1990).

DOSING

The dose and administration schedule for a BZD in the management of anxiety depend on (1) the clinical presentation (e.g., chronic and persistent anxiety, anxiety limited to episodes lasting days to weeks with full recovery between episodes, or transient anxiety associated with a particular stimulus), (2) the age and sex of the patient, (3) concurrent liver disease, (4) whether the patient smokes, and (5) the pharmacokinetic profile of the BZD (Hollister, 1986).

In GAD diazepam has been shown to be effective in the standard recommended daily dose range of 5 to 40 mg. The median dose used was 30 mg/d (Hoehn-Saric et al., 1988). Treatment with alprazolam is initiated with 0.25 or 0.5 mg b.i.d. or t.i.d. Dosages may be increased every several days. Most patients require 3 to 6 mg/d to respond, but 10 mg/d may be required. Some patients report the antipanic effects last only 4 to 6 hours, thereby necessitating multiple daily dosing. Mean doses of other BZDs are lorazepam 7.5 mg/d and clonazepam 2 mg/d.

In panic disorder the recommended daily dose range for diazepam is 5 to 40 mg. In one study the median effective dose was 30 mg/d. Treatment with alprazolam is initiated with 0.25 or 0.5 mg b.i.d. or t.i.d. (Noyes et al., 1984). Dosages may be increased every several days. Most patients require 3 to 6 mg/d for response, but 10 mg/d may be necessary in some patients. Clonazepam has been effective in the majority of patients at a mean dose of 1.9 mg/d, although some patients require up to 4 mg/d (Spier et al., 1986; Shebak et al., 1990). Clonazepam treatment is initiated with 0.5 mg bid.

The duration of action of a single dose of a BZD is determined largely by the volume of distribution and absorption rate of the drug rather than the elimination $t_{1/2}$ (Greenblatt et al., 1983). Diazepam is a very lipid-soluble drug and is rapidly and extensively taken up by fatty tissue. Although its $t_{1/2}$ is quite long, the duration of action of a single dose is very short because of its large volume of distribution. Furthermore, it has been noted that a drug with a short $t_{1/2}$, such as lorazepam, may have longer lasting clinical effects after a single dose than might be expected based on its $t_{1/2}$. A single dose of lorazepam 2.5 mg PO produced significant impairment of psychomotor skills and visual functions related to driving for 24 hours in 10 healthy volunteers (Greenblatt, 1980). In comparison, the impairment in performance after diazepam 10 mg lasted 5 to 7 hours. The slow disappearance of lorazepam from the serum (still 50 percent of peak value at 12 hours) coincided with its long duration of action (Seppala et al., 1976).

The major distinction to be made for multiple-dose treatment is between drugs with active metabolites and those with no active metabolites. BZDs fall into two classes depending on their biotransformation pathways. One group includes those which are transformed primarily by oxidative pathways (*N*-dealkylation, *N*-demethylation, or aliphatic hydroxylation) to active metabolites. These include chlordiazepoxide, clorazepate, diazepam, halazepam, and prazepam. The half-life of the parent compound and active metabolites often exceeds 48 hours. The other group includes those which are metabolized by conjugation to water-soluble glucuronides (subsequently excreted in the urine), which are pharmacologically inactive. These have half-lives that range from 6 to 20 hours and include alprazolam, lorazepam, and oxazepam. BZDs with active metabolites will accumulate in the body and not reach steady state until days or weeks of continuous dosing. Therefore, the full therapeutic or adverse effects may not be apparent until 5 to 10 days. For the same reason, clinical effects may persist for several days after the drug is discontinued (Greenblatt, 1980); thus these drugs may be administered in a once- or twice-a-day schedule (Greenblatt et al., 1978). BZDs with no active metabolites, however, accumulate rapidly and reach steady-state concentrations in 2 to 4 days. This potential benefit of this class of BZDs may be offset by the fact that if the patient misses a dose or a day of treatment, blood concentrations will decline rapidly to zero. This is not so critical with the BZDs with active metabolites and long $t_{1/2}$.

In many clinical situations, multiple daily dosing of available BZDs is not necessary for adequate effect, and daily or twice-daily dosing should be considered. The daily dose can be given at night, and if needed, a smaller dose can be given during the day. This will eliminate the need for a separate hypnotic in those patients with anxiety accompanied by sleep disturbance.

Absorption of chlordiazepoxide or diazepam from a gluteal IM injection site is slow and may be incomplete, possibly leading to unpredictable and unsatisfactory clinical effects. However, absorption of diazepam and lorazepam from a deltoid IM injection site is rapid and nearly complete. Lorazepam causes injection-site pain to the same extent as that associated with chlordiazepoxide and diazepam (Greenblatt et al., 1978).

After an IV bolus injection of diazepam, serum concentrations decline very rapidly over a period of several minutes to several hours, owing to rapid and extensive drug distribution. This reduction is generally accompanied by rapid diminution or termination of the desired sedative, anticonvulsant, or amnestic effects. With lorazepam, drug distribution is less rapid and extensive, thereby prolonging the clinical effects. Anterograde amnesia lasting up to several hours is consistently reported to follow injection of lorazepam 4 mg, whereas amnesia after diazepam may last 30 minutes (Greenblatt et al., 1978).

Although drug metabolism declines in patients with liver disease, drugs that are transformed by oxidation are affected to a greater extent than those which are conjugated. It is expected that other BZDs metabolized primarily by oxidation, although not specifically studied, would be similarly affected. It is important to remember that because the margin of safety of all BZDs is large, the choice of the particular BZD is not as important as is gradual dose titration and close monitoring (Greenblatt, 1980).

BZDs can produce greater effects on the central nervous system in the elderly than in younger patients. This is due partly to increased target-organ sensitivity to BZDs and partly to changes in drug disposition in the elderly (Reidenberg et al., 1978). All BZDs, given in repeated doses, will accumulate to some degree and may produce adverse effects (Thompson et al., 1983). The BZDs with a longer $t_{1/2}$ (e.g., diazepam, chlordiazepoxide, clorazepate, prazepam, halazepam) should be prescribed for the elderly in smaller doses (at least 50 percent of usual dose) and at more widely spaced intervals (once and twice daily versus twice and three times daily) than is recommended for younger patients. The BZDs with a shorter $t_{1/2}$ (e.g., oxazepam, lorazepam, alprazolam) also require decreased doses. However, because the pharmacokinetics of these drugs with relatively shorter $t_{1/2}$ are not greatly changed in the elderly, the dosage administration schedule can be more similar to that in younger patients.

ADVERSE EFFECTS

BZDs have few pharmacologic effects outside the central nervous system (CNS). The majority of adverse effects are mediated through the CNS. A wide range of other non-CNS adverse effects have been attributed to BZDs. However, their reported incidence is <1 percent (Cole et al., 1981).

ALLERGIC. There have been few documented allergies to BZDs. The effects of BZDs on blood pressure, heart rate, and cardiac output are minimal. Occasionally, transient episodes of bradycardia and hypotension are noted after rapid IV injection of diazepam.

CENTRAL NERVOUS SYSTEM. Excessive *CNS depression* (drowsiness, muscle weakness, ataxia, nystagmus, and dysarthria) is the most common adverse effect attributed to BZDs. It has been reported in 4 to 12 percent of patients taking diazepam or chlordiazepoxide. These adverse effects are dose-dependent and remit when the dose is lowered or the drug is discontinued. There is evidence to suggest that the central depressant effects of BZDs tend to decline as the duration of exposure increases, thereby reducing the sedative effects of chronic exposure and of drug accumulation (Cole et al., 1981). Elderly individuals and patients with low serum albumin levels are more likely to experience these adverse effects. Cigarette smokers are less likely to experience CNS depression than are nonsmokers. This interaction between nicotine and BZDs probably occurs in the CNS, since BZD metabolism has been shown not to be affected by smoking.

The BZDs have a risk for abuse and physical dependence (Busto et al., 1986; Perry et al., 1986). The incidence of major abstinence reactions is unknown, although it is thought to be low in comparison with older anxiolytics. It is recommended that patients who have been taking BZDs regularly for more than 1 month have the drug gradually withdrawn.

The BZDs have been demonstrated in the laboratory to impair *reaction time, motor coordination, and intellectual functioning* in a dose-related fashion. A study of long-term BZD users suggests that tolerance develops to these effects (Hoehn-Saric et al., 1988; Shebak et al., 1990; Lucki et al., 1985).

It has been shown that patients with anxiety may become better drivers while being treated with a BZD because of a reduction of anxiety (Katcher, 1978). Most studies, unfortunately, use normal controls and/or subjects who are given only a single dose of the drug. One study, using patients, administered diazepam 15 to 30 mg/d or placebo for 2 weeks. The differences between the diazepam and placebo groups decreased over the 2-week period even though blood concentrations of diazepam were continually rising. Apparently, familiarity with the test and drug effect improved performance. However, the risk of being involved in a traffic accident is increased fivefold if a driver is receiving a BZD, possibly because intermittent use does not produce tolerance to the sedative effect of the drug (Dubovsky, 1990). The use of ethanol increases this risk. Because BZDs may impair driving performance in some patients, all patients should be cautioned about driving and operating machinery, especially during the first few weeks of treatment (Katcher, 1978).

Amnesia may occur with all BZDs (Gelenberg, 1985). Parenteral administration has been most commonly reported to produce this effect, but it is now commonly reported with oral use. BZDs exert their primary effect in impairing acquisition of new information but do not appear to affect a person's ability to retain acquired information. The clinical effect of BZDs taken over a long period of time remains to be investigated. However, patients should avoid taking BZDs shortly before studying, making important decisions, or performing other tasks dependent on an intact memory.

Chlordiazepoxide, diazepam, and lorazepam IM injections are painful because of precipitated particles or the propylene glycol solvent, and they cause elevations in serum creatine phosphokinase (Cole et al., 1981). Diazepam, the most commonly used parenteral BZD, causes local pain in about 5 to 7 percent of patients receiving it IV. To avoid these problems, the rate of injection should not exceed 5 mg (1 ml) per minute, large veins should be used, injection sites should be alternated, and the veins should be flushed well after each injection (Katcher, 1978).

Like ethanol and barbiturates, BZDs have been reported to produce *paradoxical excitement*, hostility, rage, and even violent, destructive behavior. These adverse effects are infrequent, although the exact incidence rate is unknown (Katcher, 1978).

PULMONARY. BZDs are relatively benign in comparison with other anxiolytic/hypnotics in their effects on respiration. Even though overdoses with BZDs are frequent, serious sequelae are rare because of minimal respiratory depressant effects. However, in patients with compromised pulmonary function, BZDs may produce clinically significant respiratory depressant effects. All anxiolytic/hypnotics should be used with caution in patients with reduced pulmonary function (Katcher, 1978).

TERATOGENIC. Studies have indicated that diazepam and its metabolites are excreted into breast milk in levels sufficient to produce pharmacologic effects in newborns (i.e., sedation). Milk levels have been reported to be 8 to 50 percent of serum levels. Infant serum concentrations have been noted to be initially high; the fact that they fall by 6 days is probably due to the increased ability for hepatic conjugation, an elimination pathway necessary for all BZDs. Accumulation of BZDs may occur.

Although some studies have suggested an association between ingestion of a BZD and an increased risk of congenital anomalies, this has not been a consistent finding (Gelenberg, 1987). If malformations were reported, the BZDs often were ingested during the first trimester of pregnancy, and the malformations consisted mainly of oral clefts. Even though the data have not conclusively indicated an association between BZDs and teratogenicity, benefit/risk considerations are such that their use during pregnancy should almost always be avoided because their use is rarely urgent. If a woman has ingested a BZD during the first trimester of pregnancy, the relative risk of cleft lip (with or without cleft palate) is increased; however, the absolute increased risk is low (Cole et al., 1981).

Reports have indicated that a neonate may experience a BZD withdrawal syndrome if the mother ingests BZDs during pregnancy (Katcher, 1978). This observation has lead to the recommendation that the BZD should be gradually tapered during the last month of pregnancy.

Antidepressants

EFFICACY

Short-term, controlled studies reported imipramine (two studies) and doxepin (one study) to be as effective as chlordiazepoxide, diazepam, and alprazolam, respectively, in the treatment of GAD (Kahn et al., 1986; Haskell et al., 1978).

The pharmacologic management of panic disorder and agoraphobia with panic attacks was originally investigated in the early 1960s with monoamine oxidase inhibitors (MAOIs) and with tricyclic antidepressants (TCAs) (Noyes et al., 1989; Ballenger, 1986; Jann, 1987; Dommisse et al., 1987).

Seven of nine controlled trials with imipramine have demonstrated its efficacy versus placebo in panic disorder and agoraphobia. Results from the four largest studies indicate moderate to marked improvement in phobic symptoms and secondary disability in 70 to 90 percent of patients (Noyes et al., 1989). Response to imipramine may occur within the first or second week of treatment, but maximum effect may take 6 to 10 weeks.

The other available TCAs have not been as widely studied as imipramine. Limited evidence has suggested that desipramine, nortriptyline, doxepin, and amitriptyline are clinically effective (Ballenger, 1986). Clomipramine has been shown to be effective in suppressing panic attacks and phobic symptoms in uncontrolled trials. One uncontrolled trial reported complete cessation of panic attacks in 13 of 17 patients and a marked reduction in attacks in the remaining 4 (Perry et al., 1990; Golger et al., 1989). Comparison studies with TCAs are needed to determine their relative efficacy.

Data suggest that the antidepressants are roughly equivalent in efficacy to the BZDs (Ballenger, 1986). BZDs may be used in patients to achieve a rapid control of symptoms while antidepressant treatment is being initiated. Antidepressants, compared with the BZDs, are the preferred treatment in patients with panic disorder who are significantly depressed or have a history of major depressive disorder. Because of necessary dietary restrictions with MAOIs, TCAs often are the treatment class of choice.

Although no studies directly compare beta blockers with antidepressants for the treatment of panic attacks, antidepressants are reported to be more effective than beta blockers (Ballenger, 1986).

The question of efficacy of pharmacologic versus behavioral treatment is not answered because of research limitations. A controlled study and a literature review of three studies reported that imipramine was an effective antipanic and antiphobic agent when used alone (Noyes et al., 1989; Mavissakalian et al., 1989). One study reported that the combination of imipramine and behavior therapy provided the greatest response rate (Mavissakalian et al., 1983).

If an adequate trial with one treatment (e.g., antidepressant, BZD) fails, then another treatment should be tried. Though not well studied, combination treatment with various agents has been reported to succeed when individual drugs fail (Jann et al., 1987).

Evidence from controlled trials shows that patients continue to improve for up to 6 months with pharmacologic management (Zitrin et al., 1983). Some clinicians report that patients continue to improve over most of the first year of treatment. As a general rule, regardless of whether the patient has been treated successfully, approximately 50 to 95 percent of patients will relapse (Coryell et al., 1983). It appears that a large percentage of patients can remain off medications during the second year of treatment, but some will require long-term treatment. Therefore, after 6 to 12 months of successful treatment, it is reasonable to consider discontinuing medications (Pecknold et al., 1988).

It is recommended that any of the three classes (e.g., BZD, TCAs, MAOIs) of treatment be tapered gradually over 1 to 3 months to allow early detection of relapse. Tapering of BZDs should be done very slowly to avoid significant withdrawal symptoms, especially if higher doses are being used (Pecknold et al., 1988). If the patient relapses after the first taper, then reinstitution of treatment often achieves clinical control. It is recommended that tapering be tried again in 3 to 6 months.

Experience with second-generation antidepressants in the treatment of GAD and panic disorder is limited. In panic disorder, maprotiline has been reported to be effective in open trials. A double-blind trial reported maprotiline was ineffective in preventing panic attacks (Den Boer et al., 1988). Trazodone has been reported to be effective in panic disorder and agoraphobia with panic attacks in two studies (Mavissakalian et al., 1987; Sheehan, 1982). One controlled, blind trial found no effect, but the dose and duration of treatment may have been inadequate to produce a response (Charney et al., 1986). In a single-blind, placebo-controlled trial, bupropion was shown to be an ineffective treatment (Sheehan et al., 1983). Fluoxetine produced a 44 percent response in 16 patients treated with 80 mg/d (Gorman et al., 1987). However, 8 patients discontinued treatment because of adverse effects of restlessness, agitation, jitteriness, diarrhea, and insomnia. The efficacy of lower doses needs to be investigated. Amoxapine has not been studied in the treatment of panic disorder.

Six placebo-controlled trials (five using phenelzine) reported that MAOIs are effective in 65 to 70 percent of patients (Ballenger, 1986; Buigues et al., 1987). Although the overall response rate with MAOIs is slightly less than that with the TCAs, this finding may be because the MAOI studies used smaller samples, a mixed group of patients, and very low doses of drugs. An open trial using average phenelzine doses of 55 mg/d reported that panic attacks were blocked in 100 percent of panic disorder patients and 95 percent of agoraphobic patients. Avoidance behavior improved in 74 percent of subjects, which was not statistically significant (Buigues et al., 1987).

The time for symptomatic response in the studies was 2 to 6 weeks, although some patients may take longer to respond. Duration of antidepressant treatment in a newly diagnosed patient may be 1 year. Attempts to discontinue the drug should be made periodically to determine continuing need (Ballenger, 1986). It is important to note that some patients require behavioral treatment to achieve symptom relief after the panic attacks are pharmacologically controlled (Ballenger, 1986).

DOSING

Dosage recommendations in panic disorder are given for the most widely studied antidepressants, imipramine and phenelzine. Several reports have indicated that although some patients may respond to imipramine doses of 25 mg/d, most patients require >150 mg/d to achieve a satisfactory response. Some patients may require that the dose be increased to 400 mg/d (Ballenger, 1986). Imipramine doses should be initiated at 10 to 25 mg/d, which can be increased to 100 to 200 mg/d over a 2- to 4-week period. If a response is not seen in 2 to 6 weeks, the dose may be increased to 400 mg/d. Doses of antidepressants other than imipramine in the management of panic disorder are typically in the antidepressant range.

Research investigating the relationship between imipramine serum concentrations and clinical response has been reviewed (Mavissakalian et al., 1989). Because of inconsistency of the findings, no therapeutic range has been established for panic disorder or agoraphobia. Routine serum level monitoring in management of panic attacks is not recommended.

Over 75 percent of patients with agoraphobia with panic attacks responded to phenelzine 45 mg/d. Some individuals may require 60 to 90 mg/d to achieve a response (Ballenger, 1986). Treatment with phenelzine is usually initiated at 15 mg/d and increased by 15 mg/d q3–4d until 60 mg/d is reached. Doses may be increased further if a response does not occur within 2 to 6 weeks.

ADVERSE EFFECTS

TCAs in panic patients have been associated with typical adverse effects (e.g., anticholinergic effects, orthostatic hypotension, weight gain, sedation), which occurred in 35 percent of patients discontinuing treatment (Noyes et al., 1989).

A reaction that appears almost exclusively in panic patients is the jitteriness syndrome or hypersensitivity reaction. Forty-nine of 158 patients (30 percent) with panic disorder developed this reaction in one retrospective study (Pohl et al., 1988). Symptoms included jitteriness, shakiness, increased anxiety, and insomnia. Although TCA doses usually were started at 10 mg/d, symptoms still occurred. It appeared with initial doses, and tolerance developed over 7 to 10 days (Pohl et al., 1988; Zitrin et al., 1983). If tolerance does not develop within this time period, it is unlikely to occur. Desipramine was reported to be more likely to produce this adverse effect than imipramine, based on retrospective data (Pohl et al., 1988).

Buspirone

EFFICACY

Buspirone is a member of a new class of agents known as *azaspirodecanediones* and is the first non-BZD anxiolytic to be introduced in the United States. The drug is not a controlled substance.

Buspirone is indicated for the short-term treatment of GAD, when symptoms are rated as mild to moderate in severity (Goldberg, 1984; Dommisse et al., 1985). Studies of patients with a primary anxiety disorder have reported that accompanying depressive symptoms may improve with buspirone. However, an uncontrolled 4-week trial of buspirone in DSM-III–diagnosed major depressive disorder reported the drug to be ineffective in melancholic depression. In nonmelancholic depression, moderate to marked improvement occurred in 55 percent of the patients receiving a dose of 40 to 60 mg/d. The role of buspirone in depression remains to be determined.

Seven clinical studies evaluating the anxiolytic efficacy of buspirone in GAD have been reported in the literature. All were double-blind, outpatient studies comparing the efficacy of buspirone with placebo and/or a BZD (diazepam, alprazolam, or clorazepate). Although the studies differed in methodology, the preliminary conclusion was that buspirone is superior to placebo and is as efficacious as the reference BZDs in the treatment of anxiety states.

One study reported that a prior history of BZD exposure predicted a lower response rate to buspirone as compared with patients without a past history of use (Schweizer et al., 1986). The clinical implication of this finding awaits further investigation and experience with buspirone.

Several reports indicated that maximum therapeutic benefit from buspirone may not occur until 4 to 6 weeks of treatment and that women may respond better than men. This delayed onset prevents the prn use of buspirone.

Buspirone was compared with clorazepate in a 6-month study. After 1 month of treatment with buspirone, 45 percent of the patients discontinued treatment because of lack of efficacy and another 26 percent discontinued the drug during the next 5 months (Rickels et al., 1988). This compares to 26 and 17 percent, respectively, for clorazepate. This study requires duplication, but its results are not encouraging for the utility of buspirone.

One controlled trial comparing buspirone, imipramine, and placebo reported buspirone to be less effective than imipramine and equal to placebo (33 percent response rate) in panic disorder (Sheehan, 1987). Another study reported that imipramine and buspirone were not better than placebo in a double-blind trial (Pohl et al., 1989). At this time it appears that buspirone may have some utility in patients unable to take BZDs (i.e., those displaying disinhibition) or those with a history of anxiolytic/hypnotic abuse.

DOSING

The usual anxiolytic dose is 15 to 45 mg/d. Initial starting dose is 15 mg/d divided 2 to 3 times per day. The dose may be increased by 5 mg/d, and the maximum recommended daily dose is 60 mg (Dommisse et al., 1985).

ADVERSE EFFECTS

All reviews of the overall adverse effect profile of buspirone have concluded that the drug (45 percent) has more adverse effects than placebo (33 percent) but fewer than the BZDs (45 to 60 percent) (Newton et al., 1982). Dizziness, drowsiness, and headache occurred in 12, 10, and 6 percent of buspirone-treated patients, respectively. These adverse effects are more common with doses >20 mg/d. Dizziness was reported to occur 30 to 60 minutes after buspirone was administered, especially when subjects were walking or standing.

Dysphoria has been reported, primarily with doses >30 mg/d. Initial studies indicated that buspirone <20 mg/d produced less psychomotor impairment than the BZDs. The effects of buspirone in combination with ethanol were compared with lorazepam plus ethanol (two studies) of diazepam plus ethanol (one study) (Seppala et al., 1982; Moskorvitz et al., 1982; Matilla et al., 1982). All three studies demonstrated that in healthy subjects receiving buspirone plus ethanol, objective performances were impaired significantly less than in those subjects receiving lorazepam or diazepam. Interestingly, normal subjects reported some drowsiness, weakness, and faintness after buspirone plus ethanol, although their objective performance was not impaired. However, after lorazepam plus ethanol, the subjects did not perceive adverse effects that were associated with psychomotor impairment.

Studies of the abuse potential of buspirone in animals and recreational sedative users demonstrated no overt sedative or euphoric effects (Goldberg, 1984; Dommisse et al., 1985). It is important to note that buspirone is not cross-tolerant with standard anxiolytic/hypnotics (i.e., BZDs, barbiturates). Therefore, buspirone will not prevent withdrawal signs and symptoms that may occur if a patient is abruptly changed from one of these drugs to buspirone. Likewise, buspirone will not treat anxiolytic/hypnotic withdrawal symptoms.

Nausea was the most common gastrointestinal adverse effect, occurring in 8 percent of patients. Use of buspirone during pregnancy or while breast feeding is not recommended because it has not been adequately investigated.

Barbiturates

EFFICACY

The first barbiturate was synthesized in 1903. In short-term studies, barbiturates have been demonstrated to be more effective than placebo in the treatment of anxiety. They have been shown to be equal in efficacy to the BZDs and more effective than propanediols (Rall, 1990a, 1990b).

DOSING

As with all anxiolytics, dosage must be individualized on the basis of therapeutic and adverse effects. These drugs have usually been administered on a multiple-daily dose basis despite their long $t_{1/2}$ (see product list for individual doses) (Rall, 1990b).

ADVERSE EFFECTS

CENTRAL NERVOUS SYSTEM. Repeated daily use of barbiturates may lead to tolerance and dependence. The severity of the abstinence syndrome relates to the duration of drug use and dose (Rall, 1990b). Hangover occurs with the barbiturates, especially phenobarbital. They also give rise to confusional states or delirium, to which the elderly are especially prone. Dosages of these drugs that do not produce drowsiness may impair psychomotor skills, including those involved in driving (Rall, 1990b). Paradoxical excitement, as reported with other anxiolytics, also occurs with barbiturates (Rall, 1990b).

PULMONARY. Patients with severe pulmonary diseases are unusually sensitive to the respiratory depressant action of these drugs. Studies have indicated significant decreases in minute volume, oxygen saturation, and blood pH after low doses of phenobarbital. These agents are to be avoided or used with extreme caution in patients with respiratory difficulties. In overdoses with barbiturates, the respiratory depressant effects are more pronounced. In healthy individuals, anxiolytic or hypnotic doses of barbiturates involve no more depression of respiration than normal sleep (Rall, 1990b).

TERATOGENICITY. Most barbiturates readily pass the placental barrier. A study indicated that more mothers of children with brain tumors used barbiturates during pregnancy than did mothers of normal controls or mothers of cancer controls. The use of barbiturates for anxiety during pregnancy is not recommended. Barbiturates produce metabolic changes, such as liver enzyme induction, in the fetus. All barbiturates discussed appear in breast milk. Drowsiness has been reported in infants whose breast feeding mothers were taking barbiturates.

SUMMARY

Barbiturates are not recommended in the routine treatment of anxiety. They are as effective as other anxiolytics but possess the disadvantages of enzyme induction, which leads to tolerance and drug interactions and respiratory depressant properties, making the risk of suicide greater with these agents than with the BZDs.

Propanediols

EFFICACY

The propanediol class of anxiolytics was introduced in the United States in 1955 with meprobamate. In a review of meprobamate, only 5 of 26 studies reported that the drug was more effective than placebo, and in only 1 of 10 studies was it clearly more effective than a barbiturate (Greenblatt et al., 1971). Due to questionable efficacy and greater potential for adverse effects, the propanediols have been replaced by the BZDs in the general management of anxiety.

DOSING

The usual dosage of meprobamate is 400 to 1200 mg/d. The doses usually are administered on a split daily-dose schedule (Rall, 1990a).

ADVERSE EFFECTS

CENTRAL NERVOUS SYSTEM. Meprobamate may cause significant withdrawal signs and symptoms after abrupt discontinuation of 3.2 to 6.4 g/d for ≥40 days.

Sedation is the main adverse effect at therapeutic doses. This is sometimes accompanied by ataxia and hypotension. Lowering of the daily dose is recommended. Doses of 1600 mg/d may impair learning, motor coordination, and reaction time (Rall, 1990a).

As reported with other anxiolytics, meprobamate can cause paradoxical excitement. The incidence of this adverse effect is not known. If suspected, the drug should be discontinued (Rall, 1990a).

TERATOGENICITY. In a retrospective study involving 19,000 live births, the rate of anomalies when meprobamate was prescribed during the first 6 weeks of pregnancy was higher (12.1 per 100,000) than when no drug was given (2.6 per 100,000). The finding indicated that 5 of 8 anomalies involved heart deformities. When meprobamate was given later in pregnancy, no differences in anomalies were seen. Meprobamate use during pregnancy is not recommended (Anon, 1975). In a single-dose study using meprobamate 800 mg, the peak milk level of the drug occurred at 4 hours, 2 hours after the peak plasma concentration. The effect of meprobamate on the nursing infant is unknown.

Beta-Adrenergic Blocking Drugs

EFFICACY

Of the beta-adrenergic receptor blocking agents available in the United States, propranolol is the most extensively studied in the management of anxiety. It is not approved by the FDA for use as an anxiolytic.

The anxiolytic effect of propranolol was first examined in 1966. The majority of six controlled studies show propranolol to be only slightly more effective than placebo in the treatment of GAD (Lader, 1988). Several studies report response rates of 60 to 70 percent; however, placebo response may be as high as 35 percent (Kathol et al., 1980). According to most studies, propranolol produces the greatest improvement in patients with primarily somatic complaints (e.g., palpitations, tremor, sweating); psychological symptoms (e.g., apprehension, irritability, tension) respond less well. One study reported improvement in both psychological and somatic symptomatology (Kathol et al., 1980). There are no established guidelines for the use of propranolol in the treatment of GAD. Unsatisfactory classification of anxiety states, as well as variation in study design, dose of the drug used, and assessment instruments, makes specific recommendations difficult. Beta blockers are considered second-line drugs in the treatment of GAD until further studies are performed.

No conclusive statement can be made about the comparative efficacy of propranolol versus BZDs because of the limited number of trials performed. However, most published studies reported BZDs to be superior to propranolol in anxiety disorders (Ballenger, 1986; Noyes et al., 1984).

In an open trial, 10 patients with panic disorder were treated with propranolol 20 to 80 mg/d, and 8 patients were reported to respond (Lader, 1988). In a double-blind, placebo-controlled trial, propranolol 160 mg/d was significantly more effective than placebo. Nine of 17 patients showed moderate to marked clinical improvement (Kathol et al., 1980). In a 2-week study, propranolol produced only a 33 percent response rate in prevention of panic attacks when compared with diazepam (Noyes et al., 1984). Another study reported propranolol to be less effective than alprazolam in the treatment of panic attacks and agoraphobia with panic attacks (Munjack et al., 1989). Propranolol 160 mg/d was as effective as imipramine in 23 patients with panic disorder (Lader, 1988).

Beta blockers appear to be effective in the treatment of acute situational anxiety (Lader, 1988). The drugs appear to be most effective when somatic symptoms predominate (Shuckit, 1981). Beta blockers have improved performance in students taking examinations, decreased tachycardia and lipid response to the stresses of race car driving, decreased somatic symptoms during the stress induced by public speaking, reduced tremor in string instrument players, and reduced symptoms of anxiety related to stress in anxious outpatients (Lader, 1988).

Beta blockers have not been investigated in the treatment of simple phobia (Noyes et al., 1986; Dommisse et al., 1987). However, they are reported to be beneficial in social phobia (Dommisse et al., 1987).

DOSING

There is no well-defined dosage range for propranolol in the treatment of GAD. Previous trials have suggested that ≤160 mg/d may be necessary to exert an anxiolytic effect. One study reported a positive correlation with heart rate and anxiolytic action when the heart rate was reduced to between 60 and 70 beats per minute (Kathol et al., 1980). Initial doses should be 40 to 60 mg/d. Doses may be increased 20 to 40 mg every other day depending on adverse effects. The drug usually is dosed t.i.d. or q.i.d. Once- or twice-daily dosing schedules, which have been effective in the treatment of hypertension, have not been studied in anxiety disorders.

Propranolol 40 to 80 mg has been used successfully in acute situational anxiety and for social phobia (Dommisse et al., 1987). The dose should be administered 1 to 2 hours prior to the stressful event.

ADVERSE EFFECTS

The reported incidence of adverse effects with propranolol in patients with anxiety is 25 to 40 percent (Kathol et al., 1980). This is higher than the reported 9 to 17 percent incidence of adverse effects reported in disorders other than anxiety. The explanation may be that the common adverse effects of propranolol (i.e., dizziness, fatigue, insomnia) are common complaints accompanying anxiety.

CARDIAC. Nearly 3 percent of 268 patients treated with propranolol experienced significant adverse reactions: bradycardia, impaired atrioventricular conduction, or hypotension. These reactions occur more frequently in the elderly. Long-term use of propranolol in doses of 160 to 400 mg/d resulted in a 9 percent incidence of left ventricular failure (Young et al., 1978). These effects are a result of the beta-blocking effects of the drug. All are reversible upon discontinuation of propranolol. Propranolol should be discontinued gradually in patients receiving the drug for angina because of reports of myocardial infarction associated with rapid withdrawal (Kathol et al., 1980; Young et al., 1978).

CENTRAL NERVOUS SYSTEM. Reactions such as fatigue and lethargy are frequently reported. Effects such as vivid dreams and nightmares are commonly reported; hallucinations, almost always visual and often of a hypnagogic nature, have been reported, though rarely. Toxic psychosis may occur and responds to stopping the drug temporarily and restarting at a lower dose (Erman, 1981).

Depression has been reported frequently as a complication of beta-blocker therapy; however, the true incidence is difficult to determine. The possibility of depression should be remembered in patients treated with propranolol who have a history of depression (Erman, 1981).

PULMONARY. Respiratory complications of propranolol are related to increased airway resistance that may become symptomatic in asthmatics or patients with chronic obstructive pulmonary disease. Approximately 0.5 to 2 percent of patients have developed dyspnea and wheezing after the initiation of propranolol (Young et al., 1978).

TERATOGENICITY. Propranolol use during pregnancy has been reported to cause decreased placental size, fetal growth retardation, and neonatal bradycardia and hypoglycemia. Studies in breast feeding women receiving propranolol found levels in the milk to be 50 to 100 percent of the plasma level of the mother. Adverse effects on the child are unknown (Young et al., 1978).

Miscellaneous Agents

Several additional drugs have been investigated in the treatment of panic disorder. Baclofen 30 mg/d in a double-blind trial was significantly more effective than placebo (Breslow et al., 1989). Carbamazepine produced a marked improvement in only 1 of 14 patients (Uhde et al., 1988). Valproic acid 2250 mg/d in an open trial produced moderate improvement in 6 of 10 patients treated for 7 weeks. Adverse effects included nausea and dizziness ($n = 4$); drowsiness, tremor, and diarrhea ($n = 3$); and constipation, dry mouth, and headaches ($n = 2$) (Primeau et al., 1990). In a double-blind, placebo-controlled, 5-week crossover design, verapamil 480 mg/d produced a significant reduction in panic attacks but not symptoms of agoraphobia in 11 patients. Overall, in self-ratings, patients considered themselves markedly improved ($n = 4$), marginally improved ($n = 3$), and nonresponsive ($n = 4$) (Klein et al., 1990).

OBSESSIVE-COMPULSIVE DISORDER

The pharmacologic treatment of obsessive-compulsive disorder (OCD) has improved considerably during the past few years. Until the latter half of the 1980s, there were not any medications marketed in the United States that were clearly effective for OCD. During the past few years, two effective antiobsessional agents have been marketed in the United States, namely, clomipramine and fluoxetine.

Clomipramine

EFFICACY

Clomipramine has been available outside the United States for more than 20 years. The chemical structure of clomipramine is similar to that of imipramine except for the addition of a chloride atom. Clomipramine is a specific serotonin reuptake blocker, although its metabolite, desmethylclomipramine, has effects on blocking norepinephrine reuptake.

Clomipramine has been used in therapeutic trials for a variety of disorders, including depression (Noll et al., 1985), eating disorders (Lacey and Crisp, 1988), and cataplexy (Mendelson, 1987). Use of clomipramine for OCD was first reported in the late 1960s. By 1980, several open-label studies suggested clomipramine may be effective for OCD (Ananth, 1986). During the last 10 years many controlled, double-blind investigations have demonstrated that clomipramine is more effective in the treatment of OCD than either placebo or a variety of antidepressants (Thoren et al., 1980b; Insel, 1984; Ananth, 1986; Zohar and Insel, 1987a, 1987b; Leonard et al., 1988; Murphy et al., 1989). A large multicenter trial showed a 40 percent reduction in OCD symptom ratings in 194 patients treated with clomipramine compared with only a few percent reduction in symptoms for 190 patients treated with placebo (DeVeaugh-Geiss et al., 1989).

DOSING

Twenty-five milligrams of clomipramine per day is the usual starting dose. It is most often given as a single bedtime dose to simplify compliance and reduce the impact of certain side effects such as sedation. This starting dose of 25 mg/d should be gradually increased over several days to 2 weeks as determined by side effects to a minimum dose of 150 mg/d. Patients who show no response to 150 mg/d after 4 weeks of treatment should have their dose increased to 200 mg/d. If there is little or no improvement to this dose within the next 2 or 3 weeks, the dose should be increased to 250 mg/d. Some response of OCD symptoms to clomipramine may be noticed during the first several weeks of treatment, but often the maximal response occurs after 6 to 12 weeks. Some patients continue to show further gradual improvement for months after treatment initiation.

Patients not responding to a dose of 250 mg/d after 2 or 3 months of treatment should have a 12-hour blood sample for measurement of clomipramine levels. Preliminary data suggest that patients may need a plasma level of clomipramine of at least 100 to 250 ng/ml. Patients who do not achieve these levels on 250 mg/d should be asked about compliance. If the clinician is convinced that the patient is compliant, then a low plasma level could indicate the patient is metabolizing the clomipramine rapidly. A small percentage of individuals are fast metabolizers of the TCAs similar to clomipramine. Some of these rapid metabolizers appear to benefit from dosages that are greater than the recommended maximums. It would seem that the same situation would be true for the treatment of OCD with clomipramine.

If bothersome side effects make dosage increases unacceptable, the physician may decide to keep a patient on a dose lower than those recommended above. Some patients have showed improvement on dosages as low as 75 mg/d (Ananth, 1986). Patients not responding to whatever dose after a trial of several months should be classified as nonresponders and given alternative treatment.

ADVERSE EFFECTS

Side effects to clomipramine can be quite bothersome for some patients. Clomipramine side effects are similar in severity and nature to those of TCAs such as amitriptyline. Side effects include drowsiness, orthostatic hypotension, tremor, lethargy, fatigue, impaired cognition, weight gain, and a variety of anticholinergic effects such as dry mouth, constipation, and blurred vision. Sexual changes associated with clomipramine use include decreased sexual interest and anorgasmia. One report found 22 of 24 OCD patients (male and female) developed anorgasmia, usually within the first few days of clomipramine initiation (Monteiro et al., 1987).

The clinician needs to alert the patient to potential side effects prior to starting therapy. Patients should be encouraged to remain on clomipramine if side effects are mild, since there are few treatment alternatives for OCD. Furthermore, most of the side effects decrease over time. Many patients will tolerate mild to moderate side effects if they experience significant improvement. Some patients who respond to clomipramine can maintain the same level of improvement on slightly reduced dosages of medication (Pato and Zohar, 1991). At times, modest dosage reductions can alleviate some side effects.

Fluoxetine

EFFICACY

Fluoxetine is another medication that effects improvement in OCD, although treatment of OCD is not yet an approved indication. During the past several years, several anecdotal and nonblind studies have suggested that fluoxetine is efficacious for OCD. Ten OCD patients treated with fluoxetine 20 to 80 mg/d showed improvement in a single-blind, placebo-controlled study (Turner et al., 1985), as did 61 OCD patients in an open-label trial (Jenike et al., 1989) and 50 OCD patients in a third study (60 to 100 mg/d) (Fontaine and Chouinard, 1989). Another nonblind study of 7 OCD patients showed 6 responded to doses of 60 to 90 mg/d (Fontaine and Chouinard, 1985). This response was similar to that found for clomipramine, which had previously been prescribed to these patients.

A crossover study (Pigott, 1991) of 32 OCD patients treated with fluoxetine 80 mg/d, clomipramine 200 mg/d, or placebo revealed the following: (1) fluoxetine and clomipramine were equally effective and significantly better than placebo, (2) both drugs required significant time lags (i.e., many weeks) to show improvement, (3) side effects were significantly more common with clomipramine, (4) responders to clomipramine treatment were often responders to fluoxetine treatment, and (5) relapses to both drugs occurred following placebo substitution.

DOSING

Patients should be started on a once-daily morning dose of fluoxetine 20 mg/d. This can be increased over a period of 2 or 3 weeks to 60 to 80 mg/d. Some early evidence of response to fluoxetine may be evident within the first 4 to 8 weeks after treatment initiation. Maximum benefits are often not evident for 2 to 3 months and sometimes longer. The dose of fluoxetine used in most treatment trials has been approximately 80 mg/d. Whether lower doses might be efficacious for some patients has not been rigorously tested.

ADVERSE EFFECTS

Side effects to fluoxetine are noticeably less than those of the traditional antidepressant medications. The most commonly reported side effects include nausea, insomnia, and a feeling of being restless or stimulated. These side effects tend to decrease with time. Occasionally, a patient will find one of these side effects intolerable and stop the medication. Patients bothered by side effects should first reduce their dose and then try to gradually increase the dose after a period of many days.

Conclusion

How long should fluoxetine or clomipramine be continued in responding patients? A double-blind discontinuation study of clomipramine showed 17 of 18 OCD patients relapsed after stopping medication (mean treatment time was 11 months) (Pato et al., 1988). Several anecdotal reports indicate that OCD symptoms are likely to return after stopping either clomipramine or fluoxetine (Asberg et al., 1982; Ananth, 1986; Pigott, 1991). Conversely, one discontinuation study of fluoxetine demonstrated that only 8 of 35 OCD patients relapsed within 1 year of stopping medication treatment (Fontaine and Chouinard, 1989). Because OCD is a chronic illness, it would seem that most patients would require long-term treatment with medications.

Fluvoxamine, like fluoxetine, appears to be a relatively specific serotonin reuptake blocker with little affect on other neurotransmitters or their receptors. It is marketed in several European countries but has not been approved for use in the United States yet. Several studies have found fluvoxamine to be effective in OCD (Price et al., 1987; Perse et al., 1988; Goodman et al., 1989). The time course and magnitude of response appear similar to those reported for fluoxetine and clomipramine. The side effects to fluvoxamine are similar to those of fluoxetine (Goodman and Price, 1991).

While the pharmacologic treatment of OCD has been enhanced significantly during the past several years, a sizable proportion of patients show little or no response to an adequate treatment trial of either fluoxetine or clomipramine. What should the clinician do with a nonresponding patient? For patients who have had an adequate trial of clomipramine (i.e., 200 to 250 mg/d for 10 to 12 weeks) or fluoxetine (60 to 80 mg/d for 10 to 12 weeks), there are some preliminary data to support that some patients may respond to augmentation of the fluoxetine or clomipramine with one of the following medications: lithium, clonazepam, clonidine, trazodone, buspirone, tryptophan, or pimozide (Jenike, 1991). The augmentation periods usually have been for approximately 1 month. If there is no response to the augmentation, the medications should be stopped and the patients switched to the other main agent (i.e., fluoxetine or clomipramine) and treated as though they were new patients to the medication. The rationale for the switch is that some patients appear to respond to one of these two drugs but not the other. If there is no response to an adequate trial of the second drug, then augmentation with one of the augmenting medications listed above should be tried. If there is no response to the first augmenting combination, other combinations can be considered. Nonresponding patients might next be considered for treatment with buspirone or experimental agents such as fluvoxamine, if available. Patients not re-

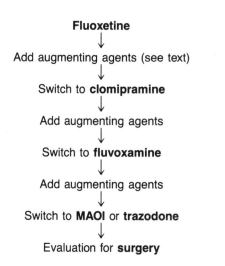

FIGURE 33-3.   *Treatment Scheme for Nonresponding OCD Patients (↓ = If No Response)*

sponding to these drugs could be switched to medications such as trazodone or imipramine or a monoamine oxidase inhibitor (Jenike, 1991). Figure 33-3 illustrates a flowchart for nonresponding patients.

The mechanism of action of drugs such as fluoxetine and clomipramine in OCD is unclear. Both drugs block the reuptake of serotonin and therefore increase synaptic levels of it. This would be consistent with a theory that in responsive patients there was too little serotonin. However, patients with high (not low) pretreatment platelet serotonin or high cerebral spinal fluid levels of 5-HIAA (a metabolite of serotonin) were found more likely to respond to clomipramine (Thoren et al., 1980a; Flament et al., 1987). Conversely, there is indirect evidence of upregulation of postsynaptic serotonin receptors which could be secondary to deficient release of serotonin (Murphy et al., 1986; Zohar et al., 1987; Hollander et al., 1989; Meltzer et al., 1988; Lesch et al., 1991). The mechanism by which clomipramine and fluoxetine improve OCD symptoms is not obvious and must await further clarification.

Electroconvulsive treatment (ECT) of OCD does not appear to be effective, although there have not been any well-controlled studies that address this issue. One review of pre-1965 studies concluded ECT was not very effective for obsessional conditions (Grimshaw, 1965). ECT combined with various other therapies has produced mixed results (Walter et al., 1972; Mellerman and Gorman, 1984).

Patients with significant OCD symptoms that have been unresponsive to several adequate medication trials may be appropriate candidates for psychosurgery. Psychosurgery may noticeably benefit

one-half or more of selected OCD patients (Jenike, 1991; Jenike et al., 1991).

In addition to the somatic therapies discussed above, there is evidence that specific behavioral therapies are effective for some OCD patients. Patients who have ritualistic or compulsive behaviors rather than primarily obsessional thoughts seem to respond best (Jenike, 1991; Steketee and Tynes, 1991).

A review of different forms of behavioral treatment suggests that exposure and response prevention are effective, whereas other treatments such as cognitive therapy, imaginal desensitization, aversion procedure, or paradoxical intention have little data supporting their effectiveness (Steketee and Tynes, 1991). Some investigators express the view that combining behavior therapy and medications may produce the best results (Jenike, 1991).

Certain factors reduced the likelihood treatment response. OCD patients with personality disorders, especially schizotypal, do poorly (Rachman and Hodgson, 1980; Jenike et al., 1986; Minichiello et al., 1987). Patients who are psychotic also have poor treatment responses (Solyom et al., 1985).

EATING DISORDERS

The eating disorders anorexia nervosa and bulimia nervosa have received increased scientific and public interest during the past decade. The prevalence of anorexia nervosa is approximately 1 percent, and bulimia nervosa is 5 to 10 percent (Crisp et al., 1976; Jones et al., 1980; Pope et al., 1984).

The pharmacologic treatment of these disorders is relatively new. There is somewhat more data about the drug treatment of bulimia nervosa than anorexia nervosa. There are still many unanswered questions about medication treatment of these two entities. For example, are antidepressants the drugs of choice? If so, is one antidepressant better than another? What is the optimal dose of these medications? How long should poor treatment response last before switching to another medication? Are combinations of medications helpful? Will the newer serotonin uptake blockers be more effective than the older antidepressants? How long should maintenance therapy last? While many unanswered questions exist, there are some data to assist the clinician in the treatment of these challenging patients.

Efficacy

ANOREXIA NERVOSA. Limited efficacy has been demonstrated for the pharmacologic treatment of anorexia nervosa with a variety of medications, including some antidepressants and cyproheptadine, a drug ordinarily used for allergic reactions. Antipsychotics also have been tried in the treatment of anorexia nervosa but without apparent success

(Dally and Sargent, 1960; Vandereycken and Pierloot, 1982; Vandereycken, 1984).

Amitriptyline has been used to treat anorexia nervosa in two placebo-controlled studies. One 5-week study (Biederman et al., 1985) produced no significant improvement in 25 completers taking a mean dose 115 mg/d, whereas an 8-week study using 40 to 160 mg/d showed some increase in the rate of weight gain in 36 completers (Halmi et al., 1986). Clomipramine used at a relatively low dose of 50 mg/d in 16 patients for 10 weeks provided no improvement in weight gain but did produce a significant increase in hunger and a decrease in obsessive-compulsive symptoms when compared with placebo (Lacey and Crisp, 1988). Lithium was superior to placebo for weight gain in a 4-week study of 16 patients (Gross et al., 1981). Three studies (131 patients) comparing placebo to cyproheptadine (12 to 32 mg/d) produced conflicting results (Vigersky and Lariaux, 1977; Goldberg et al., 1979; Halmi et al., 1982). Patients on higher doses of cyproheptadine or those with more severe anorexia nervosa appeared to gain more weight than placebo-treated patients, whereas many other active medication patients did not show this improvement.

Anorexia nervosa may result from the coalescence of several etiologic factors, one of which may be a biologic abnormality involving a serotonin. Serotonin plays an important role in the loss of appetite (Breisch et al., 1976; Leibowitz and Papadakos, 1978; Blundell, 1984a, 1984b). Various research strategies indicate that serotonin plays an important role in the loss of appetite or inhibition of food intake (Blundell, 1984a, 1984b). Injection of serotonin into the paraventricular nucleus inhibits feeding in animals (Leibowitz and Papadakos, 1978). Serotonin agonists such as m-chloro-phenylpiperazine (m-CPP) or agents that may indirectly facilitate serotonergic transmission such as fenfluramine cause a loss of appetite (Blundell, 1984a). In animals, intracerebral injection of p-chlorophenylalanine depletes serotonin and increases appetite (Breisch et al., 1976).

Serotonin activity is affected by all the medications that have shown some therapeutic benefit in treatment of anorexia nervosa (e.g., cyproheptadine, lithium, antidepressants). At present it is not known how the medications that effect improvement in anorexia nervosa work, but their effect on serotonin activity is one possibility.

A variety of other antidepressants have been used to treat anorexia nervosa in open-label trials. Some of these medications appear to be helpful to some patients (Hudson et al., 1985). Some authors have suggested that anorexia nervosa patients with coexistent depression might be more likely to respond to antidepressants (Hudson et al., 1985). However, other researchers cautioned against using the presence of depression as a criteria for administering antidepressants early in the course of treatment, believing that these symptoms often remit with weight gain (Eckert and Mitchell, 1989).

Medications should be part of comprehensive treatment strategy that may include interventions such as cognitive-behavioral therapy, family therapy, educational sessions, and dietary management (Eckert and Mitchell, 1989). Two recent articles review these nonpharmacologic treatments for anorexia nervosa (Garner and Garfinkle, 1985; Eckert and Mitchell, 1989).

BULIMIA NERVOSA. A variety of antidepressants appear to be effective for bulimia nervosa. Table 33-2 summarizes those studies which have compared placebo with active medication treatment.

TABLE 33-2. *Placebo-Controlled Medication Trials for Bulimia Nervosa*

Author	Drug	Dose	Completers (% original sample)	Results*
Pope, 1983	Imipramine	200 mg	19 (86%)	+
Sabine, 1983	Mianserin	60 mg	36 (72%)	a
Mitchell, 1984	Amitriptyline	150 mg	32 (84%)	b
Walsh, 1984	Phenelzine	60–90 mg	50 (81%)	+
Hughes, 1986	Desipramine	≥200 mg	16 (73%)	+
Agras, 1987	Imipramine	167 mg	20 (91%)	+
Barlow, 1988	Desipramine	150 mg	24 (51%)	+
Horne, 1988	Buproprion	450 mg	49 (60%)	+
Blouin, 1988	Desipramine + Fenfluramine	150 mg 60 mg	22 (61%)	+
Pope, 1989	Trazadone	200–400 mg	42 (91%)	+
Fluoxetine Group, 1992	Fluoxetine	20 or 60 mg	266 (69%)	+

* + = significant improvement of active medication vs. placebo.
  a = both groups improved.
  b = trend favoring amitriptyline vs. placebo.

The presence of depression does not appear necessary for medication improvement of bulimic behaviors. Two studies specifically excluded patients with depression and still showed a positive treatment response (Hughes et al., 1986; Horne et al., 1988).

The largest medication study to date involved 387 women treated for 8 weeks with placebo, fluoxetine 20 mg/d, or fluoxetine 60 mg/d (Fluoxetine Study Group, 1992). Fluoxetine 60 mg/d was clearly superior to placebo for reducing the number of binges and vomiting episodes. The 20 mg/d dose was modestly better than placebo.

Medications other than traditional antidepressants also may be effective for bulimia nervosa. Lithium reduced bulimia nervosa symptoms in the majority of patients in a nonblind study (Hsu, 1984). Phenytoin produced improvement in a placebo crossover study; however, the results appeared to be confounded by extension of active medication effects into the placebo phase of the trial (Wermuth et al., 1977). An open-label study of naltrexone suggested a positive therapeutic response (Jonas and Gold, 1987), but this was not confirmed in a small ($n = 14$) placebo-controlled trial that showed only a trend favoring naltrexone (Mitchell et al., 1989a).

As with the treatment of anorexia nervosa, pharmacologic treatments for bulimia nervosa need to be considered as part of an individualized treatment program that may include specific forms of psychotherapy and educational interventions. A review of controlled studies utilizing specific psychotherapies (most often cognitive-behavioral) indicate they are often effective (Mitchell et al., 1989b).

Most of the outcome research for treatments of anorexia nervosa and bulimia nervosa has been short term (i.e., weeks to months). Much less is known about the long-term efficacy of various treatments. In view of the chronicity of eating disorders, medications will probably need to be administered for long periods. Optimal dosages or treatment times for longitudinal therapy have not been established.

DEMENTIA

VASODILATORS

The only drug specifically approved by the FDA for the treatment of dementia is a compound of ergoloid mesylates (i.e., Hydergine). Unlike other ergoid alkaloids, this compound decreases rather than increases cerebral blood flow. However, it is currently believed that the vasodilatory action has nothing to do with the effect of the drug. Instead, it has been theorized that Hydergine exerts its effect simply by increasing alertness (Cooper, 1991). However, the most recent controlled trial of the drug at the suggested therapeutic dose of 3 mg/d did not find the drug to be effective (Thompson et al., 1990).

Cholinergic Agonists

The most recent pharmacotherapeutic approach in the treatment of the memory loss associated with Alzheimer's disease has been targeted at increasing the levels of acetylcholine (ACh) in the brain. It is hypothesized that the primary neuropharmacologic defect in Alzheimer's is a decrease in choline acetyltransferase (CAT) activity. This enzyme is responsible for controlling the synthesis of ACh from choline and acetyl-CoA. A direct correlation has been demonstrated between ACh synthesis and cognitive impairment. However, the issue is not quite this simple, since other neurotransmitters (norepinephrine, epinephrine, dopamine, and somatostatin) have been shown to be compromised in Alzheimer's disease. CNS concentrations of ACh can be increased pharmacologically by (1) administration of the ACh dietary precursors, e.g., lecithin and choline, (2) administration of the ACh-esterase antagonists, e.g., physostigmine and tacrine, which decrease ACh degradation, (3) use of postsynaptic ACh receptor agonists, e.g., arecoline and RS-86, and (4) stimulation of ACh production, e.g., human nerve growth factor. Intact presynaptic cholinergic neurons are required for the ACh precursors and ACh-esterase inhibitors. These agents are thought to be useful only in the early stages of Alzheimer's disease. However, the postsynaptic receptor agonists are postulated to be of benefit in the later stages of the disease. Six studies estimated the effectiveness of the ACh precursors. Choline was administered in a dose of 50 to 200 mg/kg per day for 2 weeks in one study, while lecithin was administered in a dose of 11–35 g/d for 1 week to 6 months in five other studies. Improvement was reported only in the 6-month-long lecithin study. Oral physostigmine in doses of 0.5 to 15 mg/d for 3 days to 6 weeks was effective in two of three controlled trials. Single-dose studies of the IV formulation of 0.125 to 1.0 mg produced improvement in two studies. Tacrine (tetrahydroaminoacridine, or THA), when administered orally in doses ranging from 10 to 250 mg/d for up to 8 weeks, produced two positive and three negative studies (Volger, 1991; Eagger et al., 1991). The one IV single-dose formulation study was positive. Lecithin was utilized as a concomitant medication in all the studies. The patients most likely to respond to tacrine unsurprisingly were the patients with the least advanced disease. Despite the discouraging results regarding the tacrine studies, the FDA in November of 1991 approved a treatment program involving as many as 3000 Alzheimer's patients. This was surprising since in July of 1991 an FDA advisory committee concluded that there was little evidence that the drug provided much benefit to patients. Because the drug can cause up to threefold increases in liver function tests, the maximum daily dose for subsequent studies has been reduced to 100 mg/d. Studies evaluating the effect of human nerve growth factor on the cognition of patients with dementias have not been reported at this time (Volger, 1991).

Antiaggression

There are no drugs available currently that produce improvement in the memory dysfunction of patients with dementia. Thus the pharmacotherapy of dementia is primarily targeted at improving behavior. Traditionally, neuroleptics such as haloperidol and benzodiazepines such as diazepam have been utilized as the first-line treatments to control agitated demented patients. However, treatment of aggression and agitation with drugs other than antipsychotic agents (neuroleptics) in long-term care facilities that include skilled nursing facilities and intermediate-care facilities is being mandated by the most recent revision of the Omnibus Budget Reconciliation Act (OBRA). The Health Care Financing Administration (HCFA), a government agency, recently issued revised regulations for Medicare and Medicaid recipients treatment in long-term care facilities. With respect to antipsychotic drugs, the agency now requires that a physician certify that the use of antipsychotic drugs is necessary to treat a specific condition, e.g., delusions and hallucinations associated with either dementia, schizophrenia, schizoaffective illness, schizophreniform illness, depression, or mania. It is also now mandated that neuroleptic-treated residents who use antipsychotics should receive gradual dose reductions, drug holidays, and behavioral programming to discontinue these drugs. These changes went into effect on October 1, 1990. The neuroleptics were defined as the phenothiazine, butyrophenone, thioxanthene chemical classes and the individual agents molindone and loxapine. This legislation was passed in part due to the risk of adverse effects associated with these drugs, including pseudoparkinsonism, dystonias, akathisia, tardive dyskinesia, orthostatic hypotension, and anticholinergic delirium. Thus it is important for clinicians to be cognizant of the pharmacotherapeutic alternatives for the treatment of agitation and aggression. Beta blockers, carbamazepine, benzodiazepines, and buspirone have been studied in the treatment of agitation in mental retardation, autism, dementia and organic brain syndromes. However, of these medications, only the beta blockers and carbamazepine have been studied in demented patients. In three double-blind studies, Greendyke (1986a, 1986b, 1989) demonstrated that the beta blockers propranolol and pindolol were effective in decreasing aggression, hostility, and agitation in two-thirds of the organic patients. Propranolol doses ranged from 200 to 520 mg/d, while the pindolol doses ranged from 10 to 100 mg/d. Of the two drugs, pindolol was preferred because it produced no hypotension and bradycardia in the patients, whereas propranolol caused these adverse effects in 13 to 78 percent of patients. Generally, a 2-week trial of pindolol 40 to 60 mg/d PO is regarded as sufficient to determine whether the drug will be effective. The data evaluating the effectiveness of carbamazepine in the treatment of dementias are considerably less robust in contrast to that for the beta blockers. There are three open trials (Patterson, 1987, 1988; Gleason and Schneider, 1990) in which carbamazepine was administered in doses of 200 to 1000 mg/d or doses that produced blood levels between 8 and 12 μg/ml. The overall response rate in the treatment of aggression and agitation in these patients was 80 percent. Given the paucity and low quality of these data, a therapeutic carbamazepine trial of at least 2 weeks is justified to treat aggression and agitation only if the patient had failed on a trial beta blocker. The only adverse effect problems mentioned in these studies included diplopia and ataxia. There were no occurrences of hematologic complications.

REFERENCES

Agras WS, Dorian B, Kirkley BG, et al: Imipramine in the treatment of bulimia: double-blind controlled study. Int J Eating Disord 6:29–38, 1987.

Alexander B: Antipsychotics: How strict the formulary? Drug Intell Clin Pharmacol 22:324–326, 1988.

Ananth J: Clomipramine an antiobsessive drug. Can J Psychiatry 31:253–258, 1986.

Angst J: Clinical indications for a prophylactic treatment of depression. Adv Biol Psychiatry 7:218–229, 1981.

Anonymous: Teratogenicity of minor tranquilizers. FDA Drug Bull 5:14–15, 1975.

Asberg M, Thoren P, Bertilsson L: Clomipramine treatment of obsessive disorder: Biochemical and clinical aspects. Psychopharmacol Bull 18:13–21, 1982.

Aubree JC, Lader MH: High and very high dosage anti-psychotics: A critical review. J Clin Psychiatry 41:341–350, 1980.

Avery D, Lubrano A: Depression treated with imipramine and ECT: The De Carolis study reconsidered. Am J Psychiatry 136:559–562, 1979.

Awad AG: Drug therapy in schizophrenia: Variability of outcome and prediction of response. Can J Psychiatry 34:711–720, 1989.

Baldessarini RJ, Cohen BM, Teicher MH: Significance of neuroleptic dose and plasma level in the pharmacological treatment of psychoses. Arch Gen Psychiatry 45:79–91, 1988.

Ballenger JC: Pharmacotherapy of the panic disorders. J Clin Psychiatry 6(suppl):27–32, 1986.

Ballenger JC, Burrows GD, DuPont RL Jr, et al: Alprazolam in panic disorder and agoraphobia: Results from a multicenter trial: I. Efficacy in short-term treatment. Arch Gen Psychiatry 45:413–422, 1988.

Ballenger JC, Post RM: Carbamazepine in manic-depressive illness: A new treatment. Am J Psychiatry 137:782–790, 1980.

Barlow J, Blouin J, Blouin A, et al: Treatment of bulimia with desipramine: Double-blind crossover study. Can J Psychiatry 33:129–133, 1988.

Baskin SI, Esdale A: Is chlordiazepoxide the rational choice among benzodiazepines? Pharmacotherapy 12:110–119, 1982.

Beresford R, Ward A: Haloperidol decanoate: A preliminary review of its pharmacodynamic and pharmacokinetic properties and therapeutic use in psychosis. Drugs 33:31–49, 1987.

Bergen JA, Eyland EA, Campbell JA, et al: The course of tardive dyskinesia in patients on long-term neuroleptics. Br J Psychiatry 154:523–528, 1989.

Bertilsson L, Tomson T: Clinical pharmacokinetics and pharmacological effects of carbamazepine and carbamazepine-10-11-epoxide. Clin Pharmacokinet 11:177–198, 1986.

Beumont PJV, Corker CS, Friesen HG, et al: The effects of phenothiazines on endocrine function: II. Effects in men and post-menopausal women. Br J Psychiatry 124:420–430, 1974.

Biederman J, Herzog DB. Rivinus TM: Amitriptyline in the treatment of anorexia nervosa: A double-blind placebo-controlled study. J Clin Psychopharmacol 5:10–16, 1985.

Bielski RJ, Fiedel DO: Prediction of tricyclic antidepressant response: A critical review. Arch Gen Psychiatry 33:1479–1489, 1976.

Black JL, Richelson E, Richardson JW: Antipsychotic agents: A clinical update. Mayo Clin Proc 60:777–789, 1985.

Blouin AG, Blouin JH, Perez EL, et al: Treatment of bulimia with fenfluramine and desipramine. J Clin Psychopharmacol 8:261–269, 1988.

Blundell JE: Serotonin and appetite. Neuropharmacology 23:1537–1551, 1984a.

Blundell JE: Systems and interactions: An approach to the pharmacology of eating and hunger. In Stunkard AJ, Stellar E (eds): Eating and Its Disorders. New York, Raven Press, 1984b, pp 39–65.

Breier A, Wolkowitz OM, Doran AR, et al: Neuroleptic responsivity of negative and positive symptoms in schizophrenia. Am J Psychiatry 144:1549–1555, 1987.

Breisch ST, Zemlan FP, Hoebel BG: Hyperphagia and obesity following serotonin depletion by intraventricular parachlorophenylalanine. Science 192:382–385, 1976.

Brennan M, Sandyk R, Borsook D: Use of sodium valproate in the management of affective disorders: Basic and clinical aspects. In Emrich HM, Okuma T, Muller AA (eds): Anticonvulsants in Affective Disorders. Amsterdam, Exerpta Medica, 1984, pp 56–65.

Breslow MF, Fankhauser MP, Potter RL, et al: Role of gamma-aminobutyric acid in antipanic drug efficacy. Am J Psychiatry 146:353–356, 1989.

Buigues J, Vallejo J: Therapeutic response to phenelzine in patients with panic disorder and agoraphobia with panic attacks. J Clin Psychiatry 48:55–59, 1987.

Busto U, Sellers, EM, Naranjo CA, et al: Withdrawal reactions after long-term therapeutic use of benzodiazepines. N Engl J Med 315:854–859, 1986.

Butler G, Gelder M, Hibbert G, et al: Anxiety management: Developing effective strategies. Behav Res Ther 25:517–522, 1987.

Calabrese JR, Gulledge AD: Psychotropics during pregnancy and lactation: A review. Psychosomatics 26:413–426, 1985.

Carpenter WT, Heinrichs DW, Hanlan TE: A comparative trial of pharmacologic strategies in schizophrenia. Am J Psychiatry 144:1466–1470, 1987.

Casey DE, Povlsen UJ, Meidahl B, et al: Neuroleptic-induced tardive dyskinesia and parkinsonism: Changes during several years of continuing treatment. Psychopharmacol Bull 22:250–253, 1986.

Chan J, Alldredge BK, Baskin LS: Perphenazine-induced priapism. DICP Ann Pharmacother 24:246–249, 1990.

Chandler J, Winokur G: How antipsychotic are the antipsychotics? A clinical study of the subjective antipsychotic effects of the antipsychotics in chronic schizophrenia. Ann Clin Psychiatry 1:215–220, 1989.

Charney DS, Woods SW, Goodman WK, et al: Drug treatment of panic disorder: The comparative efficacy of imipramine, alprazolam, and trazodone. J Clin Psychiatry 47:580–586, 1986.

Chouinard G, Annable L, Campbell W: A randomized clinical trial of haloperidol decanoate and fluphenazine decanoate in the outpatient treatment of schizophrenia. J Clin Psychopharmacol 9:247–253, 1989.

Chouinard G, Annable L, Fontaine R, et al: Alprazolam in the treatment of generalized anxiety and panic disorders: A double-blind, placebo-controlled study. Psychopharmacology 77:229–233, 1982.

Cohen S, Chiles J, MacNaughton A: Weight gain associated with clozapine. Am J Psychiatry 147:503–504, 1990.

Cole JO, Haskell DS, Orzack MH: Problems with benzodiazepines: An assessment of the available evidence. McLean Hosp J 6:46–74, 1981.

Consensus Development Panel: NIMH/NIH Consensus Development Conference Statement: Mood disorders: Pharmacologic prevention of recurrences. Am J Psychiatry 142:469–476, 1985.

Cooper JK: Drug treatment of Alzheimer's disease. Arch Intern Med 151:245–249, 1991.

Coryell W, Noyes R, Clancy J: Panic disorder and primary unipolar depression: A comparison of background and outcome. J Affective Disord 5:311–317, 1983.

Crisp AH, Palmer RL, Kalucy RS, et al: How common is anorexia nervosa? A prevalence study. Br J Psychiatry 128:549–554, 1976.

Dally PJ, Sargent W: A new treatment of anorexia nervosa. Br Med J 1:1770–1773, 1960.

Davis JM, Casper R: Antipsychotic drugs: Clinical pharmacology and therapeutic use. Drugs 14:260–282, 1977.

Davis JM, Schyve PM, Pavkovic I: Clinical and legal issues in neuroleptic use. Clin Neuropharmacol 6:117–128, 1983.

Degivity R: Extrapyramidal motor disorders following long-term treatment with neuroleptic drugs. In Grave GE, Gardner R (eds): Psychotropic Drugs and Dysfunctions of the Basal Ganglion (Public Health Service Publication 1938). Bethesda, MD, National Institute of Mental Health, 1969, pp 22–32.

Del Giudice J, Clark WG, Gocka EF: Prevention of recidivism of schizophrenics treated with fluphenazine enanthate. Psychosomatics 16:32–36, 1975.

Delva NJ, Letemendia FJJ: Lithium treatment in schizophrenia and schizoaffective disorders. Br J Psychiatry 141:387–400, 1982.

Den Boer JA, Westenberg GM: Effect of a serotonin and noradrenaline uptake inhibitor in panic disorder: A double-blind comparative study with fluvoxamine and maprotiline. Int Clin Psychopharmacol 3:59–74, 1988.

DeVeaugh-Geiss J, Landau P, Katz R: Treatment of obsessive-compulsive disorder with clomipramine. Psychiatr Ann 19:97–101, 1989.

Dommisse CS, DeVane CL: Buspirone: A new type of anxiolytic. Drug Intell Clin Pharmacol 19:624–628, 1985.

Dommisse CS, Hayes PE: Current concepts in clinical therapeutics: Anxiety disorders, part 2. Clin Pharmacol 6:196–215, 1987.

Dose M, Emrich HM, Cording-Tommel C, von Zerssen D: Use of calcium antagonists in mania. Psychoneuroendocrinology 11:241–243, 1986.

Dubovsky SL: Generalized anxiety disorder: New concepts and psychopharmacologic therapies. J Clin Psychiatry 51(suppl):3–10, 1990.

Dubovsky SL, Franks RD, Allen S, Murphy J: Calcium antagonists in mania: A double-blind study of verapamil. Psychiatry Res 18:309–320, 1986.

Dubovsky SL, Franks RD, Lifschitz M, Coen P: Effectiveness of verapamil in the treatment of a manic patient. Am J Psychiatry 139:502–504, 1982.

Dunner DL, Ishiki D, Avery DH, et al: Effect of alprazolam and diazepam on anxiety and panic attacks in panic disorder: A controlled study. J Clin Psychiatry 47:458–460, 1986.

Eagger SA, Levy R, Sahakian BJ: Tacrine in Alzheimer's disease. Lancet 337:989–992, 1991.

Eckert ED, Mitchell JE: An overview of the treatment of anorexia nervosa. Psychiatr Med 7:293–315, 1989.

El-Mallakh RS: Acute lithium neurotoxicity. Psychiatr Dev 4:311–328, 1986.

Emrich HM, Dose M, von Zerssen D: The use of sodium valproate, carbamazepine, and oxycarbamazepine in patients with affective disorders. J Affective Disord 18:243–250, 1985.

Ereshefsky L, Saklad SR: Haloperidol decanoate loading doses and pharmacokinetics. Presented at the New Clinical Drug Evaluation Unit Annual Meeting. Key Biscayne, FL, June 4, 1989a.

Ereshefsky L, Watanabe MD, Tran-Johnson TK: Clozapine: An atypical antipsychotic agent. Clin Pharmacol 8:691–709, 1989b.

Ereshefsky L, Saklad SR, Jann MW, et al: Future of depot neuroleptic therapy: Pharmacokinetic and pharmacodynamic approaches. J Clin Psychiatry 45(5, sec 2):50–59, 1984.

Erman MK, Gruggenheim FG: Psychiatric side effects of commonly used drugs. Drug Ther 11:117–126, 1981.

Feinberg SS, Halbreich U: The association between the definition and reported prevalence of treatment-resistant depression. In Halbreich U, Feinberg SS (eds): Psychosocial Aspects of Nonresponse to Antidepressant Drugs. Washington, American Psychiatric Press, 1986, pp 5–34.

Flament MF, Rapoport JL, Murphy DL, et al: Biochemical changes during clomipramine treatment of childhood obsessive-compulsive disorder. Arch Gen Psychiatry 44:219–225, 1987.

Fleischhacker WW, Roth SD, Kane JM: The pharmacologic treatment of neuroleptic-induced akathisia. J Clin Psychopharmacol 10:12–21, 1990.

Fluoxetine Bulimia Nervosa Collaborative Group: Fluoxetine in the treatment of bulimia nervosa. Arch Gen Psychiatry 49:139–147, 1992.

Fontaine R, Chouinard G: Fluoxetine in the treatment of obsessive-compulsive disorder. Prog Neuropsychopharmacol Biol Psychiatry 9:605–608, 1985.

Fontaine R, Chouinard G: Fluoxetine in the long-term maintenance treatment of obsessive-compulsive disorder. Psychiatr Ann 19:88–91, 1989.

Freeman TW, Clothier JL, Pazzaglia P, et al: A double-blind comparison of valproate and lithium in the treatment of acute mania. Am J Psychiatry 149:108–111, 1992.

Garner DM, Garfinkel PE (eds): Handbook of Psychotherapy for Anorexia and Bulimia. New York, Guilford Press, 1985, pp 107–147.

Gelenberg AJ: Amnesia and benzodiazepines. Bio Ther Psychiatry 8:27, 1985.

Gelenberg AJ: Lorazepam (Ativan): Antipsychotic adjunct? Biol Ther Psychiatry 9:37–40, 1986.

Gelenberg AJ: Benzodiazepines in pregnancy. Biol Ther Psychiatry 10:18–19, 1987.

Giannini AJ, Houser WL, Loiselle RH, et al: Antimanic effects of verapamil. Am J Psychiatry 1141:1602–1603, 1984.

Giannini AJ, Loiselle RH, Price WA, et al: Comparison of antimanic efficacy of clonidine and verapamil. J Clin Pharmacol 25:307–308, 1985.

Giannini AJ, Taraszewski R, Loiselle RH: Verapamil and lithium in maintenance therapy of manic patients. J Clin Pharmacol 27:980–982, 1987.

Gitlin MJ, Midha KK, Fogeson D, et al: Persistence of fluphenazine in plasma after decanoate withdrawal. J Clin Psychopharmacol 8:53–56, 1988.

Gitlin MJ, Winer H, Fairbank L, et al: Failure of T_3 to potentiate tricyclic antidepressant response. J Affective Disord 13:267–272, 1987.

Gleason RP, Schneider LS: Carbamazepine treatment of agitation in Alzheimer's outpatients refractory to neuroleptics. J Clin Psychiatry 51:115–118, 1990.

Gloger S, Brunhaus L, Gladic D, et al: Panic attacks and agoraphobia: Low dose clomipramine treatment. J Clin Psychopharmacol 9:28–32, 1989.

Goldberg HL: Buspirone hydrochloride: A unique new anxiolytic agent. Pharmacotherapy 4:314–324, 1984.

Goldberg SC, Halmi KA, Eckert ED, et al: Cyproheptadine in anorexia nervosa. Br J Psychiatry 134:67–70, 1979.

Goodman WK, Price LH: Fluvoxamine in the treatment of obsessive-compulsive disorder. In Pato MT, Zohar J (eds): Current Treatments of Obsessive-Compulsive Disorder. Washington, American Psychiatric Press, 1991, pp 45–59.

Goodman WK, Price LH, Rasmussen SA, et al: Efficacy of fluvoxamine in obsessive-compulsive disorder: A double-blind comparison with placebo Arch Gen Psychiatry 46:36–44, 1989.

Goodnick PJ, Meltzer HY: Treatment of schizoaffective disorders. Schizophr Bull 10:30–48, 1984.

Goodwin FK, Zis AP: Lithium in the treatment of mania: Comparison with neuroleptics. Arch Gen Psychiatry 36:840–844, 1979.

Gorman JM, Liebowitz MR, Fyer AJ, et al: An open trial of fluoxetine in the treatment of panic attacks. J Clin Psychopharmacol 7:258–260, 1985.

Greenblatt DJ: Benzodiazepines 1980: Current update. Psychosomatics 21(suppl):9–14, 1980a.

Greenblatt DJ: Benzodiazepines 1980: Current update. Psychosomatics 21(suppl):26–31, 1980b.

Greenblatt DJ, Shader RI: Meprobamate: A study of irrational drug use. Am J Psychiatry 127:1297–1303, 1971.

Greenblatt DJ, Shader RI: Prazepam and lorazepam, two new benzodiazepines. N Engl J Med 299:1342–1344, 1978.

Greenblatt DJ, Shader RI, Abernathy DR: Current status of benzodiazepines (first of two parts). N Engl J Med 309:354–358, 1983.

Greendyke RM, Kanter DR: Therapeutic effects of pindolol on behavioral disturbances associated with organic brain disease: A double blind study. J Clin Psychiatry 47:423–426, 1986.

Greendyke RM, Schuester DB, Wooton JA: Propranolol in the treatment of assaultive patient with organic brain disease. J Clin Psychopharmacol 4:282–285, 1984.

Greendyke RM, Berkner, Webster JC, et al: Treatment of behavioral problems with pindolol. Psychosomatics 30:161–165, 1989.

Greendyke RM, Kanter DR, Schuster DB, et al: Propranolol treatment of assaultive patients with organic brain disease. J Nerv Ment Dis 174:290–294, 1986.

Grimshaw L: The outcome of obsessional disorder: A follow-up study of 100 cases. Br J Psychiatry 111:1051–1056, 1965.

Gross HA, Ebert MH, Faden VB, et al: A double-blind controlled trial of lithium carbonate in primary anorexia nervosa. J Clin Psychopharmacol 1:376–381, 1981.

Grossi E, Sacchetti E, Vita A, et al: Carbamazepine vs chlorpromazine in mania: A double-blind trial. In Emrich HM, Okuma T, Muller AA (eds): Anticonvulsants in Affective Disorders. Amsterdam, Excerpta Medica, 1986, pp 177–187.

Groves JE, Mandel MR: The long-acting phenothiazines. Arch Gen Psychiatry 32:893–900, 1975.

Guerrero RM, Shifrar KA: Diagnosis and treatment of neuroleptic malignant syndrome. Clin Pharmacol 7:697–701, 1988.

Halmi KA, Eckert E, Ladu T, et al: Anorexia nervosa: Treatment efficacy of cyproheptadine and amitriptyline. Arch Gen Psychiatry 43:177–181, 1986.

Halmi KA, Eckert ED, Falk JR: Cyproheptadine for anorexia nervosa. Lancet 1:1358–1376, 1982.

Haskell DS, Gambill JD, Gardos G, et al: Doxepin or diazepam for anxious and anxious-depressed outpatients. J Clin Psychiatry 39:135–139, 1978.

Herz MI: Intermittent medication and schizophrenia. In Kane JM (ed): Drug Maintenance Strategies in Schizophrenia. Washington, American Psychiatric Press, 1984, pp 51–68.

Hoehn-Saric R, McLeod DR, Zimmerli WD: Differential effects of alprazolam and imipramine in generalized anxiety disorder: Somatic versus psychic symptoms. J Clin Psychiatry 49:293–301, 1988.

Hollander E, DeCaria C, Cooper T, et al: Neuroendocrine sensitivity in obsessive-compulsive disorder. Biol Psychiatry 25(suppl) 5A, 1989.

Hollister LE: Pharmacotherapeutic considerations in anxiety disorders. J Clin Psychiatry 47(suppl):33–36, 1986.

Hollister LE, Kanter SL, Wright A: Comparison of intramuscular and oral administration of chlorpromazine and thioridazine. Arch Int Pharmacodyn Ther 144:571–578, 1963.

Holstad SG, Perry PJ, Kathol RG, et al: The effects of intravenous theophylline infusion versus sodium bicarbonate infusion on lithium clearance in normal subjects. Psychiatry Res 25:203–211, 1988.

Honigfeld G, Patin J: A two-year clinical and economic follow-up of patients on clozapine. Hosp Commun Psychiatry 41:882–825, 1990.

Horne RL, Ferguson JM, Pope HG, et al: Treatment of bulimia with bupropion: Multicenter controlled trial. J Clin Psychiatry 49:262–266, 1988.

Howarth BG, Grace MGA: Depression, drugs, and delusions. Arch Gen Psychiatry 42:1145–1147, 1985.

Hsu LKG: Treatment of bulimia with lithium. Am J Psychiatry 141:1260–1262, 1984.

Hudson JI, Pope HG, Jonas JM, et al: Treatment of anorexia nervosa with antidepressants. J Clin Psychopharmacol 5:10–16, 1985.

Hughes PL, Wells LA, Cunningham CJ, et al: Treating bulimia with desipramine. Arch Gen Psychiatry 43:182–186, 1986.

Inoue H, Hazama H, Ogura C, et al: Neuroendocrinological study of amenorrhea induced by antipsychotic drugs (letter). Folia Psychiatr Neurol (Jpn) 34:181, 1980.

Insel TR: New Findings in Obsessive-Compulsive Disorder. Washington, American Psychiatry Press, 1984.

Jacobs SC, Nelson JC, Zisook S: Treating depression of bereavements with antidepressants: A pilot study. Psychiatr Clin North Am 110:501–510, 1987.

Janicak PG, Pandey GN, Davis JM, et al: Response of psychotic and nonpsychotic depression to phenelzine. Am J Psychiatry 145:93–95, 1988.

Jann MW, Kurtz NM: Treatment of panic and phobic disorders. Clin Pharmacol 6:947–962, 1987.

Jeavons PM: Sodium valproate and neural tube defects. Lancet 12:1282–1283, 1982.

Jenike MA: Management of patients with treatment-resistant obsessive-compulsive disorder. In Pato MT, Zohar J (eds): Current Treatments of Obsessive-Compulsive Disorder. Washington, American Psychiatric Press, 1991, pp 135–155.

Jenike MA, Baer L, Minichiello WE, et al: Concomitant obsessive-compulsive disorder and schizotypal personality disorder. Am J Psychiatry 143:530–532, 1986.

Jenike MA, Buttolph L, Baer L, et al: Open trial of fluoxetine in obsessive-compulsive disorder. Am J Psychiatry 146:909–911, 1989.

Jenike MA, Baer L, Ballatine T, et al: Cingulotomy for refractory obsessive-compulsive disorder. Arch Gen Psychiatry 48:548–555, 1991.

Jester DV, Potkin SG, Sinka S, et al: Tardive dyskinesia-reversible and persistent. Arch Gen Psychiatry 36:585–590, 1979.

Johnson DAW: Observations on the dose regime of fluphenazine decanoate in maintenance treatment of schizophrenia. Br J Psychiatry 126:457–461, 1975.

Johnson DAW: Observations of the use of long-acting depot neuroleptic injections in the maintenance therapy of schizophrenia. J Clin Psychiatry 45(5, sec 2):13–21, 1984.

Johnson DAW: Antipsychotic medication: Clinical guidelines for maintenance therapy. J Clin Psychiatry 46(suppl):6–15, 1985.

Jolly AG, Hirsch SR, McRink A, et al: Trial of brief intermittent neuroleptic prophylaxis for selected schizophrenic outpatients: Clinical outcome at one year. Br Med J 298:985–991, 1989.

Jonas JM, Gold MS: Treatment of bulimia with the opiate antagonist naltrexone: Preliminary data and theoretical implications. In Hudson Jl, Pope HG (eds): Psychobiology of Bulimia. Washington, APA Press, 1987.

Jones DJ, Fox MM, Babigiar HM, et al: Epidemiology of anorexia nervosa in Monroe Co., New York: 1960–1979. Psychosom Med 42:558–561, 1980.

Jones KL, Lacro RV, Johnson KA, et al: Pattern of malformations in the children of women treated with carbamazepine during pregnancy. N Engl J Med 320:1661–1666, 1989.

Kahn RJ, McNair DM, Lipman RS, et al: Imipramine and chlordiazepoxide in depressive and anxiety disorders: II. Efficacy in anxious outpatients. Arch Gen Psychiatry 43:79–85, 1986.

Kahne GJ: Rebound psychoses following the discontinuation of a high potency antipsychotic. Can J Psychiatry 34:227–229, 1989.

Kane JM: The use of depot neuroleptics: Clinical experience in the United States. J Clin Psychiatry 45(5, sec 2):5–12, 1984.

Kane JM: Dosage strategies with long-acting injectable neuroleptics including haloperidol decanoate. J Clin Psychopharmacol 6(suppl):20–23, 1986.

Kane JM: The current status of neuroleptic therapy. J Clin Psychiatry 50:322–328, 1989.

Kane JM, Borenstein M: Compliance in the long-term treatment of schizophrenia. Psychopharmacol Bull 21:23–27, 1985.

Kane JM, Honigfeld G, Singer J, et al: Clozaril Collaborative Study Group. Clozapine for the treatment-resistant schizophrenic: A double-blind comparison with chlorpromazine. Arch Gen Psychiatry 45:789–796, 1988.

Katcher BS: General care: Anxiety and insomnia. In Koda-Kimble MA, Katcher BS, Young LY (eds): Applied Therapeutics for Clinical Pharmacists, 2d ed. San Francisco, Applied Therapeutics, 1978, pp 71–85.

Kathol RG, Noyes R, Slymen DJ, et al: Propranolol in chronic anxiety disorders. Arch Gen Psychiatry 37:1361–1365, 1980.

Kay SR, Singh MM: The positive-negative distinction in drug-free schizophrenic symptoms. Arch Gen Psychiatry 46:711–718, 1989.

Keck PE, Cohen BM, Baldessarini RJ, et al: Time course of antipsychotic effects of neuroleptic drugs. Am J Psychiatry 146:1289–1292, 1989a.

Keck PE, Sebastianelli J, Pope HG, et al: Frequency and presentation of neuroleptic malignant syndrome in a state psychiatric hospital. J Clin Psychiatry 50:352–355, 1989b.

Kim HR, Delva NJ, Lawson JS: Prophylactic medication for unipolar depressive illness: The place of lithium carbonate in combination with antidepressant medication. Can J Psychiatry 35:107–114, 1990.

Kissling W, Moller HJ, Walter K, et al: Double-blind comparison of haloperidol decanoate and fluphenazine decanoate effectiveness, side effects, dosage and serum levels during a six-month treatment for relapse prevention. Pharmacopsychiatry 18:240–245, 1985.

Klein E, Uhde TW: Controlled study of verapamil for treatment of panic disorder. Am J Psychiatry 145:431–434, 1990.

Klerman GL, Cole JO: Clinical pharmacology of imipramine and related antidepressant compounds. Pharmacol Rev 17:101–141, 1965.

Lacey JH, Crisp AH: Hunger, food intake, and weight: The impact of clomipramine on a refeeding anorexia nervosa population. Postgrad Med 56:79–85, 1980.

Lader M: Beta-adrenoceptor antagonists in neuropsychiatry: An update. J Clin Psychiatry 49:213–223, 1988.

Lee A: Treatment of drug-induced dystonic reactions. Journal of American College of Emergency Physicians 8:453–457, 1979.

Leibowitz SF, Papadakos PJ: Serotonin-norepinephrine interactions in the paraventricular nucleus: Antagonistic effects on feeding behavior in the rat. Neurosci Abstr 4:452, 1978.

Leonard H, Swedo S, Rapoport JL, et al: Treatment of childhood obsessive-compulsive disorder with clomipramine and desmethylimipramine: A double-blind crossover comparison. Psychopharmacol Bull 24:93–95, 1988.

Lerer B, Moore N, Meyendorf E, et al: Carbamazepine versus lithium in mania. J Clin Psychiatry 48:89–93, 1987.

Lesch KP, Hoh A, Disselkamp-Tietze J, et al: 5-Hydroxytryptamine$_{1a}$ receptor responsivity in obsessive-compulsive disorder. Arch Gen Psychiatry 48:540–547, 1991.

Lieberman JA, Kane JM, Johns CA: Clozapine: Guidelines for clinical management. J Clin Psychiatry 50:329–338, 1989.

Lindstrom LH: The effect of long-term treatment with clozapine in schizophrenia: A retrospective study in 96 patients treated with clozapine for up to 13 years. Acta Psychiatr Scand 77:524–529, 1988.

Lister RG: The amnesic action of benzodiazepines in man. Neurosci Biobehav Rev 9:87–94, 1985.

Livingston S, Pauli L, Berman W: Carbamazepine in epilepsy: Nine-year follow-up with special emphasis on untoward reactions. Dis Nerv Syst 35:103–107, 1974.

Lucki I, Rickels K, Geller AM: Psychomotor performance following the long-term use of benzodiazepines. Psychopharmacol Bull 21:93–96, 1985.

Lusznat RM, Murphy DP, Numm MH: Carbamazepine versus lithium in mania: A double-blind study. Br J Psychiatry 153:198–204, 1988.

Lyskowski J, Nasrallah HA: Slow-release lithium: A review and a comparative study. J Clin Psychopharmacol 1:406–408, 1981.

Marder SR, Van Putten T: Who should receive clozapine? Arch Gen Psychiatry 45:865–867, 1988.

Marken PA, Wells BG, Brown CS: Treatment of psychosis in pregnancy. DICP Ann Pharmacother 23:598–599, 1989.

Marriott P, Pansa M, Hiep A: Intervals between long acting neuroleptics: Outcome and re-admission variables. Prog Neuropsychopharmacol Biol Psychiatry 8:109–114, 1984.

Matilla MJ, Aranko K, Seppala T: Acute effects of buspirone and alcohol on psychomotor skills. J Clin Psychiatry 43:56–60, 1982.

Mavissakalian M, Perel J, Bowler K, et al: Trazodone in the treatment of panic disorder and agoraphobia with panic attacks. Am J Psychiatry 144:785–787, 1987.

Mavissakalian MR, Michelson L, Dealy RS: Pharmacologic treatment of agoraphobia: Imipramine vs imipramine with programmed practice. Br J Psychiatry 143:348–355, 1983.

Mavissakalian MR, Perel JM: Imipramine dose-response relationship in panic disorder with agoraphobia. Arch Gen Psychiatry 46:127–131, 1989.

McCabe MS, Norris B: Electroconvulsive therapy versus chlorpromazine in mania. Biol Psychiatry 12:245–254, 1977.

McGreadie RG, Dingwall JM, Wiles DH, et al: Intermittent pimozide versus fluphenazine decanoate as maintenance therapy for chronic schizophrenia. Br J Psychiatry 137:510–517, 1980.

McIntyre IM, Gershon S: Interpatient variations in anti-psychotic therapy. J Clin Psychiatry 46(suppl):3–5, 1985.

Mellerman LA, Gorman JM: Successful treatment of obsessive-compulsive disorder with ECT. Am J Psychiatry 144:596–597, 1984.

Meltzer HY: Duration of a clozapine trial in neuroleptic-resistant schizophrenia (letter). Arch Gen Psychiatry 46:672, 1989.

Meltzer HY, Nash JF Jr: Serotonin and mood: Neuroendocrine aspects. In Ganten F, Pfaff D, Fuxe F (eds): Current Topics in Neuroendocrinology. New York, Springer-Verlag, 1988, pp 183–210.

Mendelson WB: Medications in the treatment of sleep disorders. In Meltzer HY (ed): Psychopharmacology: A Generation of Progress. New York, Raven Press, 1987, pp 1305–1311.

Minichiello WE, Baer L, Jenike MA: Schizotypal personality disorder: A poor prognostic indicator for behavior therapy in the treatment of obsessive-compulsive disorder. J Anxiety Disord 1:273–276, 1987.

Mitchell JE, Groat R: A placebo-controlled, double-blind trial of amitriptyline in bulimia. J Clin Psychopharmacol 4:186–193, 1984.

Mitchell JE, Hoberman H, Pyle RL: An overview of the treatment of bulimia nervosa. Psychiatr Med 7:317–332, 1989a.

Mitchell JE, Christenson G, Jennings J, et al: A placebo-controlled double-blind crossover study of naltrexone hydrochloride in outpatients with normal weight bulimia. J Clin Psychopharmacol 9:94–97, 1989b.

Monteiro WO, Noshirvani HF, Marks IM, et al: Anorgasmia from clomipramine in obsessive-compulsive disorder: A controlled trial. Br J Psychiatry 151:107–112, 1987.

Morris JB, Beck AT: The efficacy of antidepressant drugs: A review of research (1958 to 1972). Arch Gen Psychiatry 30:667–674, 1974.

Moskorvitz H, Smiley A: Effects of chronically administered buspirone and diazepam on driving-related skills performance. J Clin Psychiatry 43:45–56, 1982.

Munetz MR, Benjamin S: How to examine patients using the abnormal involuntary movement scale. Hosp Commun Psychiatry 39:1172–1177, 1988.

Munjack DJ, Baltazar PL, Bohn PB, et al: Clonazepam in the treatment of social phobia: a pilot study. J Clin Psychiatry 51(suppl):35–40, 1990.

Munjack DJ, Crocker B, Cabe D, et al: Alprazolam, propranolol, and placebo in the treatment of panic disorder and agoraphobia with panic attacks. J Clin Psychopharmacol 9:22–27, 1989.

Murphy DL, Mueller EA, Garrick NA, et al: Use of serotonergic agents in the clinical assessment of central serotonin function. J Clin Psychiatry 47:9–15, 1987.

Murphy DL, Zohar J, Benkelfat C, et al: Obsessive-compulsive disorder as a serotonin subsystem-related behavioral disorder. Br J Psychiatry 155(suppl 8):15–24, 1989.

Murphy SM, Owen R, Tyrer P: Comparative assessment of efficacy and withdrawal symptoms after 6 and 12 weeks' treatment with diazepam or buspirone. Br J Psychiatry 154:529–534, 1989.

Nair NPV, Suranyi-Cadotte B, Schwartz G, et al: A clinical trial comparing intramuscular haloperidol decanoate and oral haloperidol in chronic schizophrenic patients: Efficacy, safety, and dosage equivalence. J Clin Psychopharmacol 6(suppl):30–37, 1986.

Nayak RK, Doose DR, Nair NPV: The bioavailability and pharmacokinetics of oral and depot intramuscular haloperidol in schizophrenic patients. J Clin Pharmacol 27:144–150, 1987.

Newton RE, Casten GP, Alms DR, et al: The side effect profile of buspirone in comparison to active controls and placebo. J Clin Psychiatry 43:100–102, 1982.

Nies A: Differential response patterns to MAO inhibitors and tricyclics. J Clin Psychiatry 45(sec. 2):70–77, 1984.

Noll KM, Davis JM, DeLeon-Jones F: Medical and somatic therapies in the treatment of depression. In Beckham EE, Leber WR (eds): Handbook of Depression. Homewood, IL, Dorsey Press, 1985, pp 184–203.

Noyes R Jr, Garvey MJ, Cook BL, et al: Problems with tricyclic antidepressant use in patients with panic disorder or agoraphobia: Results of a naturalistic follow-up study. J Clin Psychiatry 50:163–169, 1989.

Noyes R, Anderson D, Clancy J: Diazepam and propranolol in panic disorder and agoraphobia. Arch Gen Psychiatry 41:287–292, 1984.

Noyes R, Chaudry DR, Domingo DV: Pharmacologic treatment of phobic disorders. J Clin Psychiatry 47:445–452, 1986.

Noyes R, Garvey MJ, Cook BL, et al: Problems with tricyclic antidepressant use in patients with panic disorder or agoraphobia: Results of a naturalistic follow-up study. J Clin Psychiatry 50:163–169, 1989.

O'Brien RA, Young GB: Neuroleptic malignant syndrome: A review. Can Fam Physician 35:1119–1122, 1989.

Okuma T, Inanga K, Otsuki S, et al: Comparison of the antimanic efficacy of carbamazepine and chlorpromazine: A double-blind controlled study. Psychopharmacology 66:211–217, 1979.

Okuma T, Yamashita I, Takahashi R et al: Comparison of the antimanic efficacy of carbamazepine and lithium carbonate by double-blind controlled study. Pharmacopsychiatry 23:143–150, 1990.

Ortiz A, Gershon S: The future of neuroleptic psychopharmacology. J Clin Psychiatry 47(suppl):3–11, 1986.

Overall JE: Prior psychiatric treatment and the development of breast cancer. Arch Gen Psychiatry 35:898–899, 1978.

Parent MM, Roy S, Sramek J, et al: Effect of molindone on weight change in hospitalized schizophrenic patients. Drug Intell Clin Pharmacol 20:873–875, 1986.

Pasternak R-E, Reynolds CF, Schlernitzauer M, et al: Acute open-trial nortriptyline therapy of bereavement-related depression in late life. J Clin Psychiatry 52:307–310, 1991.

Pato MT, Zohar J: Clomipramine in the treatment of obsessive-compulsive disorder. In Pato MT, Zohar J (eds): Current Treatments of Obsessive-Compulsive Disorder. Washington, American Psychiatric Press, 1991, pp 13–28.

Pato MT, Zohar-Kadouch R, Zohar J, et al: Return of symptoms after discontinuation of clomipramine in patients with obsessive-compulsive disorder. Am J Psychiatry 145:1521–1525, 1988.

Patterson JF: A preliminary study of carbamazepine in the treatment of assaultive patients with dementia. J Geriatr Psychiatry Neurol 1:21–23, 1988.

Patterson JF: Carbamazepine for assaultive patients with organic brain disease. Psychosomatics 28:579–581, 1987.

Pecknold JC, Swinson RP, Kuch K, et al: Alprazolam in panic disorder and agoraphobia: Results from a multicenter trial. Arch Gen Psychiatry 45:429–436, 1988.

Perry PJ, Alexander B: Sedative/hypnotic dependence: Patient stabilization, tolerance testing, and withdrawal. Drug Intell Clin Pharmacol 20:532–537, 1986.

Perry PJ, Alexander B, Liskow BI: Psychotropic Drug Handbook, 6th ed. Cincinnati, Whitney Books, 1991.

Perry PJ, Alexander B, Prince RA, et al: A single point dosing protocol for predicting steady state lithium levels. Br J Psychiatry 148:401–405, 1986.

Perry PJ, Garvey M, Noyes R: Benzodiazepine treatment of generalized anxiety disorder. In Noyes R, Roth M, Burrows GD (eds): Handbook of Anxiety: Treatment of Anxiety, vol 4. Amsterdam, Elsevier, 1990, pp 111–124.

Perry PJ, Pfohl BM, Holstad SG: The relationship between antidepressant response and tricyclic antidepressant plasma concentrations: A retrospective analysis of the literature using logistic regression analysis. Clin Pharmacokinet 13:381–392, 1987.

Perry PJ, Browne JL, Alexander B, et al: Two prospective dosing methods for nortriptyline. Clin Pharmacokinet 9:555–563, 1984.

Perse TL. Greist JH, Jefferson JW, et al: Fluvoxamine treatment of obsessive-compulsive disorder. Am J Psychiatry 144: 1543–1548, 1988.

Pigott TA: Fluoxetine in the treatment of obessive-compulsive disorder. In Pato MT, Zohar J (eds): Current Treatments of Obsessive-Compulsive Disorder. Washington, American Psychiatric Press, 1991, pp 29–44.

Placidi GF, Lenzi A, Lazzerini F, et al: The comparative efficacy and safety of carbamazepine versus lithium: A randomized, double-blind 3-year trial in 83 patients. J Clin Psychiatry 47:490–494, 1986.

Pohl R, Balon R, Yeragani VK, et al: Serotonergic anxiolytics in the treatment of panic disorder: A controlled study with buspirone. Psychopathology 2(suppl):S60–S67, 1989.

Pohl R, Yeragani VK, Balon R, et al: The jitteriness syndrome in panic disorder patients treated with antidepressants. J Clin Psychiatry 49:100–104, 1988.

Pollack MH: Long-term management of panic disorder. J Clin Psychiatry 51(suppl):11–13, 1990.

Pope HG Jr, Hudson JI, Jonas JM, et al: Bulimia treated with imipramine: A placebo-controlled, double-blind study. Am J Psychiatry 140:554–558, 1983.

Pope HG, Hudson J, Yurgium-Todd D: Anorexia nervosa and bulimia among 300 women shoppers. Am J Psychiatry 141:292–294, 1984.

Pope HG, Keck PE Jr, McElroy SM, Hudson JI: A placebo-controlled, study of trazodone in bulimia nervosa. J Clin Psychopharmacol 9:254–259, 1989.

Pope HG, McElroy SL, Keck PE, et al: Valproate in the treatment of acute mania: A placebo-controlled study. Arch Gen Psychiatry 48:62–68, 1991.

Post RM: Time course of clinical effects of carbamazepine: Implications for mechanisms of action. J Clin Psychiatry 49 (suppl):35–46, 1988.

Post RM, Berrettini W, Uhde TW, et al: Selective response to the anticonvulsant carbamazepine in manic-depressive illness: a case study. J Clin Psychopharmacol 14:178–185, 1984.

Post RM, Uhde TW: Carbamazepine in bipolar illness. Psychopharmacol Bull 21:10–17, 1985.

Price LH, Goodman WK, Charney DS, et al: Treatment of severe obsessive-compulsive disorder with fluvoxamine. Am J Psychiatry 144:1059–1061, 1987.

Prien RF, Caffey EM, Klett CJ: Relationship between serum lithium level and clinical response in acute mania treated with lithium. Br J Psychiatry 120:409–414, 1971.

Prien RF, Klett CJ, Caffey EM: Lithium carbonate and imipramine in prevention of affective episodes: A comparison in recurrent affective illness. Arch Gen Psychiatry 29:420–425, 1973.

Prien RF, Kupfer DJ: Continuation drug therapy for major depressive episodes: How long should it be maintained? Am J Psychiatry 143:18–23, 1986.

Primeau F, Fontaine R, Beauclair L: Valproic acid and panic disorder. Can J Psychiatry 35:248–250, 1990.

Rabkin J, Quitkin F, Harrison W, et al: Adverse reactions to monoamine oxidase inhibitors: I. A comparative study. J Clin Psychopharmacol 4:270–278, 1984.

Rachman SJ, Hodgson RJ: Obsessions and Compulsions. Englewood-Cliffs, NJ, Prentice-Hall, 1980.

Rall TW: Hypnotics and sedatives: Ethanol. In Gilman AG, Rall TW, Nies AS, Taylor P (eds): Goodman and Gilman's The Pharmacological Basis of Therapeutics, 8th ed. New York, Pergamon Press, 1990a, pp 366–367.

Rall TW: Hypnotics and sedatives: Ethanol. In Gilman AG, Rall TW, Nies AS, Taylor P (eds): Goodman and Gilman's The Pharmacological Basis of Therapeutics, 8th ed. New York, Pergamon Press, 1990b, pp 358–365.

Raskind MA, Risse SC: Antipsychotic drugs and the elderly. J Clin Psychiatry 47(suppl):17–22, 1986.

Reidenberg MM, Levy M, Warner H, et al: Relationship between diazepam dose, plasma level, age, and central nervous system depression. Clin Pharmacol Ther 23:371–374, 1978.

Remington G: Pharmacotherapy of schizophrenia. Can J Psychiatry 34:211–216, 1989 (erratum 34:457–461).

Rhoades HM, Overall JE: Side effect potentials of different antipsychotic and antidepressant drugs. Psychopharmacol Bull 20:83–88, 1984.

Richelson E, Nelson A: Antagonism by antidepressants of neurotransmitter receptors of normal human brain in vitro. J Pharmacol Exp Ther 230:94–102, 1984.

Rickels K, Case G, Downing RW, et al: Long-term diazepam therapy and clinical outcome. JAMA 250:767–771, 1983.

Rickels K, Schweizer E, Csanalosi I, et al: Long-term treatment of anxiety and risk of withdrawal: Prospective comparison of clorazepate and buspirone. Arch Gen Psychiatry 45:444–450, 1988.

Rosenberg MR, Green M: Neuroleptic malignant syndrome. Arch Intern Med 149:1927–1931, 1989.

Sabine EJ, Yonace A. Farrington AJ, et al: Bulimia nervosa: A placebo-controlled double-blind therapeutic trial of mianserin. Br J Clin Pharmacol 15:195S–202S, 1983.

Satel SL, Nelson JC: Stimulants in the treatment of depression: A critical overview. J Clin Psychiatry 50:241–249, 1989.

Schweizer E, Fox I, Case G, et al: Lorazepam vs alprazolam in the treatment of panic disorder. Psychopharmacol Bull 24:224–227, 1988.

Schweizer E, Rickels K, Lucki I: Resistance to the anti-anxiety effect of buspirone in patients with a history of benzodiazepine use (letter). N Engl J Med 314:719–720, 1986.

Segraves RT: Effects of psychotropic drugs on human erection and ejaculation. Arch Gen Psychiatry 46:275–284, 1989.

Seppala T, Aranko K, Matilla MJ, et al: Effects of alcohol on buspirone and lorazepam actions. Clin Pharmacol Ther 32:201–207, 1982.

Seppala T, Kortilla K, Hakkinen S, et al: Residual effects and skills related to driving after a single oral administration of diazepam, medazepam or lorazepam. Br J Clin Pharmacol 3:831–841, 1976.

Shader RI, DiMascio A (eds): Psychotropic Drug Side Effects: Clinical and Theoretical Perspectives. Baltimore, Williams & Wilkins, 1970, pp 4–9, 63–85, 92–106, 116–123, 149–174, 175–198.

Shalev A, Hermesh H, Munitz H: Mortality from neuroleptic malignant syndrome. J Clin Psychiatry 50:18–25, 1989.

Shapiro AK, Stuening EL, Shapiro E, et al: Diazepam: how much better than placebo? J Psychiatr Res 17:51–73, 1983.

Shebak S, Cameron A, Levander S: Clonazepam and imipramine in the treatment of panic attacks: A double-blind comparison of efficacy and side effects. J Clin Psychiatry 51 (suppl)14–17, 1990.

Sheehan DV: Current views in the treatment of panic attacks and phobias. Drug Ther 12:179–187, 1982.

Sheehan DV: Is buspirone effective in the treatment of panic disorder? Presented at the New Clinical Drug Evaluation Unit annual meeting, Key Biscayne, FL, May 28, 1987.

Sheehan DV, Coleman JH, Greenblatt DJ, et al: Some biochemical correlates of panic attacks with agoraphobia and their response to a new treatment. J Clin Psychopharmacol 4:66–75, 1984.

Sheehan DV, Davidson J, Manschreck T, et al: Lack of efficacy of a new antidepressant (bupropion) in the treatment of panic disorder with phobias. J Clin Psychopharmacol 3:28–31, 1983.

Shenoy RS, Sadler AG, Goldberg SC, et al: Effects of a six-week drug holiday on symptom status, relapse, and tardive dyskinesia in chronic schizophrenics. J Clin Psychopharmacol 1:141–145, 1981.

Shuckit MA: Current therapeutic options in the management of typical anxiety. J Clin Psychiatry 142(sec 2):15–26, 1981.

Simpson GM, Pi EH, Sramek JJ: Adverse effects of antipsychotic agents. Drugs 21:138–151, 1981.

Small JC, Klapper MH, Milstein V, et al: Carbamazepine compared with lithium in the treatment of mania. Arch Gen Psychiatry 48:915–921, 1991.

Sobotka JL, Alexander B, Cook BL: A review of carbamazepine's hematologic reactions and monitoring recommendations. DICP Ann Pharmacother 24:1214–1219, 1990.

Solyom L, DiNicola VF, Phil M, et al: Is there an obsessive psychosis? Aetiological and prognostic factors of an atypical form of obsessive-compulsive neurosis. Can J Psychiatry 30:372–380, 1985.

Sovner R, DiMascio A: Extrapyramidal syndromes and other neurological side effects of psychotropic drugs. In Lipton MA, DiMascio A, Killam KF (eds): Psychopharmacology: A Generation of Progress. New York, Raven Press, 1021–1032, 1978.

Spier SA, Tesar GE, Rosenbaum JF, et al: Treatment of panic disorder and agoraphobia with clonazepam. J Clin Psychiatry 47:238–242, 1986.

Spiker DG, Dealy RS, Hanin I, et al: Treating delusional depressives with amitriptyline. J Clin Psychiatry 147:243–246, 1986.

Spiker DG, Weiss JC, Dealy RS, et al: The pharmacological treatment of delusional depression. Am J Psychiatry 142:430–436, 1985.

Steketee G, Tynes LL: Behavioral treatment of obsessive-compulsive disorder. In Pato MT, Zohar J (eds): Current Treatments of Obsessive-Compulsive Disorder. Washington, American Psychiatric Press, 1991, pp 61–86.

Stewart JW, Harrison W, Ouitkin F, et al: Phenelzine-induce pyridosine deficiency. J Clin Psychopharmacol 4:225–226, 1984.

Stromgren LSM, Boller S: Carbamazepine in treatment and prophylaxis of manic-depressive disorder. Psychiatr Dev 4:349–367, 1985.

Stuppaeck C, Barnas C, Miller C, et al: Carbamazepine in the prophylaxis of mood disorders. J Clin Psychopharmacol 10:39–42, 1990.

Susman VL, Addonizio G: Recurrence of neuroleptic malignant syndrome. J Nerv Ment Dis 176:234–240, 1988.

Tandon R, Greden JF: Cholinergic hyperactivity and negative schizophrenic symptoms. Arch Gen Psychiatry 46:745–753, 1989.

Taylor CB, Hayward C, King R, et al: Cardiovascular and symptomatic reduction effects of alprazolam and imipramine in patients with panic disorder: Results of a double-blind, placebo-controlled trial. J Clin Psychopharmacol 10:112–118, 1990.

Tesar GE, Rosenbaum JF, Pollack MH, et al: Clonazepam versus alprazolam in the treatment of panic disorder: interim analysis of data from a prospective, double-blind, placebo-controlled trial. J Clin Psychiatry 48(suppl):S16–S19, 1987.

Thompson TL, Moran MG, Nies AS: Drug therapy: Psychotropic drug use in the elderly (first of two parts). N Engl J Med 308:134–138, 1983.

Thompson TL, Filley CM, Mitchell WD, et al: Lack of efficacy of hydergin in patients with Alzheimer's disease. N Engl J Med 323:445–448, 1990.

Thoren P, Asberg M, Bertilsson L, et al: Clomipramine treatment of obsessive-compulsive disorder: II. Biochemical aspects. Arch Gen Psychiatry 37:1289–1294, 1980a.

Thoren P, Asberg M, Cronholm B, et al: Clomipramine treatment of obsessive-compulsive disorder: I. A controlled clinical trial. Arch Gen Psychiatry 37:1281–1285, 1980b.

Thornhill DP, Field SP: Distribution of lithium elimination rates in a selected population of psychiatric patients. Eur J Clin Pharmacol 21:351–354, 1982.

Turner SM, Jacob RG, Beidel DC, et al: Fluoxetine treatment of obsessive-compulsive disorder. J Clin Psychopharmacol 5:207–212, 1985.

Uhde TW, Stein MB, Post RM: Lack of efficacy of carbamazepine in the treatment of panic disorder. Am J Psychiatry 145:1104–1109, 1988.

Vallejo J, Gasto C, Salamero M: Double-blind study of imipramine versus phenelzine in melancholias and dysthymic disorders. Br J Psychiatry 1151:639–642, 1987.

Van Pragg HM, Dols LCW: Fluphenazine enanthate and decanoate: A comparison of their duration of action and motor side effects. Am J Psychiatry 130:801–804, 1973.

Van Putten T, May PRA, Marder SA: Akathisia with haloperidol and thiothixene. Arch Gen Psychiatry 41:1036–1039, 1984.

Vandereycken W: Neuroleptics in the short-term treatment of anorexia nervosa: A double-blind placebo-controlled study with sulpiride. Br J Psychiatry 144:288–292, 1984.

Vandereycken W, Pierloot R: Pimozide combined with behavioral therapy in the short-term treatment of anorexia nervosa. Acta Psychiatr Scand 66:445–450, 1982.

Vestergaard P, Amdisen A, Schou M: Clinically significant side effects of lithium treatment: A survey of 237 patients in long-term treatment. Acta Psychiatr Scand 162:193–200, 1980.

Vigersky RA, Loriaux DL: The effect of cyproheptadine in anorexia nervosa: A double blind trial. In Vigersky RA (ed): Anorexia Nervosa. New York, Raven Press, 1977, pp 349–356.

Volger BW: Alternatives in the treatment of memory loss in patients with Alzheimer's disease. Clin Pharm 10:447–456, 1991.

Walsh BT, Gladis M, Roose SP, et al: Phenelzine vs placebo in 50 patients with bulimia. Arch Gen Psychiatry 45:471–475, 1984.

Walter CJS, Mitchell-Heggs N, Sargant W: Modified narcosis, ECT, and antidepressant drugs: A review of technique and immediate outcome. Br J Psychiatry 120:651–662, 1972.

Wells AJ, Sommi RW, Crismon ML: Neuroleptic rechallenge after neuroleptic malignant syndrome: Case report and literature review. Drug Intell Clin Pharm 22:475–479, 1988.

Wermuth BM, David KL, Hollister LE, et al: Phenytoin treatment of the binge eating syndrome. Am J Psychiatry 134:1249–1254, 1977.

Whalley LJ: Drug treatment of dementia. Br J Psychiatry 155:595–611, 1989.

Wirshing WC, Freidenberg DL, Cummings JL, et al: Effects of anticholinergic agents on patients with tardive dyskinesia and concomitant drug-induced parkinsonism. J Clin Psychopharmacol 9:407–411, 1989.

Wistedt B, Persson T, Hellborn E: A clinical double-blind comparison between haloperidol decanoate and fluphenazine decanoate. Curr Ther Res 53:804–814, 1984.

Wistedt B, Wiles DH, Kolakowska T: Slow decline of plasma drug and prolactin levels after discontinuation of chronic treatment with depot neuroleptics (letter). Lancet: Vol. 1 1163, 1981.

Yadalam KG, Simpson GM: Changing from oral to depot fluphenazine. J Clin Psychiatry 49:346–348, 1988.

Young LY, Riddiough MA: Essential hypertension. In Koda-Kimble MA, Katcher BS, Young LY (eds): Applied Therapeutics for Clinical Pharmacists, 2d ed. San Francisco, Applied Therapeutics, 1978, pp 146–147, 240–242.

Zito J, Sofair JB, Jaeger J: Self-reported neuroendocrine effects of antipsychotics in women: A pilot study. DICP Ann Pharmacother 24:176–180, 1990.

Zitrin CM, Klein DF, Woerner MG, et al: Treatment of phobia: I. Comparison of imipramine hydrochloride and placebo. Arch Gen Psychiatry 40:125–138, 1983.

Zohar J, Insel TR: Drug treatment of obsessive-compulsive disorder. J Affective Disord 13:193–202, 1987a.

Zohar J, Insel TR: Obsessive-compulsive disorder: Psychobiologic approaches to diagnosis, treatment, and pathophysiology. Biol Psychiatry 22:667–687, 1987b.

Zohar J, Mueller EA, Insel TR, et al: Serotonergic responsivity in obsessive-compulsive disorder: comparison of patients and healthy controls. Arch Gen Psychiatry 44:946–951, 1987c.

Index

Page numbers followed by f represent figures; those followed by t represent tables.

Acceleration, psychomotor, 7
Acetylcholine, metabolism of, 448–449
  neurons containing, 448
  storage, release, and uptake of, 449
Acute immunodeficiency syndrome (AIDS), psychiatric
  manifestations of, 501
Acute intermittent porphyria (AIP), 177
  psychiatric manifestations of, 501
ADD. See *Attention deficit disorder (ADD).*
Addison's disease, psychiatric manifestations of,
  498–499
ADHD. See *Attention deficit disorder (ADD).*
Adjustment disorder, case history of, 274
  clinical picture of, 273–274
  course of, 274–275
  defined, 273, 274t
  differential diagnosis of, 275–276
  epidemiology of, 273, 274t
  etiology of, 275
  prevalence of, 274t
  treatment of, 276
Adolescence, depression in, 301, 305–306, 305t, 308
  illness in, epidemiology of, 518–519
  suicide attempts in, 310–312
  suicide in, 309–310, 535
Adoption studies, 460–461
  of alcoholism, 229, 231
  of antisocial personality, 205–206
  of bipolar illness, 49–50
  of personality disorders, 430
  of schizophrenia, 97–98
  of suicide incidence, 536
Adrenaline, structure of, 444f
Adrenocortical insufficiency, psychiatric manifestations
  of, 498–499
Affect, as indicator of mental status, 8
  defined, 89, 365
  disturbances of, 13–14
Affective delusions, 10
Affective disorders, adoption studies of, 464–465
  biologic markers for, 467, 482t

Affective disorder *Continued*
  distinguished from Briquet's syndrome, 178
  distinguished from delusional disorders, 136
  distinguished from disruptive behavior disorders in
    children, 292
  etiologic markers for, 467–468
  family studies of, 464t, 465, 466t
  in children and adolescents, 312, 317
    clinical picture of, 305–306, 305t
    course of, 306
    defined, 302–303
    differential diagnosis of, 308
    epidemiology of, 304–305
    etiology of, 303–304, 303t
    failed suicide in, 310–312
    laboratory findings in, 306–308, 307t
    suicide in, 309–310
  laboratory findings in, 497, 504–505, 506
  mode of transmission of, 465–466, 466t
  motor abnormalities in, 419
  neurobiology of, 451–453
  spectrum disorders of, 482t
  suicide in, 533, 537, 539
  twin studies of, 463–464, 463t
Affective incontinence, 13
Age, as demographic factor, 523–524
Agitation, psychomotor, 7
Agoraphobia, 142, 381. See also *Panic disorder.*
  childhood trauma and, 522
  family studies of, 479
  panic attacks in, 389, 390
AIDS (acute immunodeficiency syndrome), psychiatric
  manifestations of, 501
AIP (acute intermittent porphyria), 177
  psychiatric manifestations of, 501
Akathisia, 422, 550
  as side effect of neuroleptics, 106
Alanine aminotransferase (ALT) values, in alcoholism,
  225
Alcohol abuse. See also *Alcoholism.*
  compared with steroid misuse, 282–284, 282t
  distinguished from bipolar illness, 59

Alcohol abuse *Continued*
    in antisocial personality, 205–206, 210–211, 212t,
        214, 216
    induced depression in, 79
    relapse rate for, 249t
    trauma and, 522
Alcohol withdrawal, generalized anxiety disorder in,
    147
Alcoholism. See also *Alcohol abuse.*
    adoption studies of, 474–475
    anxiety disorders and, 387
    biologic markers for, 476–477, 482t
    case study of, 224–225
    causing dementia, 25, 26t
    clinical picture of, 223–224
    coupled with thiamine deficiency, causing amnestic
        syndrome, 39, 41, 42, 44
    course of, 226–228
    defined, 219–220
    differential diagnosis of, 228–229
    distinguished from schizophrenia, 93
    epidemiology of, 220–223
    etiologic markers for, 477
    etiology of, 229–231
    family studies of, 475–476
    in childhood affective disorders, 309
    laboratory findings in, 225–226
    mode of transmission of, 476
    morbidity and mortality associated with, 221, 228
    spectrum of, 476
    suicide in, 537–538, 538t
    treatment of, 231–233
    twin studies of, 474
    types of, 230
Alexithymia, 187
Aluminum toxicity, 23
Alzheimer's disease, causing amnestic syndrome,
    39, 41
    clinical picture of, 27
    course of, 27–28
    defined, 22
    dementia in, 404
    diagnosis of, 25t
    differential diagnosis of, 28–29
    distinguished from delirium, 21–22
    epidemiology of, 24, 26t
    etiology and pathogenesis of, 23
    hereditary, 23
    laboratory findings in, 28
    neurobiology of, 453–454
    pathology of, 25
    sexual dysfunction and, 255
    treatment of, 29, treatment of, 581
Amenorrhea, in anorexia nervosa, 197
Amino acids, as neurotransmitters, 449–450
Amnesia, anterograde, 39, 42
    of psychogenic origin, 44
    retrograde, 39, 42
Amnestic syndrome, case study of, 43–44
    clinical picture of, 41–44
    defined, 39
    differential diagnosis of, 44–45
    etiology and pathogenesis of, 39
    laboratory findings in, 44
    pathology of, 39–41, 41f
    treatment of, 45
Amok, 284t
Amoxapine, 560, 561

Amphetamine abuse, anxiety as symptom of, 386
    distinguished from schizophrenia, 93
    pathology of, 242
Amphetamine crash, distinguished from schizoaffective
    disorder, 124
Amyl nitrate intoxication, anxiety as symptom of, 386
Anabolic steroid misuse, addiction hypothesis of, 282
    epidemiology of, 280
    psychiatric effects of, 280–282
Anaclitic depression, 301
Anergy, physical, as symptom of schizophrenia, 89
Anger, defined, 8
Angina pectoris, anxiety as symptom of, 382–383
    distinguished from anxiety disorders, 143
Anhedonia, 13
    in depressive syndrome, 367
Animal phobia, 150
Anorexia nervosa, clinical picture of, 195–196
    compared with bulimia, 194t, 198, 201
    course of, 196
    differential diagnosis of, 198
    drug treatment of, 579–580
    epidemiology of, 195
    etiology and pathogenesis of, 193–195
    family studies of, 466–467
    in depression, 308
    laboratory findings in, 505
    medical complications of, 197–198, 197t
    treatment of, 198–199
Anoxemia, cerebral, causing amnestic syndrome, 39
Anterograde amnesia, 39, 42
Antiaggression drugs, 582
Antidepressants, 82–83. See also *Monoamine oxidase
    (MAO) inhibitors; Second-generation antidepressants;
    Tricyclic antidepressants.*
    pediatric use of, 314t–316t
Antipsychotics, adverse effects of, 548–552
    dosages of, 546–548
    efficacy of, 543–546
Antisocial personality, adoption studies of, 478
    biologic markers for, 478–479, 482t
    clinical picture of, 206–212, 210t
    course of, 212–213
    defined, 205
    diagnostic criteria for, 207t
    differential diagnosis of, 213–214
    distinguished from bipolar illness, 59
    distinguished from Briquet's syndrome, 179
    epidemiology of, 206
    etiology of, 205–206, 206t
    family studies of, 478
    in adolescents, 205, 207–208, 208t
    in adults, 208–209, 209t
    mode of transmission of, 478
    somatic symptoms of, 211t
    spectrum disorders of, 482t
    treatment of, 214–216
    twin studies of, 477
Antisocial personality disorder, 426
Anxiety, 381
    defined, 8
    distinguished from depressive syndrome, 371–372,
        372t
    organic syndromes of, 382
    physical conditions causing, 382–387, 382t
    psychological conditions causing, 387–390
Anxiety attacks, 71
Anxiety disorders. See also *Panic disorder.*
    agoraphobia, 142

Anxiety disorders *Continued*
   childhood trauma and, 522
   distinguished from adjustment disorder, 275
   distinguished from antisocial personality, 213
   distinguished from Briquet's syndrome, 178
   distinguished from disruptive behavior disorders in
     children, 292
   drug treatment of, 568–577
   due to medical conditions, 31
   etiology of, 521
   family studies of, 479
   generalized, 144–148. See also *Generalized anxiety
     disorder.*
   in brain disease, 413–414
   laboratory findings in, 497
   motor abnormalities in, 419
   neurobiology of, 457–458
   of childhood, clinical picture of, 351–352
     defined, 349
     differential diagnosis of, 356
     epidemiology of, 351
     etiology of, 350
     outcome of, 352
     treatment of, 357–359
   personality disorders coexisting with, 428–429
Anxiety symptom management, 147
Aphasia, defined, 8–9
   jargon, 397
   Wernicke's, 397
Appearance, as indicator of mental status, 6–7
Appetite, in depressive syndrome, 368
Arguing voices, as symptom of schizophrenia, 88
Arousal, disorders of, 20
Aspartate aminotransferase (AST) values, in alcohol-
   ism, 225
Asperger syndrome, 334–335
Assistance, delusions of, 10
Association(s), loose, 14
   as symptom of schizophrenia, 89
Association studies, 467, 472, 483
Asthenia, neurocirculatory, 283t
Asthma, anxiety as symptom of, 384–385
Attention deficit disorder (ADD), clinical picture
   of, 290
   course and outcome of, 295–296
   differential diagnosis of, 292–293
   distinguished from depression and hypomania, 308
   epidemiology of, 293
   etiology of, 294
   motor abnormalities in, 419–420
   speech and language disorders in, 291
   treatment of, 297–298
Attention deficit hyperactivity disorder (ADHD). See
   Attention deficit disorder (ADD).
Attention span, disturbances of, 20
   indicating mental status, 12
Attitude, as indicator of mental status, 7
Atypical autism, 334
Atypical depression, 372
Atypical paraphilia, course of, 265t
   diagnosis of, 263t
Audible thoughts, as symptom of schizophrenia, 88
Auditory hallucinations, 10
Autism. See also *Autistic disorder.*
   atypical, 334
   Bleuler's definition of, 8
Autistic disorder, biochemical factors in, 327–329
   clinical features of, 331–334
   course and prognosis of, 334

Autistic disorder *Continued*
   defined, 321
   diagnostic criteria for, 322–323
   differential diagnosis of, 334–336
   distinguished from disruptive behavior disorders in
     children, 292
   distinguished from schizophrenia, 337–338, 342
   epidemiology of, 330–331, 330t
   etiology of, 323–330
   genetic factors in, 324–325
   immunologic factors in, 329
   neuroanatomic factors in, 326–327
   neurologic aspects of, 326
   neurophysiologic factors in, 327
   obstetric factors in, 325–326
   prevalence of, 330, 330t
   psychogenic factors in, 323
   treatment of, 338–340
Autoscopy, 11
Aversion, sexual, 254t
Avoidant disorder, clinical picture of, 353–354
   defined, 349
   differential diagnosis of, 356
   epidemiology of, 351
   etiology of, 350
   outcome of, 354
   treatment of, 357–359
Avoidant personality disorder, 426
   social phobia in, 152
Awareness, disturbances of, 20
Azaspirodecanediones, 573

Barbiturates, adverse effects of, 574–575
   dosages of, 574
   efficacy of, 573–574
Basal ganglia, calcification of, motor abnormalities
   in, 421
BEAM (brain electrical activity mapping), 508
Behavior, as indicator of mental status, 6–7
   overt, recording of, 5
Behavioral family therapy, for schizophrenia, 108
Behavioral therapy, for schizophrenia, 108
Belle indifférence, 14
Benzodiazepine receptors, 238
Benzodiazepines, adverse effects of, 570–572
   dosages of, 569–570
   efficacy of, 568–569
   motoric side effects of, 422–423
   pediatric use of, 359
   withdrawal from, anxiety as symptom of, 386
     obsessive-compulsive neurosis in, 162
Beta-adrenergic blockers, 575–576
Binge-eating disorder, 201
Biological markers, studies of, 462–463
Bipolar disorder. See also *Cyclothymia.*
   biochemistry of, 50–51
   case study of, 55–56
   clinical picture of, 54–56
   complications of, 57–58
   course of, 56–57
   defined, 47–48, 365
   depression in, 55
   differential diagnosis of, 58–59
   distinguished from disruptive behavior disorders in
     children, 292
   distinguished from schizophrenia, 374–375, 374t
   electrophysiologic factors of, 51–52
   epidemiology of, 53
   etiology of, 48–53

Bipolar disorder *Continued*
  genetics of, 48–50
  in adolescents, 306
  in brain disease, 412
  in children, 306
    distinguished from disruptive behavior disorders,
      292
  mania in, 52–53, 55
  risk factors for, 53–54
  treatment of, 59–63
Bipolar II disorder, 376
  defined, 366
Bipolar III disorder, 376
Birth, season of, as demographic factor, 526
Blepharospasm, 420
Blindness, peripheral, distinguished from autistic
  disorder, 336
Blocking, 396
  as symptom of schizophrenia, 89
Blood alcohol level values, in alcoholism, 225
Blood phobia, 150
Blunted affect, 13
  as symptom of schizophrenia, 89
Blunting, defined, 8
Body dysmorphic disorder, distinguished from
  obsessive-compulsive neurosis, 165
Borderline personality disorder, 426
  childhood trauma and, 522
  distinguished from bipolar illness, 59
  distinguished from factitious disorder, 278–279
  distinguished from schizophrenia, 94
  etiology of, 429, 431
Brain, anatomy of, 439–441, 440f
  imaging of, 507–508
  trauma to, depression in, 406
Brain electrical activity mapping (BEAM), 508
Brief reactive psychosis, distinguished from schizophrenia, 94
Briquet's syndrome, clinical picture of, 176–177
  course of, 177
  defined, 169–172
  differential diagnosis of, 170t, 177–178
  epidemiology of, 174–176
  etiology of, 172, 173t, 174
  laboratory findings in, 177
  symptoms of, 170t
  treatment of, 179–181
Broadcasting, thought, as symptom of schizophrenia, 88
  defined, 9
Brucellosis, distinguished from Briquet's syndrome, 178
Bulimia nervosa, clinical picture of, 200
  compared with anorexia, 194t, 198, 201
  course of, 200
  defined, 199
  differential diagnosis of, 201
  drug treatment of, 580–581, 580t
  epidemiology of, 199
  etiology and pathogenesis of, 199
  laxative abuse in, 200
  medical complications of, 197t, 200–201
  treatment of, 201
Bupropion, 560, 561, 562
Buspirone, adverse effects of, 574
  dosages of, 574
  efficacy of, 573–574

Caffeine, abuse of, pathology of, 243
  intoxication, anxiety as symptom of, 385
  generalized anxiety disorder in, 147

Cannabis, abuse of, 238
  pathology of, 242
  intoxication, anxiety as symptom of, 386
Capgras delusion, 283t
Carbamazepine (CBZ), 566–567
  therapeutic monitoring of, 502
Cardiac diseases, anxiety as symptom of, 382
Cardiac dysrhythmias, anxiety as symptom of,
  383–384
Catalepsy, 7
Catatonia, 418–419
  differential diagnosis of, 419t
  evaluation of, 124
  symptoms of, 419t
Catatonic excitement, as symptom of schizophrenia, 89
Catatonic schizophrenia, distinguished from bipolar
  illness, 59
Catatonic stupor, in schizophrenia, 90
Catecholamines, structure of, 444f
CBZ (carbamazepine), 566–567
  therapeutic monitoring of, 502
CD. See *Conduct disorder (CD)*.
Central nervous system, cytology of, 441–442
  focal lesions of, motor abnormalities in, 421–422
  tumors of, causing dementia, 25, 26t
Cerebral anoxemia, causing amnestic syndrome, 39
Cerebral infarcts, 23
  causing amnestic syndrome, 39, 40
CET (computerized electroencephalographic topog-
  raphy), 508
Chagas' disease, distinguished from Briquet's syn-
  drome, 178
Childhood autism. See *Autistic disorder*.
Childhood schizophrenia, distinguished from schizo-
  phrenia in childhood, 340
Children. See also under names of individual diseases.
  anxiety disorders of, 349–359
  illness in, epidemiology of, 518–519
Cholinergic agonists, 581–582
Cholinergic REM induction, 468
Chronic idiopathic pain. See *Psychogenic pain*.
Chronic systemic disorders, causing psychiatric condi-
  tions, 501
Circular insanity. See *Bipolar illness*.
Circumstantiality, defined, 8
Clang association, defined, 8
Clanging, 398
Classic conditioning, prepared, 149
Claustrophobia, 150
Clerambault's delusion, 283t
Clomipramine, 577–578
Clozapine, adverse effects of, 553–554
  efficacy of, 552–553
Cocaine, abuse of, anxiety as symptom of, 386
  compared with steroid misuse, 282t
  pathology of, 242
  intoxication with, obsessive-compulsive neurosis in,
    162
Cognitive behavioral therapy, 154, 267–268
Cognitive impairment disorders, as proposed classifi-
  cation, 17
Combined systemic disease, anxiety as symptom of,
  385
Commenting voices, as symptom of schizophrenia, 88
Compulsion, defined, 9, 161
Computed tomography (CT), 507
Computerized electroencephalographic topography
  (CET), 508
Concentration, as indicator of mental status, 12
Concrete thinking, assessment of, 14

Conditioning, prepared classic, 149
Conduct disorder (CD), clinical picture of, 290–291
  course and outcome of, 295
  differential diagnosis of, 293
  epidemiology of, 293
  etiology of, 293–294
  treatment of, 296–297
Confabulation, 13
Conjugal paranoia, 134
Content of speech, poverty of, 395, 396
  as symptom of schizophrenia, 89
Control, delusions of, defined, 9
Conversion reaction, clinical picture of, 183–184
  course of, 184
  defined, 181
  differential diagnosis of, 184–185, 184t
  distinguished from amnestic syndrome, 45
  epidemiology of, 182–183
  etiology of, 181–182
  laboratory findings in, 184
  treatment of, 185–186
Cotard's delusion, 283t
Couvade syndrome, 283t
Creutzfeldt-Jakob disease, 22, 24, 25
Crisis intervention, 157
CT (computed tomography), 507
Cushing's syndrome, psychiatric manifestations of, 498
Cyclothymia, 376. See also *Bipolar illness.*
  clinical features of, 376t
  defined, 366
  family studies of, 467

DaCosta's syndrome, 283t
DeClerambault's syndrome, 134
Déjà entendu, 11
Déjà vu, 11
Delirium, 135, 405
  caused by tricyclics, 558
  causes of, 495t
  clinical picture of, 20–21
  course of, 21
  defined, 18–19
  differential diagnosis of, 21–22
  distinguished from dementia, 21–22
  epidemiology of, 19–20
  etiology and pathogenesis of, 19
  laboratory findings in, 21, 495–496
  pathology of, 20
  treatment of, 22
Delusional disorders, cases of, 134–135
  clinical picture of, 133–134
  course of, 135, 135t
  defined, 131
  differential diagnosis of, 135–136
  distinguished from schizophrenia, 133, 136
  epidemiology of, 132, 132t
  etiology of, 131–132
  family history in, 132–133, 132t
  genetic factors in, 480
  in brain disease, 412–413
  laboratory examinations for, 136
  prevalence of, 132, 132t
  subtypes of, 133–135
  treatment of, 136
Delusional mood, 10
Delusional perception, 10
  as symptom of schizophrenia, 89

Delusions, affective, 10
  assessment of, 14
  defined, 9
  distinguished from obsessions, 164–165
  in depression, 71
  mood-congruent, 72
  mood-incongruent, 72
  morbid, 10
  of control, defined, 9
  of influence, defined, 9
  secondary, 10
Dementia, 135
  Alzheimer's. See *Alzheimer's disease.*
  clinical picture of, 27
  course of, 27–28
  defined, 22–23, 403
  diagnosis of, 25t, 403–404
  differential diagnosis of, 28–29, 405
  diseases causing, 24
  distinguished from delirium, 21–22
  distinguished from depression, 369t
  drug treatment of, 581–582
  epidemiology of, 24–25, 26t
  etiology and pathogenesis of, 23–24
  in Huntington's disease, 420
  laboratory findings in, 28, 495t, 496–497, 496t
  multiple-infarct, 404
  pathology of, 25, 27
  treatment of, 29
  vascular, 404
Dementia infantilis, 335
"Dementia praecox," 87
Demographic factors, described, 523–526
Dental phobias, 150
Dependent personality disorder, 426–427
Depersonalization, 11
Depression. See also *Depressive syndrome; Unipolar depression.*
  anaclitic, 301
  anorexia nervosa in, 308
  atypical, 372
  brain lesions in, 407–409, 408t
  defined, 8
  distinguished from anorexia nervosa, 198
  distinguished from antisocial personality, 213
  distinguished from anxiety disorders, 143
  distinguished from dementia, 369t
  distinguished from obsessive-compulsive neurosis, 165
  distinguished from schizophrenia, 13, 93
  double, 75
  drug treatment of, 554–562
  drugs causing, 366t
  dysthymic, 405
  endogenous, 72, 76, 367
  endogenous-psychotic, 80
  etiology of, 521
  flat affect after medication in, 13
  in adolescents, 301, 305–306, 305t, 308
  in bipolar illness, 55
  in brain disease, 406–411
    correlated with physical and cognitive impairment, 409–410
    diagnosis of, 406
    duration of, 406–407
    etiology of, 406
    treatment of, 410–411

Depression *Continued*
  in children. See *Affective disorders, in children and adolescents.*
  in obsessive-compulsive neurosis, 164
  in Parkinson's disease, 420
  in schizophrenia, 105
  medical conditions associated with, 366t
  neurotic-reactive, 72, 76, 79–80
  panic attacks in, 388
  personality disorders coexisting with, 428–429
  postpsychotic, 107
  schizoaffective, 120, 124
  secondary, 30, 79
Depression spectrum disease, 78, 79
  suicide in, 533, 537, 539
  thought disorder in, 398–399, 399t
  trauma and, 522
Depressive disease, pure, 78
  sporadic, 78
Depressive personality disorder, 427
Depressive syndrome. See also *Depression.*
  anxiety in, 371–372, 372t
  cognitive disturbances in, 369–370
  defined, 366–367
  mood change in, 367
  psychomotor disturbances in, 369
  vegetative disturbances in, 367–369
Derailment, 14, 394, 396–397
  as symptom of schizophrenia, 89
  defined, 8
Derealization, 11
Dereistic, defined, 8
Developmental language disorder, receptive type, 336
Developmental learning disabilities of the right hemisphere, 336
Dexamethasone suppression test, diagnostic use of, 504–505
  in childhood depression, 307
  in obsessive-compulsive neurosis, 164
  in schizoaffective disorder, 123–124
  in unipolar depression, 80, 81t
Dhat, 284t
Diagnosis, laboratory tests for, 3
  of medical conditions, 493–501
  mental status examination in, 3–4
  of psychiatric conditions, 504–508
Disintegrative disorders, 335
Disruptive behavior disorders. See *Attention deficit disorder (ADD); Conduct disorder (CD); Oppositional defiant disorder (ODD).*
Dissociation, defined, 182
Dissociative reaction, clinical picture of, 183–184
  course of, 184
  defined, 181
  differential diagnosis of, 184–185, 184t
  epidemiology of, 182–183
  etiology of, 181–182
  laboratory findings in, 184
  treatment of, 185–186
Distractible speech, 398
Diurnal variation, defined, 71
Dopa, structure of, 444f
Dopamine, in autistic disorder, 328
  in schizophrenia, 101–102
  metabolism of, 447
  release and uptake of, 447
  structure of, 444f
  system anatomy of, 447

Dopamine agonist studies, diagnostic use of, 505
Doppelganger, 11
Double depression, 75
Double-bind situation, 102
Double-form insanity. See *Bipolar illness.*
Drug abuse. See also *Alcoholism; names of specific drugs.*
  agent factors in, 239
  clinical picture of, 243–244
  coexistent with alcoholism, 228
  course of, 244, 246
  defined, 237–238
  demographics of, 241
  differential diagnosis of, 249–250
  distinguished from bipolar illness, 59
  distinguished from schizophrenia, 93
  epidemiology of, 240–241
  etiology and pathogenesis of, 238–240
  illicit steroid use, 280–284
  in antisocial personality, 210–211, 214, 216
  in childhood affective disorders, 309
  laboratory findings in, 246–249, 497
  laws against, 240
  pathology of, 241
  phases of, 246t, 247t, 248t
  rates of, 240–241
  social influences and, 240
  suicide in, 533, 537–538, 539–540
  symptoms of, 245t
  trauma and, 522
  treatment of, 248t, 250–251
Drug overdose, 250
Drug toxicity, causing dementia, 25, 26t
Dyskinesia, spontaneous (nontardive), 418
  tardive, 422–423, 551
    as side effect of neuroleptics, 106
Dysmegalopsia, 11
Dysmorphic delusions, 135
Dyspareunia, 254t
Dysrhythmias, anxiety as symptom of, 383–384
Dysthymia, 405
  aspects of, 372–373
  defined, 365–366
Dystonia, as side effect of neuroleptics, 106
  drug-induced, 422, 550
  motor abnormalities in, 420
  tardive, 551

Early-morning awakening, 71
Eating disorders. See *Anorexia nervosa; Bulimia nervosa.*
écho de pensée, 10
Echolalia, defined, 8
Echopraxia, as indicator of mental instability, 7
ECT (electroconvulsive therapy), 83–84
Effectors, 442
Ejaculation, premature, 254t, 255, 256
  treatment of, 256
Elation, 13
Elderly, suicide in, 536
Elective mutism, distinguished from autistic disorder, 337
Electroconvulsive therapy (ECT), 83–84
Embolism, pulmonary, anxiety as symptom of, 384
Encapsulation, defined, 133
Encephalitis, causing amnestic syndrome, 39, 40
  causing dementia, 25
  personality change due to, 31
Encephalopathy, hepatic, causing dementia, 26t
Endocrine diseases, anxiety as symptom of, 384
  causing psychiatric conditions, 497–500, 504

Endogenous depression, 72, 76, 367
Endogenous-psychotic depression, 80
Endorphins, 238
Epidemiology, analytic, 511, 519–520
    defined, 511
    descriptive, 511, 515–519
    diagnostic instruments of, 514–515
    experimental, 511, 520–526
    methodological issues in, 511
    primary measurements for, 511–514
    psychiatric applications of, 511
Epilepsy, grand mal, anxiety as symptom of, 385
    obsessive-compulsive neurosis in, 162
    sexual dysfunction and, 255
    temporal lobe, causing amnestic syndrome, 39, 44
        distinguished from conversion reaction, 185
        distinguished from schizoaffective disorder, 124
        distinguished from schizophrenia, 93
Epinephrine, in autistic disorder, 328
Erectile disorder, 254t, 256–257
    treatment of, 256
Erotic delusional disorder, 134–135
Erotomania, 134
    pure, 283t
Estrogen deficiency, psychiatric manifestations of, 499
Ethnicity, as demographic factor, 524
Euphoria, 13
    defined, 8
Euthymia, defined, 8
Excitement, catatonic, as symptom of schizo-
    phrenia, 89
Exhibitionism, course of, 265t
    diagnosis of, 263t
Extension, of delusional disorders, 133
Extracampine hallucinations, 11

Factitious disorder, case history of, 277–278
    clinical picture of, 277
    course of, 278
    defined, 276–277
    differential diagnosis of, 278–279
    epidemiology of, 277
    in antisocial personality, 214
    laboratory tests in, 279
    prevalence of, 277t
    treatment of, 279
Fahr's disease, motor abnormalities in, 421
Failed suicide, 310–311
Familial pure depressive disease, 78
Family studies, 461, 483
    of autism, 324–325
    of bipolar illness, 48–49
    of depression, 77, 77t
    of personality disorders, 430
    of schizophrenia, 96–97, 97t, 105–106
Family therapy, behavioral, 108–109
Fear, childhood, 354
Feelings, made, as symptom of schizophrenia, 88
Female sexual arousal disorder, 254t
Flat affect, 13
    as symptom of schizophrenia, 89
Flattening, defined, 8
Flight of ideas, 14, 396
    defined, 8
Fluoxetine, to treat depression, 560, 561, 562
    to treat obsessive-compulsive neurosis, 578–579
Fluvoxamine, 578

Focal striatal abnormalities, obsessive-compulsive neu-
    rosis in, 162
Folie à deux, 131
Formication, 11
Fregoil's delusion, 283t
Frontal lobe, abnormalities of, motor abnormalities in,
    421–422
        obsessive-compulsive neurosis in, 162
Frotteurism, course of, 265t
    diagnosis of, 263t
Fugue, defined, 181
    distinguished from amnestic syndrome, 45
Fungal infection, causing dementia, 26t

Gamma glutamyl transpeptidase (GGTP) values, in al-
    coholism, 225
Gamma-aminobutyric acid (GABA) system, 449–450
Ganser's delusion, 283t
    distinguished from amnestic syndrome, 44
Gender identity disorders, assessment of, 260–261
    classification of, 259t
    course of, 260
    defined, 258
    differential diagnosis of, 260
    etiology of, 260
    prevalence of, 258–260
    treatment of, 261–262
Generalized anxiety disorder, childhood trauma and,
    522
    classification of, 144–145
    clinical picture of, 146
    course of, 146–147
    defined, 144
    differential diagnosis of, 143, 147
    epidemiology of, 146
    etiology of, 145–146
    treatment of, 147–148
Genetic counseling, 480–482
    empirical data for, 481t
Genetics, adoption studies in, 460–461
    association studies in, 467, 472, 483
    biologic markers in, 467, 472, 476, 478–479
    etiologic markers in, 467–468, 473–474, 477–478
    family studies in, 461, 483
    high-risk studies in, 461–462, 468–469, 483
    linkage studies in, 467, 472, 483
    pharmacogenetic studies in, 483
    twin studies in, 460
GGTP (gamma glutamyl transpeptidase) values, in al-
    coholism, 225
Grand mal epilepsy, anxiety as symptom of, 385
Grandiose delusional disorder, 135
Grandiose delusions, 10
Graves' disease, psychiatric manifestations of, 498
Grief, distinguished from melancholia, 370–371
    medication for, 555
Guilt, delusions of, 10

Hallucinations, defined, 10
    in brain disease, 412–413
    types of, 10–11
Hallucinogens, pathology of, 243
Haptic hallucinations, 11
Head injury, obsessive-compulsive neurosis in, 162
Headaches, distinguished from psychogenic pain, 188
Hebephrenic schizophrenia, 91, 91t
Hematoma, subdural, causing dementia, 25, 26t
Hepatic encephalopathy, causing dementia, 26t

Hepatolenticular degeneration, motor abnormalities in, 420–421
Herpes virus infections, psychiatric manifestations of, 501
High-risk studies, 461–462, 468–469, 483
History, of patient, 5
Histrionic personality disorder, 426
    distinguished from Briquet's syndrome, 179
    distinguished from schizophrenia, 94
Homicidal ideation and threats, 9
Homosexuality, 260
    male, genetic factors in, 480
Hopelessness, defined, 9
Hormones, in treatment of paraphilias, 268
Huntington's chorea, 22, 24, 25
    anxiety as symptom of, 385
    motor abnormalities in, 420
    psychiatric manifestations of, 500
Hydrocarbons, psychotoxic, pathology of, 243
Hydrocephalus, normal-pressure, 22, 25, 26t
Hyperactivity. See Attention deficit disorder (ADD).
Hypercalcemia, distinguished from Briquet's syndrome, 178
Hyperdynamic beta-adrenergic state, anxiety as symptom of, 383
Hyperesthesia, 11
Hyperparathyroidism, psychiatric manifestations of, 499
Hyperthymia, defined, 366
Hyperthymic disorder, 377
Hyperthyroidism, anxiety as symptom of, 384
    causing dementia, 26t
    generalized anxiety disorder in, 147
    psychiatric manifestations of, 498
Hyperventilation, 140
Hypesthesia, 11
Hypnagogic hallucinations, 11
Hypnopompic hallucinations, 11
Hypoactive sexual desire disorder, 254t
Hypocalcemia, psychiatric manifestations of, 499
Hypochondria, distinguished from periodic paralysis, 421
Hypochondriacal delusions, 10
Hypochondriacal neurosis, 189
Hypochondriasis, 150, 189–190
    distinguished from delusional disorders, 136
    distinguished from obsessive-compulsive neurosis, 165
    panic attacks in, 388
Hypoglycemia, anxiety as symptom of, 384
    distinguished from anxiety disorders, 143
    psychiatric manifestations of, 499–500
Hypomania, chronic, 377
    defined, 366, 375
    in bipolar disorders, 375–376, 375t
Hypoparathyroidism, anxiety in, 143, 384
    psychiatric manifestations of, 499
Hypothyroidism, causing dementia, 26t, 34
    psychiatric manifestations of, 497–498
Hysteria, acute. See Conversion reaction.
    chronic. See Briquet's syndrome.
    mass, 182
Hysterical pseudodementia, 283t

Ideas, flight of, 14
Idiopathic pain. See Psychogenic pain.
Illness phobia, 149
    distinguished from obsessive-compulsive neurosis, 165

Illogicality, 397
Impaired memory, 10
Impotence, 255
Imprinting, 150
Impulses, made, as symptom of schizophrenia, 89
Inappropriate affect, as symptom of schizophrenia, 89
    defined, 8
Incidence, epidemiological studies of, 515
Incoherence, 394, 397
Incongruent affect, 13
    defined, 8
Induced depressive syndrome, 79
Infantile autism. See Autistic disorder.
Infection, causing psychiatric conditions, 501
Influence, delusions of, defined, 9
Influenza, as possible etiologic agent for schizophrenia, 103
Inhibited female orgasm, 254t, 256
Inhibited male orgasm, 254t, 256
Insight, as indicator of mental status, 12–13
Insomnia, terminal, 71
Intelligence, as indicator of mental status, 12
Intoxication(s), anxiety as symptom of, 385–386
    with cocaine, 162
Involutional melancholia, 371
Irritability, defined, 8
Isoniazid toxicity, obsessive-compulsive neurosis in, 162

Jealous delusional disorder, 134
Jealousy, delusions of, 10
Judgment, as indicator of mental status, 12–13
Juvenile unmasculinity, 260

Kaleidoscopic hallucinations, 11
Khat intoxication, anxiety as symptom of, 386
Kindling, 155
Kleine-Levin syndrome, 283t
    distinguished from bulimia nervosa, 201
Klüver-Bucy syndrome, 283t
    distinguished from bulimia nervosa, 201
Koro, 284t
Korsakoff syndrome, 39, 40, 44

Labile affect, 13
Lability, defined, 8
Laboratory, in diagnosis of medical conditions, 493–501
    in diagnosis of psychiatric conditions, 504–508
    therapeutic drug monitoring by, 501–504
Latah, 284t
Latency of response, increased, as symptom of schizophrenia, 89
Lead toxicity, causing dementia, 26t
Learned helplessness, in childhood depression, 304
    in posttraumatic stress disorder, 155
Learning disabilities, distinguished from autistic disorder, 336
Leyton inventory, 163
Linkage studies, 467, 472, 483
    defined, 99
Lithium, adverse effects of, 564–566
    dosages of, 563–564
    efficacy of, 562–563
    motoric side effects of, 422–423
    side effects of, 62–63
    therapeutic monitoring of, 502
    transport of, 468

Loose associations, 14
  as symptom of schizophrenia, 89
  defined, 8
LSD intoxication, anxiety as symptom of, 386
Lupus erythematosus (SLE), psychiatric manifestations of, 501
Lyme disease, psychiatric manifestations of, 501

Macropsia, 11
Made feelings, as symptom of schizophrenia, 88
Made impulses, as symptom of schizophrenia, 89
Made volitional acts, as symptom of schizophrenia, 89
Magnetic resonance imaging (MRI), 507
Major depression. See *Depression.*
Major depressive disorder. See *Depression; Unipolar depression.*
Male erectile disorder, 254t, 256–257
  treatment of, 256
Malingering, 389
  distinguished from amnestic syndrome, 45
  distinguished from factitious disorder, 278–279
  in antisocial personality, 214
Mania, 47
  distinguished from antisocial personality, 213
  distinguished from schizophrenia, 93
  drug treatment of, 562–568
  drugs causing, 373t
  in brain disease, 411–412
  medical conditions associated with, 373t
  secondary, 52–53, 55
  thought disorder in, 398–399, 399t
Manic syndrome, cognitive disturbances in, 374
  defined, 373
  mood change in, 373
  panic attacks in, 388
  psychomotor disturbances in, 374
  vegetative disturbances in, 373–374
Manic-depressive disease. See *Bipolar illness.*
Mannerisms, as indicator of mental instability, 7
  in schizophrenia, 90
Maprotiline, 560, 561
Marital schism, 102
Masochism, course of, 265t
  diagnosis of, 263t
Mass hysteria, 182
Maudsley inventory, 163
Mean corpuscular volume values, in alcoholism, 225
Meige's syndrome, motor abnormalities in, 420
Melancholia, 47, 72, 367
  distinguished from grief, 370–371
Melatonin, light suppression of, 468
Memory, as indicator of mental status, 12
  impairment of, 10
    in delirium, 21
    in dementia, 22
  in amnestic syndrome, 39
Menopausal syndrome, 499
Mental disorders
  due to a general medical condition, 17
    clinical picture and course of, 33–34
    defined, 29
    diagnosis of, 29–30
    differential diagnosis of, 34
    epidemiology of, 31–32
    etiology of, 31
    laboratory findings in, 34
    pathology of, 32–33
    treatment of, 34–35

Mental retardation, distinguished from antisocial personality, 213
  distinguished from autistic disorder, 336
  distinguished from disruptive behavior disorders in children, 292
  distinguished from thought disorder, 395
Mental status examination, 3
  areas covered by, 6–13
  criteria for, 6–13
  errors in, 13–15
  procedures for, 6, 6t
  signs and symptoms in, 4
Metabolic disorders, causing psychiatric conditions, 500–501
Methylxanthine intoxication, anxiety as symptom of, 385
MHPG, in autistic disorder, 328
Micropsia, 11
Migration, as demographic factor, 525
Mimicry, panic attacks in, 388–389
Minor depression. See *Dysthymia.*
Mitral valve prolapse, anxiety as symptom of, 383
Monoamine oxidase (MAO) inhibitors, 83
  adverse effects of, 559–560, 559t
  dosages of, 559
  efficacy of, 558–559
  motoric side effects of, 422–423
  withdrawal from, 560
Mood, as indicator of mental status, 8
  defined, 365
  disturbance of, 367, 373
    clinical settings of, 377–378
Mood disorder, 30
  distinguished from adjustment disorder, 275
  distinguished from anxiety disorders, 143
  distinguished from schizophrenia, 93
Mood-congruent, defined, 93
Mood-congruent delusions, 72
Mood-incongruent, defined, 93
Mood-incongruent delusions, 72
Morbid affective states, 10
Motor activity, in delirium, 21
Motor symptoms, drug-induced, 422–423
  movement abnormalities as, 417–422
MRI (magnetic resonance imaging), 507
Multiple personality, distinguished from amnestic syndrome, 45
Multiple sclerosis (MS), obsessive-compulsive neurosis in, 162
  psychiatric manifestations of, 500
Munchausen syndrome, 277
  by proxy, 277
  prognosis of, 278
Musculorum deformans, motor abnormalities in, 420
Mutism, as symptom of schizophrenia, 89
  defined, 8
  elective, distinguished from autistic disorder, 337
Myasthenia gravis, distinguished from conversion reaction, 184
  motor abnormalities in, 421
Myocardial infarction, anxiety as symptom of, 382
  depression in, 406
Myofascial pain syndromes, distinguished from psychogenic pain, 188
Myoglobinuria, distinguished from conversion reaction, 184
Myopathies, distinguished from conversion reaction, 184

Narcissistic personality disorder, 426
Negativism, as indicator of mental instability, 7
  as symptom of schizophrenia, 89
Negativistic personality disorder, 427
Neologisms, 398
Neoplasia, causing psychiatric conditions, 500
Neuritis, optic, distinguished from conversion reaction, 185
Neurocirculatory asthenia, 283t
Neuroendocrine system, defined, 504
Neuroleptic malignant syndrome, 423, 549–550
  as side effect of neuroleptics, 106
Neuroleptics, adverse effects of, 106
  therapeutic monitoring of, 504
Neurologic diseases, anxiety as symptom of, 385
  causing psychiatric conditions, 500
Neurons, structure of, 441–442
Neuropeptides, 450t
  role of, 450
  synthesis and metabolism of, 451
Neurosyphilis, personality change due to, 31
  psychiatric manifestations of, 501
Neurotic-reactive depression, 72, 76, 79–80
Neurotransmitters, 238, 442
  amino acid, 449–450
  anatomy and biochemistry of, 442–449
  in autistic disorder, 327–329
  schizophrenia related to, 101–102
  studies of, diagnostic use of, 505–507
Nihilistic delusions, 10
Nontardive dyskinesia, 418
Noradrenaline, structure of, 444f
Noradrenergic system, of panic patients, 141
Norepinephrine, 442
  in autistic disorder, 328
  metabolism of, 444–446
  neurons containing, 442–444
  release and uptake of, 446–447

Obsession, defined, 9, 161
Obsessive-compulsive disorder. See *Obsessive-compulsive neurosis.*
Obsessive-compulsive neurosis, clinical picture of, 162–163
  course of, 163–164
  defined, 161
  differential diagnosis of, 164–165
  distinguished from antisocial personality, 213
  distinguished from autistic disorder, 337
  distinguished from depression, 165
  drug treatment of, 577–579, 579t
  epidemiology of, 162
  etiology of, 161–162
  in children, clinical picture of, 354–355
    differential diagnosis of, 356–357
    epidemiology of, 355
    laboratory findings in, 357
    outcome of, 355–356
  laboratory findings in, 164
  personality disorders coexisting with, 428–429
  related to anorexia nervosa, 194
  trauma and, 522
  treatment of, 165–166
  variants of, 165
Obsessive-compulsive personality disorder, 427
  social phobia in, 152
Occupation, as demographic factor, 525
OCD. See *Obsessive-compulsive neurosis.*
OCD variants, 165

ODD. See *Oppositional defiant disorder (ODD).*
Olfactory hallucinations, 11
Operant conditioning, as treatment for schizophrenia, 108
Opioid abuse, pathology of, 241
  relapse rate for, 249t
  withdrawal from, 238
Oppositional defiant disorder (ODD)
  clinical picture of, 291
  course and outcome of, 296
  differential diagnosis of, 293
  epidemiology of, 293
  etiology of, 294
  treatment of, 296
Optic neuritis, distinguished from conversion reaction, 185
Organic anxiety syndromes, 382
Organic brain syndromes, 18–29. See also *Delirium; Dementia.*
  distinguished from schizophrenia, 93
  suicide in, 534, 538
Organic delusional syndromes, 136
Organic mental disorders, defined, 17–18, 403
  distinguished from bipolar illness, 59
Organic mental syndromes, defined, 403
Organic stupor, 11
Orgasm, disorders of, 254t
  inhibited female, 254t, 256
  inhibited male, 254t, 256
Orientation, as indicator of mental status, 11
Othello's delusion, 283t
Overanxious disorder, clinical picture of, 352–353
  defined, 349
  differential diagnosis of, 356
  epidemiology of, 351
  etiology of, 350
  outcome of, 353
  treatment of, 357–359
Overinclusive, defined, 8
Overt behavior, recording, 5
Overvalued ideas, defined, 9

Pain, chronic idiopathic. See *Psychogenic pain.*
  psychogenic. See *Psychogenic pain.*
Panic, defined, 8
Panic attacks, 381–382. See also *Agoraphobia; Anxiety disorders; Panic disorder.*
  in mental disorders, 387–390
Panic disorder, 381, 390. See also *Agoraphobia; Anxiety disorders.*
  childhood trauma and, 522
  classification of, 139–140
  clinical picture of, 142
  complications of, 142–143
  course of, 142
  differential diagnosis of, 143
  distinguished from antisocial personality, 213
  drug treatment of, 568–577
  epidemiology of, 141
  etiology of, 140
  family studies of, 479
  spectrum disorders of, 482
  suicide in, 534
  treatment of, 143–144
Paragrammatism, 397
Paralysis, periodic, distinguished from conversion reaction, 185
  motor abnormalities in, 421

Paranoia. See *Delusional disorders; Paranoid disorder*.
Paranoid, defined, 14
Paranoid disorder, distinguished from psychotic disor-
    der due to medical condition, 34
    distinguished from schizophrenia, 94
Paranoid personality disorder, 426
Paranoid schizophrenia, 91, 91t
    defined, 14
    distinguished from bipolar illness, 59
Paraphilias, assessment of, 265–266
    course of, 264–265
    defined, 262
    differential diagnosis of, 266–267
    etiology of, 263–264
    prevalence of, 262–263
    treatment of, 267–269
Paraphrenia, 131
Parathyroid disorders, psychiatric manifestations of,
    499
Paresis, causing dementia, 25, 26t
Parietal lobe, lesions of, motor abnormalities in,
    421–422
Parkinson's disease, causing dementia, 25
    depression in, 406
    motor abnormalities in, 420
    psychiatric manifestations of, 500
Passive-aggressive personality disorder, 427
    distinguished from antisocial personality, 213
Passivity, 9
    somatic, as symptom of schizophrenia, 88
Patient history, taking, 5
PCP (phencyclidine), pathology of, 243
Pedophilia, course of, 265t
    diagnosis of, 263t
    treatment of, 267–269, 267t
Peptides, in autistic disorder, 329
Perception, abnormalities of, in delirium, 20
    as indicator of mental status, 10–11
    delusional, as symptom of schizophrenia, 89
    disturbances of, 10–11, 394
Periodic paralysis, distinguished from conversion
    reaction, 185
    motor abnormalities in, 421
Peripheral blindness, distinguished from autistic
    disorder, 336
Persecutory delusional disorder, 133, 134
Persecutory delusions, 10
Perseveration, 396
    defined, 8
Personality, change of, due to medical condition, 31
    dimensions of, 427
Personality disorders, assessment of, 427–428
    categories of, 425–427
    defined, 425
    differential diagnosis of, 432
    distinguished from adjustment disorder, 275
    distinguished from antisocial personality, 213
    distinguished from bipolar illness, 59
    distinguished from Briquet's syndrome, 179
    distinguished from factitious disorder, 278–279
    distinguished from schizophrenia, 94
    etiology of, 429
    genetic factors in, 430
    neurobiological abnormalities in, 431–432
    secondary to Axis I disorders, 428–429
    suicide in, 534, 538
    treatment of, 433–434
PET (positron-emission tomography), 507–508

Pharmacogenetic studies, 483
Phencyclidine (PCP) intoxication, distinguished from
    schizoaffective disorder, 124
    pathology of, 243
Phenomenology, 3–4
    problems in, 4–5
Pheochromocytoma, 147
    anxiety as symptom of, 384
    psychiatric manifestations of, 499
Phobias, defined, 9, 164
    illness. See *Illness phobia*.
    in children, clinical picture of, 354
        differential diagnosis of, 356
        outcome of, 354
    simple, 148–151. See also *Simple phobia*.
    social, 151–154. See also *Social phobia*.
Phobic disorder, distinguished from antisocial person-
    ality, 213
    distinguished from anxiety disorders, 143
    panic attacks in, 389
Phobic stimulus, 148
Physical anergy, as symptom of schizophrenia, 89
Physiologic monitoring, as part of mental status exam-
    ination, 5
Piblokto, 284t
Pica, distinguished from disruptive behavior disorders
    in children, 292
Pick's bodies, 25
Polymyositis, distinguished from conversion reaction,
    184
Porphyria, acute intermittent, psychiatric manifestations
    of, 501
        distinguished from Briquet's syndrome, 177
Positron-emission tomography (PET), 507–508
Posterolateral sclerosis, anxiety as symptom of, 385
Posthysterectomy syndrome, 499
    psychiatric manifestations of, 499
Postpsychotic depression, 107
Posttraumatic stress disorder (PTSD), 522–523
    anxiety in, 143
    classification of, 154–155
    clinical picture of, 156
    course and complications of, 157
    defined, 154
    distinguished from adjustment disorder, 275
    epidemiology of, 156
    etiology, 155–156
    panic attacks in, 389
    treatment of, 157–158
Posturing, as indicator of mental instability, 7
    in schizophrenia, 90
Poverty, delusions of, 10
    of content, 395, 396
        as symptom of schizophrenia, 89
    of speech, 395–396
        as symptom of schizophrenia, 89
Poverty of thought, defined, 8
Prader-Willi syndrome, distinguished from bulimia
    nervosa, 201
Pregnancy, complications of, related to schizophrenia,
    102–103
Premature ejaculation, 254t, 255, 256
    treatment of, 256
Premenstrual syndrome, 499
Prepared classic conditioning, 149
Presence, hallucinations of, 11
Pressure of speech, 14, 398
    defined, 8

Prevalence, epidemiological studies of, 516–519
Primary psychopaths, 212
Prodromal, defined, 90
Progressive supranuclear palsy (PSP), motor abnormalities in, 421
Prolonged psychosis, 93
Propanediols, 575
Pseudocyesis, 181
Pseudodementia, 12, 28
    hysterical, 283t
Pseudologia fantastica, 13, 278
Pseudoparkinsonism, as side effect of neuroleptics, 106, 550
Psychogenic pain, clinical picture of, 187–188, 188t
    course of, 188
    defined, 186
    differential diagnosis of, 188
    epidemiology of, 187
    etiology of, 186–187
    laboratory findings in, 188
    pathology of, 187
    treatment of, 188–189
Psychological autopsy, 532
Psychomotor acceleration, 7
Psychomotor activity, as indicator of mental status, 7
Psychomotor agitation, 7
Psychomotor retardation, 7
Psychopaths, primary vs. secondary, 212, 216
Psychopharmacology, principles of, 107
Psychosis, laboratory findings in, 497
    prolonged, 93
    reactive, distinguished from schizophrenia, 94
Psychosis NOS, distinguished from schizophrenia, 94
Psychosocial deprivation, in autistic disorder, 337
Psychotherapy, for schizophrenia, 107–108
Psychotic disorder due to a general medical condition, 30
PTSD. See *Posttraumatic stress disorder* (*PTSD*).
Pulmonary embolism, anxiety as symptom of, 384
Pure erotomania, 283t

Rabbit syndrome, 550
Reactive psychosis, brief, distinguished from schizophrenia, 94
Reading disability, specific, 480
Receptors, 442
    subtypes of, 443t
Reference, delusions of, 10
Reliability, as indicator of mental status, 12–13
REM latency, in sleep, 468
Repression, defined, 182
Residual, defined, 90
Respiratory diseases, anxiety as symptom of, 384
Response acquisition, 108
Retardation, mental. See *Mental retardation*.
    psychomotor, 7
Retrograde amnesia, 39, 42
Retrospective falsification, 13
Rett syndrome, 335
Ritual, defined, 161

Sadism, course of, 265t
    diagnosis of, 263t
Sadistic personality disorder, 427
Schizoaffective disorder, clinical picture of, 120
    compared with schizophrenia, 116, 118–119
    course of, 120, 121t-122t, 122–123
    defined, 115

Schizoaffective disorder *Continued*
    depression in, 120, 124
    differential diagnosis of, 124
    distinguished from bipolar illness, 59
    distinguished from schizophrenia, 94
    epidemiology of, 119–120
    etiology of, 115–116, 117t-118t, 118–119
    laboratory findings in, 123–124
    treatment of, 122, 124–125
    twin studies of, 466
Schizoid personality disorder, 426
Schizophrenia, adoption studies of, 97–98, 469–470
    as brain disease, 99–102
    biologic markers for, 472, 482t
    case histories of, 109–110
    childhood, 340
    compared with schizoaffective disorder, 116, 118–119
    course and outcome of, 103–106, 104t
    depression in, 105
    diagnosis of, 90–91
    diagnostic criteria for, 90t
    differential diagnosis of, 92–95
    distinguished from anorexia nervosa, 198
    distinguished from antisocial personality, 213
    distinguished from autistic disorder, 337–338, 342
    distinguished from bipolar disorder, 58–59, 374–375, 374t
    distinguished from Briquet's syndrome, 179
    distinguished from delusional disorders, 133, 136
    distinguished from depression, 13
    distinguished from psychotic disorder due to medical condition, 34
    drug treatment of, 545–554
    environment and, 102–103
    epidemiology of, 95–96
    etiologic markers for, 472–474
    etiology and pathophysiology of, 96–103
    family studies of, 96–97, 97t, 105–106, 470–471
    following obsessive-compulsive neurosis, 164
    genetic transmission of, 96–99
    hebephrenic, 91, 91t
    historical view of, 87
    in childhood, 292, 340
        clinical features of, 340–341
        course and prognosis of, 341–342
        differential diagnosis of, 342
        etiology of, 340
        treatment of, 342
    in mentally retarded patients, 94
    incidence of, 88, 95, 96t
    laboratory findings in, 506–507
    mode of transmission of, 471–472
    motor abnormalities in, 417–419, 418t
    negative symptoms of, 89–90
    neurobiology of, 454–457
    neurotransmitter theories of, 101–102
    panic attacks in, 387–388
    paranoid, 91, 91t. See also *Paranoid schizophrenia*.
        defined, 14
        distinguished from bipolar illness, 59
    paraphilias in, 266–267
    positive symptoms of, 88–89
    prevalence of, 95–96, 95t, 96t
    prodromal and residual symptoms of, 90t
    spectrum disorders of, 472, 482t
    suicide in, 533–534, 538, 540
    thought disorder in, 399–400, 399t, 400t
    treatment of, 106–109

Schizophrenia *Continued*
  twin studies of, 97, 469, 469t
  types of, 91–92, 91t
  viral theory of, 103
Schizophrenic syndrome of childhood, distinguished
  from schizophrenia in childhood, 340
Schizophreniform disorder, distinguished from schizoaffective disorder, 125, 126t, 127
  distinguished from schizophrenia, 94, 125, 126t, 127
"Schizophrenogenic mother," 102
Schizotypal personality disorder, 426
  distinguished from schizophrenia, 94
Sclerosis, multiple. See *Multiple sclerosis.*
  posterolateral, anxiety as symptom of, 385
Season of birth, as demographic factor, 526
Second-generation antidepressants, adverse effects of,
  561–562
  dosages of, 561
  efficacy of, 560–561
Secondary depression, 30, 79
Secondary gain, defined, 181
Secondary mania, 52–53
Secondary psychopaths, 212
Sedatives, abuse of, 241–242
  anxiety as symptom of, 387
  withdrawal from, 238
  anxiety as symptom of, 386
Seizures. See also *Epilepsy.*
  antipsychotics and, 551
  distinguished from panic disorders, 143
  tricyclics and, 558
Self-defeating personality disorder, 427
Sensorium, clear, 11
Separation anxiety disorder, clinical picture of,
  351–352
  defined, 349
  differential diagnosis of, 356
  epidemiology of, 351
  etiology of, 350
  laboratory findings in, 357
  outcome of, 352
  treatment of, 357–359
Serotonin, 447
  in autistic disorder, 328
  in pineal gland, 448
  in schizophrenia, 102
  metabolism of, 448, 456f
  neurons containing, 447–448
  release and uptake of, 448
  structure of, 445f
Sex, as demographic factor, 523
Sexual arousal disorders, 254t
Sexual aversion disorder, 254t
Sexual desire disorders, 254t
Sexual dysfunctions, assessment of, 256–257
  classification of, 254t
  course of, 255–256
  defined, 253
  differential diagnosis of, 257
  etiology of, 254–255
  incidence of, 253–254
  prevalence of, 253
  in males, 255t
  treatment of, 256
Sexual masochism, course of, 265t
  diagnosis of, 263t
Sexual pain disorders, 254t
Sexual sadism, course of, 265t
  diagnosis of, 263t
Shallow affect, 13

Simple phobia, classification of, 148–149
  clinical picture of, 149–150
  course of, 150
  defined, 148
  differential diagnosis of, 150
  epidemiology of, 149
  etiology of, 149
  in children, clinical picture of, 354
    differential diagnosis of, 356
    outcome of, 354
  treatment of, 150–151
Sinfulness, delusions of, 10
Single-photon-emission computed tomography
  (SPECT), 508
Skewed relationship, 102
Sleep, in depression, 51–52, 80–81
  in depressive syndrome, 368, 368t
  REM latency in, 468
Sleep-wake cycle, disturbances of, 20
Social class, as demographic factor, 524–525
Social phobia, avoidant personality disorder and, 426
  childhood trauma and, 522
  classification of, 151
  clinical picture of, 152–153
  course of, 153
  defined, 151
  differential diagnosis of, 150
  epidemiology of, 152
  etiology of, 151–152
  panic attacks in, 389
  treatment of, 153–154
Social skills training, 108, 154
Social-emotional learning disability, distinguished from
  autistic disorder, 336
Sociopathy. See *Antisocial personality.*
Somatic delusions, 10
Somatic delusional disorders, 135
Somatic passivity, as symptom of schizophrenia, 88
Somatization disorder. See also *Briquet's syndrome.*
  childhood trauma and, 522
  distinguished from factitious disorder, 279
  panic attacks in, 388
Somatoform disorders, 169. See also *Briquet's syndrome;*
  Conversion reactions; Hypochondriasis; Psychogenic pain.
Spasmophilia, panic attacks in, 389–390
Specific reading disability, 480
SPECT (single-photon-emission computed tomogra-
  phy), 508
Speech, as indicator of mental status, 8–10
  content of, poverty of, 395, 396
  distractible, 398
  poverty of, 395–396
    as symptom of schizophrenia, 89
  pressure of, 8, 14, 398
Spinal cord injury, depression in, 406
Spontaneous dyskinesia, 418
Sporadic depressive disease, 78
Steele-Richardson syndrome, motor abnormalities in,
  421
Stereotyped movements, as indicator of mental insta-
  bility, 7
Stereotypies, in schizophrenia, 90
Steroids, illicit use of, 280–284
Stimulants, abuse of, 242
  psychosis induced by, 3
  treatment of depression with, 562
  withdrawal from, 238
Stimulus, phobic, 148

Stress, epidemiological studies of, 521
Stroke, depression in, 406, 407t
Stupor, 7
    catatonic, in schizophrenia, 90
    organic, 11
Subaffective disorders, defined, 366
Subdural hematoma, causing dementia, 25, 26t
Substance abuse. See *Drug abuse.*
Subtype concordance, 91–92
Suicidal ideation, 9
Suicide, attempters of, 59
    demographics of, 529–530, 530t-531t, 532t
    executive, 540
    genetic factors in, 536
    in anorexia nervosa, 196
    in bipolar illness, 57–58
    in childhood affective disorders, 309–310
    in schizophrenia, 105
    in unipolar depression, 75–76, 76t
    method of, 530–532
    pathogenesis of, 311t, 532–536
    prediction of, 536–537
    prevention of, 539–540
    risk factors for, 537–539
Suicide attempt, clinical picture of, 542
    defined, 310, 540
    epidemiology of, 541–542
    etiology and pathogenesis of, 540–541
    methodologies of, 312t
    patient management after, 542–543
Suicide gesture, defined, 310
Sundowning, 20
Supersensitivity psychosis, 552
Sydenham's chorea, motor abnormalities in, 421
    obsessive-compulsive neurosis in, 161
Sympathetic reflex dystrophies, distinguished from psychogenic pain, 188
Sympathomimetic abuse, anxiety as symptom of, 386
Synesthesia, 10
Syphilis, psychiatric manifestations of, 501
Systematized, defined, 133
Systemic disorders, causing psychiatric conditions, 501
Systemic lupus erythematosus (SLE), psychiatric manifestations of, 501

Tachycardia, distinguished from panic attack, 383
Tactile hallucinations, 11
Talking past the point, as symptom of schizophrenia, 89
Tangentiality, 394, 396, 397
    as symptom of schizophrenia, 89
Tardive dyskinesia, 422–423, 551
    as side effect of neuroleptics, 106
Tardive dystonia, 551
Tedium vitae, defined, 9
Temporal lobe epilepsy, causing amnestic syndrome, 39, 44
    distinguished from conversion reaction, 185
    distinguished from schizoaffective disorder, 124
    distinguished from schizophrenia, 93
Tension, defined, 8
Tension headaches, distinguished from psychogenic pain, 188
Terminal insomnia, 71
Terminal medical illness, suicide in, 534–535
Theobromine intoxication, anxiety as symptom of, 385
Theophylline intoxication, anxiety as symptom of, 385
Therapeutic drug monitoring (TDM), 501–504

Thought, abnormalities of, in delirium, 20–21
    in dementia, 22
    as indicator of mental status, 14
    audible, as symptom of schizophrenia, 88
    concrete, assessment of, 14
    poverty of, 8
Thought block, defined, 8
Thought broadcasting, as symptom of schizophrenia, 88
    defined, 9
Thought disorder, defined, 393
    diagnostic and prognostic significance of, 398–399, 399t
    distinguished from creativity, 394–395
    distinguished from pedantry, 395
    inaccuracy of terminology of, 14
    negative, 395–396
    positive, 396–397
    types of, 394, 395–398
Thought insertion, as symptom of schizophrenia, 88
    defined, 9
Thought process, as indicator of mental status, 8–10
Thought withdrawal, as symptom of schizophrenia, 88
    defined, 9
Thyroid disorders, anxiety as symptom of, 384
    causing dementia, 25, 26t
    psychiatric manifestations of, 497–498
Thyroid-releasing hormone stimulation test, diagnostic use of, 505
    in schizoaffective disorder, 123
Tic disorders, motor abnormalities in, 419
Tobacco abuse, causing dependence, 238
    pathology of, 242–243
    relapse rate for, 249t
Torticollis, 420
Tourette syndrome, distinguished from autistic disorder, 337
    distinguished from disruptive behavior disorders in children, 292
    genetic basis of, 479–480
    obsessive-compulsive neurosis in, 161, 165
Transient ischemic attacks, anxiety as symptom of, 385
Transsexuality, 259, 259t, 260
    diagnosis of, 261
    surgery and, 262
Transvestism, 259
    diagnosis of, 263t
Trauma, as etiologic agent, 522
    causing amnestic syndrome, 39, 40, 44
    causing dementia, 25
    causing depression, 406
Trazodone, 560, 561–562
Trichotillomania, 165
Tricyclic antidepressants, 82–83
    motoric side effects of, 422–423
    pediatric use of, 314t-316t, 358–359
    therapeutic monitoring of, 503–504
    to treat depression, adverse effects of, 557–558
        dosages of, 555–557
        efficacy of, 554–555
    to treat panic disorders, adverse effects of, 573
        dosages of, 573
        efficacy of, 572–573
Trypanosomiasis, distinguished from Briquet's syndrome, 178
Tryptophan, metabolism of, 456f
    structure of, 445f
Tumors, causing amnestic syndrome, 39

Twin studies, 460
    of affective disorder, 304
    of alcoholism, 229–230, 231
    of anorexia nervosa, 195
    of autism, 324–325
    of bipolar illness, 49
    of depression, 77
    of generalized anxiety disorder, 145
    of panic disorder, 140
    of personality disorders, 430
    of schizophrenia, 97
    of simple phobias, 149
    of suicide incidence, 536
Tyrosine, structure of, 444f

Unipolar depression, 47
    case histories of, 73–74
    clinical picture of, 70–74
    course of, 74–76, 75t
    defined, 69, 365
    differential diagnosis of, 79–80
    epidemiology of, 53, 69–70, 70t
    etiology of, 76–79
    laboratory findings in, 80–81
    mental status in, 72t
    symptoms of, 71t, 72t
    treatment of, 81–84
Unipolar II disorder, 375–376
    defined, 366
Urbanization, as demographic factor, 526
Uric acid values, in alcoholism, 225

Vaginismus, 254t
Valproic acid, 568
    therapeutic monitoring of, 502–503
Vascular dementia, clinical picture of, 27
    course of, 27–28
    defined, 22–23
    diagnosis of, 25t
    differential diagnosis of, 28–29
    distinguished from delirium, 21–22

Vascular dementia *Continued*
    epidemiology of, 24–25, 26t
    etiology and pathogenesis of, 23–24
    laboratory findings in, 28
    pathology of, 25, 27
    treatment of, 29
Vasodilators, to treat dementia, 581
Verapamil, 567–568
Vestibular function, of panic patients, 140–141
Vestibular hallucinations, 11
Visual hallucinations, 11
Voices, as symptom of schizophrenia, 88
Volatile hydrocarbon abuse, pathology of, 243
Volitional acts, as symptom of schizophrenia, 89
Voodoo, 284t
Vorbeireden, 14
Voyeurism, course of, 265t
    diagnosis of, 263t

Wakefulness, disorders of, 20
Waxy flexibility, as indicator of mental instability, 7
    in schizophrenia, 90
Wernicke's aphasia, 397
Wernicke's encephalopathy, 39, 41, 42, 44
Wernicke-Korsakoff syndrome, 39, 44
Wilson's disease, motor abnormalities in, 420–421
    psychiatric manifestations of, 500
Windingo, 284t
Withdrawal, generalized anxiety disorder in, 147
    thought, as symptom of schizophrenia, 88
        defined, 9
Witzelsucht, 13
Word approximations, 398
Word salad, 14, 397
    as symptom of schizophrenia, 89

Yale-Brown Obsessive Compulsive Scale, 163
Yohimbine intoxication, anxiety as symptom of, 386

Zoophilia, course of, 265t
    diagnosis of, 263t

ISBN 0-7216-6484-9

90038